The Shoulder

Edited by

CHARLES A. ROCKWOOD, JR., M.D.
Professor and Chairman Emeritus
Department of Orthopaedics
The University of Texas
Health Science Center at San Antonio
San Antonio, Texas

FREDERICK A. MATSEN III, M.D.
Professor and Chairman
Department of Orthopaedics
University of Washington
School of Medicine
Seattle, Washington

VOLUME 1

1990
W.B. SAUNDERS COMPANY
Harcourt Brace Jovanovich, Inc.
Philadelphia London Toronto Montreal Sydney Tokyo

W. B. SAUNDERS COMPANY
Harcourt Brace Jovanovich, Inc.

The Curtis Center
Independence Square West
Philadelphia, PA 19106

Library of Congress Cataloging-in-Publication Data

The Shoulder/[edited by] Charles A. Rockwood, Jr., Frederick A.
Matsen III.

p. cm.

ISBN 0–7216–2828–1 (set).

1. Shoulder—Diseases.   I. Rockwood, Charles A., 1936–
II. Matsen, Frederick A.
[DNLM: 1. Shoulder.   2. Shoulder Joint.   WE 810 S55861]

RC939.S484   1990

617.5′72–dc20

DNLM/DLC   89–24221

Editor: Lewis Reines
Designer: Karen O'Keefe
Production Manager: Carolyn Naylor
Manuscript Editor: Tom Gibbons
Illustration Coordinators: Brett MacNaughton and Ceil Kunkle
Indexer: Ann Cassar
Cover Designer: Ellen Bodner

ISBN 0–7216–2829–x Volume 1
0–7216–2830–3 Volume 2
0–7216–2828–1 Set

THE SHOULDER

Printed in the United States of America.

Last digit is the print number: 9   8   7   6   5   4   3   2   1

We dedicate these volumes to Anne, Patsy, and our families who support us

and

To all the past, present, and future generations of clinicians and investigators interested in unraveling the mysteries of the shoulder.

Contributors

David W. Altchek, M.D.
Assistant Professor of Surgery (Orthopaedics), Cornell University Medical College; Assistant Attending Orthopaedic Surgeon, The Hospital for Special Surgery, New York, New York

Kai-Nan An, Ph.D.
Professor of Bioengineering, Mayo Medical School; Consultant, Orthopedic Biomechanics Laboratory, Mayo Clinic, Rochester, Minnesota

Gunnar B. J. Andersson, M.D., Ph.D.
Professor of Orthopedic Surgery, Rush Medical College; Senior Attending and Associate Chairman, Department of Orthopedic Surgery, Rush-Presbyterian–St. Luke's Medical Center, Chicago, Illinois

Steven P. Arnoczky, D.V.M.
Associate Professor of Surgery (Comparative Orthopaedics), Cornell University Medical College; Director, Laboratory for Comparative Orthopaedic Research, The Hospital for Special Surgery, New York, New York

Craig T. Arntz, M.D.
Acting Instructor, Department of Orthopaedics, University of Washington School of Medicine, Seattle, Washington; Associate Staff, Valley Medical Center, Renton, Washington

Louis U. Bigliani, M.D.
Assistant Professor of Orthopaedic Surgery, College of Physicians and Surgeons; Assistant Attending of Orthopaedic Surgery, Columbia Presbyterian Medical Center, New York, New York

Desmond J. Bokor, M.B.
Clinical Fellow, University of Western Ontario, London, Ontario, Canada; Honorary Surgeon, University of Sydney; Orthopaedic Surgeon, Westmead Hospital, Sydney, Australia

Ernest M. Burgess, M.D.
Clinical Professor, Department of Orthopaedics, University of Washington School of Medicine; Attending, University and Affiliated Hospitals of University of Washington, Seattle, Washington

Wayne Z. Burkhead, Jr., M.D.
Clinical Assistant Professor, The University of Texas Health Science Center, Southwestern Medical School; Chief of Shoulder Service, Dallas Veterans Hospital; Attending Physician, W. B. Carrell Memorial Clinic; Associate Attending, Baylor University Medical Center, Dallas, Texas

Kenneth P. Butters, M.D.
Clinical Assistant Professor, University of Oregon Orthopedic Teaching Program; Orthopedic Surgeon, Sacred Heart Hospital, Eugene, Oregon

Michael A. Caughey, M.B., Ch.B.
Consultant Orthopaedic Surgeon, Middlemore Hospital, Auckland, New Zealand

Robert H. Cofield, M.D.
Professor of Orthopedics, Mayo Medical School; Consultant in Orthopedics, Mayo Clinic, Rochester, Minnesota

Ernest U. Conrad III, M.D.
Assistant Professor, Department of Orthopaedic Surgery, University of Washington School of Medicine; Director of Division of Musculoskeletal Oncology, University of Washington; Director of Bone Tumor Clinic, Children's Hospital and Medical Center, Seattle, Washington

Edward V. Craig, M.D.
Associate Professor of Orthopaedic Surgery, University of Minnesota Medical School; Attending Surgeon, University of Minnesota Hospital; Consultant, Veterans Administration Hospital, Minneapolis, Minnesota

Ralph J. Curtis, Jr., M.D.
Clinical Assistant Professor of Orthopaedics, Department of Orthopaedics, The University of Texas Health Science Center at San Antonio, San Antonio, Texas

Anthony G. Gristina, M.D.
Professor, Bowman Gray School of Medicine; Attending, North Carolina Baptist Hospital, Winston-Salem, North Carolina

Richard J. Hawkins, M.D.
Professor, University of Western Ontario; Attending, University Hospital, London, Ontario, Canada

Christopher M. Jobe, M.D.
Assistant Professor, Department of Orthopaedics, Loma Linda University School of Medicine; Staff, Loma Linda University Medical Center and Loma Linda Community Hospital; Consulting Staff, Veterans Administration Hospital, Loma Linda, California

Frank W. Jobe, M.D.
Clinical Professor, Department of Orthopaedics, University of Southern California School of Medicine, Los Angeles, California; Associate, Kerlan-Jobe Orthopaedic Clinic; Staff, Centinela Hospital Medical Center, Inglewood, California

Gordon Kammire, M.D.
Private Practice, Lexington, North Carolina; Formerly Chief Resident in Orthopedic Surgery, Bowman Gray School of Medicine/North Carolina Baptist Hospital, Winston-Salem, North Carolina

Stephen P. Kay, M.D.
Clinical Instructor, Division of Orthopedic Surgery, UCLA Center for Health Sciences; Attending Staff, Century City Hospital and Cedars-Sinai Medical Center, Los Angeles, California

Ronald S. Kvitne, M.D.
Assistant Clinical Professor, Department of Orthopaedics, University of Southern California School of Medicine, Los Angeles, California; Assistant Clinical Instructor, Sports Medicine and Reconstructive Service, Rancho Los Amigos Hospital, Downey, California; Staff, Centinela Hospital Medical Center, Inglewood, California; Staff, Rancho Los Amigos Hospital, Downey, California

Robert D. Leffert, M.D.
Associate Professor of Orthopaedic Surgery, Harvard Medical School; Chief of the Surgical Upper Extremity Rehabilitation Unit and the Department of Rehabilitation Medicine, Massachusetts General Hospital, Boston, Massachusetts

James V. Luck, Jr., M.D.
Associate Clinical Professor, Department of Orthopaedics, University of Southern California School of Medicine; Medical Director and Chief Operating Officer, Orthopaedic Hospital, Los Angeles, California

Leonard Marchinski, M.D.
Staff, Reading Hospital, Reading, Pennsylvania

Frederick A. Matsen III, M.D.
Professor and Chairman, Department of Orthopaedics, University of Washington School of Medicine; Chief, Shoulder and Elbow Service, University of Washington Medical Center, Seattle, Washington

Bernard F. Morrey, M.D.
Professor of Orthopedics, Mayo Medical School; Chairman, Department of Orthopedics, Mayo Clinic, Rochester, Minnesota

J. Patrick Murnaghan, B.Sc., M.D.
Assistant Professor, Division of Orthopaedic Surgery, University of Ottawa; Staff Orthopaedic Surgeon, Ottawa Civic Hospital; Consultant, Royal Ottawa Hospital and Ottawa Cancer Foundation, Ottawa, Ontario, Canada

Stephen J. O'Brien, M.D.
Assistant Professor of Surgery (Orthopaedics), Cornell University Medical College; Assistant Attending Orthopaedic Surgeon—HSS Assistant Scientist, The Hospital for Special Surgery; Assistant Attending Orthopaedic Surgeon, The New York Hospital, New York, New York

L. Brian Ready, M.D.
Associate Professor of Anesthesiology, University of Washington School of Medicine; Chief, Division of Regional Anesthesia, and Director, Acute Pain Service, University Hospital, Seattle, Washington

Charles A. Rockwood, Jr., M.D.
Professor and Chairman Emeritus, Department of Orthopaedics, The University of Texas Health Science Center at San Antonio, San Antonio, Texas

Robert L. Romano, M.D.
Clinical Professor, University of Washington School of Medicine; Staff, Providence Hospital, Swedish Hospital, and Children's Orthopedic Hospital, Seattle, Washington

S. Robert Rozbruch, B.A.
Cornell University Medical College, New York, New York

Kiriti Sarkar, M.D.
Professor, Department of Pathology, University of Ottawa, Ottawa, Ontario, Canada

Michael J. Skyhar, M.D.
Assistant Clinical Professor, University of California, San Diego; Assistant Attending Orthopaedic Surgeon, Scripps Memorial Hospital, San Diego, California

Elizabeth A. Szalay, M.D.
Active Staff, St. Elizabeth Hospital and Baptist Hospital of Southeast Texas, Beaumont, Texas; Courtesy Staff, Beaumont Medical and Surgical Hospital, Beaumont, Texas; Clinical Staff, Shriners Hospital for Crippled Children, Houston Unit, Houston, Texas

Steven C. Thomas, M.D.
Shoulder Fellow, Department of Orthopaedics, University of Washington School of Medicine; Shoulder Fellow, University of Washington Medical Center, Seattle, Washington

James E. Tibone, M.D.
Clinical Associate Professor of Orthopaedics, University of Southern California, Los Angeles, California; Staff, Centinela Hospital Medical Center, Inglewood, California

Hans K. Uhthoff, M.D.
Professor and Chairman, Division of Orthopaedic Surgery, University of Ottawa; Active Staff, Ottawa General Hospital, Ottawa, Ontario, Canada

Anna Voytek, M.D.
Private Practice, Greensboro, North Carolina; Formerly Chief Resident in Orthopedic Surgery, Bowman Gray School of Medicine/North Carolina Baptist Hospital, Winston-Salem, North Carolina

Russell F. Warren, M.D.
Professor of Orthopaedic Surgery, Cornell University Medical College; Attending Orthopaedic Surgeon and Chief, Sports Medicine and Shoulder Services, The Hospital for Special Surgery; Attending Orthopaedic Surgeon, The New York Hospital, New York, New York

Lawrence X. Webb, M.D.
Associate Professor, Bowman Gray School of Medicine; Attending, North Carolina Baptist Hospital, Winston-Salem, North Carolina

Peter Welsh, M.B., Ch.B.
Assistant Professor, Department of Surgery, University of Toronto; Deputy Chief of Staff, Orthopaedic and Arthritic Hospital; Staff Orthopaedic Surgeon, The Wellesley Hospital; Consultant Orthopaedic Surgeon, Hillcrest Hospital and Riverdale Hospital, Toronto, Ontario, Canada

Kaye E. Wilkins, M.D.
Clinical Professor of Orthopaedics and Pediatrics, The University of Texas Health Science Center at San Antonio; Staff, Santa Rosa Children's Hospital and Southwest Texas Methodist Hospital, San Antonio, Texas

Virchel E. Wood, M.D.
Chief, Hand Surgery Service, and Professor of Orthopaedic Surgery, Loma Linda University School of Medicine; Staff, Loma Linda University Medical Center, Loma Linda Out-Patient Surgery Center, and Loma Linda Community Hospital, Loma Linda, California

D. Christopher Young, M.D.
Staff Orthopaedic Surgeon, Brooke Army Medical Center, San Antonio, Texas

Foreword

It is a privilege to write the Foreword for *The Shoulder* by Drs. Charles A. Rockwood, Jr., and Frederick A. Matsen III. Their objective when they began this work was an all-inclusive text on the shoulder that would also include all references on the subject in the English literature. Forty-six authors have contributed to this text.

The editors of *The Shoulder* are two of the leading shoulder surgeons in the United States. Dr. Rockwood was the fourth President of the American Shoulder and Elbow Surgeons, has organized the Instructional Course Lectures on the Shoulder for the Annual Meeting of the American Academy of Orthopaedic Surgeons for many years, and is a most experienced and dedicated teacher. Dr. Matsen is President-Elect of the American Shoulder and Elbow Surgeons and is an unusually talented teacher and leader. These two men, with their academic know-how and the help of their contributing authors, have organized a monumental text for surgeons in training and in practice, as well as one that can serve as an extensive reference source. They are to be commended for this superior book.

CHARLES S. NEER II, M.D.
Professor Emeritus, Orthopaedic Surgery,
Columbia University; Chief, Shoulder Service,
Columbia-Presbyterian Medical Center, New York

Preface

The past twenty years have witnessed a huge surge in interest and new knowledge concerning the shoulder. The shoulder is now recognized as one of the principal sites of pathology in sports injuries, work-related injuries, arthritis, and age-related degeneration. We find ourselves in an age of discovery of the mechanisms of shoulder stability and rotator cuff degeneration and about basic mechanics of the shoulder.

Our primary goal at the outset of this project was to develop a text that would become the definitive work on the management of shoulder problems in children and in adults, encompassing developmental anatomy, biomechanics, fractures, dislocations, tumors, infections, amputations, and other related areas. The contributors, each of whom is a recognized authority in his or her field, were challenged to present an in-depth review of the current available knowledge about the shoulder for their chapters, and this they have done. Each chapter follows a logical pattern and, where applicable, contains a historical review, anatomy, classification, radiographic findings, open versus closed treatment, and finally, and of importance, the author's preferred method of treatment. In addition, each chapter includes extensive references on the subject.

We realize that it is risky to put down in print the state of the art of such a rapidly moving field: new knowledge is appearing literally every day. On the other hand, it seems important to consolidate the platform of knowledge as it exists today so that it can serve as the foundation for the addition of the knowledge of tomorrow. It is our hope that *The Shoulder* will be that foundation.

To the readers we offer our best wishes in your studies of the shoulder. It is a fascinating joint! To the contributors we express our deepest gratitude; the book would not have been possible without you. We offer our sincere appreciation and thanks to our teacher, Charles S. Neer II, M.D., of New York City. We thank Rita Mandoli and Sarah Sato at the University of Washington School of Medicine and Natalie Merryman and Carol Cafiero at the University of Texas School of Medicine in San Antonio for their unfailing energy and devotion to this work. Their perseverance and attention to detail ensured that this book would be of the highest quality.

We also acknowledge the help we received from our Shoulder Fellows, Doug Harryman and Steve Thomas from the University of Washington and Jerry Williams and Mike Mirth from the University of Texas.

CHARLES A. ROCKWOOD, JR., M.D.
FREDERICK A. MATSEN III, M.D.

Contents

VOLUME 1

CHAPTER 1

Developmental Anatomy of the Shoulder and Anatomy of the Glenohumeral Joint 1
Stephen J. O'Brien, M.D. • *Steven P. Arnoczky, D.V.M.*
Russell F. Warren, M.D. • *S. Robert Rozbruch, B.A.*

    Comparative Anatomy 1
    Embryology 6
    Adult Glenohumeral Joint 12
    Microvasculature 28
    Innervation of the Glenohumeral Joint 30

CHAPTER 2

Gross Anatomy of the Shoulder 34
Christopher M. Jobe, M.D.

    Bones and Joints 39
    Muscles 49
    Nerves 66
    Blood Vessels 76
    Bursae, Compartments, and Potential Spaces 83
    Skin 89

CHAPTER 3

Congenital Anomalies of the Shoulder 98
Virchel E. Wood, M.D. • *Leonard Marchinski, M.D.*

    Bony Abnormalities 99
    Muscular Abnormalities 124
    Neurovascular Abnormalities Associated with Congenital Anomalies ... 132

CHAPTER 4

Clinical Evaluation of Shoulder Problems 149
Richard J. Hawkins, M.D. • *Desmond J. Bokor, M.D.*

    History 149
    Physical Examination 153

Injection Techniques 174
Cervical Spine Examination 174
Cervical Spine and the Shoulder 176
Further Investigative Procedures 177
Conclusions 177

CHAPTER **5**

X-ray Evaluation of Shoulder Problems 178

Charles A. Rockwood, Jr., M.D. • Elizabeth A. Szalay, M.D. • Ralph J. Curtis, Jr., M.D.
D. Christopher Young, M.D. • Stephen P. Kay, M.D.

Disorders of the Glenohumeral Joint 178
Fractures of the Shaft of the Clavicle 189
Disorders of the Acromioclavicular Joint and Distal Clavicle 189
Disorders of the Sternoclavicular Joint and Medial Clavicle 193
Evaluation of the Impingement Syndrome and the Rotator Cuff 196
Evaluation of Scapular Injuries 200
Evaluation of Calcific Tendinitis 200
Evaluation of Biceps Tendinitis 200
Tumors and Inflammatory Problems 200

CHAPTER **6**

Biomechanics of the Shoulder 208

Bernard F. Morrey, M.D. • Kai-Nan An, Ph.D.

The Shoulder Complex 208
Glenohumeral and Scapulothoracic Joint Motion 213
Shoulder Motion 218
Constraints 226
Muscle and Joint Forces 234

CHAPTER **7**

Anesthesia for Shoulder Procedures 246

L. Brian Ready, M.D.

Preoperative Considerations 246
Intraoperative Considerations 248
Choice of Anesthetics—Regional Versus General 249
Techniques for Regional Anesthesia 249
Special Considerations 255
Postoperative Anesthetic Care 255
Postoperative Pain Management 256
Summary 256

CHAPTER **8**

Shoulder Arthroscopy 258

David W. Altchek, M.D. • Russell F. Warren, M.D. • Michael J. Skyhar, M.D.

History 258
Arthroscopic Anatomy of the Glenohumeral Joint and
Subacromial Space 258

Intra-articular Anatomy 259
Indications 262
Technique 264
Anthroscopic Technique 266
Arthroscopic Procedures for the Shoulder 268
Results 276

CHAPTER **9**

Fractures of the Proximal Humerus 278
Louis U. Bigliani, M.D.

Anatomy 279
Classification 281
Incidence 284
Mechanism of Injury 284
Clinical Presentation 285
Differential Diagnosis 286
Radiographic Evaluation 286
Complications 289
Methods of Treatment 291
Surgical Approaches 305
Author's Preferred Method of Treatment 309

CHAPTER **10**

The Scapula 335
Kenneth P. Butters, M.D.

Anatomy 335
Classification of Fractures of the Scapula 336
Clinical Presentation 338
Associated Injuries and Complications 338
Differential Diagnosis 339
Types of Fractures and Methods of Treatment 343
Results of Treatment 359
Author's Preferred Method of Treatment 360
Other Disorders 361

CHAPTER **11**

Fractures of the Clavicle 367
Edward V. Craig, M.D.

Historical Review 367
Anatomy 368
Function of the Clavicle 370
Classification of Clavicular Fractures 372
Mechanism of Injury 376
Clinical Presentation 377
X-ray Evaluation 383
Differential Diagnosis 386
Complications 387

Treatment 392
Postoperative Care 397
Author's Preferred Method of Treatment 398

CHAPTER 12

Disorders of the Acromioclavicular Joint 413
Charles A. Rockwood, Jr., M.D. • D. Christopher Young, M.D.

Historical Review 413
Surgical Anatomy 413
Mechanism of Injury 420
Classification of Injury 422
Incidence of Injury 425
Signs and Symptoms of Injury 425
X-ray Evaluation 426
Treatment of Injuries 434
Authors' Preferred Method of Treatment of Injuries 447
Prognosis 463
Complications of Injuries to the Acromioclavicular
Joint 463
Degenerative Arthritis of the Acromioclavicular Joint ... 467
Rheumatoid Arthritis of the Acromioclavicular Joint 467
Septic Arthritis of the Acromioclavicular Joint 468
Cysts of the Acromioclavicular Joint 468

CHAPTER 13

Disorders of the Sternoclavicular Joint 477
Charles A. Rockwood, Jr., M.D.

Historical Review 477
Surgical Anatomy 477
Mechanism of Injury 483
Classification of Problems of the Sternoclavicular Joint .. 486
Incidence of Injury to the Sternoclavicular Joint 489
Signs and Symptoms of Injuries to the
Sternoclavicular Joint 491
X-ray Findings of Injury to the Sternoclavicular Joint ... 491
Treatment 495
Author's Preferred Method of Treatment 507
Complications of Injuries to the Sternoclavicular Joint ... 517
Complications of Operative Procedures 519

CHAPTER 14

Anterior Glenohumeral Instability 526
Frederick A. Matsen III, M.D. • Steven C. Thomas, M.D. • Charles A. Rockwood, Jr., M.D.

Historical Review 526
Anatomy of the Glenohumeral Joint 531
Classification of Glenohumeral Instability 541
Incidence and Mechanism of Injury 543
Clinical Presentation 544

Radiographic and Laboratory Evaluation 551
Complications of Injury 562
Differential Diagnosis 569
Treatment 569

VOLUME 2

CHAPTER **15**

Subacromial Impingement 623
Frederick A. Matsen III, M.D. • Craig T. Arntz, M.D.

Definition and Historical Review 623
Anatomy 624
Classification 626
Incidence and Mechanisms of Injury 626
Clinical Presentation 629
Cuff Imaging Techniques 629
Complications 632
Differential Diagnosis 632
Methods of Treatment 633
Authors' Preferred Method of Treatment 636

CHAPTER **16**

Rotator Cuff Tendon Failure 647
Frederick A. Matsen III, M.D. • Craig T. Arntz, M.D.

Historical Review 647
Anatomy and Function 647
Classification of Injury 650
Incidence and Mechanism of Injury 650
Associated Pathology 654
Clinical Presentation 654
Imaging Evaluation 656
Complications 660
Differential Diagnosis 661
Methods of Treatment 662
Results 664
Authors' Preferred Method of Treatment 665

CHAPTER **17**

Degenerative and Arthritic Problems of the Glenohumeral Joint 678
Robert H. Cofield, M.D.

Historical Review 678
Surgical Indications 686
Disease Characteristics 687
Clinical Evaluation 701

Methods of Surgical Treatment 703
Operative Techniques 718
Postoperative Rehabilitation 735
Results 736
Complications 740
Revision Surgery 742

CHAPTER 18

Neurological Problems
.... 750

Robert D. Leffert, M.D.

Clinical Presentation 751
X-ray and Laboratory Evaluation 751
Pathology and Classification 755
Methods of Treatment of Kinesiological Abnormalities of
the Shoulder 758

CHAPTER 19

Calcifying Tendinitis
.... 774

Hans K. Uhthoff, M.D. • Kiriti Sarkar, M.D.

Historical Review 774
Anatomy 774
Incidence 775
Classification 776
Pathology 776
Pathogenesis 778
Clinical Presentation 781
Radiology 783
Laboratory Investigations 785
Complications 785
Differential Diagnosis 785
Treatment 785
Authors' Preferred Method of Treatment 787
Concluding Remarks 788

CHAPTER 20

The Biceps Tendon
.... 791

Wayne Z. Burkhead, Jr., M.D.

Historical Review 791
Anatomy 793
Osseous Pathoanatomy 799
Function of the Biceps Tendon 805
Classification of Bicipital Lesions 808
Incidence 810
Etiology 811
Prevention 811
Clinical Presentation of Bicipital Lesions 812
Associated Conditions 816

Diagnostic Tests 816
Complications 820
Differential Diagnosis 821
Treatment of Bicipital Lesions: Review of Conservative Treatment 824
Results of Nonoperative Treatment of Biceps Rupture 824
Review of Operative Treatment 824
Author's Preferred Methods of Treatment 827
Summary 832

CHAPTER 21

Frozen Shoulder

Frozen Shoulder 837

J. Patrick Murnaghan, M.D.

Historical Review 837
Anatomy 839
Pathology 840
Diagnostic Criteria 841
Classification 842
Incidence 843
Mechanism of Injury 844
Predisposing Factors 844
Clinical Examination 845
Clinical Presentation 846
Investigations 849
Complications 851
Differential Diagnosis 851
Treatment 853
Author's Preferred Method of Treatment 858

CHAPTER 22

Muscle Ruptures Affecting the Shoulder Girdle

Muscle Ruptures Affecting the Shoulder Girdle 863

Michael A. Caughey, M.B. • Peter Welsh, M.B

General Principles of Rupture of the Musculotendinous Unit 863
Rupture of the Pectoralis Major 864
Rupture of the Deltoid 866
Rupture of the Triceps 867
Rupture of the Biceps 869
Rupture of the Serratus Anterior 871
Rupture of the Coracobrachialis 871
Rupture of the Subscapularis 872
Conclusion 872

CHAPTER 23

Tumors and Related Conditions

Tumors and Related Conditions 874

Ernest U. Conrad III, M.D.

Historical Review 874
Anatomy 875
Staging and Classification of Tumors 877

Incidence of Neoplasms 892
Clinical Presentation 895
X-ray and Laboratory Evaluation 897
Complications of Tumors 898
Differential Diagnosis 899
Biopsy, Resections, Reconstructions, and the Management of Specific
Lesions 901
Author's Preferred Methods of Treatment 913

CHAPTER **24**

Sepsis of the Shoulder: Molecular Mechanisms and Pathogenesis 920

Anthony G. Gristina, M.D. • Gordon Kammire, M.D. • Anna Voytek, M.D.
Lawrence X. Webb, M.D.

History 920
Septic Anatomy of the Shoulder 921
Classification 923
Incidence and Pathogenic Mechanisms of Septic Arthritis
and Osteomyelitis 924
Microbial Adhesion and Intra-articular Sepsis 926
Bacterial Pathogens 928
Clinical Presentation 929
Laboratory and X-ray Evaluation 930
Complications 932
Treatment 932
Authors' Preferred Method of Treatment 936

CHAPTER **25**

Amputations and Prosthetic Replacement 940

Robert L. Romano, M.D. • Ernest M. Burgess, M.D.

Types of Amputations 940
Precipitating Factors 941
Specific Procedures 941
Prosthetic Rehabilitation 952

CHAPTER **26**

The Shoulder in Sports 961

Frank W. Jobe, M.D. • James E. Tibone, M.D. • Christopher M. Jobe, M.D.
Ronald S. Kvitne, M.D.

Biomechanics of the Throwing Shoulder 961
Impingement and Instability in the Athlete 963
Posterior Shoulder Problems in the Athlete 983
Acromioclavicular Joint Problems 986
Neurological Problems 987
Vascular Problems 987
The Shoulder in Swimming 988
Conclusion 989

CHAPTER **27**

Fractures and Dislocations of the Shoulder in Children 991
Ralph J. Curtis, Jr., M.D. • Charles A. Rockwood, Jr., M.D.

Fractures of the Proximal Humerus 991
Glenohumeral Subluxation and Dislocation 1002
Fractures of the Clavicle and Injuries to the
Sternoclavicular and Acromioclavicular Joints 1007
Scapula 1025

CHAPTER **28**

Special Problems with the Child's Shoulder 1033
Kaye E. Wilkins, M.D.

Brachial Plexus Injuries 1033
Torticollis 1055
The Shoulder in Arthrogryposis 1072
Bone and Joint Infections 1074

CHAPTER **29**

Occupational Shoulder Disorders 1088
James V. Luck, Jr., M.D. • Gunnar B. J. Andersson, M.D., Ph.D.

Occupational Cervicobrachial Disorder 1088
Shoulder Tendinitis 1093
Degenerative Arthritis 1095
Prevention 1095
Treatment 1100
Evaluation of Impairment 1103
Index i

The Shoulder

Developmental Anatomy of the Shoulder and Anatomy of the Glenohumeral Joint

Stephen J. O'Brien, M.D.
Steven P. Arnoczky, D.V.M.
Russell F. Warren, M.D.
S. Robert Rozbruch, B.A.

When humans assumed the erect position, it triggered a series of complex adaptive changes that make the study of the shoulder and its appendages both exciting and at the same time humbling. Stability was exchanged for mobility in an effort to facilitate prehension and to comply with the demands of the orthograde posture.

In this chapter, we will focus on the developmental anatomy of the shoulder, from phylogenetic to embryological changes, and then to the anatomy of the adult glenohumeral joint. The following chapter will then discuss in detail the gross anatomy of the remainder of the pectoral girdle.

Comparative Anatomy

GENERAL DEVELOPMENT

The forelimb in humans is a paired appendage derived originally from longitudinal lateral folds of epidermis in fish, extending caudad from the region just behind the gills to the anus (Fig. 1–1). The pectoral and pelvic fins developed from the proximal and distal portions, respectively (Fig. 1–2).[61]

Muscle buds, along with spinal nerves, migrated into these pectoral fins, allowing for movement. Peripheral nerve fibers repeatedly divided to form a plexus of nerves, and different regions of muscle tissue often combined or segmented as function evolved.

Cartilage rays called radials (Fig. 1–3) arose between muscle buds to form a support structure, and the

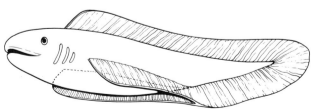

Figure 1–1. Paired lateral longitudinal forms of epidermis of the fish, extending caudad from the region just posterior to the gills to the anus.

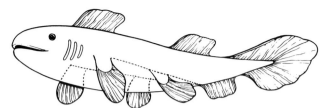

Figure 1–2. The pectoral and pelvic fins from the proximal and distal portions of the paired longitudinal lateral folds. These are the precursors of the upper and lower limbs.

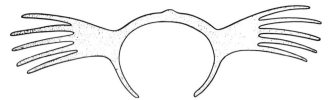

Figure 1–4. The paired basilia come together in the midline to form the primitive pectoral girdle. As these basilia migrate, they form a bar that is the precursor to the paired clavicles.

proximal portions of these radials coalesced to form basal cartilages, or basilia. This formed the primitive pectoral girdle (Fig. 1–4). These paired basilia eventually migrated ventrally toward the midline anteriorly to form a ventral bar, which was the precursor of the paired clavicles. The basilia also projected dorsally over the thorax to form the precursor of the scapula. Articulations within the basilia eventually developed at the junction of the ventral and dorsal segments (glenoid fossa) with the remainder of the pectoral fin, which eventually became the glenohumeral joint (Fig. 1–5).

Through the amphibian stages, the head was eventually freed from its attachments to the pectoral girdle, and in the reptile, the pectoral girdle migrated a considerable distance caudally. The cleitrum, a membranous bone that previously attached the pectoral girdle to the skull, disappeared entirely in this reptilian stage.

The basic mammalian pattern developed with articulations arising between a well-developed clavicle and sternum medially and a flat, fairly wide scapula laterally. The coracoid enlarged during this period, and also the scapular spine developed in response to new functional demands (Fig. 1–6). Four main variations on the scheme are seen.[7] Mammals adapted for running

have lost their clavicle to further mobilize the scapula, and the scapula is relatively narrowed. Mammals adapted for swimming also have lost their clavicle, although the scapula is wider, permitting more varied function. Shoulder girdles modified for flying have a large, long, well-developed clavicle with a small, narrow, curved scapula. Finally, shoulders modified for brachiating (including man) developed a strong clavicle, a large coracoid, and a widened, strong scapula.

Other adaptations in the erect posture were the relative flattening of the thorax in the anteroposterior dimension, leaving the scapula approximately 45 degrees to the midline (Fig. 1–7), and the evolution of the pentadactyl limb, with a strong, mobile thumb and four ulnar digits. This pentadactyl limb formed the basic blueprint for the human arm as we know it.

In approaching the more human form, we will now discuss the evolution of the different regions of the shoulder and pectoral girdle separately.

DEVELOPMENT OF INDIVIDUAL REGIONS

The Scapula

The scapula in humans is suspended by muscles alone and reflects clearly the adaptive development of the shoulder. It has shifted caudally from the cervical position in lower animals, freeing the shoulder from the head and neck to serve as a base or platform to facilitate arm movement. The most striking modification in the development of the bone of the scapula itself is in the relationship between the length (measured along the base of the spine) and the breadth (measured from the superior to the inferior angle) of the scapula, or the scapular index (Fig. 1–8).[46] This index is extremely high in the pronograde with a long, narrow scapula. In the primates and humans the scapula broadens, with the most pronounced changes confined to the infraspinous fossa. This has been referred to as an increase in the infraspinous index.

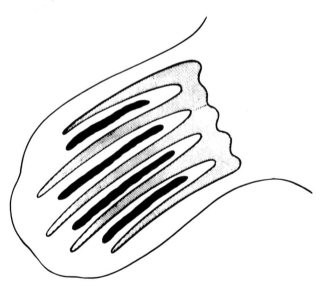

Figure 1–3. Cartilage rays called radials arise between muscle buds formed as a support structure for the limb. The proximal portions of these radials coalesce to form basal cartilages or basilia.

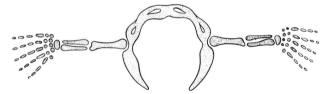

Figure 1–5. Articulations within the basilia develop at the junction of the ventral and dorsal segments, which form the primitive glenoid fossa.

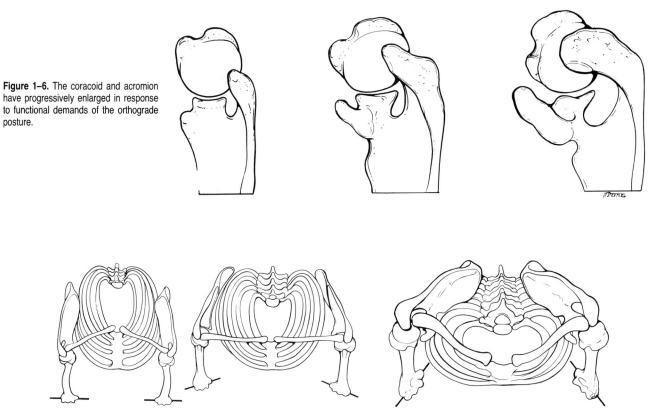

Figure 1–6. The coracoid and acromion have progressively enlarged in response to functional demands of the orthograde posture.

Figure 1–7. The anteroposterior dimension of the thoracic cage has decreased over time, with the scapula approximately 45 degrees to the midline. The scapula and the glenoid fossa also assumed a more dorsal position in the thoracic cage. This led to the glenoid fossa being directed laterally. Consequently, a relative external rotation of the humeral head and an internal rotation of the shaft occurred.

Figure 1–8. The size of the infraspinous fossa has gradually enlarged over time relative to the length of the scapular spine. This has led to a decrease in the scapular index.

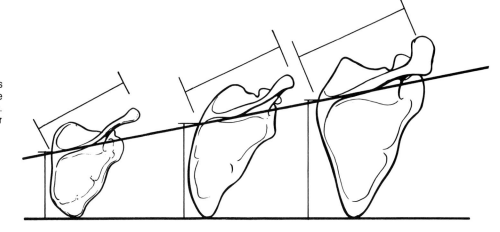

Broadening of the infraspinous fossa results in a change in the vector of muscle pull from the axillary border of the scapula to the glenoid fossa and consequently alters the action of the attached musculature. This allows the infraspinatus and teres minor to be more effective in their roles as depressors and external rotators of the humeral head. The supraspinous fossa and muscle have seen relatively little change in size or shape over time.

The acromion process, which is an extension of the spine of the scapula (see Fig. 1–6), is also enlarging over time.[46] In pronograde animals, the acromion process is insignificant; in humans, however, it is a massive structure overlying the humeral head. This change reflects the increasing role of the deltoid muscle in shoulder function. By broadening its attachment on the acromion and shifting distally its insertion on the humerus, it increases its mechanical advantage in shoulder motion.

The coracoid process has also seen an increase in its size over time (see Fig. 1–6).[46] In addition to forming an important origin and insertion site for pectoral musculature, recent biomechanical studies we have performed with the shoulder abducted 90 degrees show that the overlap of the coracoid over the glenohumeral joint may limit anterior excursion and take stress off the anterior capsule. In one shoulder we tested following sectioning of the capsule, the shoulder would not dislocate anteriorly in full abduction until after the coracoid process was removed (Fig. 1–9).

The Humerus

Like the scapula, the humerus has undergone significant morphological changes. As mentioned previously, the insertion site of the deltoid has migrated distally to improve the lever arm of the deltoid muscle (Fig. 1–10).[46, 49]

Another important change is in the development of

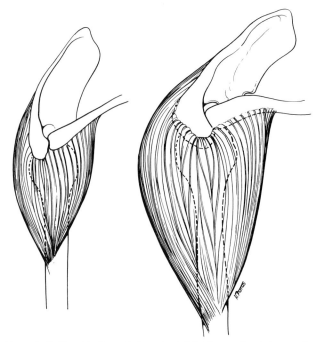

Figure 1–10. The deltoid muscle has migrated distally over time to improve the lever arm on the humerus.

torsion in the humeral shaft.[46] As the thoracic cage flattened in the anteroposterior plane, the scapula and glenoid fossa assumed a more dorsal position in the thoracic cage. This led to the glenoid fossa being directed more laterally (see Fig. 1–7). Consequent to this, a relative external rotation of the humeral head and internal rotation of the shaft relative to it occurred, leading to a medial displacement of the intertubercular groove and decreased size of the lesser tuberosity relative to the greater tuberosity. The resultant retroversion of the humeral head is approximately 30 degrees with the epicondyles of the elbow in the coronal plane. This, however, is variable.

The other effect of the torsion on the humerus is that the biceps, which was previously a strong elevator of the arm, is rendered biomechanically ineffective unless the arm is externally rotated. In this fashion, it can be used as an abductor, which is often seen in infantile paralysis.

The Clavicle

The clavicle is not present in horses or other animals that use their forelimbs for standing. In animals that use their upper limbs for holding, grasping, and climbing, however, the clavicle allows the scapula and humerus to be held away from the body to help the limb move free of the axial skeleton. In humans it also provides a means of transmitting the supporting force of the trapezius to the scapula through the coracoclavicular ligaments, a bony framework for muscle attachments, and a mechanism for increasing range of motion at the glenohumeral joint.

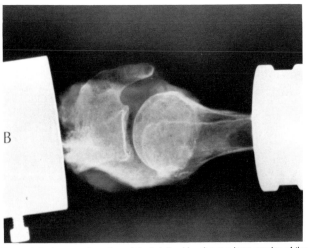

Figure 1–9. An x-ray view of an abducted shoulder shows a large overlap of the coracoid over the glenohumeral joint, which may restrict anterior translation.

The Scapulohumeral Muscles

These muscles include the supraspinatus, infraspinatus, teres minor, subscapularis, deltoid, and teres major. The supraspinatus has remained relatively static morphologically but has progressively decreased in relative mass (Fig. 1–11).[49] The deltoid, on the other hand, has more than doubled in proportional representation and constitutes approximately 41 per cent of the scapulohumeral muscle mass. This increase in size also increases the overall strength of the deltoid. In lower animals, a portion of the deltoid attaches to the inferior angle of the scapula. In humans, this portion of the deltoid separated distally and formed the teres minor muscle. This would explain the identical innervation in these two muscles.

The infraspinatus is absent in lower species; however, in humans, it makes up approximately 5 per cent of the mass of the scapulohumeral muscles. The subscapularis has undergone no significant changes, except for a slight increase in the number of fasciculi concomitant with the elongation of the scapula, and makes up approximately 20 per cent of the mass of the scapulohumeral group. This adaptation allows the lower part of the muscle to pull in a downward direction and assists the infraspinatus and teres minor to act as a group to function as depressors as well as stabilizers of the head of the humerus against the glenoid during arm elevation.

The Axioscapular Muscles

The axioscapular muscles include the serratus anterior, rhomboids, levator scapulae, and trapezius. All of these muscles except the trapezius originate from one complex of muscle fibers arising from the first eight ribs and the transverse processes of the cervical vertebrae and inserting into the vertebral border of the scapula. As differentiation occurred, the fibers concerned with dorsal scapular motion became the rhomboid muscles. The fibers controlling ventral motion evolved into the serratus anterior muscle. Finally, the levator scapulae evolved to control the cranial displacement of the scapula. The trapezius has undergone little morphological change throughout primate development.

This group of muscles acts to anchor the scapula on the thoracic cage while allowing freedom of motion. The serratus anterior provides horizontal stability and prevents winging of the scapula.

The Axiohumeral Muscles

The axiohumeral muscles connect the humerus to the trunk and consist of the pectoralis major, pectoralis minor, and latissimus dorsi. The pectoral muscles originate from a single muscle mass which divides into a superficial and a deep layer. The superficial layer becomes the pectoralis major, and the deep layer gives rise to the pectoralis minor. The pectoralis minor in lower forms is attached to the humerus, while in humans it has undergone transference to the coracoid process.

The Muscles of the Upper Arm

The biceps in more primitive animals has a single origin and often assists the supraspinatus in limb elevation. In humans, the biceps has two origins and, because of torsional changes in the humerus, is ineffective in shoulder elevation unless the arm is fully externally rotated.

The triceps has not undergone significant morphological changes, but the size of the long head of the triceps has been progressively decreasing.

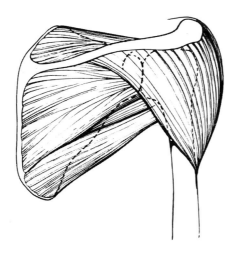
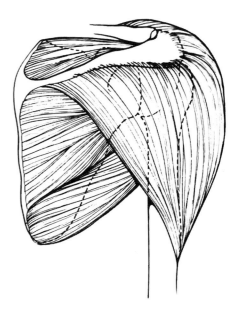

Figure 1–11. The supraspinatus muscle has remained relatively static morphologically but has progressively decreased in relative mass to the infraspinous muscles, although the enlarged deltoid muscle can be appreciated. The increased importance of the deltoid is evidenced by its increase in relative size.

Embryology

PRENATAL DEVELOPMENT

Prenatal human embryological development can be divided into two major periods, the embryonic and the fetal. The *embryonic* period comprises the first eight weeks of development, and the *fetal* period is the remainder of the prenatal period until term. The embryonic period is very important because all the major external and internal organs develop during this time, and by the end of this period, differentiation is practically completed. All the bones and joints will have a form and arrangement characteristic of the adult. Exposure to the teratogens during this period may cause major congenital malformations. During the fetal period, growth and maturation of the limbs occur with a continual remodeling and reconstructive process which enables a bone to maintain its characteristic shape. In the skeleton in general, increments of growth in individual bones are in precise relationship to those of the skeleton as a whole. Ligaments show an increase in collagen content, bursae develop, tendinous attachments shift to accommodate growth, and epiphyseal cartilages become vascularized.

The three germ layers give rise to all the tissues and organs of the body. The cells of each germ layer divide, migrate, aggregate, and differentiate in rather precise patterns as they form various organ systems. The three germ layers are the *ectoderm,* which gives rise to the central nervous system, peripheral nervous system, the epidermis and its appendages, the mammary glands, the pituitary gland, and the subcutaneous glands; the *mesoderm,* which gives rise to the cartilage, bone, connective tissue, striated and smooth muscle, blood cells, the kidneys, the gonads, the spleen, and the serous membrane lining of the body cavities; and the *endoderm,* which gives rise to the epithelial lining of the gastrointestinal, respiratory, and urinary tracts, the lining of the auditory canal, and the parenchyma of the tonsils, thyroid glands, parathyroid gland, thymus, liver, and pancreas. Development of the embryo requires a coordinated interaction of these germ layers, orchestrated by genetic and environmental factors under the influence of basic induction and regulatory mechanisms.

Embryonic Period

The limb buds are first seen as small elevations on the ventrolateral body wall at the end of the fourth week of gestation.[59] The upper limb buds appear first at a few days and maintain a growth advantage over the lower limbs throughout development. Because development of the head and neck occurs in advance of the rest of the embryo, the upper limb buds appear disproportionately low on the embryo's trunk (Fig. 1–12). During the early stages of limb development, the

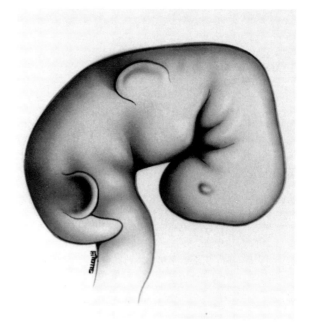

Figure 1–12. Development of the head and neck occurs in advance of the rest of the embryo, resulting in disproportionately low positions of the upper and lower limb buds on the embryo's trunk.

upper and lower extremities develop in similar fashion, with the upper limb bud developing opposite the lower six cervical and first and second thoracic segments.

At four weeks, the upper limb is a sac of ectoderm filled with mesoderm and is approximately 3 mm long. Each limb bud is delineated dorsally by a sulcus and ventrally by a pit. The pit for the upper limb bud is called the fossa axillaris. The mesoderm in the upper limb bud is developed from somatic mesoderm and consists of a mass of mesenchyme, which is a loosely organized embryonic connective tissue. Mesenchymal cells have the ability to differentiate in many different ways, i.e., into fibroblasts, chondroblasts, or osteoblasts (Fig. 1–13). Most bones first appear as condensations of these mesenchymal cells that form a longitudinal core called the blastema.[59, 102] This is orchestrated by the apical ectodermal ridge (Fig. 1–14)[59] which exerts an inductive influence on the limb mesenchyme that promotes growth and development.

During the fifth week, a number of developments occur simultaneously. The peripheral nerves grow from the brachial plexus into the mesenchyme of the limb buds. This stimulates the development of the limb musculature, where *in situ* somatic limb mesoderm aggregates and differentiates into myoblasts and the discrete muscle units. This is different from the development of axial musculature, which develops from myotomic regions of somites, which are segments of two longitudinal columns of paraxial mesoderm (Fig. 1–15). Also, at this time, the central core of the humerus begins to chondrify, although the shoulder joint is not yet formed. There is an area in the blastema called the interzone which has not undergone chondri-

Figure 1–13. The mesoderm in the upper limb bud is developed from somatic mesoderm and consists of a mass of mesenchyme (loosely organized embryonic connective tissue). It eventually differentiates into fibroblastic, chondroblastic, and osteoblastic tissue. The apical ectodermal ridge exerts an inductive influence on the limb to promote growth and development.

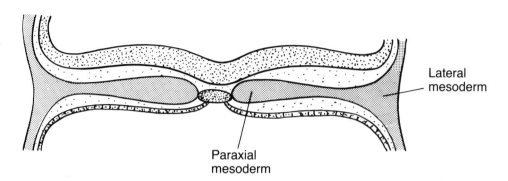

Lateral mesoderm

Paraxial mesoderm

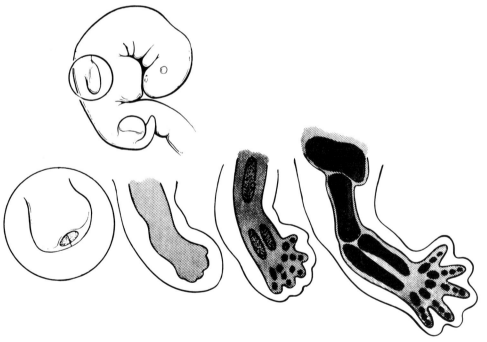

Figure 1–14. The apical ectodermal ridge exerts an inductive influence on the development of the upper limb.

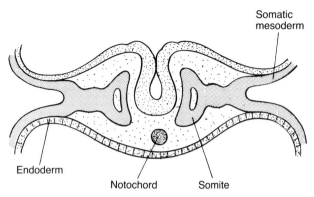

Figure 1–15. The development of the axial musculature comes from myotomic regions of somites, which are segments of two longitudinal columns of paraxial mesoderm. This differs from somatic mesoderm, from which the limb develops.

fication and is the precursor of the shoulder joint (Fig. 1–16). The scapula at this time lies at the level of C4 and C5 (Fig. 1–17),[52] and the clavicle is beginning to ossify (which along with the mandible is the first bone to begin to ossify).

During the sixth week, the mesenchymal tissue in the periphery of the hand plates condenses to form digital rays. The mesodermal cells of the limb bud rearrange themselves to form a deep layer, an intermediate layer, and a superficial layer. This layering is brought on by a differential in growth rates.[102] This differential growth in the limb also stimulates bending

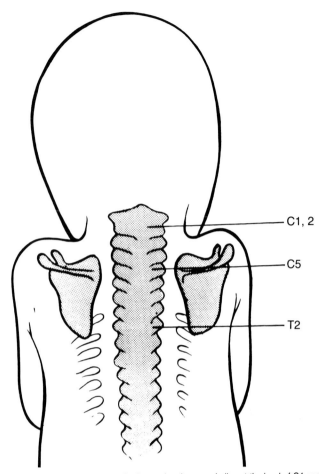

Figure 1–17. By the fifth week of gestation the scapula lies at the level of C4 and C5. It gradually descends with development. Failure of the scapula to descend is termed Sprengel's deformity.

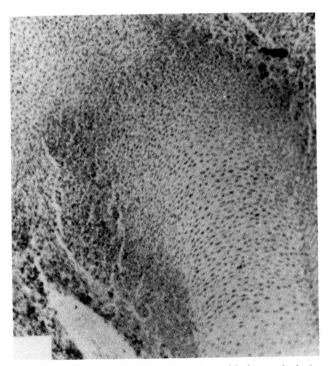

Figure 1–16. At five weeks of gestation the central core of the humerus begins to chondrify, but a homogeneous interzone remains between the scapula and the humerus. (Reproduced with permission from Gardner E, and Gray DJ: Prenatal development of the human shoulder and acromio-clavicular joint. Am J Anat 92:219, 1953.)

at the elbow, as the cells on the ventral side grow faster than those on the dorsal side, which stretches to accommodate the ventral growth. The muscle groups divide into dorsal extensors and ventral flexors, and the individual muscles migrate caudally as the limb bud develops. In the shoulder joint, the interzone assumes a three-layered configuration, with a chondrogenic layer on either side of a loose layer of cells.[42] At this time, the glenoid lip is discernible (Fig. 1–18), although cavitation or joint formation has not occurred. Initial bone formation in the primary ossification center of the humerus begins. The scapula at this time undergoes marked enlargement and extends from C4 to approximately T7.

Early in the seventh week, the limbs extend ventrally and the upper and lower limb buds rotate in opposite directions (Fig. 1–19). The upper limbs rotate laterally through 90 degrees on their longitudinal axes, with the elbow facing posteriorly and the extensor muscles facing laterally and posteriorly.[59] The lower limbs rotate medially through almost 90 degrees, with the knee and extensor musculature facing anteriorly. The final result is that the radius is in a lateral position in the

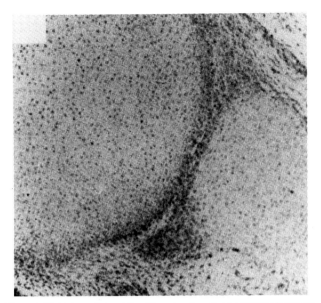

Figure 1–18. At six weeks' gestation (21 mm), a three-layered interzone is present and the beginning of the development of the glenoid labrum can be seen. (Reproduced with permission from Gardner E, and Gray DJ: Prenatal development of the human shoulder and acromio-clavicular joint. Am J Anat 92:219, 1953.)

upper limb and the tibia is in a medial position in the lower limb, although they are homologous bones. The ulna and fibula are also homologous bones, and the thumb and great toe are homologous digits. The shoulder joint is now well formed, with the middle zone of the three-layered interzone becoming less and less dense with increasing cavitation (Fig. 1–20). The scapula has now descended and spans from just below the

level of the first rib to the level of the fifth rib.[52] The brachial plexus has also migrated caudally and lies over the first rib. The final few degrees of downward displacement of the scapula occur later when the anterior rib cage drops obliquely downward.

By the eighth week, the embryo is about 23 mm long, and through growth of the upper limb, the hands are stretched with arms pronated (Fig. 1–21). The musculature of the limb is now also clearly defined. The shoulder joint has the form of the adult glenohumeral joint, and the glenohumeral ligaments are now able to be visualized as thickenings in the shoulder capsule.[47, 59]

Although certain toxins and other environmental factors can still cause limb deformities (for example, affecting the vascular supply), it is the embryonic period that is most vulnerable to congenital malformations, with the type of abnormality depending on the time at which the orderly sequence of differentiation was interrupted. One important factor in gross limb abnormalities, such as amelia, involves injuries to the apical ectodermal ridge, which, as mentioned before, has a strong inductive influence over the limb mesoderm. This will be discussed in more detail in the chapter on limb malformations. However, knowledge of the timing of embryological development is critical to understanding anomalies and malformations.

Fetal Period

Fetal development is mostly concerned with the expansion in size of the structures developed during the embryonic period. By the end of the 12th week,

Figure 1–19. *A,* Following the seventh week of gestation, the limbs extend ventrally and the upper and lower limb buds rotate in opposite directions. *B,* As a result, the radius occupies a lateral position in the upper limb while the tibia assumes a medial position in the lower limb, although they are homologous bones.

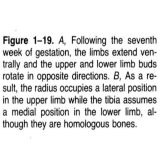
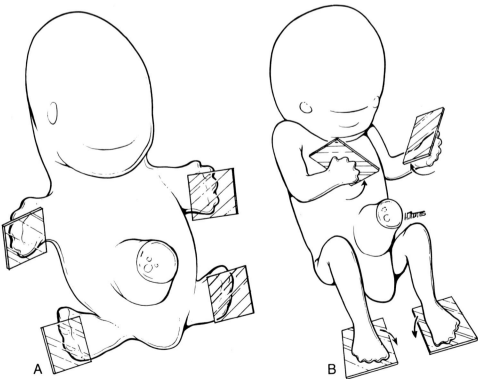

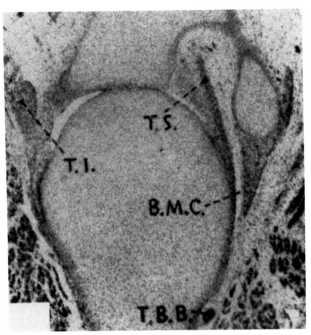

Figure 1–20. By the seventh week the glenohumeral joint is now well formed, with the middle zone of the three-layered interzone becoming less and less dense with increasing cavitation. The tendons of the infraspinatus (T.I.), subscapularis (T.S.), and biceps (T.B.B.) are clearly seen, as is the bursa of the coracobrachialis (B.M.C.). (Reproduced with permission from Gardner E, and Gray DJ: Prenatal development of the human shoulder and acromio-clavicular joint. Am J Anat 92:219, 1953.)

the upper limbs have almost reached their final length. Ossification proceeds rapidly during this period, especially during the 13th to 16th weeks. The first indication of ossification in the cartilaginous model of a long bone is visible near the center of the shaft. Primary centers appear at different times in different bones, but usually between the 7th and 12th weeks. The part of the bone ossified from the primary center is called the diaphysis. Secondary centers of ossification form what is called the epiphysis. The physeal plate separates these two centers of ossification until the bone grows to its adult height. From the 12th to the 16th week, the epiphyses are invaded by a vascular network, and in the shoulder joint, the epiphysis and part of the metaphysis are intracapsular.

The tendons, ligaments, and joint capsule around the shoulder are also penetrated by a rich vascular network during the same time in the fetal period, i.e., the third to fourth month of gestation. Most of the bursae of the shoulder, including the subdeltoid, subcoracoid, and subscapularis bursae, develop during this time. The glenoid labrum also develops prior to birth, with the majority of the tissue consisting of dense fibrous and some elastic tissue, but not fibrocartilage as seen in the menisci of the knee. The acromioclavicular joint develops in a manner different from that of the shoulder joint. Its development begins well into the fetal period, not the embryonic period, and a three-layered interzone is not seen as it is in the glenohumeral joint (Fig. 1–22).

POSTNATAL DEVELOPMENT

Postnatal development of the shoulder is mainly concerned with the appearance and development of the secondary centers of ossification, as the soft tissue changes only in size following birth. The development of the individual bones will be discussed separately.

Clavicle

As mentioned previously, the clavicle, along with the mandible, is the first bone in the body to ossify during the fifth week of gestation. Most bones in the body develop by endochondral ossification, in which condensations of mesenchymal tissue become cartilage and then undergo ossification. The major portion of the clavicle forms by intramembranous ossification, in which the mesenchymal cells are mineralized directly into bone. There are two separate ossification centers that form during the fifth week, the lateral and the medial. The lateral center is usually more prominent than the medial center, and the two masses form a long mass of bone. The cells at the acromial and sternal

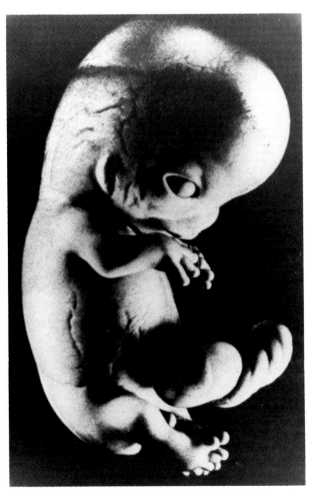

Figure 1–21. At the eighth week of gestation the embryo is about 23 mm long; through growth of the upper limb, the hands are stretched with the arms pronated. The firm musculature is now clearly defined.

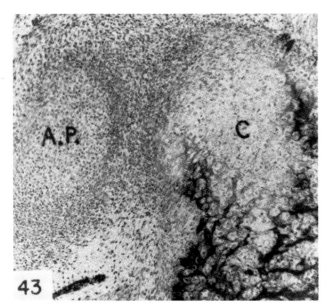

Figure 1–22. The acromioclavicular joint develops in a manner different from that of the shoulder joint. A three-layered interzone is not present as it is in the glenohumeral joint. (A.P. = acromion process; C = clavicle.)

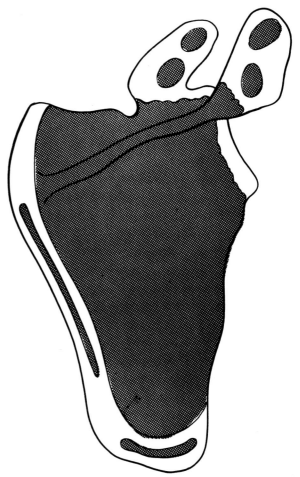

Figure 1–24. The coracoid process has two and sometimes three centers of ossification. A third inconsistent ossific center may appear at the tip of the coracoid process during puberty and occasionally fails to fuse with the coracoid. It may be confused with a fracture. The acromion has two and occasionally three ossification centers as well; unfused apophysis is not an uncommon finding and often presents with impingement syndrome.

ends of the clavicle take on a cartilaginous pattern to form the sternoclavicular and acromioclavicular joints. Therefore, the clavicle increases in diameter by intramembranous ossification of the periosteum and grows in length through endochondral activity at the cartilaginous ends. The medial clavicular epiphysis (Fig. 1–23) is responsible for the majority of longitudinal growth. It begins to ossify at age 18 and fuses with the clavicle between the ages of 22 and 25. The lateral epiphysis is less constant and often may appear as a wafer-like edge of bone just proximal to the acromioclavicular joint and can be confused with a fracture.

Scapula

The majority of the scapula also forms by intramembranous ossification. At birth, the body and the spine of the scapula have ossified, but not the coracoid, glenoid, acromion, and vertebral border and inferior angle of the scapula. The coracoid process has two, and occasionally three, centers of ossification (Fig. 1–

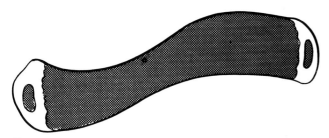

Figure 1–23. The medial clavicular epiphysis is responsible for most of the longitudinal growth of the clavicle. It fuses at ages 22 to 25. The lateral epiphysis is less constant; it often appears as a wafer-like edge of bone and may be confused with a fracture.

24). The first appears during the first year of life in the center of the coracoid process. The second arises around age 10 and appears at the base of the coracoid process. The second ossific nucleus also contributes to the formation of the superior portion of the glenoid cavity. These two centers unite with the scapula around age 15. A third inconsistent ossific center may appear at the tip of the coracoid process during puberty and occasionally fails to fuse with the coracoid. This may often be confused with a fracture, just like the distal clavicular epiphysis.

The acromion has two, and occasionally three, ossification centers as well. They arise during puberty and fuse together around age 22. This may again be confused with a fracture when, on axillary view, an unfused apophysis, most often a mesoacromion, presents itself. This is not an uncommon finding and often is seen in patients presenting with impingement syndrome.

The glenoid fossa has two ossification centers. The first appears at the base of the coracoid around age 10 and fuses around age 15, contributing as well to the superior portion of the glenoid cavity and the base of the coracoid process. The second ossification center is a horseshoe-shaped center arising from the inferior portion of the glenoid during puberty and forms the lower three-fourths of the glenoid.

The vertebral border and inferior angle of the scapula each have one ossification center, both of which appear at puberty and fuse around age 22.

Proximal Humerus

There are three ossification centers in the proximal humerus (Fig. 1–25): one for the head of the humerus, one for the greater tuberosity, and one for the lesser tuberosity. The ossification center in the humeral head usually appears between the fourth and sixth months, although it has been reported in *Gray's Anatomy*[41] to be present in 20 per cent of newborns. Without this radiographic landmark, it is often quite difficult to diagnose birth injuries. The ossification center for the greater tuberosity arises during the third year, and the center for the lesser tuberosity during the fifth year. The epiphyses for the tuberosities fuse together during the fifth year as well, and they in turn fuse with the center for the humeral head during the seventh year. Union between the head and the shaft usually occurs around age 19.

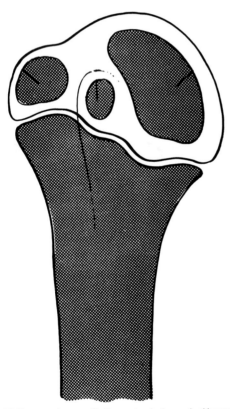

Figure 1–25. There are three ossification centers in the proximal humerus—for the head of the humerus, for the greater tuberosity, and for the lesser tuberosity.

Adult Glenohumeral Joint

BONY ANATOMY

The adult glenohumeral joint is formed by the humeral head and the glenoid surface of the scapula. Their geometrical relationship allows for remarkable ranges of motion, so important for prehensile activity. However, this is achieved with a concurrent loss of inherent biomechanical stability. The large spherical head of the humerus articulates against, and not within, a small, shallow glenoid fossa. It could best be compared to a golf ball sitting on a tee, with its stability relying on the static and dynamic soft tissue restraints acting across the joint.

The head of the humerus is a large, globular bony structure whose articular surface forms one-third of an irregular sphere which is directed medially, superiorly, and posteriorly. The head is inclined 130 to 150 degrees with relation to the shaft and has a retrotorsion angle of an average of 20 to 30 degrees (Fig. 1–26). The bicipital groove is 30 degrees medial to a line passing from the shaft through the center of the head of the humerus (Fig. 1–27). The greater tuberosity forms the lateral wall, and the lesser tuberosity the medial wall of this groove. The average vertical dimension of the surface of the articular portion of the head is 48 mm with a 25-mm radius of curvature. The average transverse dimension is 45 mm with a 22-mm radius of curvature.

The glenoid cavity is shaped like an inverted comma (Fig. 1–28). Its superior portion (tail) is narrow and the inferior portion broad. The transverse line between these two regions roughly corresponds to the epiphyseal line of the glenoid cavity.[22] It has a slightly concave articular surface covered by hyaline cartilage. In the center of the glenoid cavity there is often noted a distinct circular area of thinning which, according to DePalma,[22] was related to this region's greater contact with the humeral head and also related to age (Fig. 1–29). The average vertical dimension of the glenoid is 35 mm, and the average transverse diameter is 25 mm. In previous studies by Saha,[91, 92, 93] it had been noted that the glenoid may be either anteverted or retroverted with respect to the plane of the scapula. He found that 75 per cent of the shoulders studied had retroverted glenoid surfaces averaging 7.4 degrees, and approximately 25 per cent of the glenoid surfaces were anteverted from 2 to 10 degrees. With regard to vertical tilt, the superior portion of the superior/inferior line of the glenoid is angled an average of 15 degrees medially with regard to the scapular plane, making the glenoid surface on which the humeral head lies relatively horizontal (Fig. 1–30).

Based on contact surface studies in 20 shoulders, Saha[92] classified the glenohumeral articular surfaces into three types: Type A, in which the humeral surface has a radius of curvature smaller than that of the

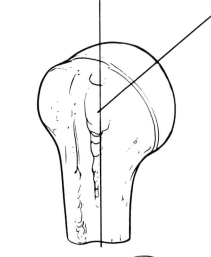

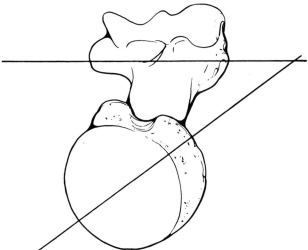

Figure 1–26. The neck and head of the humerus have an angle of inclination of 130 to 150 degrees in relation to the shaft *(top)* and a retrotorsion angle of 20 to 30 degrees *(bottom)*.

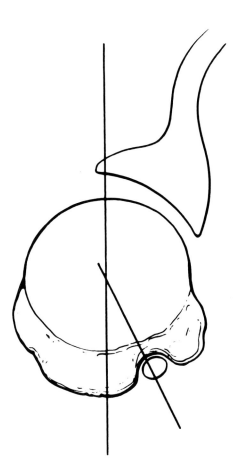

Figure 1–27. The bicipital groove is 30 degrees medial to a line that passes from the shaft through the center of the head of the humerus.

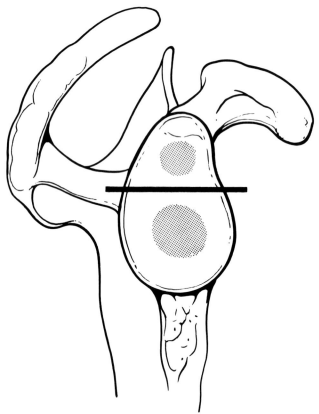

Figure 1–28. The glenoid cavity is shaped like an inverted comma. The transverse line corresponds to the epiphyseal line of the glenoid cavity.

glenoid, is therefore more curved than the corresponding glenoid, and has a small circular contact area; Type B, in which the humeral and glenoid surfaces have similar curvatures and a larger circular contact area; and Type C, in which the humeral surface has a radius

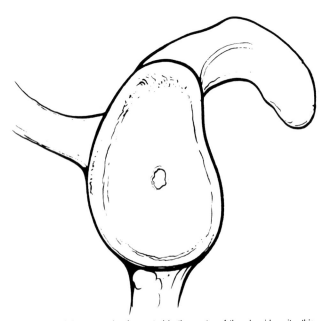

Figure 1–29. A bare area is often noted in the center of the glenoid cavity; this may be related to greater contact pressure and also to age.

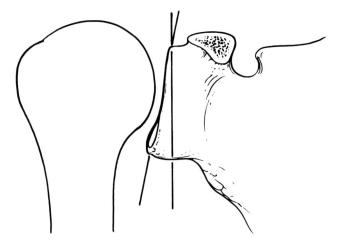

Figure 1–30. The superior portion of the superoinferior line of the glenoid is angled at an average of 15 degrees medially with regard to the scapular plane.

of curvature larger than that of the glenoid, which is more curved. The contact is limited to the periphery, and the contact surface is ring-shaped.

The glenoid labrum is a rim of fibrous tissue which is triangular in cross-section and overlies the glenoid cavity at the rim or edge (Fig. 1–31). It is variable in size and thickness, sometimes resembling the meniscus in the knee with a free inner edge projecting into the joint and sometimes being virtually absent. The labrum may also form the origin of the long head of the biceps tendon and the glenohumeral ligaments. Previously, the labrum had been likened to the fibrocartilaginous meniscus of the knee; however, Moseley and Overgaard[60] showed the labrum to be devoid of fibro-cartilage except in a small transition zone at the attachment on the osseous glenoid rim. The vast majority of the labrum consists of dense fibrous tissue with a few elastic fibers. It provides little, if any, depth to enhance stability of the shoulder, and we feel it adds little to stability unless integrally attached to the inferior glenohumeral ligament complex, which will be discussed shortly.

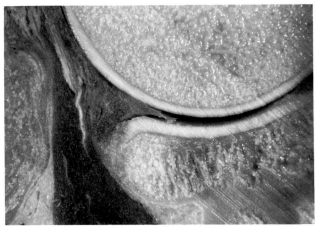

Figure 1–31. The glenoid labrum, the rim of fibrous tissue that is triangular in cross-section, overlies the glenoid cavity at the rim or edge. It may have a striking resemblance to the meniscus in the knee.

The long head of the biceps tendon inserts into the supraglenoid tubercle and is often continuous with the superior portion of the labrum. In previous studies by DePalma,[22] considerable variation may be present in this structure. It may exist as a double structure or within the fibrous capsule, or, as in one case, it may be absent from within the joint. In older patients with malfunction and degenerative changes within the rotator cuff, the biceps may undergo significant degeneration from superior migration of the humeral head. This manifests as thickening, widening, and shredding, especially in the shoulders from the fifth decade onwards, although Andrews has recently described similar changes in younger throwers.

SHOULDER CAPSULE

The shoulder capsule is large, having twice the surface area of the humeral head. A patient will normally accept approximately 10 to 15 ml of fluid; however, in pathological conditions, this will vary. For example, patients with adhesive capsulitis will only accept 5 ml or less of fluid, while patients with considerable laxity or instability will accept large volumes of fluid (>30 ml) easily.

The shoulder capsule is lined with synovium and extends from the glenoid neck (or occasionally labrum) to the anatomical neck and the proximal shaft of the humerus to varying degrees. In addition, the capsule will often extend to attach to the coracoid process superiorly (via the coracohumeral ligament) and the anterior or posterior body of the scapula (via anterior and posterior recesses) and extend down for variable lengths along the biceps tendon and intertubercular groove of the humerus.

In recent years, biochemical investigations have shown that various connective tissues in the body are endowed with several types of collagen molecules. As we know, collagen is the basic structural fiber in animals and humans, occurring in the form of fibrous (often cross-striated) supporting elements. The shoulder capsule is a good example of how varying collagen content and orientation lends static stability to this unstable joint. Various portions of the capsule take on function both according to the inherent collagen content and orientation and also according to *how* and *where* they are attached to the glenoid, labrum, and humerus. There are basically five types of collagen molecules, based on varying arrangements of three noncoaxial helical polypeptides stabilized by interchain hydrogen bonds (Fig. 1–32).[48] Type I collagen comprises two alpha 1 (I) chains and an alpha 2 (I) chain. It is the most common collagen of bone, tendon, skin, and other connective tissues. Type II collagen is seen in hyaline cartilage and comprises three alpha 1 (II) chains. Type III collagen contains three alpha 1 (III) chains and is common in aorta, infant skin, and muscular and elastic tissues. Type IV is the main constituent of basement membrane collagen. Type V collagen

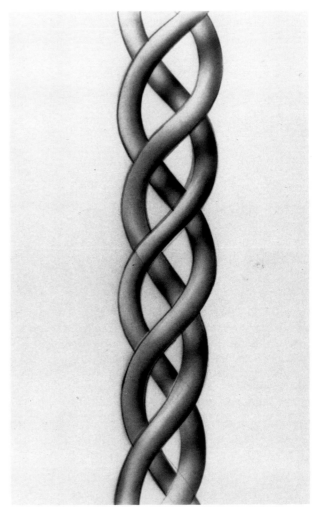

Figure 1–32. A collagen molecule has three noncoaxial helical polypeptides stabilized by interchain hydrogen bonds. The type of collagen present and its orientation determine the strength and thickness of different regions of the shoulder capsule.

consists of two different chains, alpha A and alpha B, and is present in aorta, placenta, smooth cells in culture, fibroblasts, and chondroblasts. The electrophoretic pattern of the shoulder joint capsule demonstrates the presence of Types I, III, and V collagen and is similar in this respect to other joints.

The most important and constant thickenings in the shoulder capsule are termed ligaments and show great variation in size, shape, thickness, and attachment site. The coracohumeral ligament is a rather strong band originating from the base and lateral border of the coracoid process just below the origin of the coracoacromial ligament (Fig. 1–33). It is directed transversely and inserts on the greater tuberosity. The anterior border is often distinct medially and merges with the capsule laterally. The posterior border is usually indistinct from the remaining capsule. Some authors believe that it represents phylogenetically the old insertion of the pectoralis minor, and in 15 per cent of the population, a part of the pectoralis minor

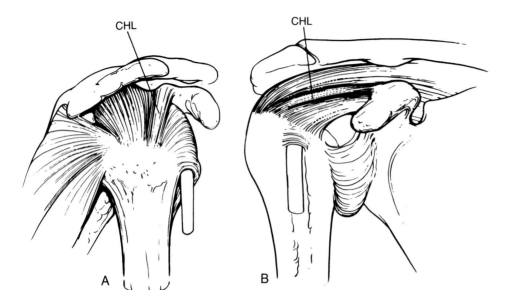

Figure 1–33. *A, B,* The coracohumeral ligament (CHL) is a strong band originating from the base of the lateral border of the coracoid process, just below the coracoacromial ligament, and merging with the capsule laterally to insert on the greater tuberosity. This ligament may have importance as a suspensory structure for the adducted arm.

crosses the coracoid process to insert on the humeral head.[41] Although the biomechanical contribution of this ligament is not yet fully known, it appears to have a static suspensory function for the humeral head in the glenoid cavity when the arm is held at the side. With abduction, it relaxes and loses its ability to support the humerus.

The transverse humeral ligament (Fig. 1–34) is composed of a few transverse fibers of the capsule extending between the greater and lesser tuberosities and helps to contain the tendon of the long head of the biceps in its groove.

On all sides of the shoulder capsule, except the inferior portion, the capsule is reinforced and strength-

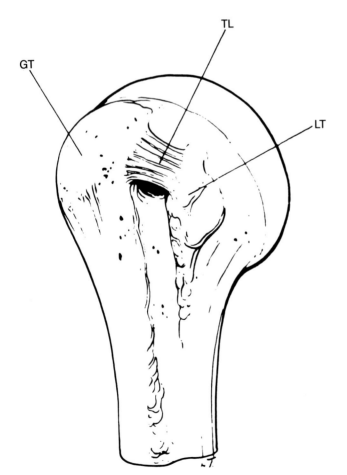

Figure 1–34. The transverse humeral ligament (TL) is composed of transverse fibers of the capsule extending between the greater tuberosity (GT) and the lesser tuberosity (LT), containing the tendon of the long head of the biceps in its groove.

RC

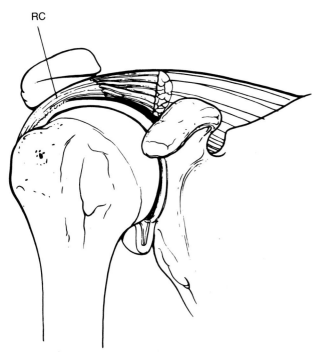

Figure 1–35. The rotator cuff (RC) musculature blends into the capsule over varying lengths (on average approximately 2.5 cm) from the insertion site of the rotator cuff on the humerus.

ened by the tendons of the rotator cuff muscles, i.e., the supraspinatus, infraspinatus, teres minor, and subscapularis (Fig. 1–35). The tendons blend into the capsule over varying lengths, averaging approximately 2.5 cm. The most prominent of these is the tendinous

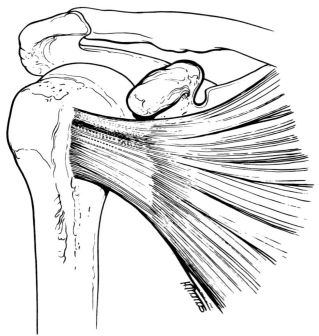

Figure 1–36. The subscapularis muscle inserts into the lesser tuberosity with the most superior portion and has a distinct thickening that may resemble a tendon.

portion of the subscapularis anteriorly (Fig. 1–36). They form the musculotendinous, or capsulotendinous, cuff.

GLENOHUMERAL LIGAMENTS

The glenohumeral ligaments are collagenous reinforcements to the shoulder capsule which are not visible on its external surface. They are best appreciated *in situ* arthroscopically without distention with air or saline (Fig. 1–37). Their function is dependent on (1) their collagenous integrity, (2) their attachment sites, and (3) the position of the arm.

Superior Glenohumeral Ligament

The superior glenohumeral ligament is a fairly constant structure, with the shoulder capsule arising just anterior to the long head of the biceps origin. Three common variations are seen in its glenoid attachment site.[22] It is either originating from a common origin with the biceps tendon, arising from the labrum just anterior to the biceps tendon, or arising with the origin of the middle glenohumeral ligament (Fig. 1–38). It inserts into the fovea capitis, lying just superior to the lesser tuberosity (Fig. 1–39).[105]

The superior glenohumeral ligament was present 97 per cent of the time in a classic anatomical study by DePalma[22] and 90 per cent of the time in a recent anatomical study we conducted at our institution.[66] Its size and integrity are quite variable, however. It may exist as a thin wisp of capsular tissue or as a thickening similar to the patellofemoral ligaments in the knee. Recent biomechanical studies we have performed show that it contributes very little to static stability of the glenohumeral joint.[96] Selective cutting of this ligament

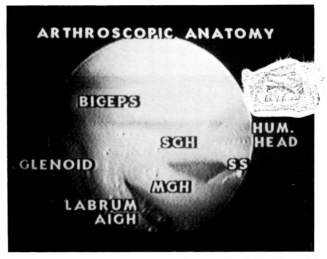

Figure 1–37. The glenohumeral ligaments are best appreciated with arthroscopic visualization without distention with air or saline. In this view, the various glenohumeral ligaments are seen as they appear from a posterior portal view.

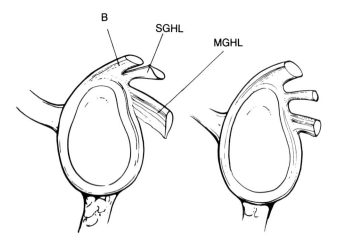
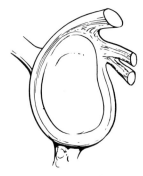

Figure 1–38. Three common variations of the origin of the superior glenohumeral ligament (SGHL). (B = biceps tendon; MGHL = middle glenohumeral ligament.)

did not significantly affect translation either anteriorly or posteriorly in the abducted shoulder. Its contribution to stability would best be demonstrated with the arm at the side, lending support to keep the humeral head suspended (along with the coracohumeral ligament and rotator cuff), and its relative contribution dependent on its thickness and collagenous integrity.

Middle Glenohumeral Ligament

The middle glenohumeral ligament shows the greatest variation in size of the glenohumeral ligaments and is not present as frequently as the other glenohumeral ligaments. In 96 shoulders studied by DePalma,[22] it was a well-formed, distinct structure in 68, poorly defined in 16, and absent in 12. We found it to be absent in approximately 27 per cent of the specimens we studied.[66] In an individual specimen, it may be either quite thin or as thick as the biceps tendon (Fig. 1–40). When present, it arises in most specimens from

the labrum immediately below the superior glenohumeral ligament or from the adjacent neck of the glenoid. It inserts into the humerus just medial to the lesser tuberosity, under the tendon of the subscapularis, to which it adheres (Fig. 1–39).[105] Other variations are seen in which the middle glenohumeral ligament has no attachment site other than the anterior portion of the capsule or it exists as two parallel thickenings in the anterior capsule. Its contribution to static stability is variable. However, when it is quite thick, it can act as an important secondary restraint to anterior translation if the anterior portion of the inferior glenohumeral ligament is damaged.[96]

Inferior Glenohumeral Ligament

The inferior glenohumeral ligament is a complex structure that is the main static stabilizer of the abducted shoulder. Originally described as a triangular-shaped structure with its apex at the labrum and its base blending with the capsule between the subscapularis and the triceps area,[22] Turkel and colleagues[105] expanded on the anatomical description of the inferior glenohumeral ligament by calling attention to the anterior superior edge of this ligament that was especially thickened, which they called the superior band of the inferior glenohumeral ligament (Fig. 1–41). In addition, they called the region between the superior band and the middle glenohumeral ligament the anterior axillary pouch, and the remainder of the capsule posterior to the superior band the posterior axillary pouch.

With the advent of arthroscopy, we have been able to study the joint *in situ* and appreciate capsular structures that earlier investigators could not. This is because arthrotomy of the shoulder disrupts important geometrical arrangements needed to appreciate parts of the capsular anatomy. By inserting the arthroscope from anterior and superior portals, in addition to traditional posterior portals, and also by observing the joint without distention by air or saline, we have observed that the inferior glenohumeral ligament is more complex than previously thought. We observed

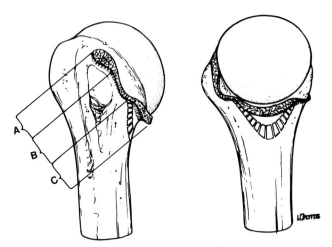

Figure 1–39. The attachment sites of the glenohumeral ligaments. *Left,* the superior glenohumeral ligament inserts into the fovea capitis line just superior to the lesser tuberosity (A). The middle glenohumeral ligament inserts into the humerus just medial to the lesser tuberosity (B). The inferior glenohumeral ligament complex has two common attachment mechanisms (C). It may attach in a collar-like fashion, or it may have a V-shaped attachment to the articular edge *(right).*

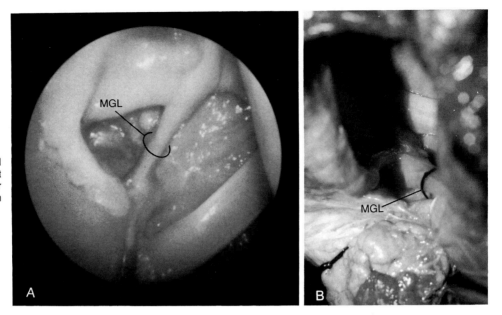

Figure 1–40. The middle glenohumeral ligament (MGL) has great variability. It may exist as a thin wisp of tissue *(A)*, or it may be as thick as the biceps tendon *(B)*.

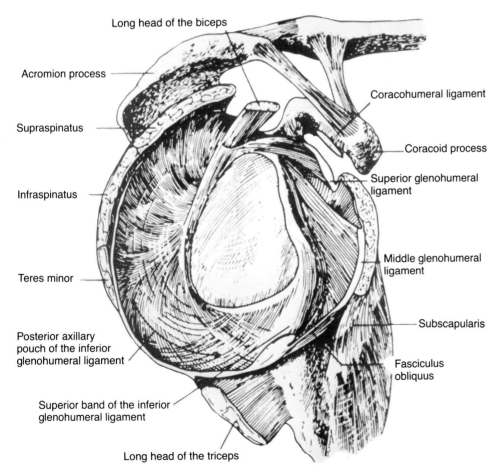

Figure 1–41. The anatomical description by Turkel and colleagues of the inferior glenohumeral ligament called attention to the anterior/superior edge of this ligament, which was especially thickened; they called this the superior band of the inferior glenohumeral ligament. However, there are no posterior structures defined. (Reproduced from Turkel SJ, Panio MW, Marshall JL, and Girgis FG: Stabilizing mechanisms preventing anterior dislocation of the glenohumeral joint. J Bone Joint Surg 63A:1208–1217, 1981.)

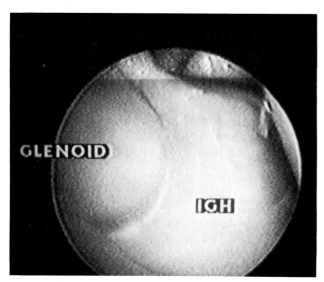

Figure 1–42. Posterior arthroscopic view of the inferior glenohumeral (IGH) ligament complex. It is a hammock-like structure originating from the glenoid and inserting onto the anatomical neck of the humerus.

that the inferior glenohumeral ligament is a hammock-like structure originating from the glenoid and inserting into the anatomical neck of the humerus (Fig. 1–42).[66] This was composed of an anterior band, a posterior band, and an axillary pouch lying in between. We have called this the inferior glenohumeral ligament complex. The anterior and posterior bands are most clearly defined with the arm abducted (Fig. 1–43). With abduction and external rotation, the anterior band fans out to support the head, and the posterior band becomes cord-like (Fig. 1–44). Conversely, with internal rotation, the posterior band fans out to support the head, and the anterior band becomes cord-like.

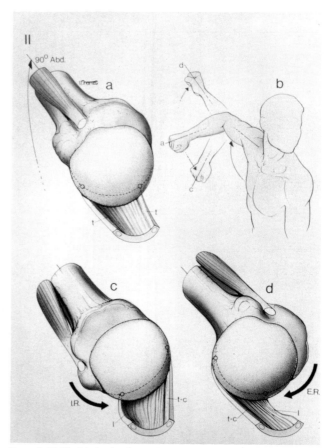

Figure 1–44. The inferior glenohumeral complex is tightened during abduction (a). During abduction and internal or external rotation different parts of the band are tightened (b). With internal rotation the posterior band fans out to support the head and the anterior band becomes cord-like or relaxed, depending on the degree of horizontal flexion or extension (c). Upon abduction and external rotation, the anterior band fans out to support the head and the posterior band becomes cord-like or relaxed, depending on the degree of horizontal flexion or extension (d).

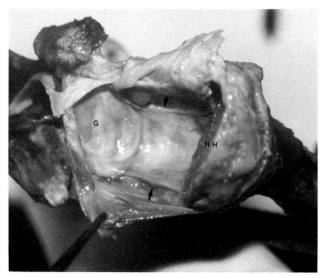

Figure 1–43. The anterior and posterior ends of the inferior glenohumeral ligament (black arrows) complex are clearly defined in this picture of an abducted shoulder specimen with the humeral head (HH) partially resected.

On gross examination, the inferior glenohumeral ligament complex takes its origin from either the glenoid labrum or the glenoid neck and inserts into the anatomical neck of the humerus. The origins of the anterior band and posterior band on the glenoid can be described in terms of the face of a clock. In a recent anatomical study we conducted (Fig. 1–45),[66] the anterior band of each specimen originated from various areas from 2:00 to 4:00, and the posterior band from 7:00 to 9:00. On the humeral head side, the inferior glenohumeral ligament complex attaches in an approximately 90-degree arc just below the articular margin of the humeral head. Two methods of attachment were noted. In some specimens, there was a collar-like attachment of varying thickness just inferior to the articular edge, being closer to the articular edge than the remainder of the capsule (Fig. 1–46). In other specimens, the inferior glenohumeral ligament complex attached in a V-shaped fashion, with the anterior band and posterior band attaching close to the articular surface, and the axillary pouch attaching to the hu-

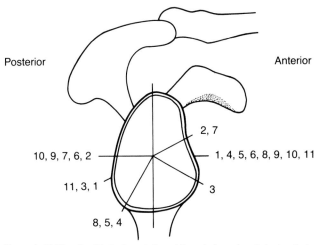

Figure 1–45. The glenoid attachment sites of the anterior and posterior bands. In 11 cadaver specimens the anterior band originated from various areas between 2:00 and 4:00, and the posterior band from areas between 7:00 and 9:00.

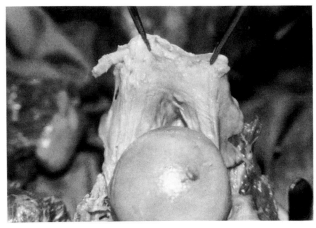

Figure 1–47. A V-shaped attachment of the inferior glenohumeral ligament complex of the humerus, with the axillary pouch attaching to the humerus at the apex of the V farther from the articular edge.

merus at the apex of the V, further from the articular edge (Fig. 1–47).

The inferior glenohumeral ligament complex is thicker than the rest of the capsule adjoining it anteriorly and posteriorly (Fig. 1–48), although considerable variation exists. The inferior glenohumeral ligament is thicker than the anterior capsule, which in turn is thicker than the posterior capsule.

The anterior and posterior bands of the inferior glenohumeral ligament complex also show great variation in thickness, but we have been able to identify them in all specimens (Figs. 1–49 and 1–50).[66] The anterior band is usually easier to distinguish than the posterior band, owing to the fact that it attaches higher on the glenoid and it is usually thicker than the posterior band. However, the anterior and posterior

bands are often of equal thickness, and occasionally, the posterior band is thicker than the anterior band. Sometimes, the anterior band and posterior band can only be visualized grossly by abducting the arm and by internally and externally rotating the arm at 90 degrees of abduction.

Histologically, the inferior glenohumeral ligament complex is distinguishable from the remainder of the shoulder capsule, and the anterior band, axillary pouch, and posterior band are distinct structures.[66] Even in cases in which the bands were not so well-defined macroscopically, they were easily distinguishable histologically. In fact, the posterior band is easier to distinguish histologically than the anterior band, owing to the more abrupt transition from the thin posterior capsule.

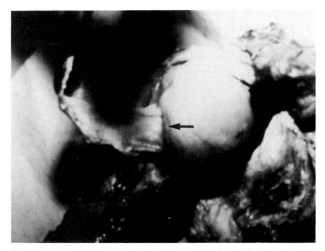

Figure 1–46. An example of a collar-like attachment of the inferior glenohumeral ligament complex just inferior to the articular edge and closer to the articular edge than the remainder of the capsule.

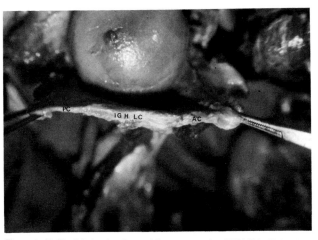

Figure 1–48. The inferior glenohumeral ligament complex (IGH LC) is thicker than both the anterior capsule (AC) and the posterior capsule (PC).

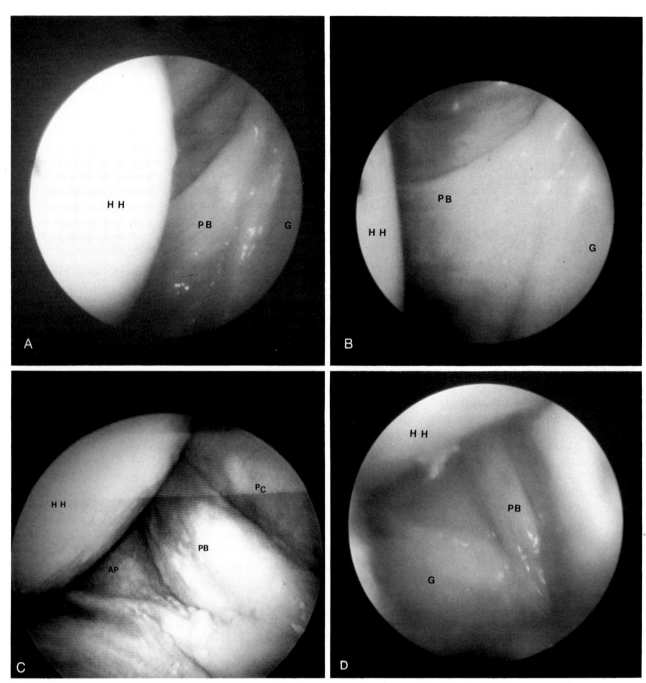

Figure 1–49. Various views of the posterior band of the inferior glenohumeral ligament complex as viewed arthroscopically from an anterior portal. *A* and *B* show the distinct configuration of the posterior band (PB) with internal and external rotation. With internal rotation, the posterior band fans out to support the humeral head (HH). *C* and *D* show two superior portal views of the posterior band, the posterior capsule (PC), the axillary pouch (AP), and the glenoid (G).

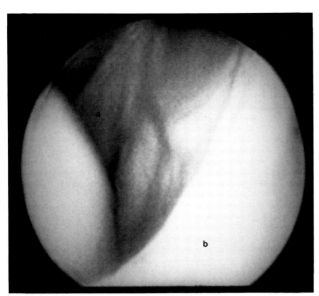

Figure 1-50. An arthroscopic view anteriorly of the inferior glenohumeral ligament complex showing the anterior and posterior bands *(a and b)* and the intervening axillary pouch.

The shoulder capsule consists of a synovial lining and three well-defined layers of collagen (Fig. 1–51). The fibers of the inner and outer layers extend in a coronal axis from the glenoid to the humerus. The middle layer of collagen extends in a sagittal direction, crossing the fibers of the other two layers. The relative thickness and the degree of intermingling of collagen fibers of the three layers vary with the different portions of the capsule.

The posterior capsule is quite thin (Fig. 1–52). The three layers of the capsule are well seen, but the outer layer is least prominent and quickly blends into a layer of loose areolar tissue outside the capsule.

The posterior band exists as an abrupt thickening in the capsule (Fig. 1–53). This is due mostly to the presence of increased, well-organized, coarse collagen bundles in the coronal plane within the inner layer, oriented at 90 degrees to the middle layer. The inner layer is displaced outward at the expense of relative thinning of the outer layer. This can be appreciated quite well in coronal views of the posterior band (Fig. 1–54).

The transition from the posterior band to the axillary pouch is less distinct, and the axillary pouch has a gradual intermingling of the coarse longitudinal inner fibers with the sagittal transverse fibers which are continuous with the transverse fibers of the middle layer (Fig. 1–55). In the axillary pouch region, the outer layer is attenuated and virtually disappears.

The anterior band also exists as an abrupt thickening of the inner layer of the anterior capsule, although the distinction histologically is not as marked as the transition with the posterior band and posterior capsule. The more precise collagen orientation, similar to the posterior band, can be seen, and in the coronal view in Figure 1–56, we can see that the histological picture is virtually identical to that seen in Figure 1–54 of the posterior band. As we again approach the axillary pouch, these bundles lose their precise organization and intermingle with the fibers of the middle layer.

The capsule anterior to the inferior glenohumeral ligament complex is qualitatively thicker than the capsule posterior to the inferior glenohumeral ligament complex, mainly owing to the relative increase in thickness of the middle layer. There is a lot of intermingling of the middle and outer layers of the capsule in this region (see Figs. 1–48 and 1–51).

This concept of the inferior glenohumeral ligament complex functioning as a hammock-like sling to support the humeral head (Fig. 1–57) gives a unifying concept to understanding anterior and posterior instability in the human shoulder and explains how damage in one

SAGITTAL SCHEMATIC OF HISTOLOGY

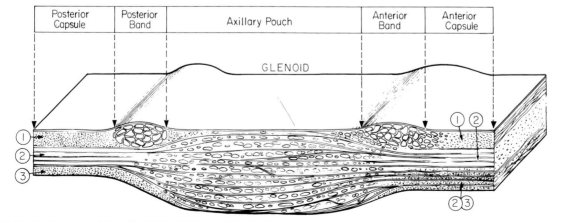

Figure 1-51. A schematic representation of the histological layers of the shoulder capsule. The capsule consists of a thin synovial lining and three well-defined layers of collagen (see text).

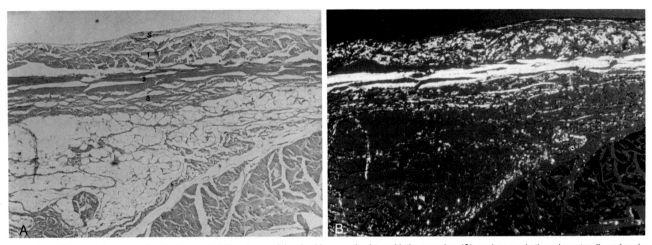

Figure 1–52. The posterior capsule is quite thin, and all three layers of the shoulder capsule along with the synovium (S) can be seen in these hematoxylin and eosin (A) and polarized light (B) views. The posterior capsule quickly blends into a layer of loose areolar tissue outside the capsule.

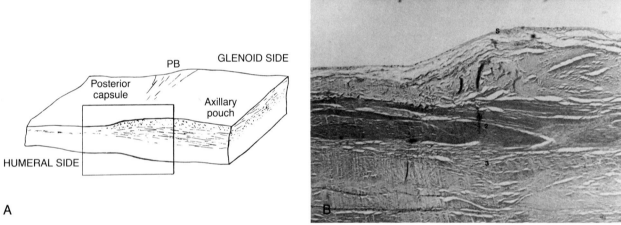

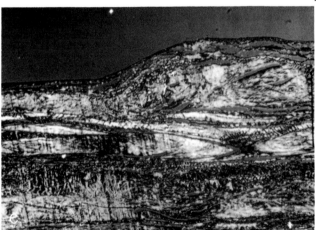

Figure 1–53. A, The posterior band exists as an abrupt thickening in the shoulder capsule. B, C, In these sagittal views, the thickening can be seen in the inner layer of the capsule.

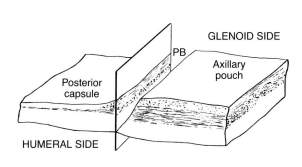

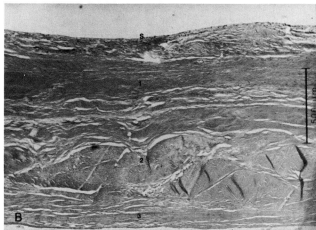

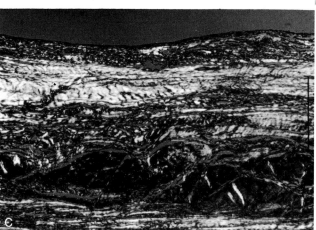

Figure 1–54. *A* shows the precise organization of the posterior band. *B, C,* The coronal views demonstrate three well-defined layers in this region.

Figure 1–55. *A, B,* The sagittal views of the axillary pouch show blending of the inner and middle layers and continuation of the outermost layer.

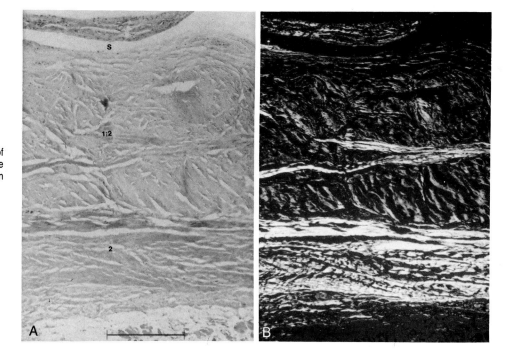

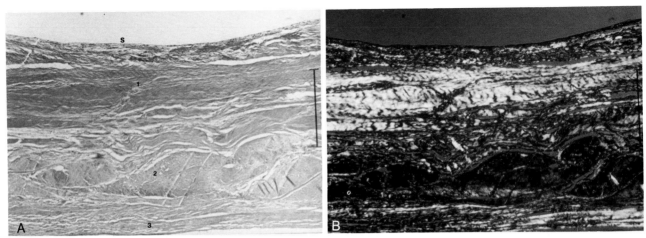

Figure 1-56. *A, B,* The more precise collagen orientation returns in the region of the anterior band, as seen in these coronal views. These are virtually identical with the views of the posterior band in Figure 1-54.

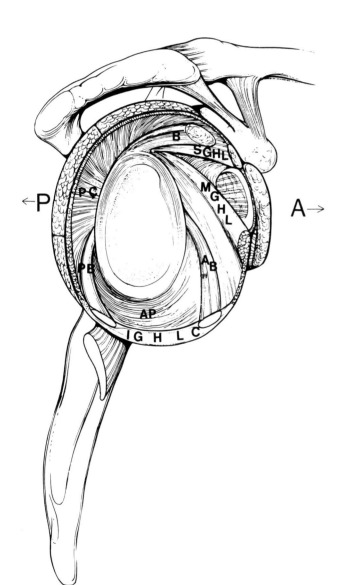

Figure 1-57. Anatomical depiction of the glenohumeral ligaments and inferior glenohumeral ligament complex (IGHLC). (P = posterior; A = anterior; SGHL = superior glenohumeral ligament; MGHL = middle glenohumeral ligament.)

portion of the shoulder capsule may have effects on the opposite side. This has clinical significance for treating instability disorders of the shoulder.

BURSAE

There are several bursae found in the shoulder region, and there are a number of recesses in the shoulder capsule formed between the glenohumeral ligaments. Two bursae in particular have clinical importance: the subacromial bursa, which will be discussed later; and the subscapular bursa. The subscapular bursa lies between the subscapularis tendon and the neck of the scapula (Fig. 1–58), and it communicates with the joint cavity between the superior and middle glenohumeral ligaments. It protects the tendon of the subscapularis where it passes under the base of the coracoid process and over the neck of the scapula. It is often involved with housing loose bodies in the shoulder, and it is also a region where synovitis of the shoulder may be most intense, where small fringes, or villi, may project into the joint cavity.

Although uncommon (and not in communication with the joint cavity), another bursa may be present between the infraspinatus muscle and the capsule. Other synovial recesses are usually in the anterior portion of the capsule. The number, size, and location of these depend on the topographical variations of the glenohumeral ligaments. DePalma[22] described six common variations or types of recesses in the anterior capsule (Fig. 1–59) which are really variations in the opening of the subscapularis bursa: Type 1 (30.2 per cent) exhibits one synovial recess above the middle

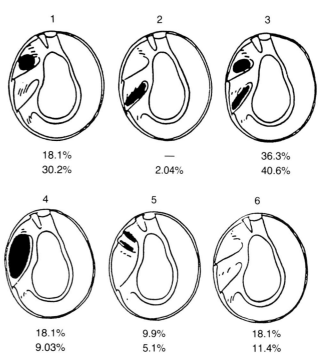

TYPES OF ARRANGEMENT OF THE SYNOVIAL RECESS
(DePalma et al, 1949)

1	2	3
18.1%	—	36.3%
30.2%	2.04%	40.6%

4	5	6
18.1%	9.9%	18.1%
9.03%	5.1%	11.4%

Figure 1–59. Variations in the types of anterior recesses in the capsule. The original percentages of DePalma are listed *(top lines)* along with percentages from more recent anatomical studies *(bottom lines)*.

glenohumeral ligament; Type 2 (2.04 per cent) presents one synovial recess below the middle glenohumeral ligament; Type 3 (40.6 per cent) discloses one recess above and one below the middle glenohumeral ligament; Type 4 (9.03 per cent) reveals one large recess above the inferior ligament with the middle glenohumeral ligament absent; Type 5 (5.1 per cent) presents the middle glenohumeral ligament as two small synovial folds; and Type 6 (11.4 per cent) has no synovial recesses, but all the ligaments are well defined. Regardless of the type in which the recesses are found, the recesses show extreme variability. DePalma felt that if the capsule arises at the labrum or glenoid border of the scapula, there are few, if any, recesses. However, if the capsule begins farther medially on the scapula or glenoid neck, the synovial recesses will be larger and more numerous. He believed that the end result of this was a thin, weakened anterior capsule that may predispose the patient to instability.

Others refer to this general area of the anterior capsule as the rotator interval,[65] which they define as the space between the superior border of the subscapularis and the supraspinatus. This interval also includes the region of the superior glenohumeral ligament and coracohumeral ligament, in addition to the middle glenohumeral ligament. Some authors believe that this area may increase instability in certain shoulders and should be surgically obliterated during stabilization procedures.[65, 89]

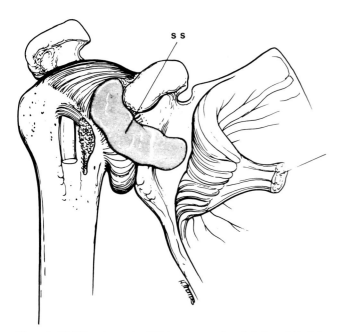

S S

Figure 1–58. This subscapular (SS) bursa connects anteriorly and inferiorly under the coracoid process in the anterior portion of the capsule. Loose bodies are often found in this region.

Microvasculature

ROTATOR CUFF

Six arteries contribute regularly to the arterial supply of the rotator cuff tendons: (1) suprascapular (100 per cent); (2) anterior circumflex humeral (100 per cent); (3) posterior circumflex humeral (100 per cent); (4) thoracoacromial (76 per cent); (5) suprahumeral (59 per cent); and (6) subscapular (38 per cent).[88] The posterior circumflex humeral and suprascapular arteries form an interlacing pattern on the posterior portion of the rotator cuff with several large anastomoses. These are the predominant arteries to the teres minor and the infraspinatus tendons (Fig. 1–60). The anterior humeral circumflex artery supplies the subscapularis muscle and tendon and anastomoses with the posterior humeral circumflex over the tendon of the long head of the biceps (Fig. 1–61). In addition, a large branch of the anterior humeral circumflex artery enters the intertubercular groove, becoming the major blood supply to the humeral head.

Branches of the acromial portion of the thoracoacromial artery supply the anterosuperior portion of the rotator cuff, particularly the supraspinatus tendon (Fig. 1–62), and frequently anastomoses with both circumflex humeral arteries. The subscapular and suprahumeral artery (named by Rothman and Parke to describe a small vessel from the third portion of the axillary artery to the anterior rotator cuff and lesser

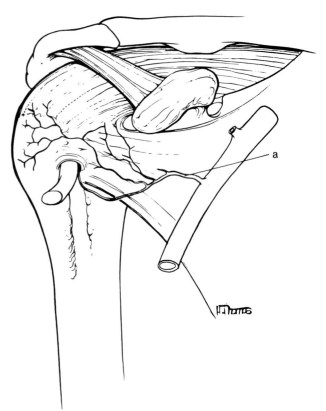

Figure 1–61. The anterior humeral circumflex artery (a) supplies the subscapularis muscle and tendon and anastomoses with the posterior humeral circumflex over the tendon of the long head of the biceps. In addition, a large branch of the anterior humeral circumflex enters the intertubercular groove, becoming the major blood supply to the head.

tuberosity) make only minimal contributions to the rotator cuff. Approximately two-thirds of shoulders will have a hypovascular zone in the tendinous portion of the supraspinatus tendon just proximal to its insertion. Less frequently, the infraspinatus (37 per cent) and the subscapularis (7 per cent) will have a hypovascular area. This area of hypovascularity corresponds to the common areas of degeneration in the rotator cuff, although these hypovascular regions may be present at birth.[82] However, a significant decrease in vascularity with aging and degeneration can be seen. Rathburn and Macnab[82] demonstrated that in this hypovascular "critical zone" in the rotator cuff, vascular filling was dependent on the position of the arm, with less filling noted with the arm in adduction (Fig. 1–63). Most likely, filling is also chronically impeded with advanced impingement, with the humeral head and rotator cuff impinging on the acromion, compressing the hypovascular zone and limiting the potential for repair of small additional tears in these locations. This, however, has never been proved.

GLENOID LABRUM

The glenoid labrum is supplied by small branches of three major vessels supplying the shoulder joint: the

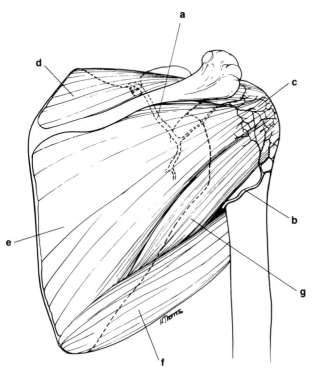

Figure 1–60. The suprascapular artery (a) and the posterior circumflex humeral artery (b) form an interlacing pattern on the posterior portion of the rotator cuff (c) with several large anastomoses. Also depicted are the supraspinatus (d), infraspinatus (e), teres major (f), and teres minor (g).

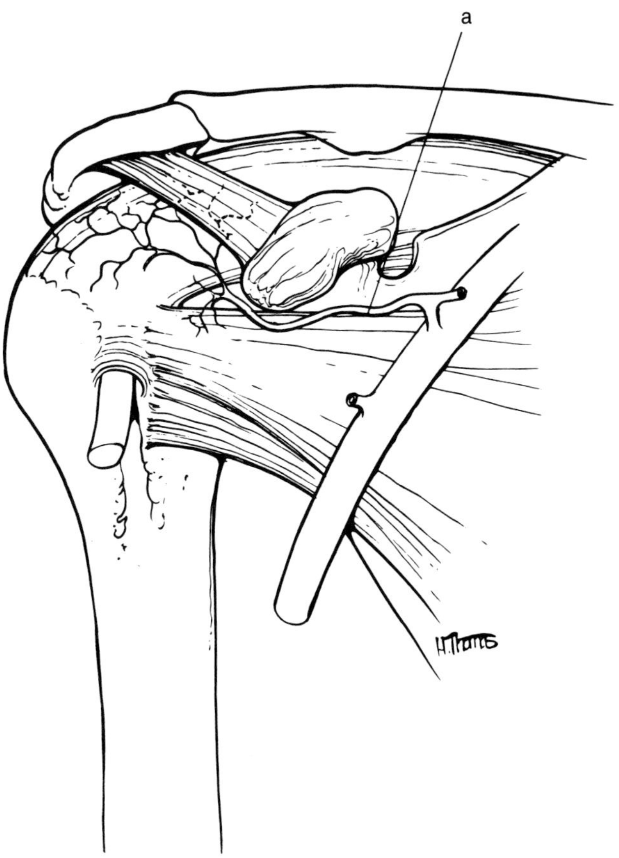

Figure 1–62. The acromial branch (a) of the thoracoacromial artery supplies the anterosuperior portion of the rotator cuff, particularly the supraspinatus tendon.

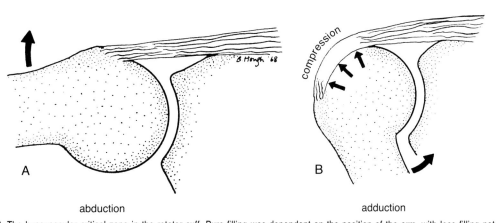

abduction   adduction

Figure 1–63. *A, B,* The hypovascular critical zone in the rotator cuff. Pure filling was dependent on the position of the arm, with less filling noted with the arm in adduction. (Reproduced with permission from Rathburn JB, and Macnab I: The microvascular pattern of the rotator cuff. J Bone Joint Surg *52-B*:540–553, 1970.)

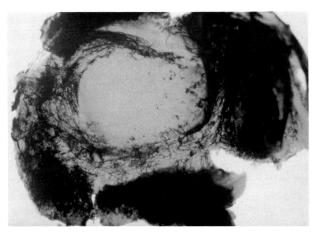

Figure 1–64. The microvasculature of the shoulder capsule and labrum. The inferior glenohumeral ligament complex has increased vascularity with regard to the remainder of the posterior capsule, which is relatively devoid of significant vasculature.

suprascapular artery, the circumflex scapular artery, and the posterior humeral circumflex artery (Fig. 1–64). These vessels supply the peripheral attachment of the labrum through small periosteal and capsular vessels (Fig. 1–65). Although the extent of these micro-

vascular patterns is variable throughout the labrum, they are usually limited to the outermost aspect of the labrum with the inner rim being devoid of vessels. This arrangement is similar to that observed in the menisci in the knee.[3]

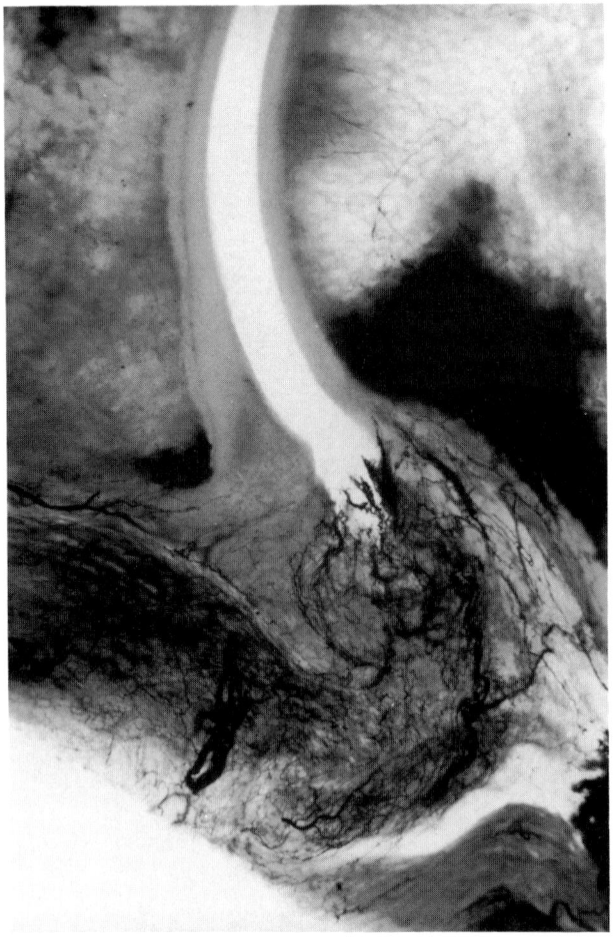

Innervation of the Glenohumeral Joint

The superficial and deep structures of the shoulder are profusely innervated by a network of nerve fibers which are mainly derived from the C5, C6, and C7 nerve roots (although the C4 root may make a minor contribution).[20, 33] The innervation of the joint itself follows Hilton's Law, which states that nerves crossing a joint give off branches to the joint and innervate it. Therefore, the nerves supplying the ligaments, capsule, and synovial membrane of the shoulder are medullary and nonmedullary fibers from the axillary, suprascapular, subscapular, and musculocutaneous nerves, in addition to occasional contributions from small branches of the posterior cord of the brachial plexus. The relative contributions of these nerves are not constant and may, in fact, be reciprocal (e.g., if the branch from the axillary nerve is large since there are several branches from the axillary nerve), and the

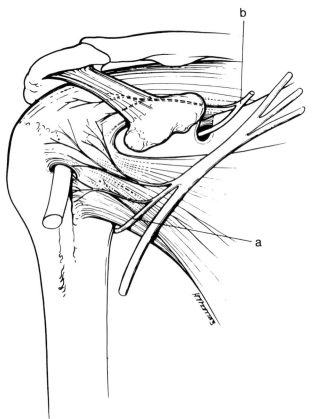

Figure 1–66. The innervation of the anterior portion of the shoulder. The axillary (a) and suprascapular (b) nerves form most of the nerve supply to the capsule and the glenohumeral joint. In some instances the musculocutaneous nerve may send some twigs to the anterosuperior portion of the joint.

Figure 1–65. The vasculature of the labrum's edge, with small periosteal and capsular vessels visible.

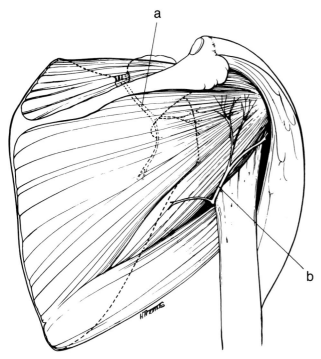

Figure 1-67. The posterior innervation of the shoulder joint. The primary nerves are the suprascapular (a) and the axillary (b).

supply from the musculocutaneous nerve may be very small or completely absent. After piercing the joint capsule, branches from these nerves form a network, or plexus, to supply the synovium.

Anteriorly, the axillary nerve and suprascapular nerve provide most of the nerve supply to the capsule and glenohumeral joint. In some instances, the musculocutaneous nerve may innervate the anterosuperior portion of the joint. In addition, the anterior capsule may be supplied by either the subscapular nerves or the posterior cord of the brachial plexus after they have pierced the subscapularis (Fig. 1–66).

Superiorly, the nerves contributing primarily are two branches of the suprascapular nerve, with one branch proceeding anteriorly as far as the coracoid process and coracoacromial ligament, while the other branch reaches the posterior aspect of the joint. Other nerves contributing to this region of the joint are the axillary nerve, musculocutaneous nerve, and branches from the lateral anterior thoracic nerve.

Posteriorly, the chief nerves are the suprascapular nerve in the upper region and the axillary nerve in the lower region (Fig. 1–67).

Inferiorly, the anterior portion is primarily supplied by the axillary nerve, and the posterior portion is supplied by a combination of the axillary nerve and lower ramifications of the suprascapular nerve.

References

1. Adler H, and Lohman B: The stability of the shoulder joint in stress radiography. Arch Orthop Trauma Surg *103*:83–84, 1984.
2. Anderson H: Histochemistry and development of the human shoulder and acromioclavicular joints with particular reference to the early development of the clavicle. Acta Anat *55*:124–165, 1963.
3. Arnoczky SP, and Allen A: The microvasculature of the glenoid labrum in the human shoulder (unpublished data).
4. Bankart AS: The pathology and treatment of recurrent dislocation of the shoulder joint. Br J Surg 23–29, 1938–1939.
5. Bardeen CR, and Lewis WH: Development of the limbs, bodywall and back in man. Am J Anat *1*:1–26, 1901.
6. Basmajian JV, Bazant FJ, and Kingston CM: Factors preventing downward dislocation of the adducted shoulder joint. J Bone Joint Surg *41-A*:1182–1186, 1959.
7. Bechtol CO: Biomechanics of the shoulder. Clin Orthop *146*:37–41, 1980.
8. Bost F, and Inman VT: The pathological changes in recurrent dislocation of the shoulder. J Bone Joint Surg *3*:595–613, 1942.
9. Bretzhe CA, Crass JR, Craig EV, and Feinberg SB: Ultrasonography of the rotator cuff: normal and pathologic anatomy. Invest Radiol *20*:311–315, May-June 1985.
10. Brooks DB, Burnstein AH, and Frankel H: The biomechanics of torsional fractures: the stress concentration effect of a dull hole. J Bone Joint Surg *52-A*:507–514, 1970.
11. Buechel FF, Pappas MJ, and DePalma AF: "Floating socket" total shoulder replacement: anatomical, biomechanical and surgical rationale. J Biomed Mat Res *12*:89–114, 1978.
12. Ciochon RL, and Corruccini RS: The coracoacromial ligament and projection index in man and other anthropoid primates. J Anat *124*:627–632, 1977.
13. Codman EA: The Shoulder: Rupture of the Supraspinatus Tendon and Other Lesions in or about the Subacromial Bursa. Brooklyn: G. Miller and Co, 1934.
14. Corruccini RS, and Ciochon RL: Morphometric affinities of the human shoulder. Am J Anat *152*:419–432, 1978.
15. Corruccini RS, and Ciochon R: Morphometric affinities of the human shoulder. Am J Phys Anthropol *45*:19–38, 1976.
16. Corruccini RS, and Ciochon R: Morphoclinical variation in the anthropoid shoulder. Am J Phys Anthropol *48*:539–542, 1978.
17. Craig EV: The posterior mechanism of acute anterior shoulder dislocation. Clin Orthop *190*:212–216, 1984.
18. Crass JR, Craig EV, and Feinberg SB: Sonography of the postoperative rotator cuff. AJR *146*:561–564, 1986.
19. Cyprien JM, Vassey MH, Burdet A, Bonvin JC, et al: Humeral retrotorsion and glenohumeral relationship in the normal shoulder and in recurrent anterior dislocation (scapulometry). Clin Orthop *175*:8–17, 1983.
20. DePalma AF: Surgery of the Shoulder, 3rd ed. Philadelphia: JB Lippincott, 1983.
21. DePalma AF: Surgical approaches to the region of the shoulder joint. Clin Orthop *20*:163–184, 1961.
22. DePalma AF, Callery G, and Bennett GA: Shoulder joint: variational anatomy and degenerative lesions of the shoulder joint. AAOS Instructional Course Lectures *6*:255–281, 1949.
23. DePalma AF, Cooke AJ, and Prabhakar M: The role of the subscapularis in recurrent anterior dislocation of the shoulder. J Bone Joint Surg *3*:595–613, 1942.
24. DeSmet AA: Arthrographic demonstration of the subcoracoid bursa. Skel Radiol *7*:275–276, 1982.
25. Deutsch AL, Resnick D, Mink JH, et al: Computed and conventional arthrotomography of the glenohumeral joint: normal anatomy and clinical experience. Radiol *153*:603–609, 1984.
26. Deutsch AL, Resnick D, and Mink JH: Computed tomography of the glenohumeral and sternoclavicular joints. Orthop Clin North Am *16*:497–511, 1985.
27. Developmental horizons in human embryos (4th Issue): a review of the histogenesis of cartilage and bone. Carnegie Institute Series on Embryology *33*:151–167, 1949.
28. Dickson JA, Humphries AW, and O'Dell HW: Recurrent Dislocation of the Shoulder. Baltimore: Williams and Wilkins, 1953.
29. Edwards H: Congenital displacement of the shoulder joint. J Anat *62*:177–182, 1937–1938.
30. Engin AE: On the biomechanics of the shoulder complex. J Biomechan *13*:575–590, 1980.

31. Freedman L, and Munro RR: Abduction of the arm in the scapular plane: scapular and glenohumeral movements. J Bone Joint Surg 48-A:1503–1510, 1966.

32. Gardner E: The embryology of the clavicle. Clin Orthop 58:9–16, 1968.

33. Gardner E: The innervation of the shoulder joint. Anat Rec 102:1–18, 1948.

34. Gardner E, and Gray DJ: Prenatal development of the human shoulder and acromioclavicular joints. Am J Anat 92:219–276, 1953.

35. Garn SD, and McCreey LD: Variability of postnatal ossification timing and evidence for a "dosage" effect. Am J Phys Anthropol 32:139–144, 1979.

36. Garn SD, Rohmann CG, and Blumenthal T: Ossification sequence polymorphism and sexual demorphism in skeletal development. Am J Phys Anthropol 24:101–116, 1966.

37. Garn SD, Rohmann CG, Blumenthal T, and Kaplan CS: Developmental communalities of homologous and non-homologous body joints. Am J Phys Anthropol 25:147–152, 1966.

38. Garn SD, Rohmann CG, Blumenthal T, and Silverman FN: Ossification communalities of the hand and other body parts: their implication to skeletal assessment. Am J Phys Anthropol 27:75–82, 1967.

39. Gay S, Gay E, and Miller EJ: The collagens of the joint. Arth Rheum 23:937–941, 1980.

40. Gerber C, and Ganz R: Clinical assessment of instability of the shoulder, with special reference to anterior and posterior drawer tests. J Bone Joint Surg 66-B:551–556, 1984.

41. Williams PL, and Warwick R (eds): Gray's Anatomy, 36th ed. Philadelphia: WB Saunders, 1980.

42. Haines RW: The Development of Joints. J Anat 81:3–55, 1947.

43. Hollinshead HW: Anatomy for Surgeons: Volume 3. The Back and Limbs, 3rd ed. Philadelphia: Harper & Row, 1982.

44. Hovelius L, Lind B, and Thorling J: Primary dislocation of the shoulder: factors affecting the two year prognosis. Clin Orthop 176:181–185, 1983.

45. Huber DJ, Sauter R, Mueller E, et al: MR imaging of the normal shoulder. Radiol 158:405–408, 1986.

46. Inman VT, Saunders M, and Abbott LC: Observations on the function of the shoulder joint. J Bone Joint Surg 26:1–29, 1944.

47. Johnston TB: The movements of the shoulder joint: a plea for the use of the "plane of the scapula" as the plane of reference for movements occurring at the humero-scapular joint. Br J Surg 25:252–260, 1937–1938.

48. Kaltsas DS: Comparative study of the properties of the shoulder joint capsule with those of other joint capsules. Clin Orthop 173:20–26, 1983.

49. Kent BE: Functional anatomy of the shoulder complex. Phys Ther 51:867–887, 1970.

50. Keibel F, and Mall FP (eds): Manual of Human Embryology. J.B. Lippincott, Philadelphia: 1912, pp 379–391.

50a. Krieft GJ, Bloem JL, Obermann WR, et al: Normal shoulder: MR imaging. Radiology 159:741–745, 1986.

51. Kummel BM: Spectrum of lesions of the anterior capsular mechanism of the shoulder. Am J Sport Med 7:111–120, 1979.

52. Lewis WH: The development of the arm in man. Am J Anat 1:144–184, 1901.

53. Ljunggren AE: Clavicular function. Acta Orthop Scand 50:261–268, 1979.

54. Lucas GB: Biomechanics of the shoulder joint. Arch Surg 107:425–432, 1973.

55. McLaughlin HL: Recurrent anterior dislocation of the shoulder. Am J Surg 99:628–632, 1960.

56. McLaughlin HL, and MacLellan DI: Recurrent anterior dislocation of the shoulder, II. A comparative study. J Trauma 7:191–201, 1967.

57. Middleton WD, Reinus WR, Melson GL, et al: Pitfalls of rotator cuff sonography. AJR 146:555–560, 1986.

58. Mink JH, Richardson A, and Grant TT: Evaluation of glenoid labrum by double contrast shoulder arthrography. AJR 133:883–887, 1979.

59. Moore KL: The Developing Human. Philadelphia: WB Saunders, 1982.

60. Moseley HF, and Overgaard B: The anterior capsular mechanism in recurrent anterior dislocation of the shoulder. J Bone Joint Surg 44-B:913–927, 1962.

61. Neal HV, and Rand HW: Chordate Anatomy. Philadelphia: Blakiston, 1936.

62. Nelson CL, and Razzano CD: Arthrography of the shoulder: a review. J Trauma 13:136–141, 1973.

63. Neviaser JS: Adhesive capsulitis of the shoulder. AAOS Instruction Course Lectures VI:281–291, 1949.

64. Neviaser RJ: Anatomical considerations and examination of the shoulder. Orthop Clin North Am 11:187–195, 1980.

65. Nobuhara K, and Ikedda H: Rotator interval lesion. Clin Orthop 223:44–50, 1987.

66. O'Brien SJ, Neves MC, Rozbuck RS, et al: The anatomy and histology of the inferior glenohumeral ligament complex of the shoulder. Paper presented at the annual meeting of the Shoulder and Elbow Society, February 1989, Las Vegas.

67. O'Brien SJ, Warren RF, and Schwartz E: Anterior shoulder instability. Orthop Clin North Am 18:395–408, 1987.

68. Odgers SL, and Hark FW: Habitual dislocation of the shoulder joint. Surg Gynecol Obstet 75:229–234, 1942.

69. Oveson J, and Nielson S: Anterior posterior shoulder instability: a cadaver study. Acta Orthop Scand 57:324–327, 1986.

70. Oveson J, and Nielson S: Experimental distal subluxation in the glenohumeral joint. Arch Orthop Trauma Surg 104:78–81, 1985.

71. Oveson J, and Sojbjerg JO: Lesions in different types of anterior glenohumeral joint dislocation: an experimental study. Arch Orthop Trauma Surg 105:216–218, 1986.

72. Oxnard CE: Morphometric affinities of the human shoulder. Am J Phys Anthropol 46:367–374, 1977.

73. Palmer L, and Blakely RL: Documentation of medial rotation accompanying shoulder flexion: a case report. Phys Ther 66:55–58, 1986.

74. Pappas AM, Goss T, and Kleinman PK: Symptomatic shoulder instability due to lesions of the glenoid labrum. Am J Sports Med 11:279–288, 1983.

75. Peat M: Functional anatomy of the shoulder complex. Phys Ther 66:12:1855–1865, 1986.

76. Peterson CJ: Degeneration of the gleno-humeral joint. Acta Orthop Scand 54:277–283, 1983.

77. Peterson CJ, and Redlund-Johnell I: Joint space on normal gleno-humeral radiographs. Acta Orthop Scand 54:274–276, 1983.

78. Poppen NK, and Walker PS: Normal and abnormal motion of the shoulder. J Bone Joint Surg 58-A:195–201, 1976.

79. Poppen NK, and Walker PS: Forces at the glenohumeral joint in abduction. Clin Orthop 135:165–170, 1978.

80. Post M: The Shoulder: Surgical and Nonsurgical Management, 2nd ed. Philadelphia: Lea & Febiger, 1988.

81. Last RJ: Anatomy, 6th ed. New York: Churchill Livingstone, 1978.

82. Rathbun JB, and Macnab I: The microvascular pattern of the rotator cuff. J Bone Joint Surg 52-B:540–553, 1970.

83. Reeves B: Experiments in the tensile strength of the anterior capsular structures of the shoulder in man. J Bone Joint Surg 50-B:858–865, 1968.

84. Resnick D: Shoulder arthrography. Radiol Clin North Am 19:243–253, 1981.

85. Rockwood CAJ, and Green DP: Fractures in Adults, Volume I. Philadelphia: JB Lippincott, 1983.

86. Rothman RH, Marvel JP, Jr, and Heppenstall BR: Anatomic considerations in the glenohumeral joint. Orthop Clin North Am 6:341–352, 1975.

87. Rothman RH, Marvel JP, Jr, and Heppenstall, BR: Recurrent anterior dislocation of the shoulder. Orthop Clin North Am 6(2):415–422, 1975.

88. Rothman RH, and Parke WW: The vascular anatomy of the rotator cuff. Clin Orthop Rel Res 41:176–186, 1965.

89. Rowe CR: The Shoulder. New York: Churchill Livingstone, 1988.

90. Rowe CR, and Sakellarides HT: Factors related to recurrence of anterior dislocations of the shoulder. Clin Orthop 20:40–47, 1961.

91. Saha AK: Dynamic stability of the glenohumeral joint. Acta Orthop Scand *42*:491–505, 1971.
92. Saha AK: Theory of Shoulder Mechanism: Descriptive and Applied. Springfield: Charles C Thomas, 1961.
93. Saha AK: Mechanism of shoulder movements and a plea for the recognition of "zero position" of glenohumeral joint. Clin Orthop *173*:3–10, 1983.
94. Samuelson RL: Congenital and developmental anomalies of the shoulder girdle. Orthop Clin North Am *11*:219–231, 1980.
95. Sarrafian SK: Gross and functional anatomy of the shoulder. Clin Orthop *173*:11–19, 1983.
96. Schwartz RE, O'Brien SJ, Warren RF, et al: Capsular restraints to anterior-posterior motion of the abducted shoulder: a biomechanical study. Orthop Trans *12*(3):727, 1988.
97. Schwartz E, Warren RF, O'Brien SJ, and Froneck J: Posterior shoulder instability. Orthop Clin North Am *18*:409–419, 1987.
98. Seltzer SE, Finberg HJ, and Weissman BN: Arthrosonographic technique: sonographic anatomy and pathology. Invest Radiol *5*:19–28, 1980.
99. Seltzer SE, Finberg HJ, Weissman BN, et al: Arthrosonography: Gray scale ultrasound evaluation of the shoulder. Personal communication.
100. Seltzer S, and Weissman BN: CT findings in normal and dislocating shoulders. J Canad Assoc Radiol *36*:41–46, 1985.
101. Singleton MC: Functional anatomy of the shoulder. J Am Phys Ther Assoc *46*:1043–1051, 1966.
102. Streeter W: Developmental horizons in human embryology. Carnegie Series on Embryology *33*:151, 1949.
103. Symeonides PP: The significance of the subscapularis muscle on the pathogenesis of recurrent anterior dislocation of the shoulder. J Bone Joint Surg *54-B*:476–483, 1972.
104. Townley CO: The capsular mechanism in recurrent dislocation of the shoulder. J Bone Joint Surg *32-A*:370–380, 1950.
105. Turkel SJ, Panio MW, Marshall JL, and Girgis FG: Stabilizing mechanisms preventing anterior dislocation of the glenohumeral joint. J Bone Joint Surg *63-A*:1208–1217, 1981.
106. Vasseur PB, Moore D, Brown SS, and Eng D: Stability of the canine shoulder joint: an in vitro analysis. Am J Vet Res *43*:352–355, 1982.
107. Warren RF, Kornblatt IB, and Marchand R: Static factors affecting posterior shoulder stability. Orthop Trans *8*(1):89, 1984.
108. Wolpert L: Mechanism of limb development and malformation. Br Med Bull *32*:65–70, 1976.

Gross Anatomy of the Shoulder

Christopher M. Jobe, M.D.

During the Renaissance a unique style of painting called glazing was developed. The artist applied to the canvas thin, transparent coats of different colors. The deep layers of paint viewed through the more superficial layers yielded a color variant and perception of depth not attainable with a single layer of paint. El Greco, Titian, and Rubens were among those artists who used glazing.

A study of the history of shoulder anatomy reveals that our current picture of the shoulder was constructed in a similarly layered fashion. Much of what we know about the shoulder was worked out in significant detail in the classical age. The earliest studies of the present era cited in this chapter refer to structures defined by prior workers. I have found that subsequent studies do not deflect from earlier work but serve to explain or bring into sharper focus certain elements of those studies. Rarely does later work obliterate the significance of earlier works.

The stimulus for research and publication comes from three sources: the discovery of a new disease, the invention of a new treatment, or the arrival of a new method of studying anatomy. Perpetuation of knowledge gained depends upon the philosophical outlook and interest of the time and place in which it was nascent.

Before the Renaissance, the main barriers to anatomical study were religious and personal proscriptions against the dissection of human cadavers and different philosophical ideas regarding the laws of nature. Because of these prejudices early contributions were not advanced and, since they were not reconfirmed, were lost to mankind. In a dialogue written in the Warring States Period (fifth century B.C.), Huang Ti described the unidirectional flow of blood in arteries and veins. Huang Ti, the Yellow Emperor of China who lived around 2600 B.C., is the mythological father of Chinese medicine.[11, 12, 14] This and other indications of anatomical study were buried in a heavily philosophical treatise on the yin and yang influences on the human body. (Recent work in traditional Chinese medicine correlates the yang acupuncture meridians with the course of postaxial nerve branches of the posterior cord and the yin meridians with the preaxial nerve branches of the medial and lateral cords.[7]) This Daoist orientation led, over the centuries, to a de-emphasis on surgical anatomy and a resultant prejudice against surgery. Although Chinese anatomical observations were subsequently carried out by physicians who witnessed executions, the "death of a thousand cuts," and bodies disinterred by dogs following an epidemic, the philosophical climate was unfavorable for propagation and use of this information.[11] Therefore, a lasting description of circulation awaited rediscovery by John Harvey in the more receptive atmosphere of the 17th century some 2000 years later.

The handling of dead bodies was prohibited in India, except when preparing them for cremation, but Sustruta, in the sixth century B.C., devised a frame through which flesh was dissected away from the deeper layers with stiff brooms.[10, 18] He then correctly described the two shoulder bones, at a time when the West thought of the acromion as a separate bone. In the same era, Atroya fully described the bones of humans. Alcmaeon performed animal dissection around 500 B.C. in Greece.[18] The significance of these discoveries was lost because further study was not done.

Hippocrates was probably the first physician whose ideas regarding shoulder anatomy were perpetuated.[19] Writing in the fifth century B.C., his discussion of articulations began with the shoulder and much of his work focused on this joint. His writings applied to clinical rather than basic science. Although Hippocrates referred to "the unpleasant if not cruel task" of dissecting cadavers, we must assume that he witnessed dissections because he gave explicit instructions for obtaining exposure of portions of the shoulder anatomy in order to prove a clinical point.[9, 18] He also described the position of nerves of the axilla in discussing his burning technique for treatment of anterior dislocation of the shoulder and, in his assessment of the patient, noted that some individuals have a "predisposing constitution" to dislocation. He demonstrated knowledge of the acromioclavicular separation, palsies of the shoulder, and growth plate fractures.[9]

Herophilus (circa 300 B.C.), the father of anatomy, dissected some 600 cadavers at the medical school in Alexandria and started an osteology collection. This is the first recorded evidence of what might be called a scientific approach in that he dissected more than just a few cadavers and did his dissections for description rather than pathological analysis.[18] Early authors such as Celsus accused him of vivisection, but this is unjustified.[18] His permanent anatomical collections, particularly of bones, contributed to the medical knowledge of the late Greek and early Roman eras. In the late Republic and early Empire, new proscriptions against dissection, some of which were written into law, stemmed the progress that had been made. Celsus (30 B.C.–A.D.41), who was not a physician but an encyclopedist, collected the medical knowledge of the day and advocated allowing human dissection, but the prohibition continued.[14, 18]

Despite such barriers to the study of human anatomy, advances were made sporadically by gifted physicians in unique situations. Galen, a Greco-Roman physician who practiced in Pergamum and then Rome during the second century A.D., contributed greatly to the early knowledge of anatomy. He is the father of the study of clinical anatomy and, because he was surgeon to the gladiators in Pergamum, might also be considered the father of sports medicine.[8] His writings on the usefulness of the human body parts contain the earliest effort at a detailed anatomy of the shoulder. In discussing the bones and joints of the shoulder, he described the thin ligaments of the glenohumeral joint and observed that the rim of the glenoid was frequently broken with dislocation. Galen attributed the frequency of dislocation of the shoulder, in comparison with other joints, to an "antagonism between diversity of movement and safety of construction." He described the anatomical principle of placing joints in a series to increase motion so that "the additional articulation might supply the deficiency of the first articulation." He also provided a complete description of all the muscles and their subdivisions, although he did not apply the Latin names used today.[8]

In describing the nerves, Galen referred to a sympathetic trunk and a plexus but did not apply names or recognize a standard construction of the brachial plexus. Instead, he considered the plexus to be a necessary method of strengthening support to the nerves. He described terminal branches of the brachial plexus including the dorsal scapular, axillary, median, ulnar, and radial nerves. He also described the accessory spinal nerve. He noted the axillary artery, the carotid artery, and the lymph glands about the shoulder.[8] In short, he provided an impressive outline of shoulder anatomy, even by 20th-century standards.

Many differences between Galen's writings and modern descriptions relate to the fact that he performed only animal dissection. He perpetuated the erroneous idea that the acromion is a separate bone, a concept that continued into the Renaissance. Also, his writings on the acromium probably do not refer to the acromium as we know it but to the acromioclavicular joint.[8]

Shortly after Galen's time Christianity became dominant in the Roman empire, leading to the intensification of pre-existing laws against cadaveric dissection.[14] For centuries, no anatomical studies were performed on human material in Europe or in the Moslem empire. Although the Moslems were more successful at preserving the Galenic writings, their religion prohibited illustration. Perhaps the very completeness of Galen's studies contributed to the suppression of anatomical studies. Centuries passed with no new knowledge of human anatomy being acquired.[18]

When Greek and Roman literature was reintroduced from the East, scholasticism was the dominant academic philosophy in the West. The scholastic philosophers, Abelard and St. Thomas Aquinas, depended heavily upon deductive reasoning for any original contributions they made and did not use observation or experimentation.[14, 18] Considering the rich sources that reappeared from the East, one can understand how a scholar could absorb a much larger volume of information from ancient writings than from the slow and laborious process of experimentation.

Finally, during the Black Plague of 1348, the papacy allowed necropsy to be performed for the first time to elucidate cause of death from the plague, not for anatomical study. Interestingly, when dissection for the purpose of teaching anatomy was reintroduced, it was not investigational but simply demonstrated the precepts of Galen.[18]

One of the greatest leaps in anatomical illustration occurred among Renaissance painters interested in accurate representation, some of whom dissected in secret and became serious students of anatomy (Fig. 2–1). Although their purpose was illustration and not new discovery, the increase in accuracy of illustrations from older anatomical textbooks to the notebooks of Leonardo da Vinci is quite remarkable.[18] Leonardo, in his early notebooks, was seeking to illustrate ideas from Mondino's dissection manual which Mondino derived from Galen. The bulk of his drawing, however, is made up of his own observations, often independent of Galen.[4] Leonardo also recognized the value of dissecting multiple specimens:

And you who say that it is better to look at an anatomical demonstration than to see these drawings, you might be right, if it were possible to observe all the details shown in these drawings in a single figure, in which with all your ability you will not see . . . nor acquire a knowledge . . . while in order to obtain an exact and complete knowledge of these . . . I have dissected more than ten human bodies.[4]

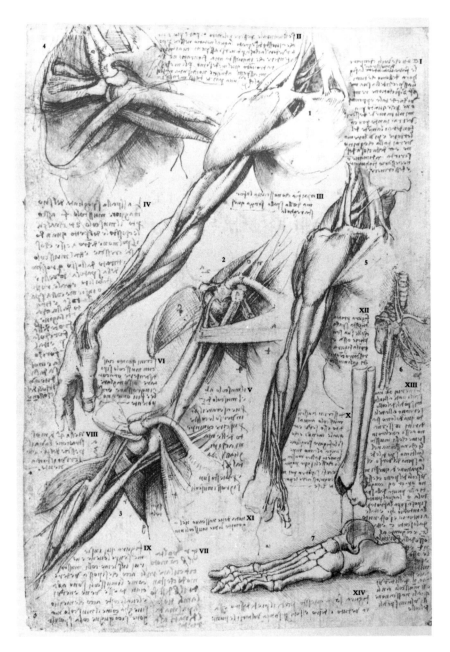

Figure 2–1. A page from Leonardo da Vinci's *Notebooks from Anatomical Study*. In comparison with other illustrations of the time, the accuracy is striking. This particular dissection is interesting because the acromion is shown as a bone separate from the rest of the scapula. Other illustrations in the *Notebooks* show the acromion united. In Leonardo's accompanying notes neither the fused nor the unfused state is stated to be normal. (Windsor Castle, Royal Library © 1990, Her Majesty Queen Elizabeth II.)

In his shoulder illustrations, he shows fused and unfused acromions without notation as to which was abnormal. His notations are largely instructions to himself—"draw the shoulder then the acromion," rather than observations of incidences of variations.[4]

Anatomical study with clear illustration steadily increased over the next century. In 1537, Pope Clement VII endorsed the teaching of anatomy, and in 1543, Vesalius published his textbook, *De Fabrica Corporis Humani*[20] (Fig. 2–2). Vesalius, although criticized for questioning the work of Galen during his early teaching career, was able to correct some of Galen's misconceptions. He described the geometry of muscles and contributed the concept of the dynamic force of the body, illustrated in a vivid portrayal of progressive muscle dissection of the cadaver. In his artist's illustra-

tions, the cadaver appears to lose more tone as each muscle layer is removed until, finally, in the last picture, the cadaver has collapsed against a wall. Vesalius demonstrated the vessels of the shoulder, and his drawings include an accurate illustration of the brachial plexus. The only missing element is the posterior division of the lower trunk (Fig. 2–3). He accurately portrayed rotation of the fibers of the costal portion of the pectoralis major.[20] His drawings also include materials from comparative anatomy and indicate where these structures would lie if they were present in the human. This was the starting point of scientific anatomy.[18]

The functions of muscles were deduced early from their shortening action and their geometry. While caring for patients during an anthrax epidemic, Galen

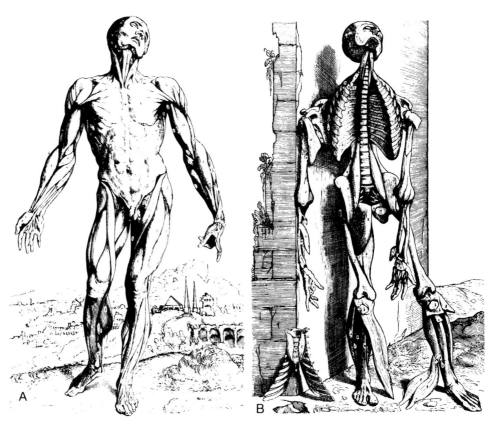

Figure 2–2. The first and last of Vesalius' series of illustrations demonstrating the dissection of the muscles of the human body. Note how his artists represent the body with dynamic strength when the muscles are intact *(A)*, and show the collapse and lack of support with the removal of the muscles *(B)*. Present-day artists who have visited the site of Vesalius' work say that many of the buildings in the background are still standing. (Vesalius A: The Illustrations from the Works of Andreas Vesalius of Brussels. Saunders JB, and O'Malley CD (eds). New York: The World Publishing Company, 1950.)

asked them to perform certain arm motions. Because of his knowledge of anatomy, he was able to determine exactly which muscle he was observing at the base of the anthrax ulcers typical of the disease, without painful probing, and how close these ulcers were to vital nerves or vessels.[18] Modern biomechanics still benefits from the study of the geometry of muscles.[17, 45]

The dynamic study of muscles was made possible with the development of electrical equipment. Emile DuBois-Reymond invented the first usable instrument for the electrical study of nerves and muscles in the early 19th century, and Herman Von Helmholtz first measured the speed of nerve conduction.[18] Duchenne studied the action of muscles using electrical stimulation of individual muscles through the skin, and like his predecessors, he began with the shoulder and emphasized that joint (Fig. 2–4). He also recognized that muscles rarely act individually and that this was a limitation on the accuracy of his method. He studied all the superficial muscles of the shoulder including the trapezius, the rhomboids, levator scapulae, serratus anterior, the deltoids, supraspinatus, infraspinatus, teres minor, subscapularis, latissimus dorsi, pectoralis major, teres major, and triceps.[1, 6, 18]

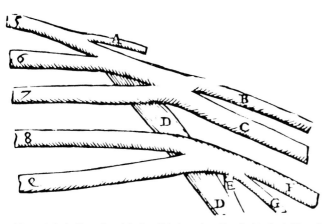

Figure 2–3. An illustration of the brachial plexus from Vesalius' textbook. There is reason to believe that Vesalius may have done this illustration himself. Note the absence of the posterior division of the inferior trunk contributing to the posterior cord. (Vesalius A: The Illustrations from the Works of Andreas Vesalius of Brussels. Saunders JB, and O'Malley CD (eds). New York: The World Publishing Company, 1950.)

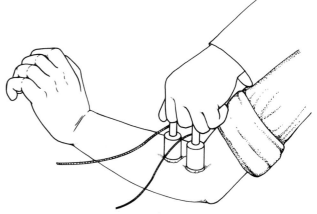

Figure 2–4. Duchenne's illustration of his technique for direct muscle stimulation. Like many of his great predecessors, he begins his text with a discussion of the shoulder. (Reprinted with permission from Duchenne GB: Physiology of Movement. Kaplan EB (trans. and ed). Philadelphia: WB Saunders, 1959.)

Subsequent developments in electromyography enabled researchers to measure activity in muscle initiated by the patient.[1]

Functional anatomy was further elucidated by the science of physics. Aristotle studied levers and geometry and wrote about the motion of animals. Galen wrote about muscle antagonists. Leonardo da Vinci discussed the concept of centers of gravity in his notebooks. However, it was Sir Isaac Newton's physics that made possible the studies we perform today. In the late 19th century, Eadweard Muybridge[16] published photographic studies of a horse in motion and later photographed human motion in rapid sequence to examine action of the various levers of the body (Fig. 2–5). It was rapid-sequence photography that elucidated the synchrony of glenohumeral and scapulothoracic motion.[13, 18] Braune and Fischer first applied Newtonian physics to functional anatomy.[2, 3] In this classic study, they used cadavers to establish the center of gravity for the entire body and for each segment of the body, the first detailed study of the physics of human motion based on such information.[19] The awareness of the great motion of the shoulder made it one of the first areas where overuse was described.[15]

The first thorough study of any joint combining all the techniques of the historical investigators was done on the shoulder by Inman, Saunders, and Abbott.[1] This landmark work used comparative anatomy, human dissection, the laws of levers and physics, photography, and the electromyogram (EMG).[44] All subsequent publications on the function of the shoulder may support or contradict findings in this study, but all cite it.[17]

Cadaveric dissection and other research continue to add to our knowledge of the shoulder and to our understanding of the findings of these early giants in the field. Exciting studies are presented at meetings and wherever the shoulder is a topic of discussion. These studies are stimulated by the same three sources that have stimulated anatomists throughout history. The first stimulus is a new disease or a new understanding of an old disease. The premiere example here would have to be the studies of impingement syndrome. The second stimulus is the invention of new technology in treatment, as when the arthroscope activated a renewed interest in variation in the labrum and ligaments of the shoulder.[5] The third is the invention of a new technique to study anatomy. In the past this has occurred with Duchenne's electrical stimulus, the EMG, and the fluoroscope.[13] More recently, biochemistry and the electron microscope have stimulated new interest. All of these have deepened the understanding of previous findings in the shoulder, rather than totally altered the picture (Fig. 2–6).

The final layer of paint in our portrait of shoulder anatomy has not been applied, and we are unlikely to see the day when further study is not required. Scholasticism appears to be creeping into medical school education. This is probably an unfortunate by-product of the information surge of the late 20th century, a phenomenon similar to the reappearance of Galen's writing in the era of scholasticism. More time is spent memorizing accumulated information at the cost of research experience. Although at present a revolution in surgical technique and technology has sent a generation of surgeons back to the anatomy laboratory,[5] we must not forget to encourage an interest in anatomy research in medical students.

In keeping with the concept of a layered portrait, the material in this chapter is arranged in a layered fashion. Discussion begins with the innermost layer, the bones and joints, the most palpable and least deformable structures of the shoulder. They are the easiest to visualize and are the best understood anatomical landmarks. We then will reveal the muscle layers that produce motion of the shoulder and the nerves that direct the muscles and provide sensation. We will discuss the vessels that control the internal environment of the tissues of the shoulder and, finally, the skin that encloses the shoulder. The central theme of the shoulder is motion. The amount of motion in the shoulder sets it apart from all other joints and accounts for the ways in which the shoulder differs from all other regions of the body.

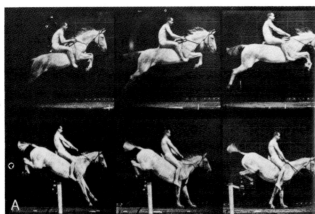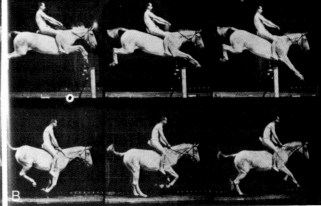

Figure 2–5. An example of the work of Eadweard Muybridge. This was the first time that high-speed photography was applied to the study of motion, both animal and human. This information, combined with the laws of Newtonian physics, brought about the birth of modern kinesiology. (Reprinted with permission from Muybridge E: In Brown LS (ed): Animals in Motion. New York: Dover, 1957.)

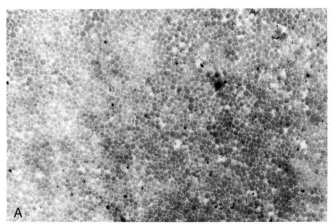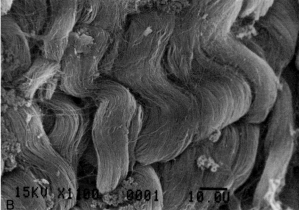

Figure 2–6. *A,* Transmission electron micrograph of collagen fibers of the subscapularis tendon. *B,* Scanning electron micrograph of the inferior glenohumeral ligament, showing collagen fibers and fiber bundles.

Bones and Joints

The orthopedic surgeon thinks of bones primarily as rigid links that are moved, secondarily as points of attachment for ligaments, muscles, and tendons, and finally as the base on which to maintain important relationships with surrounding soft tissue. Treatment of fractures has been called the treatment of soft tissues surrounding them.[71] In relation to pathology, bones are three-dimensional objects of anatomy that must be maintained or restored for joint alignment. Bones exist in a positive sense to protect soft tissues from trauma. In a negative sense they act as barriers to dissection to a surgeon trying to reach and repair a certain area of soft tissue. Loss of position of the bone may endanger soft tissue in the acute sense, and loss of alignment of the bone may endanger the longevity of the adjacent joints.

Joints have two opposing functions: to allow desired motion and to restrict undesirable motion. The stability of joints is the sum of (1) their bony congruity and stability, (2) stability of the ligaments, and (3) some additional dynamic stability obtained from adjacent muscles. The shoulder has the greatest mobility of any joint in the body and has the most predisposition to dislocation.

This great range of motion is distributed to three diarthrodial joints: the glenohumeral, the acromioclavicular, and the sternoclavicular, which, in combination with the fascial spaces between the scapula and the chest, are known collectively as the scapulothoracic articulation.[44] Because of the lack of congruence in two diarthrodial joints, i.e., acromioclavicular and sternoclavicular, motion of the scapulothoracic articulation is determined by the opposing surfaces of the thorax and scapula. About one-third of the total elevation takes place in this part of the shoulder; most motion occurs in the glenohumeral cavity. The three diarthrodial joints are constructed with little bony stability and rely mostly on their ligaments and a little on adjacent muscle.

The division of motion over these articulations has two advantages. First, it allows the muscles crossing each of these articulations to operate in the optimal portion of their length-tension curve. Second, the glenohumeral rhythm allows the glenoid to be brought underneath the humerus to bear some of the weight of the upper limb, which decreases demand on the shoulder muscles to suspend the arm. This is especially important when the muscles are operating near maximum abduction and they are at that point in their length-tension curve where they have less power.[17, 55, 68]

Study of the ultrastructure of ligaments and tendons about the shoulder is in its infancy, but preliminary studies show little difference in terms of collagen biochemistry and fiber structure.[47, 69]

Our discussion of the bones and joints will proceed from the proximal to the distal portion of the shoulder and will include the joint surfaces, ligaments, and special intra-articular structures. Joint stability and the relative importance of each of the ligaments to that stability will be elaborated. We will discuss the morphology of bones as well as their important muscle and ligament attachments. Finally, the relationship of bones and joints to other important structures in the shoulder will be demonstrated.

STERNOCLAVICULAR JOINT

The sternoclavicular joint, composed of the upper end of the sternum and the proximal end of the clavicle, is the only skeletal articulation between the upper limb and the axial skeleton.[17, 41] In both the vertical and anteroposterior dimensions, this portion of the clavicle is larger than the opposing sternum and extends superiorly and posteriorly relative to the sternum.[41, 42] The prominence of the clavicle superiorly helps create the suprasternal fossa. There is relatively little bony stability in the sternoclavicular joint, and the bony surfaces are somewhat flat. The ligamentous structures provide the stability of the joint. The proximal surface of the clavicle is convex in the coronal plane but

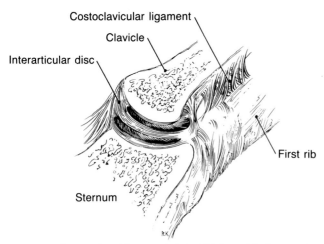

Figure 2–7. Cross-section of the sternoclavicular joint. A complete disc separates the joint into two compartments. The disc has a firm attachment to the first rib below and to the ligaments and superior border of the clavicle superiorly.

somewhat concave in the transverse plane. The joint angles posteromedially. In the coronal plane, the joint surface is angled medially toward the superior end; the joint surfaces are covered with hyaline cartilage. In 97 per cent of cadavers a complete disc is found to separate the joint into two compartments (Fig. 2–7). The disc is rarely perforated.[30, 32] The intra-articular disc is attached to the first rib below and to the superior surface of the clavicle through the interclavicular ligament superiorly. The disc rarely tears or dislocates by itself.[35]

The major ligaments in the joint are the anterior and posterior sternoclavicular or capsular ligaments (Fig. 2–8). The fibers run superiorly from their attachment to the sternum to their superior attachment on the clavicle. The most important ligament of this group, the posterior sternoclavicular ligament, is the strongest stabilizer to the inferior depression of the lateral end of the clavicle.[23] The paired sternoclavicular ligaments

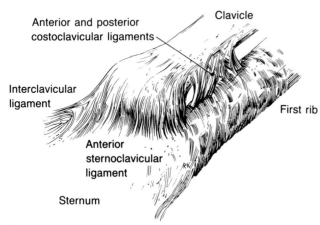

Figure 2–8. The exterior of the sternoclavicular joint. This does not show the strongest of the ligaments—the posterior sternoclavicular ligament, the posterior partner of the anterior sternoclavicular ligament. The other important ligaments are shown in their appropriate anatomical relationships.

are primary restraints so that minimal rotation occurs during depression of the clavicle.

The interclavicular ligament runs from clavicle to clavicle with attachment to the sternum and may be absent or nonpalpable in as many as 22 per cent of the population.[23] The ligament tightens as the lateral end of the clavicle is depressed, contributing to joint stability. The anterior and posterior costoclavicular ligaments attach from the first rib to the inferior surface of the clavicle. The anterior costoclavicular ligament resists lateral displacement of the clavicle on the thoracic cage, and the posterior ligament prevents medial displacement of the clavicle relative to the thoracic cage. Cave thought these ligaments act as a pivot around which much of the sternoclavicular motion takes place.[26, 30] Bearn found that they were not the fulcrum in depression until after the sternoclavicular ligaments were cut. They are the "principal limiting factor" in passive elevation of the clavicle and are a limitation on protraction and retraction.[23]

In the classic study on stability of the sternoclavicular joint, Bearn found that the posterior sternoclavicular or capsular ligament contributed most to resisting depression of the lateral end of the clavicle. He performed serial ligament releases on cadaver specimens and made careful observations on the mode of failure and the shifting of fulcra. This qualitative observation is now a useful addition to computerized assessments of joint stability.

Although reliable electromyographic studies demonstrate that the contribution of the upward rotators of the scapula is minimal in standing posture, permanent trapezius paralysis often leads to an eventual depression of the lateral end of the scapula relative to the other side, although this may be only a centimeter or two.[23] Bearn's experiment probably should be replicated using more sophisticated equipment to produce length-tension curves and to test quantitatively the response of the joint to rotational and translational loading in the transverse and vertical axes, as well as the anteroposterior axis that Bearn tested qualitatively.

Motion occurs in both sections of the sternoclavicular joint. Elevation and depression occur in the joint between the clavicle and the disc.[41] Anteroposterior motion and rotatory motion occur between the disc and the sternum. The range of motion on living specimens[44] is approximately 30 to 35 degrees of upward elevation. Movement in the anteroposterior direction is approximately 35 degrees, and rotation about the long axis is 44 to 50 degrees. Most sternoclavicular elevation occurs between 30 to 90 degrees of arm elevation.[44] Rotation occurs after 70 to 80 degrees of elevation. To estimate the range of motion by results of fusion is misleading because of secondary effects on the length-tension curve of the muscles of the glenohumeral joint and the ability of the glenoid to help support the weight of the arm. Fusion of the sternoclavicular joint limits abduction to 90 degrees.[13, 17, 71]

Blood supply to the sternoclavicular joint derives from the clavicular branch of the thoracoacromial

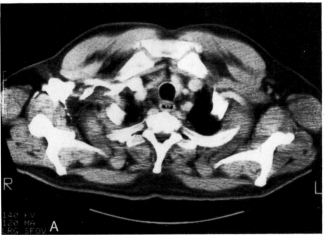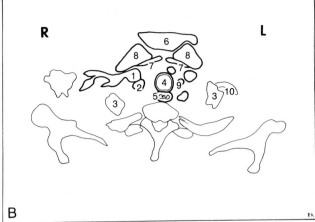

Figure 2–9. This contrast CT scan *(A)* and line drawing *(B)* illustrate some of the more important anatomical relationships of the sternoclavicular joint, including the trachea and great vessels. The structures are labeled as follows: (1) junction of subclavian and jugular veins, (2) innominate artery, (3) first rib, (4) trachea, (5) esophagus, (6) sternum, (7) sternohyoid muscle origin, (8) clavicle, (9) carotid artery, and (10) axillary artery.

artery, with additional contributions from the internal mammary and the suprascapular arteries.[41] Nerve supply to the joint arises from the nerve to subclavius with some contribution from the medial supraclavicular nerve.

Immediate relations of the joint are the origin of the sternocleidomastoid in front and the origins of the sternohyoid and sternothyroid muscles behind the joint. Of prime importance, however, are the great vessels and the trachea (Fig. 2–9), which are endangered during posterior dislocation of the clavicle on the sternum—a rare event that may precipitate a surgical emergency.[48, 71]

An open epiphysis is a structure not commonly found in adults. The epiphysis of the clavicle, however, does not ossify until the late teens and may not fuse to the remainder of the bone in men until the age of 25 years.[29, 71] Therefore, the clavicular epiphysis is a relatively normal structure within the age group at greatest risk for major trauma. The epiphysis is very thin and not prominent, which makes differentiation of physeal fractures from dislocations difficult. Instability of the sternoclavicular joint may result from trauma but, in some individuals, develops secondary to a constitutional laxity.[28]

CLAVICLE

The clavicle is a relatively straight bone when viewed anteriorly, whereas in the transverse plane it resembles an italic S[31] (Fig. 2–10). The greater radius of curvature occurs at its medial curve, which is convex anteriorly. The smaller lateral curve is convex posteriorly. The bone is somewhat rounded in its midsection and medially and relatively flat laterally. DePalma described an inverse relationship between the degree of downward facing of the lateral portion of the clavicle and the radius of curvature of the lateral curve of the clavicle.

The obvious processes of the bone include the lateral and medial articular surfaces. The medial end of the bone has a 30 per cent incidence of a rhomboid fossa on its inferior surface where the costoclavicular ligaments insert and a 2.5 per cent incidence of actual articular surface facing inferiorly toward the first rib. The middle portion of the clavicle contains the subclavian groove where the subclavius muscle has a fleshy insertion (Fig. 2–11). The lateral portion of the clavicle has the coracoclavicular process when present.

There are three bony impressions for ligament attachment to the clavicle. On the medial side is an impression for the costoclavicular ligament, which at times may be a rhomboid fossa. At the lateral end of the bone are the conoid tubercle, on the posterior portion of the lateral curve of the clavicle, and the trapezoid line, which lies in an anteroposterior direction just lateral to the conoid tubercle. The relative position of these ligament insertions is important in their function.[31, 41, 42]

Muscles that insert on the clavicle are the trapezius, on the posterior superior surface of the distal end, and the subclavius muscle, which has a fleshy insertion on the inferior surface of the middle third of the clavicle. Four muscles take origin from the clavicle. The deltoid originates on the anterior portion of the inner surface of the lateral curve. The pectoralis major takes origin over the anterior portion of the medial two-thirds. The

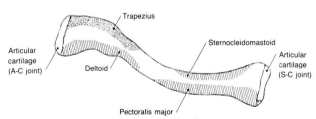

Figure 2–10. A superior view of the clavicle showing its italic S shape, the origins of the deltoid, pectoralis major, and sternocleidomastoid muscles and the insertion of the trapezius muscle. Note the breadth of the sternocleidomastoid origin.

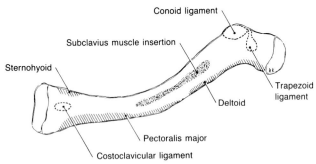

Figure 2–11. An inferior view of the clavicle showing its major ligament insertions and the origins of the deltoid, pectoralis major, and sternohyoid muscles. Also shown is the subclavian groove where the subclavius muscle has its fleshy insertion.

sternocleidomastoid has a large origin on the posterior portion of the middle third. The sternohyoid, contrary to its name, does have a small origin on the clavicle, just medial to the origin of the sternocleidomastoid.

Functionally, the clavicle acts mainly as a point of muscle attachment. Some of the literature suggests that with good repair of the muscle, the only functional consequences of surgical removal of the clavicle are with heavy overhead activity[17, 21, 52] and that therefore its function as a strut[57] is less important. This concept would seem to be supported by the relatively good function in congenital absence of the clavicle.[79] However, others have found the sudden loss of the clavicle in adulthood to have a devastating effect on shoulder function.

Important relations to the clavicle are the subclavian vein and artery and the brachial plexus posteriorly. In fact, the medial anterior curve is often described as an accommodation for these structures and does not form in Sprengel's deformity where the scapula does not descend. Therefore, the attached clavicle does not need to accommodate.[84, 85] The curve is a landmark for finding the subclavian vein.[218] This relationship is more a factor in surgery than in trauma since the bone acts as an obstruction to the surgeon in reaching the nerve or vessel tissue that he or she wishes to treat. In trauma, clavicular injury usually does not affect these structures despite their close relationship, and nonunion is rare.[45] Most cases of neurovascular trauma fall into two groups: injury to the carotid artery from the displaced medial clavicle and compression of structures over the first rib.[43]

ACROMIOCLAVICULAR JOINT

The acromioclavicular joint is the only articulation between the clavicle and the scapula, although a few individuals, as many as 1 per cent, have a coracoclavicular bar or joint.[51, 63] Lewis[51] reported in his work that about 30 per cent of cadavers had articular cartilage on their opposing coracoid and clavicular surfaces, without a bony process on the clavicle directed toward the coracoid.

The capsule of the acromioclavicular joint contains a diarthrodial joint incompletely divided by a disc which, unlike that of the sternoclavicular joint, usually has a large perforation in its center.[30, 32] The capsule tends to be thicker on its superior, anterior, and posterior surfaces than on the inferior surface. The upward and downward movement allows rotation of about 20 degrees between the acromion and clavicle, occurring in the first 20 and last 40 degrees of elevation.[44] It is estimated that many individuals have even less range of motion since, in some cases, fusion of the acromioclavicular joint does not decrease motion.[71] DePalma found degenerative changes of both the disc and articular cartilage to be the rule rather than the exception in specimens in the fourth decade or older.[32]

Blood supply to the acromioclavicular joint derives mainly from the acromial artery, a branch of the deltoid artery of the thoracoacromial axis. There are rich anastomoses between this artery, the suprascapular artery, and the posterior humeral circumflex artery. The acromial artery comes off the thoracoacromial axis anterior to the clavipectoral fascia and perforates back through the clavipectoral fascia to supply the joint. It also sends branches anteriorly up onto the acromion. Innervation of the joint is supplied by the pectoral, axillary, and suprascapular nerves.[41]

The ligaments about the acromioclavicular articulation, the trapezoid and the conoid ligaments, have been studied extensively (Fig. 2–12). Traditionally, and more recently, it has been reported that anteroposterior stability of the acromioclavicular joint was controlled by the acromioclavicular ligaments and that vertical stability was controlled by the coracoclavicular ligaments.[71, 81] Recently, a serial cutting experiment was performed using sophisticated equipment in 12 force-displacement measurements.[36] Three anatomical axes of the acromioclavicular joint were used. Translation and rotation on each axis in both directions were measured. Three of the measurements brought the clavicle and coracoid process together and, since they did not contribute useful data, were dropped from the study. Results of the experiment confirmed previously held views, particularly when displacements were large.

The acromioclavicular ligaments were found to be responsible for controlling posterior translation of the clavicle on the acromion. (In anatomical terms this is really an anterior translation of the scapula on the clavicle.) The ligaments were responsible for 90 per cent of anteroposterior stability, and 77 per cent of stability for superior translation of the clavicle (or inferior translation of the scapula) was attributed to the conoid and trapezoid ligaments. Distraction of the acromioclavicular joint was limited by the acromioclavicular ligaments (91 per cent), and compression of the joint was limited by the trapezoid ligament (75 per cent).

The unique findings of the study were the contribution in small displacements. The acromioclavicular ligaments played a much larger role in many of these

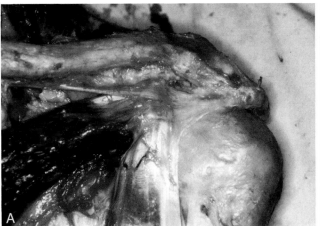
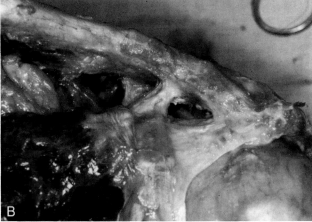

Figure 2–12. These photographs show the acromioclavicular joint complex before *(A)* and after *(B)* excision of the clavipectoral fascia, which was rather prominent in this specimen. Note the thickness of the coracoclavicular ligaments and their lines of orientation, which are consistent with their function. Note also the breadth and thickness of the coracoacromial ligament.

rotations and translations than in the larger displacements, which may reflect shorter lengths of the acromioclavicular ligaments. At shorter displacements, greater stress is being applied to the fibers of the acromioclavicular ligaments for the same displacement.

Interpretation of the stability attributed to the acromioclavicular ligament should reflect the additional role it plays in maintaining integrity of the acromioclavicular joint. While we would expect the linear arrangement of the collagen of the acromioclavicular ligament to resist distraction, it makes little sense that the acromioclavicular ligament would resist compression with these fibers, yet 12 to 16 per cent of compression stability in the study was attributed to the acromioclavicular ligament. Maintaining acromioclavicular joint integrity, particularly the position of the interarticular disc, might be the explanation. We would not expect the acromioclavicular ligament to resist superior translation of the clavicle were it not for the presence of an intact joint below it, producing a fulcrum against which these ligaments can produce a tension band effect.[36]

It is seldom that these ligaments are called upon to resist trauma, and their usual function is to control joint motion. As noted above, there is relatively little motion in this joint, and muscles controlling scapulothoracic motion insert on the scapula. To a large extent the ligaments function to guide the motions of the clavicle.[37] For example, the conoid ligament produces much of the superior rotation of the clavicle as the shoulder is elevated in flexion.[17]

There is no physeal plate on the distal end of the clavicle. Todd and D'Errico,[80] using microscopic dissection, found a small fleck of bone in some individuals that appeared to be an epiphysis, but it united within a year. I have not seen this structure at operation or by roentgenogram. Probably the articular cartilage functions in longitudinal growth as it does in an epiphysis.

SCAPULA

The scapula is a thin sheet of bone that functions mainly as a site of muscle attachment (Fig. 2–13). It is thicker at its superior and inferior angles and its lateral border, where some of the more powerful muscles are attached (Figs. 2–14 and 2–15). It also is thick in forming its processes: the coracoid, the spine, the acromion, and the glenoid. Because of the protection of overlying soft tissue, fractures usually occur in the processes via indirect trauma. The posterior surface of the scapula and presence of the spine create the supraspinatus and the infraspinatus fossae. The three processes, the spine, the coracoid, and the glenoid, create two notches in the scapula. The suprascapular notch is at the base of the coracoid, and the spinoglenoid, or greater scapular notch, is at the base of the spine. The coracoacromial and transverse scapular ligaments are two of several ligaments that attach to two parts of the same bone. Sometimes the inferior transverse scapular ligament is found in the spinoglenoid notch. Seldom studied is the coracoglenoid ligament, which originates on the coracoid between the coracoacromial and coracohumeral ligaments and inserts on the glenoid near the origin of the long head of the biceps.[82] The major ligaments that take origin from the scapula are the coracoclavicular, the coracoacromial and acromioclavicular, the glenohumeral, and the coracohumeral.

The coracoid process comes off the scapula at the base of the neck of the glenoid and passes anteriorly and laterally before hooking to a more lateral position. It functions as the origin of the short head of the biceps and the coracobrachialis tendons. It also serves as the insertion of the pectoralis minor muscle and the coracoacromial and coracoclavicular ligaments. Several anomalies of the coracoid have been described. As many as 1 per cent of the population have an abnormal connection between the coracoid and the clavicle: a

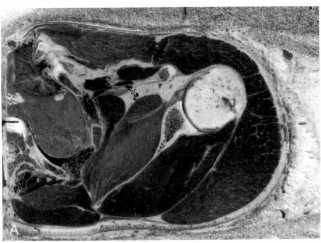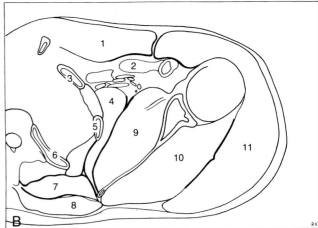

Figure 2–13. A photograph *(A)* and diagram *(B)* of a cross-section of the scapula at the midportion of the glenoid, which demonstrate the thinness of most of the scapula and its most important bony process, the glenoid. Also illustrated is the way in which the muscle and ligaments increase the stability of this inherently unstable joint by circumscribing the humeral head. Hypovascular fascial planes are emphasized. Note that the artist's line is wider than the plane depicted. The labeled structures include: (1) pectoralis major, (2) pectoralis minor, (3) first rib, (4) serratus anterior, (5) second rib, (6) third rib, (7) rhomboid, (8) trapezius, (9) subscapularis, (10) infraspinatus, and (11) deltoid.

bony bar or articulation.[63] Some surgeons have seen impingement in the interval between the head of the humerus and the deep surface of the coracoid.[33, 38, 39] The coracohumeral interval is smallest in internal rotation and forward flexion.

The spine of the scapula functions as part of the insertion of the trapezius on the scapula as well as part of the origin of the posterior deltoid. It also serves to suspend the acromion in the lateral and anterior directions to serve as a prominent lever arm for function of the deltoid. The dimensions of the spine of the scapula are regular, varying less than 1.5 cm from the mean in any dimension. Recently, a reconstruction of the mandible has been devised using the spine of the scapula. Sacrifice of the entire spine, including the acromion, has a predictable devastating effect on shoulder function.[56, 64]

Because of the amount of pathology involving the acromion and the head of the humerus, the acromion is the most studied process of the scapula.[60] Production of tendinitis and bursitis is related to impingement of the head of the humerus and the coracoacromial arch in an area called the supraspinatus outlet.[62] Viewed from the front there is a 9 to 10 mm area (6.6 to 13.8 in men, 7.1 to 11.9 in women) between acromion and humerus.[67] Recent advances in x-ray positioning allow better visualization of the outlet from the side or sagittal plane of the scapula.[62]

Several methods of describing the capaciousness of this space or its tendency toward mechanical discontinuities have been devised. Aoki and Ishii[22] have used

Figure 2–14. Anterior view of the scapula showing the muscle origins of the anterior surface *(striped pattern)* and the muscle insertions *(dotted pattern)*. Ligaments and their origins and insertions are not illustrated.

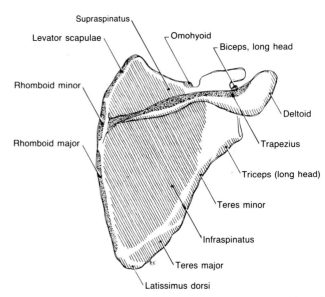

Figure 2–15. A posterior view of the scapula illustrating the muscle origins and muscle insertions.

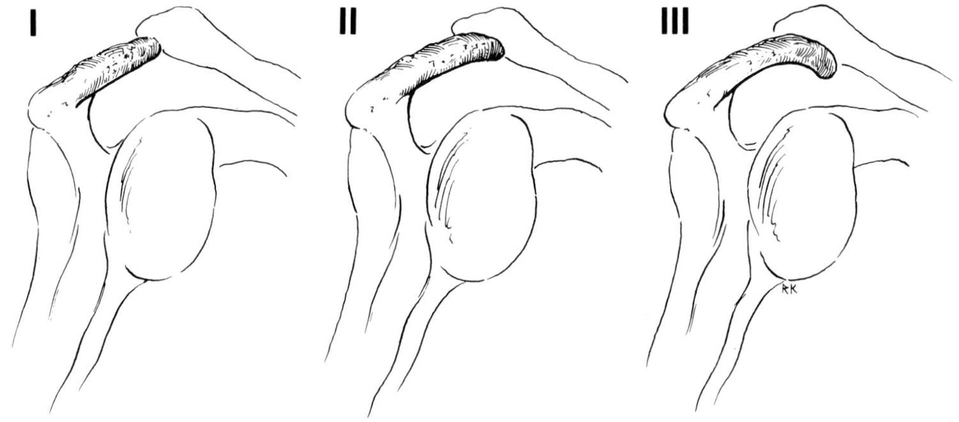

Figure 2–16. The three types of acromion morphology defined by Bigliani and Morrison. Type I, with its flat surface, provided the least compromise of the supraspinatus outlet, whereas Type III's sudden discontinuity or hook was associated with the highest rate of rotator cuff pathology in a series of cadaver dissections.

the slope of the ends of the acromion relative to a line connecting the posterior acromion with the tip of the coracoid of the scapula to determine the propensity for impingement problems. Bigliani and Morrison[24] separate acromions into three types (or classes) based on their shape, correlating occurrence of rotator cuff pathology in the cadaver with the acromion shape of the supraspinatus outlet radiographs (Fig. 2–16). Their classification is easy to use. Type I acromions are those with a flat undersurface and have the lowest risk for impingement syndrome and its sequelae. Type II have a curved undersurface, and Type III have a hooked undersurface. As one would expect, the Type III acromion with its sudden discontinuity in shape had the highest correlation with subacromial pathology. The remainder of the roof of the supraspinatus outlet is composed of the coracoacromial ligament which connects two parts of the same bone. It is broader at its base on the coracoid, tapers as it approaches the acromion, and has a narrower but still broad insertion on the undersurface of the acromion, covering a large portion of the anterior undersurface of the acromion and investing somewhat the tip of the acromion (Fig. 2–17). Because of the high incidence of impingement

in elevation and internal rotation, acromions from specimens older than the fifth decade frequently have secondary changes such as spurs or excrescences.

In addition to static deformation of the acromion, one would expect an unfused acromion epiphysis to lead to deformability of the acromion on an active basis and decrease the space of the supraspinatus outlet.[59] Neer, however, found no increased incidence of unfused epiphyses in his series of acromioplasties.[61] Liberson[53] classified the different types of unfused acromion as the pre-acromion, mes-acromion, met-acromion, and basi-acromion center (Fig. 2–18). In his series, an unfused center was found to occur in 1.4 per cent of roentgenograms and bilaterally in 62 per cent of cases. The mes-acromion–met-acromion defect was found most frequently (Fig. 2–19).

The glenoid articular surface is within 10 degrees of being perpendicular to the blade of the scapula, with the mean being 6 degrees of retroversion.[73] The more caudad portions face more anteriorly than the cephalad.[34, 75] This perpendicular relationship, combined with the complementary orientation of the scapula, and relationships determined by the ligaments of the scap-

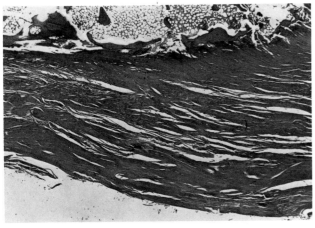

Figure 2–17. A 12× view of the insertion of the coracoacromial ligament into the undersurface of the acromion. This may continue as far as 2 cm in the posterior direction. Note the thickness of the ligament compared with the bone.

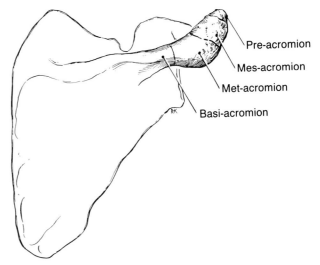

Pre-acromion

Mes-acromion

Met-acromion

Basi-acromion

Figure 2–18. The different regions of the acromion between which union may fail to occur.

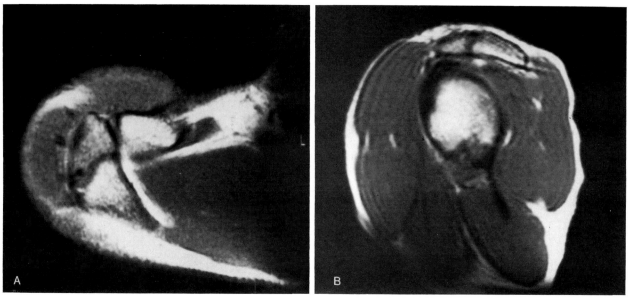

Figure 2–19. Transverse *(A)* and sagittal *(B)* MRI sections of an unfused mes-acromion.

ulohumeral orientation make the plane of the scapula the most suitable coronal plane for physical and radiological examination of the shoulder. The plane of the glenoid defines the sagittal planes, while the transverse plane remains the same.[46, 74]

Blood supply to the scapula derives from vessels in the muscles that take fleshy origin from the scapula (see section on Muscles). Vessels cross these indirect insertions (see section on Muscles) and communicate with cortical vessels. The circulation of the scapula is metaphyseal in nature; the periosteal vessels are larger than usual, and they communicate freely with the medullary vessels, rather than being limited to the outer one-third of the cortex. This may explain why subperiosteal dissection is bloodier here than over a diaphyseal bone.[25, 64] The nutrient artery of the scapula enters in the lateral suprascapular fossa[50, 64] or infrascapular fossa.[130] The subscapular, suprascapular, circumflex scapular, and acromial arteries are contributing vessels.

Other muscles that take origin from the scapula, not previously mentioned, are the rotator cuff muscles: supraspinatus, infraspinatus, teres minor, and subscapularis. At the superior and inferior poles of the glenoid are two tubercles for tendon origins, the superior for the long head of the biceps and the inferior for the long head of the triceps. At the superior angle of the scapula, immediately posterior to the medial side of the suprascapular notch, is the origin of the omohyoid, a muscle that has little significance for shoulder surgery but is an important landmark for the brachial plexus and cervical dissections. The large and powerful teres major takes origin from the lateral border of the scapula. Inserting on the scapula are all the scapulothoracic muscles: the trapezius, serratus anterior, the pectoralis minor, the levator scapulae, and the major and minor rhomboids.

HUMERUS

The articular surface of the humerus of the shoulder is spheroid with a radius of curvature of about 2.25 cm.[17] As we move down the humerus in the axis of the spheroid there is a ring of bony attachments for the ligaments and muscles that control joint stability. The ring of attachments is constructed of the two tuberosities, the intertubercular groove, and the medial surface of the neck of the humerus. Ligaments and muscles that maintain glenohumeral stability do so by contouring the humeral head so that tension in them produces a restraining force toward the center of the joint (Fig. 2–20). In this position the spheroid is always more prominent than the ligamentous or muscle attachments. For example, when the shoulder is in neutral abduction and the supraspinatus comes into play, the greater tuberosity, which is the attachment of this tendon, is less prominent than the articular surface, causing the tendon to contour the humeral head. In the abduction and external rotation position, contouring of the supraspinatus is lost. The anterior inferior glenohumeral ligament now maintains joint stability, and its attachments are now less prominent than the articulating surface.

With the arm in the anatomical position, i.e., with the epicondyles of the humerus in the coronal plane, the head of the humerus has a retroversion of approximately 30 degrees, and the intertubercular groove lies approximately 1 cm lateral to the midline of the humerus[27, 73] (Fig. 2–21). The lesser tubercle (or tuberosity) lies directly anterior, and the greater tuberosity lines up on the lateral side with the long axis of the articular surface. On the medial surface of the humerus is a smooth contour for ligamentous attachments. There are no muscle attachments on the inferior border of the joint.

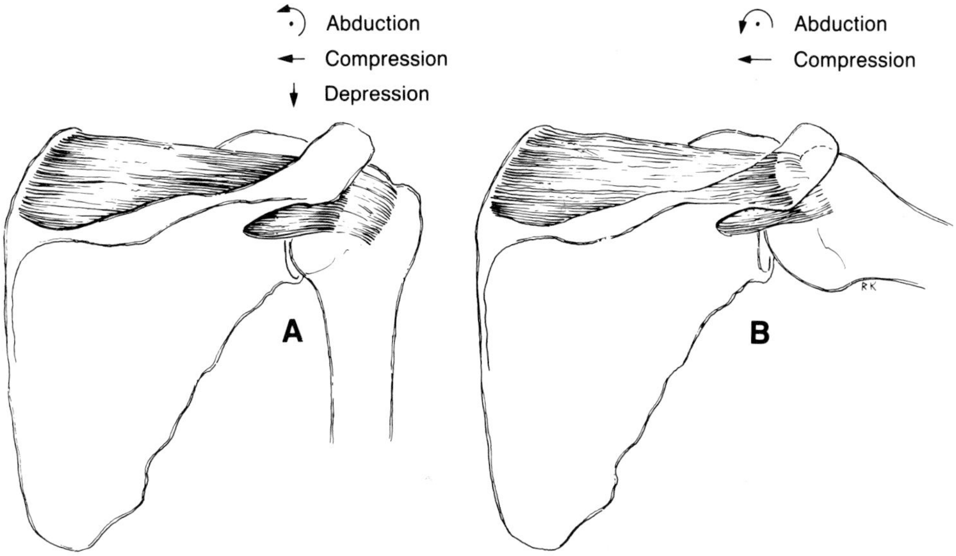

⤻) Abduction
← Compression
↓ Depression

✔·⌢ Abduction
← Compression

Figure 2–20. *A,* In neutral position, the initiation of the use of the supraspinatus muscle produces a compressing force and, because the supraspinatus circumscribes the spheroid of the humeral head, there is a head depression force. *B,* In the abducted position, when the force of the deltoid muscle does not produce as much vertical shear force, there is a loss of the prominence of the spheroid, and therefore a loss of the head-depressing force of the supraspinatus. An abduction moment and a joint compression force remain.

The space between the articular cartilage and the ligamentous and tendon attachments is referred to as the anatomical neck of the humerus (Fig. 2–22). It varies in breadth from about 1 cm on the medial, anterior, and posterior sides of the humerus to being essentially undetectable over the superior surface where there is no bone exposed between the edge of articular cartilage and the insertion of the rotator cuff. The lesser tubercle is the insertion for the subscapularis tendon, and the greater tubercle bears the insertion of the supraspinatus, infraspinatus, and teres minor in a superior to inferior order. Because of its distance from the center of rotation, the greater tubercle lengthens the lever arm of the supraspinatus as elevation increases above 30 degrees. It also acts as a pulley, increasing the lever arm of the deltoid below 60 degrees.[70] Below the level of the tubercles, the humerus narrows in a region that is referred to as the surgical neck of the humerus because of the frequent occurrence of fractures at this level.

The greater and lesser tubercles make up the boundaries of the intertubercular groove in which the long head of the biceps passes from its origin on the superior lip of the glenoid. The intertubercular groove has a peripheral roof, referred to as the intertubercular ligament or transverse humeral ligament, which has varying degrees of strength.[39, 58] Recent work has shown that the coracohumeral ligament is the primary restraint to tendon dislocation.[65, 66, 76] Because the biceps tendon is a frequent site of shoulder pathology, attempts have been made to correlate the anatomy of its intertubercular groove with predilection toward pathology (Fig. 2–23). It was thought that biceps tendinitis resulted from dislocation of the tendon because of a shallow groove or a supratubercular ridge[58] and an incompetent transverse humeral ligament. Meyer[58] attributed the greater number of dislocations of the biceps tendon on the left to activities in which the left arm is in external rotation, a position which should have been protective. Current opinion is that disloca-

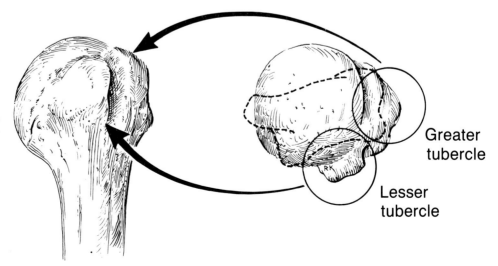

Figure 2–21. The head of the humerus has a retroversion relative to the long axis of the humerus. The bicipital groove in the neutral position lies approximately 1 cm lateral to the midline of the humerus.

Greater tubercle

Lesser tubercle

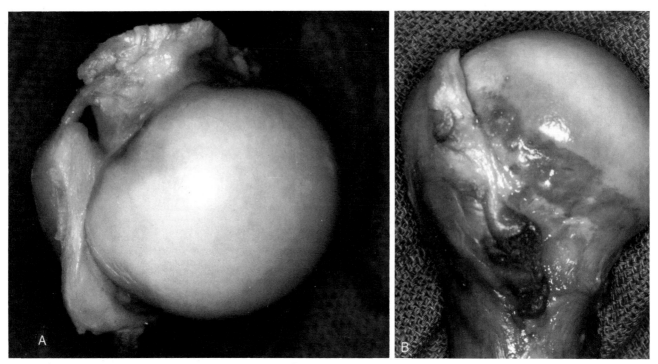

Figure 2–22. *A,* The superior surface of the humeral head, where the rotator cuff attaches immediately adjacent to the articular cartilage. The lesser tubercle is superior and the greater is to the left, with the bicipital groove and transverse humeral ligament between them. *B,* The posterior view of the humeral head and the gap between the articular surface and the attachment of the capsule and the tendon. This is the anatomical neck of the humerus.

tion of the tendon is a relatively rare etiology in bicipital tendinitis, that the vast majority of cases of bicipital tendinitis can be attributed to impingement,[67] and that dislocation of the tendon is not seen except in the presence of rotator cuff damage. It is possible that the variable depth of the intertubercular groove theory may also apply to impingement syndrome as an etiology. A shallow intertubercular groove makes the tendon of the long head of the biceps and its overlying ligaments more prominent and therefore more vulnerable to impingement damage.[61]

The intertubercular groove has a more shallow structure as it continues distally, but its boundaries, referred to as the lips of the intertubercular groove, continue to function as sites for muscle insertion. The medial lip of the intertubercular groove is the site of insertion for the latissimus dorsi and teres major, with the latissimus dorsi insertion being anterior, often on the floor of the groove. The pectoralis major has its site of insertion on the lateral lip of the bicipital groove. This area also functions as the site of entry of the major blood supply of the humeral head, the ascending

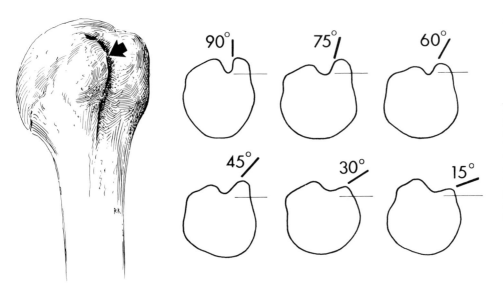

Figure 2–23. The variations in shape and depth of the intertubercular or bicipital groove. Formerly it was believed that the shallow groove combined with the supratubercular ridge of Meyer, a ridge at the top of the groove, predisposing to tendon dislocation. Bicipital disease is now thought to be the result of the impingement syndrome. (Redrawn from Hollinshead WH: Anatomy for Surgeons, Vol. 3, 3rd ed. Philadelphia: Harper & Row, 1982.)

branch of the anterior humeral circumflex artery, which enters the bone in the intertubercular groove or one of the adjacent tubercles.[49]

Two shoulder muscles insert on the humerus near its midpoint. On the lateral surface is the bony prominence of the deltoid tuberosity, over which there is a large tendinous insertion of deltoid. On the medial surface, at about the same level, is the insertion of the coracobrachialis.

The humerus, as part of the peripheral skeleton, is rarely a barrier to dissection. The essential relationships to be maintained in surgical reconstruction are the 30-degree retrograde direction of the articular surface and this surface's prominence relative to the muscle and ligamentous attachments. Longitudinal alignment should also be maintained and the distance from the head to deltoid insertion. Fractures above the insertion of the deltoid that heal creating humerus varus or in cases of birth injury causing humerus varus, the supraspinatus head depressing effect will be ineffective in the neutral position when the shear forces produced by the deltoid are maximal.[54] Interestingly, patients with congenital humerus varus rarely complain of pain but have limitation of motion.[77, 78] The important relationships to the humerus in the region of the joint are the brachial plexus structures, particularly the axillary and radial nerves, and the accompanying vessels.

Muscles

The orthopedic surgeon views muscles in several ways. First, they are producers of force. Second, they are objects of dissection in terms of repairing, transferring, or bypassing them on the way to a deeper and closely related structure. Finally, muscles are energy consuming and controllable organs for which blood and nerve supply must be maintained.

A brief review of interior anatomy is in order. The force generators within the structure of muscle are the muscle fibers, encased in a supporting collagen framework which transmits the generated force to the bony attachments. Each fiber's excursion is proportional to the sum of the sarcomeres or, in other words, its length. Muscle strength is a product of its cross-sectional area or the number of fibers.

The internal arrangements of muscle fibers can affect strength (Fig. 2–24). If all the fibers of a muscle are arranged parallel to its long axis, the muscle is called parallel and has maximum speed and excursion for size. Other muscles sacrifice this excursion and speed for strength by stacking a large number of fibers in an arrangement oblique to the long axis of the muscle, attaching to a tendon running the length of the muscle. This type of arrangement is referred to as pennate or multipennate. Strength again is the product of the number of fibers, but because of the oblique arrangement of the fibers, the strength in line with the tendon is obtained by multiplying this strength by the cosine of the angle of incidence with the desired axis of the pull. Its excursion is also a product of this cosine times the length of these shorter fibers. Some muscles, particularly the subscapularis, may have multipennate portions where excursion is so short and collagen framework so dense that the muscle acts as a passive restraint to external rotation of the glenohumeral joint (e.g., at 0 and 45 degrees of abduction).[124, 139, 142]

The complex arrangement of the shoulder into sev-

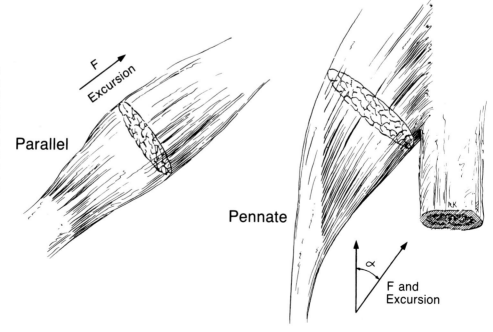

Figure 2–24. Muscles whose fibers have a parallel arrangement have maximum excursion and speed of contractility, as both force and excursion are parallel to the long axis of the muscle. In a pennate arrangement, multiple numbers of fibers with shorter length can be stacked to obtain a greater cross-sectional area. Not all of this strength is in the desired direction, nor is excursion. The effective force and excursion are projections of these vectors on the described directions, the magnitudes of which are products of the cosine of the angle times the excursion or force magnitude.

eral articulations that contribute to overall increase in mobility is also important in terms of the function of muscle. First, the multiple joint arrangement demands less excursion of the muscles that cross each articulation, allowing each joint's muscles to operate within the more effective portions of their length-tension curves. Second, joint stability requires that joint reaction forces cross the joint through the bony portions. Muscles of the shoulder serve not only to bring joint reaction forces to the glenohumeral joint in the area of the glenoid, but also to move the glenoid to meet the joint reaction forces.[102] This need for multiple muscles to function in each motion complicates diagnosis and the planning of tendon transfer.[162]

Actions of muscles have been measured in terms of standard movements such as abduction in the plane of the scapula, forward flexion of the shoulder, and internal and external rotation of the shoulder in neutral abduction. Studies have also been done on rehabilitation-associated activities such as scapular depression, an activity performed by patients using a wheelchair or walker. More complex motions of daily life and the actions of athletes are currently under research.[101] Because the upper extremity can be positioned many ways, an infinite number of studies can be performed.

A muscle performs its activity entirely by shortening its length. The action that results and the level of each muscle's activity depend on two conditions: position at the beginning of activity and the relationship of the muscle to the joint. The muscle vector of the shoulder can be divided into two components with respect to the joint surface (Fig. 2–25). One component produces shear on the joint surface, and the other produces compression and increases the stability of the joint. Muscles of the shoulder can make an additional contribution to stability by circumscribing the protruding portions of the humeral spheroid and creating compression to increase stability.[17, 119] Stability depends on the joint reaction force vector crossing the joint through cartilage and bone, the tissues designed for compression stress. A useful oversimplification of the contributions of shoulder muscles to stability is that the glenohumeral muscles strive to direct the joint reaction vector toward the glenoid and the muscles controlling the scapula move the glenoid with the force.

Externally applied resistance, including the force of gravity in the action that is being performed, is an additional determinant of which muscles will be active in a particular motion. At high levels of performance the level of training becomes important in determining how a muscle is used. People who are highly skilled may be more adept at positioning their skeletons so that they use less muscle force in retaining joint stability than the less trained. This allows more muscle force to be used in moving the limb.[103] Paradoxically, the most powerful activity of a muscle may take place during the seemingly less active phase of activity. For example, in swimming, the most active muscle in terms of its percentage of involvement is the serratus anterior, whose peak activity is in the recovery phase and not in the pull-through.[123]

Two examples illustrate the variability in muscle action in performing the same activity. First is the elevation of the scapula (Fig. 2–26). When the subject is in the anatomical position performing an elevation in the scapular plane or in forward flexion, the main elevators of the scapula are the upper fibers of the trapezius, the serratus anterior, and levator scapulae. In studies of overhead activity,[87] it was found that orientation of the throwing arm relative to the spine in different activities such as tennis, baseball, and so forth was similar, but that the arm in relationship to the ground was more vertical for heavier objects. Relationship of the humerus to the scapula and the scapula to the main axial skeleton, however, was little changed. Such a finding ought to be anticipated since these muscles are already operating within the optimum portion of Blix's curve for their activity. Further elevation is obtained by use of the contralateral trunk muscles, bending the upper trunk away from the throwing arm and creating a more vertical alignment of the throwing arm relative to the ground. Scapula rotation also begins earlier with elevation of heavier objects.[99] By producing a more level glenoid platform, this maneuver allows the glenoid to bear more of the weight of the thrown object, rather than the muscles. In a

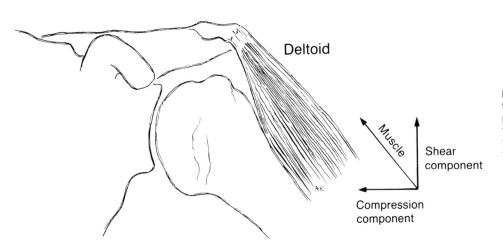

Figure 2–25. The action of muscles at the joint surface can be projected into two perpendicular vectors: a compression vector aimed directly at the articular surface, and a shear vector producing motion tangential to the joint surface.

Figure 2-26. Three different ways in which muscles produce elevation of the scapula. *A* shows pure elevation of the scapula in the scapular plane, as might be performed in a throwing motion. *B,* In throwing a heavier object, to allow the glenoid to bear extra weight more elevation of the scapula is necessary. Because the muscles of the shoulder are already operating at optimum points of their length-tension curve, further elevation must be obtained by using the contralateral trunk muscles to produce a contralateral flexion of the spine. *C,* An upward moment on the upper limb, as in the iron cross maneuver, must be resisted by a greater force in the latissimus dorsi. The resultant caudad-directed joint reaction vector must meet the bone of the glenoid. This scapular elevation is produced by the teres major.

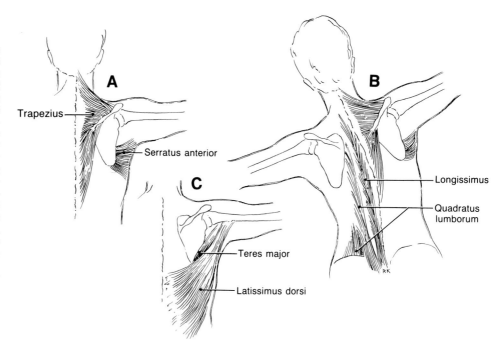

sense one might consider the contralateral trunk muscles to be elevators of the scapula.

In another athletic maneuver, the "iron cross," performed by some gymnasts, the arm is again in 90 degrees of abduction, and the entire weight is placed upon the hands. The upward force on the hands is counterbalanced by the adduction force generated by the latissimus dorsi and lower portion of the pectoralis major. Because of the shorter lever arm of these muscles, balancing forces are much greater than the upward forces upon the hands (see Chapter 6). Therefore, the joint reaction force on the humeral side will tend to run in a cephalocaudad direction. The other muscle active in this enforced adduction is the teres major which brings the lower portion of the scapula toward the humerus. In this maneuver, the hands are in a fixed position, and the teres major acts as an upward rotator of the scapula. Because the teres major is active only against strong resistance,[93] it could be postulated that scapula elevation may be the major action of the muscle.

As objects of surgical intervention, the important issues with muscles are tissue strength and resting positions that can be used to guard repairs. Muscles are also approached for the purpose of transfer. In such cases, attachment to bone, excursion of the muscle, phase activity innervation, and nutrition are important.

Recent literature reveals that tendons are attached to bone by an interlocking of the collagen of the tendon with the surface of the bone (direct insertions) or by continuation of the majority of collagen fibers into the periosteum (indirect insertions)[83] (Fig. 2-27). Direct insertions have a transition zone from the strong but pliable collagen of the tendon to the hard and unyielding calcified collagen of the bone. The transition begins on the tendon side with nonmineralized fibrocartilage, then mineralized fibrocartilage, and, finally, bone. Thus, there is no sudden transition in material properties at bone attachments, and collagen is present in amounts necessary to bear the generated stresses.

When all of the force generated by a muscle is borne by a single narrow tendon, this attachment tends to become a collagen-rich direct insertion, providing the surgeon with a firm structure to hold sutures. Where there is a wide band of attachment to bone the same layered arrangement may exist, but most of the collagen goes into periosteum in what is called indirect attachment. As the muscle force is spread over a broad area, these attachments tend to become collagen poor, or fleshy, with little collagen to hold sutures. When these areas of muscle are mobilized, a portion of contiguous periosteum should be left attached to the muscle to increase the amount of collagen available to hold sutures in reattachment. Interestingly, direct insertions are not traversed by blood vessels but indirect insertions are[83] (Fig. 2-28).

Muscles are generally approached as barriers to dissection; they overlie an area the surgeon wants to reach. When they cannot be retracted, it is more desirable to split tendons or muscles than it is to divide them. Sometimes there are limits to splitting. For example, in the deltoid, where the axillary nerve runs perpendicular to the fibers of the muscle, the amount of splitting that can be done is limited (Fig. 2-29). In the subscapularis, with its double innervation, there is also a limit to proximal splitting.

As viable structures muscles require functioning vessels and nerves. Knowledge of these structures is necessary in order to avoid damage, particularly when rather ambitious exposures or transfers are contemplated. The procedure is more complicated when the

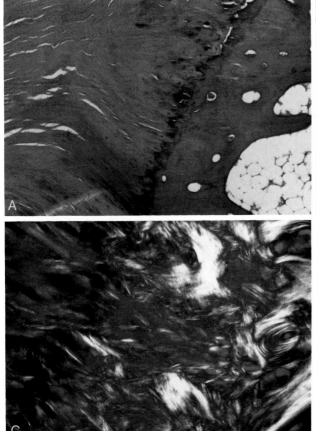

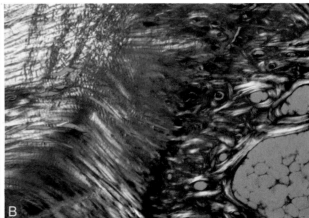

Figure 2–27. *A,* A hematoxylin and eosin section (100×) of a direct tendinous insertion (the supraspinatus). *B,* A polarized view of the same portion of the slide. *C,* A higher-power view shows the interdigitation of the collagen of the mineralized fibrocartilage of the tendon with the laminar arrangement of the collagen of the bone. Important points to note are the large amounts of collagen in this type of insertion to the complete exclusion of blood vessels crossing this transitional zone.

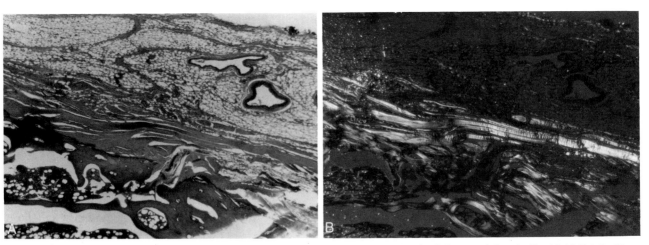

Figure 2–28. Two photomicrographs (200×) taken under direct *(A)* and polarized *(B)* light on the same section of an indirect muscle insertion (the deltoid). Note the thinner and looser arrangement of the collagen fibers. Only a minority of the fibers interdigitate with the bone, with the majority of the fibers continuing on into the collagen of the periosteum and from there into the indirect insertion of the trapezius. In an indirect attachment blood vessels cross from bone to tendon.

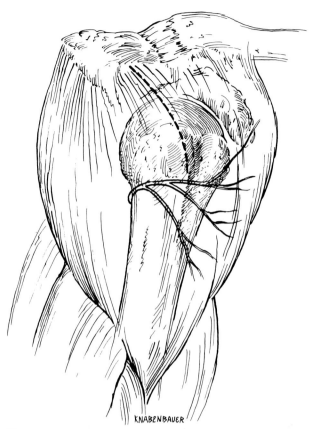

Figure 2–29. The position of the axillary nerve transverse to the fibers of the deltoid limits the extent of a deltoid-splitting incision in the anterior two-thirds of the muscle. (Reprinted from Techniques in Orthopaedics, Vol. 3, No. 4, p. 3, with permission of Aspen Publishers, Inc., © January 1989.)

surgeon wants to split a muscle or when a muscle is supplied by two separate nerves or two separate vessels.

The internal nerve and vessel arrangements in some muscles of the shoulder have been carefully studied. Much of this work was done in the 1930s by Salmon

but has not been available in the English literature.[130] Recent research has been done by microvascular surgeons[117, 118] who suggest a classification system based on the vessels of the muscle (Fig. 2–30). Type I muscle circulation has one dominant pedicle. Type II has one dominant pedicle with an additional segmental supply. Type III has two dominant pedicles. Type IV, the most problematic type, has multiple segmental arterial supplies. It is this segmental arterial supply that limits the amount of muscle that can be transferred without endangering the viability of the muscle. Several segmental vessels must be maintained in these muscles. Type V has one dominant vessel with a number of secondary supplies. A similar type of classification could be developed for the internal nerve anatomy of these muscles, since the nerves frequently follow the same connective tissue support structures into the muscle.

Perhaps the most elegant conceptualization of circulation is the idea of the angiosome.[230] As described by Taylor and Palmer, an angiosome is a block of tissue supplied by a dominant vessel.[230] The human body is then a three-dimensional jigsaw puzzle composed of these angiosomes. Each angiosome is dependent on its dominant vessel. Adjacent angiosomes have vascular connections that discourage interangiosome flow under normal circumstances but are capable of dilatation under stress. An example of an applied stress is the delaying of a flap. This allows the control vessels to dilate and "capture" adjacent tissue that might have become necrotic had the flap been moved at the first procedure.[230]

The arterial and venous angiosomes of a muscle correspond very closely, and the vessels travel together in the connective tissue framework of the muscle. The interangiosome arterial control vessels are the "choke arterioles" whose mode of function is obvious. The venous control is somewhat more complex because of the presence of valves in muscle veins which can be as

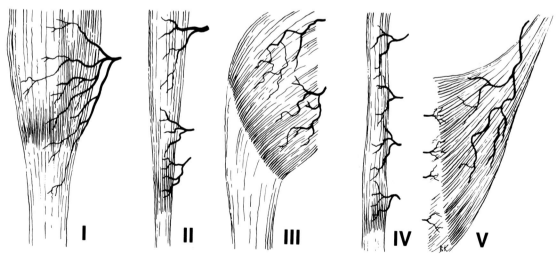

Figure 2–30. The five arrangements of blood vessels supplying muscle. Type I has one dominant vessel. Type II has a dominant vessel with one or more additional segmentally supplying vessels. Type III has two dominant pedicles. Type IV is the most difficult type to transfer because there are multiple segmental supplies rather than one or two dominant supplies on which a muscle transfer may be based. Type V has a large dominant vessel with a number of small secondary supplies. (Redrawn from Mathes SJ, and Nahai F: Classification of the vascular anatomy of muscles: experimental and clinical correlation. Plast Reconstr Surg 67:177–187, 1981.)

small as 0.2 mm in diameter.[145] These valves create unidirectional flow toward the vascular pedicle. The control veins between adjacent angiosomes are free of valves except for each end. These valves are oriented to prevent entry of blood into the control vein. Venous congestion can then lead to dilatation and valve incompetence. Because the flow in these veins can be in either direction, they are called "oscillating veins."[145]

The vessels within muscles tend to run parallel to the muscle fibers.[130, 145, 230] The exceptions to this are the main branches to the muscle which must cross perpendicularly to reach all of their smaller watersheds.[130] A knowledge of the anatomy of both the large and small vessels allows the placement of muscle splitting incisions between angiosomes while avoiding division of the main branch vessel.

Our discussion of muscles will proceed as follows. Individual muscles will be discussed in terms of origin and insertion, with comments on the type of attachment to bone. We then move on to discuss the boundaries of muscles and their function that has been described to date. Innervation of muscles will be discussed in terms of the nerve, or nerves, and the most common root representation. We then describe the vascular supply and its point of entry into the muscle, with brief mention of anomalies. The muscles are separated into four groups for purposes of discussion. First are the scapulothoracic muscles that control the motion of the scapula. The second group are the strictly glenohumeral muscles and working across that joint. Third, we discuss those muscles that cross two or more joints. Finally, we will discuss four muscles that are not directly involved with functioning of the shoulder but are important anatomical landmarks.

SCAPULOTHORACIC MUSCLES

Trapezius

The largest and most superficial of the scapulothoracic muscles is the trapezius (Fig. 2–31). This muscle takes origin from the spinous processes of C7 through T12 vertebrae.[91] The lower border can be as high as T8 or as low as L2. The upper portion of the trapezius above C7 takes its origin off the ligamentum nuchae, with two-thirds of the specimens having an upper limit of origin as high as the external occipital protuberance.[90] Insertion of the upper fibers is over the distal one-third of the clavicle. The lower cervical and upper thorax fibers have their insertion over the acromion and the spine of the scapula. The lower portion of the muscle takes insertion at the base of the scapular spine. On the anterior or deep surface, the muscle is bounded by a relatively avascular space between it and other muscles, most commonly the rhomboids. Posteriorly, the trapezius muscle is bounded by fat and skin.

As a whole, the muscle acts as a scapular retractor, with the upper fibers used mostly for elevation of the lateral angle.[122] Although some of the other fibers may

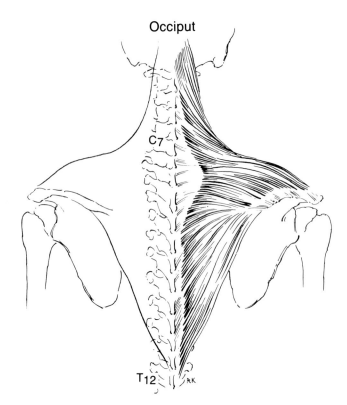

Figure 2–31. The textbook arrangement of the trapezius origins and insertions. The muscle takes its origin from the occiput, the nuchal ligament, and the dorsal spines of vertebrae C7 through T12. It inserts on the acromion, the spine of the scapula, and some distal clavicle. The trapezius is subdivided functionally into upper, middle, and lower fibers.

come into play, only the upper fibers were found by Inman to be consistently active in all upward scapular rotations.[44] The muscle follows a cephalocaudal activation as more flexion or abduction is obtained.[122] In forward flexion, the middle and lower trapezius are less active since scapular retraction is less desirable than in abduction.[44] Suspension of the scapula is supposed to be through the sternoclavicular ligaments at rest; electromyographic studies show no activity unless there is a downward tug on the shoulder.[23] The muscle must provide some intermittent relief to the ligaments of the sternoclavicular joint, however, because trapezius paralysis produces a slight depression of the clavicle, although not as much as one might expect.[23] The major deformity is protraction and downward rotation of the scapula.[13] The amount of depression may depend on the amount of downward loading of the limb with the paralyzed trapezius.[98] There appears to be a characteristic deficit seen in trapezius paralysis where, in coronal plane abduction, the shoulder can be brought up only to 90 degrees but can be brought much higher in forward flexion.[98, 107, 131] In one case of congenital absence of the trapezius and the rhomboids, the patient compensated by using forward flexion to elevate the arm and lordosis of the lumbar spine to bring the arms up. When the arms had reached the vertical position, he would then release his lumbar lordosis, holding the elevation with the serratus anterior.[134] Acquired loss of trapezius function is less well tolerated.[13, 129]

The accessory spinal nerve (CN XI) is the motor supply, with some sensory branches contributed from C2, C3, and C4. The arterial supply usually derives from the transverse cervical artery, although Salmon[130] found the dorsal scapular artery to be dominant in 75 per cent of his specimens.[130] Blood supply is described as Type II,[118] a dominant vascular pedicle with some segmental blood supply at other levels. Huelke[211] reports that the lower one-third of the trapezius is supplied by a perforator of the dorsal scapular artery and the upper fibers are supplied by arteries in the neck other than the transverse cervical artery. Other authors attribute blood supply of the lower pedicle to intercostal vessels.[145] Trapezius muscle transfers are based on supply by the transverse cervical artery.

Rhomboids

The rhomboids (Fig. 2–32) are similar in function to the midportion of the trapezius,[44] with the origin from the lower ligamentum nuchae C7 and T1 for the rhomboid minor and T2 through T5 for the rhomboid major. The rhomboid minor inserts on the posterior portion of the medial base of the spine of the scapula. The major rhomboid inserts into the posterior surface of the medial border from where the minor leaves off down to the inferior angle of the scapula. The muscle has, on its posterior surface, an avascular plane between it and the trapezius. The only crossing structure here is the transverse cervical artery. On the deep surface there is another avascular fascial space which contains only the blood vessel and nerve to the rhomboids. On the muscle's deep surface inferiorly, the rhomboid major is bounded by the latissimus at its origin. Superiorly, the rhomboid minor is bounded by the levator scapulae.

The action of the rhomboids is retraction of the scapula, and because of their oblique course, they also participate in elevation of the scapula. Innervation to the rhomboid muscle is the dorsal scapular nerve (C5) which may arise off the plexus in common with the nerve to the subclavius or with the C5 branch to the long thoracic nerve. The nerve may pass deep to, or through, the levator scapulae on its way to the rhomboids and may contain some innervation to the levator. The dorsal scapular artery provides arterial supply to the muscles on its deep surface.

Levator Scapulae and Serratus Anterior

Two muscles, the levator scapulae (Fig. 2–32) and serratus anterior, are often discussed together because of their close relationship in comparative anatomy studies. The levator scapulae takes origin from the posterior tubercles of the transverse processes from C1 through C3 and sometimes C4. It inserts into the superior angle of the scapula. The muscle is bounded in front by the scalenus medius and behind by the splenius cervicis. It is bounded laterally in the upper portion by the sternocleidomastoid and below by the

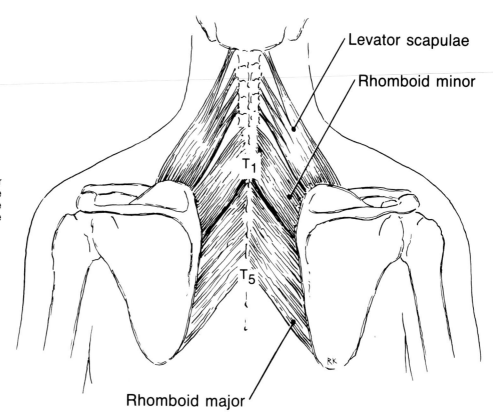

Figure 2–32. Rhomboids and the levator scapulae. The dominant orientation of the fibers of these muscles and their relative position along the medial border of the scapula are shown.

Levator scapulae

Rhomboid minor

T1

T5

Rhomboid major

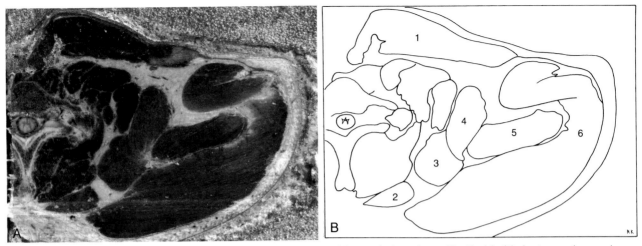

Figure 2–33. *A, B,* A transverse section at a level slightly higher than the superior angle of the scapula shows the considerable girth of the levator scapulae, seen in cross-section. Most of the other muscles noted are shown in their longitudinal section. The structures are as follows: (1) sternocleidomastoid, (2) rhomboid minor, (3) levator scapulae, (4) superior slip of serratus anterior, (5) supraspinatus, and (6) trapezius.

trapezius. The accessory nerve crosses laterally[41] in the middle section of the muscle. The dorsal scapular nerve may be deep or pass through the muscle. In specimens where the dorsal scapular comes off the transverse cervical artery, the parent transverse cervical artery splits, the dorsal scapular artery passes medial to the muscle, and the transverse cervical artery passes laterally. Ordinarily the dorsal scapular artery has a small branch that passes laterally toward the supraspinatus fossa. In at least one-third of dissections these vessels supply the levator with circulation.[210]

The levator acts to elevate the superior angle of the scapula. In conjunction with the serratus anterior, it produces upward rotation of the scapula.[17] That the levator (Fig. 2–33) has a mass larger than the upper trapezius is only illustrated properly by comparing the two muscles in cross-section; in most illustrations, it is obscured by overlying musculature.[17] Some authors speculate that this muscle may be a downward rotator of the scapula.[41] Innervation is from the deep branches of C3 and C4, and part of the C4 is contributed by the dorsal scapular nerve.

The serratus anterior (Fig. 2–34) takes origin from the ribs on the anterior lateral wall of the thoracic cage. This muscle has three divisions. The first division consists of one slip. It takes origin from ribs 1 and 2 and the intercostal space and then runs slightly upward and posteriorly to insert upon the superior angle of the scapula. The second division consists of three slips from the second, third, and fourth ribs. This division inserts along the medial anterior surface of the medial border. The lower division consists of the inferior four or five slips taking origin from ribs 5–9. They run posteriorly to insert upon the inferior angle of the scapula, giving this division the longest lever for scapular rotation.

The serratus anterior is bounded medially by the ribs and intercostal muscles and laterally by the axillary space. Anteriorly, the muscle is bounded by the exter-

nal oblique muscle with which it interdigitates, because this muscle takes origin from the same ribs.

The serratus protracts the scapula and participates in upward rotation of the scapula. It is more active in flexion than in abduction because straight abduction requires some retraction of the scapula. Scheving found that the muscle was activated by all movements of the humerus.[132] The serratus operates at a higher percentage of its maximum activity than any other shoulder

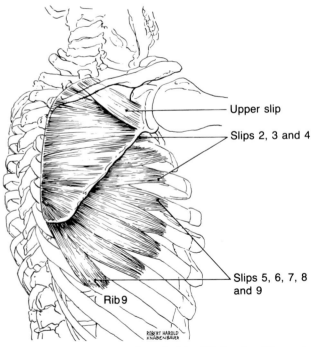

Figure 2–34. The three groups of muscles into which the slips of the serratus anterior are divided. The upper slip comes off the first two ribs and the first intercostal space, inserting at the upper edge of the medial border of the scapula. The slips coming off ribs 2, 3, and 4 insert on the broad major portion of the medial border; the slips from ribs 5, 6, 7, 8, and 9 converge on the inferior angle of the scapula.

muscle in unresisted activities.[17, 123] Absence of serratus activity, usually because of paralysis, produces a winging of the scapula with forward flexion of the arm and loss of strength in that motion.[113] Muscle transfer to replace the inferior slips restores only flexion.[100]

Innervation is supplied by the long thoracic nerve (C5, C6, and C7). Anatomy of this nerve has been studied intensely because of those events where injury has occurred. The nerve takes an angulated course across the second rib, where it can be stretched by lateral head tilt combined with depression of the shoulder.[108] Blood supply to the serratus is classically stated to be through the lateral thoracic artery.[41] There is often a large contribution from the thoracodorsal artery, especially when the lateral thoracic artery is small or absent. The lateral thoracic artery is the most frequently anomalous artery taking origin from the axillary artery.[81] The thoracodorsal artery may supply up to 50 per cent of the muscle.[130] The upper slips are supplied by the supreme thoracic artery when present.[130]

Pectoralis Minor

The pectoralis minor takes fleshy origin anteriorly on the chest wall, from the second through the fifth ribs, and has its insertion onto the base of the medial side of the coracoid (Fig. 2–35) with frequent (15 per cent) aberrant slips to the humerus, glenoid, clavicle, or scapula.[82, 111, 113, 143] The most common of the aberrant slips is the continuation across the coracoid to the humerus in the same path as the coracohumeral ligament. Its function is protraction of the scapula if the scapula is retracted and depression of the lateral angle or downward rotation of the scapula if the scapula is upwardly rotated. Innervation is from the medial pectoral nerve (C8, T1). Blood supply is through the pectoral branch of the thoracoacromial artery.[41] Taylor reported in his injection studies, however, that this vessel does not provide a constant supply to the pectoralis minor; another source is the lateral thoracic artery.[221] Salmon found multiple tiny arteries direct from the axillary which he called the posterior thoracic arteries.[130] Absence of the muscle does not seem to cause any disability.[146] This muscle was thought never to be absent when the entire pectoralis major is present,[41, 146] but Williams reports one case, verified at surgery, where the pectoralis minor was missing from beneath a normal pectoralis major.[146] Bing reports three other cases in the German literature.[92]

Subclavius

The subclavius muscle (Fig. 2–36) is included with the scapulothoracic muscles because it crosses the sternoclavicular joint where most of the scapulothoracic motion takes place. It has a tendinous origin off the first rib and cartilage and a muscular insertion on the inferior surface of the medial third of the clavicle.

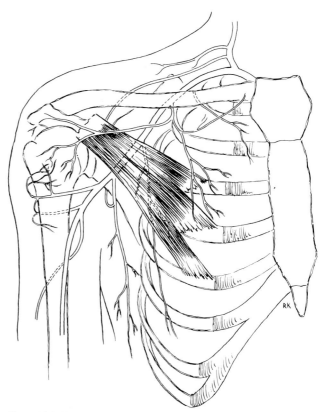

Figure 2–35. The pectoralis minor is an important landmark as an anterior border to the axillary space as well as for dividing the axillary space into its proximal, middle, and distal portions. It acts in protraction and depression of the scapula.

The tendon has a muscle that is pennate in structure. The tendon, 1 to 1.5 inches in length, lies mainly on the inferior surface of the muscle.[95] Nerve supply is the nerve to the subclavius. Blood supply is derived from the clavicular branch at the thoracoacromial artery[221] or from the suprascapular artery.[130] The action of this muscle is to stabilize the sternoclavicular joint while in motion—particularly with adduction and extension against resistance such as hanging from a bar (i.e., stabilization in intense activity).[127]

GLENOHUMERAL MUSCLES

Deltoid

The largest and most important of the glenohumeral muscles is the deltoid, consisting of three major sections: the anterior deltoid taking origin off the lateral one-third of the clavicle, the middle third of the deltoid taking origin off the acromion, and the posterior deltoid taking origin from the spine of the scapula.[86] Typical of broadly based muscles, the origin is collagen poor throughout its breadth. Insertion is on the deltoid tubercle of the humerus.

The deltoid muscle's boundary on the external side is subcutaneous fat. Because of the amount of motion involved, the bursa and fascial spaces bound the deep

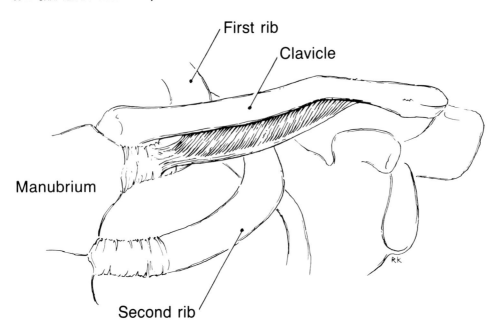

First rib

Clavicle

Manubrium

Second rib

Figure 2–36. The subclavius muscle is pennate in structure, having a long tendon on its inferior surface.

side. The axillary nerve and posterior humeral circumflex artery, the only nerve and the major blood supply of the muscle, also lie on the deep side. The pectoralis major muscle lies anteromedially. The clavicular portion of this muscle shares many functions with the anterior third of the deltoid. Within the boundary of the two muscles is the deltopectoral groove, where the cephalic vein and branches of the deltoid artery of the thoracoacromial trunk lie.

The three sections of the deltoid differ in internal structure and function (Fig. 2–37). The anterior and posterior deltoid have parallel fibers and have a longer excursion than the middle third which is multipennate and stronger and has a shorter excursion (1 cm). The middle third of the deltoid takes part in all motions of elevation of the humerus.[17] With its abundant collagen

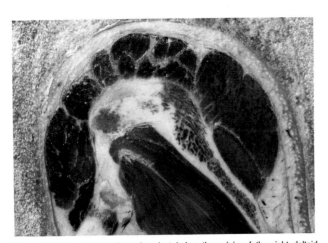

Figure 2–37. A cross-section taken just below the origin of the right deltoid demonstrates the relative positions of the three divisions of the deltoid and the differences in their internal structure. The middle deltoid, being multipennate, has an abundance of internal collagen. The anterior third (on the left) and the posterior third (on the right) tend to be parallel in structure or partially unipennate adjacent to the septum that separates them from the middle third.

it is the portion of the muscle most frequently involved with contracture.[91]

Elevation in the scapular plane is the product of the anterior and middle thirds of the deltoid, with some action by the posterior third, especially above 90 degrees.[136] Abduction in the coronal plane decreases the contribution of the anterior third and increases the contribution of the posterior deltoid. Flexion is a product of the anterior and middle thirds of the deltoid and the clavicular portion of the pectoralis major, with some contribution by the biceps (Fig. 2–38). The contribution of the last two muscles is so small as to be insufficient to hold the arm against gravity without the deltoid.[97, 138] Conversely, the deltoid contributes only 12 per cent of horizontal adduction. It was suggested that there is activity by the lower portion of the posterior deltoid in adduction. Shevlin and coworkers, however, attribute this action to providing an external rotation force on the humerus to counteract the internal rotation force of the pectoralis major, teres major, and latissimus dorsi, the major adductors of the shoulder.[136] The deltoid accounts for 60 per cent of strength in horizontal abduction.[96] The deltoid muscle's relation to the joint is such that it has its shortest leverage for elevation in the first 30 degrees,[17] although in this position leverage is increased by the prominence of the greater tubercle.[70]

The anterior third of the deltoid is bounded on its deep surface by the coracoid, the conjoint tendon of the coracobrachialis, and the short head of biceps, and above, by the coracoid and the clavipectoral fascia. The posterior portion of the deltoid is bounded on its deep surface by the infraspinatus and teres minor and by the major muscle on the other side of the avascular fascial space. The deltoid has a very dense fascia on its deep surface.[130] The axillary nerve and the posterior humeral circumflex vessels run on the muscle side of this fascia.[130]

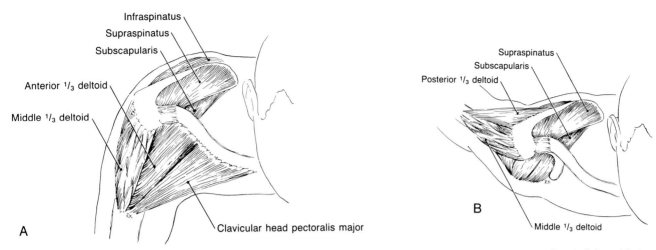

Figure 2–38. The function of the deltoid. *A,* The middle and anterior thirds of the deltoid function together, with the clavicular head of the pectoralis major in forward flexion. *B,* In horizontal abduction, the posterior third of the deltoid is active and the anterior third is inactive. The middle third of the deltoid is active in all motions of the glenohumeral joint.

Innervation of the deltoid is supplied by the axillary nerve (C5 and C6) which enters the posterior portion of the shoulder through the quadrilateral space and innervates teres minor in this position. The nerve splits in the quadrilateral space, and the nerve or nerves to the posterior third of the deltoid enter the muscle very close to their exit from the quadrilateral space, traveling in the deltoid muscle along the medial and inferior borders of the posterior deltoid. Interestingly, the posterior branch extends 6 to 8 cm in length after it leaves the quadrilateral space.[162] The branch of the axillary nerve that supplies the anterior two-thirds of the deltoid ascends superiorly and then travels anteriorly, approximately 2 inches inferior to the rim of the acromion. Paralysis of the axillary nerve produces a 50 per cent loss of strength in elevation,[96] even though the full abduction range is sometimes maintained.[137] Vascular supply is largely derived from the posterior humeral circumflex artery, which travels with the axillary nerve through the quadrilateral space to the deep surface of the muscle.[41, 42, 86, 130] The deltoid is also supplied by the deltoid branch of the thoracoacromial artery with rich anastomoses between the two vessels.[130] The deltoid artery travels in the deltopectoral groove, sending branches to the muscle.[130] The venous pedicles are identical to the arterial.[145]

Supraspinatus

The supraspinatus muscle lies on the superior portion of the scapula. It takes a fleshy origin from the supraspinatus fossa and overlying fascia and inserts into the greater tuberosity. Its tendinous insertion is in common with the infraspinatus posteriorly and the coracohumeral ligament anteriorly. Its tendon may have an asymptomatic calcium deposit in as many as 2.5 per cent of shoulders.[120] Inferiorly the muscular portion is bounded by its origin off the bone, the rim of the neck of the glenoid, and the capsule itself, which is not

divisible from the deep fibers of the tendon (Fig. 2–39).

The function of the muscle is important because it is active with any motion involving elevation.[17] Its length-tension curve exerts maximum effort at about 30 degrees of elevation.[96] Above this level, the greater tubercle increases its lever arm.[70] Because the muscle circumscribes the humeral head above and its fibers orient directly toward the glenoid, it is very important for stabilizing the glenohumeral joint. The supraspinatus, together with the other accessory muscles, the infraspinatus, subscapularis, and biceps, contrib-

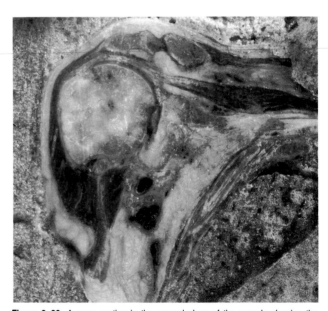

Figure 2–39. A cross-section in the coronal plane of the scapula showing the important relationships of the supraspinatus muscle. Among these are the course of the tendon that circumscribes the humeral head—essential to its head-depressing effect—and the tendon's course beneath the acromion, the acromioclavicular joint, and the indiscernible subacromial bursa. Inferiorly it is inseparable from the capsule of the joint. The subacromial bursa above the tendon, being a potential space, is indiscernible. (Compare with Fig. 2–69.)

utes equally with the deltoid in the torque of the scapular plane elevation and in forward elevation when tested by selective axillary nerve block.[17, 96, 97, 109]

Other muscles of the rotator cuff, especially the infraspinatus and subscapularis, provide further downward force on the humeral head to resist shear forces of the deltoid. If these muscles are intact, even with a small rotator cuff tear there may be enough stabilization for fairly strong abduction of the shoulder by the deltoid muscle, although endurance may be shorter.[17] Some patients may externally rotate their shoulder so that they can use their biceps for the same activity. Because the supraspinatus is confined above by the subacromial bursa and the acromion and below by the humeral head, the tendon is at risk for compression and attrition. Because of such compression, Grant's series and others indicate that 50 per cent of cadaver specimens over the age of 77 have rotator cuff tears.[104, 147] A later study by Neer shows a lower incidence.[61] The boundaries of the path of the subscapularis tendon are referred to as the supraspinatus outlet.[62] This space is decreased by internal rotation and opened by external rotation, showing the effect of the greater tubercle.[60, 116] The space is also compromised by use of the shoulder in weight bearing, as when using crutches and when doing push-ups in a wheelchair.[89] Martin and others suggest that the external rotation of the arm in elevation is produced by the coracoacromial arch acting as an inclined plane on the greater tubercle.[55, 116] Saha and others attribute this limitation of rotation in elevation to ligamentous control.[72–74]

Innervation of the supraspinatus is supplied by the suprascapular nerve (C5 with some C6). The main arterial supply is the suprascapular artery. These structures enter the muscle near its midpoint at the suprascapular notch at the base of the coracoid process. The nerve goes through the notch and is bounded above by the transverse scapular ligament. There is no motion of the nerve relative to the notch. The artery travels above this ligament. The suprascapular vessels and nerve supply the deep surface of the muscle.[130] There is also a branch between the bone of the scapular spine and the muscle. The medial portion of the muscle receives vessels from the dorsal scapular artery.[130]

Infraspinatus

The infraspinatus (Fig. 2–40) is the second most active rotator cuff muscle.[17] It takes a fleshy, collagen-poor origin off the infraspinatus fossa of the scapula, overlying dense fascia and the spine of the scapula. Its tendinous insertion is in common with the supraspinatus anterior superiorly and teres minor inferiorly at the greater tuberosity. On its superficial surface it is bounded by an avascular fascial space on the deep surface of the deltoid. The infraspinatus is one of the two main external rotators of the humerus and accounts for as much as 60 per cent of external rotation force.[96] It functions as a depressor of the humeral head.[44, 72] Even in the passive (cadaver) state it is an important

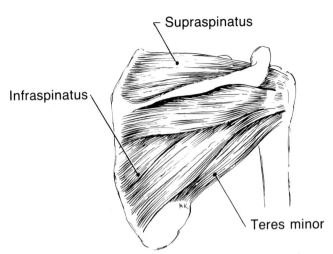

Figure 2–40. The two external rotators of the humerus, the infraspinatus and teres minor muscles, which are also the posterior wall of the rotator cuff. Note the median raphe of the infraspinatus, which is often mistaken at surgery for the border between the infraspinatus and the teres minor.

stabilizer against posterior subluxation.[125, 126] An interesting aspect of muscle action at the shoulder is that a muscle may have opposing actions in different positions. The infraspinatus muscle stabilizes the shoulder against posterior subluxation in internal rotation by circumscribing the humeral head, creating a forward force. In contradistinction it has a line of pull posteriorly, stabilizing against an anterior subluxation when the shoulder is in abduction-external rotation.[17, 94] The infraspinatus is a pennate muscle with a median raphe, often mistaken at surgery for the gap between the infraspinatus and teres minor muscles. The infraspinatus is innervated by the suprascapular nerve. Its blood supply is usually described as coming from two large branches of the suprascapular artery.[41] Salmon, however, found in two-thirds of his specimens that the subscapular artery through its dorsal or circumflex scapular branch supplied the greater portion of the circulation of the infraspinatus muscle.[130]

Teres Minor

Teres minor (Fig. 2–40) has a muscular origin from the middle portion of the lateral border of the scapula and the dense fascia of the infraspinatus. Rarely, individuals are found where the teres minor overlies the infraspinatus as far as the vertebral border of the scapula.[144] It inserts into the lower portion of the posterior greater tuberosity of the humerus. On its deep surface is the adherent posterior capsule and on the superficial surface is a fascial plane between it and the deep surface of the deltoid. On the inferior border lie the quadrilateral space laterally and the triangular space medially. In the quadrilateral space, the posterior humeral circumflex artery and axillary nerve border the teres minor. In the triangular space, the circumflex scapular artery lies just inferior to this muscle. On its deep surface, in the midportion, lies the long head of the triceps tendon, loose alveolar fat, and subscapularis. The teres minor is one of the few external rotators of the humerus. It provides up to 45 per cent of the external rotation force[96] and is important in controlling stability in the anterior direction.[94] It also probably participates in the short rotator force, coupled in abduction with the inferior portion of the subscapularis. Teres minor is innervated by the posterior branch of the axillary nerve (C5 and C6). The blood supply derives from several vessels in the area, but the branch from the posterior humeral scapular circumflex artery is the most constant.[130]

Subscapularis

The subscapularis muscle is the anterior portion of the rotator cuff. The muscle takes a fleshy origin from the subscapularis fossa which covers most of the anterior surface of the scapula. It inserts through a collagen-rich tendon into the lesser tuberosity of the humerus. The internal structure of the muscle is multipennate, and the collagen is so dense that it is considered one of the passive stabilizers of the shoulder. The muscle has been studied as a passive stabilizer in cadaver models.[124, 142, 139] It is bounded anteriorly by the axillary space and coracobrachialis bursa. Superiorly it abuts the coracoid process and the subscapularis recess, or bursa. The axillary nerve and posterior humeral circumflex artery and veins pass deep below the muscle into the quadrilateral space. The circumflex scapular artery passes into the more medial triangular space.

The subscapularis (Fig. 2–41) functions as an internal rotator and passive stabilizer to anterior subluxation and serves in its lower fibers to depress the humeral head.[44, 72] By this last function it resists the shear of the deltoid to help with elevation. Another aspect of subscapularis function is that it may vary with level of training. Among amateur pitchers the function of the subscapularis in acceleration is less than in professional throwers, implying that the less trained thrower is still adjusting his glenohumeral joint for stability while the professional can use the muscle as an internal rotator.[103] On its deep surface, in the upper portion, is the glenohumeral joint. The middle glenohumeral ligament lies beneath the middle portion of the tendon. The origin of the anterior inferior glenohumeral ligament also lies deep to the midportion. Innervation is usually supplied by two sources: the upper subscapular nerve (C5) supplies the upper portion and the lower subscapular nerve (C5, C6) supplies the lower. The upper subscapular nerve, a comparatively short nerve in the axilla, comes off the posterior cord. Because of the greater relative motion of the lower portion of the scapula, the lower subscapular nerve is longer in its course. Most of the muscle is innervated by the upper subscapular nerve. The ratio of muscle innervated by the upper nerve to that innervated by the lower is estimated to be 2:1 or 4:1. Blood supply is usually described as originating from the subscapular artery, but Bartlett and his associates found that 84 per cent of their 50 dissections had no significant vessels off the

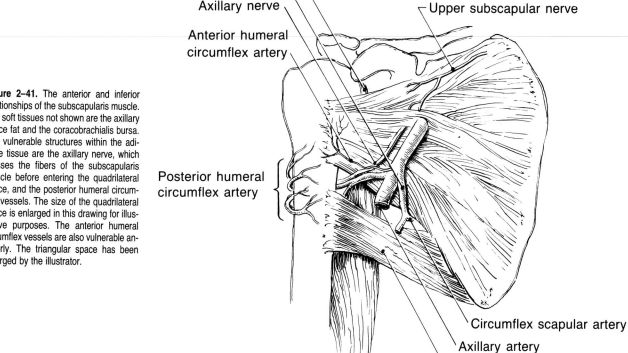

Figure 2–41. The anterior and inferior relationships of the subscapularis muscle. The soft tissues not shown are the axillary space fat and the coracobrachialis bursa. The vulnerable structures within the adipose tissue are the axillary nerve, which crosses the fibers of the subscapularis muscle before entering the quadrilateral space, and the posterior humeral circumflex vessels. The size of the quadrilateral space is enlarged in this drawing for illustrative purposes. The anterior humeral circumflex vessels are also vulnerable anteriorly. The triangular space has been enlarged by the illustrator.

Subscapular artery — Subscapularis recess

Axillary nerve — Upper subscapular nerve

Anterior humeral circumflex artery

Posterior humeral circumflex artery

Triceps muscle

Circumflex scapular artery
Axillary artery
Teres major muscle

subscapular artery prior to the bifurcation into circumflex scapular and thoracodorsal arteries.[88] This finding would increase the importance of the anterior humeral circumflex or the "upper subscapular artery" named by Huelke.[210] Salmon also describes this as a constant vessel but says it is small in caliber.[130] The major supply he found derived from the branches of subscapular artery.[130] Small branches from the dorsal scapular artery reach the medial portion of the muscle after penetrating the serratus anterior.[130] Venous drainage is via two veins to the circumflex scapular artery.[145]

Teres Major

The teres major (Fig. 2–42C) takes origin from the posterior surface of the scapula along the inferior portion of the lateral border. It has a muscular origin and a common tendinous insertion with latissimus dorsi into the humerus along the medial lip of the bicipital groove, a ridge of bone that is a continuation of the lesser tuberosity. In the course of these muscles both the latissimus dorsi and teres major undergo a 180-degree spiral, so the formerly posterior surface of the muscle is represented by fibers on the anterior surface of the tendon. Also, the relationship between the teres major and latissimus dorsi rearranges so that the formerly posterior latissimus dorsi becomes anterior to teres major. In addition to the boundaries of the latissimus dorsi, it is bounded above by the triangular and quadrilateral spaces, posteriorly by the long head

of the triceps, and anteriorly in its medial portion by the axillary space. The function of the teres major is internal rotation, adduction, and extension of the arm. It is active in these motions only against resistance.[33] There may be an additional function, upward rotation of the scapula, with activities that involve a firmly planted upper extremity such as the iron cross performed by gymnasts. Innervation is supplied by the lower subscapular nerve (C5, C6), and its blood supply derives from the branches of the subscapular artery, quite regularly a single vessel from the thoracodorsal artery.[130]

Coracobrachialis

The coracobrachialis has a fleshy and tendinous origin from the coracoid process, in common with and medial to the short head of the biceps, and inserts on the anteromedial surface in the midportion of the humerus. Laterally it is bounded by its common origin with the biceps. On the deep surface the coracobrachialis bursa lies between the two conjoint muscles and the subscapularis. The deltoid, the deltopectoral groove, and pectoralis major are on the superficial surface. These surfaces tend to be avascular or are crossed by a few small vessels. Action of the coracobrachialis is flexion and adduction of the glenohumeral joint, with innervation supplied by a small branch from the lateral cord and the musculocutaneous nerve. Most specimens have a direct nerve to the coracobrachialis

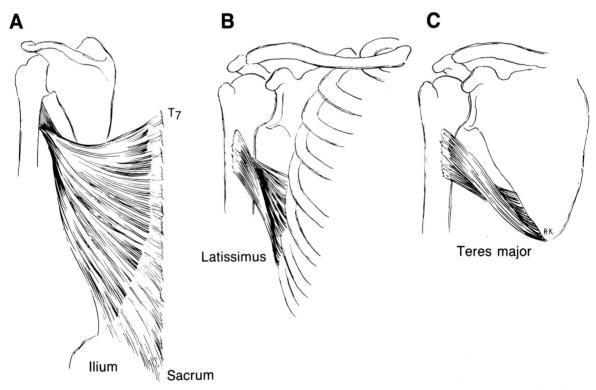

A

B

C

T7

Latissimus

Teres major

Ilium   Sacrum

Figure 2–42. Anterior and posterior views of the course of the latissimus dorsi muscle from its origin along the posterior spinous processes from T7 to the sacrum and along the iliac crest. Its insertion is along the medial lip and floor of the bicipital groove. The accompanying muscle, the teres major, with its similar fiber rotation inserts just medial to the latissimus dorsi.

from the lateral cord, in addition to the larger musculocutaneous (C5, C6) nerve. This additional nerve enters the coracobrachialis muscle on its deep surface, providing additional innervation.[158, 167] Because the larger musculocutaneous nerve's entrance to the muscle may be situated as high as 1.5 cm[149, 166] from the tip of the coracoid to as low as 7 to 8 cm, it must be located and protected during certain types of repair. The major blood supply is by a single artery, usually off the axillary. This artery may arise in common with the artery to the biceps.[130]

MULTIPLE JOINT MUSCLES

The multiple joint muscles perform action on the glenohumeral joint and one other joint, most often the scapulothoracic. Where appropriate, the action on both of these joints will be mentioned.

Pectoralis Major

The pectoralis major consists of three portions (Fig. 2–43). The upper portion takes origin from the medial one-half to two-thirds of the clavicle[221] and inserts along the lateral lip of the bicipital groove. Its fibers maintain a parallel arrangement. The middle portion takes origin from the manubrium and upper two-thirds of the body of the sternum and ribs 2–4. It inserts directly behind the clavicular portion and maintains a parallel fiber arrangement. The inferior portion of the pectoralis major takes origin from the distal body of the sternum, the fifth and sixth ribs, and the external oblique muscle fascia. It has the same insertion as the other two portions, but the fibers rotate 180 degrees so that the inferior fibers insert superiorly on the humerus. Landry noted that when a chondroepitrochlearis muscle anomaly existed, the twisted insertion was not present.[112] There is often a line of separation between the clavicular portion and the lower two portions. The superficial surface of the muscle is bounded by mammary gland and subcutaneous fat. The inferior border is the border of the axillary fold. The superior lateral border is the deltopectoral groove mentioned above. On the deep surface superior to the attachment to the ribs lies the pectoralis minor muscle, which is invested in the clavipectoral fascia.

Action of the pectoralis major depends upon its starting position. For example, the clavicular portion participates somewhat in flexion with the anterior portion of the deltoid, while the lower fibers are antagonistic. Both of these effects are lost in the coronal plane.[136] The muscle is active in internal rotation against resistance[136] and will extend the shoulder from flexion until the neutral position is reached. This muscle is also a powerful adductor of the glenohumeral joint and indirectly functions as a depressor of the lateral angle of the scapula. Loss of the sternocostal portion most noticeably affects internal rotation and scapular depression, with some loss of adduction.[115] This loss is significant only for athletics, not daily activities. The clavicular portion is most active in forward flexion and horizontal adduction.[44] Loss of pectoralis major function seems to be well tolerated.[105, 146]

Innervation of the muscle is supplied by two sources. The lateral pectoral nerve (C5, C6, and C7) innervates the clavicular portion of the muscle, probably only with C5–C6 fibers,[221] and the loop contribution from the lateral to the medial pectoral nerve carrying C7 fibers continues through or around the pectoralis minor into the upper sternal portion. The medial pectoral nerve, carrying fibers from C8 and T1, continues through pectoralis minor into the remaining portion of the pectoralis major. The major blood supply derives from two sources. The deltoid branch of the thoracoacromial artery supplies the clavicular portion, and the pectoral artery supplies the sternocostal portion of the muscle.[221] Additional blood supply is shared via the internal mammary artery, the fourth or fifth intercostal artery, and other anastomoses from the lateral thoracic artery.[130, 221] The vessel to the fourth rib area is within an additional deep origin which comes off this rib in the midclavicular line. Venous drainage laterally is through two veins to the axillary vein and medially to the internal mammary system.[145, 221] In a literature review done in 1902, Bing reported that absence of a portion or all of pectoralis major was the most commonly reported muscle defect, making up 28 per cent of the cases cited.[92]

Latissimus Dorsi

The latissimus dorsi (see Fig. 2–42A, B) takes origin by the large and broad aponeurosis from the dorsal spines of T7 through L5, a portion of the sacrum, and the crest of the ilium. Frequently there are origins on the lowest three or four ribs and the inferior angle of

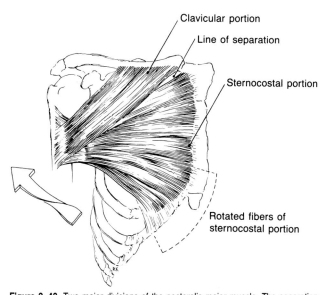

Clavicular portion

Line of separation

Sternocostal portion

Rotated fibers of sternocostal portion

Figure 2–43. Two major divisions of the pectoralis major muscle. The separation is often readily discernible. Note the 180-degree rotation of the fibers of the lower portion of the sternocostal division.

the scapula as well.[88] This muscle wraps around the teres major and inserts into the medial crest and floor of the bicipital or intertubercular groove.

On its superficial surface the muscle is bounded by subcutaneous fascia, and along the inferior border, it forms the posterior axillary fold. Anteriorly it is bounded by the axillary space, and its deep surface is bounded by ribs and the teres major. Actions of the muscle are inward rotation and adduction of the humerus, shoulder extension, and indirectly, through its pull on the humerus, downward rotation of the scapula. Scheving[132] found that this muscle is more important than the pectoralis major as an internal rotator. Ekholm found its most powerful action in the oblique motions: extension, adduction, and abduction–internal rotation.[101]

Innervation is through the thoracodorsal nerve (C6 and C7), and blood supply derives from the thoracodorsal artery with additional supply from the intercostal and lumbar perforators. The neurovascular hilum is on the inferior surface of the muscle about 2 cm medial to the muscular border.[88] Two investigators have found that this neurovascular pedicle splits inside the muscle fascia into the superomedial and inferolateral branches.[88, 141] The venous drainage mirrors the arterial supply.[145] They found that such splits are quite predictable and suggested that the muscle could be split into two separate island flaps, or free flaps.

Biceps Brachii

The biceps has its main action at the elbow rather than the shoulder. It is considered primarily an elbow muscle,[14] but it is listed here with the shoulder muscles because of its frequent involvement in shoulder pathology and its use in substitutional motions. There are two origins of the biceps muscle in the shoulder; both are collagen rich. The long head takes origin from the bicipital tubercle at the posterior rim of the glenoid and along the posterior superior rim of the glenoid and labrum, and the short head takes origin from the coracoid tip lateral to and in common with the coracobrachialis. Meyer[121] notes that much of the origin of the long head is via the superior labrum and that the size of the bicipital tubercle does not reflect the size of the biceps tendon. The muscle has two distal tendinous insertions. The lateral insertion is to the posterior part of the tuberosity of the radius, and the medial insertion is aponeurotic, passing medially across and into the deep fascia of the muscles of the volar forearm. Loss of the long head attachment expresses itself mainly as loss of supination strength (20 per cent) with a smaller loss (8 per cent) of elbow flexion strength.[114]

The relationships of the biceps tendon are most important in its role in shoulder pathology. The long head of the biceps exits the shoulder through a defect in the capsule between the greater and lesser tuberosity and passes distally in the bicipital groove. This portion of the tendon is most often involved in pathology. Many studies have been done to try to correlate construction of the groove with bicipital pathology[40, 121]

(see Fig. 2–23). It was felt that a shallow bicipital groove and a supratubercular ridge above the lesser tubercle, which is the trochlea of the tendon, would predispose the biceps tendon to dislocation with subsequent pathology of the tendon.[121] It was also noted that the intra-articular tendon is broader than that in the groove.[121] Other early authors reported no rupture of the biceps tendon in the absence of supraspinatus rupture. Recent opinion is that pathology of the tendon is related to impingement. If there is a correlation between bicipital groove morphology and the biceps tendon, it may be that a shallower groove is more likely to expose the long head of the biceps to impingement.[61] The bicipital tendon does not move up and down in the groove. Rather, the humerus moves down and up with adduction and abduction relative to the tendon. The bicipital tendon is retained within the groove by the transverse humeral ligament.

Under normal conditions the action of the biceps is flexion and supination at the elbow. In certain conditions, particularly where paralysis or rupture of the supraspinatus has occurred, patients have a hypertrophied long head of the biceps, probably because they are using the muscle as a depressor of the humeral head by placing the shoulder in external rotation.[17] One patient with a large rotator cuff tear reportedly was employed as a waiter and carried trays on the involved side with a large rotator cuff tear, a substitution maneuver commonly seen in the days of infantile paralysis.[44, 140] Lucas reports a 20 per cent loss of elevation strength in external rotation with rupture of the long head of the biceps.[55] Mariani, on the other hand, reported that loss of this head depressor effect is unlikely to worsen impingement.[114] In internal rotation there was no loss of strength, and we must remember that impingement occurs in internal rotation.[55] It should be emphasized that these are not the usual activities of the biceps in the person without shoulder pathology studied by electromyogram. Innervation of the biceps is supplied by branches of the musculocutaneous nerve (C5, C6), and the blood supply derives from a single large bicipital artery from the brachial artery (35 per cent), multiple very small arteries (40 per cent), or a combination of the two types.[130]

Triceps Brachii

The triceps is another muscle not usually considered a shoulder muscle but often involved in shoulder pathology, particularly the long head. The long head takes origin from the infraglenoid tubercle. Although this tendon is not intra-articular, like the long head of the biceps the insertion is intimately related to the labrum over a distance of 2 cm centered on the tubercle. The fibers of the tendon adjacent to the capsule radiate into the inferior capsule and reinforce it. The remaining fibers insert into bone. This reinforced capsule, a portion of the inferior glenohumeral ligament, inserts through the labrum and radiates fibers into the circular portion of the labrum.[106]

The long head origin is bounded laterally by the quadrilateral space, containing the axillary nerve and posterior humeral circumflex artery, and medially by the triangular space, containing the circumflex scapular artery. The teres major muscle passes anteriorly, and teres minor passes posteriorly. Innervation is supplied by the radial nerve with root innervation C6–C8.[41] The arterial supply is derived mainly from the profunda artery. However, near its origin, the long head receives branches from the brachial and posterior humeral circumflex arteries.

The major action of the muscle is at the elbow. The long head is felt to function in shoulder adduction against resistance to offset the shear forces generated by the primary adductors. In more violent activities such as throwing, the muscle may demonstrate 12 EMG activity up to 200 per cent of that generated by a maximal muscle test.[110] This force would be transmitted to the origin off the scapula.

LANDMARK MUSCLES

Some muscles are important to surgeons as landmarks to shoulder dissection but are not shoulder muscles in the sense of producing shoulder motion.

Sternocleidomastoid

The most obvious of these is the sternocleidomastoid muscle which, with the superior fibers of the trapezius, forms the borders of the posterior triangle of the neck.

It takes origin by tendinous head from the sternum and a broader but thin muscular head from the medial part of the clavicle.[42] The two heads unite and progress superiorly, obliquely posteriorly, and laterally to insert on the mastoid process. This muscle shares the same innervation with the trapezius, the accessory spinal nerve (CN XI). Blood supply is derived from two vascular pedicles, the superior from the occipital artery and the lower from the superior thyroid artery.

Scalenus Anterior and Medius

The anterior scalene muscle takes origin from the anterior tubercles of vertebrae C3 through C6 and has a tendinous insertion on the first rib. The middle scalene muscle, largest of the scalenes, takes its origin from all of the transverse processes in the cervical spine and also inserts into the first rib. The first rib and the two scalene muscles form a triangle (Fig. 2–44) through which the entire brachial plexus and the subclavian artery pass. The subclavian vein passes anterior to the anterior scalene and posterior to the clavicle. Innervation of these muscles is supplied from deep branches of the cervical nerves. Variations in the muscles and their relations are believed to predispose to the thoracic outlet syndrome.[128]

Omohyoid

The omohyoid muscle is seldom mentioned in the description of surgical procedures, but it divides the posterior cervical triangle into the upper occipital and

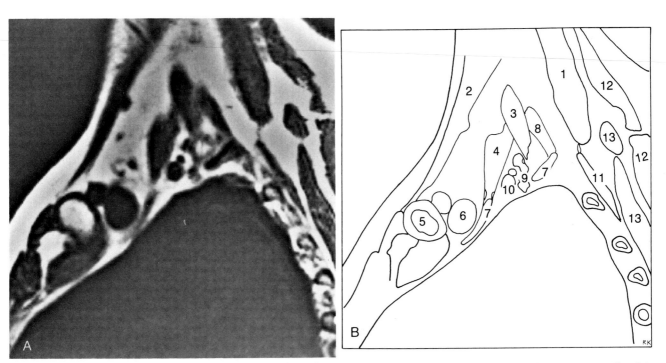

Figure 2–44. An MRI (A) and diagram (B) of the scalene triangle showing the boundaries of the scalene triangle and the relationship of the important structures. Note that the anterior tilt of the first rib places the more posterior structures at a more caudad level. Note also the greater thickness of the levator scapulae (1) compared with the trapezius (12). The labeled structures include: (1) levator scapulae, (2) sternocleidomastoid, (3) middle scalene, (4) anterior scalene, (5) clavicle, (6) subclavian vein, (7) rib 1, (8) posterior scalene, (9) brachial plexus, (10) subclavian artery, (11) serratus posterior superior, (12) trapezius, and (13) rhomboids.

lower subclavian triangles. It attaches to the superior border of the scapula just medial to the scapular notch and runs anteriorly, medially, and superiorly across the posterior cervical triangle. Deep to the sternocleidomastoid muscle there is a tendon in the midportion of the muscle belly. The muscle continues on above to an insertion on the hyoid.

CONCLUSION

Muscles of the shoulder have been studied and described in terms of simple activities, but continued research is needed for the more complex motions. Microvascular surgeons have done an admirable job in describing the circulation, nerve supply, and variations of the muscles that lie directly under the skin, but further work ought to be done on the deeper layers if we are to consider using these muscles in transfer.

Nerves

Our discussion of nerves of the shoulder includes the brachial plexus and its branches, the sympathetic nervous system, the nerves that come off the roots that form the brachial plexus, cranial nerve XI, and the supraclavicular nerves. The brachial plexus is unique in the human nervous system because of the great amount of motion involved relative to the adjacent tissues. By way of introduction we first discuss the internal anatomy of the nerves. Roots, trunks, and cords of the brachial plexus are also peripheral nerves in their cross-sectional anatomy.[185, 190, 194] We then discuss the arrangement of the peripheral nervous system relative to other structures of the limbs. As an overview, we note a uniqueness of the brachial plexus, compared with the rest of the nervous system, that is the product of increased motion of the shoulder.

We will describe the standard brachial plexus and its normal relations and then discuss nonpathological variants, variations that do not affect its function but may complicate diagnosis and surgical approaches. We also discuss cranial nerve XI, the supraclavicular nerves, and the intercostal brachial nerve.

NERVE FUNCTION AND MICROANATOMY

The principal function of the nerves is to maintain and support the axons of the efferent and afferent nerve cells. Cell bodies of these fibers are located in the dorsal root and autonomic ganglia and in the gray matter of the spinal cord. The axons are maintained somewhat by axoplasmic flow, but conduction of the nerve and its continued function have been found to be dependent on the layers surrounding the axons and their blood supply.[45, 189, 194, 200] These layers in turn are dependent upon an adequate blood supply.[184, 187, 195]

The axons in the large nerves are contained within Schwann cells either on a one-to-one ratio or, for the smaller nerve fibers, on a multiaxon-to-one Schwann cell proportion. These in turn are embedded in the endoneurium. A basal lamina separates the endoneurium from the myelin sheaths and Schwann cells.

Endoneurial tissue is mainly collagen that is closely arranged and contains capillaries and lymphatics.[175, 194, 200] The next outer tissue, referred to as the perineurium, surrounds groups of axons and serves primarily as a diffusion barrier. It also maintains intraneural pressure. The integrity of this layer is essential to function of the nerve and is the tissue most important to the surgeon. The perineurium is divided into multiple layers. The innermost layer has flat cells with tight junctions and appears to maintain the diffusion barrier. The outer layers are lamellated with interspersed collagen. The external layer of perineurium is a proven barrier to infection, while the outer layer of the nerve, the epineurium, is not.

That portion of the nerve enclosed in perineurium is referred to as a fascicle and is really the functioning portion of the nerve. All axons are contained in fascicles, and fascicles produce the necessary environment for nerve function. The size and number of fascicles vary. Fascicles tend to be larger in size and fewer in number in the spinal nerves and tend to be smaller and more numerous around branch points.[185] As a branch point is approached, fascicles bound for the branch nerve are gathered into fascicle groups.[185, 200] The variability in fascicle number and size is further complicated by the fact that fascicles travel an average distance of only 5 mm before branching or merging. This results in a plexiform internal anatomy rather than the cable form which would be more convenient for repair and grafting purposes.[185]

The epineurium is a loose alveolar tissue that is richly supplied with blood vessels and lymphatics.[200] It may compose more than 80 per cent of the cross-sectional area of the nerve or as little as 25 per cent[192, 193, 200] averaging about 40 to 50 per cent in peripheral nerves and 65 to 70 per cent in the plexus.[185]

Blood supply to the nerves has been divided into extrinsic and intrinsic vessels.[176, 177] The intrinsic are those vessels that are contained within the epineurium itself and are the arterial supply of the nerve. Terzis and Breidenbach further classified the nerves and extrinsic circulation in terms of whether all the extrinsic vessels connected to the same source artery and veins[197] for purposes of free transfer of nerve tissue. The blood vessels within the nerves are redundant and often have a convoluted course. Lundborg found that an average change of 8 per cent in length by stretching occurred before there was venous occlusion in the nerves and an average 15 per cent strain for complete cessation of arterial flow. Interestingly, function was normal in laboratory animals in which blood clots and blockages in some of the capillaries persisted even after release of tension on the nerve.[175]

Even the internal arrangement of nerves is designed

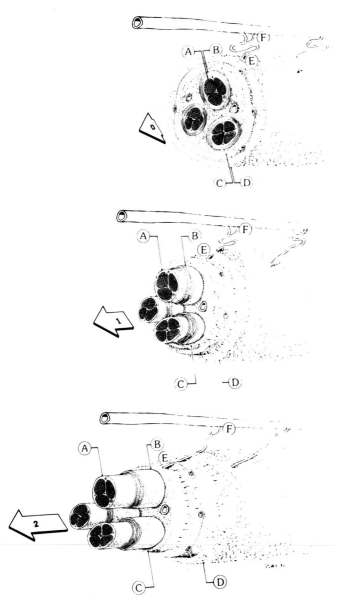

Figure 2–45. The internal anatomy of peripheral nerves and how it facilitates motion. A and B are the inner and outer layers of the perineurium; C and D are the inner and outer layers of the epineurium. E is a blood vessel within the epineurium, and F is the blood vessel of the nerve on the outside of the epineurium. Much of the cross-section of the nerve is epineurium. The various components of the soft tissue of the nerve accommodate to nerve motion. (Reprinted with permission from Lundborg G: Intraneural microcirculation. Orthop Clin North Am *19*(1):1–12, 1988.)

to accommodate motion (Fig. 2–45). Layers slide past each other and allow almost a laminar motion of the layers relative to their surroundings. The 15 per cent strain limit also has implications for the anatomical relations of nerves, particularly in the shoulder. The closer a nerve is positioned to a center of joint rotation, the less change in length of the nerve will occur with motion. There seem to be two strategies in the design of the brachial plexus that protect the nerve against overstretch. First, the location of the nerves directly behind the sternoclavicular joint protects them against stretch in elevation of the clavicle in the coronal plane. The second crucial arrangement is that the brachial

plexus in the axilla is not fixed to surrounding structures but, instead, floats freely in a quantity of fat. This allows the plexus to slide superiorly with elevation of the arm so that it moves closer to the center of rotation and necessitates less strain. The implication of this arrangement is that disruptions of the biomechanics of the shoulder may produce neurological symptoms even though original trauma or disease may not directly affect the nerves themselves. An additional protective arrangement in a joint that is so highly mobile is that most human motion is conducted forward, putting less stretch on most of the plexus. One exception to this tendency would be those nerves tightly attached to the scapula which would be stretched by scapular protraction.[168]

The extrinsic vessels to the nerve tend to have an inverse relationship between their size and number. They have a short length of 5 to 15 mm from the adjacent artery. Redundancy of the blood supply is such that a nerve, stripped of its extrinsic blood supply, will continue to function up to an 8 cm distance from the nearest arteria nervorum.[174, 175] This redundancy in blood supply is advantageous to tumor surgeons who find the epineurium to be an effective boundary in certain tumor dissections. The epineurium is sometimes sacrificed in surgery with good preservation of nerve function. Also, radiotherapy can be applied to the axilla without loss of function. The redundancy can be overcome, however, with a combination of epineurial stripping and radiation or an excessive dose of radiotherapy alone, with an adverse effect on nerve function.[157, 169]

BRACHIAL PLEXUS

Gross Anatomy

While studying the circulation of blood to the skin, Taylor and Palmer[230] identified some common elements in the distribution of blood vessels in the body which I would also apply to the arrangement of peripheral nerves. First, nerves tend to travel adjacent to either bone in intermuscular septa or other connective tissue structures. Second, the nerves travel from relatively fixed positions to relatively mobile positions. Nerves rarely cross planes where there is motion, and when they do, they cross in an oblique fashion in an area of less motion. This decreases the relative strain incurred by the nerve while crossing a mobile plane even though the actual total motion is not changed.[230]

The brachial plexus seems to contradict these tendencies. It travels from an area where it is relatively fixed at the cervical spine to an area of high mobility in the axilla, and then it returns to normal bone and intermuscular septum relationships in the arm. This is unique in the human body and is necessitated by the highly mobile nature of the shoulder and the motion of the brachial plexus nerves on their way to innervate structures in the arm and forearm. This seeming contradiction is understood when we picture the axillary sheath as the connective tissue framework for the nerves and vessels and note that it is the sheath that moves in the axillary space.

Roots

The standard brachial plexus (Fig. 2–46) is made up of the distal distribution of the anterior rami of the *spinal nerves or roots* C5, C6, C7, C8, and T1. The plexus sometimes has contributions from C4 and T1. For C4 this contribution appears in 28 to 62 per cent of specimens,[151] although in terms of neural tissue it contributes very little.[185] Bonnel found a T2 contribution in only 4 per cent of specimens.[151]

The radicles that form the spinal nerves lack a fibrous sheath[151] and obtain a significant amount of soft tissue support only when they exit the intervertebral foramina, gaining a dural sleeve. Herzberg found a postero-superior semiconic ligament at C5, C6, and C7 that attaches the spinal nerves to the transverse processes.[164] The spinal nerves C8 and T1 lack this additional protection. In most brachial plexus literature the anterior divisions of these nerves are called the roots of the brachial plexus. Herzberg and coworkers found that roots C5 and C6 could be followed proximally but failed to find a safe surgical approach to spinal nerves C8 and T1, because dissection involved particular danger to the osseous structures.[164] Other authors mention the difficulty in exposing the lower two nerves.[178]

TRUNKS, DIVISIONS, AND CORDS

The roots combine to form *trunks:* C5 and C6 form the superior trunk, C7 the middle trunk, and C8 and T1 the inferior trunk. The trunks then separate into anterior and posterior divisions. The posterior divisions combine to form the posterior cord, the anterior division of the inferior trunk forms the medial cord, and the anterior divisions of the superior and middle trunks form the lateral cord. These cords give off the remaining and largest number of the terminal nerves of the brachial plexus, and the roots from the lateral and medial cords come together to form the median nerve.

The brachial plexus leaves the cervical spine and progresses into the arm through the interval between the anterior and middle scalene muscles (Fig. 2–47). The subclavian artery follows the same course. Because of the inferior tilt of the first rib, the brachial plexus is posterior and superior to the artery at this point; only the inferior trunk is directly posterior to the artery on the rib. It is in this triangle made up of the two scalenes that nerve or vessel can be compromised by any number of abnormalities.[196] The inferior trunk forms high behind the clavicle, directly above the pleura, over a connective tissue layer referred to as Sibson's fascia. The upper two roots join to form the upper trunk at Erb's point located 2 to 3 cm above the clavicle just behind the posterior edge of the sterno-cleidomastoid muscle. The majority of plexi are penetrated by a vessel off the subclavian artery, most commonly the dorsal scapular artery, between two of the trunks.[211] The nerves between the scalene muscles become enclosed in the fascia of the scalenes, the prevertebral fascia. This interscalene sheath is important for containing and permitting the dispersal of local anesthetic about the nerves.[150]

The plexus reaches the cord level of differentiation at or before it passes below the clavicle. As the cords enter the axilla they become closely related to the axillary artery, attaining positions relative to the artery

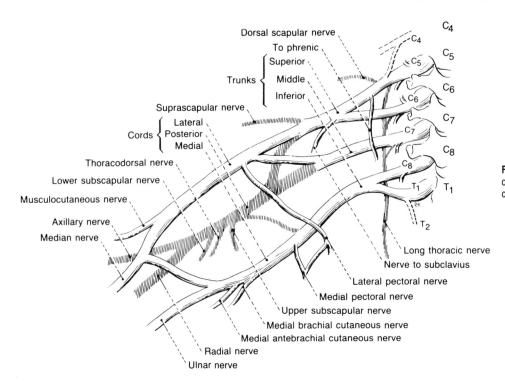

Figure 2–46. The standard arrangement of the brachial plexus and its trunks, cords, and terminal branches.

Dorsal scapular nerve
To phrenic
Superior
Middle
Inferior
Trunks
Suprascapular nerve
Lateral
Posterior
Medial
Cords
Thoracodorsal nerve
Lower subscapular nerve
Musculocutaneous nerve
Axillary nerve
Median nerve

C4
C5
C6
C7
C8
T1
T2

Long thoracic nerve
Nerve to subclavius
Lateral pectoral nerve
Medial pectoral nerve
Upper subscapular nerve
Medial brachial cutaneous nerve
Medial antebrachial cutaneous nerve
Radial nerve
Ulnar nerve

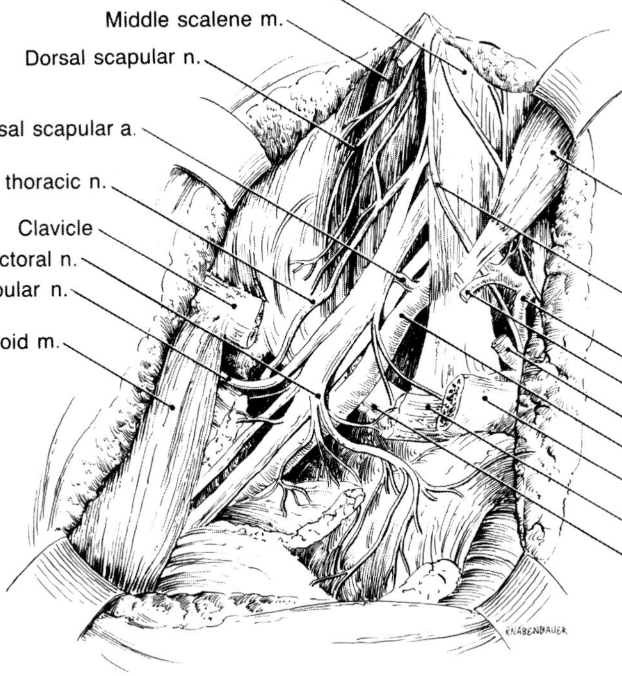

Figure 2–47. The more compressed form of the brachial plexus, found at the time of surgery, and its important anatomical relationships.

indicated by their names: lateral, posterior, and medial. The prevertebral fascia invests the plexus and vessels and forms the axillary sheath. Two other landmark arteries are the transverse cervical artery, which crosses anterior to the level of the upper two trunks,[169] and the suprascapular artery at the level of the middle trunk at the level of the clavicle.[169]

Terminal Branches

The plexus gives off some terminal branches above the clavicle. The dorsal scapular nerve comes off C5, with some C4 fibers, and penetrates the scalenus medius and levator scapulae, sometimes contributing the C4 fibers to the latter.[164] In the remaining cases the nerve to the levator is a separate nerve. It accompanies the deep branch of the transverse cervical artery or the dorsal scapular artery on the undersurface of the rhomboids and innervates them.

Rootlets come off the nerves C5, C6, and C7 immediately adjacent to the intervertebral foramina and contribute to the formation of the long thoracic nerve, which immediately passes between the middle and posterior scalene[151] or penetrates the middle scalene.[165, 169, 173] Horwitz and Tocantins report the nerve forming after the rootlets exit the muscle, with the C7 contribution not passing through muscle. They also mention that the nerve becomes more tightly fixed to muscle by branches near the distal end of the nerve.[165] This nerve may not receive a contribution from C7, but its composition is fairly regular.[165] The nerve passes behind the plexus over the prominence caused by the second rib.[180] It is felt that this nerve may be stretched by depression of the shoulder with lateral flexion of the neck in the opposite direction. Prescott and Zollinger reported two cases of injury with abduction; there may be several mechanisms of injury.[180]

The next most proximal nerve is the suprascapular nerve. It arises from the superior lateral aspect of the upper trunk shortly after its formation at Erb's point. It follows a long oblique course to its next fixed point, the suprascapular notch. This course is parallel to the inferior belly of the omohyoid. The nerve does not move relative to the notch.[182, 183, 194] The nerve passes below the transverse scapular or suprascapular ligament and enters the supraspinatus muscle, which it innervates through two branches. Both the origin off the superior trunk and the muscle attachments lie cephalad to the ligament, causing the nerve to angle around the ligament.[183] It also innervates the infraspinatus muscle through two branches after passing inferiorly around the base of the spine of the scapula.[154] The nerve also provides two articular branches: one in the supraspinatus fossa to the acromioclavicular and superior glenohumeral joints and one in the infraspinatus fossa to the posterior superior glenohumeral joint.[159] It is accompanied by the suprascapular artery which passes over the transverse scapular ligament. The surrounding bone and ligament form a foramen which may entrap the nerve. Paralysis of the nerve has profound effects on shoulder function.[188]

The small nerve to the subclavius also comes off the superior trunk. Kopell and Thompson point out an interesting relationship of this nerve. Protraction of the scapula increases the distance between the C-spine and the notch, as the scapula must move laterally around the thorax to move forward.[168] This location also predisposes the nerve to injury in scapular fractures.[156]

The lateral cord generally contains fibers of C5, C6, and C7 and gives off three terminal branches: the musculocutaneous, the lateral pectoral, and the lateral root of the median nerve. The first branch coming off the lateral cord is the lateral anterior thoracic or lateral pectoral nerve (C5–C7), which, after leaving the lateral cord, passes anterior to the first part of the axillary artery. It penetrates the clavipectoral fascia above the pectoralis minor and innervates the clavicular portion and some of the sternal portion of the pectoralis major muscle. This nerve is 4 to 6 cm in length.[162] The nerve also sends a communication to the medial pectoral nerve which carries its contribution to the remaining portion of the pectoralis major. This loop usually passes over the axillary artery just proximal to the thoracoacromial trunk.[221] Miller,[179] however, shows the artery to be more proximal. The lateral pectoral nerve also innervates the acromioclavicular joint with the suprascapular nerve.[159]

The next nerve to take origin is the musculocutaneous nerve (C5–C7) (Fig. 2–48). It takes an oblique course to where it enters the coracobrachialis, about 5 to 6 cm from the tip of the coracoid with a range of 1.5 to 9.0 cm.[149, 158, 166, 171] It originates high in the axilla. This entry point is critical because of the number of procedures that may put traction on the nerve. Kerr found nerve branches from the lateral cord or musculocutaneous nerve in slightly more than half of his specimens.[167] Flatow, Bigliani, and April specifically sought out these branches and found that they entered the muscle about 3 cm from the tip of the coracoid and were always present. One or more nerves entering the muscle in the proximal 5 cm were found in 74 per cent of shoulders.[158] The musculocutaneous nerve appears distally in the forearm as the lateral antebrachial cutaneous nerve.

The final lateral cord nerve is the lateral root (C5–C7) to the median nerve. The median nerve is formed anterior to the third portion of the axillary artery and accompanies the brachial artery and vein into the arm.

The posterior cord supplies most innervation to the muscles of the shoulder in this order: upper subscapular, thoracodorsal, lower subscapular, axillary, and radial. Because of the great range of motion of the muscles relative to the brachial plexus, nerves to the muscles in the shoulder tend to be quite long and come off quite high in relation to their destination. For this reason, and because nerves tend to segregate in neural tissue into groups of fascicles,[200] several authors report that the posterior cord is poorly formed and may be a discrete structure in only 25 per cent of cadavers.[151, 167, 199] The upper subscapular nerve (C5) takes origin off the posterior cord, entering the subscapularis muscle quite high as there is less relative motion here. It is the shortest of the nerves taking origin from this cord. It supplies two-thirds to four-fifths of the upper portion of the subscapular muscle.

The next distal nerve, the thoracodorsal nerve (C7 and C8), is the longest (12 to 18 cm)[162] of the terminal nerves coming off the brachial plexus in the axilla and is referred to as the long subscapular nerve. It is also sometimes called the long thoracic or nerve of Bell. The nerve follows the subscapular and then the thoracodorsal artery along the posterior wall of the axilla to the latissimus dorsi.[41, 167, 169] In the latissimus dorsi

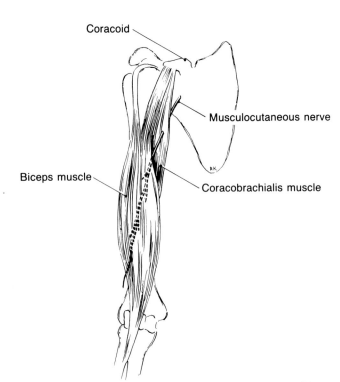

Figure 2–48. The course of the musculocutaneous nerve. This nerve originates from the lateral cord and penetrates the conjoint muscle-tendon on its deep surface. The point of penetration varies; it may be as close to the coracoid tip as 1.5 cm or as far away as 9 cm (the average is 5 cm). The nerve continues distally, innervating the long head of the biceps brachii and the brachialis muscle, and appears in the forearm as the lateral antebrachial cutaneous nerve.

muscle the nerve splits into two branches, as does the blood supply.[88]

The next branch is the lower subscapular nerve (C5 and C6) which follows a long course from its origin to entering the muscles. It innervates the lower portion of the subscapularis muscle and the teres major.

The last branch coming off the posterior cord in the shoulder area is the axillary nerve (C5 and C6) which, as it disappears into the gap between the subscapularis and teres major, is accompanied by the posterior circumflex humeral artery. They then pass lateral to the long head of the triceps and are in intimate contact with the capsule.[172] The quadrilateral shape of this space cannot be visualized from the front and, when viewed from behind, is formed by the teres minor superiorly and the teres major inferiorly (Fig. 2–49; see also Fig. 2–41). The medial border is the long head of the triceps, and the lateral border is the shaft of the humerus. It is in this space that nerve entrapment has been described.[153]

The axillary nerve divides in the space, sending a posterior branch to teres minor and the other to the posterior one-third of the deltoid. The lateral brachial cutaneous nerve, which arises with the teres minor branch, supplies the area of skin corresponding in shape and overlying the deltoid muscle, after wrapping around the posterior border of the deltoid.[86] The anterior branch comes to lie approximately 2 inches below the edge of the acromion as the nerve passes anteriorly to innervate the anterior two-thirds of the muscle. One or more small branches attach to the lower border of the posterior deltoid muscle and, unlike the anterior branch, do not proceed vertically toward the spine of the scapula but follow the inferior fibers of the muscle. The axillary nerve also supplies sensory innervation to the lower portion of the gleno-humeral joint through two articular branches. The anterior articular branch comes off before the nerve enters the quadrilateral space. The second branch comes off in the space. Together they are the major nerve supply of the joint.[159] Frequently, another branch accompanies part of the anterior humeral circumflex artery in the long head of the biceps.

The final continuation of the posterior cord is the radial nerve (C5–C8) which continues posterior to the axillary artery and, shortly after exiting the axilla, disappears into the space deep to the long head of the triceps. The nerves to the long and medial head of the triceps arise where the nerve is still in the axilla. The posterior cutaneous branch also arises in the axilla. A branch that comes off medially, referred to as the ulnar collateral nerve because of its proximity to the ulnar nerve, innervates the medial head of the triceps.

The medial cord has five branches in the following order: the medial pectoral nerve, medial brachial cutaneous, medial antebrachial cutaneous, medial root of the median nerve, and the ulnar nerve. The medial pectoral nerve (C8, T1) comes off the medial cord, which at this point has finally attained its position medial to the artery. Anteriorly, it passes between the artery and vein (the vein is the more medial structure) and enters the deep surface of the pectoralis minor. Some fibers come out anteriorly to the muscle to supply the more caudal portions of the pectoralis major. The nerve varies from 8 to 14 cm in length.[162] As mentioned above, there is a communicating branch from the

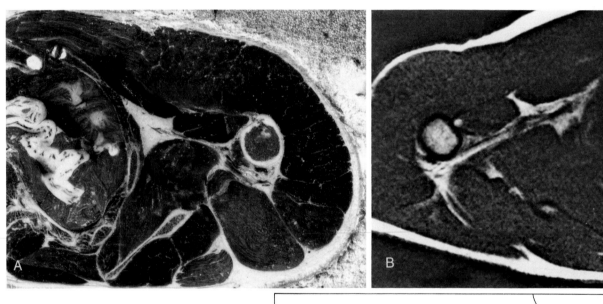
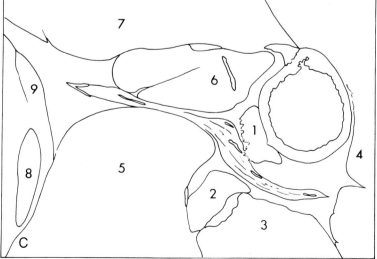

Figure 2–49. *A,* A cross-section of a right shoulder showing the quadrilateral space with the nerve and artery coming from the axillary space, passing between the conjoint and subscapularis muscles and then between the triceps and the humerus. Note how small the quadrilateral space is in comparison with the usual representations. *B,* A left shoulder MRI axial cut showing the quadrilateral space. *C,* A diagram labeling the structures shown in *A:* (1) teres major, (2) teres minor, (3) triceps long head, (4) deltoid, (5) infraspinatus, (6) coracobrachialis and short head of biceps, (7) pectoralis major and minor, (8) rib 3, and (9) serratus anterior.

lateral pectoral nerve which joins the medial pectoral before it enters the pectoralis minor muscle.

The medial brachial cutaneous contains fibers from T1 and is followed in order by the medial antebrachial cutaneous from T1 and C8. Both are cutaneous nerves that supply the area of skin indicated by their names. The medial brachial cutaneous often receives a communication from the intercostal brachial nerve. The medial root of the median nerve (C8 and T1) passes in front of the third portion of the axillary artery to join the lateral root.

The ulnar nerve is the terminal extension of the medial cord. We would expect it to have fibers of C8 and T1 alone, but researchers have found that 50 per cent of specimens have a contribution carrying fibers of C7 from the lateral cord to the ulnar nerve, usually via a nerve off of the median nerve.[151, 167, 171] The C7 fiber usually is destined for the flexor carpi ulnaris.[169] The ulnar nerve has no important branches in the shoulder area; its first branches appear as it approaches the elbow.

Like all nerves the brachial plexus receives its blood supply from adjacent arteries. Because there is little motion relative to the vessels, the arteries are short and direct. Blood supply to the brachial plexus proximally was mapped out by Abdullah and coworkers and found to originate from the subclavian artery and its branches[148] (Fig. 2–50). The vertebral artery supplies the proximal plexus along with the ascending and deep cervical arteries and the superior intercostal artery. The autonomic ganglia lying anterior near the spinal column are supplied by branches of the intercostal vessels in the thorax and branches of the vertebral artery in the cervical area. Distally, there are contributions from adjacent arteries. The relationship between the plexus and vessels is abnormal in 8 per cent of shoulders[179] (see Chapter 3) with nerves penetrated by vessels.

Autonomic Supply

All nerves of the brachial plexus carry postganglionic autonomic fibers with the largest portion (27 to 44 per cent) at C8 and the smallest portion (1 to 9 per cent) at C5.[191] A review of the common structure of the sympathetic nervous system indicates that the fibers coming from the spinal cord are myelinated and are collected in what is called the "white" rami communicantes, or Type I ramus. Fibers that leave the ganglion, the postganglionic fibers, are not myelinated and tend to be collected in the "gray" ramus. Type IIB rami are gray rami with few myelinated (preganglionic) fibers. Type III rami are mixtures of gray and white fibers. Gray or white rami may also be multiple.[190] The sympathetic supply to C5 and C6 comes through the gray rami from the middle cervical ganglion, the superior cervical ganglion, and the intervening trunks connecting these ganglia. There is a sympathetic plexus on the vertebral artery. Gray rami from the stellate ganglion are received by C7, C8, and T1. As mentioned above, the autonomic fibers mix immediately with the somatic fibers and do not travel in separate fasciculi.[190] They enter either at the convergence of the roots or proximal to them. Determination of whether a lesion is pre- or postganglionic is useful in localizing damage to the brachial plexus. The T2 nerve root is often cited as the cephalad limit of preganglionic fibers of the sympathetic nervous system, but there is indication that it may arise as high as T1[181] or C8.[190] The caudad limit of preganglionic fibers is T8 or T9.[181] The distribution of sympathetic fibers to vessels is much more prevalent in the hand than in the shoulder. The distri-

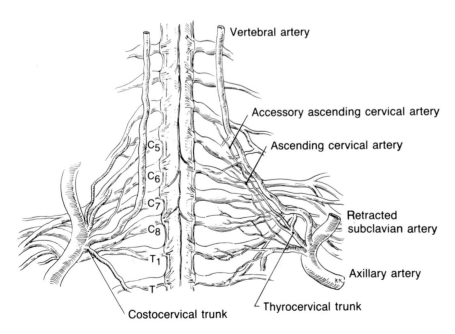

Figure 2–50. The blood supply of the proximal brachial plexus and the spinal cord. In the more distal brachial plexus, the blood supply originates from accompanying arteries and veins. (Redrawn from Abdullah S, and Bowden REM: The blood supply of the brachial plexus. Proc R Soc Med 53:203–205, 1960.)

bution of sweat and erector pili function is probably different but is still decreased in the C5 and C6 areas.[201]

Nonpathological Variants

Although most plexi basically follow the classic formation, they often differ in some small detail. For example, the axon that supplies sensation to an area of skin or stimulus to a particular muscle may take an alternate route from the spinal cord to its destination. There is no physiological means of determining this variant. Such variants are changes in three-dimensional arrangements, not in the physiology of the brachial plexus. Because it is unlikely that a physiological test will be developed to determine their existence, preoperative evaluation of these anomalies must await further refinement in imaging techniques[60] (Fig. 2–51). On computerized tomography the nerves and vessels appear as one single structure. Magnetic resonance imaging is capable of generating a much more "brachial plexus-like" picture but still not sufficient detail.

Awareness of possible plexus variants is important for several reasons. The existence of a structural anomaly may hinder diagnostic evaluation of pathological processes or complicate dissection when one attempts to find or avoid branches of the brachial plexus. An example where accurate diagnosis is confusing occurs with a prefixed brachial plexus. The myelogram or computerized tomography scan may reveal an avulsed nerve root at a level one spinal nerve higher than that indicated by physical examination. It is helpful for the diagnostician to know that this is a frequent anomaly and that the myelogram finding is not inconsistent with his or her physical examination. A prodigious number of patterns have been documented in the published series of brachial plexus dissections. To simplify matters we have grouped the more common variants together for ease in understanding anomalies.

The existence of anomalies is understandable when one considers the embryology of the limb. In the fourth week of fetal development the limb develops adjacent to the level where the relative cervical vertebrae (C5–T1) will appear. The nerves have reached the base of the limb which is now only condensed connective tissue. By the end of the fifth week, the nerves have reached the hand, but there is no muscle differentiation. As the limb migrates caudally, the muscles develop and migrate, taking their nerves with them.[170] This muscle differentiation precedes the growth of vessels whose interposition may also affect the internal arrangement of the plexus.[179] The finding of alternate routes for functioning axons is not unexpected. As they develop they tend to reach their destination before much of the intervening connective tissues mature. Walsh went so far as to state there was only one plexus arrangement and that the variants were connective tissue artifacts.[199]

Returning to our example, the prefixed brachial plexus is the most commonly cited example of what we will call a proximal take off. In this pattern, a nerve, or nerves, leave the parent neural structure more cephalad or proximal than usual. Although defined in various ways, each definition indicates that some neural tissue is exiting at a higher intervertebral foramen than is usual for those particular axons. This may not be a strict ratcheting up of the brachial plexus with all axons moving cephalad but may indicate a partial shift relative to the normal. Although authors disagree as to whether this condition actually exists or simply represents an expansion of the plexus in the proximal direction, they do agree that the nerve tissue in the spinal cord maintains the same cephalocaudad relationship from cord to cord. Such agreement helps in evaluating the patient. If there is a tendency for one group of axons to be prefixed, the other axons will be prefixed, or at least not be shifted in the opposite direction.[185]

By studying the amount of neural tissue contained in the spinal nerves which make up the brachial plexus, Slingluff, Terzis, and Edgerton[185] have come up with much more convincing evidence for the type of prefixation where all the axons move together. If confirmed by larger series of the same detailed work, it would add another dimension of predictability to brachial plexus anatomy in several ways. First, a cephalad shift of one group would mean a cephalad shift in all axons. Second (a corollary of the first), this cephalad shift would necessitate certain predictable shifts in the paths which axons would take to their respective end organs. Some of the more important shifts predicted by prefixation are listed here:

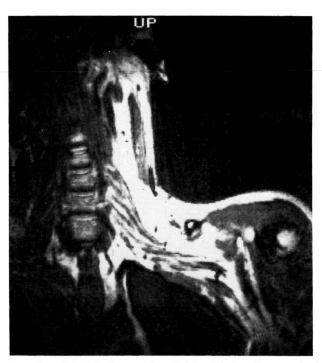

Figure 2–51. An MRI visualization of the author's brachial plexus. The current level of imaging techniques will not yet allow visualization of nonpathological variants. (Reprinted with permission from Kellman GM et al: MR imaging of the supraclavicular region: Normal anatomy. AJR *148*(1):77–82, 1987.)

1. There is less neural tissue in the T spinal nerve.
2. The upper trunk supplies more than half of posterior cord and median nerve.
3. The upper trunk supplies more than one-third of the pectoral nerve supply.
4. There is no C8 contribution to the lateral cord (loop from inferior trunk to lateral cord).
5. The ulnar nerve carries C7 fibers.

The converse would be predicted by post-fixation. That is, T1 and the lower trunk and its contributions are correspondingly larger, and C8 contributes to the lateral cord.

In this study, pre- and postfixation are circumscribed by content of neural tissue as defined by cross-sectional biopsy.

Because a prefixed brachial plexus may lead to diagnostic confusion, it would be helpful to find an alternative to biopsy of the plexus to determine presence of the abnormality. For instance, in shifting the nerves into the higher foramina, some nerve tissue destined for an ulnar nerve distribution may exit by the C7 spinal nerve, and a higher correlation of prefixation with a C7 contribution to the ulnar nerve could be predicted.[169] Such information would be helpful before extensive dissection of the brachial plexus, which requires a search for the small contribution from the lateral cord.

Let us consider the variants that may occur with a single nerve. The fasciculi that form a nerve are grouped together in the source nerve structure (cords for nerves, trunks for divisions, etc.) and frequently depart the source nerve at a more proximal level (Fig. 2–52A,B). For example, the subscapular nerve usually takes origin off the upper trunk but may originate more proximally. This is the peripheral counterpart of the prefixed brachial plexus. The medial pectoral nerve is found to come off the inferior trunk in 24 per cent of specimens, rather than the medial cord. The medial brachial cutaneous comes off the trunk in 10 per cent of cases.

Conversely, *a distal take off* (Fig. 2–52A–C) would not be unexpected. The most frequently cited example is the postfixed brachial plexus which, regardless of how it is defined, is relatively uncommon compared with the prefixed plexus. It is often found when the first thoracic rib is rudimentary.[41] Another common distal take off is the suprascapular nerve, which, in 20 per cent of cadavers, took off from the anterior division rather than the superior trunk itself.

In some cases fasciculi may leave the parent nerve prior to being joined together, resulting in a *multiple origin* (Fig. 2–52A,D) of a nerve from its parent nerve. The most common example is the lateral pectoral nerve which shows a multiple origin in 76 per cent of the specimens examined by Kerr.[167] Conversely, there also can be *substitutions* or a *common origin* (Fig. 2–52A,E). In 55 per cent of specimens no lower subscapular nerve was found, and its function was assumed by a small branch off the axillary nerve. Also, the thoracodorsal nerve was a smaller branch off the axillary or radial nerve in 11 per cent of specimens.

The brachial and antebrachial cutaneous nerves originated as a single nerve and split later in their course in 27 per cent of specimens.[167]

Another variant is *duplication of the nerve* (Fig. 2–52A,F) where axons may travel in separate nerves to a common destination. The most common example is when at least one other nerve from the lateral cord to the coracobrachialis is found in addition to the musculocutaneous, as occurs in 56 per cent of the cadavers.

Last, there are *loops* and *collaterals* (Fig. 2–52A,G). These anomalies are more complex in that the nerves involved may not have the same parent nerve. An example is the loop from the lateral pectoral nerve to the medial pectoral nerve. This is so common as to be the rule rather than the exception. The important large loops are the contribution from the lateral cord to the ulnar nerve, which Kerr found in 60 per cent of specimens, and an additional root to the median nerve coming off the musculocutaneous nerve, which occurred in 24 per cent of specimens.[167] In the latter report, there was a relative decrease in the size of the original lateral root to the median nerve, which helps indicate the existence of a musculocutaneous contribution. Slingluff and associates found a C8 contribution to the lateral cord in 14 to 29 per cent of their specimens.[185] In 60 per cent of cadavers the medial brachial cutaneous nerve and the intercostal brachial nerve formed a common nerve, and in 20 per cent of specimens, a radial nerve was formed from two roots.[167]

An interesting source of loops occurs because of an abnormal relationship with the axillary vessels and their branches. An abnormal relationship was found by Miller[179] between the nerves and arteries in 5 per cent of dissections and nerves and veins in 4 per cent.[179] One of the more common anomalies was the presence of a vessel that is splitting or diverting axons that should belong to a single structure; this occurred with the nerve cord levels.[179] Some of these altered relationships may produce pathology (see Chapter 3). Another, rarer source of plexus anomalies is an aberrant accessory muscle which entraps a portion of the plexus.[152, 158]

In summary, the majority of anomalies are understandable as alternate routes for axons to reach their normal destination, created by variations in formation of the intervening connective tissue. There are unexpected anomalies such as a single cord plexus[163] or a complete absence of C8 and T1[198] contributions to the plexus, but these are extremely rare. Even these less common anomalies would be considered normal until encountered at surgery because they do not affect physiology. Because they cannot be predicted preoperatively, awareness of the possible existence of these nonpathological variants ought to aid dissection and facilitate diagnosis.

CRANIAL NERVE XI

The spinal accessory nerve, or 11th cranial nerve, originates from the medulla and upper spinal cord through multiple rootlets. It then ascends back through the foramen magnum and exits in the middle compartment of the jugular foramen. The nerve descends between the internal jugular vein and the internal carotid artery for a short distance and then descends

laterally as it passes posteriorly, supplying the sternocleidomastoid muscle. After exiting the sternocleidomastoid, it continues in an inferior posterior direction across the posterior triangle of the neck and then supplies the trapezius muscle. In the posterior triangle

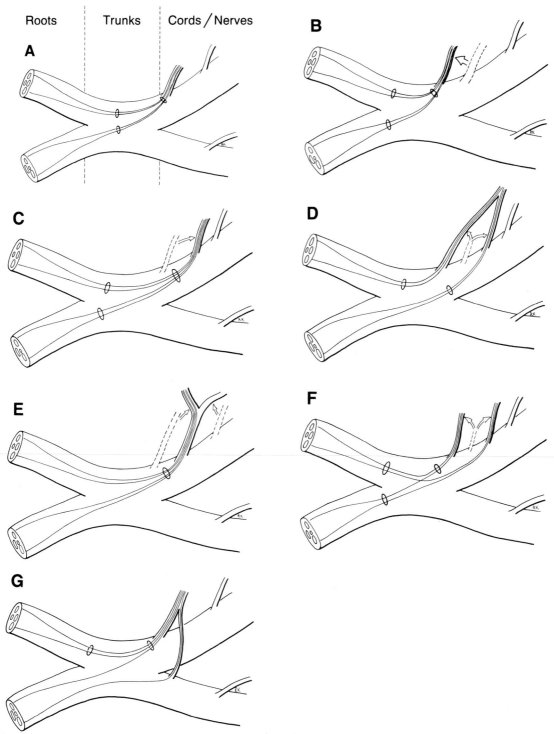

Figure 2–52. *A,* A fictitious nerve in its usual relationship to its parent structures and other nerves. The thin black lines represent axons that are normally distributed via this nerve. *B,* The circles represent fascicles, with the axons coalescing into a nerve at the more proximal level so that the nerve takes origin from the trunk. *C,* The axons leave this nerve more distally. *D,* The axons in their fascicles depart the parent nerve before joining together to form the nerve, resulting in a multiple origin. *E,* The axons of this nerve leave together with the neural material of an adjacent nerve, resulting in a common origin. Where the common origin involves two nerves of greatly different sizes, the smaller nerve may be referred to as absent and its function assumed by a branch of the larger nerve. *F,* The neural material leaves via two separate nerves, which remain separate all the way to the distal structure. This is referred to as a duplication of the nerve. *G,* Some of the neural material travels to the nerve via a small origin off different parent nerve structures, resulting in the creation of a loop.

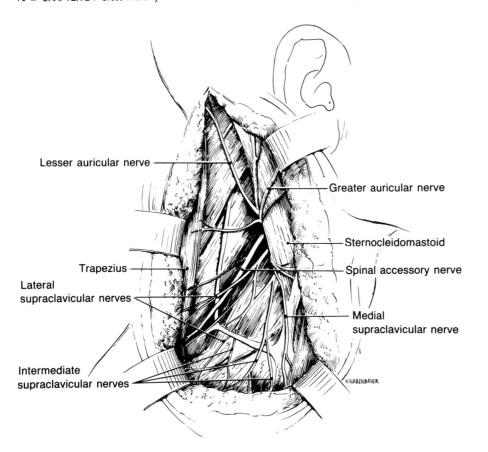

Lesser auricular nerve

Greater auricular nerve

Sternocleidomastoid

Spinal accessory nerve

Trapezius

Lateral supraclavicular nerves

Medial supraclavicular nerve

Intermediate supraclavicular nerves

K.NABENBAUER

Figure 2–53. The spinal accessory nerve and the supraclavicular nerves. The supraclavicular nerves in their three groups account for much of the cutaneous innervation of the shoulder. In the posterior triangle the spinal accessory runs from the sternocleidomastoid to the trapezius, the two superficial muscles of the neck. The spinal accessory nerve lies adjacent to the most superficial layer of deep fascia in the neck.

(Fig. 2–53), it receives afferent fibers from C2, C3, and sometimes C4.[155] Some upper fibers distribute to the sternocleidomastoid and the lower fibers to the trapezius. Because it lies so superficial in the posterior triangle, the nerve is at maximum risk for injury.

INTERCOSTAL BRACHIAL NERVE

The intercostal brachial nerve is a cutaneous branch of T2. It leaves the thorax from the second intercostal space and crosses over the dome of the axillary fossa. It sends a communication to the medial brachial cutaneous nerve (60 per cent)[167] and may supply sensation on the medial side of the arm as far as the elbow.[150, 235] Like many of the cutaneous nerves of the upper arm, it is outside the axillary sheath[150] and not anesthetized by axillary sheath injection.

SUPRACLAVICULAR NERVES

The supraclavicular nerves (see Fig. 2–53) originate from the spinal nerves C3 and C4. They are important to the shoulder surgeon because they supply sensation to the shoulder in that area described by their name, the area above the clavicle, in addition to the first two intercostal spaces anteriorly. The ventral rami of C3 to C4 emerge between the longi (colli and capitis) and scalenus medius.[42] The contributions to the supracla-

vicular nerves join and enter the posterior triangle of the neck around the posterior border of the sternocleidomastoid. They descend on the superficial surface of platysma in three groups. The medial supraclavicular nerves go to the base of the neck and the medial portion of the first two intercostal spaces. The intermediate suprascapular nerves go to the middle of the base of the posterior cervical triangle and the upper thorax in this area. The lateral suprascapular nerves cross the anterior border of the trapezius muscle and go to the tip of the shoulder.[42] The medial nerves may have an anomalous pattern where they pass through foramina in the clavicle on their way to the anterior chest.[161]

Blood Vessels

The surgeon's interest in the anatomy of blood vessels focuses on treatment of blood vessel injury and avoiding injury to these structures in the course of dissection. The main focus in the shoulder area is the axillary artery and its accompanying veins and lymphatics. These structures are more variable in their formation than the brachial plexus, but the order to their formation and arrangement makes them easier to understand. Nonpathological anomalies are more common here than in the brachial plexus. Again, nonpathological anomalies are those arrangements that have

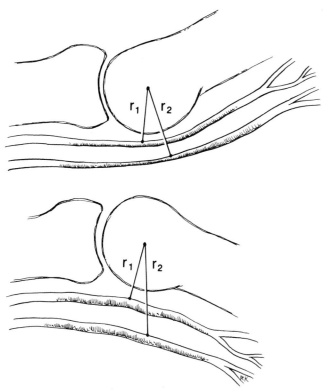

Figure 2–54. The strain on a vessel in movement is proportional to its distance from the center of rotation.

no physiological significance but are important to the surgeon because their presence may change the diagnostic picture after an injury. Also, they may affect the collateral circulation pattern or complicate a dissection by altering the position of arteries in relation to bone and tendon landmarks (see section on Nerves).

Taylor and Palmer,[230] in their extensive studies of circulation of the skin and literature review, have noted basic tendencies in the distribution of blood vessels throughout the body. They summarized these tendencies in a set of rules: (1) the blood supply of the body courses within or adjacent to a connective tissue framework, whether bone, septa, or fascia; (2) vessels course from fixed loci to mobile areas; (3) the vascular outflow is a continuous system of arteries linked predominantly by reduced caliber vessels referred to as choke arteries and arterioles; (4) because the vascular trees are linked, rather than overlapping, the body is a three-dimensional jigsaw made up of composite blocks of tissues, each of which has a main arterial supply.[230] I would add here the tendency for vessels to cross joints close to the axis of rotation so that there is less relative change in length (Fig. 2–54). This occurs particularly at the very mobile shoulder. The arteries supplying these blocks of tissue are also responsible for supplying skin and underlying tissue. These blocks and overlying skin are termed angiosomes in reference to the dominant arterial axes. A fifth tendency reiterated by Taylor and Palmer was an inverse reciprocal relationship between the size of vessels in neighboring contiguous regions, referred to as the law of equilibrium.[230]

Elaborating on these themes, they pointed out that vessels rarely cross planes where there is a great deal of movement. Their illustrations showed that when vessels do cross these planes, they have a tendency to cross at the periphery of motion planes or at the ends of muscles where there is less relative motion.[230] Also, in those cases where the vessel must cross an area of high mobility, it does so in an oblique fashion (Fig. 2–55). Such an oblique crossing is desirable because the strain (strain being the deformation expressed as a percentage of the length of the artery being performed) is greatly reduced, and yet the absolute motion between the two sides of the plane does not change.

The axillary artery and its branches may seem to be an exception to such tendencies. It comes from a fixed position adjacent to the first rib and proceeds through a very mobile area, within the axilla. It returns to another connective tissue framework adjacent to the humerus, where it becomes the brachial artery continuing into the arm. This apparent exception comes about only because of the highly mobile nature of the shoulder. I think of the axillary artery as fixed in a connective tissue structure, the axillary sheath, which has some highly mobile adjacent tissue planes—particularly so in relation to the anterior and posterior walls of the axilla. Given this relationship and the tendencies and formation of the vascular system noted above, it is predicted and found that the branches off the axillary artery going to the shoulder structures come off more proximal than they would if they followed a direct course to their destination. They tend to be long and oblique in the course of their entrance into the muscles and lie outside the axillary sheath. In addition, because structures in the shoulder move relative to each other, one would predict a number of hypovascular fascial planes.[217, 230] These planes are crossed at the periphery by a few large named vessels, rather than directly by a large number of small vessels. These hypovascular planes are frequently found between the pectoralis major and pectoralis minor, between the trapezius and rhomboids, and on the deep surface of the rhomboids (see section on Bursae, Compartments, and Potential Spaces). Taylor and Palmer mention five angiosomes of the shoulder that have a cutaneous representation: the transverse cervical artery, the thoracoacromial artery, the suprascapular artery, the posterior humeral circumflex artery, and the circumflex scapular artery.[230]

The arteries and veins are hollow structures with abundant collagen, some elastin, and layers that contain some smooth muscle. They are under the control of the autonomic nervous system. Woollard found that the distribution of sympathetic nerves to vessels appears to be more abundant in the more distal part of the limb than the proximal.[201] Also, larger arteries and veins have their own blood supply from the base of the vasa vasorum.[41]

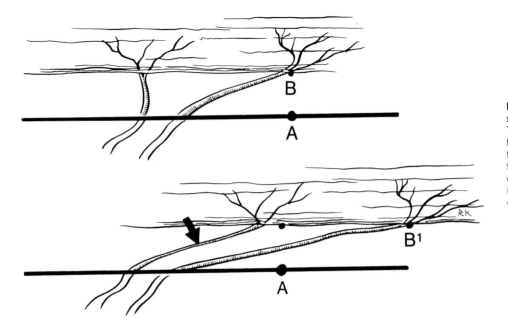

Figure 2–55. The oblique course of vessels crossing a motion plane is protective. The vessel that crosses straight across the motion plane is stretched and possibly torn *(arrow)* with the motion that is illustrated, whereas the vessel crossing obliquely has less relative stretch. Crossing at the edge of the plane of motion decreases strain even further.

ARTERIES

The arteries (Fig. 2–56) tend to be named by the watershed of the artery rather than by the main structure that comes off the axillary or subclavian artery.[231] For example, when the blood supply to the lateral wall of the axillary fossa comes from the pectoral branch of the thoracoacromial artery, it is said that the lateral thoracic artery takes origin from the pectoral artery, rather than that the lateral thoracic artery is supplanted by the pectoral artery. Huelke has reported a fairly high occurrence of branches of the axillary artery coming off in common trunks that seem to supplant each other. An interesting exception to the naming rule in the area of the subclavian artery is the dorsal scapular artery which, when it takes origin from the thyrocervical trunk, is named the deep transverse cervical artery, although Huelke has tried to correct this.[211] The dorsal scapular artery is the preferred name.

Subclavian Artery

Blood supply to the limb begins with the subclavian artery which ends at the lateral border of the first rib. It is divided into three portions in relation to the insertion of the scalenus anterior muscle. The vertebral artery takes origin in the first portion, and the costocervical trunk and thyrocervical trunk take origin in the second portion. There are usually no branches in the third portion of the artery. The artery is fairly well protected by the presence of surrounding structures. Rich and Spencer,[225] in their review of the world's literature on vascular injuries, found no large series in which the subclavian artery made up more than 1 per cent of total arterial injuries. Because they are protected, injuries affecting these arteries signify more serious trauma than injuries to other arteries remote to the great vessels.

Vertebral and Thyrocervical Trunk

The first important branch of the subclavian artery, rarely encountered by shoulder surgeons, is the vertebral artery, which supplies the proximal blood supply to the brachial plexus. The internal mammary artery is always a branch of the first.[230] Two vessels encountered more frequently by shoulder surgeons are the transverse cervical artery and the suprascapular artery which come off the thyrocervical trunk in 70 per cent of dissections.[220] In the remaining cases they may come off directly, or in common, from the subclavian artery. The transverse cervical artery divides into a superficial branch that supplies the trapezius and the deep branch (when present) that supplies the rhomboids. The suprascapular artery is somewhat more inferior and traverses the soft tissues to enter the supraspinatus muscle just superior to the transverse scapular ligament and the suprascapular nerve.

Transverse Cervical and Suprascapular

The superior of the two arteries, the transverse cervical, lies anterior to the upper and middle trunks of the brachial plexus, while the suprascapular artery lies anterior to the middle trunk just above the level of the clavicle.[169] There is a relatively high variability in the origin of these branch arteries, but the subclavian arteries themselves are rarely anomalous. The textbook arrangement is present in only 46 per cent or less of dissections.[211, 219]

Dorsal Scapular

The dorsal scapular artery is the normal artery to the rhomboids and usually comes off the subclavian but may come off the transverse cervical artery.[42, 225] Branches off the first portion of the subclavian artery, the portion between its origin and the medial border

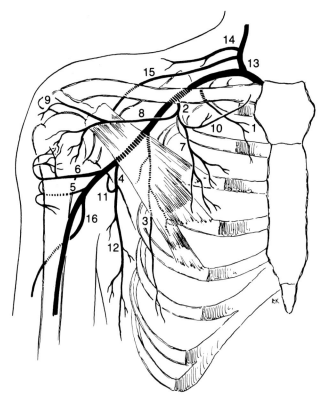

Figure 2–56. The major arterial axes of the upper limb. The major arterial axis bears three different names in its course. Medial to the lateral edge of the first rib, it is called the subclavian artery. From the lateral edge of the first rib just proximal to the take-off of the profunda brachii artery, it is termed the axillary artery, and distal to that it is known as the brachial artery. The axillary artery is divided into three portions—superior to the pectoralis minor muscle (as shown), deep to the muscle, and distal to the muscle. This drawing shows the thoracoacromial axis (2) coming off in the first part of the artery. This is a very common variation. The thoracoacromial axis usually comes off deep to the pectoralis minor. The other variant is the clavicular branch (10), shown as a branch of the pectoral artery. Most commonly it comes off the thoracoacromial axis as a trifurcation, but it may arise from any of the branches of the thoracoacromial axis or from the axillary artery itself. Note that most of the branches of the artery are deep to the pectoralis minor and its superior continuation, the clavipectoral fascia, with the exception of the thoracoacromial axis and its branches, which lie anterior to the clavipectoral fascia. The labeled branches are as follows: (1) superior thoracic artery, (2) thoracoacromial artery, (3) lateral thoracic artery, (4) subscapular artery, (5) posterior humeral circumflex artery, (6) anterior humeral circumflex artery, (7) pectoral artery, (8) deltoid artery, (9) acromial artery, (10) clavicular artery, (11) circumflex scapular artery, (12) thoracodorsal artery, (13) thyrocervical trunk, (14) transverse cervical artery, (15) suprascapular artery, and (16) profunda brachii artery.

of the scalenus anterior muscle, are the vertebral artery, the internal mammary artery, and the thyrocervical trunk. The second portion gives rise to the costocervical trunk.[225] A common anomaly that occurs in 30 per cent of individuals is where the transverse cervical artery, the suprascapular artery, or both, take origin from the subclavian artery rather than the thyrocervical trunk.[220] In the majority of cases, one of these arteries will travel between trunks of the brachial plexus to its destination.[211]

Axillary

The axillary artery is the continuation of the subclavian artery. It begins at the lateral border of the first rib and continues to the inferior border of the latissimus dorsi at which point it becomes the brachial artery. This artery is traditionally divided into three portions. The first is above the superior border of the pectoralis minor, the second is deep to pectoralis minor, and the third portion is distal to the lateral border of pectoralis minor. The usual number of branches for each of the three sections corresponds to the name of the section. There is one branch in the first section, two in the second, and three in the third.

First Portion

The first section gives off only the superior thoracic artery which supplies vessels to the first, second, and sometimes the third intercostal spaces.

Second Portion

The first branch given off in the second portion of the artery is the thoracoacromial artery, one of the suppliers of a major angiosome, as defined by Taylor and Palmer.[230] The artery has two very large branches, the deltoid and the pectoral, and two smaller branches, the acromial and clavicular. The acromial branch regularly comes off the deltoid, while the clavicular branch has a much more variable origin coming off any of the other branches, the trunk, or the axial artery (Reid and Taylor).[221] The *thoracoacromial artery* pierces the clavipectoral fascia and gives off its four branches.[41] The *pectoral branch* travels in the space between the pectoralis minor and pectoralis major. In their injections series, Reid and Taylor reported that the pectoral artery supplied the sternocostal portion of the pectoralis major muscles in every case. They found no arterial supply from the pectoral to the pectoralis minor in 46 per cent of dissections and found that the pectoralis minor received a contribution from the pectoral artery in only 14 per cent of dissections. In 34 per cent of dissections it appeared that the pectoralis minor received a direct supply from the thoracoacromial trunk.[221]

Arterial supply to the pectoralis major coincided closely with the unique nerve supply of the pectoralis minor, with the deltoid artery supplying the clavicular head and the pectoral artery the sternocostal portion.[221] The authors also found that the plane between the pectoralis major and minor was relatively avascular and that there was a rich layer of anastomoses, with the lateral thoracic artery at the lateral edges of the pectoralis major origin. Where the pectoralis major was attached over the fourth and fifth ribs an anastomotic connection around the fourth rib area was noted. The pectoral branch also supplied most of the skin anterior to the pectoralis major through vessels that came around the lateral edge of the pectoralis major.[221]

The *deltoid artery* is directed laterally and supplies the clavicular head of pectoralis major and much of the anterior deltoid. It also supplies an area of skin over the deltopectoral groove through vessels that emerge from the deltopectoral groove, including usually one large fasciocutaneous, or musculocutaneous, perforator.

The *acromial artery* is usually a branch of the deltoid artery which proceeds up to the acromioclavicular joint. The acromial artery has an anastomotic network with other portions of the deltoid, the suprascapular, and the posterior humeral circumflex arteries, and frequently has an important cutaneous branch.[221]

The *clavicular artery* often comes off the trunk or the pectoral artery and runs up to the sternoclavicular joint. Reid and Taylor noticed staining of the periosteum in the medial half of the clavicle and the skin in this area.[221] There are also anastomotic connections with the superior thoracic artery, the first perforator of the inferior mammary, and the suprascapular artery.

The second artery that comes off the second portion of the axillary artery is the *lateral thoracic,* the most variable of the arteries in the axilla in terms of origin.[210, 231] In approximately 25 per cent of specimens it takes origin from the subscapular artery.[231] At other times it originates from the pectoral branch of the thoracoacromial artery. The lateral thoracic artery runs deep to the pectoralis minor and supplies blood to the pectoralis minor, serratus anterior, and intercostal spaces 3–5. There is a rich anastomotic pattern with intercostal arteries 2–5, the pectoral artery, and the thoracodorsal branch of the subscapular artery. In some cases the thoracodorsal artery gives origin to the vessels of the lateral thoracic distribution. A variation Huelke found in 86 per cent of cadavers is an upper subscapular artery whose course parallels the upper subscapular nerve.[210] This may prove to be an important artery to subscapularis as there are no important branches off the subscapular artery before the circumflex scapular.[88]

Third Portion

The largest branch of the axillary, the *subscapular,* takes origin in the third part of the axillary artery. This artery runs caudally on the subscapularis muscle, which it reportedly supplies.[41] However, Bartlett found no important branches of the subscapular artery prior to the origin of the *circumflex scapular artery.*[88] It gives off a branch to the posterior portion of the shoulder, the circumflex scapular artery, which passes posteriorly under the inferior edge of the subscapularis and then medial to the long head of the triceps through the triangular space, where it supplies a branch to the inferior angle of the scapula and a branch to the infraspinatus fossa.[240] These two branches anastomose with the suprascapular and the transverse cervical arteries. The circumflex scapular artery has an additional large cutaneous branch which is used in an axial free flap.[240]

The continuation of the subscapular is the *thoracodorsal artery* which runs with the thoracodorsal nerve toward the latissimus dorsi on the subscapularis, teres major, and latissimus dorsi. It also has branches to the lateral thoracic wall.

The *posterior humeral circumflex* comes off poste-

riorly in the third portion and descends into the quadrilateral space with the axillary nerve. After emerging on the posterior side of the shoulder beneath teres minor, the artery divides in a fashion similar to the nerve. The anterior branch travels with the axillary nerve, approximately 2 inches below the level of the acromion, and supplies the anterior two-thirds of the deltoid. It has a small communicating branch over the acromion with the acromial branch of the thoracoacromial axis and has a communicating branch posteriorly with the deltoid branch of the profunda brachii. It also has small branches to the glenohumeral joint. This artery supplies an area of skin over the deltoid, particularly the middle third of that muscle, through connecting vessels that travel directly to the overlying skin which is firmly attached to the underlying deltoid. The posterior branch corresponds to and follows the posterior axillary nerve.

The next branch is the *anterior humeral circumflex* artery which is smaller than the posterior humeral circumflex. It is an important surgical landmark because it travels laterally at the inferior border of the subscapularis tendon. The artery has anastomoses deep to the deltoid with a posterior humeral circumflex. It supplies some branches to the subscapularis muscle and also has a branch that runs superiorly with the long head of the biceps, supplying some arterial blood to the supraspinatus tendon. The anterior ascending branch supplies most of the humeral head.[49] This branch artery crosses the subscapularis tendon anteriorly, where it is regularly encountered at anterior glenohumeral reconstruction.

Nonpathological Anomalies

The function of arteries, the delivery of blood, relates to the cross-sectional area of the delivering artery rather than the particular route the artery takes, as the arterioles are the resistance vessels.[228] Arteries are even less dependent on a straight line continuity for their function than nerves. Among the vessels, one would expect a higher rate of deviance from the anatomical norm without any physiological consequence than that of nerves, and this turns out to be the case.[178, 231] This is even more understandable when we recall that contiguous watersheds are connected by choke arteries, when the vessels in one area are large and those in the adjacent area are small.[217, 230] The types of arterial anomalies are similar to those of nerves: a change in position of origin of the artery, duplication or reduction in the number of stem arteries, and total absence of the artery with its function taken over by another artery.

The oblique route of the arteries as they course to their destination is necessitated by motion in the shoulder. As one might expect, a proximal displacement of arterial origin is more common than distal displacement. The most common example is proximal displacement of the thoracoacromial axis, found in at least one third of cadavers.[207, 210]

The next most frequently displaced arterial stem is

the subscapular artery which, in 16 to 29 per cent of cases,[210, 219] originates in the second part of the axillary artery.[207] In a small percentage of cases, the superior thoracic artery was moved proximally to take origin off the subscapular artery. Few cases of arteries being moved distally have been reported.

Another frequent variation is an increase or decrease in the number of direct branches from the axillary artery.[207, 210, 219, 231] For example, in addition to the branches discussed above, Huelke described a seventh branch that he found in 86 per cent of his dissections.[210] It is a short, direct branch accompanying the short upper subscapular nerve (and similar in anatomy), suggesting the name of upper subscapular artery.

A change in number occurs when a branch of one of the six named arterial stems coming off the axillary artery takes origin directly from the artery, or when two or more are joined in a common stem. In Huelke's series of dissections he found all seven branches in only 26.7 per cent of the dissections, six branches in 37 per cent, five branches in 16 per cent, and less than five in 11 per cent. De Garis and Swartley report as many as 11 separate branches from the axillary artery.[207] The most frequent common stems are those of the transverse cervical and suprascapular artery in a common stem off the thyrocervical trunk in as many as 28 per cent of cadavers.[220] The next common origin is the posterior humeral circumflex artery with the anterior humeral circumflex (11 per cent) or the subscapular artery (15 per cent). The opposite of consolidation may also occur when major branches of these six or seven name branches take origin directly from the axillary artery. This is seen most often in the thoracoacromial axis where the various branches may come off separately from the axillary artery, although only a small percentage of cases have been reported.

The final nonpathological anomaly is total absence of an artery and its function performed by one of the other branches. The lateral thoracic is most commonly absent, and its function is supplanted by branches off the subscapular, the pectoral branch of the thoracoacromial, or both. This variant has been seen in as many as 25 per cent of specimens.[207, 210, 231]

Collateral Circulation

A number of significant anastomoses contribute to good collateral circulation around the shoulder (Figs. 2–57, 2–58). The subclavian artery communicates with the third portion of the axillary artery through anastomosis with the transverse cervical, dorsal scapular, and suprascapular arteries and the branches of the subscapular artery. Also, there are communications between the posterior humeral circumflex with the anterior circumflex, the deltoid, the suprascapular artery, and the profunda brachii. There may be communications between the thoracoacromial artery and the intercostal arteries, particularly the fourth intercostal.

This abundant collateral circulation is both an asset

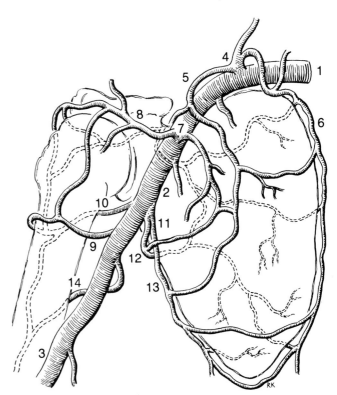

Figure 2–57. A diagram demonstrates the large amount of collateral circulation around the shoulder. Some license has been taken in depicting the dorsal scapular and suprascapular collaterals anterior to the major arterial axis. The labeled arteries are as follows: (1) subclavian, (2) axillary, (3) brachial, (4) thyrocervical trunk, (5) suprascapular, (6) dorsal scapular, (7) thoracoacromial trunk, (8) deltoid, (9) anterior humeral circumflex, (10) posterior humeral circumflex, (11) subscapular, (12) circumflex scapular, (13) thoracodorsal, and (14) profunda brachii. (Redrawn from Rich NM, and Spencer F: Vascular Trauma. Philadelphia: WB Saunders, 1978.)

to tissue viability and a disadvantage to assessment of possible arterial injury. Collateral circulation ameliorates some of the effects of an injury or sudden blockage to the axillary artery. A limb may survive on a flow pressure as low as 20 mm Hg, which would be fatal to the brain or heart.[228] In the Vietnam War, axillary artery injury had the lowest amputation rate of any of the regions of the arterial tree.[222] It may on occasion obscure the diagnosis. While collateral circulation may transmit a pulse wave (13 to 17 meters/second), it may not be sufficient to allow a flow wave (40 to 50 cm/second). This is because flow varies with the fourth power of the radius of the vessels. While the collaterals may have a total cross-sectional area close to that of the axillary artery, the resistance is greatly increased.[218, 228] Also, the same injury that interrupts the flow in the axillary or subclavian artery may injure the collateral circulation.[225]

The seriousness of a missed diagnosis in injury is demonstrated by reports on arterial ligation. Ferguson quotes Bailey as showing a 9 per cent amputation rate for subclavian artery ligation and a 9 per cent amputation rate for ligation of the axillary artery in World War I.[20] More recent battlefield statistics from DeBakey and Simeon[206] in World War II and Rich, Baugh, and Hughes in the Vietnam War reveal a much

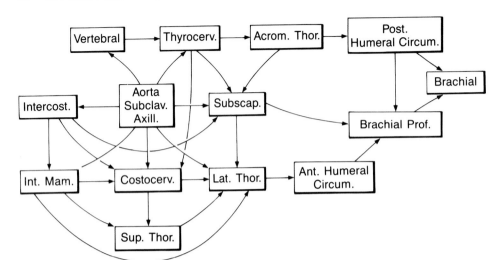

Figure 2–58. A diagram of the collateral circulation. The number of collaterals decreases in those areas where dense collagenous structures must move adjacent to each other (e.g., near the glenohumeral joint). (Adapted from Radke HM: Arterial circulation of the upper extremity. *In* Strandness DE Jr (ed): Collateral Circulation in Clinical Surgery. Philadelphia: WB Saunders, 1969, pp 294–307.)

higher amputation rate:[222] about 28.6 per cent for the subclavian artery injury in Vietnam and 43 per cent in the axillary artery in World War II.[206] An outstanding exception to this dismal report is the treatment of arteriovenous fistula and false aneurysm where ligation has a very low morbidity, perhaps because of enlarged collateral vessels.[224] Interestingly, in the 10 cases of subclavian artery ligation found in the Vietnam War registry, there were no subsequent amputations, compared with an overall rate of 28 per cent with subclavian wounds.[225] Conversely, both of the two axillary artery ligations ended in amputation.[225] Radke points out that collateral vessels are fewer in number where compact and mobile tissues span the joint.[219]

The percentages of amputation reflect the rate of gangrene necessitating amputation following ligation and ignores severe nerve pain syndromes which often occur with inadequate circulation.[225] Rich and Spencer believe that the increased gangrene rates among the military in World War II and Vietnam over World War I reflect the increasing severity of war wounds.[225] In any event, neither the old nor the modern gangrene rate is acceptable. Axillary or subclavian artery injuries need repair if possible, not ligation, and therefore require early diagnosis.[225]

VEINS

Axillary

The axillary vein begins at the inferior border of the latissimus dorsi as the continuation of the basilic vein, continues as the axillary vein to the lateral border of the first rib, and then becomes the subclavian vein.[41] It is a single structure, in contradistinction to many venae comitantes, which are often double. The subcapular vein also is a single vessel.[88] The axillary and subclavian veins usually have only one valve each,[232] whereas the muscle veins have many valves.[145] Each vein lies anterior to its artery and, especially in its proximal portion, medial or inferior to the artery. Most of the venous drainage is to the axillary vein.

Except for branches that accompany the thoracoacromial artery, more than half empty into the cephalic vein rather than continuing all the way to the axillary vein.[221] The relations of the axillary vein are the artery, which tends to be posterior and lateral, and the brachial plexus. The medial pectoral nerve emerges from the brachial plexus between the artery and the vein. The ulnar nerve comes to lie directly behind the vein as it courses down the arm. The upper limb is similar to the lower which uses a muscle pump action to aid venous return. In the upper limb, the deltoid and triceps muscles receive "afferent" veins from adjacent muscle and subcutaneous tissue.[145]

Cephalic

The cephalic vein is a superficial vein in the arm which lies deep to the deep fascia after reaching the deltopectoral groove and finally pierces the clavipectoral fascia, emptying into the axillary vein.[41] The cephalic vein may be absent in 4 per cent of cases. It receives no branches from the pectoralis major muscle in the groove.[221]

The lymph nodes of the axilla lie upon the surface of the venous structures. The axillary vein may often need to be excised to obtain an adequate node dissection. Lymphatic occlusion, rather than removal of the vein, is believed to be the cause of edema in the arm.[204, 213, 215] This might mitigate against venous repair, but Rich reports that disruptions of venous return in the lower extremity result in a higher rate of amputation.[223] Other authors have emphasized the importance of preserving a superficial vein, such as the cephalic vein, in surgery so as to cause less postoperative discomfort.[226]

LYMPHATIC DRAINAGE

Lymph drainage in the extremities is more highly developed superficially, where the lymph channels follow the superficial veins, than in the deep portion of

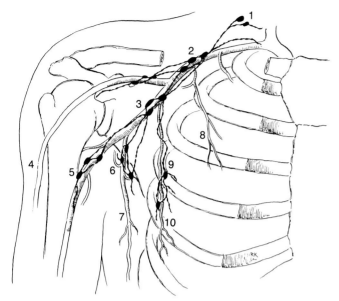

Figure 2–59. A diagram of the location of the groups of lymph glands or nodes in the axilla and some of their major interconnections. The main drainage is into the vein, but there are connections to the deep cervical nodes. Labeled nodes and vessels are as follows: (1) deep cervical, (2) apical, (3) central, (4) cephalic vein, (5) lateral, (6) subscapular, (7) thoracodorsal artery, (8) pectoral artery, (9) pectoral nodes, and (10) lateral thoracic artery.

the limb, where the lymph channels follow the arteries.[41, 42] Lymphatics in the arm generally flow to the axillary nodes (Fig. 2–59). The more radially located lymphatics in the arm may cross to the ulnar side and, hence, to the axilla or may drain consistently with the cephalic vein and deltopectoral node, bypassing the axilla into the cervical nodes.[204]

The lymph nodes are named by the area of the axillary fossa in which they lie rather than by the area to which they drain.[202] The areas they drain are rather constant, and each group of nodes receives 1 to 3 large afferents.[203] They are richly supplied with arterial blood and seem to have a constant relationship to their arteries.[202] Drainage from the breast area and anterior chest wall passes into the *pectoral nodes* (thoracic nodes) which lie on the lateral surface of ribs 2–6, deep to or within the serratus anterior fascia on both sides of the lateral thoracic artery. This group is almost contiguous with the central group. On the posterior wall of the axillary fossa are *subscapular nodes* which lie on the wall of the subscapularis muscle. They are adjacent to the thoracodorsal artery and nerve and drain lymph from this area as well as from the posterior surface of the shoulder, back, and neck. These two groups drain into the central, or largest, nodes and higher nodes. The *central nodes* also receive drainage from the lateral nodes (or brachial nodes) on the medial surface of the great vessels in the axilla and are related to the lateral thoracic and thoracodorsal arteries. All of these nodes drain into the *apical nodes* (subpectoral nodes) which may produce an afferent into the subclavian lymphatic trunk. They then join the thoracic duct on the left side and flow directly into the vein on the right. Some afferents drain into the

deep cervical nodes and have a separate entrance into the venous system through the jugular vein.

RELATIONSHIPS

The axillary artery lies in the axillary space, well cushioned by fat, and is relatively well protected from compression damage. As previously mentioned, relatively few injuries occur to the subclavian artery. It is not usually involved in thoracic outlet syndrome. A case where a normal artery is involved in a compression syndrome is in the quadrilateral space, where the posterior humeral circumflex may become compressed. Although the arteries in the shoulder are arranged around the normal mechanics, one would predict that alterations in joint mechanics might endanger the arteries, but this is not the case. Most indirect artery damage involves cases of diseased arteries, as occurs in glenohumeral dislocation.[209, 212]

Bursae, Compartments, and Potential Spaces

With any study of regional anatomy, structures that allow or restrain the spread of substances into that part of the body are an important concept. The substances may be local anesthetics, edema from trauma, infection, or tumor. The surgeon is allowed to extend his or her surgical exposure or is prevented from doing so by similar spaces and barriers. Sufficiency of the barrier is related to the speed with which the substance can spread. For example, we prefer that local anesthetics act within a few minutes. A fascial barrier that prevents this spread may be insufficient to prevent the propagation of postinjury trauma that proliferates over a period of hours. Similarly, a barrier that can contain edema, thereby causing a compartment syndrome, may be insufficient to act as a compartment barrier against the propagation of a tumor that enlarges over a period of weeks or months. We will first discuss tumor compartments and then move on to those compartments where more rapidly spreading substances are a concern.

TUMOR COMPARTMENTS

Musculoskeletal tumor surgeons have emphasized the concept of an anatomical compartment for several years. They point out that tumors grow centrifugally until they encounter a collagen barrier of fascia, tendon, or bone which limits their growth. Tumors tend to spread more rapidly in the direction in which no anatomical barriers are encountered. Therefore, a compartment is an anatomical space, bounded on all sides by a dense collagen barrier.[236]

Enneking[236] lists four compartments in the shoulder:

the scapula and its muscular envelope, the clavicle, the proximal humerus, and the deltoid. The axillary space is a primary example of a space that is, by definition, extracompartmental. It is bounded by fascia posteriorly, medially, and anteriorly and has bone along its lateral border, but there is no anatomical barrier to the spread of tumor in the proximal or distal direction.

INFECTION

Fortunately, infections in the shoulder area are rare in comparison with the hand. This is probably because there is less exposure to trauma and foreign bodies in the shoulder area. Crandon points out that a potentiating anatomical feature for development of infections in the hands is the closed space, which is infrequent in the shoulder.[233] The shoulder has three diarthrodial joints: the sternoclavicular, the acromioclavicular, and the glenohumeral. In the absence of penetrating trauma or osteomyelitis, these areas are the most likely to become infected, especially in individuals who are predisposed by a systemic disease.

COMPARTMENT SYNDROMES

Gelberman reports that shoulder area compartment syndromes are found in the biceps, triceps, and deltoid. These are secondary to drug overdose compression syndromes.[238] This occurs when the patient has been lying in one position and does not move to relieve this compression because he is so numbed by a drug overdose. The compression occurs in the most topographically prominent muscles it is possible to lie on. Compartment syndromes may also occur in severe

trauma where there is compression. Gelberman points out that the middle deltoid, because of its multipennate nature, actually consists of many small compartments in relation to the containment of edema, compared with the spread of tumor where the deltoid is a single compartment (Fig. 2–60). Therefore, decompression of the deltoid requires multiple epimysiotomy in the middle third in order to adequately release the edema (see Fig. 2–37).

REGIONAL ANESTHESIA COMPARTMENTS

The area of the shoulder most closely relevant to anesthesia is the axillary sheath, which begins in the neck as the prevertebral layer of the cervical fascia. This layer of fascia begins in the posterior midline and passes laterally deep to the trapezius. It covers the superficial surfaces of the muscles of the neck and, as it passes forward, forms the floor of the posterior triangle of the neck. It passes lateral to the scalene muscles and lateral to the upper portion of the brachial plexus, and then passes just anterior to the anterior scalene, the longus colli, and the longus capitis muscles. In this anterior position it is truly prevertebral. This layer of fascia continues laterally and distally, surrounding the brachial plexus and the axillary artery and nerve. The sheath serves the purpose of confining injected material, keeping it in contact with the nerves. In combination with the adjacent brachial fascia, it is also capable of containing the pressure of a postarteriogram hematoma enough to produce nerve compression.[242]

The interscalene position (Fig. 2–61) of the brachial plexus is quite spacious, and the appropriate anesthetic technique requires volume.[237] As the sheath proceeds

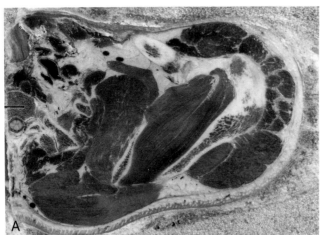
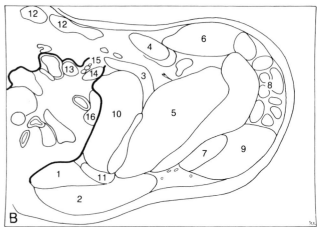

Figure 2–60. A photograph *(A)* and diagram *(B)* of a cross-section of the shoulder at the level of the acromion. Several important spaces within the shoulder are demonstrated, beginning with the *heavy line* in *B* that shows the prevertebral fascia, which contributes to the formation of the axillary sheath. In the middle portion anteriorly is a deposit of adipose tissue that is the upper end of the axillary space. Posteriorly, at the base of the spine of the scapula, there is a body of adipose tissue between the trapezius and the deltoid, wherein lie the ramifications of the cutaneous branch of the circumflex scapular artery. At the lateralmost extent can be seen the multipennate formation of the middle third of the deltoid, demonstrating why this portion of the muscle should be considered multiple compartments when treating compartment syndrome. The labeled structures are as follows: (1) rhomboid major, (2) trapezius, (3) omohyoid, (4) clavicle, (5) supraspinatus, (6) anterior third of the deltoid, (7) infraspinatus, (8) middle third of the deltoid, (9) posterior third of the deltoid, (10) serratus anterior, (11) rhomboid minor, (12) sternocleidomastoid, (13) scalenus anterior, (14) scalenus medius, (15) brachial plexus, and (16) scalenus posterior.

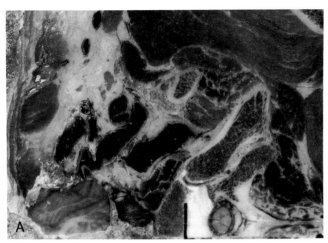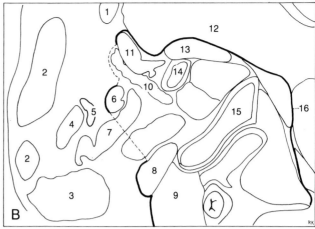

Figure 2–61. A photograph *(A)* and diagram *(B)* of a horizontal cross-section of the interscalene interval at the level where the subclavian artery is just beginning to pass behind the scalenus anterior. The *heavy line* (16) is the prevertebral fascia, which goes on to constitute the proximal axillary sheath at the proximal end. This space is so capacious that anesthesia in this area requires a dose of at least 40 ml. The labeled structures are as follows: (1) omohyoid, (2) sternocleidomastoid, (3) lung, (4) sternohyoid, (5) subclavian vein, (6) scalenus anterior, (7) subclavian artery, (8) longus colli, (9) T2 vertebra, (10) brachial plexus, (11) scalenus medius, (12) serratus anterior, (13) scalenus posterior, (14) rib 1, (15) rib 2, and (16) prevertebral fascia.

laterally toward the axilla, it is most dense proximally. Thompson and Rorie found septa (Fig. 2–62) between the various components in the sheath in anatomical dissections and tomography.[244] There were at least

three compartments. This may account for the need for multiple injections into the axillary sheath to obtain adequate brachial plexus anesthesia and may explain why axillary hematoma does not affect the entire brachial plexus at once. As we continue without pictures of the sheath as a connective tissue structure moving in relation to the adjacent structures, we should not be surprised to learn that the nerves to the shoulder and upper arm already lie outside the sheath where axillary block is performed, necessitating the use of a distal tourniquet to force the proximal migration of anesthetic solutions.

FASCIAL SPACES AND SURGICAL PLANES

The movement of surgeons through the body is greatly facilitated by planes or areas of the body that are relatively avascular and without nerves. (See sections on Nerves and Vessels for discussion.) The crossing of planes by nerve or vessel is greatly discouraged by movement across that plane. This does not mean that there are no vessels crossing, but when these planes are crossed, the vessels tend to be fewer in number and larger in size, are named, and cross in an oblique fashion to accommodate the motion. They tend to enter muscles near the points of origin or insertion and so decrease the effect of excursion of the muscle. Collateral vessels between adjacent watersheds also cross at the periphery of the planes of motion (Fig. 2–63). The shoulder is the most mobile part of the human body and, as one would expect, contains the greatest number of accommodations for that motion. Three structures specifically allow for motion: the bursae, loose alveolar tissue, and adipose tissue.

In loose alveolar tissue, the fibers and cellular elements are widely spaced. The purpose of this type of tissue is to facilitate motion between structures in relation to each other: usually muscle and muscle or

Figure 2–62. A cross-sectional diagram of the axillary sheath demonstrating the septa between the structures contained within the sheath. The labeled structures are (1) axillary artery, (2) musculocutaneous nerve, (3) vein, (4) lymph node, (5) axillary nerve, and (6) median nerve.

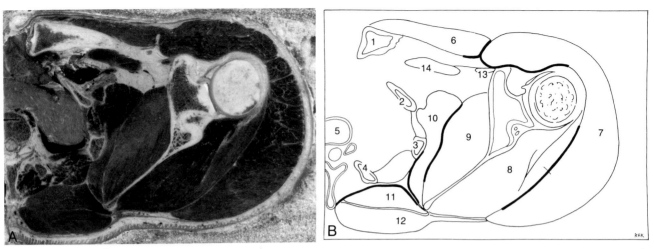

Figure 2–63. A transverse section *(A)* and diagram *(B)* showing the relationships at the level of the coracoid process. The planes where most of the motion occurs and which are most likely to be hypovascular are indicated by the *heavy lines* in *B*. The vessels that cross these planes are likely to be found at the edges of the planes of motion. For example, in the plane between the serratus anterior and the subscapularis, the vessels crossing are likely to be found close to the border of the scapula where the relative motion between these two structures is less. Also shown on this section is the proximity of the suprascapular nerve and artery to the posterior rim of the glenoid. (See Fig. 2–66 for key to diagram.)

muscle and underlying bone. These fascial spaces (Figs. 2–63 through 2–66) can be easily penetrated by pus or other unwanted fluid and yet are also useful to surgeons because of the paucity of small vessels and nerves traversing them.[230] Again, this is not to say that there are no vessels. Crossing vessels and nerves tend to be large, are named, and are usually well known and easily avoided. These fascial spaces therefore provide useful passages for dissection. The most commonly observed fascial space is seen deep to the deltopectoral groove beneath the deltoid and pectoralis major muscles, and superficial to the underlying pectoralis minor muscle and conjoint tendon. This space deep to the pectoralis major and deltoid muscles is crossed by the branches of the thoracoacromial artery close to the clavicle, with no other vessels of note crossing.

When the deltoid splitting incision is used on the posterior approach to the shoulder, a space is encountered between the deep surface of the deltoid and the outer surface of the infraspinatus and teres minor. The crossing structures are the axillary nerve and posterior circumflex artery at the inferior border of the teres minor. Deep on the costal surface of the serratus anterior, posterior to its origins, is a fascial space continuous with the loose alveolar tissue lying deep to the rhomboids. This is an avascular plane used by tumor surgeons in performing a forequarter amputation and by pediatric orthopedists in correcting an elevated scapula in a fashion that results in a less bloody dissection. Note in the illustrations that these spaces are thinner than the ink the artist used to depict them. Their existence must be borne in mind in interpreting tomograms and planning tumor margins which

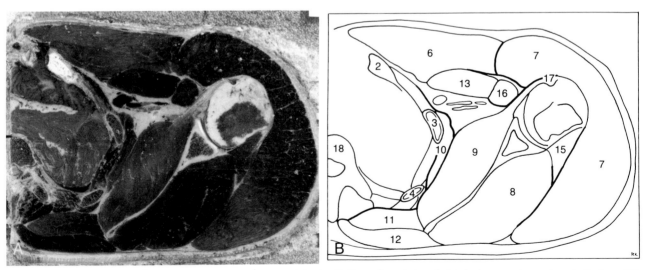

Figure 2–64. A cross-section *(A)* and diagram *(B)* slightly below the equator of the glenoid. Tissue planes that are likely to be hypovascular are shown by the *heavy lines* in *B*. (See Fig. 2–66 for key to diagram.)

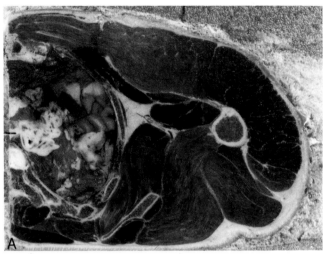 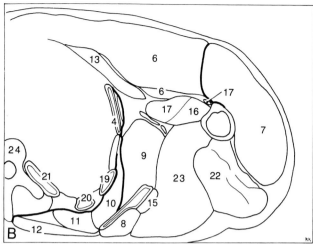

Figure 2–65. A lower cross-section *(A)* and diagram *(B)* below the level of the quadrilateral space. Careful examination of *A* shows the two layers of the pectoralis major inserting onto the lateral border of the bicipital groove. At the anterior border of the teres major, the fibers of the teres major and the latissimus dorsi moving to insert on the medial lip and floor of the bicipital groove can be seen. The position of the brachial plexus is well demarcated. (See Fig. 2–66 for key to diagram.)

may be compromised by this loose tissue. This same caveat applies to bursae.

ADIPOSE TISSUE

Adipose tissue provides the double function of cushioning nerves and vessels and allowing pulsation of arteries and dilation of veins.[230] It also allows movement of tissues in relation to each other. In the shoulder there are three deposits of adipose tissue which indicate the position of an enclosed nerve or artery. The largest of these is the axillary space which contains the brachial plexus and its branches, the

axillary artery and vein, and the major lymphatic drainage from the anterior chest wall, upper limb, and back.

The axillary space (Figs. 2–60 through 2–65, and Fig. 2–67) is bounded posteriorly by a wall of muscle, from top to bottom: the subscapularis, the teres major, and the latissimus dorsi muscles. The latissimus dorsi forms the muscle undergirding of the posterior axillary fold. These three muscles are innervated by the upper and lower subscapular nerve and the thoracodorsal nerve, formerly referred to as the middle subscapular nerve. The anterior boundary of the axillary space is the pectoralis minor muscle and the clavipectoral fascia (Fig. 2–67).

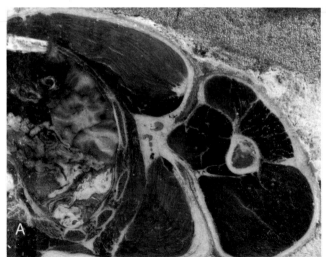 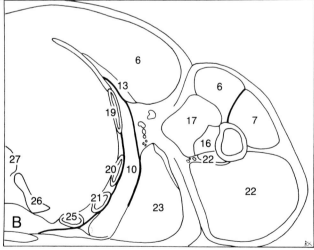

Figure 2–66. A cross-section *(A)* and diagram *(B)* only a few millimeters superior to the skin of the axillary fossa. The hypovascular planes are again emphasized. Note the large pectoral lymph nodes and the large thoracodorsal vessels. On the lateral side of the teres major, the tendon and a few remaining muscle fibers from the latissimus dorsi can be seen.

Labeled structures for Figures 2–63 through 2–66 are as follows: (1) clavicle, (2) rib 1, (3) rib 2, (4) rib 3, (5) T3 vertebra, (6) pectoralis major muscle, (7) deltoid muscle, (8) infraspinatus muscle, (9) subscapularis muscle, (10) serratus anterior muscle, (11) rhomboid muscle, (12) trapezius muscle, (13) pectoralis minor muscle, (14) subclavius muscle, (15) teres minor muscle, (16) coracobrachialis muscle, (17) biceps muscle, (18) T5 vertebra, (19) rib 4, (20) rib 5, (21) rib 6, (22) triceps muscle, (23) teres major and latissimus dorsi, (24) T6 vertebra, (25) rib 7, (26) rib 8, and (27) T8 vertebra.

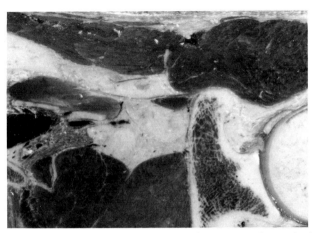

Figure 2–67. A close-up view of the axillary space demonstrates a rather prominent clavipectoral fascia starting from the tip of the coracoid and running to the left across the photograph. Just deep to this and adjacent to the coracoid lies the insertion of the pectoralis minor. The muscle to the left is the subclavius. Immediately posterior to the subclavius can be seen the brachial plexus and axillary vessels.

Superior to the pectoralis minor is a dense layer of fascia, referred to as the clavipectoral fascia, which continues medially and superiorly from the pectoralis minor. It continues medially to the first rib as the costocoracoid membrane. The pectoralis major muscle and tendon form the more definitive anterior boundary at the inferior extent of the axillary space, although there is a continuation of the clavipectoral fascia to the axilla. The medial boundary of the space is the serratus anterior muscle and the ribs. The lateral boundary is that portion of the humerus between the insertions of the teres major and latissimus dorsi and the insertion of the pectoralis major, which defines the lower extent of the intertubercular groove. In the anatomical position, the axillary space resembles a warped pyramid; its lateral border actually lies on the anterior surface of the humerus.

The next important body of adipose tissue lies posteriorly deep to the deep fascia (Fig. 2–68). It is

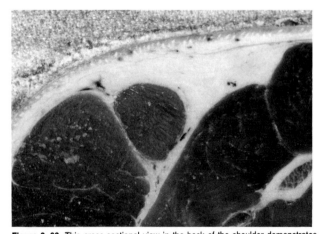

Figure 2–68. This cross-sectional view in the back of the shoulder demonstrates the pad within which the cutaneous branches of the circumflex scapular artery are located. The muscles on the left are the deltoid and the lateral head of the triceps. The teres minor is anterior, and the infraspinatus is lateral. This adipose tissue might be considered a continuation of the triangular space. Again, the presence of a body of adipose tissue is indicative of an artery or nerve.

inferomedial to the medial border of the posterior deltoid, lateral to the trapezius, and superior to the latissimus dorsi. It might be considered a continuation of the triangular space, since this tissue contains the cutaneous continuations of the circumflex scapular artery and it is here that the microvascular surgeon seeks the artery and veins of the "scapular" cutaneous flap.[240]

The third deep deposit of adipose tissue in the shoulder lies between the supraspinatus tendon and the overlying clavicle and acromioclavicular joint (see Fig. 2–39). The tissue cushions and protects the branches of the acromial artery which are frequently encountered in dissections below the acromioclavicular joint. In summary, for the purpose of dissection, adipose tissue serves to indicate the presence of vessels or nerves.

BURSAE

The last structures that facilitate motion are the bursae. Apparently, bursae form in development as a coalescence of fascial spaces.[42] Bursae tend to have incomplete linings in their normal state, but they may become quite thickened in the pathological states frequently encountered at surgery. The bursae, because they are hollow spaces, are totally avascular and can be used as spaces for dissection. Because they are the most complete of lubricating spaces, they are encountered between the most unyielding tissues: between tendon and bone or skin and bone, and occasionally between muscle and bone near a tendon insertion.

There are approximately 50 named bursae in the human body; several quite important ones are in the shoulder.[41, 42] The *subacromial bursa* and the closely related *subdeltoid bursa* are the most important. These bursae serve to lubricate motion between the rotator cuff and the overlying acromion and acromioclavicular joints. These two bursae are usually coalesced into one (Fig. 2–69). They are the most important bursae in pathological processes of the shoulder and the ones that cause the most pain when they are inflamed. Although the subacromial bursa is normally only a potential space and therefore not seen on cross-section (see Fig. 2–39) or with imaging techniques, it has a capacity of 5 to 10 ml[243] when not compromised by adhesions or edema. It normally does not communicate with the glenohumeral joint.[234]

Another frequently encountered bursa is the *subscapularis bursa,* which develops between the upper portion of the subscapularis tendon and the neck of the glenoid and, in a vast majority of cases, actually connects with the glenohumeral joint. Therefore, it is usually a recess of the glenohumeral joint rather than a separate bursa. There are fairly constant bursae near tendinous insertions between the muscle and bony insertion of several muscles including the trapezius, near the base of the scapular spine; the infraspinatus and the teres major near their attachments to the humerus; and an intermuscular bursa between the tendons of latissimus dorsi and teres major.

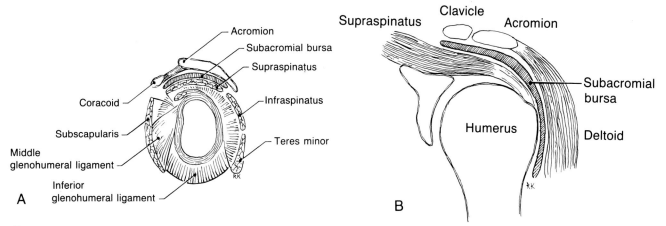

Figure 2–69. The relationships and area of distribution of the subacromial bursa. Compare these drawings with the cross-section photograph shown in Figure 2–39. In the natural state the bursa is a potential space and only exists when it is filled—e.g., with air from a surgical procedure or saline from an arthroscopy.

A less constant bursa has been found to occur between the coracoid process and *coracobrachialis muscle* and the underlying subscapularis muscle. I have seen such bursae inflamed by subcoracoid impingement processes, most often iatrogenic or post-traumatic, but two of which did not result from antecedent surgery or trauma. The coracobrachialis bursa often (20 per cent of specimens) is an extension of the subacromial bursa.[243] In such cases, the coracoid tip may be visualized through an arthroscope placed in the subacromial bursa.

Skin

Three requirements in regard to the skin should be considered in surgical planning. The first requirement is continued viability of the skin postoperatively, the second is maintenance of sensibility of the skin, and the last is cosmesis.

CIRCULATION

There are several layers of blood vessels related to the skin. A plexus of interconnecting vessels lies within the dermis itself. The largest dorsal vessels lie in the rete cutaneum, a plexus of vessels on the deep surface of the dermis.[253] There is another larger layer of vessels in the tela subcutanea, or superficial fascia.[41] The blood supply to these layers varies in different areas. Several factors relate to the arrangement of the circulation. The first factor is the relative growth of the area of the body under consideration. The number of cutaneous arteries an individual has remains constant throughout life.[248] Growth increases the distance between the skin vessels by placing greater demand upon them, which then leads to an increase in the size of the vessels.

The second factor is the path taken by the direct vessels to the skin. Direct vessels are those whose main destination is the skin. Indirect vessels are those whose main destination is some other tissue, such as bone or muscle, but which reinforce the cutaneous vessels. The paths of the direct vessels are affected by motion (Fig. 2–70) between tissues where a great deal of motion takes place between subcutaneous fat and the deep fascia. With the pectoralis major, for example, the dominant vessels cross at the edge of the plane of motion, i.e., the axilla. Some of these vessels may take direct origin off the axillary artery near its junction with the brachial artery,[202] but they mainly originate from the pectoral area.[230] The vessel travels in the subdermal plexus in the subcutaneous fascia and sends vessels to the rete cutaneum. The plane between deep fascia and subcutaneous fat is an almost bloodless field; dissection can be done without endangering the primary skin circulation.[230]

Where the skin is more fixed, the dominant vessels may lie on the superficial surface of the deep fascia, and the vessels to the dermal plexus may run more vertically than obliquely. In these areas, common on the upper arm, retaining a layer of deep fascia with skin flaps maintains another layer of circulation. The perforators to this plexus on the deep fascia travel in the intermuscular septa, rather than through the muscle where there is motion between muscle and the deep fascia. Including muscle in the flap offers no additional circulation.[230] There are a number of classifications of fasciocutaneous flaps based on how the vessels reach the deep fascia.[246, 250, 256]

On the surface, vessels tend to course from concave surfaces of the body toward convexities. Thus, they are likely to be found originating in rich supply adjacent to the borders of the axilla, and less commonly on such convexities as the breast or outer prominence of the shoulder, which are distal watersheds. As growth increases the length of limbs and the height of convexities, vessels become longer and of greater diameter, reflecting increased demand.[230]

In specialized areas of the body where dominant vessels lie just beneath the deep fascia and the skin is very well fixed, such as the palmar and plantar surfaces, the dermal vessels run straight vertically.

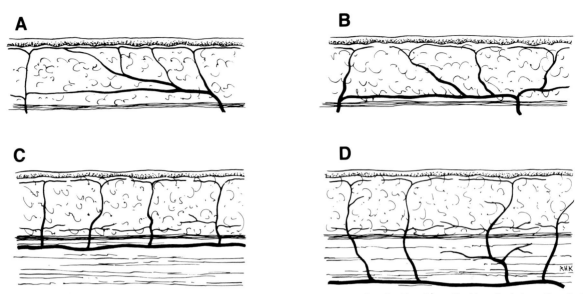

Figure 2–70. The four different types of direct circulation to the skin. Type A is found anterior to the pectoralis major. There is considerable motion between the subcutaneous fascia of the skin and the deep fascia of the muscle. The blood supply adapts to this by crossing obliquely at the edge of the plane of motion and sending a dominant vessel just deep to the tela subcutanea (subcutaneous fascia). From there the vessel sends branches to the dermal plexus. Type B occurs when there is less motion between the subcutaneous fascia and the deep fascia. In fact, there may be relative motion between the overlying deep fascia and the underlying muscle. Direct vessels branch out on the surface of the deep fascia and from there send branches to the dermal plexus. In the shoulder area this occurs over the fascia of the biceps. In Type C, the skin is very tightly attached to the underlying deep fascia, which has an artery running just below it. This is a specialized situation occurring at the palmar and plantar fascia. In Type D, the dominant vessel supplying this area of skin lies deep to the muscle and sends direct perforators to the dermal plexus. As expected, this also occurs where there is very little motion between skin and underlying muscle. (Redrawn from Taylor GI, and Palmer JH: The vascular territories (angiosomes) of the body; experimental study and clinical applications. Br J Plast Surg *40*:133–137, 1930.)

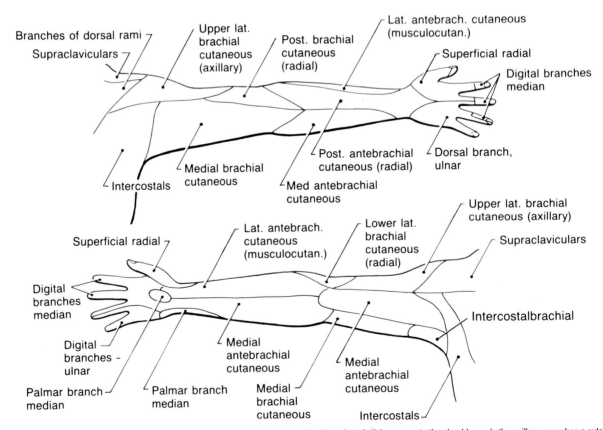

Figure 2–71. The cutaneous sensity representation of the nerves of the upper extremity. Note that of all the nerves to the shoulder, only the axillary nerve has a cutaneous representation. The remainder of the shoulder area is innervated by the supraclavicular nerves and the dorsal rami of the spinal nerves. There is not a sharp demarcation between the area of skin innervated by the intercostal brachial and medial brachial cutaneous nerves because of communication from the former. Intercostal brachial numbness following a radical mastectomy is the only cutaneous nerve sensitivity problem common in the shoulder. (Redrawn from Hollinshead WH: Anatomy for Surgeons, Vol. 3, 3rd ed. Philadelphia: Harper & Row, 1982.)

In other areas of the body, for example, over the middle third of the deltoid, the skin is extremely well fixed to underlying muscle. The dominant vessels, here the posterior humeral circumflex artery and veins,[230] actually course on the deep surface of the muscles with the direct vessels running vertically through the intramuscular septa of the deltoid muscle to the skin. Dissection on either side of the deep fascia will divide these vessels. Only a myocutaneous flap would offer additional vessels to the skin.[257]

These types of skin circulation are not mutually exclusive and may reinforce each other. Over the pectoralis major muscle, for example, direct vessels from the internal mammary vessels reinforce the Type A vessels from the axilla.[259] Over the deltopectoral groove, perforator vessels from the deltoid artery reinforce the skin circulation. Much of the deltoid muscle vessels in the tela subcutanea are reinforced by the Type D vessels from the posterior humeral circumflex. There is likely to be less overlap over the middle one-third of the deltoid, and flap development in this area should be less extensive.

SENSATION

Sensation (Fig. 2–71) related to shoulder surgery is of less concern to the surgeon and the patient than is sensation in other areas of the body. There is a low incidence of postoperative neuroma of the shoulder.

The most cephalad of nerves that innervate the skin of the shoulder and lower neck are the supraclavicular nerves. They branch from the third and fourth cervical nerve roots and then descend from the cervical plexus into the posterior triangle of the neck. They penetrate superficial fascia anterior to platysma, descend over the clavicle, and innervate the skin over the first two intercostal spaces anteriorly.[41] Interestingly, the medial supraclavicular nerves may pass through the clavicle.

The posterior portion of the shoulder and neck is innervated from cutaneous branches off the dorsal rami of the spinal nerves. In the dorsal spine, the area of skin that is innervated is usually caudad to the intervertebral foramen through which the nerve exits. For example, the C8 cutaneous representation is in line with the spine of the scapula, which is at the same height as the third or fourth thoracic vertebra.[41]

Much of the anterior chest is innervated by the anterior intercostal nerves. The first branches come forward near the midline adjacent to the sternum and innervate the anterior portion of the chest, overlapping somewhat with the lateral intercostal cutaneous branches. Interestingly, there is no anterior cutaneous branch from the first intercostal nerve.

The lateral cutaneous branches of the intercostal nerve emerge on the lateral thorax between the slips of the serratus anterior muscle and innervate the skin in this area. They also supply the larger portion of the anterior chest anteriorly including the breast.[42]

Only three nerves of the brachial plexus have cutaneous representation in the shoulder. The most proximal of these is the upper lateral brachial cutaneous nerve, a branch of the axillary nerve that innervates the lateral side of the shoulder and the skin overlying the deltoid. The upper medial side of the arm is innervated by the medial brachial cutaneous and the

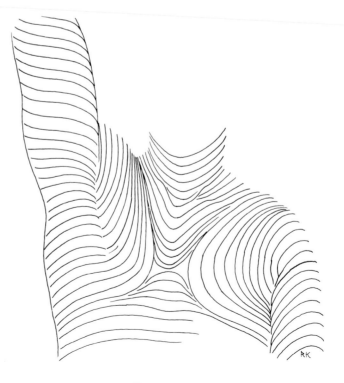

Figure 2–72. The usual locations of the relaxed skin tension lines in the male. The position of these lines varies among individuals; they should be sought for at each operation. (Redrawn from Kraissel CJ: Selection of appropriate lines for elective surgical incisions. Plast Reconstr Surg 8:1–28, 1951.)

intercostal brachial nerves combined. In the anterior portion of the arm over the biceps muscle, skin is innervated by the medial antebrachial cutaneous.[41]

RELAXED SKIN TENSION LINES

Although numerous attempts have been made over the past 200 years, and in recent years, to outline the optimum lines for incision, the best description of the basic principles is Langer's. He found that the tension in the skin is determined by the prominence of underlying structures and by motion, with underlying topography the predominant influence.[251, 252] Langer did two classic experiments. In the first he punctured cadavers with a round awl and observed the linear splits that developed because of the orientation of underlying collagen. This he called the cleavability of the skin. In the second experiment, he measured skin tension in various ways. In cadavers he would make circular incisions and observe wound retraction. He would then move the limb to look for changes in retraction. In living patients, such as women in the delivery room who were about to experience a sudden change in underlying topography, he would draw a circle on the skin with ink and observe postpartum changes.

In the 20th century cosmetic surgeons have found Langer's lines to be incorrect in certain areas of the body. Although the principles outlined by Langer are still held to be valid, newer techniques have been sought to localize the optimum lines in the living individual. These techniques have included further circular incisions, wrinkle patterns, and chemical imprints. All of these techniques agreed with the incisions empirically found to be best in some regions and not in others.

Contemporary plastic surgeons now speak of relaxed

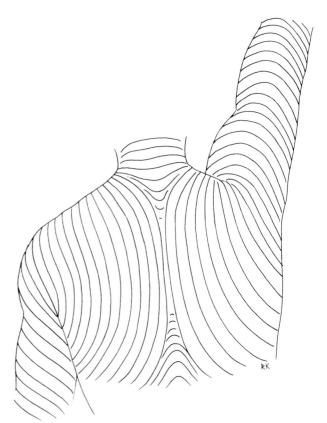

Figure 2–74. The usual position of the relaxed skin tension lines on the posterior surfaces of the shoulder region. (Redrawn from Kraissel CJ: Selection of appropriate lines for elective surgical incisions. Plast Reconstr Surg 8:1–28, 1951.)

skin tension lines (Figs. 2–72, 2–73, and 2–74). This refers to their technique of relaxing the tension on the skin between the thumb and forefinger of the surgeon and observing the pattern of fine lines in the skin. When the relation is exactly perpendicular to the optimum incision, the fine lines that form are straight and parallel. Then the skin is pinched in other directions. The line pattern is rhomboid or obscured.[245] This technique allows the surgeon to compensate for individual variability.

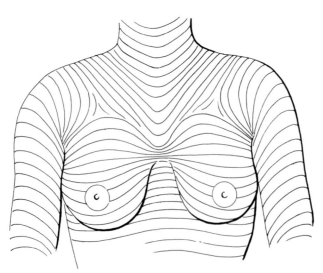

Figure 2–73. Because of the different underlying topography, the lines of skin tension in the female differ in several respects from those in the male. (Redrawn from Kraissel CJ: Selection of appropriate lines for elective surgical incisions. Plast Reconstr Surg 8:1–28, 1951.)

References

History/General

1. Basmajian JV: Muscles Alive. Their Functions Revealed by Electromyography, 4th ed. Baltimore: Williams and Wilkins, 1979.
2. Braune W, and Fischer O: On the Centre of Gravity of the Human Body. Maquet P, and Furlong R (trans). New York: Springer-Verlag, 1988.
3. Braune W, and Fischer O: The Human Gait. Maquet P, and Furlong R (trans). New York: Springer-Verlag, 1987.
4. da Vinci, Leonardo: The Drawings of Leonardo da Vinci, In the Collection of Her Majesty, The Queen, at Windsor Castle, Vols. 1–3. London: Phaedon Press Limited, 1968.
5. Detrisac DA, and Johnson LL: Arthroscopic Shoulder Anatomy. Pathologic & Surgical Implications. Thorofare, NJ: Slack Inc., 1986.
6. Duchenne GB: Physiology of Movement. Demonstrated by Means of Electrical Stimulation and Clinical Observation and

Applied to the Study of Paralysis and Deformities. Kaplan EB (trans. and ed.). Philadelphia: WB Saunders Co., 1959.

7. Dung HC: Acupuncture points of the brachial plexus. Am J Chin Med 13:49–64, 1985.
8. Galen: On the Usefulness of the Parts of the Body. May MT (trans). Ithaca, NY: Cornell University Press, 1967.
9. Hippocrates: Hippocratic Writings. Great Books of the Western World. Hutchins, RM, editor-in-chief, Pub. Enc. Brit., 1955.
10. Hoernle AFR: Studies in the Medicine of Ancient India. Part I. Osteology or the Bones of the Human Body. Oxford, England: Clarendon Press, 1907.
11. Hsieh ET: A review of ancient Chinese anatomy. Anat Rec 20:97–127, 1921.
12. Huang-Ti Nei Ching Su Wen: The Yellow Emperor's Classic of Internal Medicine. (New Edition, Ch. 1–34 translated from Chinese with Introductory Study by Ilza Veith) Los Angeles and Berkeley: University of California Press, 1966. (Original edition published 1949, Cambridge University Press.)
13. Lockhart RD: Movements of the normal shoulder joint and of a case with trapezius paralysis studied by radiogram and experiment in the living. J Anat 64:288–302, 1930.
14. McGrew R: Encyclopedia of Medical History. New York: McGraw Hill, 1985.
15. Meyer AW: Chronic functional lesions of the shoulder. Arch Surg 35:646–674, 1937.
16. Muybridge E: Animals in motion. Brown, LS (ed). New York: Dover Publications, 1957.
17. Perry J: Biomechanics of the shoulder. In Rowe, C (ed). The shoulder. New York: Churchill Livingstone, 1988.
18. Persaud TVN: Early History of Human Anatomy. From Antiquity to the Beginning of the Modern Era. Springfield, Illinois: Charles C Thomas, 1984.
19. Rasch PJ, and Burke RK: Kinesiology & Applied Anatomy: The Science of Human Movement. Philadelphia: Lea & Febiger, 1959.
20. Vesalius A: The Illustrations from the Works of Andreas Vesalius of Brussels. Saunders JB, and O'Malley CD (eds). Cleveland and New York: The World Publishing Company, 1950.

Bones and Joints

21. Abbott LS, and Lucas DB: The function of the clavicle. Its surgical significance. Ann Surg 140:583–597, 1954.
22. Aoki M, Ishii S, and Usui M: The slope of the acromion in the rotator cuff impingement. Orthop Trans 10(2):228, 1986.
23. Bearn JG: Direct observations on the function of the capsule of the sternoclavicular joint in clavicular support. J Anat 101:159–170, 1967.
24. Bigliani LU, Morrison DS, and April EW: The morphology of the acromion in its relationship to rotator cuff tears. Orthop Trans 10(2):228, 1986.
25. Brookes M: The blood supply of irregular and flat bones. In Blood Supply of the Bone. New York: Appleton-Century-Crofts, 1971, pp 47–66.
26. Cave AJE: The nature and morphology of the costoclavicular ligament. J Anat 95:170–179, 1961.
27. Cyprien JM, Vasey HM, Burdet A, et al: Humeral retrotorsion and glenohumeral relationship in the normal shoulder and in recurrent anterior dislocation (Scapulometry). Clin Orthop 175:8–17, 1983.
28. Cyriax EF: A second brief note on 'floating clavicle.' Anat Rec 52:97, 1932.
29. Denham RH, and Dingley AF, Jr: Epiphyseal separation of the medial end of the clavicle. J Bone Joint Surg 49-A:1179–1183, 1967.
30. DePalma AF, Callery G, and Bennett GA: Variational anatomy and degenerative lesions of the shoulder joint. Am Acad Orthop Surgeons Instructional Course Lectures 6:255–281, 1949.
31. DePalma AF: Surgery of the Shoulder, 3rd ed. Philadelphia: JB Lippincott, 1983.
32. DePalma AF: Surgical anatomy of acromioclavicular and sternoclavicular joints. Surg Clin North Am 43:1541–1550, 1963.
33. Dines DM, Warren RE, Inglis AE, and Pavlov H: The coracoid impingement syndrome. Orthop Trans 10:229, 1986.
34. Deutsch AL, Resnick D, and Mink JH: Computed tomography of the glenohumeral and sternoclavicular joints. Orthop Clin North Am 16(3):497–511, July 1985.
35. Duggan N: Recurrent dislocation of the sternoclavicular cartilage. J Bone Joint Surg 13:365, 1931.
36. Fukuda K, Craig EV, An K, Cofield RH, et al: Biomechanical study of the ligamentous system of the acromioclavicular joint. J Bone Joint Surg 68A:434–439, 1986.
37. Gagey O, Bonfait H, and Gillot C: Anatomic basis of ligamentous control of elevation. Surg Radiol Anat 9:19–26, 1987.
38. Gerber C, Terrier F, and Ganz R: The role of the coracoid process in the chronic impingement syndrome. J Bone Joint Surg 67B:703–708, 1985.
39. Gerber C, Terrier F, Zehnder R, and Ganz R: The subcoracoid space. An anatomic study. Clin Orthop 215:132–138, 1987.
40. Hitchcock HH, and Bechtol CO: Painful shoulder. Observations of the role of the tendon of the long head of the biceps brachii in its causation. J Bone Joint Surg 30-A:263–273, 1948.
41. Hollinshead WH: Anatomy for Surgeons, Vol. 3, 3rd ed. Philadelphia: Harper & Row, 1982.
42. Hollinshead WH: Textbook of Anatomy, 2nd ed. New York: Harper & Row, 1967.
43. Howard FM, and Shafer SJ: Injuries to the clavicle with neurovascular complications: a study of fourteen cases. J Bone Joint Surg 47-A:1335–1346, 1956.
44. Inman VT, Saunders JBDCM, and Abbott LC: Observations on the function of the shoulder joint. J Bone Joint Surg 26:1–30, 1944.
45. Johnson EW, Jr, and Collins HR: Nonunion of the clavicle. Arch Surg 87:963–966, 1963.
46. Johnston TB: The movements of the shoulder-joint: a plea for the use of the "plane of the scapula" as the plane of reference for movements occurring at the humero-scapular joint. Br J Surg 25:252–260, 1937.
47. Kaltsas DS: Comparative study of the properties of the shoulder joint capsule with those of other joints. Capsules. Clin Orthop 173:20–26, 1983.
48. Kennedy JC: Retrosternal dislocation of the clavicle. J Bone Joint Surg 31-B:74–75, 1949.
49. Laing PG: The arterial supply of the adult humerus. J Bone Joint Surg 38A:1105–1116, 1956.
50. Lexer E, and Kuliga TW: Untersuchungen uber knochenarterien. Berlin: Hirschwald, 1904, pp. 15–16.
51. Lewis OJ: The coraco-clavicular joint. J Anat 93:296–303, 1959.
52. Lewis MM, Ballet FL, Kroll PG, and Bloom N: En bloc clavicular resection: operative procedure and postoperative testing of function. Case reports. Clin Orthop 193:214–220, 1985.
53. Liberson F: Os acromiale—a contested anomaly. J Bone Joint Surg 19:683–689, 1937.
54. Lucas LS, and Gill JH: Humerus varus following birth injury to the proximal humeral epiphysis. J Bone Joint Surg 29:367–369, 1947.
55. Lucas DB: Biomechanics of the shoulder joint. Arch Surg 107:425–432, 1973.
56. Maves MD, and Philippsen LP: Surgical anatomy of the scapular spine in the trapezius-osteomuscular flap. Arch Otolaryngol Head Neck Surg 112:173–175, 1986.
57. McCally WC, and Kelly DA: Treatment of fractures of the clavicle, ribs and scapula. Am J Surg 50:558–562, 1940.
58. Meyer AW: Spontaneous dislocation and destruction of tendon of long head of biceps brachii. Fifty-nine instances. Arch Surg 17:493–506, 1928.
59. Mudge MK, Wood VE, and Frykman GK: Rotator cuff tears associated with os acromiale. J Bone Joint Surg 66A:427–429, 1984.
60. Neer CJ: Anterior acromioplasty for chronic impingement syndrome of the shoulder. J Bone Joint Surg 54-A:41–50, 1972.

61. Neer CS: Impingement lesions. Clin Orthop *173*:70–77, 1983.
62. Neer CS, and Poppen NK: Supraspinatus outlet. Orthop Trans *11*:234, 1987.
63. Nutter PD: Coracoclavicular articulations. J Bone Joint Surg *23*:177–179, 1941.
64. Panje W, and Cutting C: Trapezius osteomyocutaneous island flap for reconstruction of the anterior floor of the mouth and the mandible. Head Neck Surg *3*:66–71, 1980.
65. Paavolainen P, Slatis P, and Aalto K: Surgical pathology in chronic shoulder pain. *In* Bateman JE, and Welsh RP (eds): Surgery of the Shoulder. St. Louis: C.V. Mosby Company, 1984, pp. 313–318.
66. Petersson CJ: Spontaneous medial dislocation of the tendon of the long biceps brachii. An anatomic study of prevalence and pathomechanics. Clin Orthop *211*:224–227, 1986.
67. Petersson CJ, and Redlund-Johnell I: The subacromial space in normal shoulder radiographs. Acta Orthop Scand *55*:57–58, 1984.
68. Radin EL: Biomechanics and functional anatomy. *In* Post M (ed): The Shoulder. Surgical and Nonsurgical Management. Philadelphia: Lea & Febiger, 1978, pp. 44–49.
69. Reeves B: Experiments on the tensile strength of the anterior capsular structures of the shoulder in man. J Bone Joint Surg *50-B*:858–865, 1968.
70. Rietveld ABM, Daanen HAM, Rozing PM, and Obermann WR: The lever arm in gleno-humeral abduction after hemiarthroplasty. J Bone Joint Surg *70-B*:561–565, 1988.
71. Rockwood CA, and Green DP: Fractures in Adults. Volume 1, Part II: Subluxations and Dislocations About the Shoulder. Philadelphia: JB Lippincott, 1984, pp. 722–947.
72. Saha AK: Theory of Shoulder Mechanism: Descriptive and Applied. Springfield, IL: Charles C Thomas, 1961.
73. Saha AK: Dynamic stability of the glenohumeral joint. Acta Orthop Scand *42*:491, 1971.
74. Saha AK: Mechanism of shoulder movements and a plea for the recognition of "zero position" of the glenohumeral joint. Clin Orthop *173*:3–10, 1983.
75. Seltzer SE, and Weissman BN: CT findings in normal and dislocating shoulders. J Canad Assoc Radiol *36*:41–46, 1985.
76. Slatis P, and Aalto K: Medial dislocation of the tendon of the long head of the biceps brachii. Acta Orthop Scand *50*:73–77, 1979.
77. Tang T: Personal Communication.
78. Tang-Tian et al: Humerus varus: a report of 7 cases. Chin J Orthop *3*(3):165–170, 1983.
79. Taylor S: Clavicular dysostosis: a case report. J Bone Joint Surg *27*:710–711, 1945.
80. Todd TW, and D'Errico J, Jr: The clavicular epiphyses. Am J Anat *41*:25–50, 1928.
81. Urist MR: Follow-up notes on articles previously published in the journal: complete dislocation of the acromioclavicular joint. J Bone Joint Surg *45-A*:1750–1753, 1963.
82. Weinstabl R, Hertz H, and Firbas W: Connection of the ligamentum coracoglenoidale. Acta Anat *125*:126–131, 1986.
83. Woo S, Maynard J, Butler D, Lyon R, et al.: Ligament, Tendon, and Joint Capsule Insertions to Bone. *In* Injury & Repair of the Musculoskeletal Soft Tissues. Park Ridge, Illinois: American Academy of Orthopaedic Surgeons, 1988, pp. 133–166.
84. Wood VE, and Marchinski LM: Congenital Anomalies of the Shoulder. *In* Rockwood C, and Matsen F (eds): The shoulder. Philadelphia: WB Saunders Co., 1990.
85. Woodward, JW: Congenital elevation of the scapula: correction by release and transplantation of muscle origins. A preliminary report. J Bone Joint Surg *43-A*(2):219–228, 1961.

Muscles

86. Abbott LC, and Lucas DB: The tripartite deltoid and its surgical significance in exposure of the scapulohumeral joint. Ann Surg *136*:392–402, 1952.
87. Atwater AE: Biomechanics of overarm throwing movements and of throwing injuries. Exercise Sports Sci Rev *7*:43–85, 1979.
88. Bartlett SP, May JW, Jr, and Yaremchuk MJ: The latissimus dorsi muscle: a fresh cadaver study of the primary neurovascular pedicle. Plast Reconstr Surg *65(5)*:631–636, 1981.
89. Bayley JC, Cochran TP, and Sledge CB: The weight-bearing shoulder. The impingement syndrome in paraplegics. J Bone Joint Surg *69-A*:676–678, 1987.
90. Beaton LE, and Anson BJ: Variation of the origin of the m. trapezius. Anat Rec *83*:41–46, 1942.
91. Bhattacharyya S: Abduction contracture of the shoulder from contracture of the intermediate part of the deltoid. J Bone Joint Surg *48B*:127–131, 1966.
92. Bing R: Ueber Angeborene Muskel-defecte. Virchow's Arch B Cell Pathol *170*:175–228, 1902.
93. Broome HL, and Basmajian JV: The function of the teres major muscle: an electromyographic study. Anat Rec *170*:309–310, 1971.
94. Cain PR, Mutschler TA, Fu FH, and Lee SK: Anterior stability of the glenohumeral joint. A dynamic model. Am J Sports Med *15*:144–148, 1987.
95. Cave AJE, and Brown RW: On the tendon of the subclavius muscle. J Bone Joint Surg *34-B*:466–469, 1952.
96. Colachis SC, Jr, Strohm BR, and Brecher VL: Effects of axillary nerve block on muscle force in the upper extremity. Arch Phys Med Rehabil *50*:645–647, 1969.
97. Colachis SC, Jr, and Strohm BR: Effects of suprascapular and axillary nerve block on muscle forces in the upper extremity. Arch Phys Med Rehabil *52*:22, 1971.
98. Dewar FP, and Harris RI: Restoration of function of the shoulder following paralysis of the trapezius by fascial sling fixation and transplantation of the levator scapulae. Ann Surg *132*:1111–1115, 1950.
99. Doody SG, Freedman L, and Waterland JC: Shoulder movements during abduction in the scapular plane. Arch Phys Med Rehabil *51*:595–604, 1970.
100. Durman DC: An operation for paralysis of the serratus anterior. J Bone Joint Surg *27*:380–382, 1945.
101. Ekholm J, Arborelius UP, Hillered L, and Ortqvist A: Shoulder muscle EMG and resisting movement during diagonal exercise movements resisted by weight and pulley circuit. Scand J Rehabil Med *10*:179–185, 1978.
102. Franklin JL, Barrett WP, Jackins SE, and Matsen FA: Glenoid loosening in total shoulder arthroplasty. Association with rotator cuff deficiency. J Arthroplasty *3*:39–46, 1988.
103. Gowan ID, Jobe FW, Tibone JE, Perry J, et al: A comparative electromyographic analysis of the shoulder during pitching. Professional versus amateur pitchers. Am J Sports Med *15*:586–590, 1987.
104. Grant JCB, and Smith CG: Age incidence of rupture of the supraspinatus tendon. Anat Rec *100*:666, 1948.
105. Hayes WM: Rupture of the pectoralis major muscle: review of the literature and report of two cases. J Internat Coll Surg *14*:82–88, 1950.
106. Hertz H, Weinstabl R, Grundschober F, and Orthner E: Zur Makroskopischen und Mikroskopischen Anatomie der Schultergelenkspfanne und des Limbus Glenoidalis. Acta Anat *125*:96–100, 1986.
107. Horan FT, and Bonafede RP: Bilateral absence of the trapezius and sternal head of the pectoralis major muscles. A case report. J Bone Joint Surg *59-A*:133, 1977.
108. Horwitz MT, and Tocantins LM: Isolated paralysis of the serratus anterior (magnus) muscle. J Bone Joint Surg *20-A*:720–725, 1938b.
109. Howell SM, Imobersteg AM, Seger DH, and Marone PJ: Clarification of the role of the supraspinatus muscle in shoulder function. J Bone Joint Surg *68A*:398–404, 1986.
110. Jobe FW, Moynes DR, Tibone JE, and Perry J: An EMG analysis of the shoulder in pitching. A second report. Am J Sports Med *12*:218–220, 1984.
111. Lambert AE: A rare variation in the pectoralis minor muscle. Anat Rec *31*:193–200, 1925.
112. Landry SO, Jr: The phylogenetic significance of the chondro-epitrochlearis muscle and its accompanying pectoral abnormalities. J Anat *92*:57–61, 1958.

113. Lorhan PH: Isolated paralysis of the serratus magnus following surgical procedures. Report of a case. Arch Surg 54:656–659, 1947.
114. Mariani EM, Cofield RH, Askew LJ, Li G, et al: Rupture of the tendon of the long head of the biceps brachii. Surgical vs. nonsurgical treatment. Clin Orthop 228:233–239, March, 1988.
115. Marmor L, Bechtol CO, and Hall CB: Pectoralis major muscle. J Bone Joint Surg 43A:81–87, 1961.
116. Martin CP: The movements of the shoulder-joint, with special reference to rupture of the supraspinatus tendon. Am J Anat 66:213–234, 1940.
117. Mathes SJ, and Nahai F: Classification of the vascular anatomy of muscles: experimental and clinical correlation. Plast Reconstr Surg 67:177–187, 1981.
118. Mathes SJ, and Nahai F: Vascular anatomy of muscle: classification & application. In Clinical Applications for Muscle and Musculocutaneous Flaps. St. Louis: C. V. Mosby Co., 1982, pp. 16–94.
119. Matsen FA: Biomechanics of the shoulder. In Frankel VH, and Nordin M (eds). Basic Biomechanics of the Skeletal System. Philadelphia: Lea & Febiger, 1980, pp. 221–242.
120. McLaughlin HL: Lesions of the musculotendinous cuff of the shoulder: III. Observations on the pathology, course and treatment of calcific deposits. Ann Surg 124:354–362, 1946.
121. Meyer AW: Spontaneous dislocation and destruction of tendon of long head of the biceps brachii: fifty-nine instances. Arch Surg 17:493–506, 1928.
122. Mortensen OA, and Wiedenbauer M: An electromyographic study of the trapezius muscle. Anat Rec 112:366–367, 1952 (abstr).
123. Nuber GW, Jobe FW, Perry J, Moynes DR, et al: Fine wire electromyography analysis of muscles of the shoulder during swimming. Am J Sports Med 14:7–11, 1986.
124. Ovesen JO, and Nielsen S: Stability of the shoulder joint. Cadaver study of stabilizing structures. Acta Orthop Scand 56:149–151, 1985.
125. Ovesen JO, and Nielsen S: Anterior and posterior instability. A cadaver study. Acta Orthop Scand 57:324–327, 1986.
126. Ovesen J, and Nielsen S: Posterior instability of the shoulder. Acta Orthop Scand 57:436–439, 1986.
127. Reiss FP, De Camargo AM, Vitti M, and De Carvalho CAF: Electromyographic study of subclavius muscle. Acta Anat 105:284–290, 1979.
128. Roos DB: New concepts of thoracic outlet syndrome that explain etiology, symptoms, diagnosis and treatment. Vasc Surg 13:313–321, 1979.
129. Sakellarides HT: Injury to spinal accessory nerve with paralysis of trapezius muscle and treatment by tendon transfer. Orthop Trans 10:449, 1986.
130. Salmon M, and Dor J: Les arteres des muscles des membres et du tronc. Paris: Masson et Cie (Librairie de l'academie de medecine), 1933.
131. Saunders WH, and Johnson EW: Rehabilitation of the shoulder after radical neck dissection. Ann Otolrhinolaryngol 84:812, 1975.
132. Scheving LE, and Pauly JE: An electromyographic study of some muscles acting on the upper extremity in man. Anat Rec 135:239, 1959.
133. Seib GA: The musculus pectoralis minor in American whites and American Negroes. Am J Phys Anthropol 23:389, 1938. In Grant JCB: An Atlas of Anatomy, 5th ed. Baltimore: Williams & Wilkins Co., 1962.
134. Selden BR: Congenital absence of trapezius and rhomboideus major muscles. J Bone Joint Surg 17:1058–1061, 1935.
135. Sheehan D: Bilateral absence of trapezius. J Anat 67:180, 1932.
136. Shevlin MG, Lehmann JF, and Lucci JA: Electromyographic study of the function of some muscles crossing the glenohumeral joint. Arch Phys Med Rehabil 50:264–270, 1969.
137. Staples OS, and Watkins AL: Full active abduction in traumatic paralysis of the deltoid. J Bone Joint Surg 25:85–89, 1943.
138. Strohm BR: Shoulder dysfunction following injury to suprascapular nerve. J Am Phys Ther Assoc 45:106–111, 1965.
139. Symeonides PP: The significance of the subscapularis muscle in pathogenesis of recurrent anterior dislocation of the shoulder. J Bone Joint Surg 54-B:476–483, 1972.
140. Ting A, Jobe FW, Barto P, Ling B, et al: An EMG analysis of the lateral biceps in shoulders with rotator cuff tears. Orthop Trans 11:237, 1987.
141. Tobin GR, Schusterman M, Peterson GH, Nichols G, et al: The intramuscular, neurovascular anatomy of the latissimus dorsi muscle: the basis for splitting the flap. Plast Reconstr Surg 67:637–641, 1981.
142. Turkel SJ, Panio MW, Marshall JL, and Girgis FG: Stabilizing mechanisms preventing anterior dislocation of the glenohumeral joint. J Bone Joint Surg 63-A:1208–1217, 1981.
143. Vare AM, and Indurkar GM: Some anomalous findings in the axillary musculature. J Anat Soc India 14:34–36, 1965.
144. Waterston D: Variations in the teres minor muscle. Anat Anz 32:331–333, 1908.
145. Watterson PA, Taylor GI, and Crock JG: The venous territories of muscles: anatomical study and clinical implications. Br J Plast Surg 41:569–585, 1988.
146. Williams GA: Pectoral muscle defects: cases illustrating 3 varieties. J Bone Joint Surg 12:417, 1930.
147. Wilson CL, and Duff GL: Pathologic study of degeneration and rupture of the supraspinatus tendon. Arch Surg 47:121–135, 1943.

Nerves

148. Abdullah S, and Bowden REM: The blood supply of the brachial plexus. Proc Royal Soc Med 53:203–205, 1960.
149. Bach BR, O'Brien SJ, Warren RF, and Leighton M: An unusual neurologic complication of the Bristow procedure. J Bone Joint Surg 70-A:458–460, 1988.
150. Bonica JJ: Regional anesthesia. Clinical Anesthesia Series. Philadelphia: FA Davis Co., 1969.
151. Bonnel F: Microscopic anatomy of the adult human brachial plexus: an anatomical and histological basis for microsurgery. Microsurg 5:107–118, 1984.
152. Breisch EA: A rare human variation: the relationship of the axillary and inferior subscapular nerves to an accessory subscapularis muscle. Anat Rec 216:440–442, 1986.
153. Cahill BR, and Palmer RE: Quadrilateral space syndrome. J Hand Surg 8:65–69, 1983.
154. Clein LJ: Suprascapular entrapment neuropathy. J Neurosurg 43:337–342, 1975.
155. Corbin KB, and Harrison F: The sensory innervation of the spinal accessory and tongue musculature in the rhesus monkey. Brain 62:191–197, 1939.
156. Edeland HG, and Zachrisson BE: Fractures of the scapular notch associated with lesion of suprascapular nerve. Acta Orthop Scand 46:758–763, 1975.
157. Enneking WF: Musculoskeletal tumor surgery. New York: Churchill Livingstone, 1983, p. 212.
158. Flatow EL, Bigliani LU, and April EW: An anatomical study of the musculocutaneous nerve and its relationship to the coracoid. Clin Orthop Rel Res 244, 1989
159. Gardner E: The innervation of the shoulder joint. Anat Rec 102:1–18, 1948.
160. Gebarski KS, Glazer GM, and Gebarski SS: Brachial plexus: anatomic, radiologic, and pathologic correlation using computed tomography. J Comput Assist Tomogr 6:1058–1063, 1982.
161. Gelberman RH, Verdeck WN, and Brodhead WT: Supraclavicular nerve-entrapment syndrome. J Bone Joint Surg 57A:119, 1975.
162. Harmon PH: Surgical reconstruction of the paralytic shoulder by multiple muscle transplantations. J Bone Joint Surg 32-A:583–595, 1950.
163. Hasan M, and Narayan D: The single cord human brachial plexus. J Anat Soc India 64:103–104, 1964.
164. Herzberg G, Narakas A, Comtet JJ, Bouchet A, et al: Microsurgical relations of the roots of the brachial plexus. Practical applications. Ann Chir Main 4:120–133, 1985.
165. Horwitz MT, and Tocantins LM: An anatomical study of the role of the long thoracic nerve and the related scapular bursae

in the pathogenesis of local paralysis of the serratus anterior muscle. Anat Rec 71:375–385, 1938a.

166. Jobe CM: Unpublished data from dissections carried out at A.A.O.S. Summer Institute, 1986.

167. Kerr AT: The brachial plexus of nerves in man: the variations in its formation and branches. Am J Anat 23:285–394, 1918.

168. Kopell H, and Thompson W: Pain and the frozen shoulder. Surg Gynecol Obstet 109:92–96, 1959.

169. Leffert RD: Brachial Plexus Injuries. New York: Churchill Livingstone, 1985.

170. Lewis WH: The development of the arm in man. Am J Anat 1:145–183, 1902.

171. Linell EA: The distribution of nerves in the upper limb with reference to variabilities and their clinical significance. J Anat 55:79–112, 1921.

172. Loo RL, and Graham B: Anatomy of the axillary nerve and its relation to inferior capsular shift. Orthop Trans 11:245, 1987.

173. Lorhan PH: Isolated paralysis of the serratus magnus following surgical procedures: report of a case. Arch Surg 54:656–659, 1947.

174. Lundborg G, and Rydevik B: Effects of stretching the tibial nerve of the rabbit. A preliminary study of the intraneural circulation and the barrier function of the perineurium. J Bone Joint Surg 55-B:390–401, 1973.

175. Lundborg G: Ischemic nerve injury. Experimental studies on intraneural microvascular pathophysiology and nerve function in a limb subjected to temporary circulatory arrest. Scand J Plast Reconstr Surg (Suppl) 6:1, 1970.

176. Lundborg G: Intraneural microcirculation. Orthop Clin North Am 19(1):1–12, 1988.

177. Lundborg G, and Branemark PI: Microvascular structure and function of peripheral nerves. Vital microscopic studies of the tibial nerve in the rabbit. Adv Microcirc 1:66–88, 1968.

178. Maccarty CS: Surgical exposure of the brachial plexus. Surg Neurol 21:593–596, 1984.

179. Miller RA: Observations upon the arrangement of the axillary artery and brachial plexus. Am J Anat 64:143–159, 1939.

180. Prescott MU, and Zollinger RW: Alar scapula: an unusual surgical complication. Am J Surg 65:98–103, 1944.

181. Ray BS, Hinsey JC, and Geohegan WA: Observations on the distribution of the sympathetic nerves to the pupil and upper extremity as determined by stimulation of the anterior roots in man. Ann Surg 118:647–655, 1943.

182. Rengachary SS, Burr D, Lucas S, Hassanein KM, et al: Suprascapular entrapment neuropathy: a clinical, anatomical, and comparative study. Part 2: Anatomical study. Neurosurg 5:447–451, 1979.

183. Rengachary SS, Neff JP, Singer PA, and Brackett CE: Suprascapular entrapment neuropathy. A clinical, anatomic and comparative study. Part I. Neurosurg 5:441–446, 1979.

184. Seddon HJ: Nerve grafting. J Bone Joint Surg 45-B:447–461, 1963.

185. Slingluff CL, Terzis JK, and Edgerton MT: The quantitative microanatomy of the brachial plexus in man. Reconstructive relevance. In Terzis JK (ed): Microreconstruction of Nerve Injuries. Philadelphia: WB Saunders Co., 1987.

186. Spalteholz W: Hand Atlas of Human Anatomy, 9th ed. Philadelphia: JB Lippincott Co., 1943.

187. Strange FG St C: An operation for nerve pedicle grafting. Preliminary communication. Br J Surg 34:423, 425, 1947.

188. Strohm BR, and Colachis SC: Shoulder joint dysfunction following injury to the suprascapular nerve. Phys Ther 45:106–111, 1965.

189. Sunderland S: The anatomic foundation of peripheral nerve repair techniques. Orthop Clin North Am 12(2):245–266, 1981.

190. Sunderland S: The distribution of sympathetic fibers in the brachial plexus in man. Brain 71:88–102, 1948.

191. Sunderland S, and Bedbrook GM: The relative sympathetic contribution to individual roots of the brachial plexus in man. Brain 72:297–301, 1949.

192. Sunderland S, and Bedbrook GM: The cross sectional area of peripheral nerve trunks occupied by fibers representing individual muscular and cutaneous branches. Brain 72:613–624, 1949.

193. Sunderland SS, and Bradley KC: The cross-sectional area of peripheral nerve trunks devoted to nerve fibers. Brain 72:428–449, 1949.

194. Sunderland SS: Nerves and Nerve Injuries, 2nd ed. New York: Churchill Livingstone, 1978.

195. Tarlov IM, and Epstein JA: Nerve grafts: the importance of an adequate blood supply. J Neurosurg 2:49–71, 1945.

196. Telford ED, and Mottershead S: Pressure at the cervicobrachial junction: an operative and anatomical study. J Bone Joint Surg 30-B:249–265, 1948.

197. Terzis JK, and Breidenbach W: The anatomy of free vascularized nerve grafts. In Terzis JK (ed): Microreconstruction of Nerve Injuries. Philadelphia: WB Saunders Co., 1987.

198. Tsikaras PD, Agiabasis AS, and Hytiroglou PM: A variation in the formation of the brachial plexus characterized by the absence of C8 and T1 fibers in the trunk of the median nerve. Bull Assoc Anat 67:501–505, 1983.

199. Walsh JF: The anatomy of the brachial plexus. Am J Med Sci 74:387–399, 1887.

200. Williams HB, and Jabaley ME: The importance of internal anatomy of the peripheral nerves to nerve repair in the forearm and hand. Hand Clin 2(4):689–707, 1986.

201. Woollard HH, and Weddell G: The Composition and distribution of vascular nerves in the extremities. J Anat 69:165–176, 1935.

Blood Vessels

202. Buschmakin N: Die Lymphdrusen der Achselhohle, ihre Einteilung und Blutversorgung. Anat Anz 41:3–30, 1912.

203. Chepelenko GV: Lymphatic vessels of the upper extremity. Arkhiv Anat Gistol Embriol 89:74–81, 1985.

204. Danese C, and Howard JM: Postmastectomy lymphedema. Surg Gynecol Obstet 120:797–802, 1965.

205. Daseler EH, and Anson BJ: Surgical anatomy of the subclavian artery and its branches. Surg Gynecol Obstet 108:149–174, 1959.

206. DeBakey ME, and Simeon FA: Battle injuries of the arteries in World War II. Ann Surg 123:534–579, 1946.

207. De Garis CF, and Swartley WB: The axillary artery in white and Negro stocks. Am J Anat 41:353–397, 1928.

208. Ferguson LK, and Holt JH: Successful anastomosis of severed brachial artery. Am J Surg 79:344–347, 1950.

209. Gibson JMC: Rupture of the axillary artery. J Bone Joint Surg 44-B:114–115, 1962.

210. Huelke DF: Variation in the origins of the branches of the axillary artery. Anat Rec 135:33–41, 1959.

211. Huelke DF: A study of the transverse cervical and dorsal scapular arteries. Anat Rec 132:233, 1958.

212. Johnston GW, and Lowry JH: Rupture of the axillary artery complicating anterior dislocation of the shoulder. J Bone Joint Surg 44-B:116, 1962.

213. Kaplan T, and Katz A: Thrombosis of the axillary vein. Case report with comments on etiology, pathology and diagnosis. Am J Surg 37:326–333, 1937.

214. McKenzie AD, and Sinclair AM: Axillary artery occlusion complicating shoulder dislocation: a report of two cases. Ann Surg 148:139–141, 1958.

215. Neuhof H: Excision of the axillary vein in the radical operation for carcinoma of the breast. Ann Surg 108:15–20, 1938.

216. Nickalls RW: A new percutaneous infraclavicular approach to the axillary vein. Anaesthesia 42:151–154, 1987.

217. Palmer JH, and Taylor GI: The vascular territories of the anterior chest wall. Br J Plast Surg 39:287–299, 1986.

218. Perry MO: Vascular trauma. In Moore W (ed): Vascular Surgery. Orlando: Grune & Stratton, 1986.

219. Radke HM: Arterial circulation of the upper extremity. In Strandness DE Jr (ed): Collateral Circulation in Clinical Surgery. Philadelphia: WB Saunders, 1969, pp. 294–307.

220. Read WT, and Trotter M: The origins of transverse cervical and of transverse scapular arteries in American whites and Negroes. Am J Physiol Anthropol 28:239–247, 1941.

221. Reid CD, and Taylor GI: The vascular territory of the acromiothoracic axis. Br J Plast Surg 37:194–212, 1984.

222. Rich NM, Baugh JH, and Hughes CD: Acute arterial injury in Vietnam: 1000 cases. J Trauma *10*:359–369, 1970.
223. Rich NM, Hughes CD, and Baugh JH: Management of venous injuries. Ann Surg *171*:724–730, 1970.
224. Rich NM, Hobson RW II, and Collins GJ: Traumatic venous fistulas and false aneurysms. J Surg *78*:817–828, 1975.
225. Rich NM, and Spencer F: Vascular Trauma. Philadelphia: WB Saunders Company, 1978.
226. Rockwood CA: Keynote address to AAOS Summer Institute, San Diego, September 9, 1984.
227. Smith L, and Killeen JD: Surgical anatomy of the vascular system including related structures. *In* Moore W (ed): Vascular Surgery: A Comprehensive Review. Orlando: Grune & Stratton, 1986.
228. Strandness DE: Collateral Circulation in Clinical Surgery. Philadelphia: WB Saunders Co., 1969.
229. Strandness DE, Jr: Functional characteristics of normal and collateral circulation. *In* Strandness DE Jr (ed): Collateral Circulation in Clinical Surgery. Philadelphia: WB Saunders, 1969, pp. 2–25.
230. Taylor GI, and Palmer JH: The vascular territories (angiosomes) of the body: experimental study & clinical applications. Br J Plast Surg *40*:113–141, 1987.
231. Trotter M, Henderson JL, Gass H, Brua RS, et al: The origins of the branches of the axillary artery in whites and American Negroes. Anat Rec *46*:133–137, 1930.
232. Weathersby HT: The valves of the axillary, subclavian and internal jugular veins. Anat Rec *124*:379–380, 1956 (abstr.).

Spaces

233. Crandon JH: Infections of the hand. *In* Surgical Infectious Diseases. Simmons RL (ed). Norwalk, CT: Appleton & Lange, 1987.
234. Ellis VH: The diagnosis of shoulder lesions due to injuries of the rotator cuff. J Bone Joint Surg *35-B*:72–74, 1953.
235. Ellis H, and Feldman ST: Anatomy for Anesthetists, 3rd ed. Oxford: Blackwell Scientific Publications, 1977.
236. Enneking WF: Shoulder girdle. *In* Musculoskeletal Tumor Surgery. New York: Churchill Livingstone, 1983, pp. 355–410.
237. Evenepoel MC, and Blomme A: Interscalenic approach to the cervico-brachial plexus. Acta Anaesthesiol Belg *32*:317–322, 1981.
238. Gelberman RH: Upper extremity compartment syndromes: treatment. *In* Mubarak SJ, and Hargens AR (eds): Compartment Syndromes & Volkmann's Contracture. Philadelphia: WB Saunders Co., 1981, pp. 133–146.
239. Horwitz MT, and Tocantins LM: An anatomical study of the role of the long thoracic nerve and the related scapular bursae in the pathogenesis of local paralysis of the serratus anterior muscle. Anat Rec *71*:375–385, 1938a.
240. Mayou BJ, Whitby D, and Jones BM: The scapular flap. Br J Plast Surg *35*:8–13, 1982.
241. Moore DC, Bridenbaugh LD, and Eather KF: Block of the upper extremity: supraclavicular approach vs. axillary approach. Arch Surg *90*:68–72, 1965.
242. Smith DC, Mitchell D, Smith LL, Mera SS, et al: Anatomic considerations in neurologic injury following transaxillary angiography. Radiology, in press.
243. Strizak AM, Danzig L, Jackson DW, Greenway G, et al: Subacromial bursography. An anatomical and clinical study. J Bone Joint Surg *64*:196–201, 1982.
244. Thompson GE, and Rorie DK: Functional anatomy of the brachial plexus sheaths. Anesthesiol *59*:117–122, 1983.

Skin

245. Borges AF: The relaxed skin tension lines (RSTL) vs. other skin lines. Plast Reconstr Surg *73*:144–150, 1984.
246. Cormack GC, and Lamberty BGH: Classification of fasciocutaneous flaps according to their patterns of vascularisation. Br J Plast Surg *37*:80, 1984.
247. Courtiss EH, Longacre JJ, Destefano GA, Brizio L, et al: The placement of elective skin incisions. Plast Reconstr Surg *31*:31–44, 1963.
248. Hunter J: Quoted in Taylor GI, and Palmer JH: The vascular territories (angiosomes) of the body: experimental study and clinical applications. Br J Plast Surg *40*:113–141, 1987.
249. Kraissel CJ: Selection of appropriate lines for elective surgical incisions. Plast Reconstr Surg *8*:1–28, 1951.
250. Lamberty BGH, and Cormack GC: The forearm angiotomes. Br J Plast Surg *35*:420–429, 1982.
251. Langer K: On the anatomy and physiology of the skin: I. The cleavability of the skin. Br J Plast Surg *31*:3, 1978.
252. Langer K: On the anatomy and physiology of the skin: II. Skin tension. Br J Plast Surg *31*:93, 1978.
253. Leeson T, and Leeson CR: Histology, ed. 2. Philadelphia: WB Saunders, 1970.
254. McCormack LJ, Cauldwell EW, and Anson BJ: Brachial and antebrachial arterial patterns: a study of 750 extremities. Surg Gynecol Obstet *96*:43–54, 1953.
255. McGraw JV, Dibbell DG, and Carraway JH: Clinical definition of independent myocutaneous vascular territories. Plast Reconstr Surg *60*:341, 1977.
256. Nakajima H, Fujino T, and Adachi S: A new concept of vascular supply to the skin and classification of skin flaps according to their vascularization. Ann Plast Surg *16*:1–19, 1986.
257. Ortichocea M: The musculocutaneous flap: an immediate and heroic substitute for the method of delay. Br J Plast Surg *25*:106–110, 1972.
258. Ray RC: Force required for wound closure in scar appearance. Plast Reconstr Surg *72*:380–382, 1983.
259. Taylor GI: Personal Telephone Communication, September 1988.

Congenital Anomalies of the Shoulder

Virchel E. Wood, M.D.
Leonard Marchinski, M.D.

Congenital anomalies of the shoulder are rare. Because many shoulder anomalies are not clinically significant and do not cause great disability, they frequently go unnoticed by patient and doctor.

We classify these anomalies as bony, muscular, or neurovascular abnormalities. The outline below lists what we consider to be the important abnormalities of the shoulder.

I. Bony Abnormalities
   A. Clavicle
      1. Cleidocranial dysostosis
      2. Congenital pseudarthrosis
      3. Duplicated clavicle
      4. Middle suprascapular nerve foramina
   B. Scapula
      1. Sprengel's deformity
         a. Holt-Oram syndrome
      2. Ossified transverse scapular ligament
      3. Clasp-like cranial margin of the scapula
      4. Double acromion and coracoid processes
      5. Os acromiale (bipartite acromion)
      6. Coracoclavicular joint (or bar)
      7. Ligamentous or bony connecting bands
         a. Costocoracoid band
         b. Costocosternale vestigiale bone
         c. Costovertebral bone
      8. Infrascapular bone
      9. Notched inferior angle of the scapula
     10. Dentated glenoid
     11. Absent scapula
        a. Phocomelia
   C. Bone Abnormalities: Glenohumeral Dysplasia
      1. Humerus varus
      2. Humeral head retroversion
      3. Absent humeral head
      4. Glenoid hypoplasia
      5. Bicipital groove aberrations
      6. Congenital dislocation of the shoulder
II. Muscular Abnormalities
   A. Extra Muscles
      1. Axillopectoral muscle (Langer's axillary arch)
      2. Sternalis muscle
      3. Chondro-epitrochlear muscle
      4. Subscapularis-teres-latissimus muscle
      5. Coraco-claviculosternal muscle
   B. Fibrous contractures
      1. Deltoid muscle contracture
      2. Congenital fossa
   C. Absent Muscles
      1. Pectoralis major muscle defects
         a. Poland's syndrome
         b. Mobius' syndrome
      2. Congenital absence of the trapezius and rhomboideus
   D. Abnormal insertion of muscles
      1. Pectoralis minor insertion into the humeral head
      2. Multiple insertions of the coracobrachialis
III. Neurovascular Abnormalities Associated with Congenital Anomalies
   A. High median nerve compression
      1. Parsonage-Turner syndrome
   B. Dorsal scapular nerve compression
   C. Suprascapular nerve compression
   D. Thoracic outlet compression syndrome

Bony Abnormalities

THE CLAVICLE

Cleidocranial Dysostosis

Cleidocranial dysostosis involves malformation of the membranous and chondral portion of the clavicles, as well as abnormal cranial ossification. Marie and Sainton,[158] reporting on four patients, named this hereditary condition in 1898 and called attention to the associated irregularities in dentition, exaggerated transverse diameter of the skull, and the delayed ossification of the fontanels. Reports of clavicular defects appeared as early as 1760.[251] The first cases to be reported in the English literature, by Cutter,[53] were of a similarly affected father and daughter whose clavicles maintained the normal sternal articulation but were deficient in the outer scapular half. The condition may coexist with some more widespread anatomical errors as what has been termed "mutational dysostosis" by Soule,[235] Rhinehart,[203] Fitchet,[73] and others.

Inheritance

Soule and Fitchet found that about half of their cases occurred sporadically, while the remaining half were inherited as what usually appeared to be an autosomal dominant trait with variable expressivity. Other authors report that the condition can be transmitted through several generations, only to disappear or skip one or more generations, thus demonstrating variability in penetrance as well. Both sexes are equally affected.

Clinical Findings

In general, patients are of normal mentality and health, are slightly dwarfed and slender, and have long necks, drooped shoulders, and narrow chests.

Craniofacial Features. Perhaps the most striking feature of this condition is the appearance of the brachiocephalic head and facies. Characteristic are the enlarged transverse diameter of the skull and the marked frontal bosses separated by an open median gutter or "metopic" suture[50] (Fig. 3–1). The orbital ridges are prominent, but the inferior margins are shrunken into the small maxilla, which gives the face a flattened appearance and the jaw a relative prognathism. The palate is arched, and the eyes and ears are wide-spread. A myriad irregularities in dentition exist, including delayed or noneruption of deciduous and permanent teeth, cup-shaped teeth, double rows and crowding of teeth, and supernumerary teeth, to mention a few. Many patients require tooth extraction and dentures.

Clavicles. Many patients have reportedly gone through life, even working as manual laborers, unaware of any abnormality. Appearance can range from a kink or dimple in the skin with small defects, to the

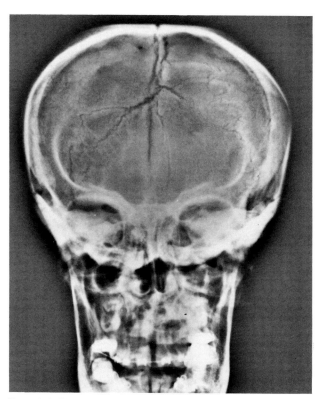

Figure 3–1. This patient with cleidocranial dysostosis shows the open median gutter or "metopic" suture.

ability voluntarily to bring both shoulders together anteriorly with large defects or absent clavicles. According to Stocks and Barrington,[239] the most common clavicular defect is the absence of the outer acromial end (Fig. 3–2). This is followed in frequency by the occurrence of two separate fragments, the sternal fragment usually being the larger (Fig. 3–3). The least common defect is the absence of the sternal end with an acromial end present. The missing segment may be represented in small defects by fibrous pseudarthrosis and in larger defects by a fibrous tether or cord. Bilaterality is the rule, with 82 to 90 per cent of cases so involved.[74, 239] As expected, there is usually an

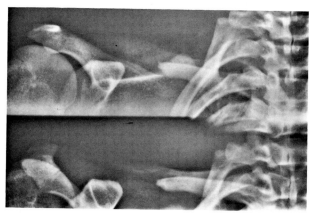

Figure 3–2. The most common clavicular defect in cleidocranial dysostosis is absence of the outer, acromial end. The sternal half is present.

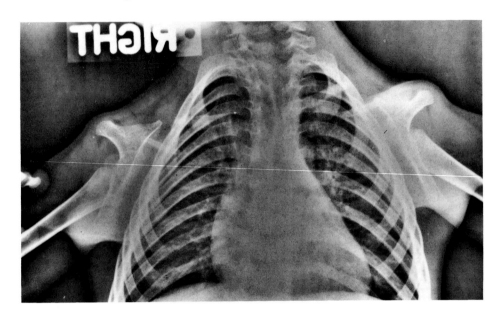

Figure 3–3. This patient with cleidocranial dysostosis shows two separate clavicular fragments, with the sternal fragment being the larger.

associated deficiency of the musculature,[74, 131] such that the more common outer clavicular defects are associated with the loss of the anterior deltoid and trapezius, while the less common sternal-end defects are associated with deficiency in the pectoralis major and sternocleidomastoid. No case of torticollis has been reported. The scapulae are usually small, high, and laterally placed, with deficiencies in the supraspinatus fossae and acromial facets when the outer half of the clavicle is absent.

Some authors have reported associated glenohumeral subluxation and dislocation,[69, 108] which are, on occasion, associated with subluxation of the radial heads and radial-ulnar synostoses.

Associated Abnormalities

Pelvis. The widened symphysis pubis was first described by Paltauf[185] in 1912, and the name "forme cleido cranio-pelvienne" was proposed for this deformity by Crouzon and Buttier.[50] Widening of several centimeters has been described in adults, although most commonly the widening results from a delay in ossification during young adulthood. The incidence of pelvic involvement is unclear, however, because the defect is not usually clinically apparent, and its diagnosis may not always have been sought. Widening of the sacroiliac joint has also been reported.[235]

Hips. Congenital or cervical coxavara has been found in up to 50 per cent of cases.[69] When present, it may contribute to the short stature of the patient.

Spine. Posterior spinal segmental defects with varying degrees of spinal dysraphism have been reported, with neurological involvement consisting of myelomeningocele and syringomyelia. Complete or partial absence of the sacrum and coccyx, as well as biconcave discs and biconvex vertebral bodies, has also been reported.

Hands and Feet. The most constant and peculiar associated abnormality is the presence of both proximal and distal epiphyses in the metacarpals and metatarsals, usually the second and fifth. The second metatarsal or metacarpal is involved prominently and, as expected, often leads to excessive growth and length. Poorly developed terminal phalanges, usually in the thumb or great toe, are common, and they give a tapered appearance to the digit. The middle and proximal phalanges, the tarsals, and carpal bones may be small and irregular.

Anatomical Pathology

Etiology. Although the cause of this condition is unknown, various theories have been put forth. Perhaps the earliest was that of Jansen[128] in 1921, who suggested that increased intrauterine and amniotic pressure was the cause. Other early reports also favored an agent extrinsic to bone, such as metabolic disturbances (e.g., rickets), thus characterizing the condition as a dystrophy. These theories have in general been abandoned in favor of one that centers on a defect intrinsic to the mesoderm or germ plasm as first suggested by Hultkrantz.[125] Such a defect leads to a faulty anlage in bone of both chondral and membranous origin and thus would represent a true dysostosis.

Embryology

The embryological and field development of the clavicle has received considerable attention.[70, 89, 90] The clavicle and mandible are the first bones to ossify in humans, and they do so like most membranous bones early in the embryonic period. The clavicle is first apparent at five weeks as a fibrocellular mesenchymal proliferation or blastema, stretching from the area of the future scapula toward the anterior midline. It is separate or discontinuous with the blastema of the upper limb and sternum. Intramembranous ossification begins as the proliferation of cells form an organic matrix that mineralizes on the connective tissue stroma to form bone that then grows as surrounding cells differentiate directly to osteoblasts. This process begins concurrently at five and a half weeks in two separate medial and lateral centers, the lateral center being more advanced. These two centers form a solid mass by six weeks. The mesenchymal cells at either end of the bone maintain their chondrogenic capacity and form a cellular hyaline-like cartilage, more noticeable at the sternal end. By six and a half weeks, cellular invasion of the solid clavicle differentiates into blood-forming and vascular elements, which form a marrow cavity with osteoblasts and osteoclasts. From seven weeks forward, the clavicle grows much like a long bone: by periosteal apposition, adding to its diameter, and by enchondral ossification at each end, adding to its length. The medial or sternal end contributes 80 per cent to the growth and length of the S-shaped clavicle. Throughout fetal development the cartilaginous ends are reduced to thin strips that vascularize and form a perichondrium, which becomes the articular facet. The sternal epiphyseal center appears in adolescence and fuses during the third decade, while the acromial epiphysis may occasionally appear during the second decade and fuse soon after its appearance.

Errors in the precursor cells that would lead to the absence of the medial or lateral ossification centers or to the failure of their union would thus explain the spectrum of clavicular defects present in cleidocranial dysostosis, as well as congenital pseudarthrosis of the clavicle.

Indications for Surgery

As mentioned above, many patients have gone through life as manual laborers unaware of any abnormality in their shoulder girdle. As well, no need has been found to recreate the strut mechanism between the upper limb and thorax.

Lewis and co-workers,[148] studying patients with isokinetic testing after *en bloc* excision of their clavicles, found subtle losses in torque production in flexion, abduction, and adduction. This may not be a fair comparison, however, as patients with the congenital condition frequently have associated muscular anomalies as outlined above. Surgical intervention is probably best reserved for patients in which excision of an offending clavicular segment would prevent interference with the underlying brachial plexus or subclavian vessels (Fig. 3–4), improve cosmesis, or prevent skin problems.

As a final note, the medical-legal aspects of this condition were first considered by Fitchet[73] in 1929 when he related "an unverified story stating that a man in England has capitalized on his deformity and makes a comfortable living by occasionally allowing his shoulder to be caught in the closing door of a public conveyance and then, with convincing x-ray evidence, collecting for his supposed injury." Fitchet noted this

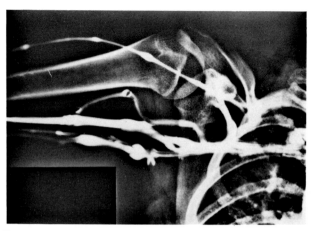

Figure 3–4. This segment of the clavicle interfered with the subclavian vein, causing thrombosis.

to be "at least worth remembering in these days of large damage and malpractice suits."

Congenital Pseudarthrosis

Congenital pseudarthrosis of the clavicle is a rare condition of unknown origins. Fitzwilliams[74] in 1910 and Saint-Pierre[218] in 1930 have been credited with first describing it as an entity distinct from birth fracture, cleidocranial dysostosis, and post-traumatic pseudarthrosis. Although fewer than 60 cases have been reported, a careful review of the literature discloses the possibility that in some series a few cases may have been misreported or misrepresented. For example, Alldred,[3] in a description of nine patients, reported a child "reluctant to move the arm after birth and with inability to push on the arm. This was attributable to the exceptional mobility of the pseudarthrosis." Perhaps this may actually have been a birth fracture. Kite,[136] describing eight patients with congenital pseudarthroses, revealed that in two "there was a normally formed clavicle which was fractured by slight trauma resulting in non union."

Clinical Findings

Congenital pseudarthrosis of the clavicle presents as a painless, nontender, mid-clavicular mass usually noted incidentally, by a parent while bathing the child, or from a routine chest x-ray. The absence of trauma, associated craniofacial anomalies, and cafe-au-lait spots differentiate it from birth fracture, cleidocranial dysostosis, and von Recklinghausen's disease, respectively.[31]

The right side is exclusively involved almost invariably (Fig. 3–5). We feel that cases of complete absence and bilateral involvement, such as described by Herman,[117] are most likely a different condition. Perhaps these cases represent the variable expressivity of cleidocranial dysostosis. Besides the cosmetic defects, most authors have agreed that the great majority of

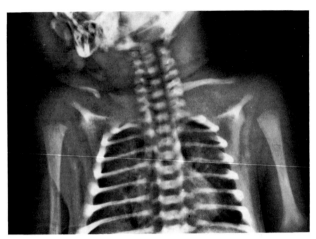

Figure 3–5. The right side is involved almost exclusively in congenital pseudarthrosis of the clavicle, except in dextrocardia.

patients are asymptomatic. The unusual patient who is symptomatic is one whose daily activities or endeavors place high demand on the shoulder in lifting and throwing, such that weakness is a complaint, as is occasional activity-related soreness. The palpable bump is the larger anterosuperiorly displaced sternal fragment that overlaps the posteroinferiorly displaced acromial fragment at the area of pseudarthrosis. This overlap classically occurs at the lateral margin of the middle third of the clavicle. When prominent, it has been described by Owen[184] as a "lanceolate deformity."

Inheritance

There is general agreement that congenital pseudarthrosis of the clavicle is not a genetic disorder.[110] However, one family with several children so affected has been reported.[130]

Associated Abnormalities

Associated skeletal abnormalities, when present, should cause one to think of cleidocranial dysostosis or mutational dysostosis as the underlying condition.[235]

Anatomical Pathology

As described by Jinkins,[130] Alldred,[3] and others,[31] the ends of the clavicle at the pseudarthrosis are smooth and capped by hyaline cartilage. Owen[184] has clearly demonstrated a diarthrodial joint in his dissections. This joint is unlike the fibrous union or cords found in cleidocranial dysostosis and lacks the exuberant callous evident radiographically and clinically with post-traumatic pseudarthrosis. Not found is the tapering or "sucked candy" appearance (Fig. 3–6) that is found in von Recklinghausen's neurofibromatosis.[2]

Embryology

The cause of this condition is unknown. It seems possible that at six weeks gestation, a local, humeral,

or mechanical factor may stop the two ossification centers from uniting.[89] The most plausible explanation is offered by Lloyd-Roberts and coworkers[151] who proposed that the pulsations of the more superior right subclavian artery cause a gradual attrition of the clavicle where the two ossification centers should coalesce. This portion of the clavicle is normally the thinnest, to accommodate the underlying great vessels as they pass between it and the first rib, theoretically making it weaker. Lending support to this explanation is the involvement of the left side in dextrocardia, as reported by Gibson and Carroll.[95]

Incidence

The incidence of congenital pseudarthrosis of the clavicle is difficult to ascertain, however, from fewer than 60 reported cases. In contrast, postfracture pseudarthrosis occurs in 4.6 per cent of clavicular fractures.

Indications for Surgery

Despite the established benign natural history of this condition and its lack of functional impairment, several authors have unilaterally proposed excision, bone grafting, and external fixation in all children under eight years of age.[3, 159, 184] Others[259] have advocated conservative management of this condition in boys, while recommending excision and bone grafting in adolescent girls for cosmesis. Nogi and colleagues[178] have excised the acromial fragment and stabilized the sternal fragment with the Weaver Dunn procedure.[260]

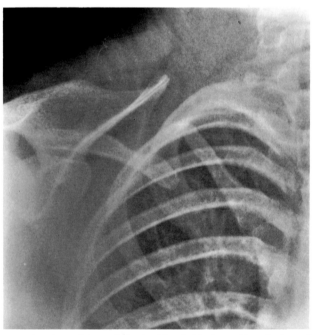

Figure 3–6. Congenital pseudarthrosis of the clavicle does not have the tapered or "sucked candy" appearance that is seen in von Recklinghausen's neurofibromatosis.

Authors' Preferred Method

We feel that surgery is best reserved for patients with a prominent deformity that causes problems with the overlying skin or is of itself cosmetically unacceptable to the patient. A direct approach, with subperiosteal dissection, excision of fibrous or cartilaginous tissue, followed by iliac corticocancellous bone grafting and internal fixation, is optimum for defects of up to 4 cm. Defects larger than 4 cm can be resected with little functional loss.

Duplicated Clavicle

Duplication of the clavicle or "os subclaviculare," is an extremely rare abnormality. It has been described only once in the literature.[97] The patient described a small painless nodule just below the left clavicle. A subcutaneous structure, which was freely movable with movements of the shoulder, was palpable. The overlying skin was somewhat elevated. Roentgenograms showed a dense osseous body approximately 7 cm by 1 cm under the normal left clavicle, which it closely resembled. The lateral end of the bone was rounded and was attached to the coracoid process of the left scapula (Fig. 3–7). The medial end did not have a bony connection, although under fluoroscopy it was found to be fixed to the coracoid process.

Embryology

The clavicle develops from a membranous connective tissue rod. At about the sixth week of intrauterine life, the rod usually has two ossification centers. If these centers do not fuse, a defective clavicle consisting of two parts results. The duplicate clavicle may result when one of the centers becomes displaced *in utero*, producing a completely separate clavicle, or perhaps

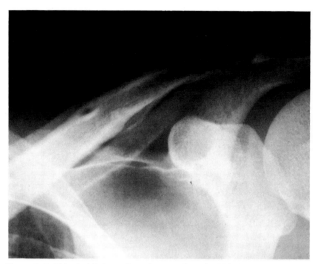

Figure 3–8. This clavicle has a large foramen through which the middle supraclavicular nerve passes.

the patient developed with two ossification centers, one of which formed the extra bone.

Treatment

This particular anomaly had no clinical significance;[161] therefore, treatment was not necessary.

Middle Supraclavicular Nerve Foramina

The middle supraclavicular nerve[138] exits through the center of the clavicle. (The clavicle is one of the few bones through which a significant large nerve travels.[231])

Figure 3–8 shows a large foramen in a clavicle through which the middle supraclavicular nerve passes. Figure 3–9 shows the path of the nerve in the neck. Any abnormality about the neck, such as a fracture, increased rotation of the clavicle, or displacement of the clavicle, can put traction on the middle supraclavicular nerve and cause neck pain.

Clinically, people with this condition have a vague discomfort about the neck. The treatment obviously would be to remove the nerve from its bony imprisonment, but we have never found this to be necessary.

THE SCAPULA

Sprengel's Deformity

No discussion of this deformity would be complete without mentioning that it would be more accurately named "Eulenburg's deformity." Indeed, Eulenburg's[66, 67, 68] first descriptions in 1863 of three cases, as well as Willet's and Walsham's[266, 267] anatomical dissection and therapeutic omovertebral bone excision in 1880 and 1883, antedate Sprengel's four cases in 1891 by several years. Kolliker[139] in 1891, reporting two cases later in the same year and in the same journal,

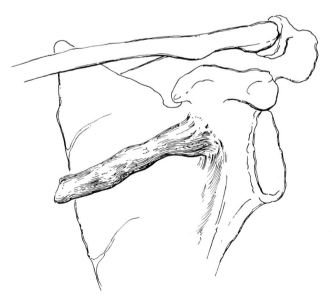

Figure 3–7. Duplication of the clavicle is an extremely rare abnormality. The lateral end of the extra clavicle attaches to the base of the coracoid process.

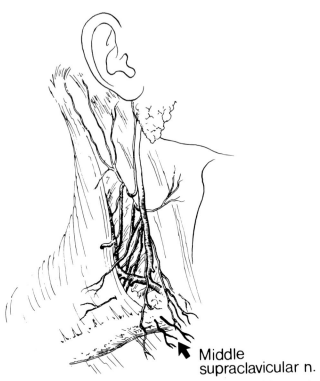

Figure 3–9. The middle supraclavicular nerve penetrates the clavicle to supply sensation to the lower neck area.

referenced Sprengel's[237] notable article in which Sprengel denied an awareness of previous descriptions of the deformity. It was in Kolliker's report that Sprengel was credited with the somewhat undeserved eponymous memorial.

Nevertheless, Sprengel, unlike those who preceded him, recognized that the deformity was caused by the failure of the scapula to descend. Subsequent reports[64, 123, 129, 196] called attention to associated anomalies, proposed corrective techniques, and advanced explanations on pathogenesis.

Clinical Findings

The varied clinical presentation of the patient with Sprengel's deformity is a composite of the deformities produced by the undescended scapula and the associated cervicothoracic abnormalities that are almost always present. For this reason, as Cavendish[34] has pointed out, the same scapular deformity, even when bilateral, "may vary widely in ugliness."

The primary "deformity" is cosmetic (Fig. 3–10). The prominent lump in the web of the apparently short neck is noted in infancy or early childhood by the parents. Occasionally, decreased abduction is observed as the child is listing when reaching forward and upward. The prominence may be masked by contralateral thoracic scoliosis or exaggerated by an ipsilateral curve. Brevicollis that accompanies the often-associated Klippel-Feil syndrome also exaggerates the deformity. Clearly, one might best think of the condition as

a deformity of the cervicothoracic spine and shoulder girdle.[86]

In its failure to descend, the scapula remains high on the posterior chest wall. Usually hypoplastic and equilaterally triangular in shape, the scapula is rotated, such that the inferior pole abuts the thoracic spinous processes, while the prominent superomedial angle curves anteriorly over the chest in the supraclavicular region. The clavicle is usually straight; its impetus to curve to accommodate the great vessels and plexus is absent without scapular descent. (The shape of the scapula is important in relocation procedures.) An omovertebral connection is present in up to 50 per cent of patients and is palpable as a chondro-osseous bar, rather than as a fibrous cord, in 20 to 30 per cent of all patients. Scapulothoracic motion is further limited by fibrous bands beneath the subscapularis, associated muscular deficiencies, scapulospinous abutment at the inferior angle, and binding of the curved superior angle over the chest.

Although glenohumeral motion is normal, the medial scapular rotation faces the glenoid downward (Fig. 3–11), such that the normal arc of abduction is similarly rotated and thus not fully available. Scapular relocation procedures can therefore be expected to improve both scapulothoracic and glenohumeral abduction.

Inheritance

Usually arising sporadically, the deformity is occasionally inherited as an autosomal dominant trait. Several familial cases have been reported. A consistent 3:1 male predominance exists. Shoulders are involved with equal incidence, and bilateral cases have been

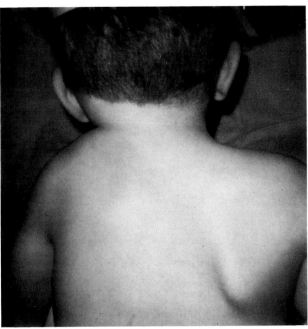

Figure 3–10. Congenital elevation of the scapula (Sprengel's deformity) is primarily a cosmetic deformity, giving the appearance of a short neck.

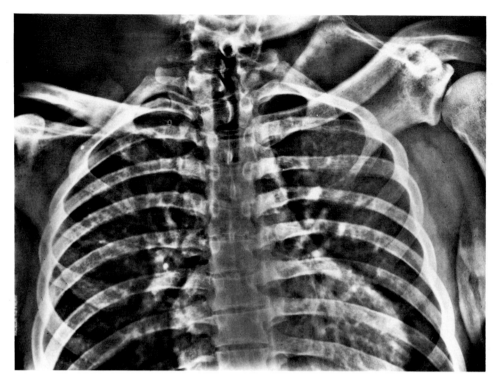

Figure 3–11. In Sprengel's deformity, medial scapular rotation forces the glenoid downward so that the normal arc of abduction is not fully available.

reported by Blair[17] and Ross.[214] Although an exact incidence is not reported, it is generally agreed that Sprengel's deformity is the most common congenital anomaly of the shoulder.

Associated Anomalies

Associated musculoskeletal abnormalities are the rule in Sprengel's deformity, occurring in from 67 to 100 per cent of the series reported.[32, 34, 107, 123, 190] In our review of the literature (Table 3–1), associated abnormalities occur in 95 per cent of patients. Scoliosis is found in nearly half (47 per cent) of the patients, with congenital scoliosis accounting for 31 per cent and idiopathic scoliosis for 16 per cent. Rib abnormalities,

including synostosis, absence, duplication, and cervical ribs, followed at 38 per cent. Klippel-Feil syndrome (Fig. 3–12) was found in 29 per cent, spina bifida in 19 per cent and diastematomyelia[8] in 3 per cent. A multitude of other abnormalities is found, including but not limited to congenital dislocated hip, talipes equinovarus, pes planus, radial club hand, congenital dislocation of the radial head, symbrachydactylia, congenital heart disease, situs inversus viscerum, absent thumb, tethered cord, and atlantoaxial instability.

The most common serious systemic condition results from renal abnormalities, with absent and ectopic kidneys reported in up to six per cent of patients. Muscular abnormalities are relatively common, occurring in 14 per cent of Cavendish's series; however, he

Table 3–1. ABNORMALITIES ASSOCIATED WITH CONGENITAL ELEVATION OF THE SCAPULA (SPRENGEL'S DEFORMITY)

Abnormalities	Author (Total Patients)				Total All Series (179)	Per Cent
	Cavendish (100)	Grogan (20)	Carson (11)	Pinsky (48)		
Scoliosis { Idiopathic	23	1	3	—	27	16
Scoliosis { Congenital	16	8	4	25	53	31
Spinal dysraphism	28	1	3	—	32	19
Diastematomyelia	3	2	—	—	5	3
Klippel-Feil syndrome	20	9	2	18	49	29
Rib cage	25	9	6	24	64	38
Muscular	14	—	1	—	15	9
CDH	1	2	—	—	3	2
Hand	4	1	1	—	6	4
Foot	6	—	—	—	6	4
Renal	0	—	2	8	10	6
Total assoc. anomalies	98	20	11	41	170	

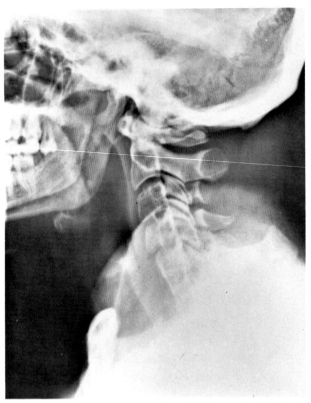

Figure 3–12. The Klippel-Feil syndrome is found in 29 per cent of children with Sprengel's deformity.

states that they were present less obviously in more patients. The most common abnormalities were the absence or hypoplasia of the pectoralis major, trapezius, rhomboids, serratus anterior, and latissimus dorsi. Shortening of the levator scapulae is inherent to the deformity.

These associated conditions are of great clinical significance for several reasons: (1) Parents and patients must be made aware of the deformities that will remain unchanged after surgical correction of the undescended scapula (such as scoliosis with Klippel-Feil syndrome) so that their expectations are realistic. (2) Tethered cord and diastematomyelia should be ruled out prior to considering scoliosis surgery. (3) Ipsilateral rib cage abnormalities may predispose these patients to thoracic outlet syndromes with scapular replantation. (4) Midline dissection should be avoided in patients with thoracic spinal dysraphism. (5) Prior to surgery renal status should be evaluated with ultrasonography, if not intravenous pyelography, because of the high incidence of associated renal abnormalities.

Anatomical Pathology

At about five weeks the fetal scapula begins to differentiate from the fourth, fifth, and sixth cervical vertebrae. By six weeks, the acromion and coracoid are recognizable as condensations of mesenchyme. The body of the scapula is precartilage and is continuous

with the bases of the acromion and coracoid. The acromion and coracoid are consistently larger than the body of the scapula, with the acromion being the larger of the two processes. By the end of the sixth week, the scapular neck can be identified, and the perichondrium has formed from tissues adjacent to the scapula. Early in the seventh week the coracoid is hook-shaped, and by the end of this week, the scapular contour resembles that of the adult. Ossification begins by the eighth week. The scapular neck is ossified at the 28-mm stage, the body and spine by 37 mm, and the base of the acromion at 60 mm. Between the 9th and 12th weeks, caudal migration to a position opposite T2 and T7 occurs. At term, the scapula is largely osseous, with only the coracoid, glenoid, vertebral border, and inferior angle remaining cartilaginous. As development proceeds, the horizontal width decreases until it is exceeded by the vertical height. By 25 years, 7 or more ossification nuclei are united. At 10 years, a subcoracoid nucleus appears to become part of the coracoid base and upper glenoid. At 15 years, one of the two acromial tip nuclei appear as the vertebral border and inferior angle ossify. The inferior glenoid center appears near puberty, and, with its growth, the volume of the glenoid fossa increases. The two remaining nuclei appear at the angle and on the tip of the coracoid.

Sprengel's deformity results from impediment of normal scapular descent and subsequent abnormal development of the bone itself, together with its surrounding musculature.

In half the patients, an omovertebral connection exists between the spinous process, lamina, or transverse process of the lower cervical spine, usually C6, and the superomedial angle of the scapula[161] (Fig. 3–13). The connection is a chondro-osseous bar (called the omovertebral bone) in 20 per cent of patients according to Cavendish[34] and in 30 per cent according to Jeannopoulos.[129] The morphology of this bone is variable, having been shown to have diarthrodial joints, cartilaginous connections, fibrous bands, and solid bony unions at either or both ends (Fig. 3–14).

Hypotheses on the origin of the omovertebral bone are as varied as its morphology. Willet and Walsham[17, 19, 266] in 1883 suggested that it represented a maldeveloped epiphysis from the vertebral border of the scapula or from the vertebrae, analogous to the suprascapular bone in the thornback skate. These same authors also theorized that it might represent an ossified intermuscular plane. Accessory ossicles have similarly been described in the levator scapulae mechanism.[85]

Horwitz[123] first proposed an environmental cause for the failure of descent, citing increased intrauterine pressure with oligo- or polyhydramnios. As well, he postulated the omovertebral connection and deficient musculature to be causative. Engel,[64] in the "bleb" theory as described by Weed,[261] suggested that the cause of the deformity was in the embryo itself. In the bleb theory, the abnormal permeability of the roof of the fourth ventricle permits cerebrospinal fluid to es-

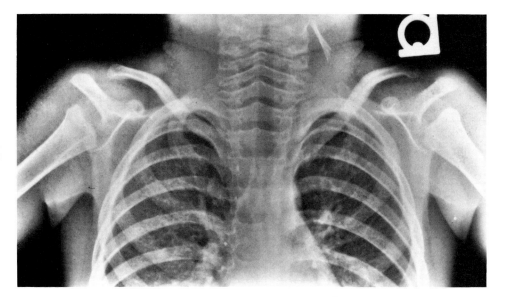

Figure 3–13. On the left side of this patient, an omovertebral bone connects the transverse process of the lower cervical spine of C6 with the superomedial angle of the scapula.

cape into the subcutis, forming "blebs" of "jelly-blood." Bonnevie[19] described a gene responsible for the "blebs," and Bagg[7] reproduced a similar deformity in mouse tribes using irradiation. The blebs, through their travel from the spine to the shoulder and upper limb bud, can thus exert their deleterious effect on the mesoderm, leading to spinal dysraphism, Klippel-Feil syndrome, scoliosis, Arnold-Chiari malformation, Sprengel's deformity, and symbrachydactylia. The theory also explains the anomalies commonly associated with the deformity.

Indications for Surgery

Cavendish,[34] discussing the surgical indications of the deformity, stated that "appearance is the usual indication for treatment and the yardstick of its success." He formulated the most commonly used grading system for the deformity on the basis of appearance. Grade I deformities are very mild. The shoulder joints are level, and the deformity is invisible or almost so when the patient is dressed. Grade II deformities are mild. Although the shoulder joints are level, or almost level, in the dressed patient the deformity is visible as a lump in the web of the neck. In Grade III, or moderate deformities, the shoulder joint is elevated 2 to 5 cm, and the deformity is easily visible. Grade IV deformities are severe. The shoulder is so elevated that the superior angle of the scapula is near the occiput, with or without neck webbing or brevicollis. Cavendish recommended that Grades II, III, and IV be treated surgically.

Carson[32] suggested that improving the function of the neck and shoulder was also an objective.

Conservative treatment has its proponents. Mercer and Duthie[163] have outlined programs that include exercises, passive stretching, and encouragement to use the unaffected shoulder. Tachdjian[248] recommended passive and active abduction of the shoulder, scapular depression and adduction, dorsal hyperextension, tra-peze hanging, and push-ups. However, exercise is of limited value in correcting a structural problem such as this. Another conservative measure is to pad the contralateral shoulder to improve symmetry when dressed.

Operations may release, resect, or relocate the scapula. Although most authors agree that the ideal surgical candidate for scapular relocation is a child between 3 and 8 years old with moderate to severe deformity, surgical correction in patients as young as 18 months and as old as 15 years has been reported. Surgery on children younger than 2 years of age is technically demanding, secondary to inherent difficulty with dissection. However, in general, early operative interven-

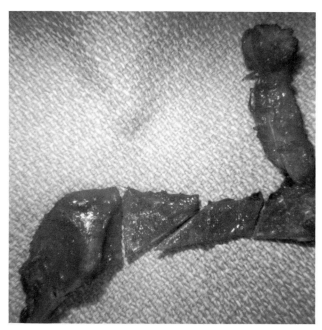

Figure 3–14. The omovertebral bone can have a diarthrodial joint, cartilaginous connections, fibrous bands, or solid bony unions at either or both ends.

tion in the more severe deformity gives the best results. Older patients with severe, fixed deformities are best served by more limited resection of the prominent superomedial angle.

As alluded to above, preoperative evaluation should include a thorough history and physical examination and a radiographic evaluation of the cervical and thoracolumbar spine, as well as renal ultrasound or intravenous pyelogram to rule out associated abnormalities. Evaluation of both shoulders should include measurements of combined glenohumeral and scapulothoracic abduction and standing anteroposterior and lateral x-rays.

Surgical Procedures

In addition to a simple excision of the omovertebral bone and superomedial angle of the scapula, we found 10 named surgical procedures for Sprengel's deformity. Below, we briefly mention those of historical merit and describe in detail those that we feel to be most clinically useful.

Excision of the omovertebral bone was first performed by Eulenburg in 1863. In 1888, McBurney[160] added conservative resection of the superomedial angle of the scapula (also advocated by Cavendish in 1972). In 1908, Putti[196] described detaching the rhomboids and trapezius insertions, omovertebral resection, relocating the scapula, and fixing the inferior angle to a lower rib. In 1926, Shrock[225, 226] modified Putti's procedure by subperiosteally resecting the combined attachments of the rhomboids and serratus anterior, as well as infraspinatus, supraspinatus, and teres major and minor, and by completely freeing the inferior angle and the lower two-thirds of the axillary border. If the shoulder then cannot be freely brought down, an osteotomy at the base of the acromion is done. The inferior angle is anchored to the lowest rib possible with heavy chromic sutures. Ober's modification, as described by Inclan[126] in 1949, used skeletal traction with a less aggressive subperiosteal dissection as a first stage, followed by soft tissue fixation of the inferior angle when the desired level was obtained.

Jeannopoulos[129] in 1952 reported a follow-up study of the Shrock procedure. He found that excessive subperiosteal stripping was ill-advised and felt it was responsible for winging of the scapula, regeneration of the resected portion, and scapulothoracic binding and scarring. Green[105] in 1957 described a procedure in which an extraperiosteal resection of the supraspinous scapula and omovertebral bone was performed along with the detachment of the insertions of the trapezius, rhomboid, levator scapulae, and latissimus from the scapula. The inferior angle is buried under the latissimus as described by Konig in 1914.[140] A three-pound spring traction wire on the scapular spine is then attached to a spica cast to achieve the desired level. The Woodward procedure,[273] discussed in detail below, was novel in its midline approach, which avoided unsightly keloid scars, and in its relocation of muscular origins, which avoided periscapular dissection and scarring.

Robinson[205] in 1967 described morcellation of the clavicle before relocation to avoid postoperative brachial plexus palsy. This procedure is now widely accepted as an adjunct to any replantation technique. Petrie[189] in 1973 noted that an osteotomy through the coracoid would allow better caudal mobilization of the scapula. Wilkinson[265] in 1980 reported on vertical displacement osteotomy at the vertebral border of the scapula, finding it to be reliable and safe.

Complications of surgical correction include unsightly keloid scars, winging of the scapula, regeneration of the superomedial angle, and brachial plexus palsy. The latter is best avoided by clavicular osteotomy and by avoiding overenthusiasm for caudal displacement. The glenohumeral joints or scapular spines, and not the inferior angles of the scapula, should be leveled for this reason (Fig. 3–15).

In a retrospective study of 77 patients, Ross and Cruess[214] found that the Woodward and Green procedures provided the most abduction at 143 degrees and 146 degrees, respectively, as opposed to the 124 degrees and 129 degrees provided by the Petrie and Shrock procedures. The Woodward procedure was also the most successful in lowering the scapula, leaving only an average of 0.8 cm residual elevation as compared with 1.8 cm, 2 cm, and 2 cm for the Green, Petrie, and Shrock procedures, respectively. In most series, 2 to 3 cm of scapular lowering was obtained, varying by the method of measurement. Carson and colleagues[32] reported an average lowering of 1.6 cm with the Woodward procedure, using the inferomedial angle as reference. Grogan and co-workers[107] reported an average scapular lowering of 2 cm using the "centrum, the mid-point of a line from the inferior to the superomedial angle, as reference."

Authors' Preferred Method

For Grade I deformities, we recommend no treatment. For Grade II and III deformities, we prefer the Woodward procedure with clavicular morcellation as described by Robinson and colleagues, ideally in children 3 to 8 years old. We recommend resecting the superomedial angle and omovertebral bone in older patients. For Grade IV deformities, we recommend the Woodward procedure with clavicular osteotomy in children under 6 years of age and resection of the superomedial angle and omovertebral bone in older children.

The Woodward Procedure. The patient is placed in lateral decubitus position with the entire arm and shoulder girdle included in the operative field. A subperiosteal exposure of the clavicle can be developed through a transverse incision above the middle third. A segment approximately 2 cm long is removed at the midportion, morcellized, then replaced in the periosteal tube, which is carefully repaired and the skin closed. The patient is then rolled into the prone

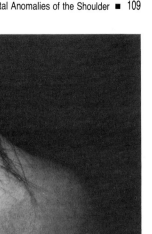

Figure 3–15. At surgery, the glenohumeral joints or scapular spines—not the inferior angles of the scapula—should be leveled.

position without redraping. The head is supported on a craniotomy headrest with the neck slightly flexed. A midline incision is then made from the C4 spinous processes to the T9 spinous process (Fig. 3–16A). The skin and subcutaneous tissues are undermined on the involved side out to the vertebral border of the scapula to allow better visualization of the musculature and to allow scapular lowering without skin tension. The lateral border of the distal trapezius is identified and should be bluntly separated from the latissimus dorsi. The origin of the trapezius is then sharply dissected from the spinous processes. The origins of the rhomboids major and minor are identified and divided. The rhomboids and the upper portion of the trapezius are separated from the serratus posterior superiorly and the sacrospinalis by the deep fascial layer. This tissue plane must be gained, as the intact aponeurosis is essential for scapular fixation (Fig. 3–16B). When this fascial layer has been removed from the spinous processes to the upper limits of the exposure, the sheet of musculature can be retracted laterally to expose the omovertebral connection, when present.

When removing an omovertebral bone, it is best to do so extraperiosteally. A bone-biting rongeur can be used to remove the bone from the scapular angle and from its connection to the cervical spine. The spinal accessory nerve on the undersurface of the trapezius and along the vertebral border of the scapula must be protected, especially when removing the omovertebral bone. The transverse cervical artery must also be protected during the dissection. The supraspinous portion of the scapula should be removed extraperiosteally when its anterior curvature limits downward caudal mobilization or when it remains as a prominence after the scapula is relocated. The shoulder girdle and combined trapezius and rhomboid muscular sheet are then

moved caudally until the spine of the scapula on the affected side comes down to the same level as the scapular spine on the uninvolved shoulder. Lowering the inferior angle to the level on the normal side is overcorrection and should be avoided.

While maintaining the position of the scapula (Fig. 3–16C), reattach the aponeurosis of the trapezius and rhomboids. The redundant tissue of the trapezius and aponeurosis is folded over and sutured in a pants-over-vest fashion. The skin and subcutaneous tissue should be closed meticulously to minimize the spreading of the scar in the superior aspect of the incision. A Velpeau bandage is then applied and worn for approximately two weeks.

Holt-Oram Syndrome

Holt and Oram[122] in 1960 reported four cases of congenital heart disease and associated skeletal malformations through four generations of a family. Their report was interesting from several perspectives. The usual inheritance for congenital heart disease is autosomal recessive with incomplete penetrance, while the reported cases were autosomal dominant. All the patients had atrial fibrillation with an atrioventricular conduction block, pulmonary hypertension, atrial septal defect, and hypoplastic peripheral vasculature. Three patients had bilateral, hypoplastic, finger-like triphalangeal thumbs with long slender carpal bones and first and second metacarpals. The left side was usually more severely involved. The fourth patient had dorsal kyphosis, sternal depression, and what was called Sprengel's deformity. X-ray evidence and a detailed description of the shoulder malformation were not presented.

Since the original 1960 report, the term Holt-Oram

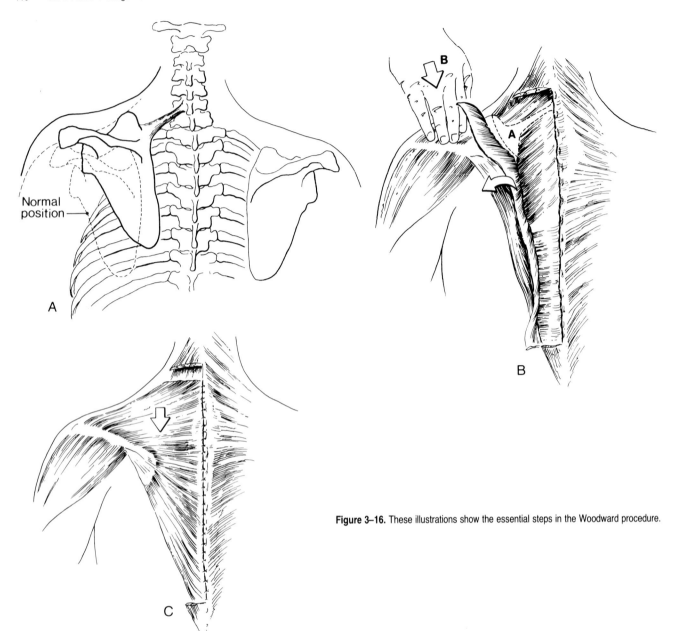

Figure 3–16. These illustrations show the essential steps in the Woodward procedure.

syndrome has been used to describe virtually any familially transmitted association of congenital heart disease (including ventricular septal defect, atrial septal defect, patent ductus, and tetralogy) in association with upper limb malformations.[121]

Clinical Findings

The most consistent shoulder anomaly is a prominent but hypoplastic and rotated scapula.[195] Patients have apparent forward sloping shoulders and difficulty with abduction.[93] Clavicular abnormalities are the next most common defect, with the clavicles having broad ends and coracoclavicular articulations. Described less frequently are deformity of the humeral head and prominent deltoid ridges, which occur in 25 per cent of cases. Os acromiale and os coracoidale have also been reported.[35, 195]

Inheritance

As mentioned, Holt-Oram syndrome is a familial condition with mendelian dominant inheritance, although sporadic cases[84] have been reported.

Incidence

Although the incidence is uncertain, musculoskeletal anomalies are the most common extracardiac anomalies associated with congenital heart disease.[264] They occur in up to 20 per cent of cases. The fingers are involved far more often than any other part.[94, 157]

Embryology

The limb bud appears in the fourth week of gestation at the same time the primitive heart tube differentiates.

In two to three weeks, the upper and lower limbs develop simultaneously with the heart. It is thought that the preferential involvement of the upper limbs occurs because they appear first and complete their development in advance of the lower limbs. The close temporal relationship in the development of the limbs, heart, and eyes supports the association of Holt-Oram syndrome with Duane's syndrome, or abducens palsy.[71]

Surgical Procedures and Indications

The indications for surgery are those outlined for Sprengel's deformity, assuming the cardiovascular status of the patient is satisfactory.

Ossified Transverse Scapular Ligament

The transverse scapular ligament may ossify.[161, 162] The suprascapular nerve passes through the scapular notch, which is sometimes converted into a foramen by ossification of the ligament. This condition can cause nerve entrapment from the hard, firm edges of the foramina and is discussed under suprascapular nerve compression.

Clasp-like Cranial Margin of the Scapula

Kohler,[138] in *Borderlands of Roentgenology,* coined the name for this anomaly of the superior scapular border because it resembles a clasp or handle. The anomaly was first described by Birkner.[16] There are no pathological clinical findings, other than that it is a congenital anomaly noted by radiologists[161] (Fig. 3–17).

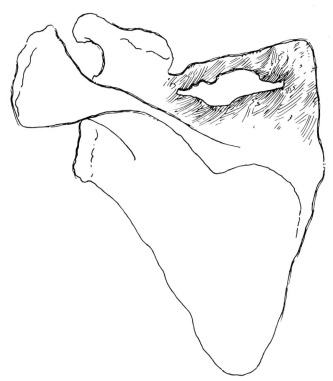

Figure 3–17. The clasp-like handle of the cranial margin of the scapula is seen.

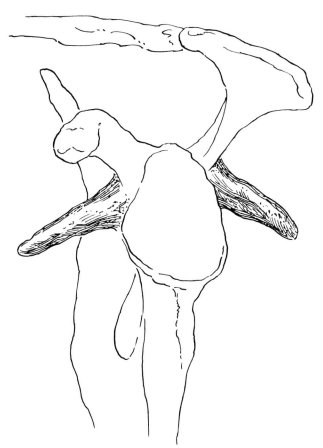

Figure 3–18. Double acromion and coracoid processes shown here have been identified only once, by McClure and Raney.[162]

Double Acromion and Coracoid Processes

This anomaly, described by McClure and Raney[162] in 1974, occurred in the left shoulder of a man who stated that the deformity had prevented him from becoming active in athletics but had not interfered with any of his duties as an engineer. Roentgenograms showed that he had a double acromion and a double coracoid process. No similar case has ever been identified.

The upper acromium seemed to articulate and was essentially within the normal relationship with the clavicle at the acromioclavicular joint, while the lower acromion had an essentially normal relationship with the humerus at the glenohumeral joint (Fig. 3–18). The eighth and ninth ribs were fused in the lateral and anterior portions.

A great deal of discussion concerning embryological aspects evolved from this case. This patient's scapular anomaly apparently was simply an ontogenetic mishap; no other conclusions could be drawn as to why this happened embryologically.

Os Acromiale (Bipartite Acromion)

Nonunion of one or more of the three ossification centers of the acromion to the rest of the scapula has been studied by several authors.[40, 137] This lack of fusion

Variations of OS Acromiale

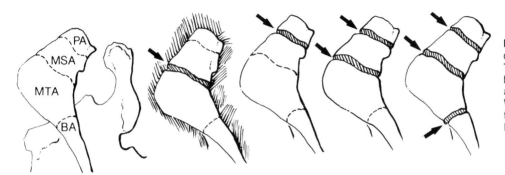

Figure 3-19. There are three separate ossification centers for the os acromiale. The most common site of nonunion is between the meso-acromion and meta-acromion. (Reproduced from Mudge MK, Wood VE, and Frykman GK: Rotator cuff tears associated with os acromiale. J Bone Joint Surg 66A:427-429, 1984.)

PA = Pre - Acromion   MTA = Met - Acromion
MSA = Mes - Acromion   BA = Basi - Acromion

of the epiphyseal centers has produced roentgenographic anomalies that have been called by many different names such as os acromiale, bipartite acromion, or meta-acromion.

Clinical Findings

Usually nonunion is regarded as an incidental finding not associated with any disability, but we have seen several patients with full-thickness rotator cuff tears who had this anomaly.[171] Therefore, we feel that nonunion contributes to an impingement mechanism that eventually involves the rotator cuff. The failure of the epiphyses to fuse has sometimes been confused with a fracture of the acromion.[150, 223] The anomaly does not seem to be inherited, and there are no associated abnormalities.

Anatomical Pathology

There are usually three separate ossification centers for the os acromion[76] (Fig. 3-19). At birth the anterior two-thirds of the acromion is pure cartilage. About the 15th or 16th year, ossification centers begin to appear anteriorly, and usually by the 25th year, fusion is complete.[176] Investigations in cadavers have shown that occasionally these epiphyses fail to fuse to the body and spine of the scapula, and the articulation of the shoulder is not perfect because of this fibrous union.[52, 102, 104, 169]

Liberson[150] reviewed the roentgenograms of 1800 shoulder girdles chosen at random and found 21 typical and 4 atypical cases of os acromiale, an incidence of 1.4 per cent. He also provided a detailed account of the ossification centers of the acromion and their variations.

Studies on the os acromiale have been completed by several German anatomists[176, 223] who note that the lesion is bilateral in up to 62 per cent of cases.[137] Others note that the incidence varies anywhere from 2 to 8

per cent after the age of 30.[102, 150] The most common site of nonunion is between the meso-acromion and meta-acromion, and this was true for all of our patients.[171]

Indications for Surgery

A rotator cuff tear may often be associated with os acromiale.[174] A patient with a suspected rotator cuff tear should be carefully studied with arthrography of the shoulder. An axillary roentgenogram (Fig. 3-20) is also important in identifying the anomaly. If an os acromiale is present, one may assume that the acromion has impinged on the rotator cuff, probably with

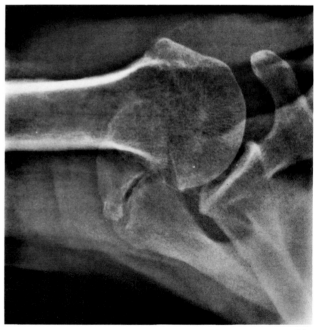

Figure 3-20. The os acromiale is best seen in the axillary roentgenogram of the shoulder.

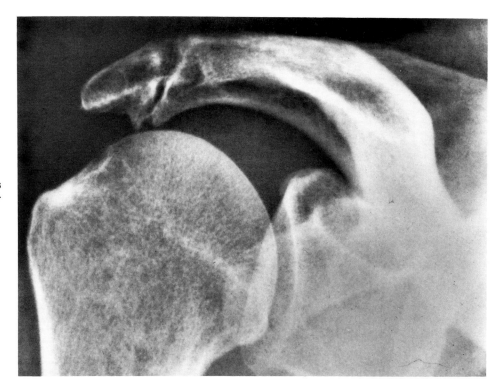

Figure 3–21. A large bone spur forms from the nonunion at the site of the shoulder impingement.

direct pressure of the irregular surface. When the deltoid contracts, the bone and any spurs apparently are driven into the rotator cuff, eventually causing the tendon to tear (Fig. 3–21). Neer[175] feels that this process represents an impingement syndrome and should change one's approach for an anterior acromioplasty.

Surgical Procedure

To correct this condition, the rotator cuff must be repaired, and this is described elsewhere. Also, an os acromiale modifies the approach for anterior acromioplasty. As for correcting the os acromiale itself, a small, unfused anterior acromioepiphysis can usually be excised (Fig. 3–22). The deltoid muscle can be reattached to the scapula. However, in the larger, unfused fragments, try to tilt the bone upward and close the epiphyseal space by curettage and local bone grafts. These fragments usually require internal fixation with a screw or threaded pin. If the fragment is freely movable, two parallel threaded pins and, occasionally, nonabsorbable sutures with local bone grafts can be used.[174] In our experience, most of the os acromiale fragments associated with rotator cuffs can be repaired by simply removing the fragment and reattaching the deltoid muscles to the remaining acromion.[171]

Coracoclavicular Joint or Bar

In this anomaly, a bar of bone may persist between the clavicle and the coracoid process, or an actual joint may be present. Usually this abnormality is discovered as an incidental finding in a routine roentgenographic examination of the chest.

Clinical Findings

This ligament, joint, or bar has been linked to compression of the neurovascular bundle[112] of the subclavian artery and brachial plexus, particularly when a coracoclavicular joint is present. Clinically, the only finding is some restriction in shoulder motion because

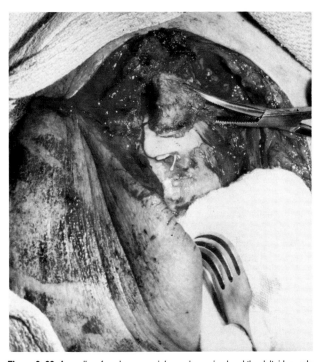

Figure 3–22. A small, unfused os acromiale can be excised and the deltoid muscle reattached to the scapula.

the bar seems to interfere with scapular rotation. Strenuous physical activity involving circumduction may irritate the neurovascular bundle. If the bar is sufficiently thick to fix the clavicle, arthritic changes may occur in the acromioclavicular joint as a result of the restricted motion that the bar imposes on the shoulder. Removing the bar has relieved the discomfort in many patients.

DePalma[56] divided this deformity into three different clinical groups: (1) patients in whom a solid bony strut connects the coracoid with the clavicle; (2) patients in whom a bony process on the inferior aspect of the outer third of the clavicle articulates with, and has an actual joint arising from, the coracoid process; and (3) patients in whom an incomplete bony bar or a bony spur projects from the inferior surface of the clavicle.

Calcification or pathological ossification of the coracoclavicular ligaments should not be confused with a true joint. Many times, after a fracture or third-degree separation of the acromioclavicular joint, one will see calcification, particularly if the patient has had surgical intervention. This calcification is a different circumstance. Most often, the extra articulation does not disturb the patient.

Frasseto[78] believed that this articulation can be a predisposing factor in fracture of the surgical neck of a humerus from a direct or indirect blow. A coracoclavicular joint prevents the two bones of the shoulder girdle from separating; normal ligaments allow some separation. Without this flexibility, the head of the humerus comes against the glenoid cavity—a particularly rigid wall—and the shoulder is not able to soften a blow that is transmitted through the humerus. This positioning imparts increased energy to the humerus and therefore increases the probability of fracture.

This articulation replaces the normal conoid and trapezoid ligaments. McClure and Raney[161] agree that a solid bone bridge in the position of the coracoid and trapezoid ligaments probably represents a more extended and severe variation of the same embryological process that created the joint. Many people have triangular bony overgrowth under the clavicle with a downwardly directed apex (Fig. 3–23). In the examination of 60 cadavers, Schlyvitch[224] found no bony contact between the clavicle and the coracoid process in 44. In eight cases he found that the two surfaces were in contact and were covered by fibrous tissue (Fig. 3–24). In only six cases did he find the coracoid projection actually covered by cartilage and in only one was a true diarthrosis surrounded by an articular capsule (Fig. 3–25). Wertheimer[262] in 1948 identified 48 coracoclavicular joints in an extensive review of the literature and added two of his own cases. Of these 50 cases, 33 were diagnosed by roentgenography and 17 during surgery or autopsy.

Wertheimer examined microscopically the bony projections that formed the joint. The projections were made of a spongy, osseous tissue containing lacunae and filled with bone marrow and covered by a thin layer of bone. Overlying this bone was a thick layer of fibrous cartilage.

Embryology

During normal development of the shoulder, the primitive mesenchymal tissue between the rudiments of the clavicle and the coracoid process usually evolve into the coracoclavicular ligaments: the coracoid and the trapezoid.[56] Defective development of this tissue can result in either a joint or a bridge.

In the lowest vertebral forms, the conoid process becomes an extensive bone bar that gradually disappears until it is represented in most mammals by a small stub and a costocoracoid ligament. This ligament varies in size and shape and may contain islands of cartilage.

The incidence of this anomaly varies greatly but most often averages from 1 to 1.2 per cent. Nutter[179] screened 1000 unselected roentgenograms of adult shoulders and found an incidence of 1.2 per cent. (Of these 12 patients, the coracoclavicular joint was bilateral in 6.) However, in a study of 2300 roentgenograms, Ponde and Silveira[193] found only 1 coracoclavicular joint. Poirier[191] found 3 cases in 10 cadavers, but we believe this is an unusually high incidence of this rare anomaly.

Indications for Surgery

In patients who have an established bony bar and persistent symptoms, pain can be relieved by surgical excision of the bar. Pain occurs because the bar interferes with scapular rotation.

Several authors[10, 262] have resected bars with excellent results. Hall[112] had a patient with numbness and tingling in the median nerve distribution of the right hand. He excised only the clavicular portion of the joint and achieved complete relief of all symptoms.

Operative Procedure

The procedure we use begins just below the clavicle through a short transverse incision. The coracoid process is identified, and the bony bar is followed from the top of the coracoid up to the clavicle. This bar can usually be easily identified by palpation. The bar and the intervening joint are excised as completely as possible.[10]

Wertheimer[262] makes a 15-cm incision over the deltopectoral groove, from the clavicle to the anterior axillary fold. He then dissects the superficial fascia down to the pectoral fascia. The deltoid muscle is detached from the clavicle and turned outward. A mass of fat fills the subclavicular space. When this fat is removed, a band of fibrous tissue resembling a true ligament is exposed. After excising this band of tissue, the bar can be seen, with one end at the union of the lateral and middle thirds of the clavicle and the other

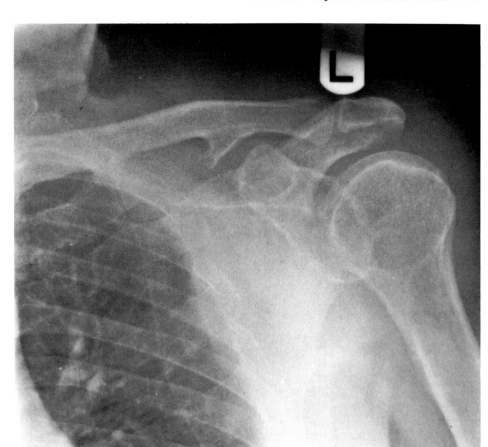

Figure 3–23. A triangular bony overgrowth under the clavicle may be present, with its apex directed down to the coracoid.

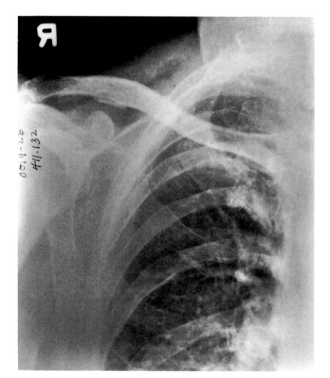

Figure 3–24. A coracoclavicular joint may consist of two contacting surfaces covered by fibrous tissue.

at the base of the coracoid process. The two joining processes are removed first, then the fibrous tissue band, and then the joint.

Only rarely will it be necessary to operate on patients with a coracoclavicular joint, but when necessary, complete relief can be expected and is easily obtained with this simple procedure.

Ligamentous or Bony Connecting Bands: Costocoracoid Band

Three ligamentous bands, similar in character, have been noted by different authors to cause severe disability in the shoulder. The first band we discuss, the costocoracoid band, was brought to our attention by Dr. Allan MacKenzie,[156] who derived his information from Dr. Robert Salter.[220]

Patients with this band have narrow and sloping shoulders, which are rigidly held forward and medially. Salter[220] called this "the congenital forward fixation of the scapula." A tight band extends from the anterior end of the first rib to the base of the coracoid process, thereby producing a forward flexion of the scapula. This fibrous band becomes ossified in adult life.

The abnormal position of the shoulders cannot be corrected during a physical examination, either actively by the patient or passively by the examiner. The band

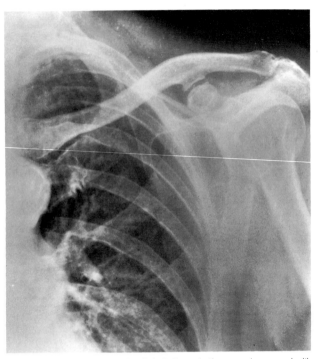

Figure 3–25. Both the coracoid and clavicular projections may be covered with cartilage, forming a true diarthrodial joint surrounded by an articular capsule.

can be palpated and is deep to the pectoralis major muscle, just inferior to the clavicle, and extends from the first costocartilage to the base of the coracoid process. Roentgenograms reveal a small ossicle medial to the coracoid process. This anomaly is probably inherited as a mendelian dominant trait because it was noted in several relatives. At the time of the communication from Salter, nine individuals had been identified as having this deformity.

Surgical Indications

Surgery on children to correct the deformity is probably justifiable, but Salter considered it unwise to try and correct the deformity in adults.[220]

At surgery, a tight fibrous band that tethers the first costocartilage to the base of the coracoid process is excised. This band is about 0.5 cm thick and prevents the backward displacement of the scapula. The band occupies the area usually occupied by the thin costocoracoid membrane that, in turn, is part of the clavipectoral fascia. The procedure works well, as all patients were completely relieved of their tight shoulders.

Coracocostosternale Vestigiale Bone

Only one congenital instance of this bone has been reported.[72] The bone was associated with spina bifida of the cervical region, congenital elevation of the right scapula, and torticollis. On physical examination, the child had a prominent right clavicle, with some twisting of the head to the left side.

Finder[72] felt that this band represented an embryological remnant, as described by Subkowitsch. Subkowitsch[240] studied embryos and found a connection between the coracoid process and the sternum. The coracoid always developed in connection with the glenoid. As the coracoid forms, a mass of mesenchymal cells appears and spreads to the mesenchymal anlage of the sternum, with which it subsequently unites. Somewhat later, the mesenchymal bar divides along its long axis into an upper and lower portion. Still later, the cephalad portion begins to disappear from its coracoid end, while the caudal layer fades from its sternal end. Probably all that remains of the mesenchymal bar in the mature fetus is the coracoclavicular ligament, composed of the coracoid and trapezoid portions. In Finder's patient, this bar was not removed, but we feel that, as with the costocoracoid band, it would be realistic to do so.

Costovertebral Bone

Goodwin and colleagues[99] reported a patient in 1984 who complained of increasing pain on the left side of the neck and of a tendency to bend the neck to the left. The patient noted that, since birth, her right shoulder had been elevated. At the age of seven she had developed scoliosis. There was no family history of any other muscular abnormality. Because of the constant pain, deformity, and restricted motion of the neck, surgical excision of the bone was indicated.

During surgery, the anomalous bone appeared to be continuous with the left bifid spinous process of the sixth cervical vertebra. It extended caudally and laterally and was embedded in the serratus posterior superior muscle to form a pseudarticulation with the posterior aspect of the left fourth rib (Fig. 3–26).

Three explanations were proposed for this particular band. The first was that a group of sclerodermal cells, brought into an abnormal position during the migratory shift of neighboring structures, developed into ectopic bone. The second postulated that a group of normally situated mesenchymal cells from the epaxial myotome differentiated into bone rather than into muscle. The third, considered to be the least likely, was that a group of damaged mesenchymal cells developed into bone within the mass of the serratus posterior superior muscle.

Whenever there are bands, either ligamentous or bony, we recommend that they be removed if possible. Even in adults, removing the band will diminish the pain and increase flexibility.

Infrascapular Bone

An accessory ossification center or actually the persistence of a normal center at the inferior angle of the scapula has been reported.[138] The center usually fuses with the scapula, but before fusion is complete, the ossification center can be confused with a fracture. Kohler and Wilk[138] recommend tne term "infrascapular bone" for this ossification center.

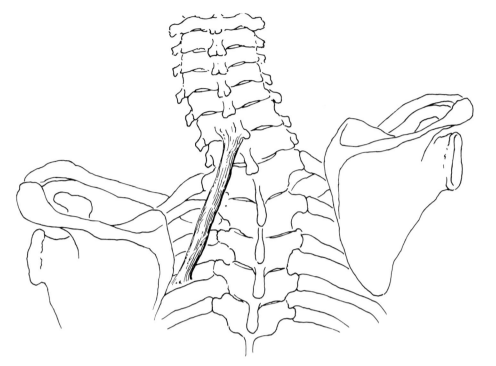

Figure 3–26. The costovertebral bone ties together the bifid spinous process of the sixth cervical vertebra and the fourth rib.

Adler[1] reported a case in which the round shadow of this ossification center was misinterpreted as a pulmonary nodule. As described by Lossen and Wegner,[152] the ossification centers are usually smooth, rounded, and bilaterally symmetrical, as shown in our patient (Fig. 3–27).

Notched Inferior Angle of the Scapula

Kohler and Wilk[138] call this particular anomaly the "swallow tail" malformation. Khoo and Kuo[135] observed under fluoroscopy a swallow-tail-like cleavage at the inferior angle of the scapula in one of their patients. Roentgenogram of the right scapula showed that the scapula was shorter than normal, owing to the absence of its inferior fourth. The most striking feature, however, was that the inferior aspect of the scapula ended in two processes, with the deep semieliptical notch between them (Fig. 3–28).

Khoo and Kuo[135] tried to correlate this anomaly with certain observations of Hrdlicka[124] and Gray,[103] who have devoted special attention to the ossification centers and anomalies of the scapula. McClure and Raney[161] postulated that this anomaly is caused by the absence of the ossification nucleus of the inferior angle of the scapula.

Dentated Glenoid

Between the ages of 8 and 13, the border of the glenoid appears rippled, or dentated.[138] The border consists of an epiphyseal annular ring that is visualized only on a radiograph taken in a certain projection (Fig. 3–29). These ridges remain only a short time because they fuse quickly with the body of the scapula. Usually,

the secondary ossification centers for the upper portion of the glenoid develop earlier; the center for the lower half develops three to four years later. The absence or immature development of the secondary ossification center in the inferior segment of the glenoid results in a dentated-shaped glenoid (Fig. 3–30), similar to the radiographic appearance of vertebral bodies in Scheuermann's disease of the vertebral column.

The abnormal contour of the glenoid may be a predisposing cause for premature development of os-

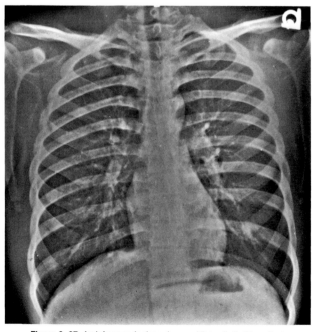

Figure 3–27. An infrascapular bone is seen bilaterally in this patient.

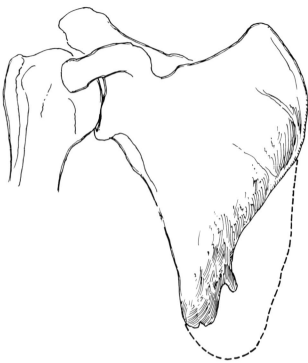

Figure 3–28. The notched inferior angle of the scapula probably represents an absence of the ossification nucleus of the inferior angle of the scapula.

teoarthritis in the glenohumeral joint. During the 18th year these epiphyses normally fuse with the body of the scapula. Nevertheless, occasionally the ossifying process persists, and these delayed fusions can often look quite alarming. Sutro[245] described two patients with dentated articular surface of the glenoid. The opposite shoulder also showed minor indentation of

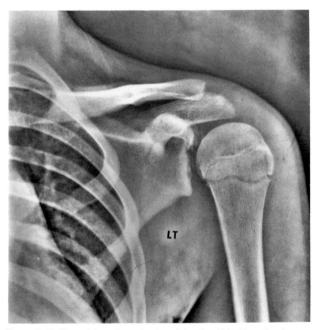

Figure 3–29. The epiphyseal annular ring of the glenoid in this patient has not fused and appears rippled or dentated.

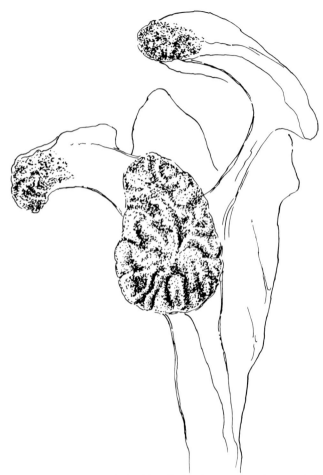

Figure 3–30. This dentated glenoid ossification ring was drawn from an actual specimen.

the glenoid. The patient we examined also showed bilateral indentation of the glenoid (Fig. 3–31).

Absent Scapula: Phocomelia

Complete absence of the scapula has not been reported except when the associated entire limb is missing.[161] This anomaly is rare.[177] One of the abnormalities associated with a complete absence of a limb is phocomelia. Phocomelia means "seal limb," in Greek, but the resemblance becomes strictly superficial. This deformity belongs to the general category of failure of formation.[247]

Clinical Findings

Intercalary deficiency leads to overall and sometimes extreme shortening of the limb. Many variations occur. Patients can have fairly well-developed shoulders and arms with hypoplastic hands and fused elbows.[60] Phocomelia seems to be classifiable into three anatomical types. In complete phocomelia, all the limb bones proximal to the hand are absent, and the hand attaches directly to the trunk. In the second type, the proximal limb bone is absent or extremely hypoplastic, so the

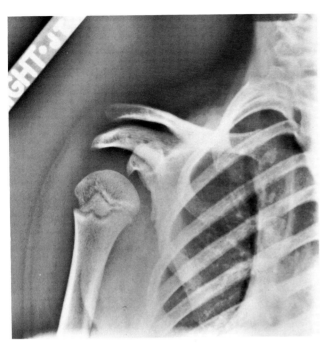

Figure 3–31. In an older individual the glenoid may be indented. The abnormal contour of the glenoid may be a predisposing cause of osteoarthritis.

activating prosthetic devices. Every effort should be made to save any portion of the functioning limb.

Occasionally, a deficient phocomelic limb can be increased in length for stability. If the tubular humerus is of sufficient size, it can be lengthened by any one of four techniques: a Z-type osteotomy, a transverse osteotomy with a sliding lengthening and bone graft with fixation, an intercalated bone graft,[60] or various mechanical devices.[58] These procedures are successful only if the humerus is of sufficient length.

Usually the humerus is short. The elbow has poor function or is absent. The upper arm can be lengthened with microvascular techniques. The fibula may be transplanted to the arm, placing the epiphysis in the glenoid fossa and attaching the distal end to the distal humeral remnant (Fig. 3–34). A reasonably stable, comfortable, and controllable elbow joint is desirable, but if one does not develop, the fibula can be fused to the glenoid at a later time to stabilize the arm.[232]

Finally, the humerus can be lengthened by mobilizing the clavicle. The sternal end is detached, and the medial two-thirds is stripped subperiosteally. The bone is then turned into the arm, where the medial end is attached to the remnant of the distal humerus and forearm.[243]

forearm or a short synostosis of the forearm segment and hand attach to the trunk. In the third type, the hand attaches directly to the humerus. Sometimes only a finger attaches to the trunk (Fig. 3–32). The usual incidence is about 0.8 per cent of all congenital upper limb abnormalities.[75]

Embryology

Phocomelia became notorious in the 1950s and early 1960s when it affected about 60 per cent of infants born to mothers who had taken thalidomide between the 38th and 54th day after conception.[250]

Anatomical Pathology

Seldom is any portion of the limb completely normal. A rudimentary distal end of the humerus is almost always present (Fig. 3–33). The wrists and fingers can function, but the muscular power is extremely weak.

Indications for Surgery

There are few indications for surgery in phocomelia. Amputation of the remnant may be indicated if it is functionless and unsightly. Occasionally, the phocomelic limb can be improved by some type of digital reconstruction, such as an osteotomy or tendon transfer, but these procedures are not pertinent to our discussion here.

An artificial limb is a poor solution, but in some children, the need for a prosthesis is great.[77] Even partial function of the terminal digits can be useful in

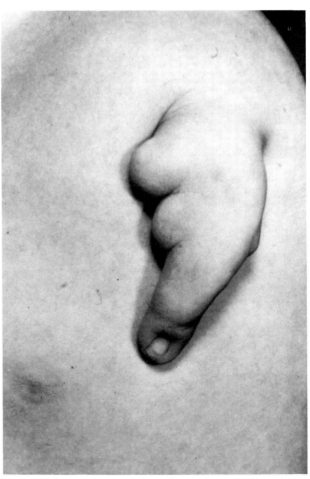

Figure 3–32. In an extreme case of phocomelia, sometimes only a finger attaches to the trunk.

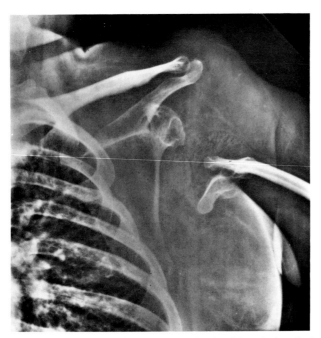

Figure 3–33. An abnormal glenoid articulates with only a deformed, short, distal end of the humerus in this patient with phocomelia.

Operative Procedure

The operative procedure is based on the transposition of the clavicle.[241, 242, 244] The skin incision is placed along the clavicle to the anterior side of the extremity. The clavicle and bony remnants of the upper extremity are carefully exposed. The clavicle is detached from the sternoclavicular joint and freed extraperiosteally for two-thirds of its length. It is then possible to turn the clavicle in the direction of the arm and elbow. In some children over one year of age, the acromion has to be cut to facilitate this procedure. In the maximally stretched arm, the clavicle is brought in contact with the rudimentary bones of the forearm. The clavicle is fixed by wire cerclage to the rudimentary humerus and to the subperiosteally exposed bony remnant of the forearm (Fig. 3–35).

On occasion the clavicle has almost disappeared by reabsorption.[244] Shifting the clavicle from its normal site has had no drawbacks in the few patients in which it has been done. In fact, with the clavicle removed, the shoulders can actually move more vertically, which improves the functioning of the very short arms.

The phocomelic arm usually has a suggestion of an elbow joint between the rudimentary humerus and the forearm. When the clavicle is transposed to this area, it must be fixed to the bony remnant of the humerus and to the bony remnant of the forearm. If the clavicle, the humerus, and the remnant of the forearm fuse, function improves.[27]

In the bilateral case, transposing the clavicle to lengthen the humerus allows the hands to be brought together in front of the body, an ability of great functional benefit.[242]

GLENOHUMERAL DYSPLASIAS

Glenohumeral dysplasias encompass a broad spectrum of conditions affecting the shoulder. Most commonly seen are the asymptomatic patients with incidental findings on routine x-rays. Infrequently, severe cases with marked deformity, stiffness, and disability are seen. These dysplastic conditions likely arise from an interplay of intrinsic and extrinsic factors that can affect the developing joint *in utero,* at birth, or during early childhood. The sequelae to this as yet undetermined injury is seen in the child or adult as glenoid hypoplasia, humerus varus, humeral retroversion, deformity, or absence of the humeral head. These may occur to varying degrees and in various combinations.

As shown by Brailsford[22] in his radiological studies,

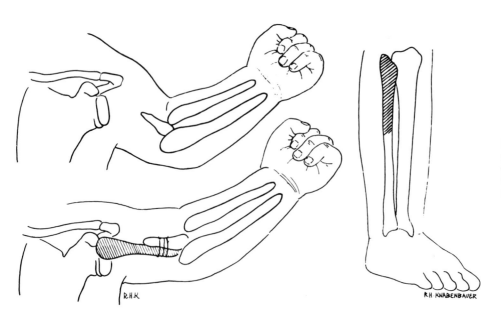

Figure 3–34. The fibula may be transplanted to the upper arm by placing the epiphysis in the glenoid fossa and attaching the distal end to the distal humeral remnant.

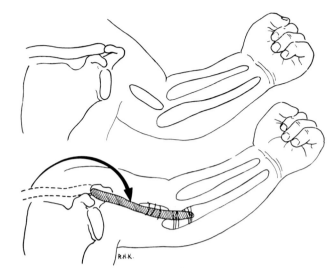

Figure 3–35. Transposition of the clavicle is accomplished by exposing it subperiosteally and using the sternal end to lengthen the humerus.

the glenoid is formed from three components: (1) the floor and the main scapular body and coracoid base, which appear by 10 years; (2) the inferior glenoid center, which appears at 13 years—its growth deepens the glenoid fossa and forms the inferior articular margin; and (3) the precartilaginous center, which is well developed *in utero*.

The humeral head is formed from a medial epiphyseal ossification center at six months, a lateral center at two years, and the lesser tuberosity center at five years.

Owen[183] theorized that dysplasia was caused by an intrinsic developmental failure of the precartilaginous inferior apophysis, as this anlagen determines the future shape of the bone. Other intrinsic conditions could include Fairbanks-type epiphyseal dysplasia, dystrophy secondary to rickets or other metabolic disturbances, and intrinsic congenital soft-tissue contractures, as seen with amyoplasia. Injury to the primordial limb bud, as in phocomelia, also affects the shoulder girdle to a variable extent.

Extrinsic factors include neuromuscular conditions, such as Erb's palsy, muscular dystrophy, and arthrogryposis, along with traumatic epiphyseal and physeal injury occurring at birth. Often, the exact cause is difficult to determine.

HUMERUS VARUS

Humerus varus, as described by Lucas,[153] has marked varus of the head in relation to the shaft. The neck distal to the physeal plate is also narrowed (Fig. 3–36). The condition likely results from physeal trauma with asymmetric, premature medial epiphysiodesis.

HUMERAL HEAD RETROVERSION

Humeral head retroversion has been described by Putti[196] and Scaglietti[222] as secondary to anterior soft-tissue contractures. The bony deformity was noted as an increased "angle of declination" or increased hu-

meral torsion.[55] Clinically, the forearm appears pronated, and the patient has decreased external rotation, abduction, and adduction. The shoulder roundness is lost, and a Putti scapular sign may be elicited with external rotation. Anterior release, as described by Sever, followed by a second-stage Putti derotational osteotomy is indicated when the deformity is severe.[222]

ABSENT HUMERAL HEAD

The late appearance of the ossific nucleus of the humeral head and varying degrees of lateral displace-

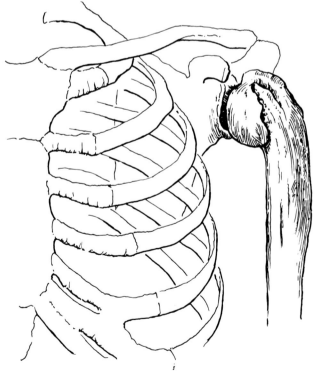

Figure 3–36. Humerus varus most likely results from physeal trauma. There is marked varus at the head in relation to the shaft and a narrowing of the neck distal to the physeal plate.

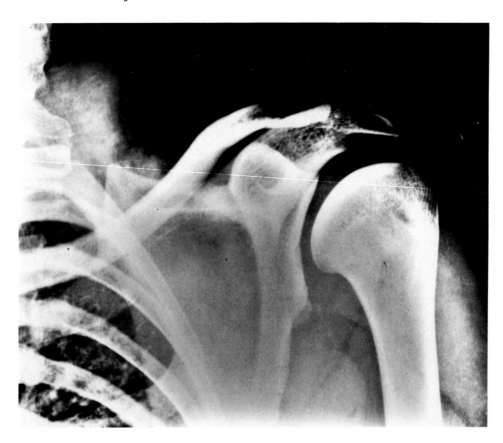

Figure 3–37. Varying degrees of glenoid flattening are seen in glenoid hypoplasia.

ment of the epiphysis have been described and are reminiscent of findings in avascular necrosis following congenital dislocation of the hip and in Perthes' disease. Complete absence of the humeral head may indeed be an extreme injury of similar etiology.[4]

GLENOID HYPOPLASIA

Glenoid hypoplasia occurs in a manner similar to the acetabular dysplasia in congenital dislocation of the hip (CDH) as the glenoid lacks the stimulus to form without a well-formed and contained humeral head. Varying degrees of glenoid flattening (Fig. 3–37) or convexity, as well as aplasia of the scapular neck (Fig. 3–38), can occur.[161] Clinically pronounced webbing of the axilla and limited abduction have been reported by Owen.[183]

Surgery and other treatment is usually not indicated in this condition.

BICIPITAL GROOVE ABERRATIONS

Hitchcock and Bechtol[119] attributed great importance to subluxation and peritendinitis of the long head of the biceps brachii tendon in the etiology of shoulder conditions. After examining 100 humeri these authors proposed that biceps tendon mechanics became faulty from a phylogenetic developmental standpoint as humans assumed an erect posture. In particular, a shallow

groove and a supratubercular ridge were thought to be predisposing factors in several pathological conditions.

The supratubercular bony ridge[164] projects immediately proximal to the medial wall of the bicipital

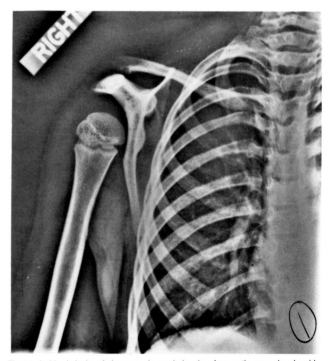

Figure 3–38. Aplasia of the scapula neck is also frequently seen in glenoid hypoplasia.

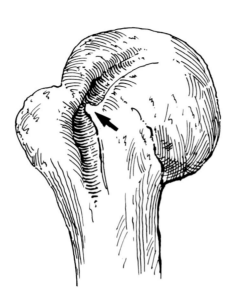

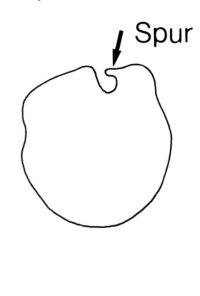

Figure 3–39. The supratubercular bony ridge of Meyer and a spur can develop secondarily to peritendinous inflammation.

groove, limiting the excursion of the tendon and forcing it against the roof of the canal or transverse humeral ligament (Fig. 3–39). This ridge was present in 17.5 per cent of Meyer's series of 200 humeri. The ridge was moderately developed in 59 per cent of Hitchcock and Bechtol's series. Bony excrescences on the lesser tuberosity also form, secondary to peritendinous inflammation.

In 92 per cent, the humeri had an intertubercular groove with medial and lateral walls between 45 to 90 degrees of each other, while in 8 per cent the medial wall of the groove was less than 45 degrees from the lateral wall[119] (Fig. 3–40). These findings closely correlated with those of Meyer's previous work, in which eight per cent of biceps tendons were dislocated medially in a fascial sling from a shallow groove.

Among other primates, only the orangutan has a shallow groove with a medial wall angle of 60 degrees. On the other hand, supratubercular ridges are common to gorillas, chimpanzees, gibbons, and orangutans.[119]

Anteroposterior flattening of the thorax with dorsal rotation of the scapula will laterally displace the glenohumeral joint and provide an additional subluxation force that pushes the humerus lateral in relation to the fixed tendon.[119]

Surgical correction of the instability and subsequent inflammation and attrition includes fixing the tendon in the groove and associated debridement.[49, 59, 180] This procedure is addressed in Chapter 20.

CONGENITAL DISLOCATION OF THE SHOULDER

Cozen[47] called attention to the fact that many glenohumeral dislocations reported as congenital are actually intrauterine, paralytic, or possibly obstetrical in origin. He maintained that dislocation resulting from paralysis or trauma at birth may be distinguished from congenital dislocation by a history of dystocia or forceps delivery, muscle paralysis, and the absence of other congenital anomalies. Frosch,[81] Greig,[106] and Whitman[263] supported this idea, agreeing that it is difficult to determine the etiological factor in "congenital shoulder dislocations" and the exact cause-effect relationship with Erb's palsy. Several authors[47, 263, 269] have reported patients with shoulder dislocations occurring as one of multiple congenital malformations. Similarly, we have seen it in conjunction with Holt-Oram syndrome (Fig. 3–41).

Familial occurrences have been described.[257] Similar

Wall angle of biceps groove

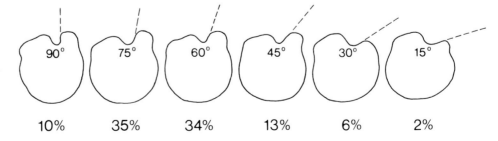

Figure 3–40. The varying degrees of angulation of the intertubercular groove, as described by Hitchcock and Bechtol.[119]

90° 75° 60° 45° 30° 15°

10% 35% 34% 13% 6% 2%

Frequency of each type of groove

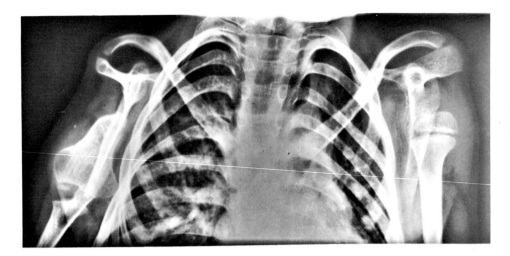

Figure 3–41. This patient with a Holt-Oram syndrome demonstrates a phocomelia on the right and congenital dislocation of the shoulder on the left.

to hip involvement, arthrogryposis multiplex congenita may present with congenital shoulder dislocations, paralytic contractures, and axillary webs.[47]

Royal Whitman[263] described a closed reduction and casting technique for correcting congenital and acquired luxations at the shoulder. However, no series of cases has been reported for the treatment of this rare condition.

Muscular Abnormalities

EXTRA MUSCLES

The Axillopectoral Muscle

The first description of this anomalous structure, as quoted by Testut,[253] is attributed to Carl Reiter von Edenberg von Langer, who reported his findings in the Uster Medix Wutchenshrift. In 1846, Langer-Oester,[145] under the name of Achselbogen, described a muscle at the lower lateral border of the axilla. This muscle became known in German as Langer's armbogen, as described by Corning in 1949.[46] In the English literature, this anomaly was called Langer's arm arch or the axillopectoral muscle.[20]

Testut[253] also quoted Malgaigne who stated that he discovered this muscle in the course of ligation of the axillary artery and at first mistook it for a brachialis.

The axillopectoral muscle is an anomalous muscle that extends from the latissimus dorsi and inserts into the pectoralis major, also overlying the neurovascular bundle in the axilla. Although rare, the aberrant muscle tissue can extend from the latissimus dorsi muscle to the coracoid process.

Clinical Findings

This muscle is made taut by abduction and elevation of the arm or by putting the arm behind the head. Boontje[20] reports on the entrapment of the axillary vein by the muscle in an 18-year-old woman who complained of pain and tiredness in the arm, which

was swollen and discolored and had an intensified venous pattern. She also complained of a heaviness and stiffness in the right arm, which had occurred gradually. Her hand was usually swollen, especially at rest, and she was unable to sleep well as a result of the discomfort. Long-standing compression of the vein by the anomalous muscle and the dependent position of the arm can lead to venous thrombosis.

Inheritance does not appear to be a factor in this anomaly.

Embryology

The latissimus dorsi muscle arises on the posterior aspect of the shoulder and migrates to its attachment on the humerus during the rotation phase of the shoulder girdle and humerus. The lengthy course of the nerve is thought to result from this migration. The anterior counterpart to the latissimus dorsi is the pectorals which develop in close relationship to the arm but in front of the chest. In this position the mass attaches in sequence to the humerus, the coracoid, the clavicle, and the upper ribs. The primitive muscle mass splits horizontally, eventually demarcating between the pectoralis major and the pectoralis minor. The pectoralis major develops from the superficial layer and remains attached to the humerus. As the humerus rotates, the muscle insertion is drawn with it and eventually is folded over on itself, thus explaining the appearance of this tendon in the adult. The pectoralis minor develops from a split in this mass, but it does not rotate as extensively, so there is no folding over of the tendon.[10]

At dissection, the band appears to be about 8 cm in length (Fig. 3–42). The origin on the latissimus dorsi is quite broad; it narrows as it inserts into the pectoralis major[134] (Fig. 3–43). The axillopectoral muscle is innervated by the nerve to the pectoralis minor.[111, 204, 219] Langer reported that this arch was present in about 4 per cent of his dissections. Haagenson[111] quotes Paul Isler who stated that the axillary pectoral muscle is present in about 7.7 per cent of subjects of European stock.

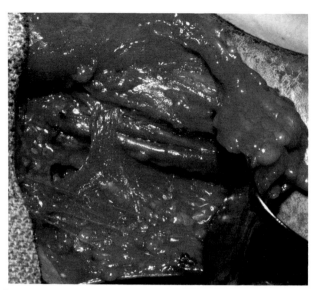

Figure 3–42. A Langer's arm arch muscle is shown at surgery causing pressure to the neurovascular bundle.

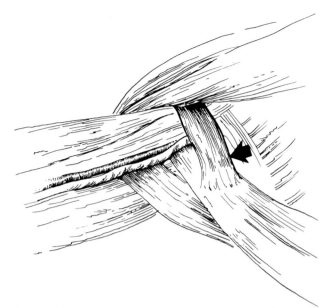

Figure 3–43. The axillopectoral muscle extends from the latissimus dorsi to insert into the pectoralis major. It overlies the neurovascular bundle in the axilla.

On occasion an axillary muscle mass may be mistaken for a tumor of the axilla.[219] Several authors[30, 61, 217, 254] have noted thrombosis of the axillary artery and vascular occlusion. A venous thrombosis and vascular occlusion with persistent, progressive pain is a clear indication for resection of the muscle.

In treating this condition, we use the transaxillary approach as described by Roos.[210] The treatment of the problem is simple—resect the aberrant muscle and eliminate the compression. Venous reconstruction can then be considered if a thrombosis is present or if the venous wall is damaged.

Sternalis Muscle

The sternalis muscle is superficial to the pectoralis major. It more or less parallels the sternum and has variable attachments to it, including the sheath of the rectus, the sternocleidomastoid muscle, and the pectoralis major (Fig. 3–44).

Turner, in 1867,[256] credited Cabriolus with the first adequate documentation in 1604 of the sternalis muscle.

Among 535 cadavers, Barlow[9] found 38 sternalis muscles in 33. The sternalis muscle occurred with equal frequency on the left, the right, bilaterally, and in both sexes. Unilateral muscles were approximately twice as frequent as bilateral muscles.

Turner[256] proposed four possible origins of the sternalis muscle: (1) an upward prolongation of the rectus abdominus; (2) a downward prolongation of the sternocleidomastoid; (3) a downward prolongation of the platysma or, more generally, a representative part of the panniculus carnosus as has been noted in some animals; and (4) a muscle *sui generis* peculiar to humans. Cunningham[51] proposed an additional origin—that it is a member of the pectoral group of muscles. Barlow, who has written the most about this

abnormality, believes that the sternalis muscle is the rudimentary muscle in man of the panniculus carnosus.

Interestingly, this muscle is innervated by both the anterior thoracic nerve and the intercostal nerve. The nerve supply is usually from one or both pectoral nerves. The incidence is in the neighborhood of 4 per cent. The sternalis seems to be more common in the darkly pigmented race,[120] although Barlow[9] disputed this idea.

According to Hollinshead,[120] this muscle can be associated with an axillary arch muscle and therefore is capable of producing median nerve symptomatology.

If the muscle compresses the nerves, it should be removed.

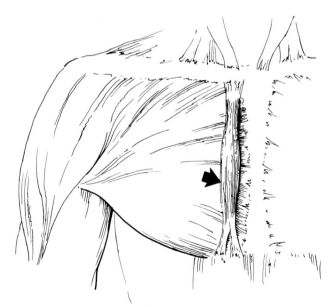

Figure 3–44. The sternalis muscle.

We have no clinical experience with this abnormality.

Chondroepitrochlear Muscle

The chondroepitrochlearis muscle originates from the pectoralis major or the costal cartilages of the aponeurosis of the external oblique and inserts on the medial epicondyle, the intermuscular septum, or the inner side of the arm into the brachial fascia.[24, 43, 147, 154, 170, 271] Classically it is described as originating from the pectoralis major and inserting on the medial epicondyle of the humerus. In 1868, Testut[252] attributed the name chondroepitrochlearis to Wood.[270]

Clinical Abnormalities

This muscle serves no known function in humans and actually limits the normal range of motion of the upper limb by restricting abduction. In addition, as a result of the large web in the axilla, it is cosmetically unpleasing. This abnormal web at the level of the anterior axillary fold appears to be musculotendinous.

This muscle can originate from the lower third of the anterior chest wall and inserts broadly along the medial aspect of the humerus, down into the medial epicondyle (Fig. 3–45). Voto and Weiner,[258] who surgically dissected this muscle in a child, described two origins at the chondrocartilage of ribs 3 through 7 and 7 through 10. These origins formed into two dense bands that traversed across the axilla and proceeded down to the elbow, to insert along the medial epicondyle. The chondroepitrochlearis is innervated by fibers from the anterior division and is derived from the ventral flexor muscle mass of the pectoralis major muscle.[29, 249]

Embryology

Wood[271] and Perrin[187] thought that the chondroepitrochlearis muscle represented in humans an aberrant insertion of the most caudal part of the pectoralis major. Tobler[255] and Ruge[216] independently suggested the same explanation. The explanation seems to be valid because the muscle's nerve supply is identical to that of the pectoralis major.

Most reports[6, 13, 38, 143] have been based on postmortem examinations of stillborn infants who had multiple congenital anomalies or on incidental findings in cadaver studies. Rarely does a patient live who has a chondroepitrochlear muscle. Chiba and co-workers[38] after an extensive study of the English literature, found only 20 cases of this rare abnormality.

Voto and Weiner[258] helped one child both functionally and cosmetically with surgery by simply removing the muscle. The muscle is superficial enough to be easily visualized and removed.

If the chondroepitrochlear muscle is present in a child with limited abduction and a large axillary web, surgery is indicated.

Subscapularis-Teres-Latissimus Muscles

Kameda,[133] in 1976, found this anomalous muscle in 10 of 190 human cadavers, an incidence of 5.2 per cent. The muscle arose near the lateral margin of the scapula, either from the surface of the subscapularis muscle, or from the border of the quadrangular tendon of the latissimus dorsi, or from both, and ran obliquely upward to fuse with the insertion of the subscapularis (Fig. 3–46).

Kameda divided this muscle abnormality into three types. In Type I the muscle crossed over the axillary and lower subscapular nerves, behind the radial nerve,

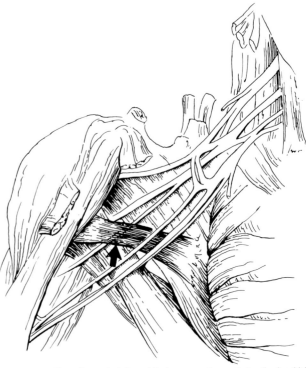

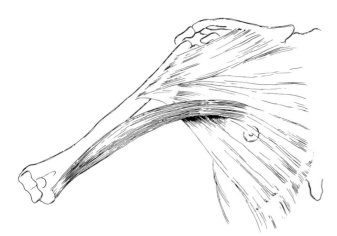

Figure 3–45. The chondroepitrochlear muscle originates on the anterior chest wall and inserts along the medial aspect of the humerus to the medial epicondyle.

Figure 3–46. The subscapularis-teres-latissimus muscle penetrates the brachial plexus and may lie on top of the axillary, lower subscapular, thoracodorsal, or radial nerve.

and was innervated by the lower subscapular nerve. In Type II the muscle penetrated the brachial plexus and separated the radial nerve into two roots: one from the posterior division of the upper trunk and one from the posterior divisions of the middle and lower trunks. Type II muscles were supplied by the radial nerve, which always originated at the same level as the origin of the thoracodorsal nerve. In Type III the muscle passed through the level of the brachial plexus and was supplied by branches from the radial and thoracodorsal nerve. The subscapular and thoracodorsal nerves also passed posterior to this anomalous muscle.

When a muscle arises from the latissimus dorsi or the subscapularis muscle and passes through the brachial plexus to insert into the vicinity of subscapularis, there can be nerve compression and vascular compression. This could be another cause of brachial neuritis.

We have not encountered this anomaly. The muscle is extremely difficult to identify preoperatively; most likely it will only be discovered when dissecting the brachial plexus.

Coracoclaviculosternal Muscle

We found only one reference to this abnormal muscle. Lane[144] describes this anomalous muscle in a powerfully built adult male. The muscle lay beneath the costocoracoid membrane and originated from the whole anterior margin of the coracoid process and from a comparatively strong coracoclavicular ligament and inserted into the lower part of the anterior margin of the clavicular facet of the sternum. The subclavius muscle and the costocoracoid membrane were all present in their normal relationships.

Because the coracosternal connection is a mesenchymatous one, the anomaly may be a muscle-tissue derivative of the embryonic structure.

No clinical symptoms are known to result from this anomaly, which we have never seen.

Deltoid Muscle Contracture

Abduction contracture of the shoulder resulting from fibrosis of the deltoid was first reported in 1965 by Sato and colleagues.[221] Then, in 1972, Roldan and Warren[207] reported a collection of 100 cases from Colombia, South America. They suggest that the condition is more common than the orthopedic literature indicates.

Clinical Findings

Abduction contracture of the shoulder is the most common finding. A simultaneous extension contracture of the shoulder is also often seen. Also frequently associated is winging of the scapula: Almost all patients develop winging from the contraction. Minami and colleagues[168] reported on 82 shoulder joints in 68 patients. Of these, 21 patients had bilateral contractures, and 19 had unilateral contractures of the left shoulder.

No patients had contractures of the right shoulder alone. Most of the children hold their shoulder in internal rotation, but besides adduction, no other movements are restricted. If the deformity has persisted for a long time, the humeral head may be flattened[40] or the shoulder dislocated.[37] Flexion contracture from fibrosis of the anterior muscles has been reported, although involvement of the posterior portion has not.

Inheritance

Wolbrink[268] reported that the mother of one such patient had a less severe form of the same condition, with a minimum abduction contracture of the arm. Aside from this, there are no reports of any abnormalities in other family members.

Anatomical Pathology

There appear to be two types of contracture: (1) congenital, with no history of injections and (2) a history of muscular injections. By far the most frequent cause of fibrotic contracture of the deltoid muscle is injection into the muscle. True congenital fibrous contracture is rare, and until 1972 only 10 cases had been reported.[98, 115, 116, 118, 167, 173] However, a mysterious report appeared from Roldan and Warren[207] from Medellin, Columbia, South America. They reported in 1972 on 100 patients with contractures of the intermediate part of the deltoid. These patients had no history of injections or vaccinations and could be considered to demonstrate pathology of the congenital variety. To date, more than 100 cases of congenital fibrosis have been reported.

Groves and Goldner[109] reported that the common denominator in their cases was the frequent intermuscular injections of a relatively large volume of fluid into the involved muscle. Numerous drugs have been associated with the development of contractures, including Talwin,[23, 48] antibiotics (particularly penicillin and lincomycin), Depo-Medrol,[65] Dramamine,[109] and an unlisted number of addictive drugs and drugs administered for the anemias. Of the reported drugs, Talwin damages tissue at the site of injection most often. Vitamin preparations, antipyretics,[113] streptomycin, and tetracycline[36] have all been incriminated in causing fibrosis of the deltoid muscle.

Minami and colleagues[168] reported that 39 of their 40 patients had histories of injections in their deltoid muscles, in most instances for a common cold, fever or asthma. The number of injections could not be confirmed accurately as a result of uncertain parental recall. The number of reported injections ranged from 3 to 60, with most patients receiving more than 10 injections. The severity of the contracture did not seem to be related to the type of drug. Correlating the incidence of the present contracture with the frequency of injections is difficult because it appears that some people have a greater sensitivity to injections than others. Bhattacharyya[14] suggested that the intermediate part of the deltoid muscle has an anatomical structure different from that of the anterior and posterior parts, with numerous fibrous septae. He suggested that it becomes fibrotic at birth or gradually undergoes fibrosis after birth. Sections taken from surgeries show collagenization but few inflammatory or ischemic changes, suggesting dermatomyositis or scleroderma. A propensity to fibrosis may add to the factor of the structure of the muscle itself. The invariable finding at surgery was a dense fibrous cord with atrophy of the surrounding muscle fibers.

Indications for Surgery

Exercises and stretching do not seem to improve this condition. Therefore, operative treatment is indicated when the abduction contracture is greater than 25 degrees. Surgery should be limited to patients who are at least five to six years of age and who have demonstrated progressive deformity during growth.

Surgical Procedure

The patient is prepped and draped in the usual manner for surgery under general anesthesia. A 5- to 6-cm skin incision is made transversely along the acromion, posterior to the spine of the scapula. The deltoid fascia and subcutaneous tissue are thoroughly and widely released. The middle fibers of the deltoid muscle are usually seen to be replaced by a thick fibrous tissue, similar in appearance to a tendon. The bands are released but not completely excised. This release is followed by manipulating the arm into adduction and forward flexion, where the scapula is held in position to correct both the lateral and posterior contractures. When a large gap occurs under the acromion, a portion of the posterior deltoid fibers must be transferred anteriorly and laterally. If the shoulder is dislocated, excision of the fibrous band is required, as is the release of the posterior third of the deltoid from its origin, to correct the abduction deformity and the dislocation.[37] In the series presented by Minami[168] 24 shoulders were treated by tenotomy, and 25 shoulders had a tenotomy and muscle transfer. The authors noted some complications, with the two most serious cosmetic complications being a keloid formation at the site of operation in 8 shoulders (16 per cent), and the absence of the middle fibers causing a staircase-like deformity from the acromion to the proximal humerus in 12 cases. This loss of tissue resulted in the loss of a natural roundness of the shoulders and became a serious cosmetic deformity, especially for young women.

Congenital Fossa

Several fossae (or "pits" or "dimples") can form around the shoulder. A clavicular fossa[10] may develop at the sternal end of the clavicle. Dimples on both

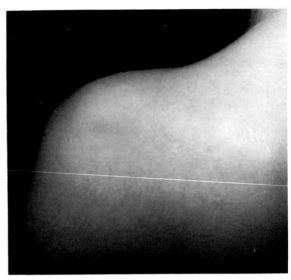

Figure 3–47. Congenital supraspinatus fossae.

sides of the clavicle out on the lateral portion are called congenital supraspinatus fossae (Fig. 3–47).

Little has been written about fossae or dimples. Browne,[28] in an exhaustive report, postulated that they resulted from the catching of tissues between a sharp bony post and the uterine wall. The skin and structures become compressed and adherent, and when the pressure is released, the surrounding parts remain tied down, forming small pits or dimples.

These abnormalities are often bilateral and are erroneously interpreted as evidence of an infectious or neoplastic process. No symptoms have been reported from this abnormality, and no treatment is usually required.

Recently, we saw a fossa in the scapular region of an infant who cried every time the arm was abducted (Fig. 3–48). We believe that this fossa probably did communicate and adhere to the scapula. In some cases we advise that the fossa be excised with the scar tissue to give free motion to the shoulder.

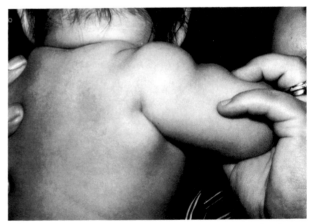

Figure 3–48. This child with a scapular fossa cried every time the arm was abducted from her side.

ABSENT MUSCLES

Pectoralis Major Muscle Defects

The association of congenital thoracic anomalies with ipsilateral syndactyly was first described by Alfred Poland[192] in 1841. His report of a detailed cadaveric dissection at Guy's Hospital as a student describes a 27-year-old male convict who lacked the left sterno-costal head of the pectoralis major and minor, with hypoplasia of the serratus anterior, external oblique, and muscles of the left arm. The syndactyly of the ipsilateral hand was incomplete, stopping at the prox-imal interphalangeal joint. The middle phalanges were absent, save for a quarter-inch ring of bone represent-ing the middle phalanx of the long finger. Clarkson,[42] in 1962, first used the term Poland's syndactyly to describe these same anomalies. In 1967, Baudine and co-workers[11] more accurately termed this group of anomalies Poland's syndrome.

Clinical Findings

The right side is most commonly involved. The pectoralis major or its sternocostal head is missing, creating a loss of the normally distinct anterior axillary fold. Occasionally, the pectoralis minor is absent. When marked, this anterior deficiency allows the pos-terior axillary fold to be viewed from the front. Only 13.5 per cent of patients with pectoralis major muscle defect have Poland's syndrome.[15]

Associated with this defect are varying degrees of deficiency in the overlying fascia, fat, breast, hair, and underlying ribs. The defect in the chest cage is variable, with the absence or only rudimentary development of the anterior portions of the second to the fifth ribs and costal cartilages. The sternum is without deformity. Instability of the deficient portion of the chest wall, consisting of a fibromuscular membrane and skin, is minor when present. Lung herniation can be demon-strated, usually with forceful expiratory or Valsalva's maneuver. As the thoracic cage enlarges with age, the deformity becomes more pronounced, but the defect of the chest wall becomes more stable.[62] With no associated incapacity there is no need for surgical correction.[25] The above-mentioned anomalies give rise to the characteristic chest flatness and high, supernu-merary, or absent nipple (Fig. 3–49).

Approximately 10 per cent of patients have a con-tracted axillary band of fibrous tissue formed in the web over the anterior surface of the axilla, limiting abduction.[92] The ipsilateral clavicle is usually short, and the scapula is elevated or winged from the serratus anterior deficiency. The ipsilateral upper extremity is hypoplastic in up to 40 per cent of patients.[12] Arm and forearm atrophy was initially thought to be secondary to disuse atrophy.[202] The hand is always hypoplastic, the forearm is usually so, and the arm is less frequently so.[127]

The syndactyly is generally simple and incomplete. All the fingers are usually involved, and the first web

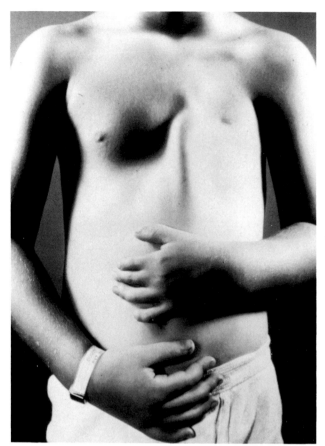

Figure 3–49. A typical patient with Poland's syndrome.

space is shallow, thus forming the "mitten hand." The thumb is in the same plane as the fingers and is usually malrotated and disproportionally small. The bony anomaly is usually limited to the area of webbing or syndactyly, which is characteristically out to the middle phalanges. The middle phalanges are aplastic or dis-proportionately hypoplastic, such that there is effec-tively only one phalangeal joint. These are most cor-rectly termed ectrodactyly and brachydactylia, respectively.[230] According to Gausewitz,[91] the rare pa-tient with radial ray deficiency and absence of the thumb has the most extensive shoulder girdle involve-ment. A specific dermatoglyphic pattern has also been established for Poland's syndrome.[54, 79]

Inheritance

Poland's syndrome arises sporadically, with only one report of a familial occurrence.[82] This point is important in regard to genetic counseling when Poland's syndac-tyly is compared with cleft hand[63] and an associated pectoralis major muscle defect, as this may be inherited in an autosomal dominant pattern.

Associated Abnormalities

Gausewitz and colleagues[91] presented a report of severe limb deficiencies in Poland's syndrome from the

UCLA Children Amputees Prosthetic Project. Only 1 of 10 patients had syndactyly. We consider this stretching the use of the term Poland's syndrome and again call to mind that only 1 of 10 patients with pectoralis major muscle defects have the syndrome.

Associated Anomalies

Associated anomalies, excluding those in the thorax and ipsilateral upper extremity, include:
1. Musculoskeletal: contralateral syndactyly, club foot, toe syndactyly, hemivertebrae, and scoliosis.[155]
2. Genitourinary: renal aplasia, hypospadias, and inguinal hernia.
3. Gastrointestinal: situs inversus.
4. Hematopoietic: spherocytosis and acute lymphoblastic and myelogenous leukemia.[5, 18]

Some authors[79, 146, 166] believe that leukemia occurs more frequently when capillary hemangiomas are present in Poland's syndrome patients, in a manner similar to the association of leukemia with ataxia-telangiectasia.

Anatomical Pathology

Embryology. The main obstacle for the dysmorphogenetic hypothesis of Poland's syndrome lies in the lack of knowledge about embryological origin and development of the shoulder girdle.[33] Between the sixth and seventh weeks of gestation, the pectoral premuscle mass separates into major and minor primordium, while the hand differentiates into five distinct rays. According to Lewis,[148] this primordial mass fails to attach to the ribs and sternum, and thus the muscles and the underlying ribs do not develop. This failure of attachment may be caused by a predisposition of patients to overreact to teratogenic environmental factors, such that maternal drug use,[54] viral illness, hormonal manipulation,[33, 54] or vascular insufficiency[21] may produce the developmental field complex of Poland's syndrome.[182]

Incidence

The incidence of Poland's syndrome ranges from 1 in 25,000 to 1 in 49,000 cases, as compared to pectoralis major muscle defect, which occurs in 1 in 11,000 to 1 in 22,000 cases.[33] The incidence of Poland's syndrome in patients with syndactyly ranges between 2.5 and 13.5 per cent.[127]

Surgical Treatment

The absence of the pectoralis major produces little disability and requires no treatment.[234] Indeed, Brown and McDowell[26] described a professional fencer, and Christopher[39] described a pitcher, both with involvement of their dominant sides.

Relative to the shoulder girdle, the prime surgical concern is the anterior axillary fold contracture, secondary to the fibrous remnant of the pectoral muscles, which often limits abduction and extension of the shoulder. Motion can be improved by excising the fibrous remnant and closing with a Z-plasty. Breast reconstruction by augmentation (mammoplasty) is a cosmetic benefit to many female patients[188] (Fig. 3–50).

Mobius Syndrome

The Mobius syndrome,[100, 132] consisting of facial paralysis, abducens, and other cranial nerve palsies; anomalies of the brachial and thoracic musculature; and similar associated muscoloskeletal anomalies as seen in Poland's syndrome, may be an extreme expression of the developmental field complex theory previously mentioned.

Congenital Absence of the Trapezius and Rhomboideus

Congenital absence of muscles about the shoulder is rare. Sheehan[233] and Schulze-Gocht[227] reported a congenital absence of the trapezius. In 1935, Selden[229] reported on the collective absence of the trapezius and

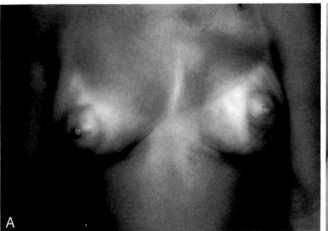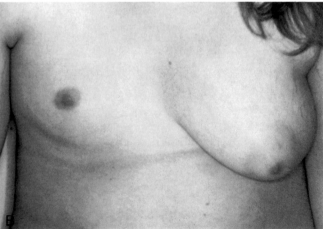

Figure 3–50. A, B, Breast augmentation mammoplasty is of cosmetic benefit to many female patients with Poland's syndrome.

rhomboid major muscles. Patients without these muscles normally learn to function well.

The first muscles connected to the shoulder girdle develop from a sheet of primitive tissue growing caudad from the occiput to the arm bud. This sheet splits to form the trapezius posteriorly and the sternomastoid anteriorly, becoming the posterior triangle of the neck in adults. The nerve supply of the trapezius and sternomastoid follows these muscles as they migrate from the occiput to the base of the bud arm, which explains why the course of the spinal accessory nerve is so extensive.

The sternomastoid muscle develops as a strap-like layer extending from the mastoid process to the sternum and the inner end of the clavicle. We previously discussed the origin of the sternalis muscle; this information adds validity to that discussion.

ABNORMAL INSERTION OF MUSCLES

Pectoralis Minor Insertion into the Humeral Head

Gantzer,[87] in 1813, was the first to report the insertion of the pectoralis minor into the shoulder joint capsule. Foltz,[80] in 1863, reported a case in which "the pectoralis minor did not insert into the coracoid process but passed over the superior surface of this process with the aid of a bursa and inserted into the humerus, medial to the greater tubercle, inferior to the supraspinatus, and fused with the articular capsule." (This is also the earliest reference to a bursa intervening between the abnormal tendon and the coracoid.) Grant,[101] in 1962, noted this abnormal insertion in 15 per cent of the upper extremities that he dissected.

DePalma[56] and Rowe[215] both report the abnormal insertion of the pectoralis minor into the humeral head in the region of the coracohumeral ligament. The tendon of the pectoralis minor, when inserting into the humeral head, usually passes over the coracoid process and between the two limbs of the coracoacromial ligament (Fig. 3–51). Rowe[215] noted the abnormal insertion of the pectoralis minor on two occasions. In his cases, the pectoralis minor originated on the medial aspect of the coracoid process. The entire tendon extended over the coracoid, passed between the two limbs of the coracoacromial ligament, and inserted into the coracohumeral ligament and the greater tuberosity of the humerus. In one case, a bursa was present under the tendon. By removing the bursa and reattaching the tendon to its normal insertion, complete relief from an impingement syndrome was obtained.

Seib[228] studied the anatomical variations of the pectoralis minor in great detail. In 15 per cent of his 1000 cases, the pectoralis minor tendon crossed over the coracoid to attach in the humeral head. The abnormal tendon had one of three insertions. In the humeral insertion, which had an incidence of 62.5 per cent, the tendon inserted directly into the coracohumeral ligament or into the immediately adjacent tendon of the supraspinatus or articular capsule (and thus into the

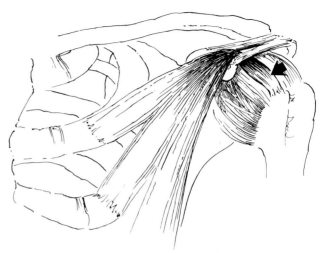

Figure 3–51. The tendon of the pectoralis minor may pass over the coracoid process to insert into the humeral head. A bursa may form under the tendon, causing an impingement syndrome.

tuberculum majus humeri), or into both of these structures. In the coracoglenoid insertion, which had an incidence of 25 per cent, the tendon inserted primarily into the articular capsule and the supraglenoid tubercle, ranging about the superior and posterior portions of the glenoid border. The third type of insertion was a combination of the humeral and coracoglenoid insertions and had an incidence of 12.5 per cent.

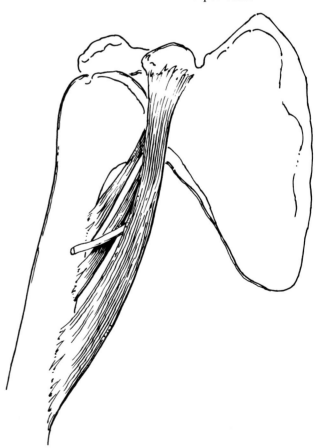

Figure 3–52. The coracobrachialis may present with two or even three muscle bellies through which the musculocutaneous nerve may be forced to pass.

An abnormal tendon insertion into the humeral head will produce a symptomatic bursa and grooving of the coracoid process. The abnormal insertion and the bursa may not have been identified in the occasional patient with an impingement syndrome who has not responded to surgery. For such patients, simply removing the bursa and moving the tendon to its normal insertion will bring relief.

Multiple Insertions of the Coracobrachialis

The coracobrachialis usually has only one muscle belly. However, the belly may split into two or even into three parts, with the musculocutaneous nerve passing between them[56] (Fig. 3–52). This abnormality is neither clinically significant nor disabling.

Neurovascular Abnormalities Associated with Congenital Anomalies

The final group of congenital shoulder anomalies involves neurovascular compression syndromes caused by abnormalities in the embryo or with associated congenital syndromes.

HIGH MEDIAN NERVE COMPRESSION, COMPLETE OR PARTIAL

Parsonage-Turner Syndrome

A group of lesions categorized as idiopathic or cryptogenic brachial plexus neuritis actually represents a spontaneous entrapment in the brachial plexus. Many of these lesions fall into the category of what Spinner[236] called the Parsonage-Turner syndrome.

Clinical Findings

Patients present with pain in and about the shoulder and with partial or complete high median nerve paralysis involving the peripheral nerve and muscles. In the hand these lesions usually produce a loss of flexion of the thumb and of the distal phalanx of the index finger, similar to that caused by an anterior interosseous nerve syndrome. Parsonage and Turner[186] described many years ago a neuritis characterized by the absence of flexion of the distal phalanx of the thumb and by variable weakness of the scapular muscles. (Paralysis of the proximal limb muscles distinguishes this syndrome from a localized entrapment of the median nerve in the forearm or hand.) This combination became known as the Parsonage-Turner syndrome. Most of the following congenital abnormalities fall into this type of neuritis.

Spinner[181] treated six patients who had partial or complete median nerve paralysis caused by anomalous vascular proliferations or vascular arches that compressed or tethered the median nerve in the axilla. The associated vascular anomalies can be either arterial or venous.

When the lesion is partial, sensation remains unaffected, while the forearm muscles, which are innervated by the median nerve, are paralyzed. In isolated cases, only a single muscle, such as the flexor pollicis longus, may be paralyzed. Most often, the flexor pollicis longus, pronator teres, pronator quadratus, flexor carpi radialis, and palmaris longus are nonfunctional, while the remaining intrinsic and extrinsic muscles innervated by the median nerve are uninvolved clinically or have negative EMG results. When the flexor pollicis longus alone is paralyzed, the diagnosis must be differentiated from an anterior interosseous nerve paralysis or an isolated rupture of the flexor pollicis longus tendon.

Spinner[181] recommended subclavian arteriography and venography with the arm abducted and adducted. With the arm at the side, the arterial tree is visualized; in abduction, the vessel with an aberrant course does not fill and cannot be seen. Brachial venography with similar positioning of the arm may reveal the pathology when the major vein perforates the nerve. Venography can be performed using the basilic rather than cephalic vein to visualize the details of region.

Anatomical Pathology

In three of Spinner's six cases, the median nerve, or the lateral root of the median nerve, was penetrated by the posterior humeral circumflex artery and vein. The subclavian arteriogram with the arm at the side revealed a segmental narrowing and a waviness of the posterior humeral circumflex artery. With the arm abducted, this artery was occluded, while the anterior humeral circumflex vessels were still easily visualized.

While the posterior humeral circumflex artery or vein seems to be the most common vessel to perforate the median nerve, the subscapular and anterior thoracic vessels have also been reported to follow anomalous paths.[120]

In an extensive study by Miller[165] of 480 human cadavers he demonstrated an aberrant relationship between the axillary artery and its major branches and the elements of the brachial plexus. In 8 of the 480 extremities, Miller reported 15 instances in which the median nerve below the union of its two roots was penetrated and divided by a branch of the axillary artery (Fig. 3–53A). The subscapular artery was involved in 10 instances, a stem common to both humeral circumflex arteries in 4, and the deep branch in 1. She also found three cases in which a common stem from the humeral circumflex arteries divided the lateral root of the median nerve (Fig. 3–53B) and one case in which the artery divided the lateral cord (Fig. 3–53C). In two bodies the lateral thoracic artery divided the median cord in four instances. In two cases there was a communication between the musculocutaneous and median nerves around the common stem of the hu-

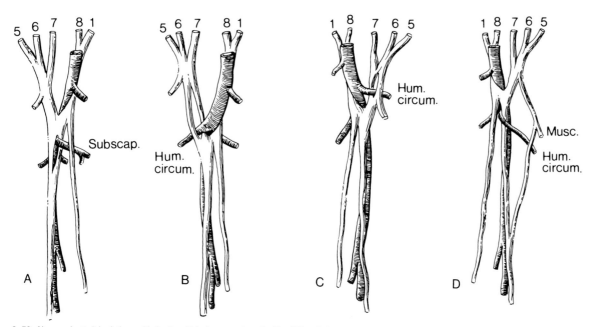

Figure 3–53. Abnormal arterial relations with the brachial plexus as described by Miller: *A,* the median nerve is penetrated and divided by a branch of the axillary artery; *B,* a common stem from the humeral circumflex artery divides the lateral root of the median nerve; *C,* the common stem may divide the lateral cord; *D,* there may be a communication between the musculocutaneous and median nerves around the humeral circumflex arteries.

meral circumflex arteries (Fig. 3–53D). In one instance she found a communication between the lateral thoracic and ulnar nerves around the axillary artery, and, in another instance, a communication between the median and ulnar nerves around the subscapular artery.

In Miller's series 8 per cent of the bodies had some type of anomalous plexus-artery relationship. In addition, 4 per cent showed anomalies of the plexus associated with veins, but she did not describe them.

Indications for Surgery

Patients who repeatedly abduct the shoulder, tethering these neurological elements, may develop an extensive paralysis about the shoulder and in the median-innervated muscles of the forearm and hand. Some cases of brachial plexus neuritis, previously considered to be idiopathic or viral in nature, may also be caused by abduction. Therefore, if a patient displays symptoms of median nerve paralysis with shoulder girdle paralysis, an arteriovenogram should be obtained with the arm adducted and abducted.

Spinner and others have performed surgery on patients in which they tied off this anomalous vessel reinnervating the nerve. The pain in the shoulder was immediately relieved. The recovery from paralysis followed both neurapractic and axonotmetric patterns, as some of the muscles involved recovered within a few days after surgery, although they remained weak, while others recovered well after two months and recovered fully by nine months.

Therefore, whenever brachial plexus and median nerve paralysis occur together, think of the Parsonage-Turner syndrome and consider both arteriography and the ultimate elimination of these aberrant vessels.

Dorsal Scapular Nerve Compression

This syndrome is rarely seen and probably more rarely diagnosed.[141] The dorsal scapular nerve comes from the C5 root and is a motor nerve supplying only the rhomboid major and minor and the levator scapulae. This nerve arises just above the upper trunk and passes almost immediately through the scalenus medius muscle (Fig. 3–54). Because this nerve enters the scalenus medius muscle, it is easy to see how many situations could compress the nerve inside this muscle.[142]

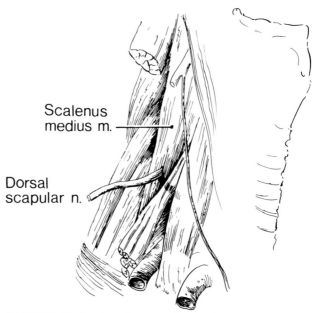

Figure 3–54. The dorsal scapular nerve arises just above the upper trunk and passes almost immediately through the body of the scalenus medius muscle.

Clinical symptoms can be caused by hypertrophy or spasm of the neck muscles. Chronic spasm can lead to hypertrophy. The brachial plexus, as it passes laterally from its spinous origin, can be angulated or kinked over the firm edge of the scalenus medius. The greater the muscle is hypertrophied, the more the brachial plexus is altered.

Certain arm and head motions will increase the muscular pressure against the nerve. In addition, the nerve can be compressed by an abnormal fibrotic muscle, such as an abnormal fibrotic scalenus medius muscle, or by an abnormal insertion of the scalenus medius muscle laterally on the first rib. The scalenus minimus muscle, particularly if it is fibrotic, can also compress the dorsal scapular nerve.

Clinical Findings

Patients complain of an aching pain and soreness in the levator scapulae and rhomboids. When seen by their general practitioner they are often diagnosed as having myofibrositis of the vertebral scapular musculature. The pain is most marked along the medial border of the scapula on the affected side. A diffuse pain radiates down the lateral surface of the arm and sometimes into the forearm. The rhomboid musculature may be extremely tender to deep palpation. If the compression continues, scapular winging will develop.

The patients characteristically complain of pain when turning the head to the affected side. Pressure on the back of the neck directly over the nerve will aggravate the pain, whereas pressure on top of the head will relieve the pain. As a result, these patients frequently press their hands on top of their heads to relieve the pain. This compression syndrome is often accompanied by an abnormally large C7 transverse process (Fig. 3–55).

Treatment

Treatment involves physical therapy, traction of the neck, sedation, and muscle relaxants. If these measures fail, however, surgical neurolysis is indicated.

The usual incision for an anterior scalenectomy runs parallel to the clavicle, but to expose the scalenus medius at the entrapment point, the posterior portion of the incision must be extended upward so that the entire incision is shaped like a hockey stick. When releasing the scalenus medius it becomes important to have a nerve stimulator to identify the nerve. Care must be taken when cutting across the muscle not to sever any of the branches of the dorsal scapular nerve, which are embedded deep in the muscle. The muscle should be teased piecemeal, using the nerve stimulator ahead of the knife, until the scalenus medius is completely relieved and the nerve is released.

Sectioning the scalenus medius does not produce any postoperative late disability, and it seems to cause little difficulty.

Suprascapular Nerve Compression

Suprascapular nerve entrapment was first described by Kopell and Thompson[141] in 1959 as a cause of frozen

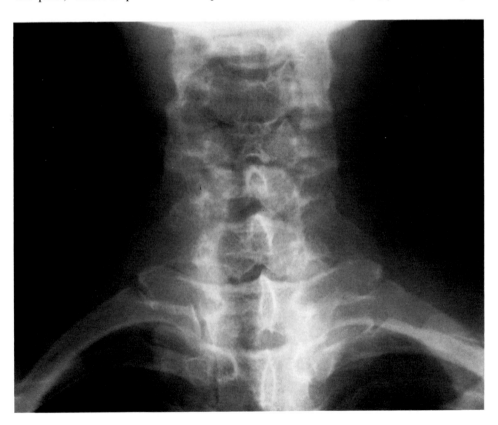

Figure 3–55. The dorsal scapular nerve compression syndrome often includes an abnormally large C7 transverse process. (Reproduced from Wood VE, Twito RS, and Verska JM: Thoracic outlet syndrome: the results of first rib resection in 100 patients. Orthop Clin North Am *19*:131–146, 1988.)

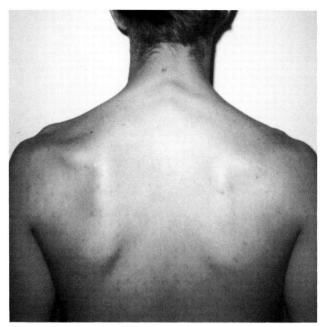

Figure 3–56. Compression of the suprascapular nerve produces weakness and atrophy of the supraspinatus and infraspinatus muscles.

shoulder. In this report, resection of the transverse scapular ligament was proposed as treatment. Today, suprascapular nerve entrapment is well recognized but infrequently observed, with fewer than 25 cases reported in the literature.

Clinical Findings

Clinically, compressive lesions of this mixed nerve produce weakness and atrophy of the supraspinatus and infraspinatus muscles (Fig. 3–56) and a deep, vague, and diffuse aching pain along the posterior aspect of the shoulder and scapula. Occasionally, the pain radiates to the neck, anterior chest wall, and arm. Adduction of the extended arm may exacerbate the pain, and palpation in the area of the suprascapular notch may reveal exquisite tenderness. Electrodiagnostic findings of denervation potentials and prolonged distal motor latencies, as well as relief with local injection, support the clinical diagnosis.[198] Bilateral cases have been reported.[88]

Anatomical Pathology

The suprascapular nerve is derived from the upper trunks of the brachial plexus, formed primarily by C5 and C6. The nerve passes posteriorly and caudally behind the plexus, along the omohyoid, and beneath the trapezius. It then enters the supraspinous fossa through the suprascapular notch, passing through the tunnel formed by the bony confines of the notch and the overlying transverse scapular ligament (Fig. 3–57). The nerve innervates the supraspinatus muscle and sends sensory branches to the posterior glenohumeral

and acromioclavicular joints and to the rotator cuff. It then passes laterally around the edge of the scapular spine in the spinoglenoid notch to innervate the infraspinatus muscle.

Suprascapular neuropathy may result from direct trauma, fracture with secondary callus and bleeding, tumor, and traction.

From a congenital or developmental perspective, certain variations in the dimension of the fibro-osseous tunnel may predispose patients to an encroachment syndrome with overuse or minimal trauma.

In their clinical, anatomical, and comparative study of this area, Rengachary and colleagues[199, 200, 201] define six specific types of suprascapular notch configurations (Fig. 3–58). The width of the suprascapular ligament paralleled the notch size.

Type I   Notch had a wide depression in the superior border of the scapula and occurred in 8 per cent of the sample.

Type II   Notch had a wide, blunted, V-shape and occurred in 31 per cent of the sample.

Type III Notch had a symmetrical U-shape and occurred in 48 per cent of the sample.

Type IV   Notch had a very small V-shape, frequently with an adjacent shallow groove for a nerve, and occurred in 3 per cent of the sample.

Type V   Notch had a partially ossified medial ligament with a minimal diameter along the superior border of the scapula and occurred in 6 per cent of the sample.

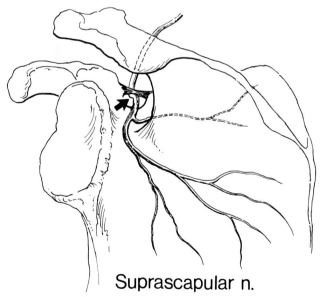

Suprascapular n.

Figure 3–57. The suprascapular nerve passes through the suprascapular notch, where it may be trapped by bone or by the overlying transverse scapular ligament.

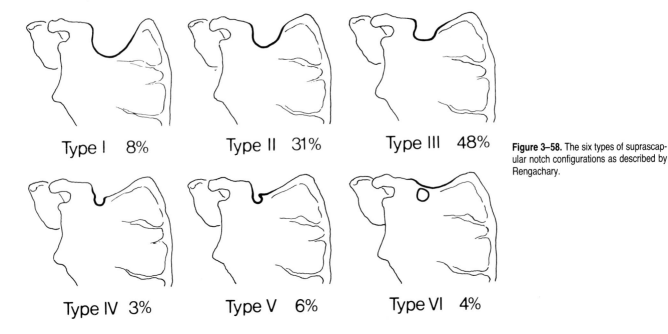

Type I 8%   Type II 31%   Type III 48%

Type IV 3%   Type V 6%   Type VI 4%

Figure 3–58. The six types of suprascapular notch configurations as described by Rengachary.

Type VI Notch had a completely ossified ligament with small bony foramen and occurred in 4 per cent of the sample.

By the nature of their study, the authors were unable to prove any association between a particular notch configuration and an entrapment syndrome. However, they felt that the notch size may have predictive value in determining a predisposition to the syndrome. Their study further demonstrated that the nerve does not undergo translational motion through the foramen. Instead, and of greater significance, the nerve undergoes angular deformation as it passes under the ligament from a higher plane of origin to the lower plane of insertion. This they termed the "sling effect," the kinking of the nerve against the ligament at the foramen.[200]

Surgical Treatment

Once the diagnosis is confirmed, the notch is evaluated by an anteroposterior x-ray with 20-degree caudal tilt. If a Type IV, V, or VI suprascapular notch is identified, it is reasonable to enlarge the notch as an adjunct to releasing the transverse scapular ligament.[200] The notch should be enlarged as well if, at the time of exploration and ligament release, the nerve does not appear to lie freely.[194, 246] This procedure is best performed through a posterior approach, beginning parallel to and just above the scapular spine. The trapezius muscle is elevated from the spine of the scapula to expose the supraspinatus and transverse scapular ligament. The transverse scapular ligament is released or excised, and a 45-degree rongeur is used to perform the notch plasty. Early motion is encouraged.

Thoracic Outlet Compression Syndrome

The thoracic outlet syndrome (TOS) is incompletely understood, difficult to diagnose, and often poorly managed.

The earliest reference to this syndrome dates back to 1627 and is found in the third chapter of William Harvey's *de Motu cordis*.[114] Harvey believed his patient had diminished blood flow in the involved arm as a result of intussusception by an aneurysm. In 1821 Sir Ashley Cooper[44] first described the symptom complex considered to be TOS.

Anatomical Pathology

The first rib is unique in that its superior surface is almost flat. On its middle anterior portion there are two transverse grooves separated by the anterior scalene tubercle. The subclavian vein rests in the groove of the rib anterior to the scalenus anterior. Posterior to the scalenus anterior lies the subclavian artery and brachial plexus. The scalenus medius inserts into the first rib posterior to the artery and the nerves. At the point where the subclavian artery and the lower trunk of the brachial plexus traverse the rib, the clavicle immediately overrides the neurovascular structures. As the clavicle swings posteriorly, the vein, artery, and nerves can be progressively squeezed like a "nut in a nutcracker," causing the symptoms now recognized as TOS.

Gage, in 1947,[83] observed that the cords of the brachial plexus may pass through the fibers of the anterior scalene muscle rather than behind them. Roos[209] observed that 98 per cent of his patients with TOS had anomalous fibrous muscular bands near the brachial plexus that predisposed them to neurological irritation or compression involving the plexus. Roos also stated that these muscle and fascial bands are functionally similar to cervical ribs and described nine different clinical types of bands[209] now believed to be common.

Type 1 is a taut, fibrous ligamentous band extending from the anterior tip of the incomplete cervical rib to the middle of the first thoracic rib posterior to the scalene tubercle (Fig. 3–59).

Type 2 is similar to Type 1, but the band comes from an elongated transverse process (Fig. 3–60). Type 3 is a taut, sharp-edged fibromuscular structure situated slightly lower in the thoracic outlet, originating on the neck of the first rib and passing horizontally across the outlet to lie between the T1 root of the plexus and the subclavian artery (Fig. 3–61). Type 4 is a fibrous string-like structure located on the anterior edge of the middle scalene muscle. It can form a sling connecting the middle and anterior scalene muscles into a common tendon (Fig. 3–62). Type 5 is a scalenus minimus muscle. It lies between the plexus and subclavian artery and attaches to the first rib (Fig. 3–63). Type 6 is a scalenus minimus muscle that attaches not to the rib but to Sibson's fascia over the lung and pleura. It may remain intact after the rib is resected (Fig. 3–64).

Type 7 is a fibrous cord attaching to the anterior surface of the anterior scalene, passing under the subclavian vein, to attach to the posterior surface of the sternum (Fig. 3–65). This cord may cause thrombosis of the vein known as a Paget-Schroetter syndrome or effort vein thrombosis (Fig. 3–66). Type 8 is similar to Type 7, but the band arises from the anterior surface of the scalenus medius, passing under the brachial plexus artery and vein, to attach to the posterior sternum (Fig. 3–67). Type 9 is a taut web of muscle and fascia that fills the inside posterior curve of the first rib (Fig. 3–68).

We have seen these abnormalities often in our dissections.[272] Roos[212] believes that a Type 3 band is most frequently seen.

Clinical Findings

In our cases[272] problems with the ulnar nerve alone was the most common symptom, followed by problems of the artery, and, finally, the median nerve alone. There were many combinations of symptoms. Two of our patients were admitted to the hospital for heart attack, and two others had Raynaud's phenomenon. Three women had severe breast pain and each of the three had one swollen breast.

The diagnosis of TOS is based on a detailed history and a thorough physical examination with appropriate tests. The patient may present with symptoms that are entirely neurological, arterial, or venous. Any combination of these symptoms may be present; therefore, the diagnosis of TOS can be difficult. Arterial manifestations include a decrease or absence of the radial pulse on abduction; a drop in blood pressure of 20 mm

Hg on abduction; or a systolic bruit.[197] Gilroy and Meyer[96] found that supraclavicular bruits are present in 69 per cent of normal subjects. In our examination of 120 patients, we found only 3 who had an arterial bruit. Wright,[274] in his series of 150 asymptomatic normal subjects, found that 92.6 per cent had obliteration of the radial pulse in at least one upper extremity tested in the elevated position.

In our experience, the best objective test to diagnose TOS is that described by Roos.[212] With the shoulders and arms abducted 90 degrees, the patient opens and closes the hand slowly for three minutes. Those patients with TOS will be unable to keep their arms and hands elevated because of ischemic-type pain. Pain with direct pressure on the brachial plexus, or Spurling's sign, is our second most reliable objective test.

The surgical treatment of TOS was introduced more than 100 years ago with the first reported excision of a cervical rib by Coote[45] at St. Bartholomew's Hospital in 1861. Because appreciation of this syndrome was slow to develop, 29 years passed before the second, similar operation was reported. In 1910, Thomas Murphy[172] was the first to remove a normal first thoracic rib as a result of this syndrome. He reported complete postoperative relief.

In 1927, Adson and Coffey[2] advocated simply dividing the anterior scalene muscle rather than removing a cervical or first rib. Their revolutionary technique changed the surgical treatment of this syndrome. In the 1930s, Rosati and Lord[213] added the complete removal of the clavicle and the sectioning of the subclavius muscle to scalenotomy. However, because of disappointing scalenotomy results, in 1962, Clagett[41] resurrected the concept of first rib resection, using the posterior approach to decompress the thoracic outlet.

Adson[2] advised a simple anterior scalenotomy, which is a simple operation with few complications. Stallworth and associates[238] assessed and followed, over a period of 5 to 15 years, 150 patients in whom scalenus anterior, pectoralis major and minor muscles, and cervical rib resections had been performed. They found a 60 per cent recurrence rate, with 40 per cent of these patients requiring a second operation. Roos' experience[212] demonstrated that in patients who required first-rib resection after a scalenotomy, the scalenus anterior had reattached itself to the scalene tubercle of the first rib.

Surgical Technique

Roos describes the operative technique for the trans-axillary approach in several articles and gives many valuable pointers for success.[208, 210, 211] We will briefly describe our current technique, which is modified from Roos'.

The patient is placed on a table (usually covered with an air cushion) with the hips in a straight lateral position, the thorax tilted 60 degrees, and with sandbags supporting the back for easy manipulation of the

Text continued on page 143

Type 1

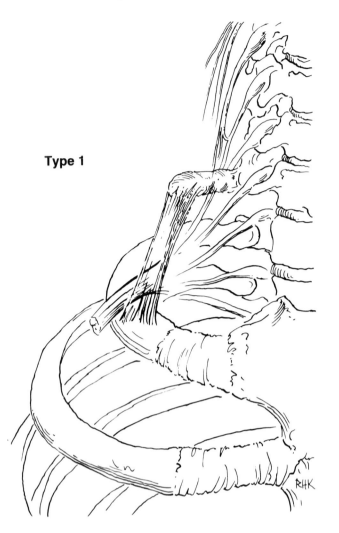

Figure 3–59. A Type 1 fibrous band (appearing in thoracic outlet syndrome).

Type 2

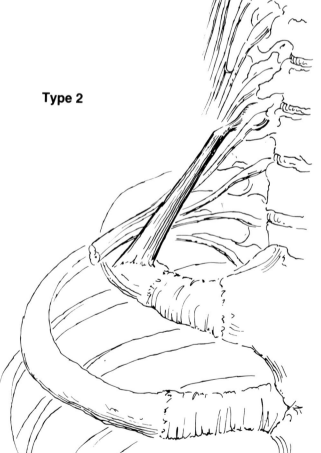

Figure 3–60. A Type 2 fibrous band (appearing in thoracic outlet syndrome).

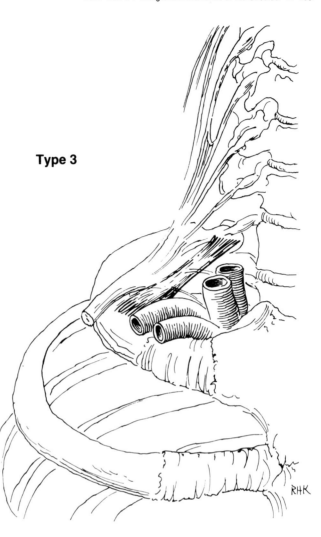

Type 3

Figure 3–61. A Type 3 is the most frequent type of anomalous band encountered in thoracic outlet syndrome.

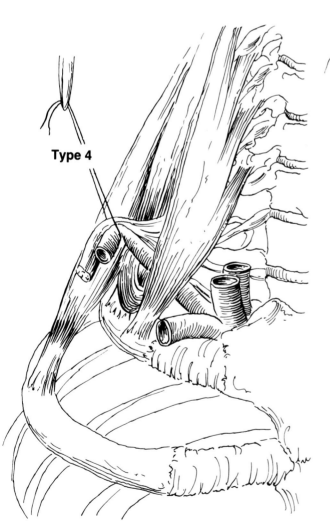

Type 4

Figure 3–62. A Type 4 fibrous sling (found in thoracic outlet syndrome).

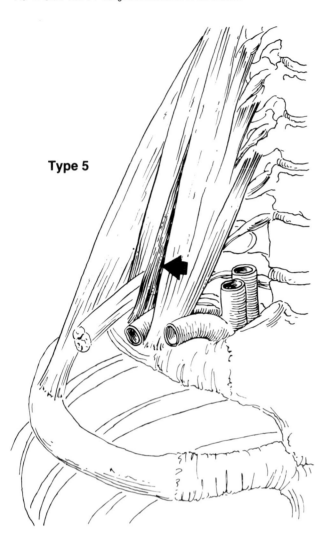

Type 5

Figure 3–63. A Type 5 band found in thoracic outlet syndrome is an abnormal scalenus minimus muscle.

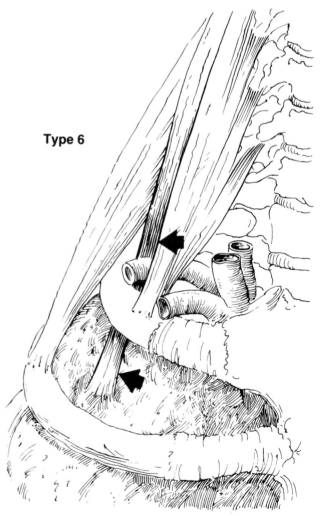

Type 6

Figure 3–64. A Type 6 band found in thoracic outlet syndrome inserts onto Sibson's fascia and must be released separately.

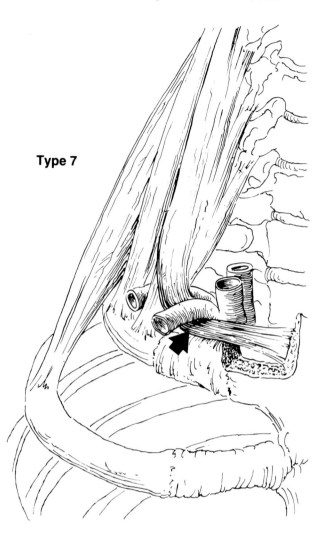

Type 7

Figure 3–65. A Type 7 band found in thoracic outlet syndrome may cause venous thrombosis.

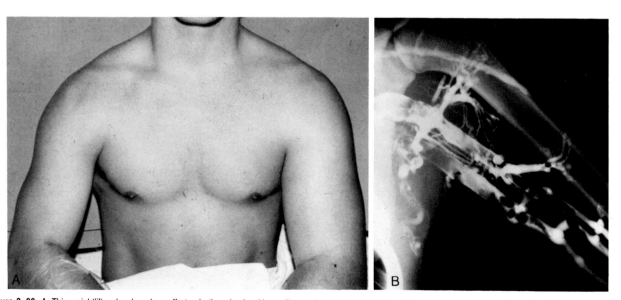

Figure 3–66. *A,* This weightlifter developed an effort vein thrombosis with swelling and pain in the left arm. *B,* The venogram shows multiple clots. This has been called Paget-Schroetter syndrome in the older literature. (Reproduced from Wood VE, Twito RS, and Verska JM: Thoracic outlet syndrome: the results of first rib resection in 100 patients. Orthop Clin North Am *19:*131–146, 1988.)

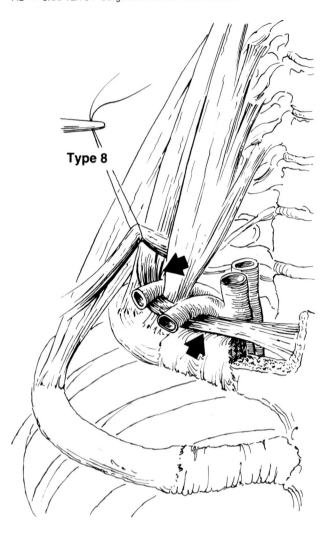

Type 8

Figure 3–67. *A* Type 8 fibrous band. (Reproduced from Wood VE, Twito RS, and Verska JM: Thoracic outlet syndrome: the results of first rib resection in 100 patients. Orthop Clin North Am *19:*131–146, 1988.)

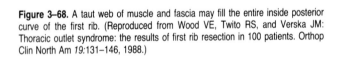

Figure 3–68. A taut web of muscle and fascia may fill the entire inside posterior curve of the first rib. (Reproduced from Wood VE, Twito RS, and Verska JM: Thoracic outlet syndrome: the results of first rib resection in 100 patients. Orthop Clin North Am *19:*131–146, 1988.)

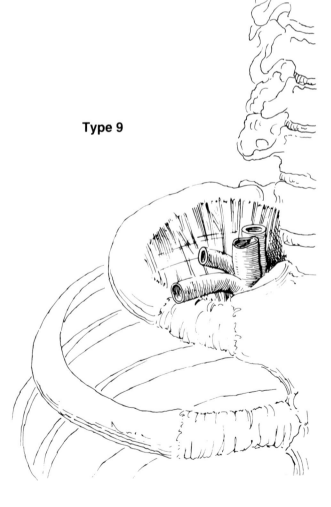

Type 9

arm. The buttocks are taped in a criss-cross fashion for stability, a pillow is placed between the legs, and the legs are strapped to the table.

The incision is made transversely in the axilla at the point where the hairline first breaks from the rib cage up to the axilla when the arm and shoulder are properly elevated toward the ceiling. If one gets too high in the axilla, the fat and lymph nodes from axillary fat make dissection impossible. If one gets below the third rib, the hole becomes extremely deep, making dissection difficult. The transverse incision is slightly curved in the shape of a smile so that it lies in the axillary skin lines, thus becoming almost imperceptible after six months.

One of the first structures encountered is the intercostal brachial nerve in the midfield coming from the second intercostal space. Even though this may be thought to be a blood vessel, it should *not* be ligated. It is best protected by dissecting it free along with a bit of fat tissue.

The arm position is extremely important. The wrist lock prevents nerve damage and is the only way to get exposure. This procedure is well described by Roos.[210] One dissects immediately to the chest wall, at which point all of the structures fall away until the first rib becomes visible. Often, the superior thoracic artery lies in the field near the first rib. The artery is easily ligated using vascular clamps. We use a Cobb elevator to remove the soft tissues from the anterior inferior surface of the first rib. When the soft tissues are dissected free, the Cobb elevator is directed posteriorly under the first rib to open up the surrounding field. Theoretically, removing the rib subperiosteally invites recurrence. However, we, as have others[57] have not found this to be a problem, but resecting it extraperiosteally invites almost certain damage to the pleura.

We next take a right-angle clamp and carefully tease all of the structures from the superior surface of the rib, including the scalenus anterior, subclavius, and a bit of the ligament between the first rib and the anterior clavicle (although this is easier cut with a knife). All of the abnormal muscle structures inserting on the first rib are teased free, with the muscle fibers carefully spread and the pleura protected at all times. The scalenus medius muscle is then teased from the first rib.

At this point, one can remove the first rib safely; a special rib cutter and a nerve root retractor (designed by Roos) are indispensable at this point. We have modified his rib cutter to one that is smaller and cuts at a 60-degree angle. The rib cutter is placed as far posterior as possible so that the T1 nerve root is immediately deep to the tips of the rib cutter. The posterior part of the rib is then cut, and using two Kocher clamps, the rib is gently pulled from the rib cage. Particularly in women, the rib can be avulsed by a gentle pull from the sternocostal junction. If it is impossible to remove the rib from the sternocostal junction, it can be cut anteriorly with the rib cutter. With these maneuvers one can obtain, in most cases,

the entire first rib except for the posterior stump. The stump should be cut and left short so that it lies posterior to the T1 cervical root; the remaining first rib should be less than 2 cm in length. A box rongeur is used to trim the first rib back to the level of the transverse process of the seventh cervical vertebra. If a cervical rib is 2 cm or less, resection is usually not necessary, but the muscles coming from its tip should be removed.

At this point the lung is carefully checked for holes by putting saline into the chest and overinflating the lungs. If a pneumothorax is found, a chest tube is placed into the hole. The skin is simply reapproximated with a subcutaneous and subcuticular stitch, and the wound is left undrained, as there have been few problems with infection.

Removal of the first rib is a surgical procedure that must be carefully thought out and meticulously executed, as it is a procedure often associated with malpractice suits. The TOS is not a procedure that lends itself well to teaching, nor is it a procedure easily mastered.[206] It is also a procedure requiring at least two assistants.

Bibliography

1. Adler KJ: Verwechslung der Apophyse des Angulus inferior scapulae mit linem Rundschalten. Roentgenpraxis 13:188, 1941.
2. Adson AW, and Coffey JR: Cervical rib—a method of anterior approach for relief of symptoms by division of the scalenus anticus. Ann Surg 85:839–857, 1927.
3. Alldred AJ: Congenital pseudarthrosis of the clavicle. J Bone Joint Surg 45B:312–319, 1963.
4. Andreasen AT: Congenital absence of the humeral head. Report of two cases. J Bone Joint Surg 30B:333–337, 1948.
5. Armendares S: Absence of pectoralis major muscle in two sisters associated with leukemia in one of them. Letter to the editor. J Pediatr 85:436–437, 1974.
6. Aziz MA: Anatomical defects in a case of trisomy 13 with a D/D translocation. Teratology 22:217–237, 1980.
7. Bagg HJ, and Halter CR: Further studies on the inheritance of structural defects in the descendants of mice exposed to roentgen-ray irradiation. (Abstract of article read by title.) Anat Rec 37:183, 1927.
8. Banniza von Bazan U: The association between congenital elevation of the scapula and diastematomyelia. A preliminary report. J Bone Joint Surg 61B:59–63, 1979.
9. Barlow RN: The sternalis muscle in American whites and Negroes. Anat Rec 61B:413–426, 1935.
10. Bateman JE: Evolution, Embryology and Congenital Anomalies. Philadelphia: WB Saunders, 1972, pp 5–38.
11. Baudine P, Bovy GL, and Wasterlain A: Un cas de syndrome de Poland. Acta Paediatr Belgica 32:407–410, 1967.
12. Beals RK, and Crawford S: Congenital absence of the pectoral muscles. A review of twenty-five patients. Clin Orthop 119:166–171, 1976.
13. Bersu ET, and Ramirez-Castro JJ: Anatomical analysis of the developmental effect of aneuploidy in man. The 18 Trisomy syndrome: anomalies of the head and neck. Am J Med Genet 1:173–193, 1977.
14. Bhattacharyya S: Abduction contracture of the shoulder from contracture of the intermediate part of the deltoid. J Bone Joint Surg 48B:127–131, 1966.
15. Bing R: Weber angeborene Muskeldefekte. Virchows Arch [A] 170:175, 1902.
16. Birkner R: Fortschr. Rontgenstr. 82:695, 1935.

17. Blair JD, and Wells PO: Bilateral undescended scapula associated with omovertebral bone. J Bone Joint Surg 39A:201–206, 1957.
18. Boaz D, Mace JW, and Gotlin RW: Poland's syndrome and leukemia. Lancet 1:349–350, 1971.
19. Bonnevie K: Embryological analysis of gene manifestation in Little and Bagg's abnormal mouse tribe. J Exp Zool 67:443, 1934.
20. Boontje AH: Axillary vein entrapment. Br J Surg 66:331–332, 1979.
21. Bouvet JP, Leveque D, Bernetieres F, and Gros JJ: Vascular origin of Poland syndrome? Eur J Pediatr 128:17, 1978.
22. Brailsford JE: The Radiology of Bones and Joints, 5th ed. Baltimore: Williams & Wilkins, 1953, pp 133, 135–137.
23. Branick RL, Robert JL, Glynn JJ, and Beatie JC: Talwin induced deltoid contracture. J Bone Joint Surg 58:279, 1976.
24. Brash JC: Muscles of upper limb. In Cunningham's Textbook of Anatomy, 9th ed. London: Oxford University Press, 1951, p 479.
25. Brooksaler FS, and Graivier L: Poland's syndrome. Am J Dis Child 121:263–264, 1971.
26. Brown JB, and McDowell F: Syndactylism with absence of the pectoralis major. Surgery 7:599–601, 1940.
27. Brown LM, Robson MJ, and Sharrard WJW: The pathophysiology of arthrogryposis multiplex congenita neurologica. J Bone Joint Surg 62-B:291–296, 1980.
28. Browne D: Congenital deformities of mechanical origin. Proc Roy Soc Med 29:1409–1431, 1936.
29. Bryce T: Note on a group of varieties of the pectoral sheet of muscle. J Anat 34:75–83, 1899.
30. Campbell CB, Chandler JG, Tegtmeyer CJ, et al.: Axillary, subclavian & brachiocephalic vein obstruction. Surgery 82:816–826, 1977.
31. Carpenter EB, and Garrett RG: Congenital pseudarthrosis of the clavicle. J Bone Joint Surg 42A:337–340, 1960.
32. Carson WG, Lovell WW, and Whitesides TE: Congenital elevation of the scapula. J Bone Joint Surg 63A:1199–1207, 1981.
33. Castilla EE, Paz JE, and Orioli IM: Pectoralis major muscle defect and Poland complex. Am J Med Genet 4:263–269, 1979.
34. Cavendish ME: Congenital elevation of the scapula. J Bone Joint Surg 54B:395–408, 1972.
35. Chang CJ: Holt-Oram syndrome. Radiology 88:479–483, 1967.
36. Chatterjee P, and Gupta SK: Deltoid contracture in children of central Calcutta. J Pediatr Orthop 3:380–383, 1983.
37. Chiari PR, Rao VY, and Rao BK: Congenital abduction contracture with dislocation of the shoulder in children: a report of two cases. Aust NZ J Surg 49:105–106, 1979.
38. Chiba S, Suzuki T, and Kasi T: A rare anomaly of the pectoralis major—the chondroepitrochlearis. Folia Anat (Japan) 60(2–3):175–186, 1983.
39. Christopher F: Congenital absence of the pectoral muscles. Case report. J Bone Joint Surg 10:350–351, 1928.
40. Chung SMK, and Nissenbaum MM: Congenital & developmental defects of the shoulder. Orthop Clin North Am 6:381–392, 1975.
41. Clagett OT: Presidential address: research & prosearch. J Thorac Cardiovasc Surg 44:153–166, 1962.
42. Clarkson P: Poland's syndactyly. Guy's Hosp Rep 111:335–346, 1962.
43. Clemente C (ed): Gray's Anatomy. Anatomy of the Human Body, 13th ed. Philadelphia: Lea & Febiger, 1985, p 520.
44. Cooper A: On exostosis. In Cooper BB, Cooper A, and Traverse B (eds): Surgical Essays. Philadelphia: James Webster, 1821, p 128.
45. Coote H: Exostosis of the left transverse process of the seventh cervical vertebra surrounded by blood vessels and nerves: Successful removal. Lancet 1:360, 1861.
46. Corning HK: Lehrbuch der Topographischen Anatomie, 24th ed. Munich: Bergmann, 1949, p 635.
47. Cozen L: Congenital dislocation of the shoulder and other anomalies. Report of a case and review of the literature. Arch Surg 35:956–966, 1937.
48. Cozen LN: Pentazocine injection as a causative factor in dislocation of the shoulder. A case report. J Bone Joint Surg 59:979–980, 1977.
49. Crenshaw AH, and Kilgore WE: Surgical treatment of bicipital tenosynovitis. J Bone Joint Surg 48A:1496–1502, 1966.
50. Crouzon O, and Buttier H: Sur une forme Particuliere, de la Dysostosis Cleidocranienine de Pierre Marie et Sainton (Forme Cleido-cranio-pelvienne). Bull Mem Soc Dilale Hop 45:972, 1099, 1921.
51. Cunningham DJ: The musculus sternalis. J Anat Physiol 22:391, 1888.
52. Cunningham's Text-Book of Anatomy, 5th ed. Robinson A, ed. New York: William Wood, 1921.
53. Cutter E.: Descriptive catalogue of the Warren anatomical museum. (JBS Jackson) 217:21, 1870.
54. David TJ: Nature and etiology of the Poland anomaly. N Engl J Med 287:487–489, 1972.
55. Debevoise NT, Hyatt GW, and Townsend GB: Humeral torsion in recurrent shoulder dislocations. Clin Orthop 76:87–93, 1971.
56. DePalma AF: Origin and comparative anatomy of the pectoral limb. In Surgery of the Shoulder, 3rd ed. Philadelphia: JB Lippincott, 1983, pp 1–33.
57. Derkash RS, Goldberg VM, and Mendelson H, et al: The results of first rib resection in thoracic outlet syndrome. Orthopedics 4:1025–1029, 1981.
58. Dick HM, and Tietjen R: Humeral lengthening for septic neonatal growth arrest: case report. J Bone Joint Surg 60:1138, 1978.
59. Dines D, Warren RF, and Inglis AE: Surgical treatment of lesions of the long head of the biceps. Clin Orthop 164:165–171, 1982.
60. Dobyns JH: Phocomelia. In Green DP (ed): Operative Hand Surgery, Vol. 1. New York: Churchill Livingstone, 1982, pp 216–219.
61. Dodd H, and Cockett FB: The Pathology and Surgery of the Veins of the Lower Limb, 2nd ed. Edinburgh: Churchill Livingstone, 1976, pp 206–207.
62. Ehrenhaft JL, Rossi NP, and Lawrence MS: Developmental chest wall defects. Ann Thorac Surg 2:384–398, 1966.
63. Engber WD: Cleft hand and pectoral aplasia. J Hand Surg 6:574–577, 1981.
64. Engel D: The etiology of the undescended scapula and related syndromes. J Bone Joint Surg 25:613–625, 1943.
65. Enna CD: Bilateral abduction contracture of shoulder girdle, case report. Orthop Rev II(9):111–113, 1982.
66. Eulenburg M: Casuistische Mittheilungen aus dem Begiete der Orthopadie. Arch Klin Chir 4:301, 1863.
67. Eulenburg M: Hochgradige Dislocation der Scapula, bedingt durch Retraction des M. levator anguli, und des oberen Theiles des M. cucullaris. Heilung mittelst subcutaner Durchschneidung beider Muskeln und entsprechender Nachbehandlung. Arch Klin Chir 4:304–311, 1863a.
68. Eulenburg M: Beitrag zur Dislocation der Scapula. Amtlicher Bericht über die Versammlung deutscher Naturforscher und Artze, 37:291–294, 1863b.
69. Fairbank HAT: Cranio-Cleido-Dysostosis. J Bone Joint Surg 31B:608–617, 1949.
70. Fawcett: The development and ossification of the human clavicle. J Anat 47:225–234, 1913.
71. Ferrell RL, Jones B, and Lucas RV: Simultaneous occurrence of the Holt-Oram and the Duane syndromes. J Pediatr 69:630–634, 1966.
72. Finder JG: Congenital anomaly of the coracoid. Os coracocosternale vestigiale. J Bone Joint Surg 18A:14–152, 1936.
73. Fitchet SM: Cleidocranial dysostosis: hereditary and familial. J Bone Joint Surg 11:838–866, 1929.
74. Fitzwilliams DCL: Hereditary cranio-cleido-dysostosis. Lancet 2:1466, 1910.
75. Flatt AE: The Care of Congenital Hand Anomalies. St. Louis: CV Mosby, 1977, p 51.
76. Folliasson A: Un cas d'os Acromial. Rev Orthop 20:533–538, 1933.
77. Frantz CH, and O'Rahilly R: Congenital skeletal limb deficiencies. J Bone Joint Surg 43:1202, 1961.

78. Frasseto F: Tre Casi Di articolazione Coraco-clavicolare osservati Radiograficamente Sul Vivente. Nota Antropologica E Clinica. Chir Org Movimento 5:116–124, 1921.
79. Freire-Maia N, Chautard EA, Opitz JM, Freire-Maia A, et al.: The Poland syndrome—clinical and genealogical data, dermatoglyphic analysis, and incidence. Hum Hered 23:97–104, 1973.
80. Foltz: Homologie des membres pelviens et thoraciques de l'homme. J Physiol Homme Animaux 6:48–81, 1863.
81. Frosch L: Congenital subluxation of shoulders. Klin Wochenschr 4:701, 1925.
82. Fuhrmann W, Mosseler U, and Neuss H: Zur Klinik und Genetik des Poland-Syndroms. Dtsch Med Wochenschr 96:1076–1078, 1971.
83. Gage M, and Parnell H: Scalenus anticus syndrome. Am J Surg 73:252–268, 1947.
84. Gall JC, Jr, Stern AM, Cohen MM, Adams, MS, et al.: Holt-Oram syndrome: clinical and genetic study of a large family. Am J Hum Genet 18:187–200, 1966.
85. Gallien R: Accessory bone at the insertion of the levator scapulae muscle in a Sprengel deformity. J Pediatr Orthop 5:352–353, 1985.
86. Galpin RD, and Birch JG: Congenital elevation of the scapula (Sprengel's deformity). Pediatr Orthop 10:965–970, 1987.
87. Gantzer: Dissertatio anatomica musculorum varietatis. Cited by Hecker, 1923, 1813.
88. Garcia G, and McQueen D: Bilateral suprascapular-nerve entrapment syndrome. Case report and review of the literature. J Bone Joint Surg 63A:491–494, 1981.
89. Gardner E: The embryology of the clavicle. Clin Orthop 58:9–16, 1968.
90. Gardner E, and Gray DJ: Prenatal development of the human shoulder and acromioclavicular joint. Am J Anat 92:219–276, 1953.
91. Gausewitz SH, Meals RA, and Setoguchi Y: Severe limb deficiency in Poland's syndrome. Clin Orthop 185:9–13, 1984.
92. Gellis SS, and Feingold M: Denouement and discussion of Poland's syndactyly. Am J Dis Child 110:85–86, 1965.
93. Gellis SS, and Feingold M: Denouement and discussion. Holt-Oram syndrome. Am J Dis Child, 112:465–466, 1966.
94. Gibson S, and Clifton WM: Congenital heart disease: clinical and postmortem study of 105 cases. Am J Dis Child 55:761–767, 1938.
95. Gibson DA, and Carroll N: Congenital pseudarthrosis of the clavicle. J Bone Joint Surg 52A:629–643, 1970.
96. Gilroy J, and Meyer JS: Compression of the subclavian artery as a cause of ischemic brachial neuropathy. Brain 86:733, 1963.
97. Golthamer CR: Duplication of the clavicle ("Os subclaviculare"). Radiology 68:576–578, 1957.
98. Goodfellow JW, and Nade S: Flexion contracture of the shoulder joint from fibrosis of the anterior part of the deltoid muscle. J Bone Joint Surg 51B:356–358, 1969.
99. Goodwin CB, Simmons EH, and Taylor I: Cervical vertebral-costal process (costovertebral bone)—a previously unreported anomaly. J Bone Joint Surg 66A:1477–1479, 1984.
100. Gorlin RJ, and Sedano H: Moebius syndrome. Mod Med 110–111, September 4, 1972.
101. Grant BJC: An Atlas of Anatomy, 5th ed. Baltimore: Williams & Wilkins, 1972.
102. Grant BJC: Grant's Atlas of Anatomy, 6th ed. Baltimore: Williams & Wilkins, 1972.
103. Gray DJ: Variations in human scapulae. Am J Physiol Anthropol 29:57–72, 1942.
104. Gray's Anatomy of the Human Body, 22nd ed. Lewis, WH ed. Philadelphia: Lea & Febiger, 1930.
105. Green WT: The surgical correction of congenital elevation of the scapula (Sprengel's deformity). J Bone Joint Surg 39A:1439, 1957.
106. Greig DM: True congenital dislocation of shoulder. Edinburgh Med J 30:157–175, 1923.
107. Grogan DP, Stanley EA, and Bobechko WP: The congenital undescended scapula. Surgical correction by the Woodward procedure. J Bone Joint Surg 65B:598–605, 1983.
108. Gross A: Uber angeborenen Mangel der Schlusselbeine. Munch Med Wochenschr 1:1151, 1903.
109. Groves J, and Goldner JL: Contracture of the deltoid muscle in the adult after intramuscular injections. J Bone Joint Surg 56A:817–820, 1974.
110. Gruenberg H: The genesis of skeletal abnormalities. Second International Conference on Congenital Malformations, pg 219, New York, The International Medical Congress, Ltd, 1963.
111. Haagenson CD: Diseases of the Breast. Philadelphia: WB Saunders, 1953, p 607.
112. Hall FJS: Coracoclavicular joint: a rare condition treated successfully by operation. Br Med J 1:766–768, 1950.
113. Hang Y: Contracture of the hip secondary to fibrosis of the gluteus maximus muscle. J Bone Joint Surg 61:52–55, 1979.
114. Harvey W: Exercitatio Anatomica de motu cordis et Sanguinis in Animalibus (1627), 5th ed. Leake CD (trans.) Springfield, IL: Charles C Thomas, 1970, p 36.
115. Hashimoto M: A case of the congenital deltoid contracture. Orthop Surg (Tokyo) 19:1259–1260, 1968.
116. Hayashi T, and Sugiura Y: Three cases of the deltoid contracture. Arch Orthop Trauma Surg 15:383–390, 1970.
117. Herman S: Congenital bilateral pseudarthrosis of the clavicle. Clin Orthop 91:162–163, 1973.
118. Hill NA, Liebler WA, Wilson HJ, and Rosenthal E: Abduction contractures of both glenohumeral joints and extension contracture of one knee secondary to partial muscle fibrosis. A case report. J Bone Joint Surg 49A:961–964, 1967.
119. Hitchcock HH, and Bechtol CO: Painful shoulder. Observations on the role of the tendon of the long head of the biceps brachii in its causation. J Bone Joint Surg 30A:263–273, 1948.
120. Hollinshead WH: The back and limbs. In Anatomy for Surgeons, Vol. 3, 2nd ed. New York: Harper & Row, 1969, pp 231, 286–288.
121. Holmes LB: Congenital heart disease and upper-extremity deformities. A report of two families. N Engl J Med 272:437–444, 1965.
122. Holt M, and Oram S: Familial heart disease with skeletal malformations. Br Heart J 22:236–242, 1960.
123. Horwitz AE: Congenital elevation of the scapula—Sprengel's deformity. Am J Orthop Surg 6:260, 1908.
124. Hrdlicka A: The scapula: visual observations. 73–94. The adult scapula. Additional observations and measurements. 363–415. The juvenile scapula. Further observations 287–310, Am J Physiol Anthropol 29, 1942.
125. Hultkrantz JW: Uber congenitalen Schlusselbeindefect und damit verbundene Schadelanomalien. Anat Anz 15:237, 1898.
126. Inclan A: Congenital elevation of the scapula or Sprengel's deformity: two clinical cases treated with Ober's operation. Circ Ortop Traum (Habana) 15:1, 1949.
127. Ireland DC; Takayama N, and Flatt AE: Poland's syndrome. A review of forty-three cases. J Bone Joint Surg 58A:52–58, 1976.
128. Jansen M: Feebleness of growth and congenital dwarfism. London: H. Froude, Horder and Stoughton, 1921.
129. Jeannopoulos CL: Congenital elevation of the scapula. J Bone Joint Surg 34A:883–892, 1952.
130. Jinkins WJ: Congenital pseudarthrosis of the clavicle. Clin Orthop 62:183–186, 1969.
131. Jones HW: Cleido-cranial dysostosis. St. Thomas Hospital Gazette 36:193–201, 1937.
132. Jorgenson RJ: V—Moebius syndrome, ectrodactyly, hypoplasia of tongue and pectoral muscles. Birth Defects 7(7):283–284, 1971.
133. Kameda Y: An anomalous muscle (accessory subscapularis teres latissimus muscle) in the axilla penetrating the brachial plexus in man. Acta Anat 96:513–533, 1976.
134. Kaplan EB: Surgical anatomy: Langer's muscles of the axilla. Bull Hosp Joint Dis 6:78–79, 1945.
135. Khoo FY, and Kuo CL: An unusual anomaly of the inferior portion of the scapula. J Bone Joint Surg 30A:1010–1011, 1948.
136. Kite JH: Congenital pseudarthrosis of the clavicle. South Med J 61:703–710, 1968.
137. Kohler A: Roentgenology: The Borderlands of the Normal and

Early Pathological in the Skiagram, 5th ed. Turnbull, A (trans and ed). New York: William Wood, 1928.

138. Kohler A and Wilk S: Borderlands of the Normal and Early Pathologic in Skeletal Roentgenology, 3rd ed. New York: Grune & Stratton, 1968, p 163.

139. Kolliker T: Mittheilungen aus der Chirurgische Casuistik und Kleinere Mittheilung. Bemerkungen zum Aufsatze von Dr. Sprengel. "Die Angeborene Vershiebung dies Schulter Blattes Nach Oben." Arch Klin Chir 42:925, 1891.

140. Konig F: Eine neue Operation des angeborenen Schulterblatt-hochstandes. Beitr Klin Chir 94:530, 537, 1914.

141. Kopell H, and Thompson W: Pain and the frozen shoulder. Surg Gynecol Obstet 109:92–96, 1959.

142. Kopell HP, and Thompson WAL: Peripheral Entrapment Neuropathies. Huntington, NY: Robert E. Krieger, 1976, pp 161–170.

143. Landry SO: The phylogenetic significance of the chondro epitrochlearis muscle and its accompanying pectoral abnormalities. J Anat 92:57–61, 1958.

144. Lane WA: A coraco-clavicular sternal muscle. J Anat Physiol 21:673, 1886–1887.

145. Langer-Oester: Med Wochenschr 15:6, 1846.

146. Lanzkowsky P: Absence of pectoralis major muscle in association with acute leukemia. Letter to the editor. J Pediatr 86:817–818, 1975.

147. Ledouble AF: Muscles des Parois de la Poitrine. Traite des Variations du Systeme Musculaire de l'homme, Vol. 1. Paris: Schleicher Freres, 1897, pp 243–258.

148. Lewis MM, Ballet FL, Kroll PG, and Bloom N: En bloc clavicular resection: operative procedure and postoperative testing of function. Case reports. Clin Orthop 193:214–220, 1985.

149. Lewis WH: Observations on the pectoralis major muscle in man. Johns Hopkins Bull 12:172, 1901.

150. Liberson F: Os acromiale—a contested anomaly. J Bone Joint Surg 19:683–689, 1937.

151. Lloyd-Roberts GC, Apley AG, and Owen R: Reflections upon the aetiology of congenital pseudarthrosis of the clavicle. J Bone Joint Surg 57B:24–29, 1975.

152. Lossen H, and Wegner RN: Die knockenkene der scapula, rontgenodogisch und verglerchend-anatomish behachtet. Fortschr Geb Rontgenstr 53:443, 1936.

153. Lucas LS, and Gill JH: Humerus varus following birth injury to the proximal humeral epiphysis. J Bone Joint Surg 29:367–369, 1947.

154. Macalister A: Additional observations on muscular anomalies in human anatomy (3rd series), with a catalogue of the principal muscular variations hitherto published. Trans Roy Ir Acad 25:1–134, 1875.

155. Mace JW, Kaplan JM, Schanberger JE, and Gotlin RW: Poland's syndrome. Report of seven cases and review of the literature. Clin Pediatr 11:98–102, 1972.

156. MacKenzie DM: Congenital forward fixation of the scapula. Personal Communication.

157. MacMahon B, McKeown T, and Record RG: Incidence and life expectation of children with congenital heart disease. Br Heart J 15:121–129, 1953.

158. Marie P, and Sainton P: On hereditary cleido-cranial dysostosis. Clin Orthop 58:5–7, 1968.

159. Marmor L: Repair of congenital pseudarthrosis of the clavicle. Clin Orthop May–June:111–113, 1966.

160. McBurney S: Congenital deformity due to malposition of the scapula. NY Med J 47:582–583, 1888.

161. McClure JG, and Raney RB: Anomalies of the scapula. Clin Orthop 110:22–31, 1975.

162. McClure JG, and Raney RB: Double acromion and coracoid processes. Case report of an anomaly of the scapula. J Bone Joint Surg 56A:830–832, 1974.

163. Mercer W, and Duthie RB: Orthopaedic Surgery, 6th ed. London: Edward Arnold, 1964, p 104.

164. Meyer AW: Spontaneous dislocation and destruction of tendon of long head of biceps brachii. Fifty-nine instances. Arch Surg 17:493–506, 1928.

165. Miller RA: Observations upon the arrangement of the axillary artery and brachial plexus. Am J Anat 64:143–163, 1939.

166. Miller RA, and Miller DR: Congenital absence of the pectoralis major muscle with acute lymphoblastic leukemia and genitourinary anomalies. J Pediatr 87:146–147, 1975.

167. Minami M, Ishii S, Usui M, and Terashima Y: The deltoid contracture. Clin Orthop Surg (Tokyo) 11:493–501, 1976.

168. Minami M, Yamazaki J, Minami A, and Ishii S: A postoperative long-term study of the deltoid contracture in children. J Pediatr Orthop 4:609–613, 1984.

169. Morris' Human Anatomy, 12th ed. Anson, BJ (ed). New York: Blakiston, 1966.

170. Mortensen OA, and Pettersen JC: The musculature. In Anson BJ (ed): Morris' Human Anatomy, 12th ed. New York: McGraw-Hill, 1966, p 459.

171. Mudge MK, Wood VE, and Frykman GK: Rotator cuff tears associated with os acromiale. J Bone Joint Surg 66A:427–429, 1984.

172. Murphy T: Brachial neuritis caused by pressure of first rib. Aust Med J 15:582, 1910.

173. Nakaya M, Kumon Y, and Fujiwara M: Two cases of the congenital deltoid contracture. Orthop Surg (Tokyo) 22:814–818, 1971.

174. Neer CS II, Craig EV, and Fukuda H: Cuff tear arthropathy. Orthop Trans 1:111, 1977.

175. Neer CS: Impingement lesions. Clin Orthop 173:70–77, 1983.

176. Neumann W: Uber das "Os Acromiale." Fortschr Geb Rontgenstr 25:180–191, 1918.

177. Neviaser RJ: Injuries to and developmental deformities of the shoulder. In Bora, FW: The Pediatric Upper Extremity: Diagnosis and Management. Philadelphia: WB Saunders, 1986, p 238.

178. Nogi J, Heckman JD, Hakala M, and Sweet DE: Non-union of the clavicle in a child. Clin Orthop 110:19–21, 1975.

179. Nutter PD: Coracoclavicular articulations. J Bone Joint Surg 23:177–179, 1941.

180. O'Donoghue DH: Subluxing biceps tendon in the athlete. Clin Orthop 164:26–29, 1982.

181. Omer G, and Spinner M: Management of Peripheral Nerve Problems. Philadelphia: WB Saunders, 1980, pp 582–592.

182. Opitz JM, Herrmann J, and Dieker H: The study of malformation syndromes in man. Birth defects: Orig Art Ser 5(2):1–10, 1969.

183. Owen R: Bilateral glenoid hypoplasia. Report of five cases. J Bone Joint Surg 35B:262–267, 1953.

184. Owen R: Congenital pseudarthrosis of the clavicle. J Bone Joint Surg 52B:644–652, 1970.

185. Paltauf R: Demonstration eines Skelettes von einem Falle von Dysostosis Cleidocranialis. Verh Dtsch Ges Pathol 15:337, 1912.

186. Parsonage MJ, and Turner JWA: Neurologic amyotrophy. The shoulder—girdle syndrome. Lancet 1:973–978, 1948.

187. Perrin JB: Notes on some variations of the pectoralis major, with its associate muscles seen during sessions 1866–69, 1869–70, at King's College, London. J Anat Physiol 5:233–240, 1871.

188. Pers M: Aplasias of the anterior thoracic wall, the pectoral muscles, and the breast. Scand J Plast Reconstr Surg 2:125–135, 1968.

189. Petrie JG: Congenital elevation of the scapula. J Bone Joint Surg 55B:441, 1973.

190. Pinsky HA, Pizutillo FD, and MacEwen GD: Congenital elevation of the scapula. Orthop Trans 4:288–289, 1980.

191. Poirer P: La Clavicle et ses Articulations. Bourses séreuses des ligaments costo-claviculaire. J Anat Physiol 26:81–103, 1890.

192. Poland A: Deficiency of the pectoralis muscles. Guy's Hosp Rep 6:191, 1841.

193. Ponde A, and Silveira J: Estudos Radiológicos da Articulacao Coraco-clavicular. J Clin 22:325–328, 1930.

194. Post M, and Mayer J: Suprascapular nerve entrapment. Diagnosis and treatment. Clin Orthop 223:126–136, 1987.

195. Poznanski AK, Gall JC, and Stern AM: Skeletal manifestations of the Holt-Oram syndrome. Radiology 94:45–53, 1970.

196. Putti V: Beitrag zur Atiologie, Pathogenese und Behandlung

des angeborenen Hochstandes des Schulterblattes. Fortschr Rontgenstr *12:*328, 1908.

197. Rainer GW, Vigor W, and Newby JP: Surgical treatment of thoracic outlet compression. Am J Surg *116:*704–707, 1968.

198. Rask MR: Suprascapular nerve entrapment. A report of two cases treated with suprascapular notch resection. Clin Orthop *123:*73–75, 1977.

199. Rengachary SS, Neff JP, Singer PA, and Brackett CE: Suprascapular entrapment neuropathy: a clinical, anatomical, and comparative study. Part 1: Clinical study. Neurosurgery *5:*441–455, 1979.

200. Rengachary SS, Burr D, Lucas S, Hassanein KM, et al.: Suprascapular entrapment neuropathy: a clinical, anatomical, and comparative study. Part 2: Anatomical study. Neurosurgery *5:*447–451, 1979.

201. Rengachary SS, Burr D, Lucas S, and Brackett CE: Suprascapular entrapment neuropathy: A clinical, anatomical, and comparative study. Part 3: Comparative study. Neurosurgery *5:*452–455, 1979.

202. Resnick E: Congenital unilateral absence of the pectoral muscles often associated with syndactylism. J Bone Joint Surg *24:*925–928, 1942.

203. Rhinehart BA: Cleidocranial dysostosis (mutational dysostosis) with a case report. Radiology *26:*741–748, 1936.

204. Rob C, and May AG: Neurovascular compression syndromes. *In* Advances in Surgery, Vol. 9. Chicago: Year Book Medical Publishers, 1975.

205. Robinson A, Braun RM, Mack P, and Zadek R: The surgical importance of the clavicular component of Sprengel's deformity. J Bone Joint Surg *49A:*1481, 1967.

206. Roeder DK, Mills M, McHale JJ, et al.: First rib resection in the treatment of thoracic outlet syndrome: transaxillary and posterior thoracoplasty approaches. Ann Surg *178:*49–52, 1973.

207. Roldan R, and Warren D: Abduction deformity of the shoulder secondary to fibrosis of the central portion of the deltoid muscle. *In* Proceedings of the American Academy of Orthopedic Surgeons. J Bone Joint Surg *54A:*1332, 1972.

208. Roos DB: Experience with first rib resection for thoracic outlet syndrome. Ann Surg *173:*429–442, 1971.

209. Roos DB: New concepts of thoracic outlet syndrome that explain etiology, symptoms, diagnosis and treatment. Vasc Surg *13:*313–321, 1979.

210. Roos DB: Transaxillary approach for first rib resection to relieve thoracic outlet syndrome. Ann Surg *163:*354–358, 1966.

211. Roos DB: Essentials and safeguards of surgery for thoracic outlet syndrome. Angiology *32:*187–197, 1981.

212. Roos DB: Congenital anomalies associated with thoracic outlet syndrome. Anatomy, symptoms, diagnosis and treatment. Am J Surg *132:*771–778, 1976.

213. Rosati LM, and Lord JW: Neurovascular compression syndromes of the shoulder girdle. *In* Modern Surgical Monographs. New York: Grune & Stratton, 1968.

214. Ross DM, and Cruess RL: The surgical correction of congenital elevation of the scapula. A review of seventy-seven cases. Clin Orthop *125:*17–23, 1977.

215. Rowe CR: Unusual Shoulder Conditions. New York: Churchill Livingstone, 1988, pp 639–646.

216. Ruge G: Ein Rest des Haut-rumpf-muskels in der Achselgegend des Meschen—Achselbogen. Morphol Jahrb *41:*519–538, 1910.

217. Sachatello CR: The axillopectoral muscle (Langer's axillary arch): a cause of axillary vein obstruction. Surgery *81*(5):610–612, 1977.

218. Saint-Pierre L: Pseudarthrose Congenitale de la Clavicule Droite, Annales d'Anatomie. Pathologique *7:*466, 1930.

219. Saitta GF, and Baum V: Langer's axillary arch, an unusual cause of axillary mass. JAMA *180:*122, 1962.

220. Salter RB: Congenital forward fixation of the scapula. Personal Communication.

221. Sato M, Hondo S, and Inoue H: Three cases of abduction contracture of the shoulder joint caused by fibrosis of the deltoid muscle. Orthop Surg (Tokyo) *16:*1052–1056, 1965.

222. Scaglietti O: The obstetrical shoulder trauma. Surg Gynecol Obstet *66:*868, 1938.

223. Schar W, and Zweifel C: Das Os Acromiale und Seine Klinische Bedeutung. Bruns' Beitr Klin Chir *164:*101–124, 1936.

224. Schlyvitch B: Uber den Articulus Coracoclavicularis. Anat Anz *85:*89–93, 1937.

225. Schrock RD: Congenital abnormalities at the cervicothoracic level. AAOS Instructional Course Lectures *6:*231–236, 1949.

226. Schrock RD: Congenital elevation of the scapula. J Bone Joint Surg *8:*207, 1926.

227. Schulze-Gocht: Uber den Trapeziusdefekt. Zugleich ein Beitrag zur Frage der Skoliosenentstehung. Arch Orthop Chir *26:*302–307, 1928.

228. Seib GA: The musculus pectoralis minor in American whites and American Negroes. Am J Physiol Anthropol *4*(23):389, 1938.

229. Selden BR: Congenital absence of trapezius and rhomboideus major muscles. J Bone Joint Surg *17:*1058–1059, 1935.

230. Senrui H, Egawa T, and Horiki A: Anatomical findings in the hands of patients with Poland's syndrome. J Bone Joint Surg *64A:*1079–1082, 1982.

231. Sharby HG: Acta Radiol (Stockholm) *17:*397, 1936.

232. Sharrard WJW: Paediatric Orthopaedics and Fractures. Oxford: Blackwell Scientific Publications, 1971.

233. Sheehan D: Bilateral absence of trapezius. J Anat *67:*180, 1932.

234. Soderberg BN: Congenital absence of the pectoral muscle and syndactylism: a deformity association sometimes overlooked. Plast Reconstr Surg *4:*434–436, 1949.

235. Soule AB: Mutational dysostosis (cleidocranial dysostosis). J Bone Joint Surg *28:*81–102, 1946.

236. Spinner M: Correspondence Club Newsletter 1977, p 32.

237. Sprengel RD: Die Angeborene Verschiebung des Schulterblattes Nach Oben. Arch Klin Chir *42:*545, 1891.

238. Stallworth JM, Quinn GJ, and Aiken AF: Is rib resection necessary for relief of thoracic outlet syndrome? Ann Surg *185:*581–592, 1977.

239. Stocks P, and Barrington A: Treasury of Human Inheritance, Vol 3. London: Cambridge University Press, 1925, p 121.

240. Subkowitsch EM: Zur Frage der Morphologie des Schultergurtels. I. Entwicklung und Morphologie des Processus coracoides bei Mensch und Fledermaus. Morphol Jahrb *65:*517, 1931.

241. Sulamaa M: Autotransplantation of epiphysis in neonates. Acta Chir Scand *119:*194, 1960.

242. Sulamaa M: Treatment of some skeletal deformities. Postgrad Med J *39:*67, 1963.

243. Sulamaa M, and Ryoppy S: Early treatment of congenital bone defects of the extremities: aftermath of thalidomide disaster. Lancet *1:*130, 1964.

244. Sulamaa M: Upper extremity phocomelia. A contribution to its operative treatment. Clin Pediatr *2:*251–257, 1963.

245. Sutro CJ: Dentated articular surface of the glenoid—an anomaly. Bull Hosp Joint Dis *27:*104–108, 1967.

246. Swafford AR, and Lichtman DH: Suprascapular nerve entrapment—case report. J Hand Surg *7:*57–60, 1982.

247. Swanson AB: A classification for congenital limb malformations. J Hand Surg *1:*8, 1976.

248. Tachdjian MO: Pediatric Orthopedics, Vol 1. Philadelphia: WB Saunders, 1972, pp 79–98.

249. Tachendorf F: Einige seltenere atypische Brustmuskeln des Menschen und ihre Beurteilung. Z Anat Ent *114:*216–229, 1949.

250. Taussig HB: A study of the German outbreak of phocomelia: the thalidomide syndrome. JAMA *180:*1106, 1962.

251. Terry RJ: Rudimentary clavicles and other abnormalities of the skeleton of a white woman. Anat Physiol *33:*413–422, 1899.

252. Testut L: Les Anomalies Musculaires Chez L'Homme Expliquees par L'Anatomie Comparee, Leur Importance en Anthropologie. Paris: Doin, 1884.

253. Testut L: Traite d'Anatomie Humaine, Paris: Gaston Doin & Cie, 1928, p 879.

254. Tilney NL, Griffiths HJG, and Edwards EA: Natural history of major venous thrombosis of upper extremity. Arch Surg *101:*792, 1970.

255. Tobler L: Der Achsiebogen des Menschen, ein Rudiment des Panniculus Cornosus der Mannaliev. Morphol Jahrb *30:*453–507, 1902.

256. Turner W: On the musculus sternalis. J Anat Physiol *1*:246, 1867.
257. Valentin B: Die Kongenitale. Schulterluxation, Bericht Uber Drei Falle in Einer Familie. Z Orthop Chir *55*:229–240, 1931.
258. Voto SJ, and Weiner DS: The chondroepitrochlearis muscle. Case report. J Pediatr Orthop *7*:213–214, 1987.
259. Wall JJ: Congenital pseudarthrosis of the clavicle. J Bone Joint Surg *52A*:1003–1009, 1970.
260. Weaver JK, and Dunn HK: Treatment of acromioclavicular injuries, especially complete acromioclavicular separation. J Bone Joint Surg *54A*:1187, 1972.
261. Weed LH: The development of the cerebrospinal spaces (Contribution to Embryology No. 14). Publication 225. Carnegie Institute of Washington, 1916.
262. Wertheimer LG: Coracoclavicular joint. J Bone Joint Surg *30A*:570–578, 1948.
263. Whitman R: The treatment of congenital and acquired luxations at the shoulder in childhood. Ann Surg *42*:110–115, 1905.
264. Wiland OK: Extracardiac anomalies in association with congenital heart disease: analysis of 200 necropsy cases. Lab Invest *5*:380–388, 1956.
265. Wilkinson JA, and Campbell D: Scapular osteotomy for Sprengel's shoulder. J Bone Joint Surg *62B*:486–490, 1980.
266. Willet A, and Walsham WJ: A second case of malformation of the left shoulder girdle, with remarks on the probable nature of the deformity. Br Med J *1*:513–514, 1883.
267. Willet A, and Walsham WJ: An account of the dissection of the parts removed after death from the body of a woman. The subject of congenital malformations of the spinal column, bony thorax, and left scapular arch. Proc Roy Med Chir Soc *8*:503–506, 1880.
268. Wolbrink AJ, Hsu Z, and Bianco AJ: Abduction contracture of the shoulders and hips secondary to fibrous bands. J Bone Joint Surg *55A*:844–846, 1973.
269. Wolff G: Ueber Einen Fall Von Kongenitaler Schulterluxation. Z Orthop Chir *51*:199–209, 1929.
270. Wood J: Variations in human myology observed during the winter session of 1867–68 at King's College, London. Proc Roy Soc *17*:483–525, 1868.
271. Wood J: Variations in human myology observed during the winter session of 1865–66 at King's College, London. Proc Roy Soc *15*:229–244, 1866.
272. Wood VE, Twito RS, and Verska JM: Thoracic outlet syndrome. Orthop Clin North Am *19*(1):1–16, 1988.
273. Woodward JW: Congenital elevation of the scapula. Correction by release and transplantation of muscle origins—a preliminary report. J Bone Joint Surg *43A*:219–228, 1961.
274. Wright IS: The neurovascular syndrome produced by hyperabduction of the arms. Am Heart J *157*:1, 1945.

4

Clinical Evaluation of Shoulder Problems

Richard J. Hawkins, M.D.
Desmond J. Bokor, M.D.

The successful treatment of any condition of the shoulder requires an accurate diagnosis. To achieve this, all pieces of information pertaining to the patient's complaint need to be collected and analyzed. It is often easy to overlook the most basic clinical skills of history and physical examination, relying instead on high-powered investigative aids. These procedures play a role in confirming an established diagnosis or occasionally assist in the challenging presentation. In the vast majority of cases, a working diagnosis can be reached following an appropriate history and careful physical examination.

Clinical assessment should avoid focusing too quickly on the shoulder complaint for fear of missing a generalized disorder which might influence diagnosis, treatment, and expectations. For example, adhesive capsulitis can occur in patients with diabetes, often with a more refractory course; both physician and patient should be aware of this.[2] Similarly, the steroid-dependent patient with rheumatoid arthritis has a higher risk of complications following surgery, often related to healing because of poor tissue quality.

Expectations and lifestyle relating to work, sport, and leisure are important factors to consider when deciding on management. Treatment of a rotator cuff tear is quite different in an 80 year old whose leisure activity involves playing chess compared with a 50 year old whose job is manual labor.

History

NATURE OF INTERVIEW

Two important facts that play a major role in establishing a diagnosis are the patient's chief complaint and age. For example, the commonest cause of shoulder pain in a 70 year old is rotator cuff pathology, whereas the usual cause of the shoulder "coming out" in an 18 year old is anterior unidirectional instability. In questioning a patient with regard to a clinical problem, two distinct areas are explored: the specific problem related to the shoulder and how this problem interacts with the patient's general health and environment. In addition to the chief complaint and age, the patient's occupation, marital status, handedness, sports, leisure activities, and any history of trauma are documented. This portion of the introduction provides the physician with an impression of the patient and serves as an informal discussion to help relax the patient, facilitating the remainder of the interview and examination. Early on it is important to appreciate whether the situation is related to worker's compensation or litigation.

The examination follows the pattern of questioning the patient relating to chief complaint and considers past history and general medical health, along with medications and family history. The order in which these features are approached depends upon the presenting circumstances and physician preference.

At the outset of the interview it is important to establish the predominant presenting symptom(s). The direction of the interview is carefully guided by the physician, although there should be appropriate time to allow the patient to speak freely. As in physical examination, the approach to historical interview is clear, organized, and comprehensive.

Patients may present with a chief complaint related to a chronic shoulder problem, or soon after an acute injury. In the former situation, the most common chief complaints referable to the shoulder are pain and instability. Other complaints are usually present as secondary symptoms but occasionally are primary and occur in isolation, such as weakness, loss of motion, functional disability, deformity, catching, and crepitus.

Once the primary complaint is established, the physician must next endeavor to take the patient's recollection back to its onset. Patients may be unclear as to how symptoms started, or they may clearly describe a spontaneous commencement of symptoms. Onset is often related to trauma, through work or an accident, to overuse, or to a change in the pattern of activities in the days or weeks leading up to its onset. This may be related to a change in the type of work, necessitating excessive overhead use of the arm in such activities as painting a house or pitching a baseball. If trauma was responsible, the mechanism and events surrounding the accident are considered. Once the circumstances surrounding the onset are established, the clinical course of the complaint is determined from its inception to the present time. During this course, the effects and timing of any treatments must be carefully considered. Any response to treatment, even if only temporary, is important as time progresses. The course of the complaint is carefully developed to determine whether it is improving, worsening, or remaining the same. This sequence of questioning eventually returns the physician and patient to the current status of the presenting symptom. A careful analysis is then made of its present character, intensity, and interference with activities of daily living, work, and sport.

TECHNIQUE OF PRESENTATION

The general presentation in this format may be as follows: A 50-year-old male farmer presents with a chief complaint of shoulder pain. His history dates back 10 years when he fell from a silo directly onto his shoulder. Since that time he has had increasing pain and been treated with physiotherapy, anti-inflammatory medication, and analgesia with little effect. An injection placed into the front of the shoulder gave him dramatic relief for three days. That brings us to the present in which his pain precludes him from doing his farming work, keeps him awake at night time, interferes with daily activities such as combing his hair, shaving, and feeding, and requires six Tylenol No. 3 tablets per day. He rates the intensity of his pain as 7 out of 10.

PAIN AS THE CHIEF COMPLAINT

Pain is the most common presenting symptom about the shoulder. Knowing the age of the patient and the nature and course of the pain will often lead to the diagnosis. It is important to note its onset, periodicity, site, character, radiation, associated symptoms, and aggravating or relieving factors. These features will likely suggest its origin. Pain may be due to local musculoskeletal pathology about the shoulder or referred from a distance such as the cervical spine. The patient is often rather vague in localizing the specific area of pathology. For example, the patient with primary shoulder pathology such as supraspinatus tendinitis will often localize his pain over the deltoid region, whereas the patient with pain referred from the cervical spine may localize his pain over the top of the shoulder. Rather than pointing to shoulder pain with one finger, patients often use their open hand to describe the location of pain (Fig. 4–1). The quality of pain is variable with different pathological presentations. Radicular pain from the cervical spine to the shoulder is often of a lancinating quality, occasionally in a nerve root pattern. The pain of shoulder tendinitis is often diffuse, dull, and aching in nature.

Pain is a subjective complaint and as such eludes objective assessment. It is, however, important for the treating physician to gain insight into its intensity and the associated degree of functional limitations. There are several parameters by which we can attempt some objective determination of pain.

1. Presence of night pain.
2. Analgesic requirement and its effect.
3. Other treatment requirements and their effects.
4. Degree of interference with work, sport, and activities of daily living.
5. Effect on lifestyle and personality.
6. An estimate on a linear scale by the patient of the amount of pain.

It is especially helpful to elaborate on the nature and extent of night pain. As the intensity of pain increases, it tends to occur both at rest and at night. At first the patient may awaken only at night when he rolls onto the affected side, but later, pain may develop as a more constant ache which disturbs sleep, even preventing him from getting to sleep. Patients may get up at night, walk about, and rub their shoulders in an attempt to ease their discomfort. Some patients go so far as to take a hot shower or attempt sleeping in a sitting position. Others require analgesia during the night. Such severe pain is typical in a patient with rotator cuff pathology. Less common conditions, such as arthritis, infection, and tumor, may also cause night pain.

The amount and type of analgesic consumed by the patient provides some appreciation of the degree of pain. The significance and interpretation of analgesic requirements in those with chronic pain can be confusing. The need for sleeping sedation may be similarly significant.

Further insight is gained by questioning patients about any restriction of activities. The pain may be intermittent and only activity related. As the degree of irritation and inflammation increases, there may be loss of ability to participate in work, sport, and even some daily activities. The degree to which patients are able to participate in work and sport is an important measure of degree of pain. Many patients present with pain related only to certain activities such as athletic performance. This can be subdivided into whether it interferes with peak performance or actually precludes

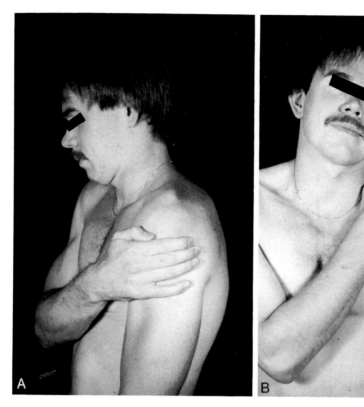

Figure 4–1. *A,* Localization of primary shoulder pain. The patient with primary shoulder pathology often localizes the pain with the open hand over the deltoid area. *B,* Localization of shoulder pain referred from cervical spine pathology. Referred pain to the shoulder, such as might be seen with cervical spine pathosis, is usually localized by the patient with an open hand over the top of the shoulder.

athletes from participating in their chosen endeavours. Obviously, the patient who has difficulty with daily activities such as feeding, shaving, and dressing is significantly disabled.

It is helpful to ask patients to grade the intensity of their pain on a scale of 1 to 10, with 10 being the most severe. This will give at least some subjective indication of the amount of pain patients are experiencing. Some people however have difficulty conceptualizing pain in terms of a linear scale, while others have a low pain threshold and will overdramatize their pain. The physician should also formulate a linear analog pain scale. The degree of pain and the duration of the complaint will aid in diagnosis and help direct management.

INSTABILITY AS THE CHIEF COMPLAINT

The next most common complaint particularly in office practice or clinic setting relates to instability. The spectrum of symptomatology in this group of patients is wide. In many cases, instability of the shoulder is readily perceived and described by the patient who often states "my shoulder comes out." In others, it may not be so obvious, especially when their instability is masked with "pain." If we consider the two main groups of instability patients as described by Matsen using the acronyms TUBS (*t*raumatic *u*nidirectional with a *B*ankart lesion responding to *s*urgery) and AMBRI (*a*traumatic *m*ultidirectional with *b*ilateral shoulder findings responsive to *r*ehabilitation and, if surgery is to be undertaken, it is an *i*nferior capsular

shift), it will allow us a better appreciation of the variation in symptomatic presentation of these patients.

A history of a significant injury causing a dislocation requiring manipulative reduction and subsequent recurrent dislocations will direct the physician toward the TUBS category. The AMBRI patients often present without any history of trauma and may perceive instability, pain, or discomfort with activities or certain arm positions. They may avoid certain activities or sports and not fully understand that their shoulder "comes out of joint." There are some patients with injuries that lie between these extremes, often with overlapping symptoms.

In questioning a patient with instability the aim is to ascertain the degree (subluxation, dislocation), its onset (traumatic, atraumatic, overuse), and direction(s) (anterior, posterior, multidirectional).

A dislocation has probably occurred if the shoulder was felt to go out of joint and stay out, for at least a few seconds. Most patients require manipulation for reduction, some by adopting a particular maneuver on their own, while others require the assistance of a physician. In most instances this sequence of events suggests anterior unidirectional instability.

With a subluxation the patient may have feelings of the shoulder "partially slipping out of joint" momentarily but quickly reducing, usually spontaneously. Like dislocation, subluxation may be posterior or multidirectional. Patients with anterior subluxation may occasionally experience a "dead arm syndrome," a complaint of tingling or numbness in the arm, particularly in the provocative position of external rotation and abduction. Others experience apprehension or pain associated with the feeling that the shoulder may come out if a particular activity is performed. Apprehension may be a feature in patients who have recurrent dislocation or subluxation and because of a fear of impending instability, these patients may refuse to put their arms in the provocative position. There is obviously overlap in these symptoms of dislocation, subluxation, and apprehension so that at times it may be difficult to be sure of the degree of instability.

Next it is important to determine the nature of the onset of the instability. Was it associated with trauma and what was the degree of violence or energy which precipitated the initial episode? It is then helpful to determine the frequency and the ease of subsequent subluxation and dislocation episodes as well as the ease of reduction of these episodes. In traumatic recurrent instability, the shoulder usually displaces anteriorly and rarely posteriorly, whereas in the atraumatic group, multidirectional and posterior displacement is much more frequent.

It is also important to relate whether these instability episodes are voluntary or involuntary. These descriptive terms more frequently apply to posterior instability. The patient who can perform the act with muscular contraction should be categorized as a voluntary subluxator. Those that have instability precipitated by arm positioning should be considered involuntary. While the voluntary subluxator or dislocator may be capable of reproducing his instability, most have an accompanying element of involuntary or unintentional instability associated with certain movements. There are patients in the voluntary category who have a conscious or unconscious desire to reproduce their shoulder instability. Recognition of this subgroup of patients with personality disorders is important since these patients may frustrate attempts at stabilization, whether operative or nonoperative. The most common category of patient with posterior instability is the involuntary subluxator where activities related to arm positioning produce the subluxation.

The direction of instability, whether anterior, posterior, inferior, or multidirectional, should be ascertained. The most common instability pattern is anterior and unidirectional. Questioning these patients may reveal apprehension with activities involving abduction and external rotation of the shoulder. The patient may describe the feeling of the shoulder moving forward or the sensation of anterior or axillary fullness. The diagnosis can be confirmed with a radiographically documented anterior dislocation or suggested with anterior glenoid rim changes or a Hill-Sachs lesion.

Posterior instability is usually demonstrable by the patient.[9] The patient may have feelings of the joint's being out when the arm is internally rotated in the forward flexed position but more commonly feels the clunk of reduction as the arm is brought toward the coronal plane of the body.

While posterior instability, like anterior instability, may occur in isolation, it can often be associated with inferior instability and therefore be multidirectional.[20] Symptomatically, the patients complain of a "loose feeling" in their shoulders with further apprehension, insecurity, or subluxation on loading the shoulder inferiorly, as occurs on lifting a suitcase. Many of these patients complain of pain which can make the diagnosis challenging.

Having ascertained all the features of the patient's instability, the final step is to formulate an overview of the disability as it relates to the instability. While the frequency of instability will be important, the ease with which these episodes occur and the ease of reduction may be of greater significance. The patient who sustains painful dislocations requiring difficult reductions at the hospital every few weeks is obviously much more disabled than the patient who has one dislocation easily reduced every three years. Any intervening complaints relating to subluxation and apprehension contribute to an understanding of the degree of disability. Further insight into the patient's disability is gained by questioning about avoidance of certain activities. The patient may be fearful of undertaking certain tasks to the degree that it may interfere with his performance at sports, leisure activities, or employment. At the extreme level there may be interference with the patient's ability to cope with activities of daily living such as putting on a coat or reaching for an object.

The final indication of disability is the degree of associated pain which can occur, related to either the instability episodes or the associated pain of tendinitis, the latter of which usually occurs in patients with underlying multidirectional instability. These patients often present with a primary complaint of diffuse, poorly localized pain which can progress to become disabling at rest and even interfere with sleep. Most of these patients detect an underlying instability problem within their shoulders often with associated tingling, paresthesias, or weakness of the upper extremity. This group of patients presents a diagnostic and therapeutic challenge. Remember, they usually represent the AMBRI group; the TUBS group usually remain comfortable between episodes of instability.

OTHER SYMPTOMS AS THE CHIEF COMPLAINT

A number of other shoulder symptoms may be present, occasionally in isolation but more often in association with the common complaints of pain and instability. These include stiffness, weakness, catching, crepitus, deformity, or paresthesias.

Stiffness of the shoulder is often associated with pain. Unfortunately, the presence of pain that causes a diminished range of motion can make a diagnosis of underlying pathology difficult. The two aspects to sort out are those with an apparent stiff shoulder and a limited range of motion owing to pain and those with a true stiff shoulder and limited motion. True reduction of shoulder motion may be related to either bony or soft tissue restraint. An adhesive capsulitis with fibrosis and contracture of the shoulder joint capsule is the most common condition limiting motion. A family history of diabetes, connective tissue disorder, or vascular disturbances related to sympathetic dystrophy may reveal such an underlying relationship. Other conditions that should be considered are post-traumatic fibrosis or altered bony architecture related to previous fractures about the shoulder girdle. A missed or locked posterior dislocation should be considered, particularly where external rotation is markedly restricted and there is a history of injury.[12] The nature of onset of shoulder stiffness, whether it is related to trauma or overuse, the age and sex of the patient, and the patient's occupation frequently lead to a diagnosis of underlying pathology. For example, the idiopathic adhesive capsulitis which is the most common cause of a frozen shoulder often occurs in the middle-aged housewife, comes on spontaneously, and progresses initially from pain alone, to pain and stiffness, and then stiffness alone. It usually has a self-limiting course.

Weakness about the shoulder as a presenting complaint can be confusing, particularly in the presence of pain. True weakness is related to either a neurological or musculotendinous deficiency. The most common cause of shoulder weakness alone is rotator cuff deficiency. Patients with rotator cuff tears may have little pain. There may be a history of trauma or a previous painful tendinitis to indicate a cuff tear as the etiology for weakness. With a cuff tear, there is often associated crunching or crepitation on shoulder movement, although this can also occur in chronic tendinitis with an intact cuff. Neurological symptoms may suggest a cervical root or a peripheral nerve pattern, supported by specific individual muscle weakness or global weakness. Generalized neurological problems such as multiple sclerosis or motor neuron disease also cause weakness.

Complaints of catching or pseudolocking, sometimes related to labral tears or loose bodies may occur, particularly in the throwing shoulder. While these problems may not be of great concern to some, the high performance athlete or worker may note significant interference with activity. With these presentations there may be associated features of instability.

Deformity as a primary presenting complaint is unusual but, if present, is often related to previous trauma, such as an acromioclavicular joint dislocation or fractures about the clavicle (Fig. 4–2). Congenital problems such as Sprengel's deformity or pseudarthrosis of the clavicle may also be of enough cosmetic concern to the patient to bring them to the physician. Surgical scar spreading may be an important clue to collagen deficiency, often related to surgical failure. Paresthesias, or 'tingling' down the arm, even into the hand, can occur with intrinsic shoulder pathology, for example, in multidirectional instability.

PRESENTATION AS AN ACUTE INJURY

Patients presenting with an acute injury to the shoulder pose a different situation from those who present with a chronic problem. Injuries cause pain associated with a diminished range of motion (e.g., the patient who presents with an acute anterior dislocation of the shoulder will be supporting the arm in the 'protected position' across the abdomen, demonstrating significant discomfort). Associated deformity and swelling may be present. The mechanism of injury and the degree of trauma may be important clues to appreciate the potential amount of soft tissue and bone damage. One should also inquire about other injuries such as cervical spine, ipsilateral elbow or hand, or involvement of noncontiguous areas such as the trunk. Knowledge of employment, social circumstance, disability insurance, and possible associated litigation will assist in planning treatment and rehabilitation.

Injuries to the shoulder can vary from a simple muscular strain or contusion to a significant fracture sometimes associated with dislocation. The above details will establish appropriate treatment and clearly indicate to the patient the expectations and duration of recovery. It is important to emphasize that in the patient who presents with a significant shoulder injury related to an event such as a motor vehicle accident, the most critical determination related to the extremity is the vascular integrity of the limb. Neurological integrity is of secondary importance.

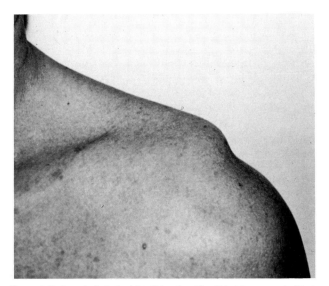

Figure 4–2. Acromioclavicular joint dislocation. The high-riding outer clavicle in acromioclavicular joint dislocation causes a step deformity on the superior aspect of the shoulder.

Physical Examination

INTRODUCTION

The technique of physical examination is both a skill and an art, mastered only by study and experience. If

Table 4-1. GENERAL FORMAT FOR EXAMINATION OF THE SHOULDER

1. Initial cursory impression
2. Inspection
3. Palpation
4. Range of motion
5. Neurological assessment
6. Stability assessment
7. Special tests
8. Vascular assessment
9. General physical examination

undertaken conscientiously, it will yield maximum benefits in leading the physician to a diagnosis as well as instilling confidence in the patient. This examination must be meticulous to avoid missing subtle changes which might otherwise be overlooked. It is often stated that more mistakes are made in medicine because of not looking than for lack of knowledge. While most techniques used in examining the shoulder are straightforward, others require practice and care in their performance and interpretation. To maximize efficiency and completeness, a systematic approach is helpful.

While the individual physician may modify certain aspects of the examination to suit circumstances, the basic three steps in physical assessment remain: look, feel, and move. In this section we will expand on this basic triad and offer an ordered format to the clinical assessment of shoulder problems (Table 4-1). An initial impression of the patient is followed by inspection and palpation of the shoulder girdle. Following this, active and passive ranges of motion are recorded, along with strength testing followed by an appropriate neurological examination. Next comes the assessment of stability and, if appropriate, special tests as applied to the shoulder such as Yergason's or Speed's sign, indicative of bicipital pathology, or the impingement sign. Assessment of the vascular status of the upper limb which may relate to shoulder problems, especially in an acute injury, may require special attention.

Throughout this examination, one should simultaneously evaluate the joints above (i.e., the cervical spine) and below (i.e., the elbow and wrist). By this stage a working diagnosis should be established and any further investigations or ongoing treatments can then be appropriately instituted. With modification, this format can be applied to examining any joint or part.[7, 9]

INITIAL IMPRESSION

Physical examination of the patient begins upon presentation as the patient enters the physician's office, hospital clinic, or even the emergency department. At this time, an initial impression is gained about the patient. This can be divided into static and dynamic. The static assessment would consider the following features:

1. Generalized diseases (e.g., rheumatoid arthritis).

2. Physiological age and appearance (e.g., athlete vs. accountant).
3. Body habitus.
4. Generalized distress (i.e., well or unwell).
5. Distress related to the shoulder.

Dynamic assessment would include:
1. Generalized distress with movement.
2. Shoulder distress with movement.
3. Performance of simple tasks and associated disability (e.g., shaking hands, disrobing).
4. Other features (e.g., gait abnormalities).

Static Factors

Signs and stigmata of generalized diseases may suggest that the shoulder problem relates to a systemic disease, such as rheumatoid arthritis, or to a congenital disorder such as Klippel-Feil syndrome with an associated Sprengel's deformity. Attention is paid to the patient's body habitus and the consistency between chronologic and physiological age. Note is taken of any general distress such as shortness of breath, as well as the degree of distress related to the affected part manifested as pain. The older patient with a chronic rotator cuff tear may show only mild pain arising from the shoulder but still be quite distressed because of significant functional disability. In contrast to this, the patient with an acute anterior dislocation of the shoulder would be in severe pain, clutching the arm against the body preventing any movement. The initial impression and possible diagnoses suggest which part of the subsequent examination should receive emphasis, i.e., range of movement, neurological assessment, or stability.

Dynamic Factors

The dynamic phase is observed twice, initially while the patient ambulates and disrobes, and later during the assessment of range of motion. As the patient enters the office, attention is directed to his gait. During normal gait, the upper extremity swings in tandem with the contralateral lower extremity. The patient with a neurological problem, such as a stroke or brachial plexus palsy or pain, will lose coordination between upper and lower limbs. The manner in which the upper limb is carried may reveal an Erb's palsy accompanied by internal rotation of the humerus. In contrast, the patient with severe generalized shoulder pain will not allow any movement of the arm and so use his opposite extremity to support the pathological side. While the patient is removing his or her clothes, attention should be paid to the pattern and quality of this act. Normally, disrobing has a smooth, flowing pattern; however, in an attempt to compensate for an inefficient movement or to avoid a painful position, the patient may substitute an abnormal jerking motion. A patient with a painful shoulder disrobes by taking the involved extremity out of the shirt or coat last and

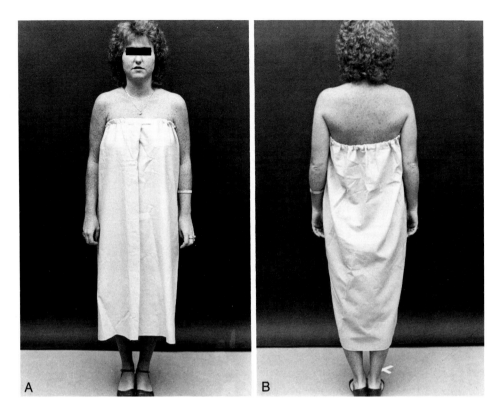

Figure 4–3. *A,* Patient in examining gown, anterior view. *B,* Patient in examining gown, posterior view. For a female patient, an appropriate gown allows exposure of all regions about the shoulder, facilitating a complete examination.

when dressing places the affected limb into the sleeve first.

Before adequate inspection of the shoulder can be undertaken, an appropriate exposure of both upper limbs is essential. Males should have removed all their clothing down to the waist. In order to allay anxiety and preserve modesty in females, adequate exposure of both shoulders may be assisted with a modified patient gown (Fig. 4–3). For those women with long hair, clips or elastic bands will help improve exposure of the neck and shoulders.

INSPECTION

One should inspect the shoulder and the upper extremity for:
1. Attitude.
2. Muscle features, particularly wasting.
3. Deformities (e.g., scars, lumps, bumps).
4. Swelling.
5. Skin manifestations and color.

To facilitate a methodical inspection, the shoulder should be divided into areas and visualized from the anterior, lateral, posterior, and superior aspects.

Attitude

Asymmetry of the shoulder with abnormalities of general contour may suggest underlying pathology. Many patients with a painful shoulder hold it higher than the opposite side. The presence of a short neck may be associated with a Klippel-Feil syndrome. The attitude of the entire upper extremity in neurological birth palsies, such as Klumpke's or Erb's, has a characteristic abnormal posture. The person with a very painful shoulder holds the arm in the 'protected position' (i.e., with the arm adducted across the abdomen, often cradled with the opposite extremity). In bilateral pathology, asymmetry may not be present.

Muscle Features

Muscle wasting may be evident around the shoulder or may involve peripheral muscle groups. Patients who have associated cervical spine complaints may have prominent trapezius and paracervical muscles owing to spasm. Root involvement from the cervical spine may be manifest as distal muscle wasting, for example, the interossei of the hand. Important muscles to observe for wasting about the shoulder are infraspinatus, deltoid, and supraspinatus. Deltoid wasting is best visualized from the anterior aspect as squaring off of the shoulder. If the spinati are wasted, there is excessive prominence of the spine of the scapula (Fig. 4–4). It is difficult to be sure of mild or moderate degrees of supraspinatus wasting because it is sheltered deep in its fossa by the overlying trapezius. Infraspinatus wasting is more easily seen. The most common cause of spinati wasting is a rotator cuff tear; however, other diagnoses such as suprascapular nerve entrapment,[25] C5 root compression, or, rarely, myopathy should be

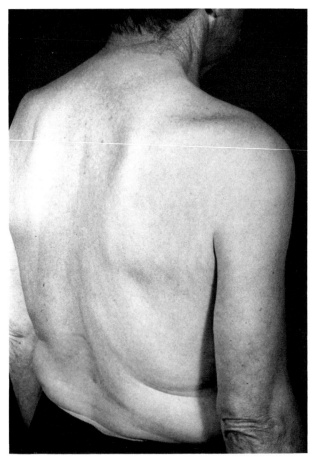

Figure 4–4. Supraspinatus/infraspinatus wasting. Marked wasting of the spinatii, in this man due to a large rotator cuff tear, results in prominence of the spine of the scapula.

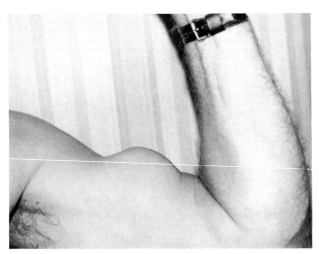

Figure 4–5. Ruptured long head of biceps brachii. The patient was asked to flex the elbow, demonstrating a 'popeye' appearance of the biceps muscle belly, classic for rupture of the long head of the biceps. This patient also has a rotator cuff tear.

der. Swelling is not common but may be associated with subacromial bursitis, frequently found in rheumatoid arthritis (Fig. 4–7). The patient with a massive cuff defect may have a synovial fluid leak through the deltoid muscle and present with a fluid-filled swelling of the bursal area.

considered. The patient should be asked to contract the biceps to reveal a rupture of its long head tendon (Fig. 4–5).

Deformities

A high-riding outer clavicle suggests pathology associated with a previous acromioclavicular joint dislocation (see Fig. 4–2). Winging of the scapula may be due to weakness of its major stabilizers, serratus anterior and trapezius. The position of the scapula may indicate which of its major stabilizing muscles is not functioning. With paralysis of the serratus anterior, the scapula tends to migrate proximally and its inferior angle moves medially (Fig. 4–6). In contrast, if the trapezius is paralyzed, the scapula migrates downward with its inferior angle moving laterally. This winging is more easily seen if the patient is asked to flex his shoulder against resistance or push against a wall. The presence of a scar from previous surgery may suggest the diagnosis of iatrogenic nerve injury.

Swelling

Swelling about the shoulder may arise from the joint, subacromial space, or other tissues around the shoul-

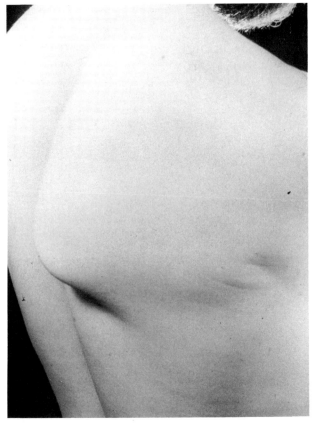

Figure 4–6. Winging of right scapula. Palsy of right serratus anterior muscle leads to migration of the scapula superiorly, with the inferior angle moving medially and protruding.

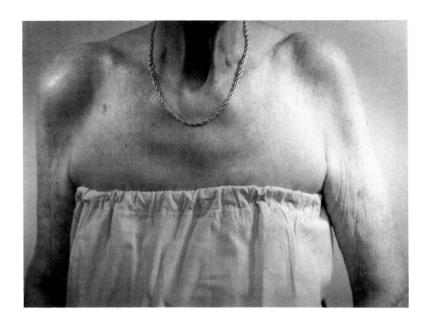

Figure 4–7. Right shoulder swelling related to rheumatoid arthritis. This patient has cystic swelling palpable through the anterior deltoid.

Skin Manifestations and Color

Inspection is made of the condition of the skin, noting any areas of discoloration or blemishes that may indicate underlying pathology. An inflammatory reaction or infection causes redness around the shoulder. Occasional yellow or bluish discoloration, often tracking down the upper arm, is secondary to hemorrhage which may be related to a rotator cuff rupture or a fracture. The scaling, red lesions of psoriasis or the café-au-lait spots of von Recklinghausen's disease will offer further insight into a general disease process. Scars and incisions are surgical archeology and offer information about previous treatment. For example, the pitting irregular scar of an old infected sinus should warn the surgeon of previous sepsis and caution about possible future difficulties with management.

PALPATION

It is helpful to regionalize the palpation of the shoulder by considering anterior, lateral, posterior, and superior aspects. It may also be helpful to divide palpation into superficial and deep and bone versus soft tissue. It is important to know the location and variation of anatomical landmarks and how they may change with different shoulder positions. Such an understanding will help to relate the physical findings to the correct pathology.

During palpation several features are considered simultaneously. These include (1) tenderness, (2) swelling, (3) temperature changes, (4) deformities, both obvious and hidden, (5) muscle characteristics, and (6) the relationships of various structures.

The most easily identifiable landmarks are bony prominences and associated joints. These include the sternoclavicular joint, clavicle, acromioclavicular joint, anterior and lateral acromion, greater tuberosity, and

bicipital region. There is little value in palpating the coracoid process since tenderness, even in the normal shoulder, is a common feature. It is, however, an important landmark to identify. The sternoclavicular joint is readily identified just lateral to the suprasternal notch and may reveal displacement, swelling, or tenderness (Fig. 4–8). The patient with recurrent subluxation or dislocation of this joint may have localized tenderness. Palpation along the clavicle will reveal any local deformities which may be tender, such as an ununited clavicular fracture. The acromioclavicular joint is readily identified on the superior aspect of the shoulder, at the distal end of the clavicle. Clinical arthritis of this joint is unusual without joint tenderness.[21] Just lateral to the acromioclavicular joint is the anterior acromion. Palpation of the superior surface of this bone may elicit tenderness in some patients with impingement or those with reflex sympathetic dystrophy about their shoulders. In identifying landmarks about the shoulder, it is helpful to initially identify the clavicle anteriorly and the spine of the scapula posteriorly. By following these laterally, one can usually identify the lateral and anterior acromion.

Tenderness of the greater tuberosity is best demonstrated by extending and internally rotating the arm. Palpation of the prominent portion of the head of the humerus, just distal to the anterolateral border of the acromion, locates the site of the greater tuberosity (Fig. 4–9). Tenderness is usually due to supraspinatus tendinitis, an acute cuff tear, or a fracture involving the greater tuberosity. Rarely, a defect in the rotator cuff can actually be palpated over the greater tuberosity.

Except in the very thin individual, palpation of the biceps tendon is not possible. Tenderness in the area of the biceps tendon as it lies in the bicipital groove is an indicator of biceps tendinitis. This tendon faces anteriorly when the arm is in 10 degrees of internal

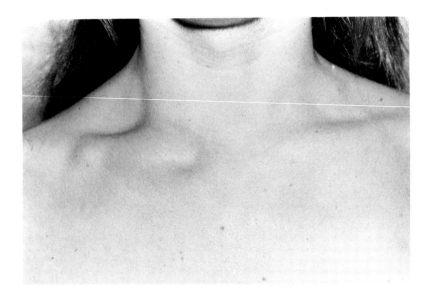

Figure 4–8. Dislocated right sternoclavicular joint. Deformity of the proximal end of the right clavicle at the sternoclavicular joint suggests a fixed anterior dislocation or an old fracture.

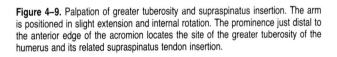

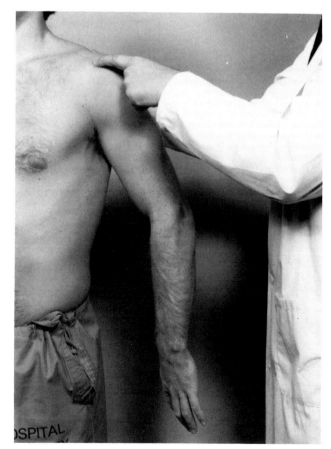

Figure 4–9. Palpation of greater tuberosity and supraspinatus insertion. The arm is positioned in slight extension and internal rotation. The prominence just distal to the anterior edge of the acromion locates the site of the greater tuberosity of the humerus and its related supraspinatus tendon insertion.

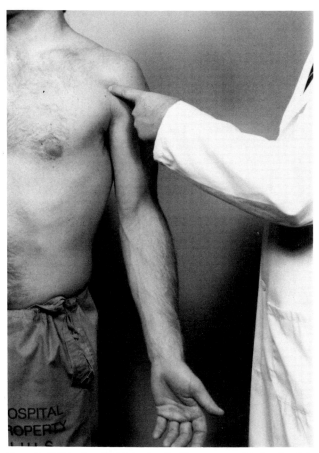

Figure 4–10. Palpation of bicipital region. The biceps groove points directly anterior when the arm is in 10 degrees of internal rotation. Although one can roll the edge of the deltoid beneath the finger (as shown here), it must not be confused with the biceps tendon.

rotation. The anterior edge of the deltoid should not be confused with the biceps tendon (Fig. 4–10).

Other bony landmarks include the spine and vertebral border of the scapula. This enables the physician to detect the orientation of the scapula on the chest wall. Whereas the sternoclavicular and acromioclavicular joints are readily palpable, the glenohumeral joint is located deep to a number of muscle layers. Patients with arthritis of the glenohumeral joint often reveal posterior joint line tenderness below the posterior acromion.

Assessment of the soft tissues and muscles should not be forgotten. The patient with "loose shoulders" and hyperelastic skin may have a collagen disorder such as Ehlers-Danlos syndrome. The presence of hard, rubbery periarticular swelling in the tissues about the shoulder may suggest amyloid arthropathy.[18]

The major muscle groups are palpated with attention directed to the presence of tenderness, tone, and consistency. When evaluating muscles, ask the patient to contract that muscle to note alteration in contour. A ruptured long head of the biceps has a characteristic deformity with bunching of the muscle belly in the distal upper arm, visible especially with contraction (see Fig. 4–5). A ruptured pectoralis major may show

loss of contour of the anterior axillary fold. Denervation may cause muscles to develop a flabby, atonic consistency, in contrast to the woody sensation that occurs with polymyositis. Diffuse swelling may occur with cellulitis of the subcutaneous tissues. Increased local temperature may be present with an underlying inflammatory process such as rheumatoid arthritis or infection.

JOINT MOTION

Assessment of motion of the shoulder joint involves not only documenting range but also noting the quality of movement. As the most mobile joint in the body, its multiplanar range of motion is due to contributions from sternoclavicular, acromioclavicular, and glenohumeral joints and the scapulothoracic articulation. Loss of motion in the shoulder can be due to several causes, the most common of which is pain. It is critical to determine the degree of pain in association with motion and where within the arc it occurs.

Quality of Movement

The ease of movement of the upper limb will have already been noted while the patient was undressing. With the shoulder fully exposed, a more detailed observation is made. Elevation of the arm should be smooth and continuous, with synchronous contributions from all four articulations. Attention is paid to the relationship between the scapulothoracic and glenohumeral articulations and how each contributes to overall elevation. Various reports in the literature indicate that the ratio between glenohumeral and scapulothoracic movement varies from 2:1 to 5:4, with the scapulothoracic component increasing with elevation.[15, 22] Diseases such as osteoarthritis or adhesive capsulitis of the glenohumeral articulation will affect this ratio so that motion is provided mostly by the scapulothoracic articulation. Rotator cuff tears or labral pathology may cause catching pain and result in a jerky, hesitant glenohumeral rhythm. The glenohumeral component of motion can be estimated by monitoring the movement of the inferior angle of the scapula with elevation of the arm (Fig. 4–11).

RANGE OF MOTION

The shoulder may be examined both upright and supine. In the standing position, compensatory actions of the spine and pelvis may mislead the examiner in assessing shoulder motion, especially where there is limitation of the full range. Some of these compensatory movements can be diminished by having the patient sit. Abduction and internal rotation are best documented with the patient upright, preferably sitting. A simple bar stool with no back facilitates an easy examination. The supine position allows for an

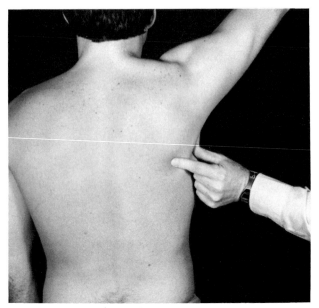

Figure 4–11. Estimation of glenohumeral versus scapulothoracic motion. In cases with loss of shoulder motion, an estimate of the amount of glenohumeral versus scapular motion can be determined by noting the movement of the inferior angle of the scapula and estimating the range of movement of each of these components.

accurate measurement of passive forward elevation and external rotation by diminishing compensatory movements of the spine. In the supine position, only 180 degrees of elevation is possible, and should a greater arc be present, it may be missed.

Active range always requires documentation. Passive testing need only be documented when active motion is incomplete. Differences between active and passive ranges may be due to musculotendinous deficiency, neurological deficit, or pain. Pain at the extremes of motion is also documented.

The American Academy of Orthopedic Surgeons has recommended the following principles for measuring and recording joint motion, especially as pertaining to the shoulder (Table 4–2):[2]

1. "All motions of a joint are measured from a defined Zero Starting Position (ZSP). Thus, the degrees of motion of a joint are added in the direction the joint moves from the ZSP." For the shoulder, this is with the patient standing erect, the arms at the side of the body in neutral rotation with palms facing the thighs.

2. "The motion of the extremity being examined should be compared to that of the opposite extremity.

Table 4–2. PRINCIPLES OF MEASURING AND RECORDING
JOINT MOTION*

1. All joint motion measured from a defined zero starting position.
2. Compare range with opposite normal side.
3. Compare range with average motion of individual of similar age, sex, and physical build (if opposite side not normal).
4. Motion is defined as active or passive.
5. If possible, examine extremity with patient in position of greatest comfort.

*As described by The American Academy of Orthopedic Surgeons.[1]

The difference may be expressed in degrees of motion as compared to the opposite extremity, or in percentages of loss of motion in comparison with the opposite extremity." Academically it is appropriate to start at 0 and give the range on both sides. In oral presentation, it is acceptable to present loss of motion compared with the opposite normal extremity.

3. "If the opposite extremity is not present or pathological, the motion should be compared to the average motion of an individual of similar age and physical build."

4. "Motion is defined as active or passive."

5. "A more accurate estimate of motion may be obtained if the extremity is examined in the position of greater comfort to the patient."

6. "The use of a goniometer is optional and should be used according to the surgeon's discretion."

Because of the global nature of shoulder motion, a multitude of ranges could be documented. In the past, this has been cumbersome, time consuming, and confusing. Historically, there have been many ways to document elevation in different planes. Elevation has been documented in the sagittal, coronal, and scapular planes and recently described in the frontal plane or midway between the sagittal and scapular planes (i.e., total elevation). While these motions map out the sphere of shoulder movement, only total elevation records the maximum elevation that can be achieved.

The Society of American Shoulder and Elbow Surgeons recommends recording the following arcs of motion for documentation. The Society has agreed that this represents a standard protocol, is simple, reproducible, and the minimum that need be recorded (Table 4–3).

1. Total elevation (active and passive).

2. External rotation with the arm at the side (active and passive).

3. External rotation in the 90-degree abduction position (when this can be reached by the patient).

4. Internal rotation, active or passive (as both are much the same).

Total Elevation

Total elevation is a more functional measurement than forward flexion in the sagittal or abduction in the coronal planes. Because of capsular tightening, the patient may have limitation of forward flexion and abduction. When the patient is allowed to find the most comfortable arc of motion, he gains an additional 15 to 20 degrees of elevation. The plane of this motion occurs somewhere between the coronal and sagittal planes, usually about 20 to 30 degrees from the sagittal plane, but may be influenced by the nature of the shoulder pathology (Fig. 4–12). The reference points for documentation of this angle are the axis of the thorax and the upper arm when viewed from the lateral projection. It is usual to record active total elevation in the upright position. Passive elevation is conveniently measured with the patient supine (Fig. 4–13).

Table 4–3. THE SOCIETY OF AMERICAN SHOULDER AND ELBOW SURGEONS BASIC SHOULDER EVALUATION FORM

Shoulder: R/L

Name _____ Hospital No. _____

Date of Examination: _____

(Circle choice)

I. Pain: (5 = none, 4 = slight, 3 = after unusual activity, 2 = moderate, 1 = marked, 0 = complete disability, and NA = not available) _____
II. Motion
  A. Patient sitting (enter motion or NA if not measured):
    1. Active total elevation of arm: _____degrees
    2. Passive internal rotation:
      (Circle segment of posterior anatomy reached by thumb)
      (Enter NA if reach restricted by limited elbow flexion)

1 = Less than trochanter	8 = L2	15 = T7
2 = Trochanter	9 = L1	16 = T6
3 = Gluteal	10 = T12	17 = T5
4 = Sacrum	11 = T11	18 = T4
5 = L5	12 = T10	19 = T3
6 = L4	13 = T9	20 = T2
7 = L3	14 = T8	21 = T1

    3. Active external rotation with arm at side: _____ degrees.
    4. Passive external rotation at 90° abduction: _____ degrees.
      (enter "NA" if cannot achieve 90° of abduction)
  B. Patient supine:
    1. Passive total elevation of arm: _____ degrees.*
    2. Passive external rotation with arm at side: _____ degrees.

III. Strength (5 = normal, 4 = good, 3 = fair, 2 = poor, 1 = trace, 0 = paralysis, and NA = not available) (Enter numbers below)
  A. Anterior deltoid _____
  B. Middle deltoid _____
  C. External rotation _____
  D. Internal rotation _____

IV. Stability (5 = normal, 4 = apprehension, 3 = rare subluxation, 2 = recurrent subluxation, 1 = recurrent dislocation, 0 = fixed dislocation, and NA = not available)
(Enter numbers below)
  A. Anterior _____
  B. Posterior _____
  C. Inferior _____

V. Function (4 = normal, 3 = mild compromise, 2 = difficulty, 1 = with aid, 0 = unable, and NA = not available) (Enter numbers below)
  A. Use back pocket (if male); fasten bra (if female) _____
  B. Perineal care _____
  C. Wash opposite axilla _____
  D. Eat with utensil _____
  E. Comb hair _____
  F. Use hand with arm at shoulder level _____
  G. Carry 10 to 15 lb with arm at side _____
  H. Dress _____
  I. Sleep on affected side _____
  J. Pulling _____
  K. Use hand overhead _____
  L. Throwing _____
  M. Lifting _____
  N. Do usual work _____ (Specify type of work) _____
  O. Do usual sport _____ (Specify sport) _____

VI. Patient Response:
(Circle choice)
(3 = much better, 2 = better, 1 = same, 0 = worse, and NA = not available/applicable)

*Total elevation of the arm is measured by viewing the patient from the side and using a goniometer to determine the angle between the arm and the thorax.

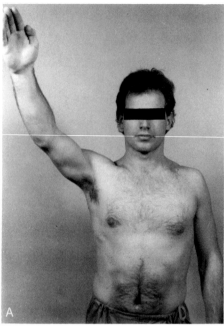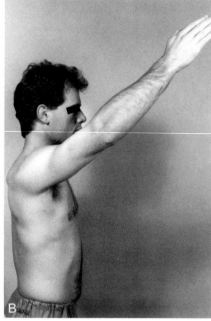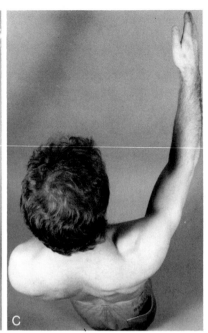

Figure 4–12. Total active elevation of the shoulder. *A*, Anterior view. *B*, Lateral view. *C*, Superior view. The patient is raising his right arm in a plane about 20 degrees from the sagittal. Reference points for measuring the angle of elevation are the axis of the thorax and the arm determined from the lateral view.

Rotation with the Arm at the Side

For recording external rotation, the arm should be resting at the side, elbow flexed to 90 degrees, and the forearm in the sagittal plane. Active and passive motion should be noted. To eliminate the effects of gravity it is preferable to record active external rotation in the upright posture. To minimize compensatory thoracic motion and provide relaxation, passive motion can be recorded supine (Fig. 4–14). It should be remembered that there is great variability among patients in total external rotation and so comparison with the opposite normal side is necessary.

External Rotation in Abduction

In selected circumstances, recording external rotation in 90 degrees of abduction is informative. In the presence of an old fracture of the greater tuberosity, there may be a difference in external rotation at 90 degrees of abduction compared with neutral. With throwing athletes, any limitation of external rotation in abduction may significantly impede peak performance. In these circumstances documentation of external rotation at 90 degrees of abduction provides useful information (Fig. 4–15).

Internal Rotation

Documentation of internal rotation is awkward because the trunk obstructs the normal arc. It is helpful to have the patient in an upright sitting position on a stool. Some shoulder extension is necessary to allow completion of the internal rotation arc. As the range increases, the position reached by the outstretched

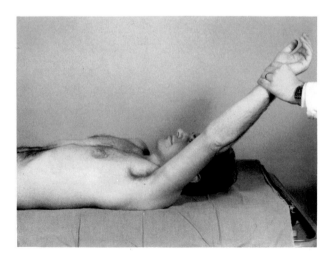

Figure 4–13. Passive elevation. With the patient supine, the limb to be examined is grasped by the physician and gently moved to maximize elevation.

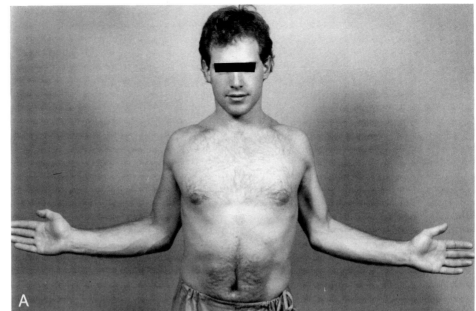

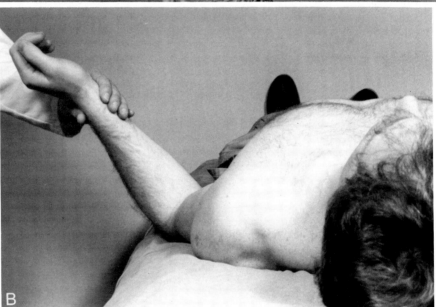

Figure 4–14. *A,* Active external rotation. The arm is resting at the side with the elbow flexed to 90 degrees. Active external rotation is measured with the patient erect. *B,* Passive external rotation. The patient is supine with the elbow held by his side. The arm is externally rotated for recording maximal passive range.

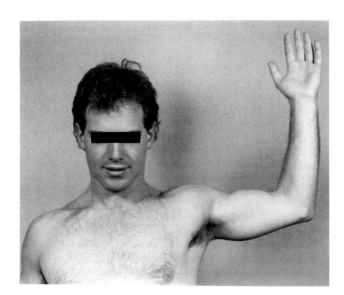

Figure 4–15. External rotation at 90-degree abduction. In special circumstances, such as the throwing athlete, the range of external rotation with the arm abducted to 90 degrees should be recorded (active and passive).

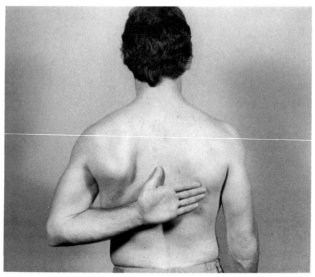

Figure 4–16. Internal rotation. Internal rotation is recorded by noting the position of the "hitch-hiker's thumb" referenced to the posterior anatomy. Here, the subject has internal rotation to T7.

Table 4–4. PRINCIPLES TO BE APPLIED FOR MUSCLE TESTING

1. Muscle to be assessed should be given the mechanical advantage.
2. Strength may vary through an arc of movement, so strength rating may need to be related to a specific arc.
3. Feel and see muscle during testing.
4. Apply resistance gradually and assign grade (0–5).
5. Always compare with the opposite normal side.
6. In the presence of significant pain, muscle strength recording is usually inaccurate.

hitch-hiking thumb in reference to the posterior anatomy is recorded (Fig. 4–16). All patients should be able to reach the greater trochanter of the ipsilateral hip. In an ascending plane, the common reference points are the greater trochanter, buttock, superior gluteal fold, and various spinous processes of the lumbar and thoracic vertebrae. Any pain with stressing at the extremes of motion should be recorded.

Abduction

This motion is not routinely documented but may provide useful information, particularly relating to impingement and strength. When assessing abduction, it should be determined in the upright position with the arc slightly posterior to the coronal plane. As the patient abducts to 90 degrees, external rotation of the humerus may occur, allowing the greater tuberosity to clear the acromion and thereby completing the arc of abduction. Pain between 90 and 120 degrees of abduction is a reliable indicator of tendinitis owing to impingement (the 'painful arc') (see Fig. 4–25D). The pain is often increased when resistance is applied.

MUSCLE TESTING

As the shoulder is put through these ranges, muscle strengths should be assessed. Muscle strength testing about the shoulder enables the physician to evaluate the integrity of the musculotendinous unit and the function of its neurological elements. It is important to distinguish root verses peripheral innervation of these muscle groups as they pertain to functional arcs of movement of the shoulder. The degree to which a detailed neurological examination is pursued is determined by the nature of the complaint and the patient's general status. This will be discussed subsequently

under a separate heading. The older patient with combined neck and shoulder pain will require detailed neurological examination relating to the cervical spine and upper extremities. The severely affected patient with rheumatoid arthritis will require a more extensive examination, even of the lower extremities, looking for evidence of long tract signs owing to atlantoaxial instability. While findings related to these situations may not relate directly to the shoulder problem, they may be crucial to the overall assessment.

Principles of Muscle Testing

When testing a muscle, it is necessary to have a reproducible technique which takes into consideration the factors that may give a reproducible estimate of strength. The following should be used as general guidelines for the physical examination (Table 4–4):

1. The individual muscle to be assessed should be given the mechanical advantage. This may be accomplished by appropriate positioning of the joint. For example, testing elbow flexion is most reliably performed at 90 degrees.

2. When testing muscle groups, the strength rating may vary throughout the arc of movement owing to recruitment of different muscles. Hence, it is necessary to break down the strength rating into the component parts of the arc. For example, abduction at 90 degrees may be more powerful than abduction at the side and reflects more muscles working at a better mechanical advantage.

3. After the limb is appropriately positioned, the examiner should always attempt to feel and see the muscle contraction.

4. Gradual resistance should be applied and a grade assigned ranging from 0 to 5. Usually the 0 to 5 grading system is employed with the addition of pluses or minuses to indicate more subtle variations, especially at the higher grades (Table 4–5).

5. Always compare the opposite side if normal. In a body builder, for example, subtle weakness may be missed if the muscle power is compared with another patient with average strength.

6. In the presence of significant pain, the recording of muscle strength may be unreliable.

Functional Strength Testing

The majority of problems around the shoulder seen by the orthopedist are musculotendinous, and as such, it is necessary to document functional arcs of motion.

Table 4–5. GRADING OF MUSCLE STRENGTH USING 0–5 SYSTEM

Grade	Degree of Muscle Strength	
0 = Zero	No palpable contraction.	(Nothing)
1 = Trace	Muscle contracts, but part normally motorized does not move, even without gravity.	(Trace)
2 = Poor	Muscle moves the part but not against gravity.	(With gravity eliminated)
3 = Fair	Muscle moves part through a range against gravity.	(Against gravity)
4 = Good	Muscle moves part even against added resistance; variations in resistance are graded plus or minus.	(Near normal)
5 = Excellent	Normal strength against full resistance is present.	(Normal)

The most common and significant strength movements to be tested include forward elevation, external rotation, and abduction. A large rotator cuff tear is frequently associated with weakness of elevation, abduction, and external rotation.

Flexion

The chief flexor of the shoulder is the anterior part of the deltoid muscle (axillary nerve, C5–C6). This is assisted by the clavicular portion of the pectoralis major muscle (lateral pectoral nerve, C5–C6). Minor accessory flexors include biceps and coracobrachialis muscles (musculocutaneous nerve, C5–C7). The flexors of the shoulder are tested applying resistance at approximately 90 degrees of elevation.

Abduction

Abduction in the coronal plane is mainly accomplished by the middle portion of the deltoid muscle (axillary nerve, C5–C6) and the supraspinatus muscle (suprascapular nerve, C5). Assistance may come from the long head of biceps (musculocutaneous nerve, C5–6C). Some physicians prefer to assess strength with the arm abducted to 90 degrees, with the forearm maximally pronated and the arm position 30 degrees forward of the coronal plane or in the plane of the scapula.[17] In this position it may be that the supraspinatus muscle is better isolated (Fig. 4–17).

External Rotation

The major muscles providing external rotation are the infraspinatus (suprascapular nerve, C5–C6) and the teres minor (axillary nerve, C5–C6). The posterior portion of the deltoid is an accessory muscle for external rotation (axillary nerve, C5–C6). External rotation is assessed with the arms at the side in a neutral position. Resistance is then applied and compared with the opposite side. External rotation can also be assessed at 90 degrees of abduction.

Other Strength Measurements

Movements such as internal rotation of the shoulder, elbow flexion, and extension or shoulder elevation can also be tested and recorded as indicated by the clinical situation. Since strength testing is part of the neurological examination, it would be appropriate at this stage to complete the neurological evaluation. Brachial plexus lesions and cervical root lesions may require very extensive muscle testing about the shoulder.

NEUROLOGICAL EXAMINATION OF THE UPPER LIMB

The neurological examination of the upper limb includes detailed muscle testing to define radicular or

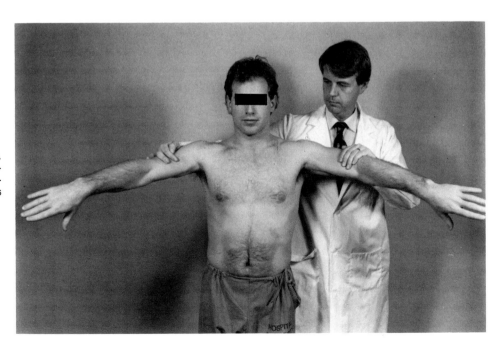

Figure 4–17. Testing the supraspinatus. Resistance is applied with the arm abducted 90 degrees, forward-flexed 30 degrees, and pronated. This position helps to isolate the supraspinatus.

Table 4–6. MUSCLE TESTING CHART

Muscle	Innervation	Myotomes	Technique for Testing
Shoulder			
Trapezius	Spinal accessory	C2–C4	Patient shrugs shoulders against resistance.
Sternomastoid	Spinal accessory	C2–C4	Patient turns head to one side with resistance over opposite temporal area.
Serratus Anterior	Long thoracic	C5–C7	Patient pushes against wall with outstretched arm. Scapular winging is observed.
Latissimus Dorsi	Thoracodorsal	C7–C8	Downward/backward pressure of arm against resistance. Muscle palpable at inf. angle of scapula during cough.
Rhomboids	Dorsal	(C4) C5*	Hands on hips pushing elbows backward against resistance.
Levator Scapulae	Scapular		
Subclavius	Nerve to subclavius	C5–C6	None
Teres Major	Subscapular (lower)	C5–C6	Similar to lat. dorsi.; muscle palpable at lower border of scapula.
Deltoid	Axillary	C5–C6 (C7)	With arm abducted 90°, downward pressure is applied. Anterior and posterior fibers may be tested in slight flexion and extension.
Subscapularis	Subscapular (upper)	C5	Arm at side with elbow flexed to 90°. Examiner resists internal rotation.
Supraspinatus	Suprascapular	C5 (C6)	Arm abducted against resistance (not isolated). With arm pronated and elevated 90° in plane of scapula, downward pressure is applied.
Infraspinatus	Suprascapular	C5 (C6)	Arm at side with elbow flexed 90°. Examiner resists external rotation.
Teres minor	Axillary	C5–C6 (C7)	Same as for infraspinatus
Pectoralis major	Medial and lateral pectoral	C5–T1	With arm flexed 30° in front of body, patient adducts against resistance.
Pectoralis minor	Medial pectoral	C8, T1	None
Coracobrachialis	Musculocutaneous	(C4) C5–C6 (C7)	None
Biceps brachii	Musculocutaneous	(C4) C5–C6 (C7)	Flexion of the supinated forearm against resistance.
Triceps	Radial	(C5) C6–C8	Resistance to extension of elbow from varying position of flexion.

*Numbers in parentheses indicate a variable but not rare contribution.

peripheral nerve function, sensory evaluation, and the testing of reflex arcs. The neurological examination should include evaluation of the sympathetic chain for findings suggestive of dystrophy. The extent of the neurological examination depends upon the clinical presentation.

Muscle Testing

A detailed knowledge of the anatomy and variations of the brachial plexus and its contributing cervical and thoracic roots is necessary to fully evaluate muscle deficits following injury or disease to localize the lesion. In a patient with a brachial plexus lesion, this examination will need to be quite detailed (Table 4–6). By contrast, the patient with degenerative cervical disc disease with encroachment on one nerve root will have more localized findings (Table 4–7).

Sensory Testing

The loss of skin sensation may be due to either peripheral nerve damage or encroachment on cervical nerve roots. The pattern of peripheral nerve cutaneous innervation is well documented, and denervation has an easily definable area. In contrast, selective cervical root involvement is less easily defined owing to der-matomal overlap. Dermatomal maps have been formulated, either by sectioning nerves above and below the segmental level (Foerster's charts) or by selectively dividing cervical nerve roots and looking at the area of altered sensation (Keegan's map).[13] A simplified pattern of dermatomes is C5—lateral deltoid; C6—thumb; C7—middle finger; C8—little finger; and T1—inner aspect proximal arm.

Reflexes

A number of reflexes around the shoulder are available for testing the integrity of neural arcs. Some are

Table 4–7. NEUROLOGICAL LEVELS IN THE UPPER LIMB/NECK

Level	Motor	Sensory	Reflex
C5	Deltoid Biceps (partial)	Lateral deltoid	Biceps
C6	Biceps ECRL and ECRB	Thumb	Brachioradialis Biceps
C7	Triceps Wrist flexors Finger extension	Middle finger	Triceps
C8	Finger flexors	Ulnar border Little finger	—
T1	Intrinsics	Medial side Proximal arm	—

specific, such as the biceps jerk, while others are testing more gross motion responses (e.g., clavicular reflex). The quality of the reflex should also be noted: Is it brisk as might occur in thyrotoxicosis, or is it sluggish as in myxedema?

Biceps Reflex

The patient's arm is flexed at the elbow. The examiner's thumb is over the biceps tendon insertion, and this is tapped with the hammer. The biceps muscle normally contracts. The neurological level is C5, but mostly C6. The peripheral nerve is the musculocutaneous.

Triceps Reflex

The patient's arm is supported with the elbow flexed to 90 degrees. The triceps insertion is struck with a hammer, and an extensor response evoked. The myotomes are C6–C8, with predominant representation of C7. The peripheral nerve is the radial.

Brachioradialis Reflex

With the forearm relaxed in neutral position, the tendon of the brachioradialis is struck approximately 2 to 3 cm proximal to the radial styloid. In response to this, a contraction with associated elbow or wrist flexion occurs. Its peripheral innervation is from the radial nerve and C5–C6 root components.

Pectoralis Reflex

The patient's arm is abducted 20 to 30 degrees and supported by the examiner. The thumb of the physician is placed over the distal tendon of the pectoralis major muscle, and this is tapped with a hammer. Contraction of the muscle is seen and felt and causes the arm to adduct and slightly internally rotate. The pectoralis major is innervated by both medial and lateral pectoral nerves and has myotomes from C5–C7 supplying the clavicular and manubrial portions; C8–T1 supplies the lower sternal portions.

Scapular Reflex

The patient stands with the arm abducted 15 to 20 degrees. The inferior angle of the scapula is tapped, the scapula moves medially, and the arm adducts owing to the action of the rhomboids and other muscles. In a very muscular individual, this test may be difficult to interpret and a negative response insignificant.

Clavicular Reflex

Tapping the lateral portion of the clavicle may result in contraction of various muscles in the arm. It can be used for demonstrating differences in irritability of deep reflexes between the two upper limbs.

Moro Reflex

This reflex is useful in evaluating gross motor responses in an infant. The reflex is present at birth but disappears between 10 to 20 weeks. The infant is laid supine and the head supported in the slightly flexed position. The head is dropped quickly but gently into slight extension; in response to this, the upper limbs show slight abduction, extension, and circumduction with flexion of the lower limbs, i.e., a startled response. If there is a brachial plexus lesion, fractured clavicle, or hemiparesis in one limb, this reflex will be absent or asymmetrical.

Horner's Syndrome

Injury or disease at the base of the neck may cause damage to the cervical sympathetic chain at the sixth cervical level. Here there is ipsilateral miosis, ptosis, and anhydrosis.

STABILITY ASSESSMENT

The assessment of stability of the glenohumeral joint requires consideration of two components: first, to document the amount of passive translation possible between the humeral head and glenoid fossa when stressed by the examiner; second, to attempt reproduction of symptoms of subluxation and apprehension by placing and stressing the shoulder in positions of compromise. The global mobility of the shoulder can allow instability of the shoulder to occur in at least three possible directions; anterior, posterior, or inferior. Instability may also be multidirectional.

Glenohumeral Translation (Load and Shift Test)

Glenohumeral translation should be examined in both the upright and supine positions. The mobility of the scapula on the thoracic wall can make assessment of this translation difficult. Although the scapula can be fixed to some degree to provide an appreciation of translation, it should not be rigidly fixed. This is comparable to the pivot shift maneuver in the knee, where both tibia and femur must have some independence of movement for an appropriate shifting assessment. With practice, the clinician will develop an appreciation and feel for glenohumeral translation.

It is important when assessing the amount of translation to ensure that the humeral head is reduced concentrically into the glenoid fossa. In patients with multidirectional laxity or in those with scarring from previous surgery the humeral head may have a resting position which is not concentric but sitting anterior, posterior, or inferior. Hence, at the commencement of any stress testing, the humeral head must be grasped and pushed into the glenoid fossa to ensure its reduction to the neutral position. Once the humeral head is "loaded," directional stresses may be applied. As the

GRADE   GLENOHUMERAL   CLINICAL
               TRANSLATION

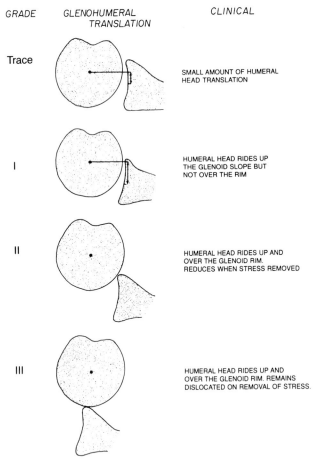

Trace

SMALL AMOUNT OF HUMERAL
HEAD TRANSLATION

I

HUMERAL HEAD RIDES UP
THE GLENOID SLOPE BUT
NOT OVER THE RIM

II

HUMERAL HEAD RIDES UP AND
OVER THE GLENOID RIM.
REDUCES WHEN STRESS REMOVED

III

HUMERAL HEAD RIDES UP AND
OVER THE GLENOID RIM. REMAINS
DISLOCATED ON REMOVAL OF STRESS.

Figure 4–18. Clinical evaluation of translation of the humeral head within the glenoid fossa, utilizing the load and shift test.

stress is increased, the head may be felt to ride up to and sometimes over the glenoid rim. This may be difficult to appreciate since there is usually associated movement of the shoulder girdle. For recording this translation, we have found a combination of a per-

centage and grading system to be helpful. This is described as the "load and shift test" (Fig. 4–18).

The technique for this part of the exam initially involves assessment with the patient sitting and the examiner located just beside and behind the side to be examined (Fig. 4–19). It is always best to examine the normal or asymptomatic shoulder first to provide a baseline assessment and demonstrate the maneuver to the patient to allay possible anxieties. The examiner places the hand over the shoulder and scapula to steady the limb girdle and then, with the opposite hand, grasps the humeral head. The head is loaded and then both an anterior and posterior stress is applied, noting the amount of translation. Next the elbow is grasped and inferior traction applied. The area adjacent to the acromion is observed and dimpling of the skin may indicate a "sulcus sign."[20] The acromion and then the space underneath it is palpated to gain an impression of the amount of inferior humeral translation (Fig. 4–20).

Glenohumeral translation is again assessed with the patient supine (Fig. 4–21). Here the arm is grasped and positioned in approximately 20 degrees abduction and forward flexion. The humeral head is again loaded then posterior and anterior stresses applied. Similarly, inferior stress is applied again noting the "sulcus sign." The accuracy of these tests will depend both on the examiner's skill and the ability of the patient to relax. In some patients with associated tendinitis it is too painful to grasp the humeral head between the thumb and fingers. In this situation, grasping the upper arm distal to the shoulder may be the only method of assessing translation but is less reliable.

In the relaxed or anesthetized patient it is important to remember that most normal shoulders allow some translation of the humeral head in the glenoid fossa. Many shoulders can be translated posteriorly up to half the width of the glenoid fossa. We have applied a grading system, and under anesthesia, it would be our interpretation that normal shoulders can be translated

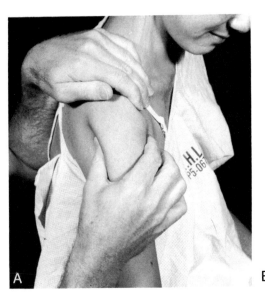

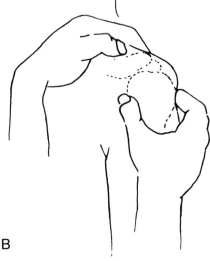

Figure 4–19. Position of sitting patient and examiner during shoulder translation determination. *A,* Both patient and examiner are seated with the physician behind the patient. Here the right hand of the examiner is used to stabilize the scapula, while the left hand grasps the humeral head to apply a load and shift test. *B,* Schematic representation of the positions of the examiner's hands during load and shift test.

A   B

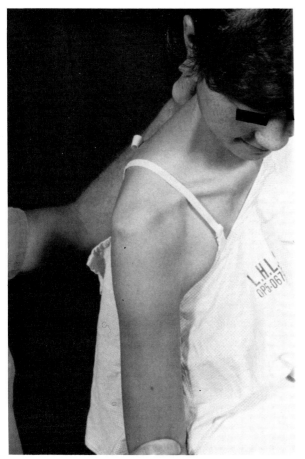

Figure 4–20. Sulcus sign. With the elbow grasped, inferior traction is applied. Dimpling of the skin below the acromion may be seen. Palpation reveals widening of the subacromial space between the acromion and humeral head.

posteriorly up to the rim of the glenoid (Grade II). Anterior and inferior translations are less (Grade I or trace) in the normal shoulder. In most patients, especially if they are relaxed, there is a good correlation of examination awake and under anesthesia.

Having determined the degree of glenohumeral joint translation it is important to correlate these findings with the patient's symptoms.

Apprehension Tests and Symptomatic Translation

The next phase of the stability assessment is either to reproduce the symptom complex of instability with translation or elicit apprehension with certain positions of impending subluxation or dislocation.

The most common direction of instability is anterior. The usual position of the arm when subluxation or dislocation occurs is abduction and external rotation. The apprehension test for anterior instability can be performed both in the upright and supine positions, though maximal muscle relaxation is best achieved with the patient supine.

With the patient sitting, the examiner stands behind the shoulder to be examined. To assess the patient's left shoulder, the examiner raises the arm to 90 degrees of abduction and begins to externally rotate the humerus. The right hand of the examiner is placed over the humeral head with the thumb pushing from posterior for extra leverage; however, the fingers are anterior to control any sudden instability episode that may occur. With increasing external rotation and gentle forward pressure exerted against the humeral head and the appropriate control, an impending feeling of anterior instability may be produced (i.e., an apprehension sign) (Fig. 4–22). This may be referred to as the 'crank test.' An apprehensive look may appear on the patient's face (he may resist with muscular contraction), or he may volunteer that if the stress is continued, his shoulder "will come out." Pain alone is not a positive apprehension sign, although it is often present.

This test can be repeated with the patient supine. The shoulder to be examined is positioned so that the scapula is supported by the edge of the examining table, and the proximal humerus is then stressed in

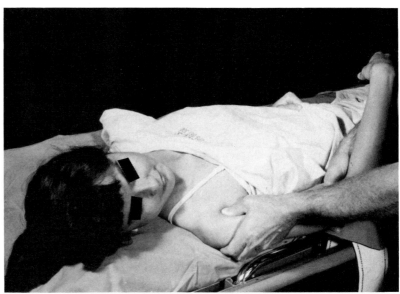

Figure 4–21. Stability assessment with the patient supine. With the patient supine, the arm is abducted and flexed approximately 20 degrees. Anterior, then posterior loads are applied. Here, the degree of posterior translation is being assessed.

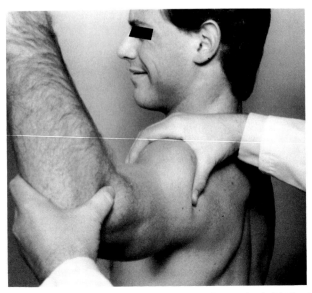

Figure 4–22. Apprehension test—sitting (crank test). The examiner's right thumb is applying anterior leverage as the patient's arm is abducted and externally rotated. The examiner's index and middle fingers are positioned on the anterior aspect of the shoulder to protect against any sudden dislocation.

varying degrees of abduction and external rotation, again attempting to reproduce impending instability (Fig. 4–23). In the supine position, the body acts as the counterweight, the edge of the table the fulcrum, and the arm the lever. When the apprehensive position is located, note is taken of the amount of external rotation. With the arm in this position, a posterior stress may be exerted on the proximal humerus and the apprehension may disappear with more external humeral rotation being possible before re-emergence of the apprehension sign. This occurs for one of two reasons: At the apprehension point, the humeral head is slightly subluxed, and pushing it posteriorly causes reduction; or the posteriorly directed pressure acts as a supportive buttress anteriorly to give the patient more confidence, thereby preventing the apprehension (Fig. 4–24).

Posterior instability is often a subluxation rather than a dislocation and, if recurrent, can often be demonstrated by the patient, either by arm position in forward elevation or by selective muscular control in various positions of elevation with applied internal rotation. Having ascertained the compromising maneuver, the examiner may attempt to reproduce the instability by manually duplicating the stresses. Since this is usually a painless subluxation which easily reduces, posterior apprehension is not commonly present and therefore not a reliable sign. In posterior instability, the patient who cannot demonstrate the instability may present a diagnostic challenge. It is perhaps in these patients that posterior translation of the humeral head on the glenoid and obvious reproduction of the symptom complex may provide the only clue to the diagnosis (see Fig. 4–19B). Patients with inferior instability may say that distal traction on the arm reproduces their

symptom complex, and this suggests underlying multidirectional instability.

SPECIAL TESTS

Impingement Tests

As an aid in the diagnosis of shoulder pain caused by tendinitis, Neer and Welch popularized the "impingement sign" and "impingement test."[19] Forcible elevation of the arm causes the critical area of the supraspinatus tendon to be impinged against the anterior inferior acromion. If the tendon is inflamed this maneuver produces the pain and often elicits a grimacing facial expression. This is the "impingement sign" (Fig. 4–25A).

An alternative method for demonstrating impingement of the supraspinatus tendon against the coracoacromial ligament is to forward flex the humerus to 90 degrees and then forcibly internally rotate the shoulder (Fig. 4–25B).

The "impingement test" documents the patient's response to an injection of lidocaine (Xylocaine) (10 ml of 1 per cent) into the subacromial bursa (Fig. 4–25C). Following introduction of the local anaesthetic under the acromion the impingement sign is repeated. If there is significant reduction or abolition of the patient's pain, this is a positive impingement test.

An additional impingement sign, although not classically described as such, consists of the traditional "painful arc." In the patient with impingement tendinitis and rotator cuff pathology, abduction in the coronal plane causes pain between 60 and 100 degrees, maximal at 90 degrees (Fig. 4–25D). This pain is often

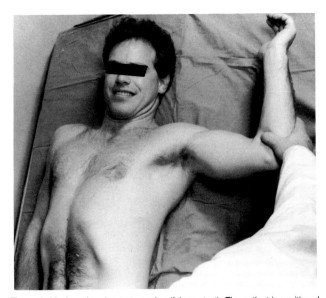

Figure 4–23. Apprehension test—supine (fulcrum test). The patient is positioned with the scapula supported by the edge of the examining table. The arm is positioned in abduction and external rotation, which produces a feeling of impending anterior instability, accompanied by apprehension on the part of the patient.

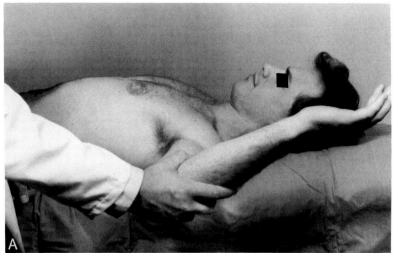

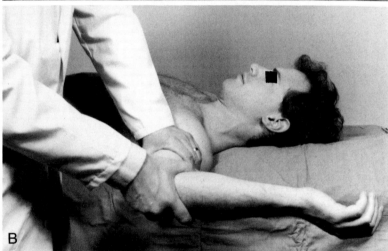

Figure 4-24. "Relocation" test. *A,* The patient, in the supine position, expresses apprehension as his arm is abducted and externally rotated. Note is taken of the amount of external rotation at this point. *B,* The examiner applies a posterior stress on the proximal arm. The patient loses his apprehension, and further external rotation of the arm is possible before re-emergence of his apprehension.

increased with resistance applied at 90 degrees of abduction. Patients sometimes externally rotate in this position to clear the greater tuberosity posteriorly under the acromion, diminishing this pain and allowing greater elevation in the coronal plane.

Biceps Evaluation

The biceps tendon is usually not palpable. Hence, examination of the biceps is largely by palpation in the region of the bicipital groove and with the use of specific provocative tests. While numerous tests have been reported, their reliability value in everyday practice is questionable. In most circumstances the examining physician will palpate the bicipital region and then apply one or two stress tests to confirm localized pathosis.

Yergason's Test

The elbow is flexed to 90 degrees, and the forearm is pronated. With the examining physician holding the patient's wrist, the patient is directed to actively supinate against resistance. If there is pain localized to the bicipital groove area, this suggests pathology in the long head of the biceps tendon in its sheath[30] (Fig. 4-26).

Speed's Test

With the elbow extended and forearm supinated, forward elevation of the humerus to approximately 60 degrees is resisted. A positive test elicits pain localized to the bicipital groove area.

Ludington's Test

With this test the patient places both palms on the top of the head with fingers interlocked and then contracts and relaxes the biceps muscles. Active disease of the biceps tendon will cause pain with this maneuver. If at the same time the biceps muscle belly is palpated and is felt to contract weakly or not at all, this may indicate bicipital tendon rupture.

Although these various bicipital tests are described, the most useful is reproduction of pain in the area of the bicipital groove with resisted forward elevation of the extremity (Speed's test).

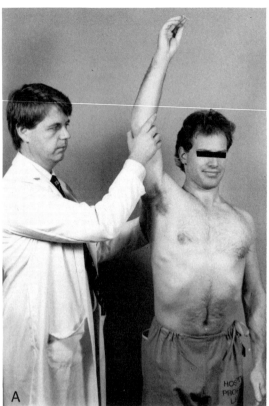

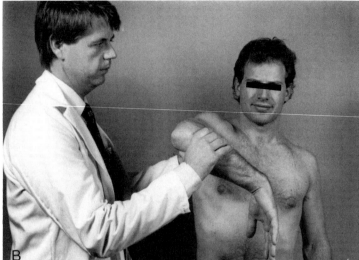

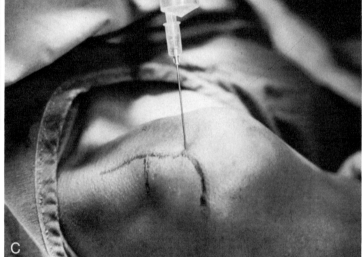

Figure 4–25. Impingement signs and test. *A,* Stressing at maximal elevation causes pain, the classic impingement sign. *B,* With the arm forward-flexed 90 degrees, forcible internal rotation causes pain owing to impingement of the supraspinatus tendon against the coracoacromial ligament. *C,* Impingement test. Ten ml of 1% lidocaine (Xylocaine) is injected into the subacromial space. Repetition of the impingement sign should elicit no or minimal pain, which is considered a positive test. *D,* Painful arc. Abduction in the coronal plane causes pain between 60 and 100 degrees.

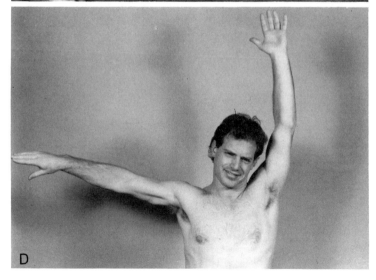

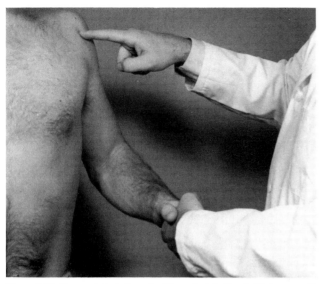

Figure 4–26. Yergason's test. The patient flexes the left elbow to 90 degrees, with the forearm pronated. The patient is requested to supinate against resistance; this maneuver elicits pain in the region of the bicipital groove, indicated by the examiner's right index finger.

VASCULAR EXAMINATION

The vascular evaluation involves assessment of a wide scope of manifestations in the upper limb. General skin texture, color, temperature, hair growth, and alteration in sensation may relate to changes in the vascular system. Checking all pulses (radial, ulnar, brachial, axillary, and subclavian) and listening for bruits with a stethoscope may be indicated, especially when significant trauma has occurred to the upper limb. Evaluation of the autonomic nervous system is important to exclude reflex sympathetic dystrophy (shoulder-hand syndrome). There are a number of tests that help detect the presence of neurovascular compression in the neck known as thoracic outlet syndromes. The reliability of any of these tests is not high, so caution should be exercised in their interpretations. If positive, these various tests may suggest different areas of pathology. Vascular compression, especially from the thoracic outlet, can give shoulder pain.

Adson's Maneuver

The examiner palpates the radial pulse. With the patient sitting, the patient is requested to extend the shoulder and arm and rotate the head toward the side being examined. Next, the patient is instructed to take a deep breath and hold while the examiner notes any diminution of the radial pulse.[5] Any decrease or obliteration of the pulse is recorded as a positive test. A few modifications of this test have been reported. They involve rotating the head to the opposite side, with the arm on the side being examined abducted to 90 degrees, extended, and externally rotated (Fig. 4–27).

Hyperabduction Syndrome Test

While the patient is sitting, both radial pulses are palpated with arms hyperabducted and the radial pulses palpated. A decrease in pulse occurs in approximately 20 per cent of normal individuals, but asymmetry may be significant. During the maneuver the neurovascular bundle is brought tightly under the coracoid process and pectoralis major muscle. With partial vascular obstruction as the arm is hyperabducted, auscultation over the clavicle or in the axilla may reveal a bruit.

Halstead's Test

The patient extends the neck and turns the head to the opposite shoulder. With downward traction on the affected arm, the pulse is palpated. If the pulse is oblitered, the test is positive. With incomplete vascular compression, auscultation over the clavicle and base of the neck may reveal the presence of a bruit.

Provocative Elevation Testing

The patient elevates both arms above the horizontal and is instructed to rapidly open and close the hands approximately 15 times. If fatigue, cramping, or tingling occurs in the hands and forearm, particularly toward the end of these repetitions, it is suggestive of vascular insufficiency and the presence of a thoracic outlet syndrome.

GENERAL PHYSICAL EXAMINATION

A general physical examination is required to complete the overall evaluation. Occasionally, findings on

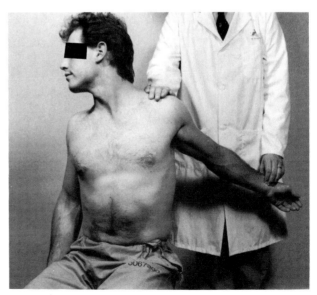

Figure 4–27. Modified Adson's maneuver. Diminution of the radial pulse with arm slightly abducted and extended and neck looking away is suggestive of vascular compression.

the general physical exam may relate to the specific shoulder complaint; for example, chest findings with an underlying Pancoast's tumor that has presented with shoulder pain. There are many disease processes such as rheumatoid arthritis, diabetes, and neurofibromatosis that can be related to problems of the shoulder. Any abnormalities relating to the cardiovascular and respiratory systems are very important in the patient considered for surgery. Limited neck range of motion or limited jaw opening may alter the anesthesiologist's approach.

Injection Techniques

In selected patients injection tests are not only diagnostic but also can be therapeutic. Owing to the close proximity and interrelationship of a multitude of structures about the shoulder, a clear diagnosis may often be difficult. Distinguishing between pain arising from the acromioclavicular joint, supraspinatus tendon, and long head of the biceps may pose a problem for the examining physician. In these circumstances there may be benefit from using selective local anesthetic injection techniques. The areas that may be injected include subacromial space (see Fig. 4–25C), acromioclavicular joint, glenohumeral joint, bicipital groove, suprascapular nerve, and various trigger areas along the trapezius and rhomboids, especially in the patient with difficult neck-shoulder pain. Strict asepsis is mandatory to minimize the risk of infection with these techniques.

SUBACROMIAL SPACE

This is the most common site to inject, providing helpful diagnostic information; it may also have a therapeutic effect. This is the impingement test, previously described (see Fig. 4–25C). The space can be most easily entered from the front. Introduction of the needle may be assisted by gentle longitudinal traction on the arm to increase the gap between the acromion and humeral head.

ACROMIOCLAVICULAR JOINT

Because it is a subcutaneous joint, the acromioclavicular is fairly easy to enter with a needle. Patients with arthritis and radiological changes have varying degrees of symptoms emanating from this joint. It is usually in conjunction with an impingement problem, and injection selectively into this joint compared with injection subacromially may clarify the degree of pain related to this joint and guide the surgeon toward or away from local surgery.

GLENOHUMERAL JOINT

The patient with an intra-articular problem may experience significant relief following injection of a local anesthetic into the joint. Since the joint is deep and is surrounded by a number of muscle layers, it may be difficult to be sure that the needle is within the joint. If there is any doubt, the position of the needle may be confirmed during fluoroscopy with insertion of radiopaque dye.

BICIPITAL GROOVE

Local pathosis of the long head of biceps may be confirmed by relief of pain with infiltration in the region of the bicipital groove. The injection should not be directly into the tendon, but rather around the tendon sheath.

SUPRASCAPULAR NERVE

In patients with posterior shoulder pain, especially those with supraspinatus and infraspinatus muscle wasting, entrapment of the suprascapular nerve may be the cause.[25] Local anesthetic injected into the region of the suprascapular notch may relieve symptoms and confirm the diagnosis.[27] Further confirmation may be obtained from EMG studies using a coaxial needle.

OTHER INJECTION SITES

In patients with exquisite localized tenderness or trigger areas, local infiltration of anesthetic may assist in the evaluation of their pain. Patients with neck pain are particularly prone to develop trigger areas in the rhomboids and trapezius, and injection often provides diagnostic information and therapeutic relief. Unusual nerve entrapments, such as supraclavicular nerves passing through osseous canals of the clavicle, may be evaluated with the aid of local anesthetics.[6]

Cervical Spine Examination

In conjunction with the shoulder assessment, examination of the cervical spine should be undertaken. Coexistent pathosis in the neck and shoulder is common, and appreciation of this fact is critical to understanding the contribution of each to the patient's overall complaint. In addition, cervical spine problems, especially those originating in a cervical root, can cause referred pain and sometimes referred findings to the shoulder. The format to be followed is the same as with the shoulder: look, feel, and move. Examination of the cervical spine is coordinated and integrated with examination of the shoulder. For example, when performing range of motion of the shoulder, it is simple to simultaneously examine range of motion of the neck.

INSPECTION

Inspection should be systematic and comprehensive, analyzing the cervical spine from anterior, posterior, and lateral perspectives.

With the neck and shoulders appropriately displayed, note is made of the posture or attitude of the cervical spine and head. The neck may be short or webbed as occurs in congenital problems such as Klippel-Feil or Turner's syndrome. The head may be held to the side, or it may be thrust forward. Observation of the paracervical musculature may show asymmetry, suggesting muscle spasm and hypertrophy. Analysis of the distal extremity looking for muscle wasting may suggest root involvement. There may be associated pathology such as thoracolumbar scoliosis or kyphosis in other areas of the spine.

PALPATION

Palpation of the neck should proceed in an orderly sequence, dividing the neck into appropriate areas, and should include soft tissue versus bone and superficial versus deep palpation. Patients with cervical spondylosis invariably have localized tenderness along the involved posterior cervical spines. Muscle spasm and tenderness with frequently associated trigger areas along the trapezius and rhomboid muscles are often present. Examination of the supraclavicular region may reveal hidden masses such as a Pancoast tumor. Gentle percussion over the brachial plexus trunks may elicit tenderness or Tinel's sign, indicating plexus inflammation or damage.

RANGE OF MOTION

Starting with the head upright, there are three ranges of motion to record:
1. *Flexion/extension.* This can be described in degrees, but for practical purposes, flexion is described as finger-breadths from sternum to chin. Extension is measured by a subjective estimation of percentage of limitation.
2. *Lateral flexion.* With a sagittal reference point, lateral flexion is more appropriately measured in degrees.
3. *Rotation.* Rotation of the cervical spine is estimated in degrees from the neutral position.

Accurate clinical measurement of cervical motion is difficult, and the use of a goniometer is often impractical. Practice and attention on the part of the clinician will enable reproducible results to be recorded. It is unusual to have significant discrepancies between passive and active ranges of motion in the neck. However, at the extremes of movement, the neck should have a gentle stress applied to see if this reproduces any pain. Strength testing of the neck muscles is of little value.

NEUROLOGICAL EXAMINATION

The neurological examination will be guided by the history and clinical findings in the patient. A thorough examination of the upper limb looks for evidence of root radiculopathy or peripheral nerve lesions. Evidence of myelopathy with lower and upper extremity long tract signs may occur and should be sought in conditions such as rheumatoid arthritis.

SPECIAL TESTS

Special tests applied to cervical spine examination include compression, distraction, and Spurling's tests and Valsalva's maneuvers.

Compression Test

This is a provocative test where downward pressure, perhaps with a jarring effect, is placed on the patient's head while the neck is in slight extension. With narrowing of the neural foramen or facet joint irritation, pain may occur, sometimes radiating into the arms mimicking the patient's symptoms. In axial pain caused by spondylosis, this test may cause reproduction of discomfort (Fig. 4–28A).

Distraction Test

Placing the hands on either side of the patient's head at the angle of the mandible, the examiner gently lifts the head in slight flexion. The neural foramen may be slightly increased in size or the facet joints separated, and the patient may experience some relief of pain (Fig. 4–28B).

Spurling's Test

The neck is stressed in lateral flexion and rotation with some compression to elicit pain. Positioning the neck in this manner causes encroachment on cervical nerve roots as they exit the neural foramina; it also stresses the facet joints[28] (Fig. 4–28C). It is a fairly nonspecific maneuver.

Valsalva's Maneuver

Valsalva's maneuver raises intrathecal pressure. In the presence of a space-occupying lesion such as a herniated disc, the patient develops pain which may

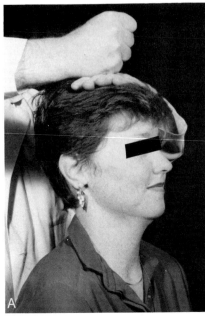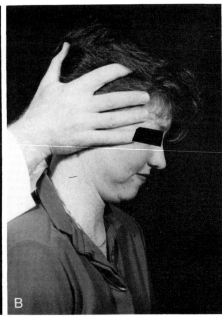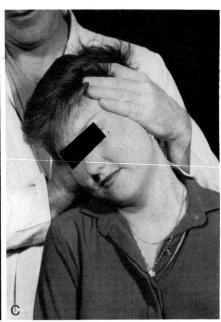

Figure 4–28. Special tests for examining the cervical spine. *A,* Compression test: With the neck slightly extended, a downward pressure is placed on the patient's head. *B,* Distraction test: With the neck in slight flexion, the examiner places his hands on either side of the patient's head and lifts, reducing symptoms. *C,* Spurling's test: The neck is stressed in lateral flexion, rotation, and some compression. Pain occurs on the side to which the head is tilted.

radiate to the dermatomal distribution and corresponds to the neurological level of the lesion.

Cervical Spine and the Shoulder

A significant number of patients present with both shoulder and neck pain.[10] The major difficulty in this group of patients is sorting out accurately the predominant source of pain. Shoulder pain as it relates to the cervical spine may present in one of five ways:

1. A cervical spine lesion with root involvement may produce referred pain to the shoulder.
2. As a result of a cervical spine lesion, a "frozen shoulder" may develop.
3. Neck pain and pathology may initiate a tendinitis in the shoulder.
4. Cervical spine pathology may occur concomitantly with shoulder pathology, particularly cervical spondylosis and tendinitis.
5. Primary shoulder pathology may cause pain to radiate into the neck.

Detailed questioning about the site and nature of the pain will help alert the physician to the possibility of a complex clinical problem. Referred pain in the shoulder from cervical pathology is often maximal over the top of the shoulder and may be associated with radicular pain with or without paresthesia below the elbow. This pain is frequently relieved by rest or a collar and often lessens at night. In contrast, patients with shoulder problems such as rotator cuff pathology have pain around the shoulder and over the deltoid

insertion. For these patients, sleep is often disturbed owing to worsening of the pain at night. It should be remembered that primary shoulder pathology can also give rise to radiating paresthesias below the elbow.

Physical examination of the cervical spine reveals midline tenderness over the posterior cervical spines and a diminished range of motion. There may be associated muscle spasm and tenderness with trigger areas over the trapezius and rhomboid muscles. Positive compression and distraction tests and pain reproduced by Spurling's test will further suggest significant cervical pathosis. A neurological examination suggesting specific root compression will confirm the neck findings. Even though shoulder pain may be present, local findings in the shoulder will be variable. In some patients there will be few if any positive findings from the shoulder; for example, there will be no local tenderness and a negative impingement sign, while in others, especially those with significant concomitant shoulder pathology, classic localized findings will also be evident.

To help clarify the diagnostic dilemma, a number of investigative techniques may prove helpful. These include plain roentgenograms of neck and shoulder, selective injection techniques, shoulder arthrography, myelography, discography, CT scanning, electromyographic studies, ultrasonography, and magnetic resonance imaging. The details and interpretation of these investigations will be expanded upon in later sections. If there is still doubt as to the exact primary pathology, a period of observation and conservative/nonoperative treatment should be undertaken to enable the physician and patient to develop a better appreciation of the problem.

Further Investigative Procedures

It is not within the domain of this chapter to discuss further investigative procedures in the evaluation of a shoulder problem. We have concentrated mainly on history, physical examination, and some specialized investigative techniques, such as selective injections. Obviously, in many patients, such as those with a rotator cuff deficiency, the investigator would proceed to plain x-rays and possibly either ultrasound or shoulder arthrography to assess the rotator cuff. The application of routine and specialized blood investigations, plain x-rays, arthrograms, ultrasound, and nuclear magnetic resonance, among many other techniques, will be elaborated upon elsewhere. Often the diagnosis is established before implementation of these tests.

Conclusions

In the majority of cases, a detailed history and careful physical examination will suggest a diagnosis. Special investigative techniques can be applied selectively, more to confirm but occasionally to diagnose in challenging cases. The physician should have an organized, comprehensive, and permanent record which can provide the necessary details for later review. The surgeon will need to develop his own particular means of recording these details. The Society of American Shoulder and Elbow Surgeons has suggested a Basic Shoulder Evaluation Form, which is included as a table (Table 4–3).

References

1. American Academy of Orthopaedic Surgeons: Joint Motion: Method of Measuring and Recording. Chicago: American Academy of Orthopaedic Surgeons, 1965.
2. Bridgman JF: Periarthritis of the shoulder and diabetes mellitus. Ann Rheum Dis 31:69–71, 1972.
3. DeGowin EL, and DeGowin RL. Bedside Diagnostic Examination, 5th ed. New York: Macmillan Publishing Company, 1987.
4. DePalma AF: Surgery of the Shoulder, 3rd ed. Philadelphia: JB Lippincott, 1983.
5. Fielding JW, Francis WR, and Hensinger RN: The cervical and thoracic spine. In Cruess RJ, and Rennie, WRJ (eds): Adult Orthopaedics, Vol. 2. New York: Churchill Livingstone, 1984, pp 747–841.
6. Gelberman RH, Verdeck WN, and Brodhead WT: Supraclavic-ular nerve entrapment syndrome. J Bone Joint Surg 57A:119, 1975.
7. Hawkins RJ, and Hobeika P: Physical examination of the shoulder. Orthopedics 6(10):1270–1278, 1983.
8. Hawkins RJ: Surgical management of rotator cuff tears. In Bateman JE, and Welsh RP (eds): Surgery of the Shoulder. Burlington, Ontario: BC Decker Inc., 1984.
9. Hawkins RJ and Murnaghan JP: The shoulder. In Cruess RL, and Rennie, WRJ (eds): Adult Orthopaedics, Vol. 2. New York: Churchill Livingstone, 1984, pp 945–1054.
10. Hawkins RJ: Cervical spine and the shoulder. In Instructional Course Lectures AAOS, Vol. 34, Chapter 17, 1985, pp 191–195.
11. Hawkins RJ, and Bell RH: Shoulder instability—diagnosis and management. Can J Sport Sci 12:67–70, 1987.
12. Hawkins RJ, Neer CS, Pianta RM, and Mendosa F: Locked posterior dislocation of the shoulder. J Bone Joint Surg 69A:9–18, 1987.
13. Hollingshead WH: Anatomy for Surgeons, Vol. 3. The Back and Limbs, 3rd ed. Philadelphia: Harper & Row Publishers, 1982.
14. Hoppenfeld S: Physical Examination of the Spine and Extremities. Norwalk, CT: Appleton-Century-Crofts, 1976.
15. Inman VT, Saunders JB, and Abbott LC: Observation of the function of the shoulder joint. J Bone Joint Surg 26A:1–30, 1944.
16. Ivey FM, Calhoun JH, Rusche K, and Bierschenk J: Isokinetic testing of shoulder strength. Normal values. Arch Phys Med Rehabil 66:384–386, 1985.
17. Jobe FW, Moynes DR, and Brewster CE: Rehabilitation of shoulder joint instabilities. Orthop Clin North Am 18:473–482, 1987.
18. Katz GA, Peters JP, Pearson CM, and Adams WS: The shoulder-pad sign: a diagnostic feature of amyloid arthropathy. N Engl J Med 288:354–355, 1973.
19. Neer CS, and Welsh RP: The shoulder in sports. Orthop Clin North Am 8:583–591, 1977.
20. Neer CS, and Foster CR: Inferior capsular shift for involuntary inferior and multidirectional instability of the shoulder. J Bone Joint Surg 62A:897–908, 1980.
21. Petersson CJ: The acromioclavicular joint in rheumatoid arthritis. Clin Orthop 223:86–93, 1987.
22. Poppen NK, and Walker PS: Normal and abnormal motion of the shoulder. J Bone Joint Surg 58A:195–201, 1976.
23. Post M: The Shoulder. Surgical and Nonsurgical Management. Philadelphia: Lea & Febiger, 1978.
24. Post M: Physical Examination of the Musculoskeletal System. Chicago: Year Book Medical Publishers Inc., 1987.
25. Post M, and Mayer J: Suprascapular nerve entrapment. Diagnosis and treatment. Clin Orthop 223:126–136, 1987.
26. Rockwood CA, and Green DP: Fractures in Adults. Philadelphia: JB Lippincott, 1984.
27. Rose DL, and Kelly CK: Shoulder pain. Suprascapular nerve block in shoulder pain. J Kans Med Soc 70:135–136, 1969.
28. Spurling RG, and Scoville WB: Lateral rupture of the cervical intervertebral discs. A common cause of shoulder and arm pain. Surg Gynecol Obstet 78:350–358, 1944.
29. Turek S: Orthopaedics. Principles and Their Application, 4th ed. Philadelphia: JB Lippincott, 1984.
30. Yergason RM: Supination sign. J Bone Joint Surg 13160, 1931.

X-ray Evaluation of Shoulder Problems

Charles A. Rockwood, Jr., M.D.
Elizabeth A. Szalay, M.D.
Ralph J. Curtis, Jr., M.D.
D. Christopher Young, M.D.
Stephen P. Kay, M.D.

The appropriate use of x-rays for the diagnosis of pathology in the musculoskeletal system requires a minimum of two x-rays of the area in question that are perpendicular to each other. Although this time-honored orthopedic principle is widely acknowledged, it is often forgotten when evaluating the shoulder.

The shoulder is a complicated anatomical unit made up of numerous bony landmarks, projections, and joints. It is impossible for all of these parts and joints to be visualized by two anteroposterior x-rays taken in the *usual* internal and external rotation views. Orthopedists do not diagnose and treat injuries in any other part of the body on the basis of a one-plane radiographic evaluation. At a minimum, anteroposterior and lateral views are always obtained, and in many instances oblique views are also obtained. All too commonly, x-rays of the shoulder include only the two anteroposterior views of the rotated proximal humerus, which are taken perpendicular to the frontal axis of the *thorax*. With the exception of localizing rotator cuff calcium deposits, these two traditional views by themselves are wholly inadequate to evaluate injuries and disorders of the shoulder joint. The scapula, which lies on the posterolateral portion of the rib cage, is actually at an angle of approximately 45 degrees to the frontal plane of the thorax. Thus, the plane of the glenohumeral joint is not the plane of the thorax, and x-rays taken in the anteroposterior plane of the thorax provide oblique views of the shoulder joint (Fig. 5–1). In addition, the rotation of the humerus into internal and external rotation does not change the orientation of the scapula to the x-ray beam. Therefore, the two traditional anteroposterior views of the shoulder in internal and external rotation provide two different views of the proximal humerus, but only one oblique view of the scapula and the shoulder joint.

Disorders of the Glenohumeral Joint

FRACTURES, SUBLUXATIONS, AND DISLOCATIONS

The Trauma Series of X-rays

Recommended Views. ■ *A true anteroposterior view and an axillary lateral or a true scapulolateral. Modified axillary laterals or a computed tomographic (CT) scan may be required.*

X-rays of the injured shoulder in two planes, i.e., anteroposterior, axillary lateral or scapular lateral, are absolutely essential to the evaluation of the acutely injured shoulder.

McLaughlin,[174] Neer,[187, 188] Neviaser,[193] DePalma,[64] Rockwood,[233] Post,[212] Rowe,[239] Bateman,[15] and many others have recognized the shortcomings of the usual two anteroposterior x-rays of the shoulder and have recommended anteroposterior *and* lateral views to properly assess shoulder problems. The x-rays used to evaluate traumatic shoulder problems have been referred to as the trauma series. The trauma series of x-rays can also be used as baseline x-rays to evaluate many of the chronic shoulder problems as well. The recommended x-rays for the trauma series include:

AP Thorax

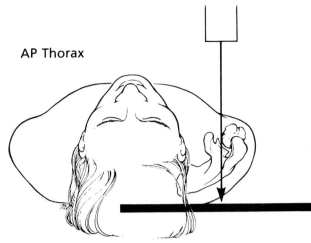

Figure 5–1. Anteroposterior x-ray of the shoulder taken in the plane of the thorax. Note that the film is actually an oblique view of the glenohumeral joint.

1. A true anteroposterior view in the plane of the scapula.

2. An axillary lateral. *If* the axillary x-ray cannot be obtained, the true scapulolateral or one of the modified axillary views must be obtained.

Techniques for Taking the Trauma Series

The True Anteroposterior View. Since the scapula lies on the posterolateral aspect of the thoracic cage, the true anteroposterior view of the glenohumeral joint is obtained by angling the x-ray beam 45 degrees from medial to lateral (Figs. 5–1 and 5–2). The patient may be supine or erect, with the arm at the side or in the sling position. An alternative technique is rotating the patient until the scapula is flat against the x-ray cassette and then taking the x-ray with the beam perpendicular to the scapula. Sometimes it is difficult for the technician to properly align the patient for the view. A simple technique, developed by one of the authors

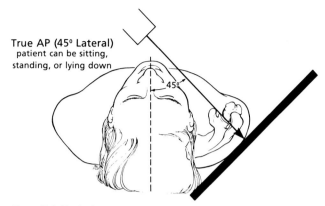

Figure 5–2. To obtain a true anteroposterior view of the glenohumeral joint, the beam must be angled 45 degrees or the patient can rotate the body until the scapula is parallel to the x-ray cassette.

(E.A.S.), has proved to be of great value in assisting the technician in positioning the patient. With a heavy marking pen, a line is drawn on the skin, along the spine of the scapula. The technician aligns the x-ray beam perpendicular to the line on the skin, directed at the cassette which is placed parallel to the line, posterior to the scapula and glenohumeral joint (Fig. 5–3). Although the scapular spine is not exactly parallel to the plane of the scapula, this technique has proved effective in clinical practice.

The advantage of the true anteroposterior view of the scapula over traditional anteroposterior views in the plane of the thorax is that the x-ray demonstrates the glenoid in profile rather than obliquely and, in the normal shoulder, clearly separates the glenoid from the humeral head (Fig. 5–4). In the true anteroposterior x-ray, the coracoid process overlaps the glenohumeral joint. If the true anteroposterior x-ray demonstrates the humeral head to be overlapping with the glenoid, the glenohumeral joint is dislocated either anteriorly or posteriorly.

The Axillary Lateral View. Initially described by

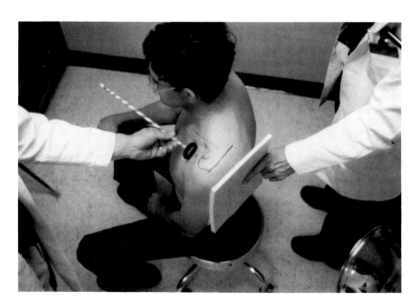

Figure 5–3. Position of the patient and the x-ray beam to obtain a true anteroposterior view of the glenohumeral joint.

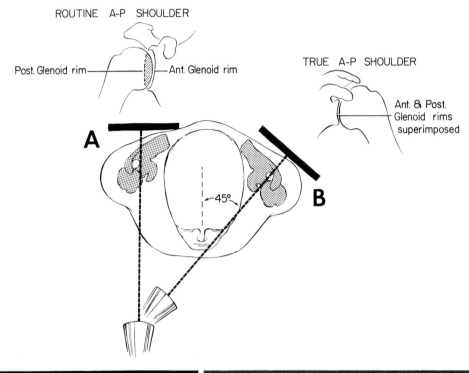

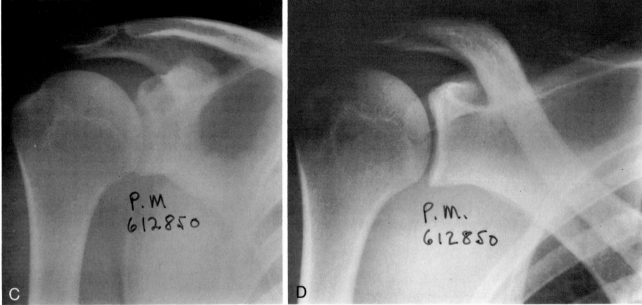

Figure 5–4. *A, B,* Note the great difference between the two angles of the x-ray beam, the placement of the cassettes, and the schematic drawings of the glenohumeral joint. *C,* An x-ray of the shoulder in the plane of the thorax. *D,* An x-ray of the shoulder taken in the plane of the scapula. (Reproduced with permission from Rockwood CA, and Green DP (eds): Fractures (3 vols), 2nd ed. Philadelphia: JB Lippincott, 1984.)

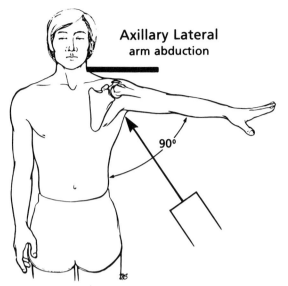

Figure 5–5. The axillary lateral x-ray. Ideally, the arm is abducted 70 to 90 degrees and the beam is directed superiorly up to the x-ray cassette.

Lawrence[152, 153] in 1915, this x-ray can be taken with the patient supine or erect. Ideally, the arm should be positioned in 70 to 90 degrees of abduction. The x-ray beam is directed into the axilla from inferior to superior, and the x-ray cassette is placed superior to the patient's shoulder (Fig. 5–5). To minimize the amount of required abduction to obtain an axillary lateral x-ray, an alternate technique was devised by Cleaves[45] in 1941. In this technique, the patient may be sitting or supine; the arm is abducted only enough to admit a *curved* x-ray cassette into the axilla. The x-ray is taken from superior to inferior through the axilla.

In some situations where abduction is severely limited to only 20 or 30 degrees, a rolled-up cardboard cassette can be substituted for the curved cassette in the axillae (Fig. 5–6).

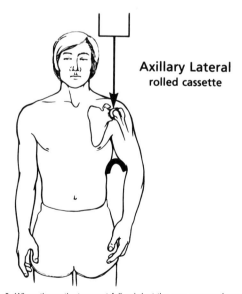

Figure 5–6. When the patient cannot fully abduct the arm, a curved cassette can be placed in the axilla and the beam directed inferiorly through the glenohumeral joint onto the cassette.

Axillary lateral x-rays provide excellent visualization of the glenoid and the humeral head and clearly delineate the spatial relationship of the two structures. Dislocations are easily identified, as are compression fractures of the humeral head and large fractures of the anterior or posterior glenoid rim (see Fig. 5–17*A, B*). Some fractures of the coracoid and the acromion and the spatial relationship of the acromioclavicular joint can also be seen on this view.

If a good quality axillary lateral x-ray can be obtained, the true scapulolateral or the modified axillary lateral views are not necessary. However, if because of pain and muscle spasm the patient will not allow enough abduction to get a good axillary view, the scapulolateral or the modified axillary laterals *must* be obtained.

Technique for the Scapulolateral X-ray

This view is sometimes known as the transscapular, the tangential lateral, or the Y lateral.[240] The position of the injured shoulder, which is in internal rotation in a sling, is left undisturbed. A marking pen (E.A.S.) is

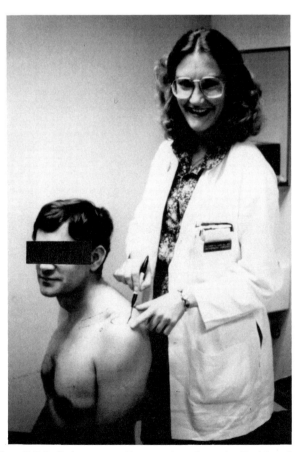

Figure 5–7. Dr. Szalay uses a marking pen to draw a line on the skin of the patient in line with the spine of the scapula. This will enable the x-ray technician to take the true anteroposterior view and the true scapulolateral x-ray. To take the true AP x-ray, the cassette is placed posterolateral, parallel to the line on the scapula, and the beam is brought perpendicular to the line. To take the true scapulolateral x-ray, the cassette is placed anterolateral, perpendicular to the line, and the beam passes down the line onto the cassette.

used to draw a heavy line over the spine of the scapula (Figs. 5–7 and 5–8*A*). The technician then aligns the x-ray beam parallel to the line on the skin, directed to the cassette which is placed perpendicular to the line at the anterolateral shoulder. The x-ray beam passes tangentially across the posterolateral chest, parallel to and down the spine of the scapula onto the x-ray cassette (Fig. 5–8*A*, *B*). The projected image is a true lateral of the scapula and, hence, a lateral of the glenohumeral joint (Fig. 5–8*B*).

A lateral projection of the scapula forms the letter Y[240] (Fig. 5–9*A, B, C*). The upper arms of the Y are formed by the coracoid process anteriorly and the

scapular spine posteriorly. The vertical portion of the Y is formed by the body of the scapula. At the intersection of the three limbs of the Y lies the glenoid fossa, and in the normal shoulder, the humeral head is located overlapping the glenoid fossa (Figs. 5–8*B* and 5–9*D*). This view is of particular help in determining the anterior or posterior relationship of the humeral head to the glenoid fossa. In anterior dislocations of the shoulder, the humeral head lies anterior to the glenoid fossa (Figs. 5–8*C* and 5–9*F*), and in posterior dislocations, it lies posterior to the glenoid fossa (Figs. 5–8*D* and 5–9*E*). The scapulolateral view will not define fractures of the anterior or posterior glenoid

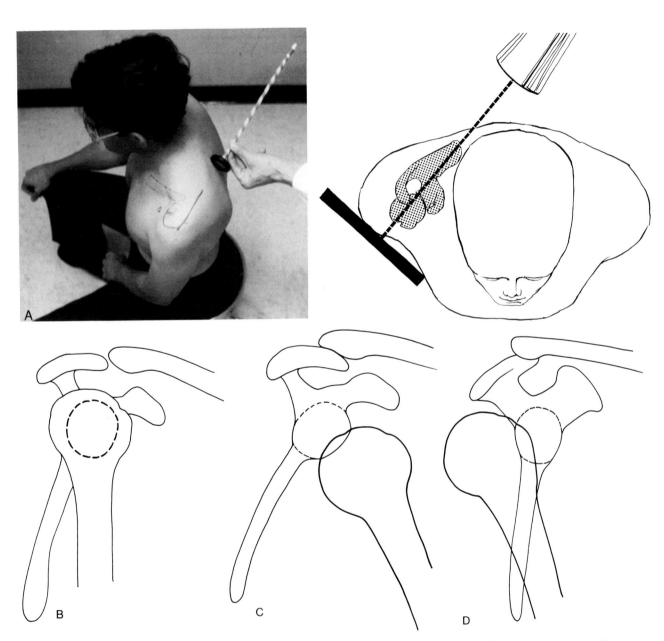

Figure 5–8. *A* demonstrates how the line marked on the skin of the shoulder helps the technician visualize the plane of the x-ray for the true scapulolateral x-ray. (Reproduced with permission from Rockwood CA, and Green DP (eds): Fractures (3 vols), 2nd ed. Philadelphia: JB Lippincott, 1984.) *B,* A schematic drawing illustrates how the humeral head on the true scapulolateral x-ray should be centered around the glenoid fossa. *C,* In anterior dislocations, the humeral head is displaced anterior to the glenoid fossa. *D,* In posterior dislocations of the shoulder, the humeral head sits posterior to the glenoid fossa.

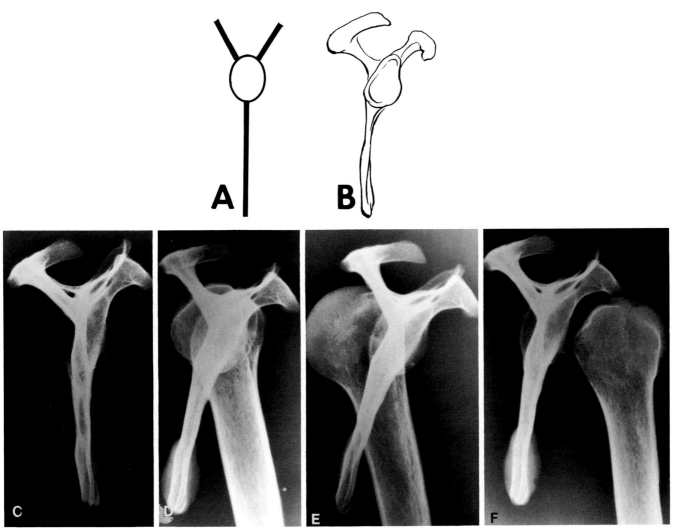

Figure 5–9. Interpretation of the true lateral x-ray of the shoulder. *A,* The schematic drawing illustrates how a lateral view of the scapula projects as the letter Y. *B,* A lateral view of the scapula. *C,* The true lateral x-ray of the scapula indicates that the glenoid fossa is located at the junction of the base of the spine and the base of the coracoid, with the body of the vertically projecting scapula. *D,* The true lateral view of the glenohumeral joint shows the humeral head well centered around the glenoid fossa. *E,* In the subacromial, posterior dislocation of the shoulder, the articular surface of the humeral head is directed posterior to the glenoid fossa. *F,* In anterior subcoracoid dislocations of the shoulder, the humeral head is anterior to the glenoid fossa. (Reproduced with permission from Rockwood CA, and Green DP (eds): Fractures (3 vols), 2nd ed. Philadelphia: JB Lippincott, 1984.)

rim but will reveal displaced fractures of the greater tuberosity. When this view is added to the true antero-posterior and the axillary lateral, they represent three views, all 90 degrees to each other, which maximizes the information.

Techniques for the Modified Axillary Views

The Velpeau Axillary Lateral. Bloom and Obata's[25] modification of the axillary lateral x-ray of the shoulder is known as the Velpeau axillary lateral because it was designed to be taken with the acutely injured shoulder still in a sling, thereby circumventing the need for abduction. With the Velpeau bandage or shoulder sling in place, the patient stands or sits at the end of the x-ray table and leans backwards 20 to 30 degrees over the table. The x-ray cassette is placed on the table directly beneath the shoulder, and the x-ray machine

is placed directly over the shoulder so that the beam passes vertically from superior to inferior, through the shoulder joint onto the cassette (Fig. 5–10). On this view, the humeral shaft appears foreshortened and the glenohumeral joint appears magnified, but otherwise, it demonstrates the relationship of the head of the humerus to the scapula.

The Stripp Axillary Lateral. The Stripp axial view, described by Horsfield,[111] is similar to the Velpeau axillary lateral view, except that the beam passes from inferior to superior and the x-ray cassette is positioned above the shoulder.

The Trauma Axillary Lateral. Another modification of the axillary lateral view has been described by Tietge and Ciullo.[43, 263] The advantage of this view over the Velpeau and Stripp views is that it can be taken while the patient is supine, as is often necessary in patients with multiple trauma. This view can be taken while

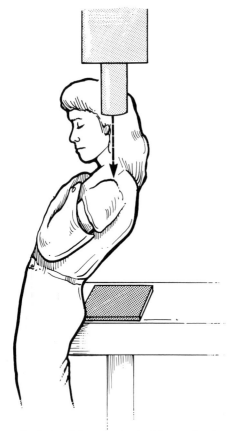

Figure 5–10. Positioning of the patient for the Velpeau axillary lateral x-ray, as described by Bloom and Obata. (Modified from Bloom MH, and Obata WG: Diagnosis of posterior dislocation of the shoulder with use of the Velpeau axillary and angled up radiographic views. J Bone Joint Surg 49A:943–949, 1967.)

the injured shoulder is still immobilized in a shoulder immobilizer dressing. To obtain this view, the patient is supine on the x-ray table, and the involved arm is supported in 20 degrees of flexion by placing radiolucent material under the elbow. The x-ray beam is directed up through the axilla to a cassette propped up against the superior aspect of the shoulder (Fig. 5–11). This view will define the relationship of the humeral head to the glenoid fossa.

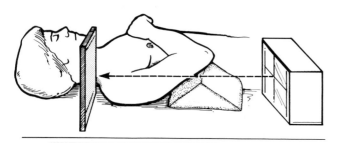

Figure 5–11. Positioning of the patient for the trauma axillary lateral x-ray. The patient is supine. The elbow is elevated by a piece of foam rubber, allowing the x-ray to pass from inferior up through the glenohumeral joint onto the x-ray cassette, which is superior to the shoulder. (Modified from Tietge RA, and Ciullo JV: The CAM axillary x-ray. Exhibit at AAOS Meeting. Orthop Trans 6:451, 1982.)

The CT Scan

Although the CT scan is not always readily available in every hospital, it will reliably demonstrate fractures, the number of fracture fragments, and fracture-dislocations of the glenohumeral joint. It is very important that the scan include *both* shoulders so that the physician can compare the anatomy of the injured shoulder with that of the normal shoulder.

ANTERIOR INSTABILITY

Recommended Views. ■ *A true anteroposterior x-ray, West Point axillary lateral, apical-oblique projection, or CT scan.*

With anterior dislocation or subluxation of the glenohumeral joint, there may be bone damage or soft tissue calcification adjacent to the anterior or, particularly, the anteroinferior rim of the glenoid. The true anteroposterior view may demonstrate a fracture of the inferior glenoid that may not be visualized on the anteroposterior views in the plane of the thorax. Although the axillary lateral may be useful to demonstrate some anterior glenoid abnormality, the West Point axillary lateral and the apical-oblique x-rays will provide more information.[224, 234] Anterior shoulder dislocations can be accompanied by fractures of the anterior glenoid rim, which may be demonstrated on a routine axillary lateral x-ray. However, in evaluating traumatic anterior subluxation, the glenoid defect almost exclusively involves the *anteroinferior glenoid,* which cannot be seen on routine axillary lateral x-rays. In many instances, the lesions seen on the anteroinferior glenoid rim may provide the only x-ray evidence of traumatic anterior shoulder subluxation. Two techniques have been described to evaluate the anteroinferior glenoid rim. They are the West Point and the apical-oblique projections.

Techniques to Evaluate Anterior Instability

The West Point Axillary Lateral. This projection was described by Rokous, Feagin, and Abbott when they were stationed at the U.S. Military Academy at West Point, New York.[234] Since 1975 the senior author has referred to this technique as the West Point view.[233] The patient is positioned prone on the x-ray table, with the involved shoulder on a pad raised approximately 8 cm from the top of the table. The head and neck are turned away from the involved side. With the cassette held against the superior aspect of the shoulder, the x-ray beam is centered at the axilla with 25 degrees downward angulation of the beam from the horizontal and 25 degrees medial angulation of the beam from the midline (Fig. 5–12A, B). The resulting x-ray is a tangential view of the anteroinferior rim of the glenoid. The usual finding seen in the traumatic anterior subluxing shoulder is soft tissue calcification located just

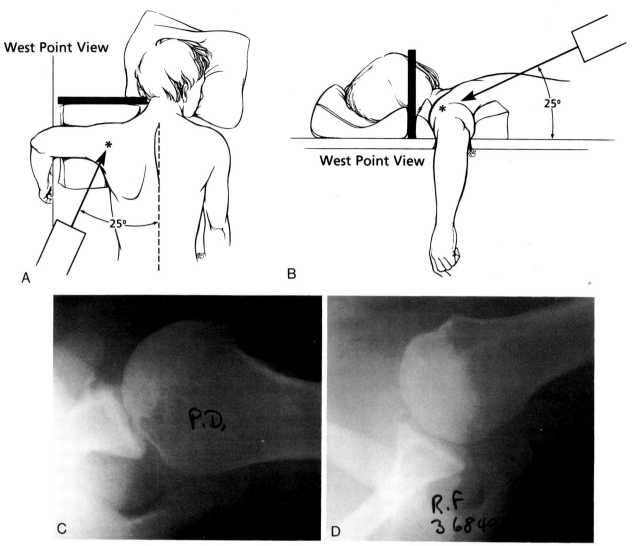

Figure 5–12. *A, B,* Positioning of the patient for the West Point x-ray to visualize the anteroinferior glenoid rim of the shoulder. (Modified from the work of Rokous JR, Feagin JA, and Abbott HG: Modified axillary roentgenogram. Clin Orthop *82:*84–86, 1972.) *C, D,* Examples of calcification on the anteroinferior glenoid rim as noted on the West Point x-ray view. (Reproduced with permission from Rockwood CA, and Green DP (eds): Fractures (3 vols), 2nd ed. Philadelphia: JB Lippincott, 1984.)

anterior to the glenoid rim (Fig. 5–12*C, D*). Occasionally, a distinct fracture fragment may be noted.

The Apical-Oblique View. Garth, Slappey, and Ochs have described an apical oblique projection, which reliably demonstrates pathology of the glenohumeral joint.[89] The patient is seated, and the arm may remain in a sling. The x-ray cassette is placed posterior, parallel to the spine of the scapula. The x-ray beam is directed through the glenohumeral joint toward the cassette at an angle of 45 degrees to the plane of the thorax, but also tipped 45 degrees caudally (Fig. 5–13*A, B*). The resultant x-ray will demonstrate anteroinferior calcification or fractures of the glenoid rim (Fig. 5–13*C, D*). Glenohumeral dislocation and posterolateral humeral head compression fractures may also be seen. Kornguth and Salazar[141] reported this to be an excellent technique.

The CT Scan and Arthro CT Scan. The CT scan may define calcification and fractures about the gle-

nohumeral joint. It is very important to remind the x-ray technician that the scan should include *both* shoulders and both arms and shoulders should be kept in the same position. In this way, the physician can compare the anatomy of the injured shoulder with that of the normal shoulder.

Evaluation of the Humeral Head Compression Fracture Associated with Anterior Dislocation

Recommended Views. ▪ *A Stryker notch view or an anteroposterior view with arm in full internal rotation.*

A frequently encountered sequela of anterior shoulder dislocation is a compression fracture of the posterolateral humeral head. This may occur during the first traumatic dislocation or following recurrent anterior dislocations. The lesion is commonly referred to as a Hill-Sachs[107] lesion and was reported by them in

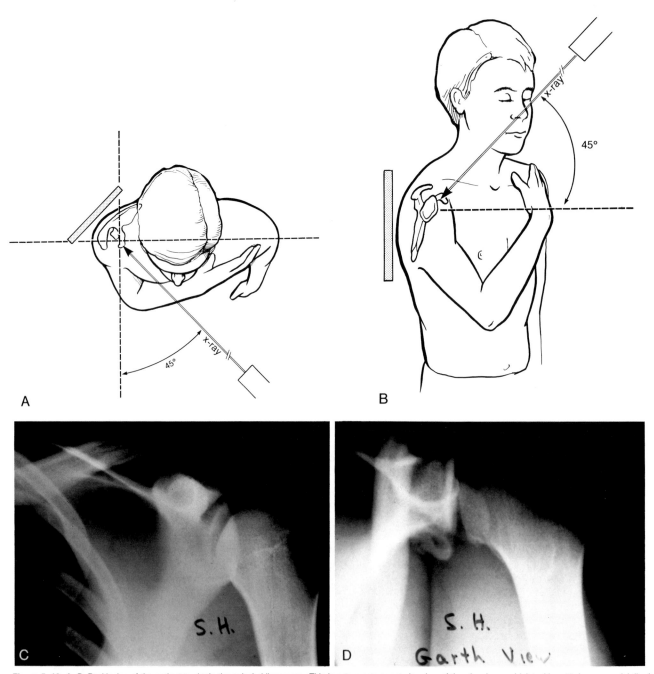

Figure 5–13. *A, B,* Positioning of the patient to obtain the apical-oblique x-ray. This is a true anteroposterior view of the glenohumeral joint with a 45-degree caudal tilt of the x-ray beam. (Modified from Garth WP Jr, Slappey CE, and Ochs CW: Radiographic demonstration of instability of the shoulder: the apical oblique projection, a technical note. J Bone Joint Surg *66A*(9):1450–1453, 1984.) *C,* An x-ray of the left shoulder in the plane of the thorax that does not reveal any significant abnormality. *D,* In the apical-oblique view, note the calcification on the anteroinferior glenoid rim. (Courtesy of Dr. Garth.)

1940 (Fig. 5–14). However, the defect was clearly described by Eve in 1880.[79] Between the report by Eve in 1880 and the report by Hill and Sachs in 1940, the defect in the humeral head was described by Malgaigne,[172] Kuster,[145] Cramer,[54] Popke,[211] Caird,[36] Broca and Hartman,[33, 34] Perthes,[209] Bankart,[13, 14] Eden,[77] Hybbinette,[114] Didiee,[73] and Hermodsson.[105] The indentation, or compression fracture, may be seen on the anteroposterior x-ray if the arm is in full internal rotation, and it may be occasionally seen on the axillary lateral view. We believe that one of the best views for identifying the compression fracture is the technique reported in 1959 by Hall, Isaac, and Booth.[102] The authors gave credit for this view to William S. Stryker, M.D., and, hence, one of us (C.A.R.) has termed it the Stryker notch view.[233]

Techniques to Evaluate the Lesion

The Stryker Notch View.[102] The patient is placed supine on the x-ray table with the cassette under the involved shoulder (Fig. 5–15A). The palm of the hand of the affected upper extremity is placed on top of the head, with the fingers toward the back of the head. The x-ray beam is tilted 10 degrees cephalad and is centered over the coracoid process. When positive, a distinct notch will be observed in the posterolateral part of the humeral head (Fig. 5–15B).

Other Views. Probably the simplest view is the one described by Adams.[4] It involves an anteroposterior view of the shoulder with the arm in full internal rotation. An indentation or compression can be seen in the posterolateral portion of the humeral head. The defect may simply appear as a vertical condensation of

bone. Pring and colleagues[214] compared the Stryker view with the internal (60 degrees) rotation view of Adams in 84 patients with anterior dislocation of the shoulder for evidence of the posterolateral defect in the humeral head. The internal rotation view was positive in 48 per cent, while the Stryker notch view was positive in 70 per cent of the patients. Other views predating the Stryker notch view have been described by Didiee[73] and Hermodsson[105] and are useful in demonstrating the presence and size of the posterolateral humeral head compression fractures. Although these techniques involve views of the proximal humerus with the arm in internal rotation, they are a bit awkward to obtain. The apical-oblique view described by Garth and colleagues[89] will also demonstrate the compression fracture. Strauss and co-workers[257] and Danzig and colleagues[58] have independently evaluated the efficacy of the various x-rays in revealing the Hill-Sachs lesion and reported that, while none of these views will always reveal the lesion in question, the Stryker notch view was probably the most effective. The presence of the compression head fracture on the x-ray confirms that the shoulder has been dislocated, whereas its absence suggests that the head may be subluxing rather than frankly dislocating.

After a study of creating lesions in the posterolateral humeral head, Danzig, Greenway, and Resnick[58] concluded that three views were optimal to define the defect; i.e., the anteroposterior view with the arm in 45 degrees of internal rotation, the Stryker notch view, and the modified Didiee view.

In a study of 120 patients, Strauss and colleagues[257] stated that a special set of x-rays could confirm the diagnosis of anterior shoulder instability with 95 per

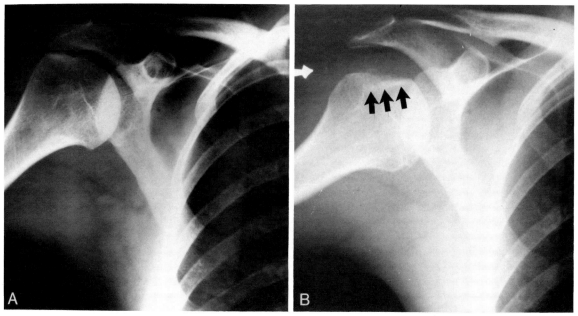

Figure 5–14. The Hill-Sachs sign. A, An anteroposterior x-ray of the right shoulder in 45 degrees of abduction and external rotation. Note that there is some sclerosis in the superior aspect of the head of the humerus. B, In full internal rotation, note the defect in the posterolateral aspect of the humeral head. Also note the dense line of bone condensation marked by the *arrows,* the so-called Hill-Sachs sign.

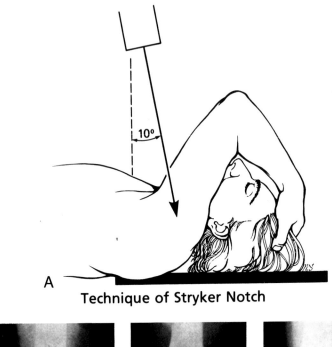

A

Technique of Stryker Notch

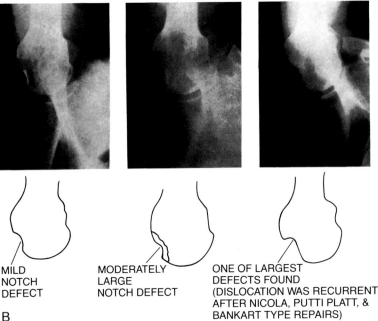

MILD
NOTCH
DEFECT

MODERATELY
LARGE
NOTCH DEFECT

ONE OF LARGEST
DEFECTS FOUND
(DISLOCATION WAS RECURRENT
AFTER NICOLA, PUTTI PLATT, &
BANKART TYPE REPAIRS)

B

Figure 5–15. *A,* The position of the patient for the Stryker notch view. The patient is supine with the cassette posterior to the shoulder. The humerus is flexed approximately 120 degrees so that the hand can be placed on top of the patient's head. Note that the angle of the x-ray tube is 10 degrees superior. *B,* Defects in the posterolateral aspect of the humeral head are seen in three different patients with recurring anterior dislocations of the shoulder. (Modified from the work of Hall RH, Isaac F, and Booth CR: Dislocation of the shoulder with special reference to accompanying small fractures. J Bone Joint Surg *41A:*489–494, 1959.)

cent accuracy. The x-rays were the anteroposterior view of the shoulder in internal rotation and the Hermodsson, axillary lateral, Stryker notch, Didiee, and West Point views.

The CT Scan. Whereas the Stryker notch view can document the presence of the compression fracture, the CT scan can be very helpful in determining the size of the compression defect.*

The Arthrogram, Arthrotomogram, and Arthro CT Scan. Occasionally, in patients with recurrent anterior or posterior dislocations and subluxations, even though there usually is significant injury to the soft tissues, bone abnormalities will not be present on the x-rays. However, in anterior dislocations, the anterior capsule

and the glenoid labrum may be stripped off the glenoid rim, as described by Perthes[209] in 1906 and by Bankart[13] in 1923. Although the arthrogram may reveal a displaced labrum with contrast material adjacent to the anterior glenoid rim and neck of the scapula, Albright,[5] Braunstein,[31] Kleinman,[138] and Pappas[203] have each demonstrated that the displaced labrum and capsular stripping can probably best be documented by arthrotomogram of the shoulder joint. Kilcoyne and Matsen[132] and Kleinman and colleagues[138] used pneumotomography to demonstrate injury to the glenoid labrum and the joint capsule. In 33 cases, they reported good correlation between the tomogram and the surgical findings. Shuman and co-workers[252] used double-contrast CT to study the glenoid labrum with a high degree of accuracy (Fig. 5–16).

---

*See references 136, 137, 175, 176, 198, 217, 218.

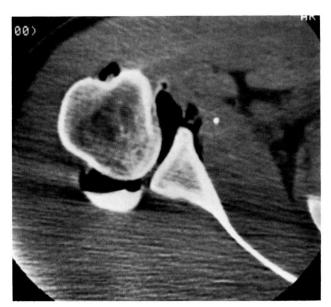

Figure 5–16. CT arthrogram of the left shoulder. Note that the labrum and capsular structures have been stripped away from the anterior glenoid rim and neck of the scapula.

POSTERIOR INSTABILITY

Recommended Views. ■ *The trauma series of x-rays, modified axillary views, or CT scan.*

Techniques to Evaluate Posterior Instability

Although posterior dislocation of the shoulder is a rare problem, i.e., 1 to 3 per cent of all dislocations about the shoulder, it is commonly misdiagnosed.[233] There are two reasons for missing the posterior displacement: first, an inadequate physical examination; and second, an inadequate x-ray examination. All too often only two anteroposterior x-rays are made with the arm in internal and external rotation. X-rays of the injured shoulder must be made in two planes, 90

degrees to each other. The diagnosis of posterior dislocation of the shoulder can always be made if the anteroposterior and one of the previously described lateral views are obtained. Occasionally, the patient will not allow enough abduction to take the true axillary view, in which case the scapulolateral, modified axillary, or the CT scan view must be obtained.

Traumatic posterior glenohumeral instability may be accompanied by damage to either the posterior glenoid rim or impaction fractures on the anteromedial surface of the humeral head, the so-called reverse Hill-Sachs lesion (Fig. 5–17). Lesions of the posterior glenoid rim can usually be noted on the axillary x-ray. The CT scan is very helpful in defining the glenoid rim fracture and in determining the size of the compression fracture of the humeral head.

Fractures of the Shaft of the Clavicle

Recommended Views. ■ *An anteroposterior x-ray, a 30-degree cephalic tilt x-ray, and a 30-degree caudal tilt x-ray.*

These three x-rays are useful for delineating the characteristics of the acute fracture and are even more helpful in following the progress of the fracture toward union. Occasionally, tomograms or CT scans are required to evaluate fracture healing (Fig. 5–18).

Disorders of the Acromioclavicular Joint and Distal Clavicle

Recommended Views. ■ *An anteroposterior view in plane of thorax, a 10-degree cephalic tilt of the acromioclavicular joint, and an axillary lateral. The true scapulolateral and stress views may be required; bone scan or CT scan may be required for special problems.*

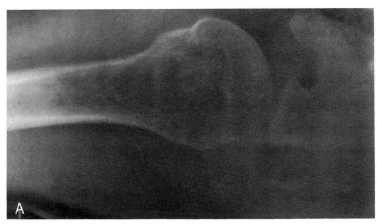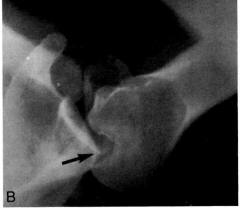

Figure 5–17. *A,* An axillary lateral view of a normal left shoulder shows the normal articulation of the humeral head with the glenoid fossa and the normal relationship of the humeral head to the coracoid process and the acromion process. *B,* The axillary lateral view of the injured right shoulder shows a large anteromedial compression fracture of the humeral head, the so-called reverse Hill-Sachs sign. The arrow indicates the posterior glenoid rim that has produced the hatchet-like defect in the humeral head. (Reproduced with permission from Rockwood CA, and Green DP (eds): Fractures (3 vols), 2nd ed. Philadelphia: JB Lippincott, 1984.)

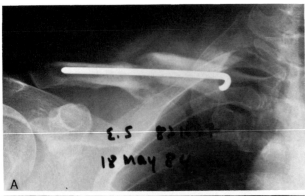

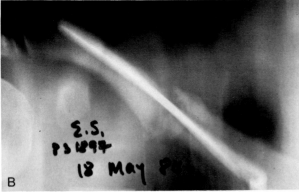

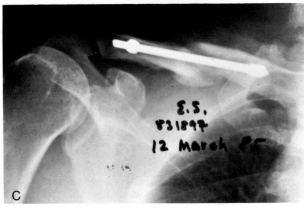

Figure 5–18. Nonunion of fracture of the right clavicle documented on tomogram. *A,* With the Rush pin in place, there appeared to be movement of the fractured right clavicle. *B,* A tomogram confirms the nonunion. *C,* A cephalic tilt x-ray eight months later confirms fracture healing.

Techniques to Evaluate the Acromioclavicular Joint and the Distal Clavicle

Reduced Voltage. The x-ray technician should specifically be requested to take films of the acromioclavicular joint and not of the "shoulder," because the technique used for the glenohumeral joint will produce a dark, overexposed x-ray of the acromioclavicular joint, which may mask traumatic or degenerative changes (Fig. 5–19*A*). The acromioclavicular joint can be clearly visualized by using 50 per cent of the x-ray voltage used in exposing an anteroposterior x-ray of the glenohumeral joint (Fig. 5–19*B*).

The Zanca View.[277] Sometimes fractures about the distal clavicle or the acromion, osteolysis of the distal clavicle, or arthritis of the acromioclavicular joint are obscured on routine anteroposterior x-rays of the joint, because the inferior portion of the distal clavicle is obscured by the overlapping shadow of the spine of the scapula. To obtain the clearest unobstructed view of the acromioclavicular joint and distal clavicle, Zanca has recommended that the x-ray beam be aimed at the acromioclavicular joint with a 10-degree cephalic tilt (Figs. 5–19*C* and 5–20*A* to *D*).

Occasionally, none of the routine x-rays will clearly delineate the extent of the pathology in this region, and tomograms, CT scan, or bone scan may be required.

The Anteroposterior Views. If the patient has an injured shoulder, it is important to compare the x-rays of the injured acromioclavicular joint with those of the normal shoulder. The x-ray may be taken with the patient either standing or sitting with the arms hanging free. If the patient is small, both shoulders may be exposed on a single horizontal 14″ × 17″ x-ray cassette, but for most adults, it is better to use separate 10″ × 12″ cassettes for each shoulder. To interpret injuries to the acromioclavicular joint, the appearance of the acromioclavicular joint and the coracoclavicular distance in the injured shoulder are compared with those seen in the normal shoulder[233] (Fig. 5–21).

It is important to determine the degree of injury to the acromioclavicular and coracoclavicular ligament. If the acromioclavicular and the coracoclavicular ligaments are both disrupted, there may be an indication for surgical correction. A full description of the various degrees of injury to these ligaments, Types I to VI, is described in Chapter 12.

The Anteroposterior Stress View. If the original x-rays of a patient with an injury to the acromioclavicular joint demonstrate a complete acromioclavicular dislocation, i.e., Types III, IV, V, or VI, stress x-rays are not required. If there is clinical suspicion of a complete dislocation of the joint, stress views of both shoulders should be taken. With the patient erect, 10 to 20 pounds of weight, depending on the size of the patient, are *strapped* around the patient's wrists while x-rays are taken of both shoulders[233] (Fig. 5–22). The patient should not grip the weights in the hands, because the muscle contractions can produce a false negative x-ray. If the stress x-rays demonstrate that the coracoclavicular distance is the same in both shoulders or has a difference of less than 25 per cent, a Type III or greater injury can be ruled out.

The Axillary Lateral View. With the arm abducted 70 to 90 degrees, the cassette should be placed superior to the shoulder and the x-ray tube placed inferior to the axilla. Obtaining this view is consistent with the basic principle of obtaining at least two x-ray views at 90 degrees to one another in evaluating musculoskeletal trauma. This view may reveal small intra-articular fractures not visualized on the anteroposterior x-ray, which indicates a worse prognosis.[189, 213] This view will also demonstrate anterior or posterior (as is seen in Type IV injuries) displacement of the clavicle and the degree of displacement of fractures of the distal clavicle.

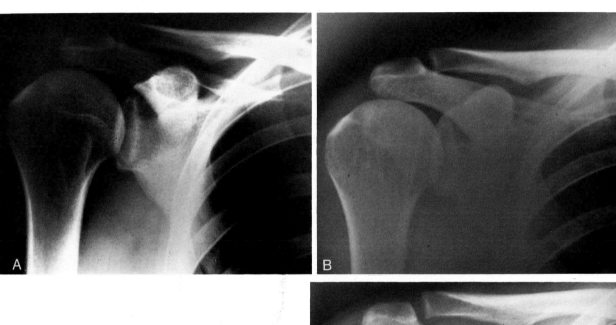

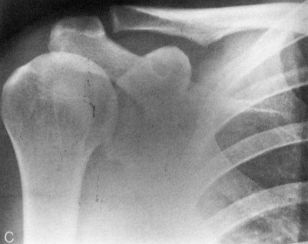

Figure 5–19. Routine x-rays of the shoulder often produce a poorly visualized acromioclavicular joint. *A,* A routine anteroposterior view of the shoulder demonstrates good visualization of the glenohumeral joint. However, the acromioclavicular joint is overpenetrated by the x-ray technique. *B,* When the exposure is decreased by 50 per cent, the acromioclavicular joint is much better visualized. However, the inferior aspect of the acromioclavicular joint is superimposed on the spine of the scapula. *C,* Using the Zanca view, tipping the tube 10 to 15 degrees superiorly provides a clear view of the glenohumeral joint. (Reproduced with permission from Rockwood CA, and Green DP (eds): Fractures (3 vols), 2nd ed. Philadelphia: JB Lippincott, 1984.)

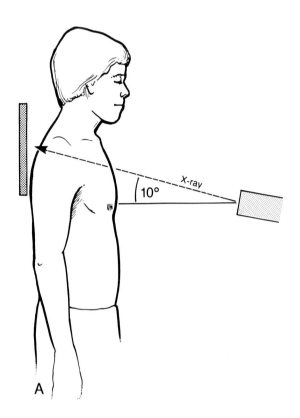

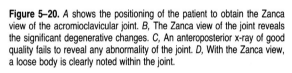

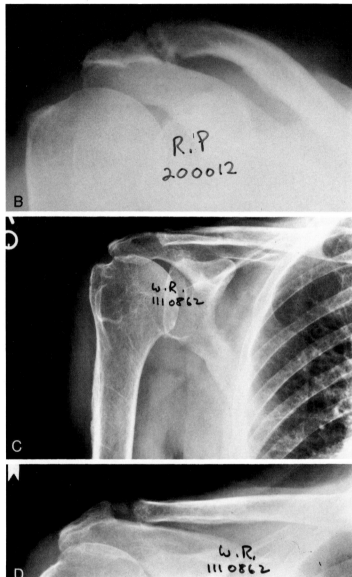

Figure 5–20. *A* shows the positioning of the patient to obtain the Zanca view of the acromioclavicular joint. *B,* The Zanca view of the joint reveals the significant degenerative changes. *C,* An anteroposterior x-ray of good quality fails to reveal any abnormality of the joint. *D,* With the Zanca view, a loose body is clearly noted within the joint.

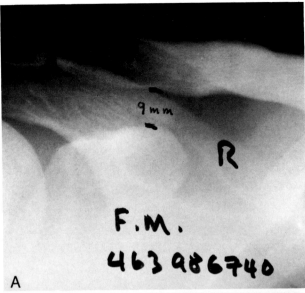

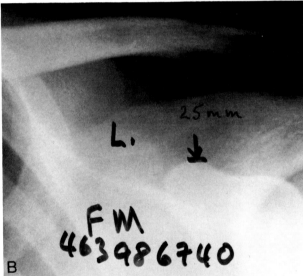

Figure 5–21. Comparison of the coracoclavicular interspace in the injured and in the normal shoulder. *A*, In the normal shoulder, the distance between the top of the coracoid and the bottom of the clavicle is 9.0 mm. *B*, In the injured shoulder, the distance between the top of the coracoid and the bottom of the clavicle is 25.0 mm, demonstrating a disruption of not only the acromioclavicular but the coracoclavicular ligament.

The Alexander View. Alexander[6, 269] described a modification of the true scapulolateral view which he found useful in evaluating injuries to the acromioclavicular joint. This is a supplemental view to demonstrate the posterior displacement of the clavicle that occurs with acromioclavicular injuries. The position of the cassette and the x-ray beam is essentially the same as for the true scapulolateral x-ray. With the patient standing or sitting, the shoulders are shrugged forward while the true scapulolateral x-ray is taken (Fig. 5–23). If there is no injury to the acromioclavicular ligament, there will be no displacement or overlap of the distal clavicle and the acromion. However, with acromioclavicular ligament disruption, the distal clav-

icle will be superiorly displaced and overlapped with the acromion.

Tomogram or CT Scan. Occasionally, none of the routine x-rays will clearly delineate the extent of the pathology of the distal clavicle or the acromioclavicular joint, and tomograms or a CT scan may be required.

Bone Scan. A bone scan will detect early evidence of degenerative arthritis, infections, and traumatic osteolysis of the distal clavicle before routine x-ray changes are noted.[255, 256, 262]

Disorders of the Sternoclavicular Joint and Medial Clavicle

Recommended Views. ■ *The anteroposterior view with a 40-degree cephalic tilt view of both clavicles, tomogram, or CT scan.*

Although some authors in the past have reported that injury of the sternoclavicular joint is purely a

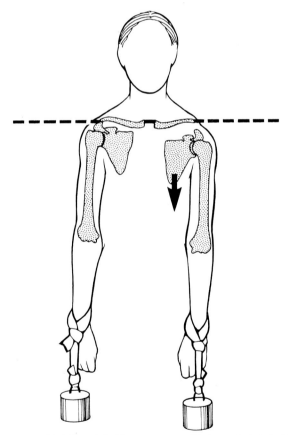

Figure 5–22. Technique of obtaining stress x-rays of both acromioclavicular joints with 10 to 15 pounds of weight hanging from the patient's wrists. The distance between the superior aspect of the coracoid and the undersurface of the clavicle is measured to determine whether or not the coracoclavicular ligaments have been disrupted. One large, horizontally placed 14-×17-inch cassette can be used in smaller patients to visualize both shoulders. In large patients, however, it is better to use two horizontally placed smaller cassettes and to take two separate x-rays for the measurements. In disruption of the coracoclavicular ligaments, note that the shoulder is displaced downward rather than the clavicle displaced upward.

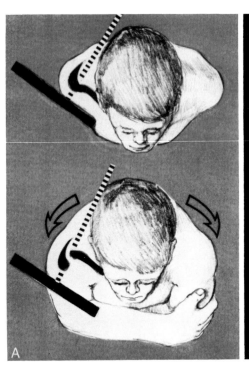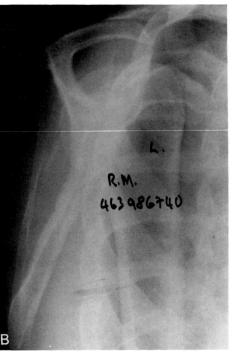

Figure 5–23. Technique of obtaining the Alexander or scapulo-lateral view of the acromioclavicular joint. A, A schematic drawing illustrates how the shoulders are thrust forward at the time the x-ray is taken. (Reproduced with permission from Rockwood CA, and Green DP (eds): Fractures (3 vols), 2nd ed. Philadelphia: JB Lippincott, 1984.) B, With the left shoulder thrust forward, note the gross displacement of the acromioclavicular joint. The clavicle is superior and posterior to the acromion.

clinical diagnosis, appropriate use of x-rays is a critical part of the work-up of this problem. Without x-rays, even the most experienced clinicians will occasionally misdiagnose injuries to the sternoclavicular joint. One cannot rely only on the clinical findings to make the proper diagnosis, because severe anterior swelling about the sternoclavicular joint, which clinically appears to be the benign anterior sternoclavicular dislocation, can be either a fracture of the medial clavicle or the very serious and dangerous posterior dislocation of the sternoclavicular joint.

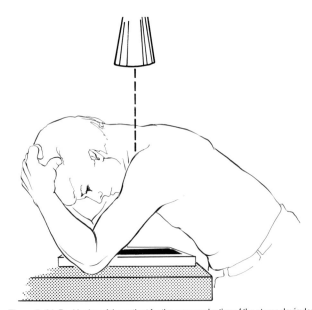

Figure 5–24. Positioning of the patient for the x-ray evaluation of the sternoclavicular joint, as recommended by Hobbs. (Modified from the work of Hobbs DW: Sternoclavicular joint, a new axial radiographic view. Radiology 90:801, 1968. Reproduced with permission from Rockwood CA, and Green DP (eds): Fractures (3 vols), 2nd ed. Philadelphia: JB Lippincott, 1984.)

Occasionally, routine anteroposterior or posteroanterior chest x-rays demonstrate asymmetry between the sternoclavicular joints, which suggests a dislocation or a fracture of the medial clavicle. The ideal view for studying this joint would be a view taken at 90 degrees to the anteroposterior lane. However, because of our anatomy, it is impossible to take a true 90-degree cephalic-to-caudal view. A lateral x-ray of the chest is difficult to interpret because of the density of the chest and the overlap of the medial ends of the clavicles with the first rib and the sternum. As a result, numerous special projections have been devised by Hobbs,[109] Kattan,[123] Kurzbauer,[144] Ritvo,[232] and Rockwood[233] (Fig. 5–24). Although most of these views are very helpful, tomograms and the CT scan offer the best information for evaluating fractures of the medial clavicle and injuries to the sternoclavicular joint. The serendipity view, i.e., a 40-degree cephalic tilt view described in 1972, is easy to obtain and is reliable for demonstrating anterior and posterior subluxations and dislocations of the sternoclavicular joint and some fractures of the medial clavicle.[233]

Techniques to Evaluate the Sternoclavicular Joint and Medial Clavicle

The Serendipity View (40-degree Cephalic Tilt View).[233] When CT scans and tomograms are not available, this view can be very helpful in determining the type of injury to the region of the sternoclavicular joint. It will certainly distinguish between the benign anterior dislocation and the dangerous posterior dislocation. The patient is positioned supine on the x-ray table with a nongrid 11″ × 14″ cassette placed under the patient's upper chest, shoulders, and neck. The

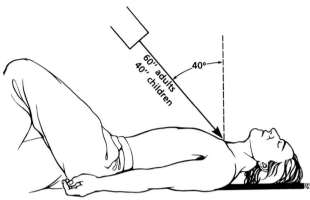

Figure 5–25. Positioning of the patient to take the "serendipity" cephalic tilt x-ray of the sternoclavicular joint. The x-ray tube is tilted 40 degrees from the vertical position and aimed directly at the manubrium. The cassette is large enough to receive the projected images of the medial halves of both clavicles. In children, the tube distance should be approximately 40 inches; in the thicker-chested adult, the distance should be 60 inches.

x-ray beam is angled 40 degrees off the vertical and is centered directly at the sternum (Fig. 5–25). The distance from the tube of the x-ray cassette is 60 inches in adults and 40 inches in children. Voltage should be the same as for an anteroposterior chest x-ray. The x-ray beam is adjusted so that it will project *both* clavicles onto the film.

To interpret this x-ray, one compares the relationship of the medial ends of the injured clavicle with the other normal clavicle. In a normal shoulder, both clavicles will be on the same horizontal plane (Fig. 5–26A). In a posterior sternoclavicular joint, the medial end of the involved dislocated clavicle will appear more inferior on the x-ray than the medial end of the normal clavicle (Fig. 5–26C). In an anterior dislocation, the injured clavicle will be more superior than the normal clavicle (Fig. 5–26B). Fractures of the medial clavicle can also be noted on this view.

Figure 5–26. Interpretation of the cephalic tilt "serendipity" view of the sternoclavicular joint. *A,* In the normal person, both clavicles appear on the same imaginary line drawn through them. *B,* In a patient with anterior dislocation of the right sternoclavicular joint, the medial end of the right clavicle is projected above an imaginary line drawn through the level of the normal left clavicle. *C,* If the patient has a posterior dislocation of the right sternoclavicular joint, the medial end of the right clavicle is displaced below the imaginary line drawn through the normal left clavicle. (Reproduced with permission from Rockwood CA, and Green DP (eds): Fractures (3 vols), 2nd ed. Philadelphia: JB Lippincott, 1984.)

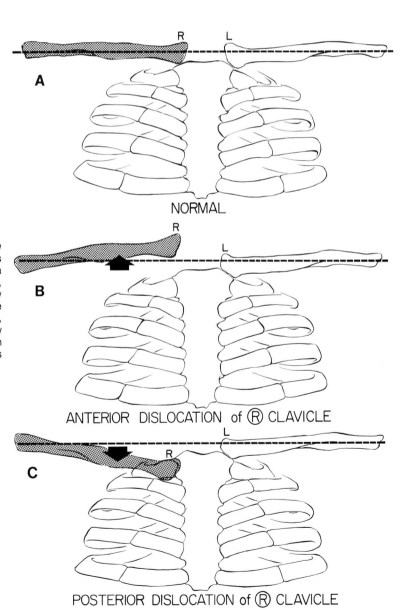

NORMAL

ANTERIOR DISLOCATION of Ⓡ CLAVICLE

POSTERIOR DISLOCATION of Ⓡ CLAVICLE

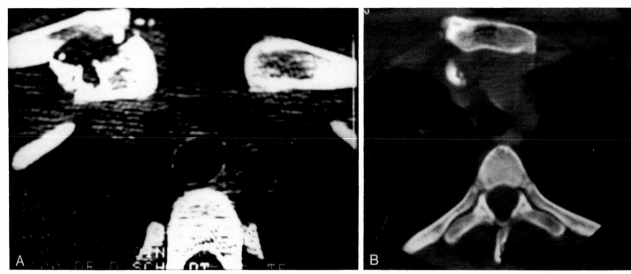

Figure 5–27. *A,* A CT scan clearly demonstrates a fracture of the medial left clavicle. *B,* A CT scan demonstrates a posterior fracture dislocation of the left sternoclavicular joint.

Tomogram and CT Scan. Tomograms are very helpful in delineating fractures of the medial clavicle,[4] in distinguishing fractures from dislocations, and in detecting arthritic problems of the sternoclavicular joint. CT scans are very valuable in demonstrating sternoclavicular subluxations, dislocations, fractures extending into the sternoclavicular joint, fractures of the medial clavicle, and arthritis of this joint.[72, 155, 164, 233] (Fig. 5–27A). In irreducible posterior dislocations, CT scans, especially if enhanced with vascular studies, accurately document the intimate juxtaposition of the displaced medial end of the clavicle to the great vessels of the mediastinum. This is an invaluable preoperative study (Fig. 5–27B).

The Bone Scan. Bone scans are helpful in detecting degenerative changes, inflammatory problems, and tumors of the sternoclavicular joint.

Evaluation of the Impingement Syndrome and the Rotator Cuff

Recommended Views. ■ *An anteroposterior, a 30-degree caudal tilt, or the scapular outlet view. An arthrogram, arthro CT scan, ultrasonography, or MRI may be used to evaluate the integrity of the rotator cuff.*

The impingement syndrome is one of the most frequent causes of pain and disability in the adult shoulder. It begins with soft tissue compromise involving the subacromial bursa and the rotator cuff, and x-rays are usually normal. As the impingement problem persists and progresses, a spur off of the anteroinferior acromion may be noted, ossification in the coracoacromial ligament may be noted,[186] or an unusual shape to the acromion may be present.[20]

Techniques to Evaluate the Impingement Syndrome

The Anteroposterior Views. Anteroposterior x-rays of the glenohumeral joint with the arm in internal and external rotation may reveal associated calcific tendinitis in the tendons of the cuff and superior migration of the humeral head under the acromion. Cystic and sclerotic changes may be noted in the greater tuberosity. Degenerative changes may also be seen in the acromioclavicular joint. Sclerotic changes secondary to anterior proliferation of the acromion may also be noted in the anterior acromion. Narrowing of the acromiohumeral interval has been frequently noted.

The 30-Degree Caudal Tilt View. Routine anteroposterior shoulder x-rays usually do not demonstrate spurs from the acromion, calcification in the coracoacromial ligament, or anteroinferior proliferation of the acromion. However, with the patient in the erect position, an anteroposterior x-ray of the shoulder taken with a 30-degree caudal tilt will adequately demonstrate the anterior acromial spur or ossification in the coracoacromial ligament (Fig. 5–28). The anteroinferior subacromial spurs can be noted on the x-rays of patients with either impingement syndrome or rotator cuff problems. The senior author (C.A.R.) has used this technique to define the spur since 1979, and has found that this view is easier to accomplish and more reliable to demonstrate spurring of the anterior acromion than the scapular outlet view (Fig. 5–29).

The Scapular Outlet View. The patient is positioned for the true scapulolateral x-ray, and the tube is angled caudally 5 to 10 degrees. This x-ray offers a view of the outlet of the supraspinatus tendon unit as it passes under the coracoacromial arch. Deformities of the anteroinferior acromion or in the acromioclavicular arch down into the outlet can be noted on this view (Fig. 5–29D). Bigliani and Morrison have identified three distinct acromial shapes on this radiologic view:

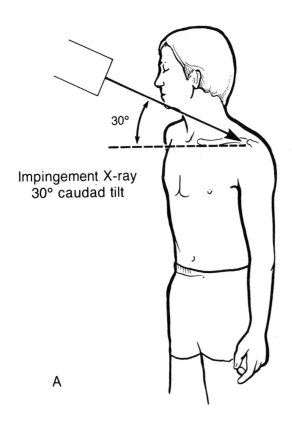

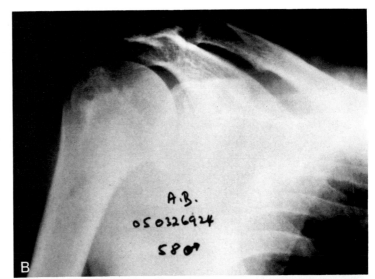

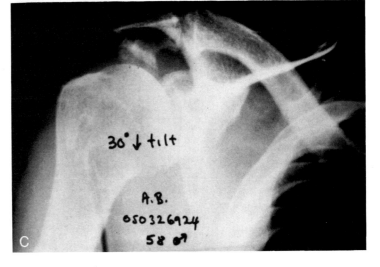

Figure 5–28. *A,* Positioning of the patient and the x-ray tube to demonstrate spurring and/or proliferation of the anteroinferior acromion, which is associated with the impingement syndrome and lesions of the rotator cuff. The patient should be erect for this evaluation. *B,* An anteroposterior x-ray of a 58-year-old patient with an impingement syndrome. The acromion does not appear to be abnormal. *C,* However, when the anteroposterior x-ray is taken with a 30-degree caudal tilt of the x-ray tube, the large, prominent, irregular spurring of the anterior acromion is easily noted.

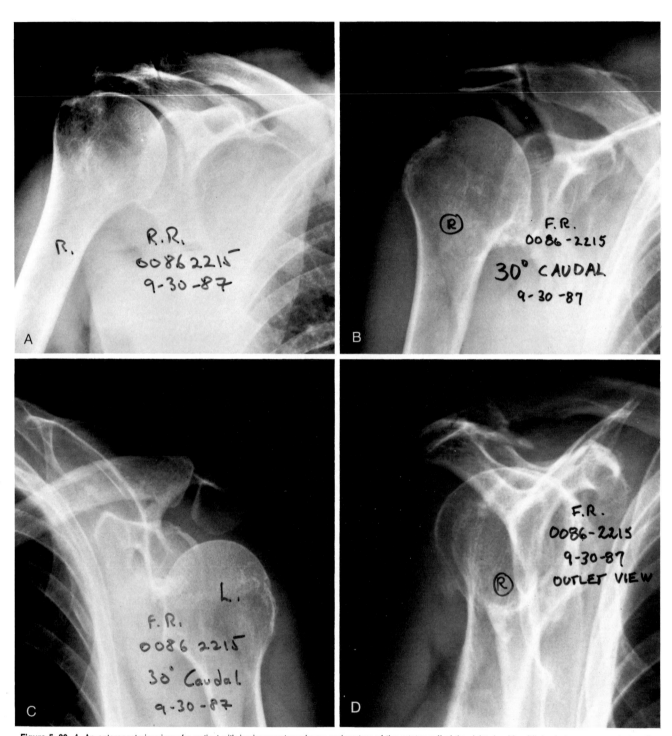

Figure 5–29. *A*, An anteroposterior view of a patient with impingement syndrome and rupture of the rotator cuff of the right shoulder. Minimal changes are noted on the anterior acromion. *B*, On the 30-degree caudal tilt view, note the large, irregularly shaped spike of bone that extends down the coracoacromial ligament into the bursa and the cuff. *C*, A 30-degree caudal tilt x-ray of the normal shoulder shows the normal relationship of the anterior acromion to the distal end of the clavicle. *D*, The scapular outlet view does reveal the spur, but there is considerable overlap with other structures.

Type I, a flat acromion; Type II, a curved acromion; and Type III, an anterior downward hook on the acromion.[20] They believe that this information may be useful in patients at risk for the impingement syndrome or rotator cuff disease.

Arthrography, Arthrotomograms, and Arthro CT Scan. The shoulder arthrogram, either single with just radiopaque material or double-contrast using air and contrast material, is extremely accurate in diagnosing full thickness tears. Deep surface partial thickness cuff tears are not always demonstrated. The presence of dye in the subacromial-subdeltoid bursa, which has escaped from the glenohumeral joint, is conclusive evidence of a defect in the rotator cuff (Fig. 5–30). The accuracy of the arthrogram is between 95 and 100 per cent. Goldman and Ghelman favor double-contrast studies, i.e., air and contrast media.[94] Although double-contrast studies may offer more information about the size of a given tear, neither technique is considered more sensitive than the other for detecting tears. Hall and colleagues[101] have demonstrated less patient discomfort following the arthrogram by using the water-soluble metrizamide contrast medium.

Combining the arthrogram with tomography or CT scans may be of help in defining the size of the defect in the rotator cuff.[132, 226, 275]

Subacromial Bursography. This has been reported by Lie and Mast,[159] Mikasa,[183] and Strizak and co-workers[260] in 1982. Strizak and co-workers studied the technique in cadavers and in patients. They reported the normal bursae would accept 5 to 10 ml of contrast medium and that patients with the impingement syndrome with thickened walls of the subacromial deltoid bursae would accept only 1 to 2 ml of medium.

Ultrasonography. Reliable demonstration of full thickness rotator cuff tears using an ultrasound scanner has been reported in the range of 92 to 95 per cent.[52, 110, 160, 169, 179, 180] In some centers, it has virtually replaced

arthrography for cuff evaluation. It is reported to be safe, rapid, noninvasive, and inexpensive and has the advantage of imaging and comparing both shoulders. The accuracy of sonographic evaluations of the cuff has increased with the experience of the ultrasonographer and in the improvements in the high resolution, linear array sonographic equipment. The spatial resolution of ultrasound images is not as great as conventional radiographic technique (including arthrography). Therefore, the sonographic examination is a "hands-on" experience, and one may not rely on the recorded images to convey the full diagnostic impact of the study. Pitfalls in the interpretation of shoulder sonograms have been described. It appears that considerable experience is necessary with sonographic technique; the equipment must have very good "near field" spatial resolution; and the anatomy of the rotator cuff must be clearly understood.

Mack and colleagues use a technique that depends upon the absence of motion in the cuff tissue when studied with "real time" ultrasound.[168, 169] Secondary signs of cuff tear, such as thinning of the cuff or abnormal echoes in the cuff, are more difficult to interpret. These latter findings may not represent complete cuff tear but may be due to incomplete tear, edema, recent steroid injection, calcifications in the cuff, surgical scar, or normal tissues in some individuals.

Kilcoyne (personal communication) believes that in order for sonography to offer a useful alternative to arthrography or arthroscopy as a screening procedure, the following criterion should be adhered to: The diagnosis of complete rotator cuff tear depends upon the absence of motion in the cuff tissue when studied sonographically. If the patient continues to have symptoms suggestive of cuff tear, an arthrogram should be performed to determine if a small cuff tear is present, a tear which can be missed by ultrasound. Using this

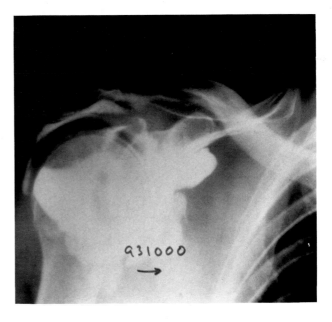

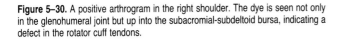

Figure 5–30. A positive arthrogram in the right shoulder. The dye is seen not only in the glenohumeral joint but up into the subacromial-subdeltoid bursa, indicating a defect in the rotator cuff tendons.

criterion, Mack and colleagues found that sonography had a sensitivity of 91 per cent, a specificity of 100 per cent, and an overall accuracy of 94 per cent.[169]

Magnetic Resonance Imaging. MRI offers an alternative, noninvasive technique for investigating lesions of the rotator cuff.* It is experimental, costly, and probably not indicated for patients with a routine cuff problem. It does require a prolonged period of time for the study inside the chamber, which cannot be tolerated by some patients with claustrophobia.

Evaluation of Scapular Injuries

Recommended Views. ■ *A true anteroposterior view of the scapula, a true scapulolateral, and an axillary lateral. Special views such as Stryker notch view, West Point view, tomograms, and CT scan may be required.*

The trauma series of x-rays will usually adequately demonstrate the fractures of the scapular body, spine, and neck. Fractures located elsewhere may require other views for optimal visualization. Glenoid rim fractures, although often visualized on the axillary lateral view of the trauma series, may be better visualized on a West Point or apical oblique view of the glenohumeral joint.[89, 234] Coracoid fractures may be visible on the axillary lateral view but are much better defined on the Stryker notch view[102] (Fig. 5–31). Acromial fractures can be seen on the axillary lateral view but may be difficult to distinguish from an os acromiale.

Finally, in determining the degree of displacement of fractures of the scapula and defining the amount of

_____
*See references 130, 131, 140, 221, 223, 246–248.

displacement in glenoid fractures, the CT scan can be of great value.

Evaluation of Calcific Tendinitis

Calcium deposits in the rotator cuff can be specifically localized in the tendons of the rotator cuff using anteroposterior x-rays of the shoulder in internal and external rotation and an axillary lateral x-ray (Fig. 5–32). More extensive radiographic workup is rarely indicated.

Evaluation of Biceps Tendinitis

Rarely is biceps tendinitis the primary cause of shoulder pain. It is usually secondarily involved as a part of the impingement syndrome or degenerative lesions of the rotator cuff. The anatomy of the groove can be evaluated by the Fisk view.[87, 177] In this view, the x-ray machine is superior to the shoulder. The image of the bicipital groove is projected down onto the cassette, which is held by the patient (Fig. 5–33). Cone, Danzig, Resnick, and Goldman[48] have extensively studied the x-ray anatomy and pathological irregularities of the bicipital groove.

Tumors and Inflammatory Problems

TUMORS

Although routine x-rays usually will define tumor problems, the use of tomograms, CT scans, and MRI

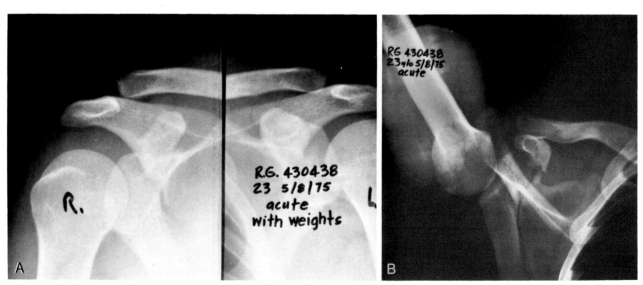

Figure 5–31. *A,* This 23-year-old patient had a traumatic injury to his right acromioclavicular joint. Note the superior displacement of the right clavicle from the acromion as compared with the left; also note that the coracoclavicular distance in both shoulders is approximately the same. The fracture at the base of the coracoid is not well visualized. *B,* The Stryker notch view reveals a fracture through the base of the coracoid.

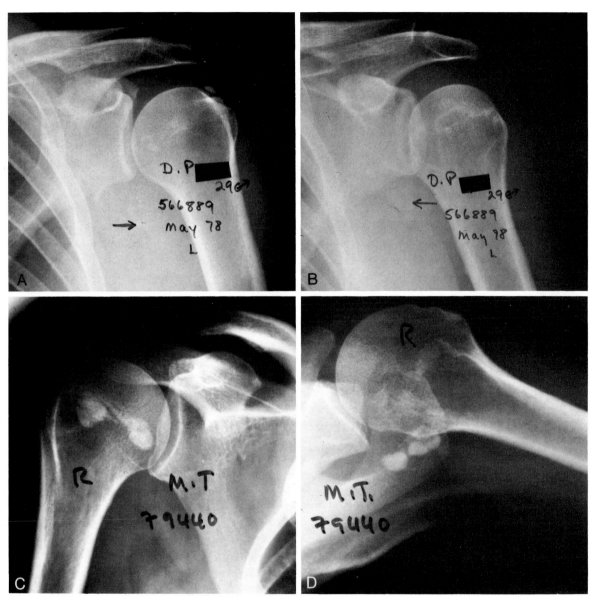

Figure 5–32. Calcific tendinitis of the left shoulder. *A,* With the arm in external rotation, the calcium deposit is visible. *B,* With the arm in internal rotation the calcium deposit is no longer visible, indicating that the calcium must be in the anterior aspect of the supraspinatus tendon. *C,* On the anteroposterior x-ray in internal and external rotation, the calcium deposit cannot be accurately localized. *D,* However, on the axillary view, the calcium deposit is quite distinct and localized either in the infraspinatus tendon or the teres minor tendon.

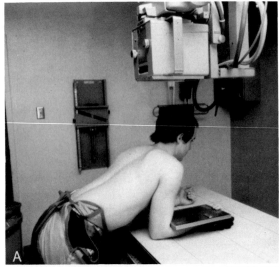

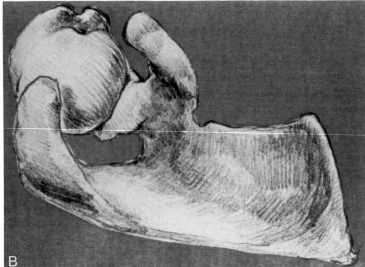

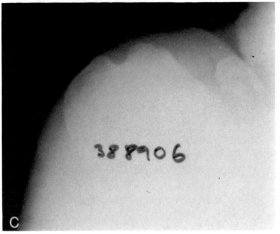

Figure 5–33. *A,* Position of the patient for the Fisk view to visualize the bicipital groove in the proximal humerus. Note that the patient is holding the cassette and leaning forward so that the beam passing down through the bicipital groove will be projected onto the cassette. *B,* Anatomy of the bicipital groove. *C,* Projection of the bicipital groove onto the x-ray film with the Fisk technique. (Modified from the work of Fisk C: Adaptation of the technique for radiography of the bicipital groove. Radiol Technol *37*:47–50, 1965.)

is often mandatory to determine the exact size of the lesion, whether the lesion has broken out of the cortex, and if certain tissue compartments have been violated. Bone scans are also helpful to determine if multiple sites of the skeleton are involved.

INFLAMMATORY PROBLEMS

Bone scans, either for bone or soft tissues, can be very helpful in diagnosing infections and inflammatory problems before they are evident on routine films. The bone scan is also helpful in diagnosing stress fractures before their appearance on routine x-rays. Tomograms, CT scans, and magnetic resonance imaging (MRI) are also helpful.

References

1. Abel MS: Symmetrical anteroposterior projections of the sternoclavicular joints with motion studies. Radiology *132*:757–759, 1979.
2. Adam P, Escude Alberge Y, Labbe JL, Kassab M, et al: Value of standard computed tomography and computed arthrography for the radiologic evaluation of injuries of the shoulder. Ann Radiol *28*(8):629–635, 1985.
3. Adams JC: Recurrent dislocation of the shoulder. J Bone Joint Surg *30B*:26–38, 1948.
4. Adams JC: The humeral head defect in recurrent anterior dislocations of the shoulder. Br J Radiol *23*:151–156, 1950.
5. Albright J, and El Khoury G: Shoulder arthrotomography in the evaluation of the injured throwing arm. *In* Zarins B, Andrews JR, and Carson WG Jr (eds): Injuries to the Throwing Arm. Philadelphia, WB Saunders, 1985, pp 66–75.
6. Alexander OM: Dislocation of the acromio-clavicular joint. Radiography *15*:260, 1949.
7. Alexander OM: Radiography of the acromioclavicular articulation. Med Radiogr Photogr *30*(2):34–39, 1954.
8. Andren L, and Lundbert BJ: Treatment of rigid shoulders by joint distension during arthrography. Acta Orthop Scand *36*:45–53, 1965.
9. Argen RJ, Wilson CH, Jr., and Wood P: Suppurative arthritis: clinical features of 42 cases. Arch Intern Med *117*:661–666, 1966.
10. Armbuster TG, Slivka J, Resnick D, Goergen TG, et al: Extraarticular manifestations of septic arthritis of the glenohumeral joint. AJR *129*:667–672, 1977.
11. Baker EC: Tomography of the sternoclavicular joint. Ohio State Med J *55*:60, 1959.
12. Baker ME, Martinez S, Kier R, and Wain S: High resolution computed tomography of the cadaveric sternoclavicular joint: findings in degenerative joint disease. J Comput Tomogr *12*(1):13–18, 1988.

13. Bankart ASB: Recurrent or habitual dislocation of the shoulder joint. Br Med J 2:1132–1133, 1923.
14. Bankart ASB: The pathology and treatment of recurrent dislocation of the shoulder joint. Br J Surg 26:23–29, 1938.
15. Bateman JE: The Shoulder and Neck, 2nd ed. Philadelphia: WB Saunders, 1978.
16. Beardon JM, Hughston JC, and Whatley GS: Acromioclavicular dislocation: method of treatment. J Sports Med 1:5–17, 1973.
17. Beck A, Papacharalampous X, Grosser G, and Milic S, et al: Importance of transthoracic x-ray in arthrography of the shoulder. Radiologe 28(2):69–72, 1988.
18. Beltran J, Gray LA, Bools JC, Zuelzer W, et al: Rotator cuff lesions of the shoulder: evaluation by direct sagittal CT arthrography. Radiology 160:161–165, 1986.
19. Berman MM, and LeMay M: Dislocation of shoulder: x-ray signs. Letter to the editor. N Engl J Med 283:600, 1970.
20. Bigliani LU, Morrison D, and April EW: The morphology of the acromion and its relationship to rotator cuff tears. Orthop Trans 10:228, 1986.
21. Binz P, Johner R, and Haertel M: Computerized axial tomography in patients with traumatic shoulder dislocation. Helv Chir Acta 49:231–234, 1982.
22. Blackett CW, and Healy TR: Roentgen studies of the shoulder. AJR 37(6):760–766, 1937.
23. Blazina ME, and Satzman JS: Recurrent anterior subluxation of the shoulder in athletics—a distinct entity (proceedings). J Bone Joint Surg 51A(5):1037–1038, 1969.
24. Blazina ME: The modified axillary roentgenogram—a useful adjunct in the diagnosis of recurrent subluxation of the shoulder. Exhibit, U.S. Military Academy, West Point, New York.
25. Bloom MH, and Obata WG: Diagnosis of posterior dislocation of the shoulder with use of Velpeau axillary and angle-up roentgenographic views. J Bone Joint Surg 49A(5):943–949, 1967.
26. Bonavita JA, and Dalinka MK: Shoulder erosions in renal osteodystrophy. Skeletal Radiol 5(2):105–108, 1980.
27. Bongartz G, Muller-Miny H, and Reiser M: Role of computed tomography in the diagnosis of shoulder joint injuries. Radiologe 28(2):73–78, 1988.
28. Bongartz G, and Peters PE: Problems associated with magnetic-resonance imaging of the shoulder (abstr). Z Rheumatol 47(4):300–301, 1988.
29. Bosworth BM: Complete acromioclavicular dislocations. N Engl J Med 241:221–225, 1949.
30. Boulis ZF, and Dick R: The greater tuberosity of the humerus: an area for mis-diagnosis. Australas Radiol 26(3):267–268, 1982.
31. Braunstein EM, and O'Connor G: Double contrast arthrotomography of the shoulder. J Bone Joint Surg 64A:192–195, 1982.
32. Bretzke CA, Crass JR, Craig EV, and Feinberg SB: Ultrasonography of the rotator cuff: normal and pathologic anatomy. Invest Radiol 20:311–315, 1985.
33. Broca A, and Hartman H: Contribution à l'étude des luxations de l'épaule (luxations dites incomplète, décollements périostiques, luxations directes et luxations indirectes). Bull Soc Anat Paris 65:312–336, 1890.
34. Broca A, and Hartman H: Contribution à l'étude des luxations de l'épaule (luxations anciennes, luxations recidivantes). Bull Soc Anat Paris 65:416–423, 1890.
35. Brower AC, and Allman RM: Pathogenesis of the neurotrophic joint: neurotraumatic vs. neurovascular. Radiology 139:349–354, 1981.
36. Caird FM: The shoulder joint in relation to certain dislocations and fractures. Edinburgh Med J 32:708–714, 1887.
37. Callaghan JJ, McNeish LM, Dehaven JP, and Savory CG, et al: A prospective comparison study of double contrast computed tomography (CT), arthrography and arthroscopy of the shoulder. Am J Sports Med 16(1):13–20, 1988.
38. Callaghan JJ, York JJ, McNeish LM, and Gillogly SD: Unusual anomaly of the scapula defined by arthroscopy and computerized tomographic arthrography. J Bone Joint Surg 70A(3):452–453, 1988.
39. Calvert PT, Packer NP, Stoker DJ, Bayley JLL, et al: Arthrography of the shoulder after operative repair of the torn rotator cuff. J Bone Joint Surg 68B(1):147–150, 1986.
40. Castagno AA, Shuman WP, Kilcoyne RF, and Haynor DR, et al: Complex fractures of the proximal humerus: role of CT in treatment. Radiology 165(3):759–762, 1987.
41. Cisternino SJ, Rogers LF, Stufflebam BC, and Kruglik GD: The trough line: a radiographic sign of posterior shoulder dislocation. AJR 130:951–954, 1978.
42. Ciullo JV, Koniuch MP, and Teitge RA: Axillary shoulder roentgenography in clinical orthopaedic practice (abstr). Orthop Trans 6:451, 1982.
43. Ciullo JV: Personal communication on axillary roentgenography exhibit presented at 1982 AAOS meeting.
44. Clark KC: Positioning in Radiography, 8th ed. New York: Grune & Stratton, 1964, p 1.
45. Cleaves EN: A new film holder for roentgen examinations of the shoulder. AJR 45:288–290, 1941.
46. Cockshott P: The coracoclavicular joint. Radiology 131(5):313–316, 1979.
47. Codman EA: The shoulder. Rupture of the supraspinatus tendon and other lesions in or about the subacromial bursa. Boston: Thomas Todd and Company, 1934, pp 18–31, 65–122.
48. Cone RO III, Danzig L, Resnick D, and Goldman AB: The bicipital groove: radiographic, anatomic, and pathologic study. AJR 141:781–788, 1983.
49. Cone RO III, Resnick D, and Danzig L: Shoulder impingement syndrome: radiographic evaluation. Radiology 150:29–33, 1984.
50. Connolly J: X-ray defects in recurrent shoulder dislocations (proceedings). J Bone Joint Surg 51A(6):1235–1236, 1969.
51. Cope R, and Riddervold HO: Posterior dislocation of the sternoclavicular joint: report of two cases, with emphasis on radiologic management and early diagnosis. Skeletal Radiol 17(4):247–50, 1988.
52. Craig EV, Crass JR, and Bretzke CL: Ultrasonography of the rotator cuff: normal anatomy and pathologic variation (abstr). Third Annual Meeting of the American Shoulder and Elbow Surgeons, Boston, November 1–4, 1984.
53. Craig EV: Importance of proper radiography in acute shoulder trauma. Minn Med, 68:109–112, 1985.
54. Cramer M: Resection des Oberarmkopfes Wegen Habitueller Luxation. Berlin Klin Wochenschr 19:21–25, 1882.
55. Crass JR, Craig EV, Thompson RG, and Feinberg SB: Ultrasonography of the rotator cuff: surgical correlation. J Clin Ultrasound 12:487–492, 1984.
56. Crass JR, and Craig EV: Noninvasive imaging of the rotator cuff. Orthopedics 11(1):57–64, 1988.
57. Cyprien JM, Vasey HM, Burdet A, Bonvin JC, et al: Humeral retrotorsion and glenohumeral relationship in the normal shoulder and in recurrent anterior dislocation. Clin Orthop 175:8–17, 1983.
58. Danzig LA, Greenway G, and Resnick D: The Hill-Sachs lesion: an experimental study. Am J Sports Med 8(5):328–332, 1980.
59. Danzig LA, Resnick D, and Greenway G: Evaluation of unstable shoulders by computed tomography. Am J Sports Med 10(3):138–141, 1982.
60. See reference 59.
61. DeAnquin CE, and DeAnquin CA: Comparative study of bone lesions in traumatic recurrent dislocation of the shoulder—their importance and treatment. In Surgery of the Shoulder, 3rd ed. Philadelphia: JB Lippincott, 1984, p 303.
62. DeAnquin CE: Recurrent dislocation of the shoulder—roentgenographic study (proceedings). J Bone Joint Surg 47A(5):1085, 1965.
63. DeHaven JP, Callaghan JJ, McNiesh LM, Savory CG, et al: A prospective comparison study of double contrast CT arthrography and shoulder arthroscopy (abstr). Am Orthop Soc Sports Med, Interim Meeting, January 21, 1987, San Francisco, CA.
64. DePalma AF: Surgery of the Shoulder, 3rd ed. Philadelphia: JB Lippincott, 1983.
65. DeSmet AA, Ting YM, and Weiss JJ: Shoulder arthrography in rheumatoid arthritis. Radiology 116:601–605, 1975.

66. DeSmet AA: Anterior oblique projection in radiography of the traumatized shoulder. AJR 134:515–518, 1980.

67. DeSmet AA: Axillary projection in radiography of the nontraumatized shoulder. AJR 134:511–514, 1980.

68. DeSouza LJ: Shoulder radiography in acute trauma: true anteroposterior and true lateral views make for better reading. Postgrad Med 73(6):234–236, 1983.

69. Deichgraber E, and Olsson B: Soft tissue radiography in painful shoulder. Acta Radiol Diagn 16(4):393–400, 1975.

70. Delgoffe C, Fery A, Regent D, Kurdziel JC, et al: Computed tomography in anterior instability of the shoulder: a review of 23 cases. J Radiol 65(11):737–745, 1984.

71. Demos TC: Radiologic case study: bilateral posterior shoulder dislocations. Orthopedics 3(9):887–897, 1980.

72. Destouet JM, Gilula LA, Murphy WA, and Sagel SS: Computed tomography of the sternoclavicular joint and sternum. Radiology 138:123–128, 1981.

73. Didiee J: Le radiodiagnostic dans la luxation recidivante de l'épaule. J Radiol Electrologie 14(4):209–218, 1930.

74. Ducrest P, and Johner R: Die Bedeutung der Ossaren Lasionen fur die Prognose der Schulterluxation. Z Unfallchir Versicherungsmed Berufskr 77(2):85–89, 1984.

75. Dyson S: Interpreting radiographs 7: radiology of the equine shoulder and elbow. Equine Vet J 18(5):352–361, 1986.

76. Eaton R, and Serletti J: Computerized axial tomography—a method of localizing Steinmann pin migration: a case report. Orthopedics 4(12):1357–1360, 1981.

77. Eden R: Zur Operation der Habituellen Schulterluxation unter Mitteilung eines nuenen Verfahrens bei Abriss am innren Pfannenrande. Dtsch Z Chir 144:269–280, 1918.

78. El-Khoury GY, Albright JP, Yousef MMA, Montgomery WJ, et al: Arthrotomography of the glenoid labrum. Radiology 131:333–337, 1979.

79. Eve FS: A case of subcoracoid dislocation of the humerus with the formation of an indentation on the posterior surface of the head. Medico-Chir Trans Soc (London) 63:317–321, 1880.

80. Faletti C, Clerico P, Indemini E, and Crova M: Standard radiography in "recurrent dislocation of the shoulder." Ital J Sports Med 7(1):33–40, 1985.

81. Fedoseev VA: Method of radiographic study of the sternoclavicular joint. Vestn Rentgenol Radiol 3:88–91, 1977.

82. Feldman F: The radiology of total shoulder prostheses. Semin Roentgenol 21(1):47–65, 1986.

83. Fery A, Lenard A, and Sommelet J: Shoulder radiographic evaluation: radiographic examination of shoulder and scapular girdle trauma. J Radiol 62(4):247–256, 1981.

84. Fery A, and Lenard A: Transsternal sternoclavicular projection: diagnostic value in sternoclavicular dislocations. J Radiol 62(3):167–170, 1981.

85. Fery A, and Sommelet J: Os acromiale. Diagnosis, pathology, and clinical significance. Twenty-eight cases including two fracture-separations. Rev Chir Orthop 74(2):160–72, 1988.

86. Figiel SJ, Figiel LS, Bardenstein MB, and Blodgett WH: Posterior dislocation of the shoulder. Radiology 87:737–740, 1966.

87. Fisk C: Adaptation of the technique for radiography of the bicipital groove. Radiol Technol 37:47–50, 1965.

88. Flinn RM, MacMillan CL Jr., Campbell DR, and Fraser DB: Optimal radiography of the acutely injured shoulder. J Can Assoc Radiol 34(2):128–132, 1983.

89. Garth WP Jr., Slappey CE, and Ochs CW: Roentgenographic demonstration of instability of the shoulder: the apical oblique projection—a technical note. J Bone Joint Surg 66A(9):1450–1453, 1984.

90. Ghelman G, and Goldman AB: The double contrast shoulder arthrogram: evaluation of rotary cuff tears. Radiology 124:251–254, 1979.

91. Glas K, Mayerhofer K, and Obletter N: Roentgenographic representation of the shoulder girdle in recidiving shoulder dislocation. Rontgenpraxis 41(4):116–120, 1988.

92. Golding FC: Radiology and orthopaedic surgery. J Bone Joint Surg 48B(2):320–332, 1966.

93. Golding FC: The shoulder—the forgotten joint. Br J Radiol 35(411):149–158, 1962.

94. Goldman AB, and Ghelman B: The double contrast shoulder arthrogram. Radiology 127:655–663, 1978.

95. Goldstone RA: Dislocation of the shoulder x-ray signs. Letter to the editor. N Engl J Med 283:600, 1970.

96. Gould R, Rosenfield AT, and Friedlaender GE: Case report: loose body within the glenohumeral joint in recurrent anterior dislocation: CT demonstration. J Comput Assist Tomogr 9(2):404–406, 1985.

97. Greenway GD, Danzig LA, Resnick D, and Haghighi P: The painful shoulder. Med Radiog Photog 58(2):22–67, 1982.

98. Griffiths HJ, and Ozer H: Changes in the medial half of the clavicle—new sign in renal osteodystrophy. J Can Assoc Radiol 24:334–336, 1973.

99. Gunson EF: Radiography of the sternoclavicular articulation. Radiog Clin Photog 19(1):20–24, 1943.

100. Gutjahr G, and Weigand H: Conventional radiographic studies of the proximal humerus. Unfallchirurgie 10(6):282–287, 1984.

101. Hall FM, Goldberg RP, Wyshak G, and Kilcoyne RF: Shoulder arthrography: comparison of morbidity after use of various contrast media. Radiology 154:339–341, 1985.

102. Hall RH, Isaac F, and Booth CR: Dislocations of the shoulder with special reference to accompanying small fractures. J Bone Joint Surg 41A(3):489–494, 1959.

103. Hardy DC, Vogler JB III, and White RH: The shoulder impingement syndrome: prevalence of radiographic findings and correlation with response to therapy. AJR 147(3):557–561, 1986.

104. Hermann G, Yeh HC, and Schwartz I: Computed tomography of soft-tissue lesions of the extremities, pelvic and shoulder girdles: sonographic and pathological correlations. Clin Radiol 35:193–202, 1984.

105. Hermodsson I: Rontgenologischen Studien über die traumatischen und habituellen Schultergelenkverrenkungen nach vorn und nach unten. Acta Radiol 20:1–173, 1934.

106. Hess F, and Schnepper E: Success and long-term results of radiotherapy for humeroscapular periarthritis. Radiologe 28(2):84–86, 1988.

107. Hill HA, and Sachs MD: The grooved defect of the humeral head: a frequently unrecognized complication of dislocations of the shoulder joint. Radiology 35:690–700, 1940.

108. Hill JA, and Tkach L: A study of glenohumeral orientation in patients with anterior recurrent shoulder dislocations using computerized axial tomography (abstr). AAOS Shoulder Meeting, Las Vegas, Nevada, January 1985.

109. Hobbs DW: Sternoclavicular joint: a new axial radiographic view. Radiology 90:801–802, 1968.

110. Hodler J, Fretz CJ, Terrier F, and Gerber C: Rotator cuff tears: correlation of sonographic and surgical findings. Radiology 169:791–794, 1988.

111. Horsfield D, and Jones SN: A useful projection in radiography of the shoulder. J Bone Joint Surg 69B(2):338, 1987.

112. Horsfield D, and Renton P: The other view in the radiography of shoulder trauma. Radiography 46(549):213–214, 1980.

113. Huber DJ, Sauter R, Mueller E, Requardt H, et al: MR Imaging of the Normal Shoulder. Radiology 158:405–408, 1986.

114. Hybbinette S: De la transplantation d'un fragment osseux pour remédier aux luxations récidivantes de l'épaule; constatations et résultats opératories. Acta Chir Scand 71:411–445, 1932.

115. Jelbert M: A pilot study of the incidence and distribution of certain skeletal and soft tissue abnormalities. Cent Afr J Med 16(2):37–40, 1970.

116. Johner R, Binz P, and Staubli HU: New diagnostic, therapeutic and prognostic aspects of shoulder dislocation. Schweiz Z Sportmed 30(2):48–52, 1982.

117. Johner R, and Burch HB: Radiologische Diagnostik bei Schulterluxation en. Internationales Symposium Uber Spezielle Fragen der Orthopadischen Chirurgie, 1984.

118. Johner R, Burch HB, Staubli HU, and Noesberger B: Radiologisches Vorgehen bei der Schulterluxation. Z Unfallchir Versicherungsmed Berufskr 77(2):79–84, 1984.

119. Johner R, Ducrest P, Staubli HU, and Burch HB: Begleitfrakturen und Prognose der Schulterluxation im Alter. Z Unfallchir Versicherungsmed Berufskr 76(4):189–193, 1983.

120. Johner R, Joz-Roland P, and Burch HB: Anterior luxation of

the shoulder: new diagnostic and therapeutic aspects. Rev Med Suisse Romande *102*(12):1143–1150, 1982.

121. Jonsson G: A method of obtaining structural pictures of the sternum. Acta Radiol *18*:336–340, 1937.

122. Kalliomaki, Viitanen SM, and Virtama P: Radiological findings of sternoclavicular joints in rheumatoid arthritis. Acta Rheum Scand *14*:233–240, 1968.

123. Kattan KR: Modified view for use in roentgen examination of the sternoclavicular joints. Radiology *108*:8, 1973.

124. Katz GA, Peter JB, Pearson CM, and Adams WS: The shoulder-pad—a diagnostic feature of amyloid arthropathy. N Engl J Med *288*(7):354–355, 1973.

125. Keats TE, and Pope TL Jr: The acromioclavicular joint: normal variation and the diagnosis of dislocation. Skeletal Radiol *17*(3):159–162, 1988.

126. Keats TE: The emergency x-ray. Emergency Medicine *19*(13):175–176, 1987.

127. Khizhko II: Supplemental (axial) roentgenography of the clavicle with patient in a sitting position. Ortop Travmatol Protez *9*:8–10, 1984.

128. Kieft GJ, Bloem JL, Obermann WR, Verbout AJ, et al: Normal shoulder: MR imaging. Radiology *159*:741–745, 1986.

129. Kieft GJ, Bloem JL, Rozing PM, and Obermann WR: Rotator cuff impingement syndrome: MR imaging. Radiology *166*(1):211–214, 1988.

130. Kieft GJ, Bloem JL, Rozing PM, and Obermann WR: MR imaging of recurrent anterior dislocation of the shoulder: comparison with CT arthrography. AJR *150*(5):1083–7, 1988.

131. Kieft GJ, Sartoris DJ, Bloem JL, Hajek PC, et al: Magnetic resonance imaging of glenohumeral joint diseases. Skeletal Radiol *16*:285–290, 1987.

132. Kilcoyne RF, and Matsen FA III: Rotator cuff tear measurement by arthropneumotomography. AJR *140*:315–318, 1983.

133. Killoran PJ, Marcove RC, and Freiberger RH: Shoulder arthrography. AJR *103*:658–668, 1968.

134. Kimberlin GE: Radiography of injuries to the region of the shoulder girdle: revisited. Radiol Technol *46*(2):69–83, 1974.

135. King JM Jr, and Holmes GW: A review of four hundred and fifty roentgen-ray examinations of the shoulder. AJR *17*(2):214–218, 1927.

136. Kinnard P, Gordon D, Levesque RY, and Bergeron D: Computerized arthrotomography in recurring shoulder dislocations and subluxations. Can J Surg *27*(5):487–488, 1984.

137. Kinnard P, Tricoir JL, Levesque RY, and Bergeron D: Assessment of the unstable shoulder by computed arthrography: a preliminary report. Am J Sports Med *11*(3):157–159, 1983.

138. Kleinman PK, Kanzaria PK, Goss TP, and Pappas AM: Axillary arthrotomography of the glenoid labrum. AJR *141*:993–999, 1984.

139. Kneeland JB, Carrera GF, Middleton WD, Campagna NF, et al: Rotator cuff tears: preliminary application of high-resolution MR imaging with counter rotating current loop-gap resonators. Radiology *160*(3):695–699, 1986.

140. Kneeland JB, Middleton WD, Carrera GF, Zeuge RC, et al: MR imaging of the shoulder: diagnosis of rotator cuff tears. AJR *149*(2):333–337, 1987.

141. Kornguth PJ, and Salazar AM: The apical oblique view of the shoulder: its usefulness in acute trauma. AJR *149*:113–116, 1987.

142. Kotzen LM: Roentgen diagnosis of rotator cuff tear: report of 48 surgically proven cases. AJR *112*:507–511, 1971.

143. Kuhlman JE, Fishman ED, Ney DR, and Magid D: Complex shoulder trauma: three dimensional CT imaging. Orthopedics *11*(11):1561–1563, 1988.

144. Kurzbauer R: The lateral projection in roentgenography of the sternoclavicular articulation. AJR *56*:104–105, 1946.

145. Kuster E: Ueber Habituelle Schulterluxation. Vehr Dtsch Ges Chir 1 *1*:112–114, 1882.

146. Lahde S, and Putkonen M: Positioning of the painful patient for the axial view of the glenohumeral joint. Rontgenblatter *38*:380–382, 1985.

147. Laing PG: The arterial supply of the adult humerus. J Bone Joint Surg *38A*:1105–1116, 1956.

148. Lams PM, and Jolles H: The scapula companion shadow. Radiology *138*(1):19–23, 1981.

149. Larde D, Benazet JP, Benameur Ch, and Ferrane J: Value of the Transscapular view in radiology of shoulder trauma. J Radiol *62*(4):227–282, 1981.

150. Larde D: Radiological Exploration of the Shoulder. Rev Prat *34*(53):2957–2969, 1984.

151. Laumann U: Disorders of the shoulder from the orthopedic point of view. Radiologe *28*(2):49–53, 1988.

152. Lawrence WS: A method of obtaining an accurate lateral roentgenogram of the shoulder joint. AJR *5*:193–194, 1918.

153. Lawrence WS: New position in radiographing the shoulder joint. AJR *2*:728–730, 1915.

154. Levine AH, Pais MJ, and Schwarts EE: Posttraumatic osteolysis of the distal clavicle with emphasis on early radiologic changes. AJR *127*:781–784, 1976.

155. Levinsohn EM, Bunnell WP, and Yuan HA: Computed tomography in the diagnosis of dislocations of the sternoclavicular joint. Clin Orthop *140*:12–16, 1979.

156. Levy M, Goldberg I, Fischel RE, Frisch E, et al: Friedrich's disease: aseptic necrosis of the sternal end of the clavicle. J Bone Joint Surg *63B*(4):539–541, 1981.

157. Liberson F: Os acromiale—contested anomaly. J Bone Joint Surg *19*:683–689, 1937.

158. Liberson F: The value and limitation of the oblique view as compared with the ordinary anteroposterior exposure of the shoulder. AJR *37*:498–509, 1937.

159. Lie S, and Mast WA: Subacromial bursography. Radiology *144*:626–630, 1982.

160. Lind T, Reinmann I, Karstrup S, and Larsen JK: Ultrasonography in the evaluation of injuries to the shoulder region (abstr). Acta Orthop Scand *58*(3):328, 1987.

161. Lindblom K: Arthrography and roentgenography in ruptures of the tendons of the shoulder joint. Acta Radiol *20*:548–562, 1939.

162. Lippmann RK: Frozen shoulder; periarthritis; bicipital tenosynovitis. Arch Surg *47*:283–296, 1943.

163. Lippmann RK: Observations concerning the calcific cuff deposit. Clin Orthop *20*:49–59, 1961.

164. Lourie JA: Tomography in the diagnosis of posterior dislocations of the sternoclavicular joint. Acta Orthop Scand *51*:579–580, 1980.

165. Lower RF, McNiesh LM, and Callaghan JJ: Computed tomographic documentation of intra-articular penetration of a screw after operations on the shoulder. J Bone Joint Surg *67A*(7):1120–1122, 1985.

166. Lusted LB, and Miller ER: Progress in indirect cineroentgenography. AJR *75*:56–62, 1956.

167. Macdonald W, Thrum CB, and Hamilton SGL: Designing an implant by CT scanning and solid modelling. J Bone Joint Surg *68B*(2):208–212, 1986.

168. Mack LA, Gannon MK, Kilcoyne RF, and Matsen FA III: Sonographic evaluation of the rotator cuff: accuracy in patients without prior surgery. Clin Orthop *234*:21–27, 1988.

169. Mack LA, Matsen FA III, Kilcoyne RF, Davies PK, et al: Ultrasonographic (US) evaluation of the rotator cuff. Radiology *157*:205–209, 1985.

170. Madler M, Mayr B, Baierl P, Klein C, et al: Value of conventional x-ray diagnosis and computerized tomography in the detection of Hill-Sachs defects and bony Bankart lesions in recurrent shoulder dislocations. ROFO *148*(4):384–389, 1988.

171. Maki NJ: Cineradiographic studies with shoulder instabilities. Am J Sports Med *16*(4):362–364, 1988.

172. Malgaigne JF: Traite des fractures et des luxations. Philadelphia: JB Lippincott Company, 1859.

173. Matsen FA III: Shoulder roentgenography. AAOS Summer Institute, 1980.

174. McLaughlin HL: Posterior dislocation of the shoulder. J Bone Joint Surg *34A*:584–590, 1952.

175. McMaster WC: Anterior glenoid labrum damage: a painful lesion in swimmers. Am J Sports Med *14*(5):383–387, 1986.

176. McNiesch LM, and Callaghan JJ: CT arthrography of the shoulder: variations of the glenoid labrum. AJR *149*:963–966, 1987.

177. Merrill V (ed): Shoulder: anteroposterior projections, postero-anterior views, glenoid fossa, Grashey position, rolled-film axial projection, Cleaves position, superoinferior axial projection, inferosuperior axial projection, Lawrence position. *In* Atlas of Roentgenographic Positions and Standard Radiologic Procedures, 4th ed. St. Louis: CV Mosby, 1975.

178. Metges PJ, Kleitz C, Tellier P, Delahaye RP, et al: Arthro-pneumotomography in recurrent dislocations and subluxations of the shoulder: methods, results, and indications in 45 cases. J Radiol *60*(12):789–796, 1979.

179. Middleton WD, Edelstein G, Reinus WR, Melson GL, et al: Ultrasonography of the rotator cuff: technique and normal anatomy. J Ultrasound Med *3*:549–551, 1984.

180. Middleton WD, Edelstein G, Reinus WR, Melson GL, et al: Sonographic detection of rotator cuff tears. AJR *144*:349–353, 1985.

181. Middleton WD, Reinus WR, Melson GL, Totty WG, et al: Pitfalls of rotator cuff sonography. AJR *146*:555–560, 1986.

182. Middleton WD, Reinus WR, Totty WG, Melson CL, et al: Ultrasonographic evaluation of the rotator cuff and biceps tendon. J Bone Joint Surg *68A*(3):440–450, 1986.

183. Mikasa M: Subacromial bursography. J Jap Orthop Assoc *53*:225–231, 1979.

184. Milbradt H, and Rosenthal H: Sonography of the shoulder joint. Techniques, sonomorphology and diagnostic significance. Radiologe *28*(2):61–68, 1988.

185. Mink JH, Richardson A, and Grant TT: Evaluation of glenoid labrum by double-contrast shoulder arthrography. AJR *133*:883–887, 1979.

186. Neer CS II: Anterior acromioplasty for the chronic impingement syndrome in the shoulder. J Bone Joint Surg *54A*:41–50, 1972.

187. Neer CS II: Displaced proximal humeral fractures. J Bone Joint Surg *52A*:1077, 1970.

188. Neer CS II: Fractures about the shoulder. *In* Rockwood CA and Green DP (eds): Fractures, 2nd ed. Philadelphia: JB Lippincott, 1984, p 679.

189. Neer CS II: Fractures of the distal clavicle with detachment of the coracoclavicular ligaments in adults. J Trauma *3*:99–110, 1963.

190. Neer CS II: Fractures of the distal third of the clavicle. Clin Orthop *58*:43–50, 1968.

191. Neer CS II: Personal communication.

192. Neviaser JS: Adhesive capsulitis of the shoulder: a study of the pathological findings in periarthritis of the shoulder. J Bone Joint Surg *27*:211–222, 1945.

192a. Neviaser JS: Adhesive capsulitis and the stiff painful shoulder. Orthop Clin North Am *11*(2):327–331, 1980.

193. Neviaser RJ: Radiologic assessment of the shoulder: plain and arthrographic. Orthop Clin North Am *18*(3):343–349, 1987.

194. Newhouse KE, El-Khoury GY, Neopola JV, and Montgomery WJ: The shoulder impingement view: a fluoroscopic technique for the detection of subacromial spurs. AJR *151*(3):539–541, 1988.

195. Nixon JD, and DiStefano V: Ruptures of the rotator cuff. Orthop Clin North Am *4*:423–447, 1975.

196. Norman A: The use of tomography in the diagnosis of skeletal disorders. Clin Orthop *107*:139–145, 1975.

197. Norwood T, and Terry GC: Shoulder posterior subluxation. Am J Sports Med *12*:25–30, 1984.

198. Nottage WM, Duge WD, and Fields WA: Computed arthro-tomography of the glenohumeral joint to evaluate anterior instability: correlation with arthroscopic findings. Arthroscopy *3*(4):273–276, 1987.

199. Ogawa K: Double contrast arthrography of the shoulder joint. Nippon Seikelgeka Gakkal Zasshi *58*(8):745–759, 1984.

200. Ogden JA, Conlogue GJ, and Bronson ML: Radiology of postnatal skeletal development: III. The clavicle. Skeletal Radiol *4*:196–203, 1979.

201. Ozonoff MB, and Ziter FMH Jr: The upper humeral notch: a normal variant in children. Radiology *113*:699–701, 1974.

202. Pancoast HK: Importance of careful roentgen-ray investigations of apical chest tumors. JAMA *83*(18):1407, 1924.

203. Pappas AM, Goss TP, and Kleinman PK: Symptomatic shoul-der instability due to lesions of the glenoid labrum. Am J Sports Med *11*:279, 1983.

204. Pavlov H, and Freibergerger RH: Fractures and dislocations about the shoulder. Semin Roentgenol *13*:85–96, 1978.

205. Pavlov H, Warren RF, Weiss CB Jr, and Dines DM: The roentgenographic evaluation of anterior shoulder instability. Clin Orthop *194*:153–158, 1985.

206. Pear BL: Bilateral posterior fracture dislocation of the shoulder—an uncommon complication of a convulsive seizure. N Engl J Med *283*:135–136, 1970.

207. Pear BL: Dislocation of the shoulder: x-ray signs. Letter to the editor. N Engl J Med *283*(20):1113, 1970.

208. Percy EC, Birbrager D, and Pitt MJ: Snapping scapula: a review of the literature and presentation of 14 patients. Can J Surg *31*(4):248–250, 1988.

209. Perthes G: Uber Operationen bei Habitueller Schulterluxation. Dtsch Z Chir *85*:199–227, 1906.

210. Petersson CJ, and Redlund-Johnell I: The subacromial space in normal shoulder radiographs. Acta Orthop Scand *55*:57–58, 1984.

211. Popke LOA: Zur Kasuistik und Therapie der Habituellen Schulterluxation. Dissertation, Halle, 1882.

212. Post M: The Shoulder. Philadelphia: Lea & Febiger, 1978.

213. Preston BJ, and Jackson JP: Investigation of shoulder disability by arthrography. Clin Radiol *28*:259–266, 1977.

214. Pring DJ, Constant O, Bayley JIL, and Stoker DJ: Radiology of the humeral head in recurrent anterior shoulder dislocations: brief report. J Bone Joint Surg *71B*(1):141–142, 1989.

215. Putkonen M, Lahde S, Puranan J, and Paivansalo M: The value of axial view in the radiography of shoulder girdle: experiences with a new modification of positioning. Rontgen-blatter *41*(4):158–162, 1988.

216. Quesada F: Technique for the roentgen diagnosis of fractures of the clavicle. Surg Gynecol Obstet *42*:424–428, 1926.

217. Rafii M, Firooznia H, Golimbu C, Minkoff J, et al: CT arthrography of capsular structures of the shoulder. AJR *146*:361–367, 1986.

218. Rafii M, Minkoff J, Bonamo J, Firooznia H, et al: Computed tomography (CT) arthrography of shoulder instabilities in athletes. Am J Sports Med *16*(4):352–361, 1988.

219. Randelli M, and Gambrioli PL: Glenohumeral osteometry by computed tomography in normal and unstable shoulders. Clin Orthop *208*:151–156, 1986.

220. Rapf Ch, Furtschegger A, and Resch H: Sonography as a new diagnostic procedure for investigating abnormalities of the shoulder. Fortschr Geb Rontgenstr Nuklearmed Erganzungs-band *145*(3):288–295, 1986.

221. Reeder JD, and Andelman S: The rotator cuff tear: MR evaluation. Magn Reson Imaging *5*:331–338, 1987.

222. Reichmann S, Astrand K, Deichgraber E, and Olsson B: Soft tissue xeroradiography of the shoulder joint. Acta Radiol Diagn *16*(6):572–576, 1975.

223. Reiser M, Erlemann R, Bongartz G, Pauly T, et al: Role of magnetic resonance imaging in the diagnosis of shoulder joint injuries. Radiologe *28*(2):79–83, 1988.

224. Resch H, Benedetto KP, Kadletz R, and Daniaux H: X-ray examination in recurrent dislocation of the shoulder—value of different techniques. Unfallchirurgie *11*(2):65–69, 1985.

225. Resch H, Helweg G, zur Nedden D, and Beck E: Double-contrast computed tomographic examination techniques in habitual and recurrent shoulder dislocation. Europ J Radiol *8*(1):6–12, 1988.

226. Resch H, Kadletz R, Beck E, and Helweg G: Simple and double-contrast CT scanning in the examination of recurrent shoulder dislocations. Unfallchirurg *89*:441–445, 1986.

227. Resnick CS, Deutsch AL, Resnick D, Mink JH, et al: Arthro-tomography of the shoulder. Radiographics *4*(6):963–976, 1984.

227a. Resnick D, and Niwayama G: Resorption of the undersurface of the distal clavicle in rheumatoid arthritis. Radiology *120*:75–77, 1976.

228. Resnick D, and Niwayama G (eds): Diagnosis of Bone and Joint Disorders, 2nd ed, Vols. 1 and 2. Philadelphia: WB Saunders Company, 1988.

229. Resnick D, and Niwayama G (eds): Anatomy of individual

joints. *In* Diagnosis of Bone and Joint Disorders, Vol. 1. Philadelphia: WB Saunders Company, 1981, pp 69–77.

230. Resnick D: Shoulder arthrography. Radiol Clin North Am *19:*243–253, 1981.

231. Richardson JB, Ramsay A, Davidson JK, and Kelly IG: Radiographs in shoulder trauma. J Bone Joint Surg *70B*(3):457–460, 1988.

232. Ritvo M, and Ritvo M: Roentgen study of the sternoclavicular region. AJR *53:*644–650, 1947.

233. Rockwood CA Jr, and Green DP (eds): Fractures, 2nd ed. Philadelphia: JB Lippincott, 1984.

234. Rokous JR, Feagin JA, and Abbott HG: Modified axillary roentgenogram. Clin Orthop *82:*84–86, 1972.

235. Rontgen WK: On a new kind of rays. Nature *53:*274–276, 1896.

236. Rosen PS: A unique shoulder lesion in ankylosing spondylitis: clinical comment (letter). J Rheumatol *7:*109–110, 1980.

237. Rosenthal H, and Galanski M: Positioning in plain film radiography of the shoulder. Radiologe *28*(2):54–60, 1988.

238. Rothman RH, Marvel JP Jr, and Heppenstall RB: Anatomic considerations in the glenohumeral joint. Orthop Clin North Am *6:*341–352, 1975.

239. Rowe CR: The Shoulder. New York: Churchill Livingstone, 1988.

240. Rubin SA, Gray RL, and Green WR: The scapular "Y": a diagnostic aid in shoulder trauma. Radiology *110:*725–726, 1974.

241. Russell AR (ed.): Medical Radiography and Photography. Rochester, NY: Eastman Kodak Company, Vol. 58, No. 2, 1982.

242. See reference 241.

243. Sackellares JC, and Swift TR: Shoulder enlargement as the presenting sign in syringomyelia: report of two cases and review of the literature. JAMA *236:*2878–2879, 1976.

244. Saha AK: Dynamic stability of the glenohumeral joint. Acta Orthop Scand *42:*491–505, 1971.

245. Sante LR: Manual of Roentgenological Technique, 9th ed. Ann Arbor, MI: Edwards Brothers, Inc., 1942, pp 160–161.

246. Seeger LL, Gold RH, Bassett LW, and Ellman H: Shoulder impingement syndrome: MR findings in 53 shoulders. AJR *150*(2):343–347, 1988.

247. Seeger LL, Gold RH, and Bassett LW: Shoulder instability: evaluation with MR imaging. Radiology *168*(3):695–697, 1988.

248. Seeger LL, Ruszkowski JT, Bassett LW, Kay SP, et al: MR imaging of the normal shoulder: Anatomic correlation. AJR *148:*83–91, 1988.

249. Seymour EQ: Osteolysis of the clavicular tip associated with repetitive minor trauma to the shoulder. Radiology *123:*56, 1977.

250. Shai G, Ring H, Costeff H, and Solzi P: Glenohumeral malalignment in the hemiplegic shoulder: an early radiologic sign. Scand J Rehab Med *16:*133–136, 1984.

251. Shenton AF: The modified axial view: an alternative radiograph in shoulder injuries (letter). Arch Emerg Med *4*(3):201–203, 1987.

252. Shuman WP, Kilcoyne RF, Matsen FA III, Rogers JV, et al: Double-contrast computed tomography of the glenoid labrum. AJR *141:*581–584, 1983.

253. Singson RD, Feldman F, Bigliani LU, and Rosenberg ZS: Recurrent shoulder dislocation after surgical repair: double-contrast CT arthrography: work in progress. Radiology *164:*425–428, 1987.

254. Slivka J, and Resnick D: An improved radiographic view of the glenohumeral joint. J Can Assoc Radiol *30:*83–85, 1979.

255. Stewart CA, Siegel ME, King D, and Moser L: Radionuclide and radiographic demonstration of condensing osteitis of the clavicle. Clin Nucl Med *13*(3):177–178, 1988.

256. Stodell MA, Nicholson R, Scott J, and Sturrock RD: Radio-

isotope scanning in the painful shoulder. Rheumatol Rehabil *19:*163–166, 1980.

257. Strauss MB, Wroble LJ, Neff RS, and Cady GW: The shrugged-off shoulder: a comparison of patients with recurrent shoulder subluxations and dislocations. Phys Sports Med *12:*85–97, 1983.

258. Strauss MB, Wroble LJ, Neff RS, et al: X-ray confirmation of anterior shoulder instability. Orthop Trans *2*(Nov):225, 1978.

259. Strauss MB: The shoulder: anatomy and mechanics. Personal communication.

260. Strizak AM, Danzig LA, Jackson DW, Greenway G, et al: Subacromial bursography: an anatomical and clinical study. J Bone Joint Surg *64A*(2):196–201, 1982.

261. Sweeney RJ (ed): A tangential projection or a lateral view of the scapula. Radiol Technol *52*(6):631–634.

262. Teates CD, Brower AC, Williamson BRJ, and Keats TE: Bone scans in condensing osteitis of the clavicle. South Med J *71*(6):736–738, 1978.

263. Tietge RA, and Ciullo JV: C.A.M. axillary x-ray. Exhibit to the Academy Meeting of the American Academy of Orthopaedic Surgeons. Orthop Trans *6:*451, 1982.

264. Tijmes J, Lloyd H, and Tullos HS: Arthrography in acute shoulder dislocations. South Med J *72*(5):564–567, 1979.

265. Treble NJ: Normal variations in radiographs of the clavicle: brief report. J Bone Joint Surg *70B*(3):490, 1988.

266. Uhthoff HK, Hammond DI, Sarkar K, Hooper GJ, et al: The role of the coracoacromial ligament in the impingement syndrome: a clinical, radiological, and histological study. Int Orthop *12*(2):97–104, 1988.

267. Usselman JA, Vint VC, and Waltz TA: CT demonstration of a brachial plexus neuroma. AJNR *1*(4):346–347, 1980.

268. ViGario GD, and Keats TE: Localization of calcific deposits in the shoulder. AJR *108:*806–811, 1970.

269. Waldrop JI, Norwood LA, and Alvarez RG: Lateral roentgenographic projections of the acromioclavicular joint. Am J Sports Med *9*(5):337–341, 1981.

270. Wallace WA, and Johnson F: Dynamic radiography in shoulder kinematics: problems and their solutions (proceedings). J Bone Joint Surg *62B:*256, 1980.

271. Weston WJ: Arthrography of the acromio-clavicular joint. Australas Radiol *18:*213–214, 1974.

272. Widner LA, and Riddervold HO: The value of the lordotic view in diagnosis of fractures of the clavicle (a technical note). Rev Interam Radiol *5*(2):69–70, 1980.

273. Woolson ST, Fellingham LL, and Vassiliadis PDA: Three-dimensional images of the elbow and shoulder from computerized tomography data (abstr). AAOS Shoulder meeting, Las Vegas, Nevada, January 1985.

274. Yang SO, Cho KJ, Kim MJ, and Ro IW: Assessment of anterior shoulder instability by CT arthrography. J Korean Med Sci *2*(3):167–171, 1987.

275. Yoh S: The value of computed tomography in the diagnosis of the rotator cuff tears, and bone and soft tissue tumors. Nippon Seikeigeka Gakkai Zasshi *58*(7):639–658, 1984.

276. Zachrisson BE, and Ejeskar A: Arthrography in dislocation of the acromioclavicular joint. Acta Radiol [Diagn] *20:*81–87, 1979.

277. Zanca P: Shoulder pain: involvement of the acromioclavicular joint: analysis of 1000 cases. AJR *112*(3):493–506, 1971.

278. Zeiger M, Dorr U, and Schulz RD: Sonography of slipped humeral epiphysis due to birth injury. Pediatr Radiol *17:*425–426, 1987.

279. Ziegler R: X-ray examination of the shoulder in suspected luxation. Z Orthop *119:*31–35, 1981.

280. Zlatkin MB, Bjorkengren AG, Gylys-Morin V, Resnick D, et al: Cross-sectional imaging of the capsular mechanism of the glenohumeral joint. AJR *150*(1):151–158, 1988.

Biomechanics of the Shoulder

Bernard F. Morrey, M.D.
Kai-Nan An, Ph.D.

Because of its component parts, a description of the biomechanics of the shoulder complex is rather involved. In order to make the subject at once comprehensive and relevant to the clinician, the structure and function of the sternoclavicular and acromioclavicular joints are dealt with first. The anatomy and biomechanics of the glenohumeral joint are then discussed in three parts according to an outline familiar to clinicians: motion, constraints, and forces across the joint (Table 6–1). By way of classification, we have adopted the increasingly accepted phrase of arm elevation rather than abduction or flexion where possible. Although this organization is somewhat artificial with some overlap, it does allow a simple approach toward understanding the entire shoulder complex.

The Shoulder Complex

The function of the shoulder girdle requires the integrated motion of the scapuloclavicular, acromioclavicular, glenohumeral, and scapulothoracic joints. This motion is created by the delicate interaction of almost 30 muscles that control the total joint complex. The discussion of biomechanics of this complex focuses first on the sternoclavicular and acromioclavicular and then the glenohumeral and scapulothoracic joints.

STERNOCLAVICULAR JOINT

Articular Surface

The sternal side of the scapuloclavicular articulation is a saddle-shaped joint surface with its long axis running from superior to inferior and the shorter axis

from anterior to posterior (Fig. 6–1).[59] This saddle-shaped joint is oriented to face slightly posterior, lateral, and upward, the posterior angulation being approximately 20 degrees.[31] On the clavicular side, a reciprocal concave-convex surface fits congruently with the sternal articulation. A small facet that articulates with the rib is present inferiorly. Inspection of the joint surfaces with the congruent superior–inferior long axis and the shorter anterior–posterior axis suggests the possibility of two directions of translation: (1) anterior-to-posterior motion and (2) superior and inferior translation. However, axial rotation of the clavicle also occurs at this articulation.

A coronal section of this joint reveals that the congruity of the surfaces is not complete.[42] Such a relationship requires the presence of a meniscus (intra-articular disc), which is present at this joint as at the acromioclavicular joint. Further stability of the joint is brought about by certain positions of the clavicle, by intrinsic forces generated by the ligaments, and by extrinsic forces supplied by the muscles.[24]

Ligamentous Constraints

The sternoclavicular joint is stabilized by a complex of four ligaments arranged about the joint anteriorly, posteriorly, superiorly, and inferiorly (Fig. 6–2). Stability is further enhanced by the intra-articular disc.[42]

Table 6–1. RELATIONSHIP OF JOINT FUNCTION AND BIOMECHANICAL MEASUREMENTS

Clinical Function	Biomechanical Description
Motion	Kinematics
Stability	Constraints
Strength	Force transmission

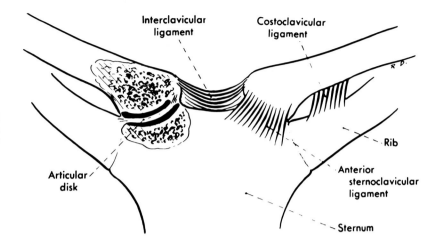

Figure 6–1. The sternoclavicular joint is a saddle-shaped joint that is oriented posterior, lateral, and upward. (Reproduced with permission from Hollinshead WH: Anatomy for Surgeons, Vol 3. New York: Harper & Row, 1969.)

Interclavicular Ligaments

The superior constraints to this joint[8] consist of two portions of the so-called interclavicular ligament. This ligament is composed of a band that connects the superomedial aspect of each clavicle with an intermediate attachment to the midportion of the manubrium. There is as well an anterior portion from the anterosuperior aspect of the manubrium to the clavicle (see Fig. 6–2A). The ligament becomes taut with arm depression and is lax with arm elevation.[86]

Sternoclavicular Ligaments

Immediately inferior and anterior to the interclavicular ligament is the anterior capsular constraint. The capsular ligament is thought to have two portions, an anterosuperior bundle that blends inferiorly to the remainder of the anterior capsule. The anterior capsular ligament is stronger than the posterior capsular ligament. In fact, the anterior bundle may be the

strongest of the sternoclavicular constraints.[11] The capsular ligaments originate from the sternal articular border and insert into the medial epiphysis of the clavicle.[86]

Costoclavicular Ligaments

The inferior aspect of the articulation is stabilized by the costoclavicular ligament, which consists of two components—anterior and posterior. This ligament courses obliquely and laterally from the first rib to the undersurface of the medial clavicle (see Fig. 6–2B). Continuing posteriorly, the costoclavicular ligament blends with the posterior sternoclavicular ligament. The dimensions and orientation are analogous to those of the coracoclavicular constraints of the lateral clavicle.[22, 86, 107] Functionally, the anterior fibers resist upward displacement while the posterior position resists downward rotation of the medial clavicle.[11] These structures assume a significant role not only in stabilizing this joint but also in restricting its motion.

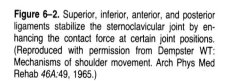

Figure 6–2. Superior, inferior, anterior, and posterior ligaments stabilize the sternoclavicular joint by enhancing the contact force at certain joint positions. (Reproduced with permission from Dempster WT: Mechanisms of shoulder movement. Arch Phys Med Rehab 46A:49, 1965.)

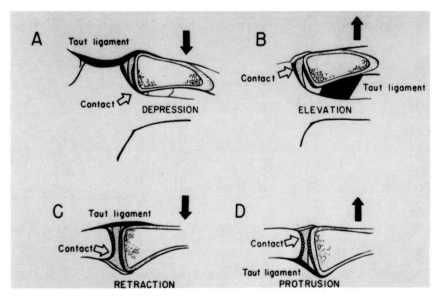

Motion and Constraint

According to Dempster, six actions occur at the sternoclavicular joint: elevation, depression, protrusion, retraction, and upward and downward rotation.[31] The amount of potential motion present at this articulation has been studied by disarticulating the scapula. Anteroposterior rotation exceeds superoinferior motion by about a two-to-one ratio.[31] In the intact and functioning extremity, the actual amount of displacement is of course limited by the attachment to the scapula; this motion will be described later. At the extremes, motion is limited by tension developed in the ligamentous complex on the opposite side of the joint. This constraint occurs in concert with increased contact pressure occurring at the articulation and the intra-articular disc ligament (see Fig. 6–2). Approximately 35 degrees of upward rotation occurs at the sternoclavicular joint.[51, 64] A similar 35 degrees of anterior and posterior rotation and up to 45 to 50 degrees of axial rotation also occur at this joint.

Anterior displacement of the distal clavicle is not affected by release of the interclavicular or costoclavicular ligaments or by the intraarticular disc.[11] Release of the capsular ligament is followed by downward displacement of the lateral clavicle.

Inferior displacement of the clavicle at the sternum is resisted by articular contact at the inferior aspect of the joint and by tautness developed in the interclavicular joint and the posterior expansion of the capsular joint.[31] Superior translation of the joint is resisted by tension developed in the entire costoclavicular complex. Little if any articular contribution assists in resisting this displacement.

Protrusion or anterior displacement of the clavicle is resisted not only by the anterior capsule but also by the posterior portion of the interclavicular ligament and the posterior sternoclavicular ligament. Conversely, posterior displacement or retraction of the medial aspect of the clavicle generates tension in the anterior portion of the inferior capsular ligaments and in the anterior sternoclavicular ligament, as well as in the anterior portion of the costoclavicular ligament. Only a limited amount of articular contact resists this displacement; this is on the posterior vertical ridge of the sternal articulation and the posterior portion of the clavicle.

Clavicular rotation causes twisting of the capsular ligaments. Only about 10 degrees of downward (forward) rotation occurs before the ligaments become taut, thus limiting further motion. With upward (backward) rotation of the clavicle, up to 45 degrees of rotation occurs before the entire complex again becomes taut, resisting further rotatory displacement.[86] Both of these actions increase compression across the sternoclavicular joint. The costoclavicular ligament is believed to be the most important single constraint in limiting motion at this joint.[59]

ACROMIOCLAVICULAR JOINT

Articular Surface

As with the sternoclavicular joint, the articular surfaces of the acromioclavicular joint are not perfectly congruent, requiring the presence of a meniscus for optimum contact and force transmission. The articular surface present on the anteromedial border of the acromion is flat or slightly convex. This joint has been classified as a "plane type" and is variously oriented but typically faces anteriorly, medially, and superiorly.

The articulation at the distal aspect of the clavicle has an inferior slope to the articular surface, which is flat or slightly convex and faces inferiorly, posteriorly, and laterally (Fig. 6–3).

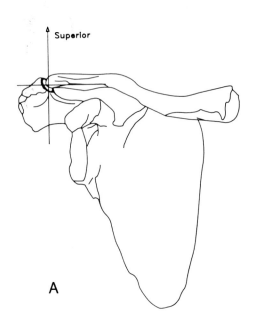

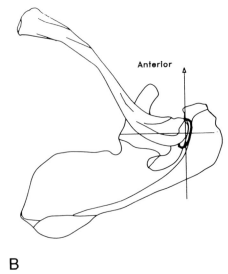

Figure 6–3. The acromioclavicular joint is oriented anterior-superior and is considered a "plane" type of joint.

A

B

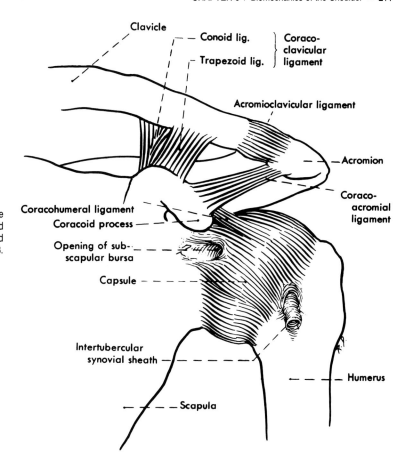

Figure 6–4. The coracohumeral ligament complex consists of the larger and heavier trapezoid ligament, which is oriented laterally, and the smaller conoid ligament, situated more medially. (Reproduced with permission from Hollinshead WH: Anatomy for Surgeons, Vol 3. New York: Harper & Row, 1969.)

Ligamentous Structure

The ligamentous anatomy of the distal clavicle is well known to the orthopedic surgeon. The all-important coracoclavicular ligaments consist of (1) the conoid ligament, which inserts into the inferior surface of the clavicle on the conoid tubercle near its posterior ridge, and (2) the trapezoid ligament, which runs obliquely, superiorly, and then laterally toward the trapezoid ridge to a roughened triangular patch situated anterolaterally on the inferior surface of the clavicle. Of the two, the trapezoid ligament is larger, longer, and stronger with a greater cross-sectional area (Fig. 6–4). The acromioclavicular capsule consists of fibers running medially, posteriorly, and upward from the acromion to the clavicle. These fibers resist anteroposterior displacement and lateral motion of the scapula from the end of the clavicle. The acromioclavicular ligament is a thickening of the superior capsule.

Motion and Constraint

The amount of possible acromioclavicular motion that is independent of the sternoclavicular link has been found to be limited by the complex arrangement of the coracoclavicular and acromioclavicular ligaments. According to most investigators, the rotation of the acromioclavicular joint takes place about three axes. These motions are variously described but can simply be termed anteroposterior rotation of the clavicle on the scapula, superoinferior rotation, and anterior (inferior) and posterior (superior) axial rotation. Of these three, the anteroposterior rotation of the clavicle with respect to the acromion is approximately three times as great as the superoinferior rotation of the intact specimen.[31] There is little documentation of the specific angular dimensions of this rotation, but significant attention has been paid to the constraining elements. Dempster noted that the conoid and trapezoid became taut with anteroposterior scapular rotation, thus serving as the constraint of this motion.[31] In a recent study by Fukuda and coworkers, however, the acromioclavicular ligament was noted to be taut in its anterior and posterior components with posterior and anterior rotation, respectively.[41] Anterior rotation of the clavicle referable to the scapula was also found to cause some tightness in the conoid and trapezoid ligaments, but this was of a magnitude approximately equal to the stretch observed in the posterior acromioclavicular ligament. Thus, the limiting factor to this motion is the posterior component of the acromioclavicular ligament. On the other hand, posterior rotation of the clavicle is restrained only by the anterior fibers of the acromioclavicular ligament, with virtually no contribution from the other structures.

Superoinferior rotation of the clavicle is quite limited at the acromioclavicular joint. Both Dempster and

Kapandji noted virtually no ligamentous contribution to resisting inferior displacement (see Fig. 6–3).[31, 59] On the other hand, superior rotation of the clavicle with respect to the acromion is limited primarily by the medial aspect of the conoid ligament, with subsequent tightening of the lateral portion of this structure. The trapezoid provides approximately the same degree of constraint as do the anterior and posterior portions of the acromioclavicular ligament complex. Once again, the magnitude of this displacement is not reported by either investigator but is said to be limited.

Anterior and posterior axial rotation (inferior–superior) was reported by Dempster and Inman to be about 20 to 30 degrees.[31, 51] Greater anterior rotation occurs than posterior, but both motions are limited by the conoid ligament. Rockwood, however, could demonstrate only 5 to 8 degrees of motion at the acromioclavicular joint.[86] Posterior axial rotation is accompanied by tightening of the trapezoid ligament, with some contribution from the medial and anterior conoid as well as from the acromioclavicular ligament complex.[41]

Dempster, on the other hand, indicates that the acromioclavicular ligament is taut in the extreme of anterior and posterior axial rotation and is a limiting factor of this motion.[31] Fukuda and colleagues have quantified the displacement as a function of the ligamentous constraints.[41] Slight displacement is limited by the acromioclavicular ligament, but large displacements are resisted by the coracoclavicular ligaments (Fig. 6–5).

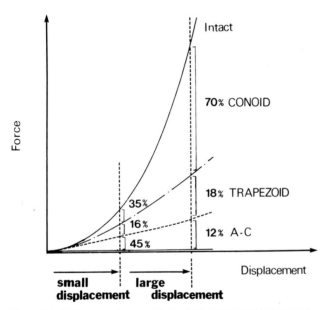

Figure 6–5. All displacements are resisted by the force generated in the acromioclavicular ligament, and large displacements are also resisted by the conoid and trapezoid structures. (Reproduced with permission from Fukuda K, Craig EV, An KN, et al: Biomechanical study of the ligamentous system of the acromioclavicular joint. J Bone Joint Surg *68A*(3):434–440, 1986.)

MOTION OF THE CLAVICLE

The potential motion present at the sternoclavicular and acromioclavicular joints exceeds that actually attained during active motion of the shoulder complex. Current data indicate that accurate demonstration of the phasic three-dimensional motion of the sternoclavicular and acromioclavicular joints that occurs with arm elevation is a complex problem.[61] During elevation of the extremity, clavicular elevation of about 30 degrees occurs with the maximum at about 130 degrees of elevation (Fig. 6–6).[51] The clavicle also rotates forward approximately 10 degrees during the first 40 degrees of elevation. There is no change during the next 90 degrees of elevation; an additional 15 to 20 degrees of forward rotation then occurs during the terminal arc. Forward elevation (flexion) demonstrates virtually the identical pattern of clavicular motion.

Axial rotation of the clavicle is reported by Inman and coworkers to be an essential and fundamental feature of shoulder motion, particularly arm elevation (Fig. 6–7). If the clavicle is not allowed to rotate, elevation of only about 110 degrees is said to be possible.[51] Superior (posterior) rotation of the clavicle begins after the arm has attained an arc of about 90 degrees of elevation and then progresses in a rather linear fashion, attaining approximately 40 degrees of rotation at full elevation (Fig. 6–7).[51] These findings have been challenged by Rockwood. Placing pins in the clavicle and acromium shows less than 10 degrees' rotation with full arm elevation.[86] This discrepancy suggests that some scapulothoracic motion was being recorded by Inman and colleagues. Clinical observation and experience supports the position of Rockwood.[59a] Fixation of the clavicle to the coracoid by a screw does not greatly limit shoulder elevation; ankylosis by ectopic bone also causes minimal loss of arm elevation.

Thus the sternoclavicular and acromioclavicular joints demonstrate rather unique articular anatomy. A significant arc of motion is present at both articulations. This linkage system provides the degrees of freedom that assist but are not essential for the proper rotation in the scapula and for full elevation of the arm. Loss of motion at the acromioclavicular joint appears to be better tolerated than fusion or loss of motion at the sternoclavicular joint.

CLINICAL RELEVANCE

Sternoclavicular Joint

The anatomy and biomechanics of this joint provide information helpful to the clinician in managing sternoclavicular instability. If displacement of the clavicle occurs posteriorly, the airway may be compromised. Since the articulation is oriented posteriorly, it allows relatively little inherent stability in the posterior direction; reconstruction of an anterior static constraint is necessary to prevent posterior displacement of the

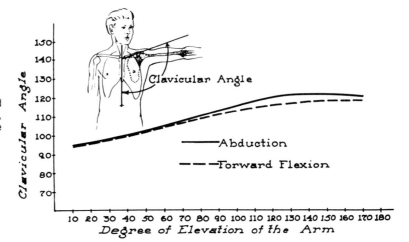

Figure 6–6. Clavicular elevation during abduction and forward flexion of the arm. (Reproduced with permission from Inman VT, Saunders M, and Abbott LC: Observations on the function of the shoulder joint. J Bone Joint Surg 26:1, 1944.)

medial end of the clavicle. Fortunately, anterior displacement of the medial end of the clavicle is more common. In this circumstance, a posteriorly directed reduction generally is quite stable.

Acromioclavicular instability is one of the most important and controversial topics clinically relevant to the shoulder. The acromioclavicular capsular ligament complex is the primary constraint for small rotational displacements at this joint. Downward force applied to the end of the scapula causes an upward elevation (Grade III injury) of the clavicle, violating the constraint provided by the conoid and trapezoid ligaments. Lesser degrees of ligamentous disruption, such as occur with Type 1 or 2 acromioclavicular sprains, demonstrate minimal or no superior migration of the clavicle. The biomechanical data have explained this finding by showing that the conoid ligament must be intact to prevent even slight displacement.

Some axial rotation of the clavicle is obligatory for arm elevation at the acromioclavicular joint. Clinical experience suggests that this requirement is minimal for normal shoulder function.[86] Spontaneous ankylosis of the acromioclavicular joint can occur owing to the formation of ectopic bone. Such a condition would not be expected to limit arm elevation to any significant degree. The patient shown in Figure 6–8 could elevate his arm to about 160 degrees.

Glenohumeral and Scapulothoracic Joint Motion

The motion of the shoulder complex is probably greater than that of any other joint in the body. The arm can move through an angle of approximately 0 to 180 degrees in elevation; internal and external rotation of approximately 150 degrees is possible; "flexion and extension" or anterior and posterior rotation in the horizontal plane is approximately 170 degrees.[98] This motion, which represents the composite motion of several joints, primarily occurs in the glenohumeral and scapulothoracic joints; extreme positions require rotation at the sternoclavicular and acromioclavicular joints.

The motion of the shoulder complex has been the topic of concern and controversy for over 100 years. The reasons for this debate are many and include the imperfect devices or means of measurement, since the soft tissue envelope makes it difficult to actually observe the skeletal motion; confusion with respect to terminology; inconsistency in defining the reference system; and an early lack of understanding of the concept of sequence-dependent serial rotation. The early investigations focused on arm motion about the

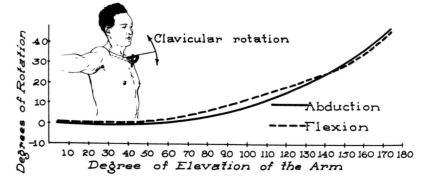

Figure 6–7. Axial rotation of the clavicle during arm elevation. (Reproduced with permission from Inman VT, Saunders M, and Abbott LC: Observations on the function of the shoulder joint. J Bone Joint Surg 26:1, 1944.)

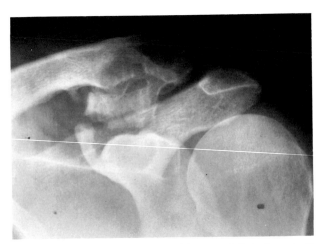

Figure 6–8. Extensive ectopic ossification of the coracoclavicular ligaments. By limiting clavicular motion, only a small portion of the full range of motion of the shoulder complex is limited.

sagittal, coronal, and transverse planes. However, since the sequence-dependent nature of rotation about orthogonal axes was not appreciated, years of debate and discussion centered on understanding and explaining the so-called "Codman's paradox."

CODMAN'S PARADOX

Codman's paradox may be easily demonstrated (Fig. 6–9). From the resting position in the anatomical posture with the medial epicondyle pointing toward the midline of the body, the arm is brought forward to 90 degrees of flexion. The arm is next abducted 90 degrees. The epicondyle is now pointing perpendicular to the coronal plane. The arm is then brought back to the side to its apparent initial position, but the medial epicondyle is now observed to be rotated anteriorly away from the body instead of medially toward the midline of the body. Yet the humerus was never axially rotated.[56]

The difficulty of understanding this phenomenon has prompted numerous discussions. The simplest explanation is that serial angular rotations are not additive and are sequence dependent. This means that 90 degrees of rotation about the x and then y axes results in a different final position than rotation about x and then z axes (Fig. 6–10). Multiple rotations about orthogonal axes must therefore be defined by the sequence of the rotation. In aerospace terms, these rotations are termed the "Eulerian angles": yaw, pitch, and roll.

The confusion is significantly resolved by the use of two reference systems. First, scapular motion is best defined referable to the classical anatomical system of the trunk. Second, humeral motion is described referable to the scapula. This issue is discussed in detail later.

TECHNIQUES TO OBSERVE AND DESCRIBE THE SHOULDER COMPLEX MOTION

Because of the complexity of this issue and the conflicting results, it is appropriate to describe various techniques that have been used to measure upper-extremity motion. The methods of observing and describing motion of the upper extremities may be broadly categorized into research and clinical efforts.

The early research efforts to describe shoulder joint (complex) motion consisted of simple (but careful) observation of cadaveric material and thus often included the observation of the ligamentous constraints.[21, 24, 34, 56] A gross description of the motion and

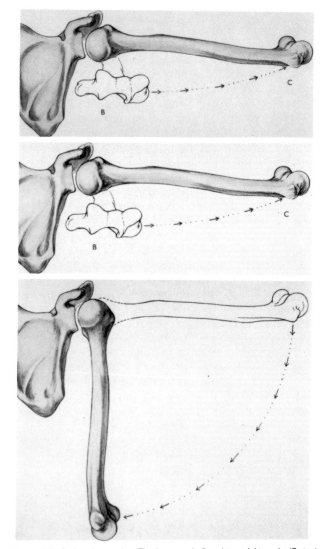

Figure 6–9. Codman's paradox. The humerus is flexed to a right angle *(B, top)*, swung backward to the plane of the scapula *(C, middle)*, and then brought back to the vertical *(bottom)*. An axial rotation position change has occurred without an actual axial rotation taking place. (Reproduced with permission from Johnston TB: The movements of the shoulder joint. A plea for the use of the "plane of the scapula" as the plane of reference for movements occurring at the humero-scapular joint. Br J Surg 25:252, 1937.)

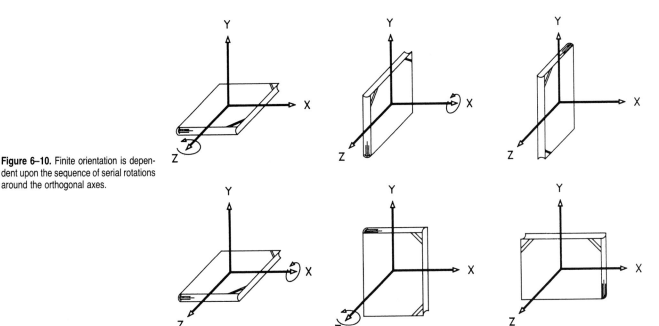

Figure 6–10. Finite orientation is dependent upon the sequence of serial rotations around the orthogonal axes.

displacement has proved to be accurate even today owing to the careful nature of these early observations. With the advent of the roentgenogram, uniplanar[28] and biplanar[39, 64, 82] plane and cineradiographs are the more common techniques employed today for both active and passive studies. These techniques are particularly attractive since they can be employed *in vivo*. By implanting metal markers, very accurate three-dimensional rotation may be measured from these radiographs.[69] More recently, with the advent of computer data manipulation, replication of motion using a complex system involving an interactive microcomputer for analyzing images with a real-time graphic display has been developed. This method and other modeling techniques are far too complex for routine use but may serve as a valuable research tool.[46, 77, 81]

Clinical measurement techniques include simple and complex goniometers. Doddy and associates have designed a goniometer to be used *in vivo* that measures both glenohumeral and scapulothoracic motion simultaneously.[34] Electrogoniometers have not been of routine clinical value but have been extensively used for basic science investigations. Unfortunately, the anatomy constraints at the shoulder limit the value of electrogoniometers. A stereometric method has also been used for three-dimensional kinematic analysis. Basically, when three non-colinear points fixed to a rigid body are defined within an inertial reference frame, the position and orientation of that rigid body can be specified and the relative rotation and translation occurring at a joint can be determined. Numerous commercial systems using light-emitting diodes, reflecting dots, and ultrasonic transducer techniques are available for such an application.

More recently, aerospace technology has provided a device that uses three mutually orthogonal magnetic fields;[5] this has proved useful as both a research and a clinical tool. This instrument may be applied to *in vivo* or *in vitro* studies and measures simultaneous three-dimensional rotational motion. In addition, translation displacement may also be calculated, thus allowing the determination of the screw axis. This defines the complete displacement characteristics of the system.

DESCRIPTION OF JOINT MOTION

The above techniques permit joint motion to be described with varying degrees of sophistication. In general, joint kinematics may be divided into two-dimensional planar motion or three-dimensional spatial motion. With planar motion, the moving segment both translates and rotates around the fixed segment. For a more unique description, however, the planar motion can be described based on a rotation around a point or axis, which is defined as the instantaneous center of rotation (ICR). Theoretically, the ICR could be determined accurately if the velocities of points on the rigid body are measurable. Practically, an alternative technique based on Rouleaux's method is commonly adopted. In this method, the instantaneous locations of two points on the moving segment are identified from two consecutive positions within a short period of time, and the intersection of the bisectors of the lines joining the same points at the two positions defines the ICR (Fig. 6–11).

Occasionally it is useful to describe the planar joint articulating motion.[3] For general planar or gliding motion of the articular surface, the terms *sliding, spinning,* and *rolling* are commonly used (Fig. 6–12).

Sliding motion is defined as the pure translation of a moving segment against the surface of a fixed seg-

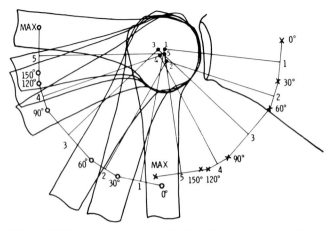

Figure 6–11. Measurement of the center of rotation of the humeral head as defined by the Rouleaux technique. (From Walker PS: Human Joints and Their Artificial Replacements. Courtesy of Charles C Thomas, Publisher, Springfield, Illinois.)

ment. The contact point of the moving segment does not change, while its mating surface has a constantly changing contact point. If the surface of the fixed segment is flat, the ICR is located at infinity; otherwise, it is at the center of the curvature of the fixed surface.

Spinning motion is the exact opposite of sliding motion; the moving segment rotates and the contact point on the fixed surface does not change. The ICR, in this case, is located at the center or curvature of the spinning body that is undergoing pure rotation.

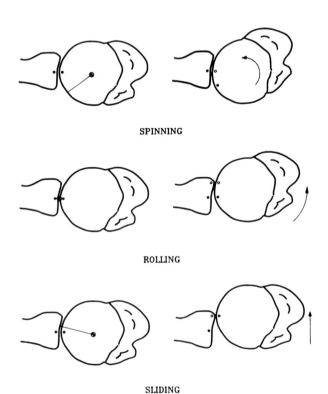

Figure 6–12. All three types of motion (spinning, rolling, and sliding) occur at the glenohumeral articulation.

Rolling motion is motion between moving and fixed segments in which the contact points on each surface are constantly changing. However, the arc length of the moving surface matches the path on the fixed surface so that the two surfaces have point-to-point contact without slippage. The relative motion of rolling is a combination of translation and rotation. The ICR is located at the contact point.

Most of the planar articulating motion can be described using a combination of any two of these three basic types of motion.

THREE-DIMENSIONAL GLENOHUMERAL JOINT MOTION

Three-dimensional analysis of the rigid body motion requires three linear and three angular coordinates to specify the location and orientation of a rigid body in space. In other words, any rigid body with unconstrained motion will have six degrees of freedom in space. Numerous methods are available to describe the spatial rigid body motion; two of the most commonly used are the Eulerian angle and the screw displacement axis descriptions.

If the glenohumeral joint is stable and the motion can be assumed as that of a ball-in-socket joint, it is then sufficient to consider only the rotation of the joint and neglect small amounts of translation. In this case, the description of three-dimensional rotation using the Eulerian angle system is most appropriate (Fig. 6–13). It should be remembered, as emphasized earlier, that the general three-dimensional rotation is sequence dependent. In other words, with the same specified amount of rotation around three axes, the final result will be different if the sequence of the axes of rotation is different. This is one of the explanations of Codman's paradox.

With the arm hanging at the side of the body, the z axis is defined to be perpendicular to the scapular plane. The y axis points out laterally and the x axis points distally along the humeral shaft axis. The rotational sequence for the Eulerian description of the glenohumeral joint rotation or the orientation of the humerus relative to the scapula is as follows: First rotate the humerus around the x axis by an amount ϕ to define the plane of elevation. Then rotate the arm around the rotated z (z') axis by an amount θ to define the arm elevation. Finally, the axial rotation of the humerus around the rotated x (x'') axis by an amount ψ.

During the circumduction motion of the humerus, for example, the corresponding Eulerian angle could be measured as shown in Figure 6–13. This description could be used clinically to describe the range of joint motion as well as the specification of joint position where any abnormality or pathological process should be documented.

In instances when a more general description of the glenohumeral joint displacement is required, the screw

1 – 3' – 1" Rotation Sequence
[Left Shoulder (PA View)]

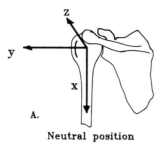

A.

Neutral position

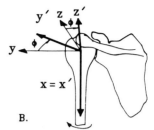

B.

1st Rotation φ :
Axial rotation about x axis
represents the plane of elevation.

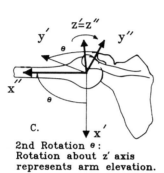

C.

2nd Rotation θ :
Rotation about z' axis
represents arm elevation.

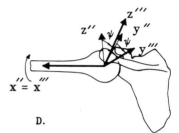

D.

3rd Rotation ψ :
Axial rotation about x″ axis
represents humeral rotation.

Figure 6–13. Three-dimensional rotation around each of the orthogonal axes is most accurately described using the Eulerian angle system. Glenohumeral motion is defined by the sequence-dependent Eulerian angles.

displacement axis (SDA) description is most appropriate. The rotation and translation components of displacement of the humerus relative to the glenoid or scapula are defined by a rotation around and translation along a unique so-called screw axis (Fig. 6–14).

In addition to incorporating a description of translation, the advantage of using the SDA method is that the orientation of SDA remains invariant regardless of the reference coordinate axes used. The SDA can be experimentally determined using various methods.

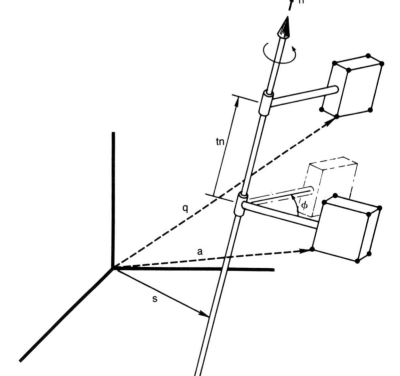

Figure 6–14. Both rotational and translational components of displacement of a rigid body may be expressed by the concept of the screw axis, which represents the shortest path around or along which the displacement can be described. (See text for description.)

With the rotational matrix describing the orientation and a positional vector from a reference point known for the rigid body, the SDA can be calculated.[23] If the coordinates of at least three reference points on the rigid body are measured, the SDA can also be calculated.[97]

Shoulder Motion

SCAPULAR MOTION

Resting Posture

The resting position of the scapula referable to the trunk is anteriorly rotated about 30 degrees[62, 98] with respect to the frontal plane as viewed from above. The scapula is also rotated (Fig. 6–15) upward about 3 degrees referable to the transverse plane as viewed from the back (Fig. 6–16). Finally, it is tilted forward (anteflexed) about 20 degrees with respect to the sagittal plane[62] when viewed from the side. Interestingly, this posture of the scapula is not influenced by an external load (up to 20 kg) applied to the extremity.[62]

GLENOHUMERAL MOTION

Resting Posture

The humeral head rests in the center of the glenoid when viewed in the plane of the glenoid surface.[37, 56] Fick refers to this relationship as *Nullmeridianebene* or dead meridian plane.[37] The humeral head and shaft are thought to lie in the plane of the scapula. The 30-degree retroversion of the articular orientation is complemented by the 30-degree anterior rotation of the scapula on the trunk. With the arm at the side, this relationship is referred to as the "zero position" by Nobuhara.[76]

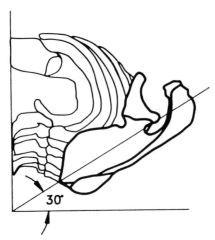

Figure 6–15. The resting position of the scapula is about 30 degrees forward with respect to the coronal plane as viewed in the transverse plane.

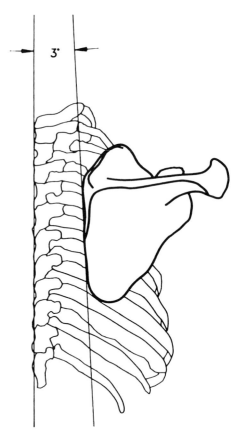

Figure 6–16. The resting position of the scapula is rotated about 3 degrees superior as viewed in the frontal plane.

ARTICULAR SURFACE AND ORIENTATION

Humerus

The articular surface of the humerus constitutes approximately one-third of the surface of a sphere with an arc of about 120 degrees. This articular surface is oriented with an upward tilt of approximately 45 degrees and is retroverted approximately 30 degrees referable to the condylar line of the distal humerus (Fig. 6–17).[25, 31, 37, 98]

Glenoid

In the coronal plane, the articular surface of the glenoid comprises an arc of approximately 75 degrees. The shape of the articulation is that of an inverted comma. The typical long axis dimension is about 3.5 to 4.0 cm. In the transverse plane, the arc of curvature of the glenoid is only about 50 degrees with a linear dimension of about 2.5 to 3.0 cm.[37] The relationship of the articular surface to the body of the scapula is difficult to precisely define owing to the difficulty of defining a frame of reference. Typically, it is accepted that the glenoid has a slight upward tilt of about 5 degrees[8] referable to the medial border of the scapula and is retroverted a mean of approximately 7 degrees,

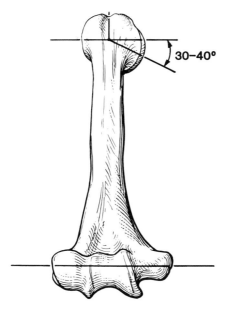

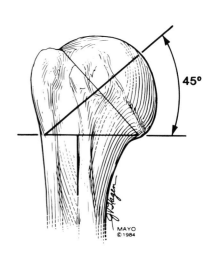

Figure 6–17. The two-dimensional orientation of the articular surface of the humerus with respect to the bicondylar axis.

although there is considerable individual variation in these measurements (Fig. 6–18).[89]

Saha has defined the relationship of the dimensions of the humeral head and the glenoid as the glenohumeral ratio. This relationship is approximately 0.8 in the coronal plane and 0.6 in the horizontal or transverse plane.[89] This is consistent with several observations that estimated that only about one-third of the surface of the humeral head is in contact with the glenoid at any given time.[98]

Arm Elevation

The most important function of the shoulder—arm elevation—has been extensively studied to determine the relationship and contribution of the glenohumeral and scapulothoracic joints, the so-called scapulotho-

racic rhythm.* Although early descriptions of the scapulothoracic rhythm have been performed referable to the coronal (frontal) plane, recent discussion has defined this motion referable to the scapular plane. Neither reference system is completely adequate to fully describe the complex rotational sequences involved in elevation of the arm, since the scapular position changes during elevation usually have not been considered.

Early descriptions of this motion defined the glenohumeral contribution as the first 90 degrees, followed by scapulothoracic rotation.[98] Subsequent discussions place the overall glenohumeral-scapulothoracic motion at a two-to-one ratio.[51, 62] More sophisticated investi-

---

*See references 24, 34, 36, 39, 48, 51, 63, 76, 82, 89.

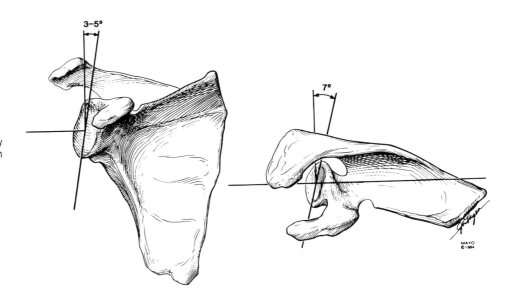

Figure 6–18. The glenoid faces slightly superior and posterior (retroverted) with respect to the body of the scapula.

gations indicate an inconsistent ratio during the first 30 degrees of elevation[39, 106] with variation by individual and even by sex.[34]

Poppen and Walker report a four-to-one glenohumeral to scapulothoracic motion ratio during the first 25 degrees of arm elevation.[82] Thereafter, an almost equal five-to-four rotation ratio occurs during subsequent elevation. The overall ratio averages about two to one.

The lack of linearity of this motion complex has also been observed by Doddy and coworkers, who showed a seven-to-one ratio of scapulothoracic to glenohumeral motion during the first 30 degrees of elevation and approximately a one-to-one ratio from 90 degrees to 150 degrees of arm elevation.[34] Others have also shown the nonlinear variation during elevation.[76] Further evaluation of the arm against resistance elicits scapulothoracic motion earlier than with passive motion alone.[34]

The various studies have been simply summarized by Bergmann.[14] During the first 30 degrees of elevation, variably greater motion occurs at the glenohumeral joint. The last 60 degrees occurs with about an equal contribution of the glenohumeral and scapulothoracic motion. The overall ratio throughout the entire arc of elevation is about two to one (Fig. 6–19).

With upward movement of the arm, a complex rotational motion of the scapula occurs (Fig. 6–20). In addition to the upward rotation described above, about 6 degrees of anterior rotation referable to the thorax occurs during the first 90 degrees of arm elevation. Posterior rotation of about 16 degrees occurs next so that the scapula comes to rest about 10 degrees posteriorly rotated compared with the original resting position.[24] Thus, an arc of about 15 degrees of anteroposterior rotation of the scapula occurs with elevation of the arm. Concurrently, about 20 degrees of forward tilt referable to the thorax also occurs during elevation.[62]

EXTERNAL ROTATION OF THE HUMERUS

Early observers noted that an "obligatory" external rotation of the humerus was necessary for maximum elevation.[56] Tuberosity impingement with the coracoacromial arch was assumed to be the mechanical constraint. External rotation clears the tuberosity posteriorly, allowing for full arm elevation (Fig. 6–21).[56] A further explanation is that with external rotation the articulation of the humerus, which is retroverted with respect to the glenoid, is rotated anteriorly into a more optimum position for articulation with the glenoid. Finally, it has been observed in our laboratory that external rotation of the humerus also loosens the inferior ligaments of the glenohumeral joint. This mechanism thus releases the inferior checkrein effect, allowing full elevation of the arm. Full elevation with maximum external rotation has also recently been shown to be a position of greater stability of the shoulder than the elevated position.[36]

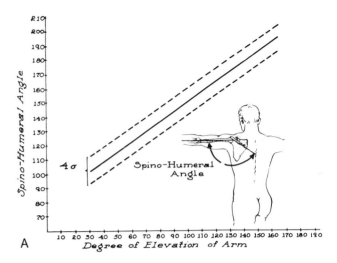

A

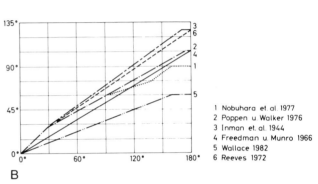

B

1	Nobuhara et. al. 1977
2	Poppen u. Walker 1976
3	Inman et. al. 1944
4	Freedman u. Munro 1966
5	Wallace 1982
6	Reeves 1972

Figure 6–19. *A,* The classic study by Inman and colleagues shows the relationship between glenohumeral and scapulothoracic motion. (Reproduced with permission from Inman VT, Saunders M, and Abbott LC: Observations on the function of the shoulder joint. J Bone Joint Surg 26:1, 1944.) *B,* Angular changes of the glenohumeral joint with respect to arm elevation were determined by several investigators. (Reproduced with permission from Bergmann G: Biomechanics and pathomechanics of the shoulder joint with reference to prosthetic joint replacement. *In* Kolbel R, et al (eds): Shoulder Replacement. Berlin, Springer-Verlag, 1987.)

The role of internal rotation and arm elevation has hardly been investigated. Experiments in our laboratory have shown that maximum glenohumeral elevation (scapula fixed) with the arm in full internal rotation occurs in a plane about 20 to 30 degrees posterior to that of the scapula and is limited to only about 115 degrees.[18]

Combining the motion of the glenohumeral and scapulothoracic joints, this complex sequence of events has been divided into four stages. First, glenohumeral motion occurs; next, sternoclavicular and then acromioclavicular rotations are observed with elevation of the scapula; finally, the scapula pivots upward around the acromioclavicular joint. This simplified analytical description is, in general, consistent with the observations of Laumann, Nobuhara, and others.[62, 76]

Joint Contact

The joint contact area and position changes during various glenohumeral motions and is difficult to accu-

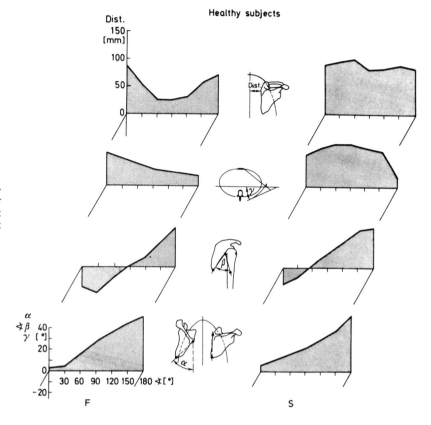

Figure 6–20. Complex three-dimensional rotation and translation of the scapula during arm elevation (see text for description). (Reproduced with permission from Laumann U: Kinesiology of the shoulder joint. *In* Kolbel R, et al (eds): Shoulder Replacement. Berlin: Springer-Verlag, 1987.)

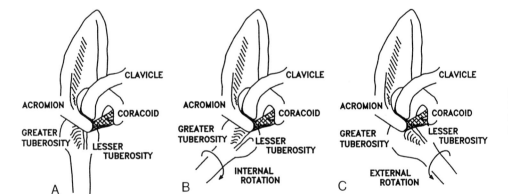

Figure 6–21. Upward elevation of the arm requires obligatory external rotation to avoid tuberosity impingement under the acromial process.

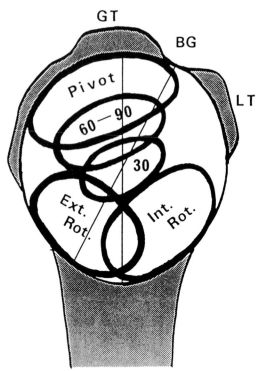

Figure 6–22. Humeral contact positions as a function of glenohumeral motion and positions. (Reproduced with permission from Nobuhara K: The Shoulder: Its Function and Clinical Aspects. Tokyo: Igaku-Shoin, 1987.)

rately measure by direct techniques. The contact point moves forward and inferior during internal rotation.[62, 89] With external rotation, the contact is just posteroinferior (Fig. 6–22). Saha reports that with elevation the contact area moves superiorly. If combined with internal and external rotation, however, the humeral head remains centered in the glenoid as viewed in the axillary plane.[48]

CENTER OF ROTATION

An accurate calculation of the instantaneous center of rotation of the humeral head is a complex problem that is much simplified if the motion is limited to a single plane.[95, 101] Such has been the assumption of most analysis. Hence, the center of rotation of the glenohumeral joint has been defined as a locus of points situated within 6.0 ± 2.0 mm of the geometric center of the humeral head (see Fig. 6–11).[82] This definition, generated by the Rouleaux technique, is considered reasonably accurate.[103] However, this particular technique for defining the center of rotation is accurate only for pure rolling motion, is subject to input-type error,[96] and is not accurate in pathological conditions in which translation is a significant component of the displacement or if there is a significant amount of nonplanar motion. This may explain why other authors have found the center to lie 8.0 mm behind and 6.0 mm below the intersection of the shaft and head axes.[53] Still others have reported that multiple centers of rotation occur during abduction.[29]

The relatively small dimension of this locus and the relative consistency of its definition as lying in the geometric center of the humeral head reflects the small amount of translation that normally occurs at this joint and is consistent with the above observations. A small amount (about 3 mm) of upward translation has been reported in the intact shoulder during the first 30 degrees of elevation; only about 1 mm of additional excursion occurs with elevation measured at greater than 30 degrees.[82] Furthermore, an increase of up to 1 cm of translation occurs with certain pathological processes such as rotator cuff deficiency.

The center of rotation of the scapula for arm elevation is situated at the tip of the acromion as viewed edge on (Fig. 6–23).

Screw Axis

The application of SDA for glenohumeral joint motion has one specific advantage. Using the concept of the intersection or the middle point of the common perpendicular between two instantaneous screw axes as the measurement of the "three-dimensional instantaneous center of rotation," the stability or laxity of the joint can be described. If the joint is tight and stable, the points of the intersections of all the screw axes will be confined within a small sphere (Fig. 6–24). On the other hand, when the joint is becoming unstable owing either to disease of the capsular-ligamentous structures or the rotator cuff, the points of the intersection of the screw axes will be more dispersed and confined in a larger sphere. This concept has the potential to be further developed as a useful clinical tool.

CLINICAL RELEVANCE

Understanding of the biomechanical features discussed above has several clinically relevant applications. The orientation of the scapula and humerus referable to the thorax and to each other has been important in designing the optimum radiographic studies to best visualize the scapulohumeral relationship. Thus, the true anteroposterior radiograph of the glenohumeral joint is taken 30 degrees oblique to the sagittal plane. Some feel that this orientation is closer to 45 degrees, as this angle produces a better true anteroposterior radiographic study.[86] The scapular view is taken at a 30-degree angle to the frontal plane; hence the anteroposterior radiograph (Fig. 6–25) that is perpendicular to this view is taken at an angle of about 60 degrees to the thorax.[74]

The relationship of coupled external rotation with maximum arm elevation helps to explain, to some extent, the limitation of elevation that is seen with the frozen shoulder. To the extent that this condition results in limitation of external rotation, an even more severe restriction of arm elevation is apt to occur. Knowledge of this coupling effect is also important with respect to prescribing the appropriate physical

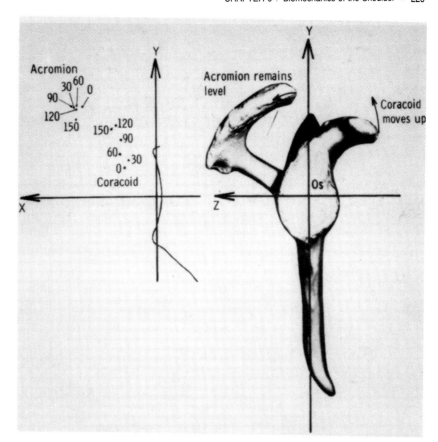

Figure 6–23. The center of rotation of the scapula for arm elevation is focused in the tip of the acromion. (Reproduced with permission from Poppen NK, and Walker PS: Normal and abnormal motion of the shoulder. J Bone Joint Surg *58A*:195, 1976.)

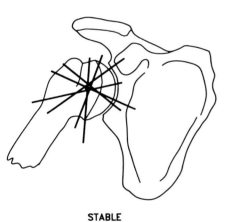

STABLE

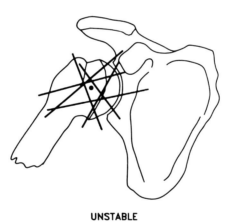

UNSTABLE

Figure 6–24. The common intersection of the screw axes creates a perfect ball-and-socket joint *(left)*. When significant translation occurs, the axes do not intersect at a single point *(right)*.

Figure 6–25. The anterior and lateral views of the glenohumeral joint were defined by Neer, based on knowledge of the scapulothoracic orientation. (Reproduced with permission from Neer CS II: Displaced proximal humeral fractures. I. Classification and evaluation. J Bone Joint Surg *52A*:1077, 1970.)

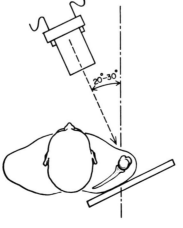

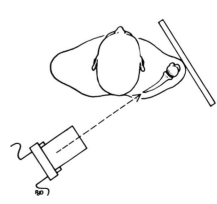

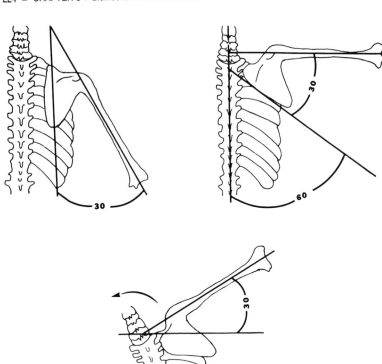

Figure 6–26. Arthrodesis of the glenohumeral joint in the optimum position allows arm elevation to and above the horizontal by scapulothoracic motion as well as by tilting of the trunk.

therapy after certain surgical procedures or pathological states.

Arthrodesis of the shoulder is an effective procedure but is most efficacious if the fusion is performed in the appropriate position.[88] Although the optimum position is debated, the basis of the selection is dependent on the normal scapulothoracic motion (Fig. 6–26). This knowledge, coupled with an understanding of the motion required for the activities of daily living, dictates the position of the fusion. This topic is discussed in more detail elsewhere in this text.

The potential for scapulothoracic motion provides an explanation of the remaining motion of the shoulder girdle present with frozen shoulder and after arthrodesis. In addition, the rotation of the scapula may be viewed as a means of providing a glenohumeral relationship that allows the deltoid muscle to remain effective even with the arm fully elevated (Fig. 6–27).

Understanding the axis of rotation is important for prosthetic replacement of the glenohumeral joint. The relative lack of translation in the intact shoulder justifies the design of an unconstrained glenoid surface. To the extent that the cuff musculature is deficient, a greater amount of translation is anticipated. This places additional requirements on the optimum glenoid design in order to accommodate the increased translation.[107] Probably more important is that, as will be discussed later, the initiation of shoulder abduction results in forces directed toward the superior rim of the glenoid; this has implications regarding the stability, force, and optimum prosthetic design and surgical implantation technique.

Finally, the well-recognized superior translation of the humeral head in the rotator cuff–deficient shoulder is explained in part by the pull of the deltoid and lack of soft tissue interposition of the rotator cuff (Fig. 6–28).[109]

Of equal and possibly greater importance in accounting for proximal migration is the superiorly directed resultant vector that occurs with initiation of abduction by the intact deltoid.

Thus, knowledge of the motion of the glenohumeral and scapulothoracic joints has numerous current clinical applications. A clear knowledge of these factors is important for the proper diagnosis and management of many shoulder conditions.

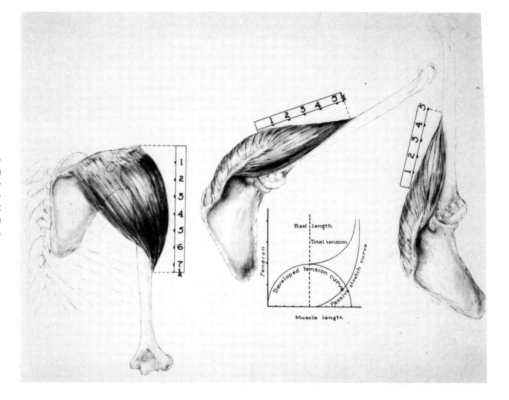

Figure 6–27. Scapulothoracic motion allows the deltoid to remain in the optimum position for effective contraction throughout the arch of arm elevation. (Reproduced with permission from Lucas DB: Biomechanics of the shoulder joint. Arch Surg *107(3):*425, 1973. Copyright 1973, American Medical Association.)

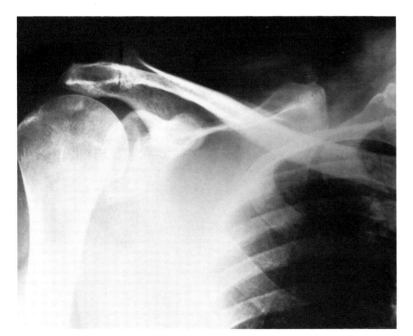

Figure 6–28. Superior migration of the humeral head in the rotator cuff–deficient shoulder is due in part to the pull of the deltoid muscle.

Constraints

It is convenient to consider the constraints of any joint as consisting of static and dynamic elements. The static contribution may be further subdivided into articular and capsular-ligamentous components (Table 6–2). Knowledge of the shoulder constraints is of particular clinical interest as it pertains to anterior dislocation and, more recently, posterior and multidirectional recurrent instability of the shoulder.[27, 75]

Early investigators focused on one element or the other. Hence, Saha emphasized the articular component of shoulder stability,[28, 89] Moseley[73] and Townley[103] focused on the capsular ligamentous complex, and DePalma and others emphasized the dynamic contribution of the interrelationship between the dynamic and the static capsular ligamentous constraints.[17, 33, 47]

STATIC CONSTRAINTS

Articular Contribution to Glenohumeral Stability

The humeral articular surface is not inherently stable. The 30-degree retroversion is obviously necessary for the proper balance of the soft tissues and normal kinematics. Most studies of the articular contribution to shoulder stability have focused on the glenoid. The glenoid articulation demonstrates a slight but definite posterior or retroverted orientation averaging about 7 degrees referable to the body of the scapula (see Fig. 6–18). Saha has emphasized that this orientation is an important contribution to the stability of the joint.[89] Although significant individual variation and degree of retroversion has been correlated with a greater tendency for recurrent dislocation of the shoulder in those with less retroversion,[89] this hypothesis has not been confirmed by subsequent investigators and is not popularly held today.

Only 25 to 30 per cent of the humeral head is covered by the glenoid surface in any given anatomical position.[17, 25, 98] The dimensional relationship between the humeral head and the glenoid reflects the inherent instability of the joint and has been referred to as the *glenohumeral index*. This is calculated as

$$\frac{\text{maximum diameter of glenoid}}{\text{maximum diameter of humeral head}}$$

Table 6–2. STATIC AND DYNAMIC CONTRIBUTIONS TO SHOULDER STABILITY

Static
Soft tissue
Glenohumeral ligaments
Labrum
Capsule
Articular surface
Dynamic
Rotator cuff muscles

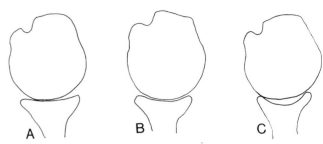

Figure 6–29. Articular stability of the glenohumeral joint is enhanced or lessened according to the variation in articular congruence: *A,* shallow glenoid surface; *B,* conforming surfaces; and *C,* excessively deepened glenoid surfaces. (Modified from Saha AK: Dynamic stability of the glenohumeral joint. Acta Orthop Scand 42:491, 1971.)

Saha calculated this ratio as approximately 0.75 in the sagittal plane and as approximately 0.6 in the more critical transverse plane.[89] More recently, this relationship has been redetermined with similar values of 0.86 and 0.58, respectively.[65] Developmental hypoplasia of the glenoid may alter this ratio and may play some role in recurrent dislocation of the shoulder, but such observations have been rather limited in the clinical literature.[71] Subtle variation of the articular anatomy of the glenoid has also been described and has been advocated as an explanation for inherent instability of the joint (Fig. 6–29). There is little clinical or basic research data to support this hypothesis. In general, according to the current literature the articular contribution to the stability of this joint is minimal, and significant variations of the articular orientation are not common.[13]

As noted, the glenoid articular surface comprises an arc of about 75 degrees.[98] Although the depth of the glenoid is minimal it is functionally deepened by the presence of the glenoid labrum. The early literature placed a major emphasis on this anatomical structure as increasing the stability offered by the glenoid articular surface. This consideration has received relatively little support in recent years. Moseley and Overgaard demonstrated that the labrum was a specialized portion of the anterior capsule.[73] With external rotation, this structure flattens and thus serves only as a source of attachment of the inferior glenohumeral ligament; hence, they conclude that the labrum itself seems to offer little to the inherent stability of the joint. However, more recent studies have placed additional importance to the labrum.[47] Howell and Galinat measured an average depth of 9.0 mm in the superior-to-inferior direction of the glenoid.[47] This is equivalent to approximately 40 per cent of the radius of a typical 44-mm humeral replacement prosthesis. The anteroposterior depth of the glenoid measured an average of only 2.5 mm. However, these investigators felt that the anterior and posterior glenoid labrum added an additional 2.5 mm of depth. Once again, these data suggest that the labrum may be effective in increasing the depth of the glenoid and hence has some contribution to articular stability. The precise role of the glenoid labrum in joint stability has yet to be defined.

The slight 5-degree superior tilt of the articular

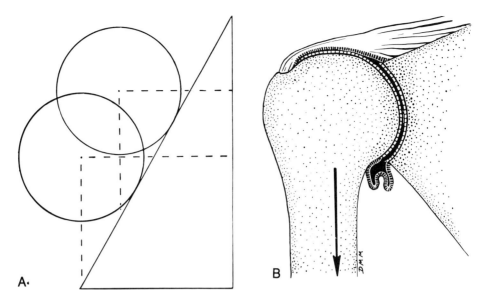

Figure 6–30. The upward tilt of the glenoid, coupled with the superior glenohumeral ligament and coracohumeral ligament, resists passive downward displacement of the humeral head. (Reproduced with permission from Basmajian JV, and Bazant FJ: Factors preventing downward dislocation of the adducted shoulder joint. J Bone Joint Surg 41A:1182, 1959.)

surface has been offered by Basmajian as a factor in preventing inferior subluxation of the humerus when combined with the effect of the superior capsule and superior glenohumeral ligament (Fig. 6–30).[8] However, a recent intensive study by Kumar and Balasubramaniam has shown that a negative pressure normally exists in the glenohumeral joint.[60] If this pressure is equalized by an arthrotomy or even by a small puncture, inferior subluxation of the shoulder readily occurs (Fig. 6–31). This effect is greater when the cuff musculature has been removed but is present in the muscle-intact specimens as well. It is of interest that a similar observation was also reported in 1930 by Lockhart.[63]

In general it might be concluded, based on the current literature, that the articular geometry as such offers minimal static stability to the shoulder.

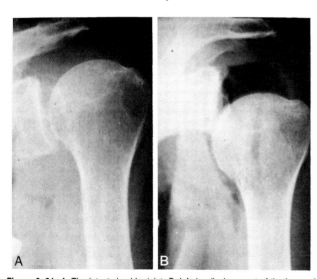

Figure 6–31. A, The intact shoulder joint. B, Inferior displacement of the humeral head occurs with loss of hydrostatic pressure of the glenohumeral joint. (Reproduced with permission from Kumar VP, and Balasubramaniam P: The role of atmospheric pressure in stabilizing the shoulder: an experimental study. J Bone Joint Surg 67B(5):719, 1985.)

Capsular and Ligamentous Contributions to Static Shoulder Stability

Little is known of the biochemical constitution of the capsule of the shoulder joint except that it is composed of Type I, III, and V collagen. In this respect (not surprisingly), its composition is qualitatively similar to that of the elbow and other joints.[58] The forces

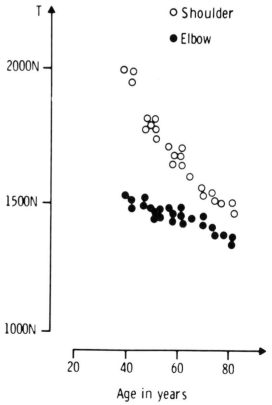

Figure 6–32. Comparison of dislocation forces at the shoulder and elbow. (Reproduced with permission from Kaltsas DS: Comparative study of the properties of the shoulder joint capsules with those of other joint capsules. Clin Orthop 173:20, 1973.)

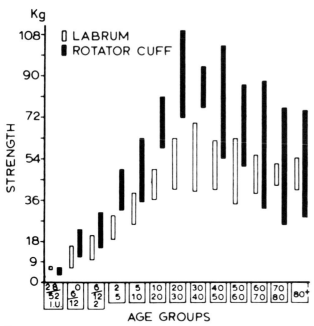

Figure 6–33. Tensile strength of the labrum, capsular complex, and rotator cuff as a function of age. (Reproduced with permission from Reeves B: Experiments on the tensile strength of the anterior capsular structures of the shoulder region. J Bone Joint Surg *50B*:858, 1968.)

required to dislocate the shoulder and elbow were studied by Kaltsas. A markedly greater force of up to 2000 newtons (N) was required to disrupt the shoulder complex, compared with the 1500 N required for the elbow in individuals under 40 years of age.[58] The force to dislocate both these joints decreases with increasing age, but the decrease is more drastic in the shoulder (Fig. 6–32). The tensile strength of the anterior capsular complex has been investigated by Reeves.[84] The cadaver specimen demonstrated a maximum tensile stress of about 70 N. Considerable variation exists with

age and from individual to individual. Less tensile resistance was noted in those under 20 and over 50 years of age (Fig. 6–33). The anterior shear force has been calculated to be about 60 kg if the arm is abducted and externally rotated (Fig. 6–34). Hence, the static constraints may potentially be exceeded under certain muscle activity or loading conditions.[70]

The shoulder capsule itself is thin and redundant. In some individuals this redundancy may be a congenital variation from the normal and hence may predispose to shoulder instability.[105] The capsule-ligament complex consists of superior, middle, and inferior portions that, together with the coracohumeral ligament, constitute the defined ligamentous structures of the anterior and superior shoulder joint (Fig. 6–35). These structures were defined and carefully depicted by Flood in 1829.[38]

Coracohumeral Ligament

The coracohumeral ligament originates from the anterior lateral base of the coracoid process and extends as two bands over the top of the shoulder to blend with the capsule and attach to the greater and lesser tuberosities.[59] This ligament is a constant finding and is considered the most consistent of the ligaments of the fibrous capsule.[32] The function of this ligament has not been studied extensively. Terry and coworkers and Basmajian and associates have demonstrated that it becomes taut in external rotation and also that it appears to contribute to resisting inferior subluxation of the joint (see Fig. 6–30).[8, 102]

Superior Glenohumeral Ligament

The superior glenohumeral ligament is a constant structure arising from the tubercle of the glenoid

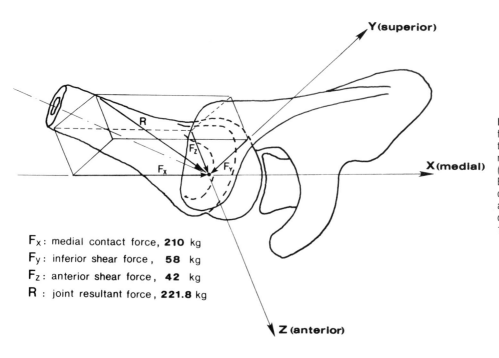

F_x: medial contact force, **210** kg
F_y: inferior shear force, **58** kg
F_z: anterior shear force, **42** kg
R : joint resultant force, **221.8** kg

Figure 6–34. A significant anterior shear force of up to 40 kg is generated when the shoulder is abducted and externally rotated and all muscles are contracting. (Reproduced with permission from Morrey BF, and Chao EYS: Recurrent anterior dislocation of the shoulder. *In* Block J, and Dumbleton JH (eds): Clinical Biomechanics. New York: Churchill Livingstone, 1981.)

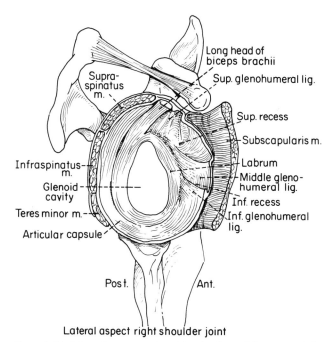

Figure 6–35. Schematic representation of the glenohumeral ligaments and the rotator cuff stabilizers of the glenohumeral joint. (Reproduced with permission from Morrey BF, and Chao EYS: Recurrent anterior dislocation of the shoulder. *In* Black J, and Dumbleton JH (eds): Clinical Biomechanics. New York: Churchill Livingstone, 1981.)

anterior to the origin of the long biceps tendon and running inferior and lateral to insert on the head of the humerus near the proximal tip of the lesser tuberosity (Fig. 6–36). Basmajian thought that the function of the superior glenohumeral ligament was, in conjunction with the superior tilt of the glenoid, to provide passive resistance to inferior subluxation or dislocation of the humerus.[102] Recent work supports this concept by showing that if this structure is intact, the shoulder does not translate posteriorly and inferiorly even in the absence of the inferior ligament and capsule.[91] When this structure is sectioned, however, the lesion created in the posterior-inferior capsule allows the humeral head to readily dislocate inferiorly.

These observations support Dempster's global concept of stability as being provided by both the anterior and posterior structures, since both are observed to force the articular surface of the humeral head against the glenoid (Fig. 6–37). Translation in one direction causes tension in the ligament on the opposite side of the joint; thus, inferior translation causes increased tension in the superior capsule and the superior glenohumeral ligament.

Middle Glenohumeral Ligament

The middle glenohumeral ligament originates from the supraglenoid tubercle at the superior aspect of the glenoid and from the anterior superior aspect of the labrum and extends laterally and inferiorly to blend with the subscapularis tendon about 2.0 cm medial to its insertion at the lesser tuberosity (see Figs. 6–35 and 6–36). The middle glenohumeral ligament is a substantial structure measuring up to 2.0 cm in width and 4.0 mm in thickness.[30] This ligament is one of the more developed of the glenohumeral ligaments and was reported by DePalma, Moseley, and others to be the major constraint to anterior humeral displacement.[32, 73] It is observed to become taut when the shoulder is abducted and externally rotated.[104] Although its origin is from the superior aspect of the labrum, this attachment is probably not often disrupted with recurrent anterior dislocation. Turkel and coworkers also observed the middle glenohumeral ligament to tighten in the position of instability when the shoulder is abducted and externally rotated (Fig. 6–38).[104] Selective sectioning of the glenohumeral ligament does allow for increased excursion but does not typically result in instability.[91] Thus, although this structure is not essential to resist anterior translation with abduction and external rotation, in this position it does nonetheless contribute to anterior stability of the glenohumeral joint.

The ligament is observed to become taut in extremes of both internal and external rotation, which is consistent with the constraint hypothesis of Dempster.

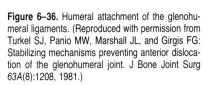

Figure 6–36. Humeral attachment of the glenohumeral ligaments. (Reproduced with permission from Turkel SJ, Panio MW, Marshall JL, and Girgis FG: Stabilizing mechanisms preventing anterior dislocation of the glenohumeral joint. J Bone Joint Surg 63A(8):1208, 1981.)

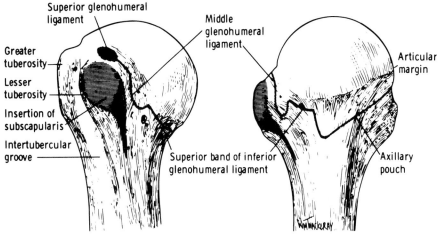

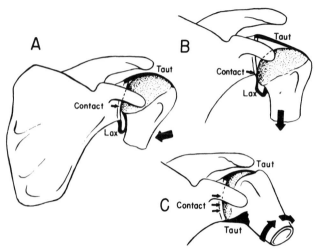

Figure 6–37. Dempster's concept of the shared contribution of the ligaments and articular surface in providing stability to a joint system. (Reproduced with permission from Dempster WT: Mechanisms of shoulder movement. Arch Phys Med Rehab 46A:49, 1965.)

Inferior Glenohumeral Ligament

DePalma believed that the inferior glenohumeral ligament was a relatively unimportant stabilizer since, in his dissections, about one-half of the specimens lacked a recognizable, discrete inferior glenohumeral ligament.[33] Recent interpretations of the anatomy of the shoulder have suggested an expanded definition of the ligament that includes the anteroinferior, inferior, and posteroinferior capsule, regardless of whether or not a discrete thickening is present (see Figs. 6–35 and 6–36).[104] On careful inspection, the origin of the inferior glenohumeral ligament is found to consist of almost the entire anterior glenoid labrum (Fig. 6–39). It then courses laterally and inferiorly to insert on the inferior margin of the humeral articular surface and then down and around the anatomical neck of the femur (see Fig. 6–36). This anatomical arrangement is consistent with the emerging data suggesting the central role and

function of this ligament in anterior and inferior glenohumeral instability.[75]

A clear understanding of the inferior glenohumeral ligaments helps to resolve some of the controversial issues regarding anterior and inferior shoulder instability. The clinical significance of a detached labrum leading to recurrent anterior dislocation is explained in view of the fact that this lesion leads to an incompetent inferior glenohumeral ligament complex.

The entire inferior capsule traditionally has been recognized as one of the contributing factors to limiting elevation of the arm.[24, 56, 79] The structure also becomes taut with internal or external rotation of the dependent humerus.[104] Release of the inferior glenohumeral ligament has been further demonstrated to allow anterior and inferior subluxation in the experimental model.[91] Of interest, however, is the fact that the greatest amount of inferior translation occurs only when the superior posterior capsule is also released. Similar observations were made by Ovesen and Nielsen, who studied the entire glenohumeral complex as a unit. Increased anterior translation occurred with posterior capsular release (Fig. 6–40).[78] Conversely, increased posterior translation was shown to increase with sectioning of the anterior capsule. The overall displacement patterns increased with inferior capsular release.

These observations also pertain to posterior translation of the humeral head.[78, 91] Release of the anterior structures increases the posterior rotation and translation of the humeral head. The patterns described relate to translation in the neutral position. Different results would be expected if the arm were fully internally or externally rotated.

In summary, the major static stabilizer of the shoulder joint consists of the capsular-ligamentous complex, with the inferior glenohumeral ligament being the most essential component of the complex. Yet the function of the other components must not be overlooked; hence the concept of "load sharing" of the soft tissue constraints. This concept states that the ligaments function in a coordinated manner to resist joint trans-

ANTERIOR-POSTERIOR VIEWS

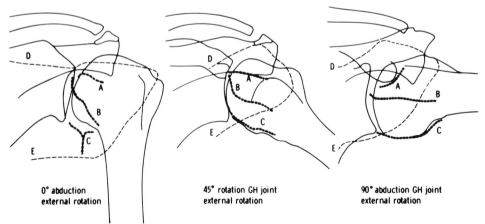

0° abduction
external rotation

45° rotation GH joint
external rotation

90° abduction GH joint
external rotation

Figure 6–38. Orientation of the glenohumeral ligaments as a function of shoulder position. A, B and C are the superior, middle, and inferior glenohumeral ligaments, respectively; D–E outlines the capsule. (Reproduced with permission from Turkel SJ, Panio MW, Marshall JL, and Girgis FG: Stabilizing mechanisms preventing anterior dislocation of the glenohumeral joint. J Bone Joint Surg 63A(8):1208, 1981.)

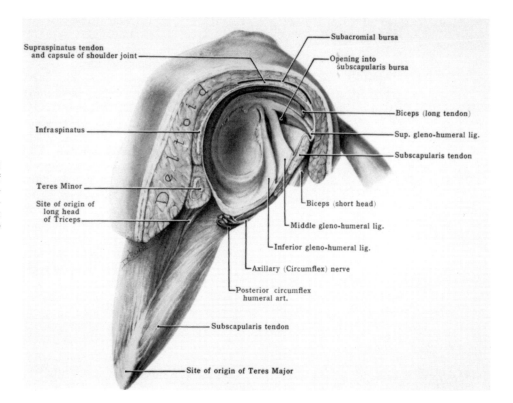

Figure 6–39. The inferior glenohumeral ligament inserts to the glenoid by way of the anterior labrum, extending more proximally than might be thought. (Reproduced with permission from Grant JCB: Method of Anatomy, 7th ed. © 1965, the Williams & Wilkins Co., Baltimore.)

lation, primarily by resisting displacement through their presence and secondarily by imparting increased joint contact pressure opposite the direction of displacement, which also increases joint stability (see Fig. 6–37).

DYNAMIC STABILIZERS

The suspensory stabilizing function of the active or passive muscle activity of the shoulder girdle is surprisingly minimal under resting conditions.[90] Electromyographic studies revealed inactivity of the deltoid, pectoralis major, serratus anterior, and latissimus dorsi muscles when the arm is hanging freely at the side. Subsequent investigations have shown no or minimal EMG activity even when the upper extremity is loaded up to 25 pounds.[10] These findings are in concert with and give further credence to the previously discussed theories that negative pressure and the articular-ligamentous constraints resist inferior subluxation of the humeral head.

Dynamic shoulder stability during activity occurs by action of the shoulder musculature. Of the 26 muscles controlling the shoulder girdle, only the four components of the rotator cuff are thought to play a significant role in the dynamic stability of this joint.[96] The contribution of the cuff muscles to joint stability may be due to (1) passive muscle tension from the bulk effect of the muscle itself;[18, 60, 102] (2) contraction causing compression of the articular surfaces; (3) joint motion

that secondarily tightens the passive ligamentous constraints; and (4) the barrier effect of the contracted muscle.

Passive Muscle Tension

The passive role played by muscle bulk in joint stability is demonstrated by the increased passive arc of motion when the muscle is removed.[18, 79] Howell and Galinat have demonstrated that when the soft tissue envelope of the skin and the muscle is removed, up to 10 mm of additional superior and inferior translation may occur.[47] Ovesen and Nielsen have also shown increased translation, both anteriorly and posteriorly, with shoulder muscle release in the cadaver specimen (Fig. 6–41).[78] Kumar and Balasubramaniam have also shown greater inferior translocation due to the effect of gravity when the muscles are removed in a cadaver preparation.[60]

Compression of the Articular Surface

By simulating active rotator cuff muscle function, an elaborate cadaver experiment has demonstrated that the humeral head is positioned in the center of the glenoid in the horizontal plane.[47] Of interest is the fact that this stabilizing effect may be largely independent of the specific simulated muscle action. Even with unequal ("unbalanced") simulated activity of the anterior and posterior cuff musculature, the function of the active cuff still brings about the centering phenom-

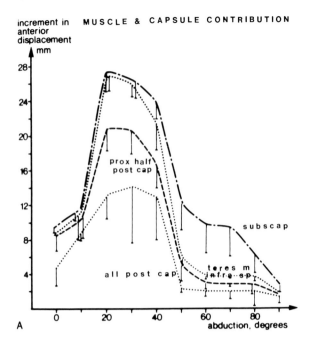

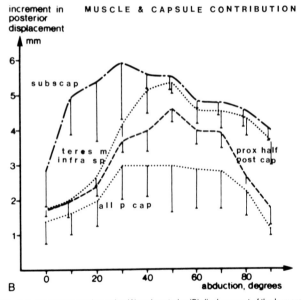

Figure 6–40. Incremental anterior *(A)* and posterior *(B)* displacement of the humeral head in millimeters as a function of serial release of the constraints on glenohumeral joint motion. (Reproduced with permission from Ovesen J, and Nielsen S: Anterior and posterior shoulder instability. Acta Orthop Scand 57:324; copyright © 1986, Munksgaard International Publishers Ltd., Copenhagen, Denmark.)

enon. It has thus been hypothesized that the centering effect of the humeral head in the glenoid is possible without balanced muscle activity and that the contact area and pressure are mediated by secondary obligatory tightening of the ligaments.

Dynamic Elements Causing Secondary Tightening of Static Constraints

Dempster has pointed out that the supraspinatus muscle simultaneously elevates and externally rotates

the arm.[31] As has been previously shown, external rotation tightens the inferior ligament and thus limits upward elevation. Thus the cuff musculature rotates the shoulder to a configuration rendered stable, at least in part, by tightening of the ligaments in the direction opposite the rotation (see Fig. 6–37).[24, 31]

Barrier Effect

The dampening effect of the shoulder musculature during active motion and the subsequent limitation of the active arc of motion have been long recognized.[24] Classically, the subscapularis muscle has been shown to be important, if not essential, as an anterior barrier to resist anterior-inferior humeral head displacement. When the subscapularis is lax or stretched, recurrent anterior dislocation occurs; hence, several procedures have been directed toward restoring or strengthening the barrier effect of the subscapularis.[33, 100] Furthermore, the cross-sectional areas of the anterior (subscapularis) and posterior (infraspinatus and teres minor) rotators are approximately equal.[9] Thus the torques generated by these groups are balanced and represent a force couple that resists both anterior and posterior humeral head translation.

CENTRAL CONCEPT OF SHOULDER STABILITY

The above observations may be summarized as follows. The glenohumeral joint enjoys a great degree of motion because of the complex interrelationship of the articular, capsular-ligamentous, and dynamic stabilizers. There is virtually no inherent stability imparted by the articular surfaces. The glenohumeral ligament complex prevents external rotation, and the inferior component is the primary restraint against anterior and inferior displacement. Translation is limited in part by the capsular-ligamentous complex situated opposite the direction of motion. The rotator cuff imparts a dynamic element to stability, directly as a barrier resisting translation and indirectly by moving the joint into a position that tightens the capsular-ligamentous complex. Both of these mechanisms cause increased compression of the articular surfaces, which further enhances the stability of the glenohumeral joint.

CLINICAL RELEVANCE

The topic of shoulder stability is covered extensively in this text, and details of the surgical procedures need not be addressed here. Suffice it to say that shoulder stability is one of the most common clinical problems. As our understanding increases and as patients' expectations expand, the problem has taken on an even greater significance and complexity than was once appreciated. An articular defect regularly occurs in the humeral head after anterior dislocation; this has been recognized for over 100 years.[21, 43] Yet the biomechanical data indicate that the articular surface offers little to stability. Thus most procedures directed at altering

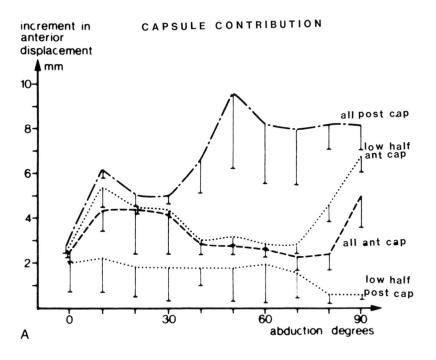

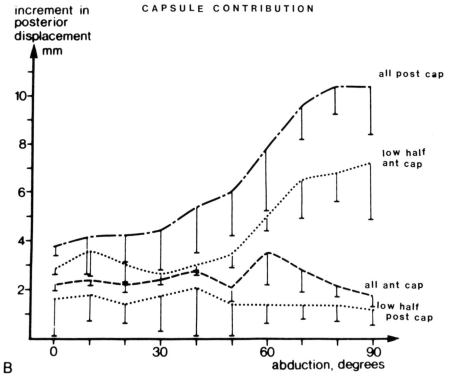

Figure 6–41. Anterior *(A)* and posterior *(B)* translation of the shoulder joint with serial constraint release as a function of glenohumeral position. Removal of the muscle envelope increases possible displacement. (Reproduced with permission from Ovesen J, and Nielsen S: Anterior and posterior shoulder instability. Acta Orthop Scand 57:324; copyright © 1986, Munksgaard International Publishers Ltd., Copenhagen, Denmark.)

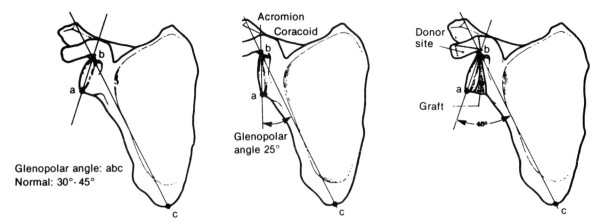

Figure 6–42. Glenoid osteotomy is the acceptable clinical option for posterior instability but not for typical anterior instability problems. (Reproduced with permission from Bestard EA, Schvene HR, and Bestard EH: Glenoplasty in the management of recurrent shoulder dislocation. Contemp Orthop 12:47, 1986.)

the articular relationship have limited benefit. The exception to this is posterior instability or those instances that relate to osseous deficiency;[15, 92] in these circumstances, glenoid osteotomy or augmentation procedures are appropriate options (Fig. 6–42). Yet the significance of these capsular mechanisms has probably not been fully appreciated.[27, 75] It is possible that more careful observation will confirm the anterior or anteroposterior capsular-ligamentous complex as important in resisting posteroinferior shoulder dislocation.[27]

Muscle-tightening procedures effectively improve stability by intentionally limiting range of motion. This causes functional limitation that is no longer an accepted clinical goal. Biomechanical data have clarified the central role of the inferior ligament complex in providing shoulder stability. With the recognition that this ligament inserts or attaches to the glenoid via the labrum, a rationale for the observation of Bankart and for the more popular current procedures—that is, those directed at restoring capsular-ligamentous integrity—is provided (Fig. 6–43).* This knowledge now allows for restoration of stability and preservation of motion.

---

*See references 6, 67, 68, 75, 78, 85, 88, 102.

Correlation of the biomechanical data of the capsular tensile strength (less than 20 kg)[84] and the anterior shear force possible from muscle contraction (60 kg)[70] may help to explain the spontaneous dislocation seen after some seizure episodes.

The stabilizing effect of negative pressure in the shoulder is not well recognized, but possibly it helps to explain the often observed phenomenon of inferior humeral head subluxation following proximal humeral fractures (Fig. 6–44). Although this finding traditionally has been thought to be related to muscle atony, this explanation is not supported by the electromyographic data, which demonstrate a limited role of active muscle contracture in resisting downward displacement of the humeral head. On the other hand, the stabilizing effect of negative pressure, which is lost when a fracture tears the capsule, does provide at least one possible explanation for this phenomenon.

Muscle and Joint Forces

Forces across the glenohumeral joint will be considered in three parts: (1) the general and specific role of the muscles crossing the joint, (2) the idealized calcu-

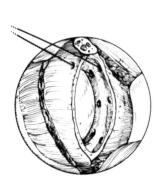

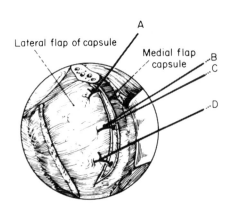

Figure 6–43. Anterior capsuloplasty provides excellent clinical results and has a sound rationale based on the biomechanics of this joint. (Reproduced with permission from Rowe CR, Patel D, and Southmayd WE: The Bankart procedure: a long-term end result study. J Bone Joint Surg 60A:1, 1978.)

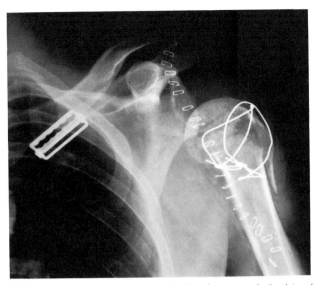

Figure 6-44. Inferior subluxation of the shoulder after open reduction–internal fixation of proximal fracture. Subluxation may be due to muscle astony and possibly also to a loss of the hydrostatic pressure of the shoulder joint.

Table 6-3. CROSS-SECTIONAL AREA AND PER CENT CONTRIBUTION OF MUSCLES CROSSING THE SHOULDER JOINT

Muscle	Area in cm² Contribution (Mean)	(%)
Biceps (LH)	2.01	(1.9)
Biceps (SH)	1.11	(2.0)
Corachobrachialis	1.60	(1.6)
Deltoid	18.17	(17.7)
Deltoid posterior	5.00	(4.9)
Infraspinatus and teres minor	13.74	(13.4)
Latissimus dorsi	12.00	(11.7)
Pectoralis major	13.34	(13.0)
Subscapularis	16.30	(15.9)
Supraspinatus	5.72	(5.6)
Teres major	8.77	(8.5)
Triceps (LH)	2.96	(3.8)

From Bassett R, Browne A, An K-N, and Morrey BF: A biomechanical analysis of shoulder muscles in the position of instability. J Biomech. Accepted for publication.

lation of the glenohumeral forces, and (3) the maximum strength characteristics for each motion function.

GENERAL OBSERVATIONS

Understanding the muscle function with regard to shoulder motion and force transmission requires consideration of three clinically recognized characteristics of that muscle: size, orientation, and activity.

Muscle Size

The effective size of a muscle, which relates to its ability to generate force, is called the *physiological cross-section*. This is not simply the area of a given muscle cross-section; it is the cross-section of the muscle fibers calculated by measuring the volume of the muscle and dividing by the fiber length. Calculation of this variable is a tedious task owing to the difficulty both in determining fiber lengths of different types of muscles and in accurately demonstrating muscle volume.[1] Yet this has been performed by several investigators (Table 6-3).[9] The proportional force per cross-sectional area of the muscle generating the force has been discussed by several authors but is not known with certainty.[50, 51, 72] Although estimates have varied considerably, our data support values of about 9.0 kg/cm².

Orientation

The accurate and precise definition of the orientation of each muscle is an essential variable in defining the forces that act on the shoulder in a given position. However, the accurate orientation of shoulder muscles is very difficult to define. Because of the great amount

of motion present and because the line of action frequently crosses close to the axis of rotation, some muscles change their function depending upon the position of the joint.[51, 62, 63, 99] Hence, the straight-line technique connecting the origin and insertion is only a first estimate that just approximates the effective moment of the muscle for a given position.[51] A more accurate determination consists of calculating the centroid of successive cross-sectional areas of the muscle as it crosses the joint. By connecting these centroids, an accurate determination of the orientation and lever arm of the muscle is possible at a given position (Fig. 6-45).[9] The limitation of this particular technique is that only a single position of the shoulder can be studied for a given specimen.[49] The effective lever arm of the shoulder muscles and the orientation of the muscle to the glenoid surface has been calculated for different positions by Poppen and Walker using radiographic techniques (Fig. 6-46).[83] A similar technique was employed by Howell and Galinat.[47] The moment arm may be analytically estimated by knowing the excursion of the muscle and the arc of motion that this muscle imparts, as well as the load required for the activity.[4, 55]

Activity

The final variable required to calculate joint force is whether a specific muscle is active during a given function and, if so, the degree of activity at a given joint position. Again, the technique to determine these data for all 26 muscles does not currently exist. The motors responsible for shoulder motion were first systematically defined by Duchenne, using galvanic stimulation.[35] These early efforts to define which muscles are active for given positions have been refined by electromyographic studies.[7, 10, 51, 93, 95]

These studies have demonstrated the important relationship of the integrated activity of the supraspinatus and deltoid muscles (Fig. 6-47).[7, 80] This is the best known and most important relationship for active

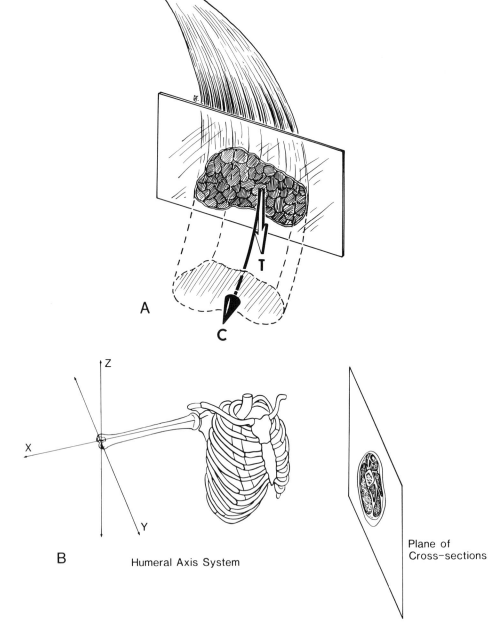

Figure 6–45. Cross-sectional studies of muscles allow an estimate of the force contributed by that muscle. *A,* The centroid estimates the location (C) and the size and magnitude (T) of the force. *B,* The technique is limited by allowing study of a single position per specimen.

A

B   Humeral Axis System

Plane of
Cross-sections

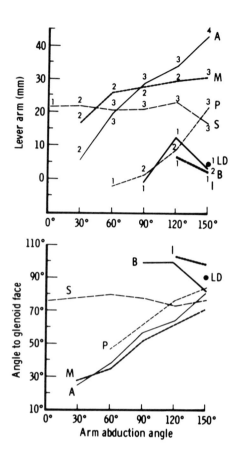

Figure 6–46. Moment arm of some of the essential shoulder muscles across the glenohumeral joint. A = anterior deltoid; P = posterior deltoid; B = subscapularis; M = middle deltoid; S = supraspinatus; LD = latissimus dorsi. (Reproduced with permission from Poppen NK, and Walker PS: Normal and abnormal motion of the shoulder. J Bone Joint Surg 58A:195, 1976.)

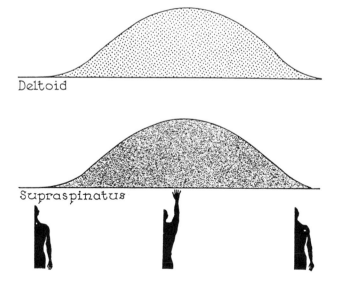

Figure 6–47. Simultaneous electromyographic activity of the deltoid and supraspinatus muscles during arm elevation and descent. (Reproduced with permission from Basmajian JV: Muscles Alive, 2nd ed. © 1967, the Williams & Wilkins Co., Baltimore.)

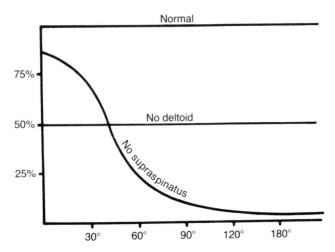

Figure 6–48. Classic representation of the relative contributions of the deltoid and supraspinatus muscles to arm elevation. (Reproduced with permission from Bechtol CO: Biomechanics of the shoulder. Clin Orthop *164*:37, 1980.)

shoulder motion. (In addition to the deltoid and supraspinatus, the rotator cuff musculature is responsible for effective arm elevation.) Although this motion is initiated by these two muscles, which are considered the primary elevators of the glenohumeral joint, their action is made possible by the stabilizing effect of the subscapularis, teres minor, and infraspinatus.[99]

Although both muscles are active with arm elevation, their specific role is debated. The classic functional relationship has been described by Bechtol (Fig. 6–48).[12] Absence of the deltoid causes a uniform decrease in abduction strength that is independent of joint position. Absence of the rotator cuff, on the other hand, allows almost normal abduction initiation strength with a rapid dropoff at elevations greater than 30 degrees.

This classic and popularly held relationship has been reassessed. Using dynamometer data and a careful dissection to accurately define the physiological cross-sectional area of the muscles, Howell and coworkers studied abduction torque in the lidocaine (Xylocaine)-induced axillary or supraspinatus nerve palsy subject.[49] Contrary to popular clinical belief, both the supraspinatus and the deltoid muscles were found to be equally responsible for generating torque during arm flexion and abduction (Fig. 6–49). Care must be taken to avoid direct clinical correlation, since Peat and Grahame[80] have shown that the electromyographic pattern of a muscle will be altered in the diseased or pathological state (Fig. 6–50). The accuracy of the data of Howell and colleagues has been confirmed by additional experimental studies and by the clinical experience of Markhede and associates, who demonstrated surprisingly good function in five patients after deltoid muscle resection.[26, 66]

Hence, the force-generating activity of a muscle for a given function varies according to its physiological cross-sectional area (PCSA), joint position, external load, rate of joint motion, and so on. The impact of these variables may be condensed by further refining the electromyographic signal through an integration technique.[29, 49, 95] However, many technical difficulties still exist when simultaneously studying the electromyographic pattern of multiple muscles.[95]

Furthermore, the position of arm elevation has been determined to be the most important factor that influences the amount of shoulder muscle load.[49, 54] In addition, loading at the hand shows greater electromyographic activity in the short rotators than in the deltoid muscle. Thus, motion of the loaded extremity is brought about by the increased activity of the cuff muscles, which stabilize the glenohumeral joint. This activity is even greater than in those muscles elevating the arm—the deltoid and the supraspinatus.

Laumann has defined what he considers the "essential" shoulder muscles for arm elevation.[62] Muscles are defined as essential if the loss of any two of them renders it impossible to elevate the arm. In addition to the deltoid and supraspinatus muscles, the trapezius

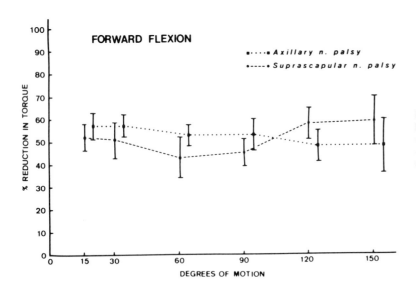

Figure 6–49. A recent study demonstrates similar contributions of both the supraspinatus and the deltoid muscles during arm flexion. (Reproduced with permission from Howell SM, Imobersteg AM, Seger DH, and Marone PJ: Clarification of the role of the supraspinatus muscle in shoulder function. J Bone Joint Surg *68A*:398, 1986.)

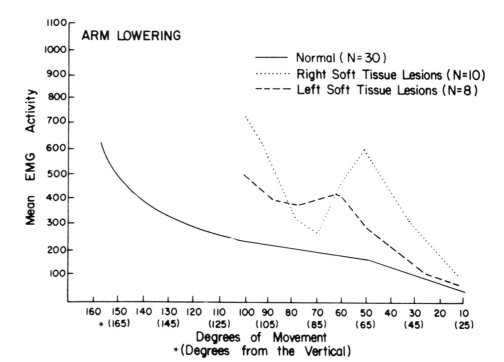

Figure 6–50. Alteration of the electromyographic pattern from the normal in individuals with a rotator cuff–deficient shoulder. (Reproduced with permission from Peat M, and Grahame RE: Electromyographic analysis of soft tissue lesions affecting shoulder function. J Phys Med 56(5):223. Copyright © by Williams & Wilkins, 1977.)

and serratus anterior are required for shoulder elevation. These findings are in accord with Duchenne's early studies showing that these muscles are active in concert with the deltoid during arm elevation.[35] The latter two (the serratus anterior and trapezius) are required to stabilize or move the scapula.

GLENOHUMERAL FORCE

Forces at the glenohumeral joint during arm elevation have been studied by several investigators. Inman, Saunders, and Abbott, in their classical observation on the function of the shoulder joint, analyzed the forces in abduction by considering the deltoid muscle force, a compressive joint force, and a "resultant rotator cuff force" acting parallel to the lateral border of the scapula.[51] A maximum compressive force of ten times and a deltoid muscle force of eight times the weight of the extremity at 90 degrees of arm abduction were formed. This is about one-half body weight. In addition, a maximum resultant rotator cuff force was calculated of nine times the weight of the extremity at 60 degrees of arm abduction (Fig. 6–51).

A simplified two-dimensional force analysis across the glenohumeral joint, similar to the model of Poppen and Walker,[83] is presented to illustrate several important concepts (Fig. 6–52). Consider the normal glenohumeral joint to be approximately a ball-and-socket joint with the center of rotation at the center of the humeral head. The muscle and joint forces involved in the elevation of the entire upper arm in the coronal plane are analyzed. Using the glenoid surface as the reference for the coordinate system, the direction and

location of the muscle forces and the external load of the upper arm can be defined. The x axis is perpendicular to the joint surface, and the y axis is parallel to the glenoid surface. A weight of 0.052 body weight (B.W.) is applied at a point 318 mm distal to the glenohumeral joint center.[83]

Free-body analysis of the entire upper arm, disarticulated at the glenohumeral joint, provides the force and moment equilibrium equations. Three groups of forces are applied to the upper arm: the weight of the arm, the muscle forces, and the reactive joint forces. The weight of the arm creates a moment around the joint, which is counterbalanced by the moment generated by the muscle forces. According to the results

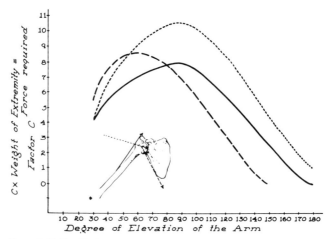

Figure 6–51. Simplified two-dimensional model has estimated up to about 0.5 times body weight compression force across the joint at 90 degrees of elevation (*dotted line*). The deltoid force (*solid line*) is about 0.4 of body weight, and an inferior "depressive" force of about 0.4 body weight (*dashed line*) was calculated.

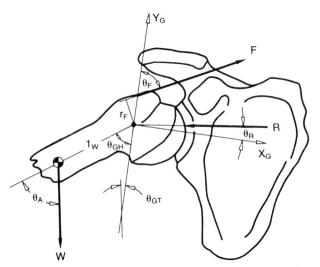

Figure 6–52. A more detailed two-dimensional model representation of the forces that cross the glenohumeral joint. (Reproduced with permission from Morrey BF, and Chao EYS: Recurrent anterior dislocation of the shoulder. *In* Black J, and Dumbleton JH (eds): Clinical Biomechanics. New York: Churchill Livingstone, 1981.)

of electromyographic studies, the deltoid and supraspinatus muscles are actively involved in arm elevation.[57] Only these two groups of muscles are considered in this example. The frictional force on the joint surface is considered to be negligible so that the reactive joint force must pass through the joint center of rotation and provide no contribution to the balance of the moment. The moment equilibrium around joint center 0 can be expressed as:

$$W \times \sin(\theta_A) \times l_W - F_d \times r_d - F_s \times r_s = 0$$

where W = the weight of the upper arm (0.052 B.W.), θ_A = the arm abduction angle, l_W = the distance between the joint center and the center of mass of the upper arm (318 mm), F_d = the deltoid muscle force, r_d = the moment arm of the deltoid muscle force, F_s = the supraspinatus muscle force, and r_s = the moment arm of the supraspinatus muscle force. Two force equilibrium equations can be obtained for the force components perpendicular (x) and parallel (y) to the glenoid surface:

$$W \times \sin(\theta_{GT}) + F_d \times \sin(\theta_d) + F_s \times \sin(\theta_s) - R \times \cos(\theta_R) = 0$$

$$-W \times \cos(\theta_{GT} + F_d \times \cos(\theta_d) + F_s \times \cos(\theta_s) - R \times \sin(\theta_R) = 0$$

where θ_{GT} = the glenothoracic angle, θ_d = the angle between the deltoid muscle line of action and the x axis, θ_s = the angle between the supraspinatus muscle line of action and the x axis, R = the reactive joint force, and θ_r = the angle between the joint force and the x axis.

With the data provided in the literature,[51, 83] the simplified muscle force and model resultant force at

the glenohumeral joint at various abduction angles could be estimated. In fact, the number of unknown muscle forces is greater than the number of available equations, so the solution to the problem becomes "indeterminate." To solve such a problem, various methods based on either reducing the number of variables (as above) or introducing additional relationships among the unknown variables have been described.[2] An assumption was made by Poppen and Walker[83] that the muscle force was proportional to the product of the integrated electromyographic activity and the cross-sectional area of the muscles. The resultant joint forces at various positions of arm elevation and rotation are shown in Figure 6–53. The maximum resultant force was about 0.9 times body weight with the arm at 90 degrees abduction. A great amount of shear force occurred between 30 degrees and 60 degrees of arm abduction.

To further illustrate the importance of coordinative efforts of the muscle action, a more refined set of three solutions was obtained for the following circumstances. First, assume that the deltoid muscle acts alone; second, that the supraspinatus muscle acts alone; and third, that both the deltoid and supraspinatus muscles act together and the relative force generated by each muscle is proportional to its physiological cross-sectional area.

The results of the joint reaction force expressed as a percentage of body weight and the angle of the reaction joint force to the x axis are illustrated in Figure 6–54A. In general, the joint reaction force is highest at about 90 degrees of arm elevation. This is simply due to the fact that the largest moment generated by the weight of the upper arm must be balanced by the muscle force that induces the large joint reaction force. According to Poppen and Walker, at lower positions of arm elevation the supraspinatus muscle has a larger moment arm and thus a greater mechanical advantage than the deltoid muscle.[83] Using the supraspinatus to counterbalance the moment at this position requires less muscle force and thus less joint reaction force. When the arm is elevated at a higher position, the deltoid muscle has a greater mechanical advantage; thus the modes that use the deltoid muscle show a lower joint force.

Since the shoulder joint is not inherently stable, the orientation and location of the joint reaction force referable to the glenoid surface is an additional important parameter for consideration. The joint articulating pressure distribution, which will be discussed in more detail later, depends not only on the available size of the articulating surface but also on the location of the joint reaction force relative to the joint surface.[44] More centrally located joint reaction forces are associated with supraspinatus activity. This is because the relative orientation of the line of action of the supraspinatus muscle is almost perpendicular to the surface of the glenoid joint throughout the range of arm motion.[9, 83] Hence, if the arm elevation is achieved by the supraspinatus muscle, the joint reaction force will be more

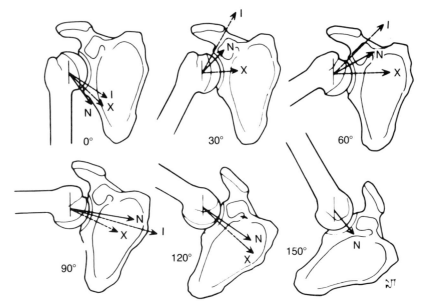

Figure 6–53. The position of the resultant force vector of the shoulder for different positions of arm elevation. (Reproduced with permission from Poppen NK, and Walker PS: Forces at the glenohumeral joint in abduction. Clin Orthop 58:165, 1978.)

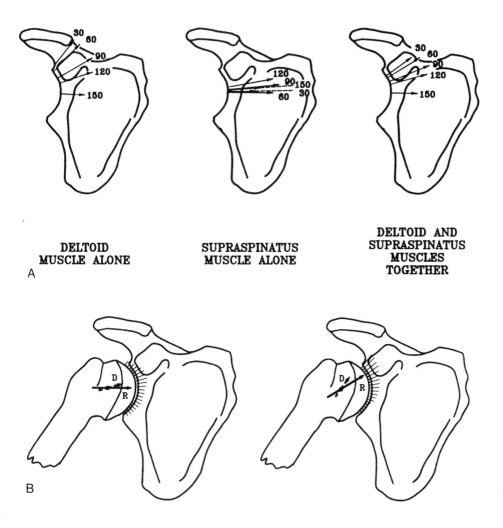

A

DELTOID MUSCLE ALONE

SUPRASPINATUS MUSCLE ALONE

DELTOID AND SUPRASPINATUS MUSCLES TOGETHER

B

Figure 6–54. *A,* Direction of the magnitude of the resultant vector for different glenohumeral joint positions as a function of different muscle activity. *B,* Resultant force across the glenohumeral joint (R) as a function of arm elevation. The direction of the humeral head is attempted displacement as shown (D). When the resultant vector is directed superiorly, the humeral head tends to sublux superiorly and causes increased superior joint pressure.

or less centrally located. On the other hand, the line of action of the deltoid muscles deviates from the surface of the glenoid joint with elevation of the arm. With the arm at less than 40 degrees of abduction, the line of action is superiorly oriented and more or less parallel to the glenoid surface. The action of the deltoid muscle will therefore result in a more off-center joint reaction force at the glenoid surface.

Considering both the magnitude and the location of the joint reaction force on the glenoid surface, it is possible to explain the electromyographic pattern and activity of both the supraspinatus and deltoid muscles at different positions of arm elevation.

Now let us consider the problem of joint articulating or contact pressure distribution. To establish the analytical and numerical model for joint pressure determination, the shapes of the articular surfaces are either mathematically or numerically described. A technique called the *rigid body spring concept* is applied. It is assumed that the bony structures of the articulating joint are relatively rigid so that, with the joint reaction force applied, the displacement or deformation takes place predominantly on the joint surface. Reaction forces between adjacent bodies are simulated by the spring system distributed over the possible contact surfaces between the two adjacent bodies. Displacement of the simulated compressive spring, normal (perpendicular) and tangential to the articular surface, can be described as a function of the displacement of a single reference point of the associated rigid body.

The capsule and ligaments are also modeled with tensile springs. Their displacement can also be described based on the displacement of the reference point of the associated rigid body. For a given joint reaction load, strain energy due to the relative displacement of the spring system can then be formulated in the quadratic function of the displacement of the reference point of the associated rigid body. By applying the principle of minimum potential energy, the stiffness equation is obtained by differentiating strain potential energy with respect to the displacement of the rigid body. A system of equations is obtained for solution of the unknown rigid body displacement. Displacement and force in the spring system, which describe the pressure distribution on articular surfaces, are then determined. In the calculation, the direction or location of the calculated rigid body displacement corresponds to the direction of possible maximum pressure and is termed *virtual* or *attempted* displacement. Factors such as the available size of the contact area and the relative location of the joint reaction force on the joint surface have been found to be important determinants not only of the magnitude but also of the uniformity of the contact pressure distribution.

For the glenohumeral joint, the same magnitude of the resultant joint reaction force R causes more uniform contact pressures when centrally loaded than when loaded toward the rim (Fig. 6–54B). The associated directions of the attempted humeral motion are

indicated by D. It has also been hypothesized that if the direction of the attempted displacement of the rigid body is within the arc of the articular surface, the joint will be stable. On the other hand, if the direction of the attempted displacement is located beyond the articulating arc, then an unstable or even a dislocated joint condition may result (see Fig. 6–53). Based on this argument, the contribution of rotator cuff muscle as a "musculotendinous glenoid" acting in conjunction with the osseous glenoid to maintain the humeral head stability has been proposed.[44]

The clinical implications of these calculations are obvious and are discussed below.

MAXIMUM TORQUE

The overall and relative working capacity of the shoulder was studied by the early German anatomists.[37, 98] Their data revealed that a balance exists between potential flexor and extensor torques.[98] However, internal rotation power exceeds external rotation by a two-to-one ratio, and the adduction force or power exceeds that of abduction by at least a two-to-one ratio.

More detailed information about maximum torque is now available from the data generated by the use of variable-resistance isokinetic devices. Using such a device, Ivey and Rusche demonstrated the following torque relationships: flexion-extension, four to five; abduction-adduction, one to two; and internal-external rotation, three to two.[52] On an absolute basis the greatest strength function is exhibited in adduction, followed by extension, flexion, abduction, internal rotation, and external rotation.[19, 52]

The magnitude and position of maximum torque generated by the shoulder muscles differ according to the strength function studied (Table 6–4). Torque data from our laboratory have revealed that the maximum torques occur at different positions, with some variation depending upon the velocity of the joint.[19] The peak torques are typically greatest at slower speeds—60 degrees per second. The maximum torque decreases for all strength functions with increasing angular test velocity (Fig. 6–55). Our data compare favorably to the relative torques described by Ivey and Rusche, but slight variations were recorded at faster joint speeds.

Table 6–4. MAXIMUM ISOKINETIC TORQUE OF THE SHOULDER AND POSITION OF OCCURRENCE AS A FUNCTION OF JOINT VELOCITY OF MALE SUBJECTS RANGING IN AGE FROM 20 TO 40 YEARS

Angular Velocity Deg/Sec	Abduction		Adduction	
	Torque/Nm	Position/Deg	Torque/Nm	Position/Deg
60	39	27	81	75
180	32	33	73	72
300	26	45	64	74

From Cahalan TD, Chao EYS, Cofield RH, and Johnson ME: Shoulder strength analysis using the Cybex II isokinetic dynamometer. Submitted for publication.

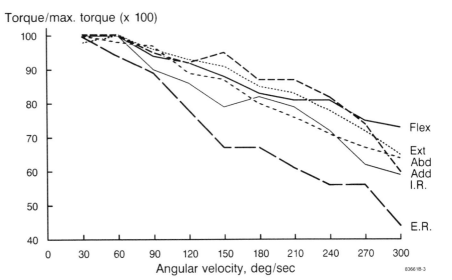

Torque/max. torque (x 100)

Flex
Ext
Abd
Add
I.R.

E.R.

Angular velocity, deg/sec

83661B-3

Figure 6–55. Torque decreases as the angular velocity of arm elevation increases for all muscle functions studied. (Reproduced with permission from Cahalan TD, Chao EYS, Cofield RH, and Johnson ME: Shoulder strength analysis using the Cybex II isokinetic dynamometer. Submitted for publication.)

The maximum torques and the position of the shoulder at the maximum torque are recorded in Table 6–4.

CLINICAL RELEVANCE

The contributions of the deltoid and supraspinatus muscles to arm elevation are easily observed clinically. In patients without a deltoid muscle, arm elevation with modest strength is possible.[66] However, the laboratory data for supraspinatus deficiency presented by Howell and colleagues and by Colachis and Strohm are contrary to clinical experience.[26, 49] The clinical experience does parallel the observations of Bechtol, although no experimental details are presented by this author (see Fig. 6–48).[12] The electromyographic data correlated with various shoulder activities closely support the role of the supraspinatus in stabilizing the humeral head in the glenoid, thus allowing the other muscles to act more effectively across this joint.

The recognition that the resultant force vector is directed superiorly during the first 60 degrees of arm elevation explains the superior migration of the humeral head in the rotator cuff–deficient shoulder (see Fig. 6–28). The orientation and magnitude are also consistent with the glenoid loosening pattern seen in some instances after shoulder joint replacement (Fig. 6–56). These force data may be further correlated with glenoid component fixation. The capacity of the glenoid bone is of limited dimensions. Hence, the fixation technique is critical (see Fig. 6–38). Appropriate design considerations can be incorporated into the glenoid compartment to take advantage of the anatomy and to resist the applied force.

Finally, the rotator cuff–deficient shoulder may also be considered to be at risk for glenoid loosening. The basis for this speculation is that arm elevation of greater than 60 degrees is often not possible with this condition. Thus, elevation that is possible loads the glenoid in a superior, nonstable configuration that exerts a downward, tilting force to the glenoid component. Thus, cuff-deficient shoulders tend to show proximal migration and, possibly, increased glenoid component loosening.

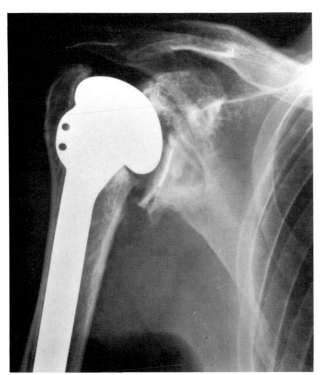

Figure 6–56. Glenoid loosening patterns are consistent with increased superior forces across the glenohumeral joint, noted particularly during the first 60 degrees of elevation.

References

1. An K-N, Hui FC, Morrey BF, et al: Muscle across the elbow joint: a biomechanical analysis. J Biomech *14:*659, 1981.

2. An K-N, Kwak BM, Chao EYS, and Morrey BF: Determination of muscle and joint forces: a new technique to solve the indeterminate problem. J Biomech Eng 106:4364, 1984a.

3. An K-N, and Chao EYS: Kinematic analysis of human movement. Ann Biomed Eng 12:585, 1984b.

4. An K-N, Takahashi K, Hanigan TP, and Chao EYS: Determination of muscle orientations and moment arms. J Biomech Eng 106:280, 1984c.

5. An K-N, Jacobsen MC, Berglund LJ, and Chao EYS: Application of a magnetic tracking device to kinesiologic studies. J Biomech 21:613, 1988.

6. Bankart ASB: The pathology and treatment of recurrent dislocation of the shoulder joint. Br J Surg 26:23, 1938.

7. Basmajian JV: Muscles Alive, 2nd ed. Baltimore: Williams & Wilkins, 1967.

8. Basmajian JV, and Bazant FJ: Factors preventing downward dislocation of the adducted shoulder joint. J Bone Joint Surg 41A:1182, 1959.

9. Bassett R, Browne A, An K-N, and Morrey BF: A biomechanical analysis of shoulder muscles in the position of instability. J Biomech. Accepted for publication.

10. Bearn JG: An electromyographic study of the trapezius, deltoid pectoralis major, biceps and triceps muscles during static loading of the upper limb. Anat Rec 140:103, 1961.

11. Bearn JG: Direct observation on the function of the capsule of the sternoclavicular joint in clavicular support. J Anat 101:159, 1967.

12. Bechtol, CO: Biomechanics of the shoulder. Clin Orthop 146:37, 1980.

13. Bergman RA, Thompson SA, and Afifi A: Catalog of Human Variation. Baltimore: Urban & Schwarzenberg, 1984.

14. Bergmann, G: Biomechanics and pathomechanics of the shoulder joint with reference to prosthetic joint replacement. In Kölbel R, et al (eds): Shoulder Replacement, Berlin: Springer-Verlag, 1987.

15. Bestard EA, Schvene HR, and Bestard EH: Glenoplasty in the management of recurrent shoulder dislocation. Contemp Orthop 12:47, 1986.

16. Borr JS, Freiberg JA, Calouna PC, and Pemberton RA: A survey of end results in stabilization of the paralytic shoulder. J Bone Joint Surg 24:699, 1942.

17. Bost FC and Inmann VTG: The pathological changes in recurrent dislocation of the shoulder. J Bone Joint Surg 24:595, 1942.

18. Browne A, Morrey BF, and An K-N: Elevation of the arm in the plane of the scapula. Submitted for publication.

19. Cahalan TD, Chao EYS, Cofield RH, and Johnson ME: Shoulder strength analysis using the Cybex II isokinetic dynamometer. Submitted for publication.

20. Caird RM: The shoulder joint in relation to certain dislocations and fractures. Edinb Med J 32:708, 1887.

21. Cathcart CW: Movements of the shoulder girdle involved in those of the arm on the trunk. Worcester Meeting, Br Med Assoc, 1882. J Anat Physiol 18:210, 1884.

22. Cave AJE: The nature and morphology of the costoclavicular ligament. J Anat 95:170, 1961.

23. Chao EYS, and An K-N: Perspectives in measurements and modeling of musculoskeletal joint dynamics. In Huiskes R, von Campen DH, and de Wijn JR (eds): Biomechanics: Principles and Applications, The Hague: Martinus Nijhoff, 1982, pp 1–18.

24. Cleland: Notes on raising the arm. J Anat Physiol 18:275, 1884.

25. Codman EA: The Shoulder. Boston: Thomas Todd, 1934.

26. Colachis SC Jr, and Strohm BR: Effect of suprascapular and axillary nerve blocks on muscle force in upper extremity. Arch Phys Med Rehabil 52:22, 1971.

27. Craig EV: The posterior mechanism of acute anterior shoulder dislocations. Clin Orthop 190:213, 1984.

28. Das SP, Ray GS, and Saha AK: Observation of the tilt of the glenoid cavity of the scapula. J Anat Soc India 15:114, 1966.

29. de Luca CJ, and Forrest WJ: Force analysis of individual muscles acting simultaneously on the shoulder joint during isometric abduction. J Biomech 6:385, 1973.

30. DeLorme D: die Hemmungs bander des Schultergelenks and ihre Deductung fur die Schulter Luxationen. Arch fur Klin Chirurg 92:79, 1910.

31. Dempster WT: Mechanisms of shoulder movement. Arch Phys Med Rehabil 46A:49, 1965.

32. DePalma AF, Callery G, and Bennett GA: Variational anatomy and degenerative lesions of the shoulder bone. AAOS Instructional Course Lecture 16:255, 1949.

33. DePalma AF, Coker AJ, and Probhaker M: The role of the subscapularis in recurrent anterior dislocation of the shoulder. Clin Orthop 54:35, 1969.

34. Doddy SG, Waterland JC, and Freedman L: Scapulohumeral goniometer. Arch Phys Med Rehabil 51:711, 1970.

35. Duchenne GBA: Physiologies des mouvements, 1867. (Kaplan EB, Trans.). Philadelphia, WB Saunders, 1949.

36. Dvir Z and Berme N: The shoulder complex in elevation of the arm: a mechanism approach. J Biomech 11:219, 1978.

37. Fick R: Spezille Gelenk and Nuskelmuchanik, Mechanik Deskniegelenkes. Jena G Fischer 111:521, 1911.

38. Flood V: Discovery of a new ligament of the shoulder. Lancet 672, 1829.

39. Freedman L, and Munro RH: Abduction of the arm in scapular plane: scapular and glenohumeral movements. J Bone Joint Surg 18A:1503, 1966.

40. Fukuda K, Chen C-M, Cofield RH, and Chao EY: Biomechanical analysis of stability and fixation strength of total shoulder prostheses. Orthopedics 11(1):141, 1988.

41. Fukuda K, Craig EV, An K-N, et al: Biomechanical study of the ligamentous system of the acromioclavicular joint. J Bone Joint Surg 68A:434, 1986.

42. Grant JCB: Method of Anatomy, 7th ed. Baltimore: Williams & Wilkins, 1965.

43. Hill HS, and Sacks MD: The grooved defect of the humeral head. A frequently unrecognized complication of dislocations of the shoulder joint. Radiology 35:690, 1940.

44. Himeno S, and Tsumra H: The role of the rotator cuff as a stabilizing mechanism of the shoulder. In Bateman J, and Welsh RP (eds): Surgery of the Shoulder. St. Louis: CV Mosby, 1984.

45. Himeno S, An K-N, Tsumura H, and Chao EYS: Pressure distribution on articular surface application to muscle force determination and joint stability evaluation. Proceedings of the North American Congress on Biomechanics 1:15, Montreal, August 25–27, 1986.

46. Hogfors C, Sigholm G, and Herberts P: Biomechanical model of the human shoulder. I. Elements. J Biomech 20:157, 1987.

47. Howell SM, and Galinat BJ: The containment mechanism: the primary stabilizer of the glenohumeral joint. Paper presented at the annual meeting of the American Academy of Orthopaedic Surgeons, San Francisco, January 23, 1987.

48. Howell SM, Galinat BJ, Renzi AJ, and Marone PJ: Normal and abnormal mechanics of the glenohumeral joint in the horizontal plane. J Bone Joint Surg 70A:227, 1988.

49. Howell SM, Imobersteg AM, Seger DH, and Marone PJ: Clarification of the role of the supraspinatus muscle in shoulder function. J Bone Joint Surg 68A:398, 1986.

50. Ikai M, and Fukunaga T: Calculation of muscle strength per unit of cross-sectional area of human muscle. A Angew Physiol Einschl Argeitsphysiol 26:26, 1968.

51. Inman VT, Saunders JR, and Abbott LC: Observations on the function of the shoulder joint. J Bone Joint Surg 26:1, 1944.

52. Ivey FM Jr, and Rusche K: Isokinetic testing of shoulder strength: normal values. Arch Phys Med Rehabil 66:384–386, 1985.

53. Jackson KM, Joseph J, and Wyard SJ: Sequential muscular contraction. J Biomech 10:97, 1977.

54. Järvholm U, Palmerud G, Styf J, et al: Intramuscular pressure in the supraspinatus muscle. J Orthop Res 6:230, 1988.

55. Jiang CC, Otis JC, Warren RF, and Wickiewicz TL: Muscle excursion measurements and moment arm definitions. J Rotator Cuff Muscles (abstract). 34th annual Orthopedic Research Society meeting, Atlanta, February 1–4, 1988.

56. Johnston TB: The movements of the shoulder joint. A plea for

the use of the "plane of the scapula" as the plane of reference for movements occurring at the humero-scapular joint. Br J Surg 25:252, 1937.

57. Jones DW Jr: The role of the shoulder muscles in the control of humeral position. Master's thesis, Case Western Reserve University, 1970.

58. Kaltsas DS: Comparative study of the properties of the shoulder joint capsules with those of other joint capsules. Clin Orthop 173:20, 1973.

59. Kapandji I: The physiology of joints, Vol 1. Baltimore: Williams & Wilkins, 1970.

59a. Kennedy JC, and Cameron H: Complete dislocation of the acromioclavicular joint. J Bone Joint Surg 36B:202, 1954.

60. Kumar VP, and Balasubramaniam P: The role of atmospheric pressure in stabilizing the shoulder: an experimental study. J Bone Joint Surg 67B:719, 1985.

61. Landon GC, Chao EY, and Cofield RH: Three dimensional analysis of angular motion of the shoulder complex. Trans Orthop Res Soc 3:297, 1978.

62. Laumann U: Kinesiology of the shoulder joint. In Kölbel R, et al (eds): Shoulder Replacement. Berlin: Springer-Verlag, 1987.

63. Lockhart RD: Movements of the normal shoulder joint and of a case with trapezius paralysis studied by radiogram and experiment in the living. J Anat 64:288, 1930.

64. Lucas DB: Biomechanics of the shoulder joint. Arch Surg 107(3):425, 1973.

65. Maki S, and Gruen T: Anthropometric study of the glenohumeral joint. Paper presented at the 22nd annual Orthopedic Research Society, New Orleans, January 28–30, 1976.

66. Markhede G, Monastyrski J, and Stener B: Shoulder function after deltoid muscle removal. Acta Orthop Scand 56:242, 1985.

67. McLaughlin HL, and Carallero WU: Primary anterior dislocation of the shoulder. I. Morbid anatomy. Am J Surg 99:628, 1960.

68. McLaughlin HL, and MacLellan DI: Recurrent anterior dislocation of the shoulder. II. A comparative study. J Trauma 7:191, 1967.

69. Morrey BF, and Chao EYS: Passive motion of the elbow joint. J Bone Joint Surg 58A:501, 1976.

70. Morrey BF, and Chao EY: Recurrent anterior dislocation of the shoulder. In Dumbleton J, and Black J (eds): Clinical Biomechanics. London: Churchill Livingstone, 1981.

71. Morrey BF, and Janes JJ: Recurrent anterior dislocation of the shoulder. Long-term follow-up of the Putti-Platt and Bankart procedures. J Bone Joint Surg 58A:252, 1976.

72. Morris CB: The measurements of the strength of muscle relative to the cross-section. Res Q Am Assoc Health Phys Ed Recreation 19:295, 1948.

73. Moseley HE, and Overgaard B: The anterior capsular mechanism in recurrent anterior dislocation of the shoulder. J Bone Joint Surg 44B:913, 1962.

74. Neer CS II: Displaced proximal humeral fractures. I. Classification and evaluation. J Bone Joint Surg 52A:1077, 1970.

75. Neer CS II, and Foster CR: Inferior capsular shift for involuntary inferior and multidirectional instability of the shoulder. J Bone Joint Surg 62A:897, 1980.

76. Nobuhara K: The Shoulder: Its Function and Clinical Aspects. Tokyo: Igaku-Shoin, 1987.

77. Ohwovoriole EN, and Mekow C: A technique for studying the kinematics of human joints. Part II: The humeroscapular joint. Orthopedics 10(3):457, 1987.

78. Ovesen J, and Nielsen S: Anterior and posterior shoulder instability. Acta Orthop Scand 57:324, 1986.

79. Partridge MJ: Joints. The limitation of their range of movement, and an explanation of certain surgical conditions. J Anat 108:346, 1923.

80. Peat M, and Grahame RE: Electromyographic analysis of soft tissue lesions affecting shoulder function. J Phys Med 56(5):223, 1977.

81. Peindl RD, and Engin AE: On the modeling of human shoulder complex II. J Biomech 20:119, 1987.

82. Poppen NK, and Walker PS: Normal and abnormal motion of the shoulder. J Bone Joint Surg 58A:195, 1976.

83. Poppen NK, and Walker PS: Forces at the glenohumeral joint in abduction. Clin Orthop 58:165, 1978.

84. Reeves B: Experiments on the tensile strength of the anterior capsular structures of the shoulder region. J Bone Joint Surg 50B:858, 1968.

85. Remmel E, and Köckerling F: Anatomical study of the capsular mechanism in dislocation of the shoulder (abstract). J Biomech 20:807, 1987.

86. Rockwood CA Jr, and Green DP (eds): Fractures in adults, 2nd ed. Philadelphia: JB Lippincott, 1984.

87. Rowe CR: Re-evaluation of the position of the arm in arthrodesis of the shoulder in the adult. J Bone Joint Surg 56A:913, 1974.

88. Rowe CR, Patel D, and Southmayd WE: The Bankart procedure: a long-term end result study. J Bone Joint Surg 60A:1, 1978.

89. Saha AK: Dynamic stability of the glenohumeral joint. Acta Orthop Scand 42:491, 1971.

90. Scheving LE, and Pauly JE: An electromyographic study of some muscles acting on the upper extremity of man. Anat Rec 135:239, 1959.

91. Schwartz E, Warren RF, O'Brien SJ, and Fronek J: Posterior shoulder instability. Orthop Clin North Am 18(3):409, 1987.

92. Scott DJ: Treatment of recurrent posterior dislocations of the shoulder by glenoplasty. J Bone Joint Surg 49A:471, 1967.

93. Shevlin MG, Lehmann JF, and Lucci JA: Electromyographic study of the function of some muscles crossing the glenohumeral joint. Arch Phys Med Rehabil 50:264, 1969.

94. Shoup TE: Optical measurement of the center of rotation for human joints. J Biomech 9:241, 1976.

95. Sigholm G, Herberts P, Almstrom C, and Kodifors R: Electromyographic analysis of shoulder muscle load. J Orthop Res 1:379, 1984.

96. Spiegelman JJ, and Woo SL-Y: A rigid-body method for finding centers of rotation and angular displacements of planar joint motion. J Biomech 20(7):715, 1987.

97. Spoor CS, and Veldpaus FE: Rigid body motion calculated from spatial co-ordinates of markers. J Bone Joint Surg 13:391, 1980.

98. Steindler A: Kinesiology of the Human Body under Normal and Pathological Conditions. Springfield, IL: Charles C Thomas, 1955.

99. Stevens JH: The action of the short rotators on the normal abduction of the arm, with a consideration of their action in some cases of subacromial bursitis and allied conditions. Am J Med Sci 136(6):871, 1909.

100. Symenoides PO: The significance of the subscapularis muscle in the pathogenesis of recurrent anterior dislocation of the shoulder. J Bone Joint Surg 54B:476, 1972.

101. Taylor CL, and Blaschke AC: Method for kinematic analysis of motions of the shoulder, arm, and hand complex. Ann NY Acad Sci 1251:19.

102. Terry GC, Hammon D, and France P: Stabilizing function of passive shoulder restraints. Unpublished data from the Hughston Orthopaedic Clinic, Columbus, GA, 1988.

103. Townley CO: The capsular mechanism in recurrent dislocation of the shoulder. J Bone Joint Surg 32A:370, 1950.

104. Turkel SJ, Panio MW, Marshall JL, and Girgis FG: Stabilizing mechanisms preventing anterior dislocation of the glenohumeral joint. J Bone Joint Surg 63A:1208, 1981.

105. Uhthoff H, and Piscopo M: Anterior capsular redundancy of the shoulder: Congenital or traumatic? J Bone Joint Surg 67B:363, 1985.

106. Walker PS: Human Joints and Their Artificial Replacements. Springfield, IL; Charles C Thomas, 1977.

107. Walker PS: Some bioengineering considerations of prosthetic replacement for the glenohumeral joint. In Inglis AE (ed): Upper Extremity Joint Replacement, 1979.

108. Warwick R, and Williams PL (eds): Gray's Anatomy, 35th ed. Philadelphia: WB Saunders, 1973.

109. Weiner DS, and MacNab I: Superior migration of the humeral head. J Bone Joint Surg 52B:524, 1970.

Anesthesia for Shoulder Procedures

L. Brian Ready, M.D.

In the fifth century B.C., Hippocrates offered surgical treatment for recurrent shoulder dislocation.[1] He described his technique in part as follows:

The cautery should be applied thus: taking hold with the hands of the skin at the armpit, it is to be drawn into the line, in which the head of the humerus is dislocated; and then the skin thus drawn aside is to be burnt to the opposite side. The burning should be performed with irons, which are not thick nor much rounded, but of an oblong form, (for thus they pass the more readily through,) and they are to be pushed forward with the hand: the cauteries should be red-hot, that they may pass through as quickly as possible.

The appearance of patients thus treated without anesthesia is left to the imagination of the reader. It was not until 1846 that William Morton demonstrated general anesthesia with ether. In 1884, Halsted injected cocaine under direct vision into the roots of the brachial plexus to produce the first regional block of the upper extremity.[2] Hirschel described the first percutaneous technique in 1911—an axillary approach that would not be expected to permit comfortable shoulder surgery.[3] In the same year, Kulenkampff described the first percutaneous supraclavicular approach.[4] An adequate volume of local anesthetic injected by his method could indeed produce satisfactory analgesia for shoulder surgery, although it is not known whether it was used for this purpose.

Appropriate and well-conducted modern anesthetics for surgical procedures involving the shoulder can optimize operating conditions, enhance safety, reduce morbidity and postoperative pain, and positively influence patients' perception of their surgical experience. To achieve these goals, patients must be considered individually with regard to the type of surgery planned, underlying medical conditions, patient preferences, and the skill and experience of the anesthesiologist. No one anesthetic technique is optimal for all patients

undergoing shoulder surgery. In this chapter, details of appropriate preoperative evaluation, intraoperative management, and postoperative anesthetic care will be considered.

Preoperative Considerations

OVERVIEW

All patients should be assessed by an anesthesiologist prior to administration of an anesthetic. For patients who are in the hospital, this should be done on the day before surgery or sooner if serious medical conditions are present. For healthy, ambulatory patients or those admitted on the day of surgery, alternatives are necessary. It may be possible for an anesthesiologist to see such patients in a clinic setting a number of days before surgery or to evaluate them early on the day of surgery. The preanesthetic visit is important for a number of reasons. A chance to meet the individual who will support and care for the patient during surgery combined with an explanation of what will be done to ensure comfort and safety is an effective means of reducing anxiety and fear. During the preoperative visit, the anesthesiologist should evaluate underlying medical conditions, allergies, and medication use. Previous anesthetic experiences should be reviewed and a physical examination completed. This should include examination of the upper airway, the chest, and the cardiovascular system. A neurological examination will exclude or document pre-existing sensory or motor deficits in the upper extremity. Laboratory studies, x-rays, and electrocardiograms, if indicated, are reviewed. A discussion of the available anesthetic options (including their respective benefits and risks) should be provided. Then, based on the evaluation, a professional recommendation for choice of technique should be made. Concerns and questions should be addressed. In general, patients should not be forced to accept an anesthetic approach they do not want.

UNDERLYING MEDICAL CONDITIONS

A population of patients scheduled for shoulder surgery will suffer a spectrum of medical conditions that are of importance in considering anesthetic management. It is our policy to delay elective surgery until the risk from any underlying medical condition is minimized. A brief discussion of a number of common examples will serve to illustrate the importance of the preoperative assessment. It is beyond the scope of this chapter to provide a detailed discussion of the evaluation and management of patients with these and other underlying conditions.

Patients with rheumatoid arthritis who require shoulder joint surgery frequently have other damaged joints. These need support and protection during surgery to avoid pain (if regional anesthesia is used) or further damage (with any type of anesthetic). Preoperative evaluation of the cervical spine and temporomandibular joints is essential in this population. Reduced range of motion in these joints may make visualization of the larynx, tracheal intubation, and ventilation difficult or impossible following induction of general anesthesia.[5, 6, 7] It is important to have an awareness that this population may also suffer extra-articular manifestations of their disease. These include cardiac, pulmonary, renal, neurological, and hematopoietic dysfunction[8, 9] and adrenal suppression secondary to chronic corticosteroid therapy.

Cardiac disease is common in patients undergoing shoulder surgery. It may include ischemic disease (angina pectoris, myocardial infarction), defective conduction (arrhythmias), restricted flow (valvular or pericardial disease), or inflammation (myocarditis). Evaluation of individual patients' symptoms, physical limitations, and appropriate diagnostic tests will facilitate optimal anesthetic management.

Hypertension is present in about 10 per cent of the population of the United States.[10] Important management goals in patients with this condition include institution or maintenance of therapy to control blood pressure throughout the perioperative period, adequate monitoring of blood pressure and myocardial function during surgery, and avoidance of marked hypo- or hypertension. Good preoperative control is important since it will reduce the risk of myocardial infarction and stroke during anesthesia and surgery. Elective procedures should be postponed until optimal control of blood pressure has been achieved. Possible interactions of anesthetic agents with antihypertensive agents must be considered in the anesthetic plan.

Pulmonary disease remains common, especially in older patients with a long smoking history. Emphysema, chronic bronchitis, asthma, or a mixed picture may be present. A history and examination including exercise limits will help define the nature and extent of disease. Pulmonary function studies and arterial blood gas analysis should be considered in patients with limited exercise tolerance. Bronchospasm should be treated with appropriate bronchodilators preoperatively. Since airway instrumentation (i.e., tracheal intubation) may trigger severe bronchospasm, it should be avoided if possible.

Diabetes mellitus is another disease present in many patients having shoulder surgery. It may give rise to multiple organ system involvement, in particular cardiovascular and renal disease. Blood glucose may be labile in the perioperative period when dietary routines must be changed. Insulin-dependent diabetics require especially careful assessment. Adjustment in insulin doses to achieve control of glucose levels, correction of acidosis and hypokalemia, and adequate hydration may be needed before surgery. Severe hypoglycemia must be avoided since it can result in brain damage. Surgery scheduled early in the morning is optimal for these patients. Regional anesthesia may have the advantage of less nausea and vomiting and permitting early resumption of a normal diet.

Obese patients represent a number of challenges to the anesthesiologist.[11, 12] Cardiac output is increased. The weighted chest enhances the elastic recoil of the thorax with a net decrease in expiratory reserve volume. Hypercarbia and hypoxemia are thus more likely to occur. Diabetes, myocardial disease, and hypertension commonly accompany obesity. Technical problems may include difficulty in establishing venous access, maintaining a clear airway, and obtaining adequate information using conventional monitors. Frequently, obese patients will have indistinct landmarks for regional anesthesia.

PREOPERATIVE DIAGNOSTIC TESTS

It has been traditional to order routine blood work, urinalysis, and chest x-rays for all patients scheduled for surgery as well as electrocardiograms for older patients. The usefulness of this approach is in question, and many anesthesiologists now support the use of only those tests indicated by history and physical examination. An 18-year-old athlete scheduled for repair of a recurrent dislocation probably will not benefit from any preoperative testing, whereas a 65-year-old obese diabetic patient who is hypertensive, has myocardial ischemia, and is taking digoxin and a diuretic will require a number of laboratory tests.

PREMEDICATION

Anesthesiologists vary considerably in their views about medicating patients before surgery. In patients who are not anxious, premedication may not be necessary. Rather, an intravenous agent may be titrated to optimal effect just before entering the operating room or placing a regional block. For anxious patients, an oral sedative/tranquilizer may be taken with a sip of water on the morning of surgery and repeated if surgery is scheduled late in the day. If a regional technique that requires a patient's reporting of paresthesias is planned, heavy preoperative sedation should be avoided. Such sedation may make determination of correct needle placement difficult and result in multiple needle passes with associated soft tissue or nerve trauma. Outpatients who need premedication should receive small doses of short-acting drugs that will not interfere with early discharge following surgery.

When it is suspected that airway management will be difficult (e.g., anatomical abnormalities, grossly obese patients, or the presence of arthritic involvement of the cervical spine and temporomandibular joints), drying of airway secretions with an intramuscular belladonna alkaloid (atropine, scopolamine) or glycopyrrolate one hour before induction of anesthesia may be useful.

Intraoperative Considerations

VENOUS ACCESS

Adequate venous access must be established before performing a regional block or induction of general anesthesia. In cases of possible rapid and extensive blood loss, a 16- or 14-gauge cannula should be placed. Since patients will use only their unoperated upper extremity during the immediate postoperative period, it is desirable to keep it as functional as possible. An intravenous cannula placed on the forearm is naturally splinted and less likely to interfere with function than a cannula placed on the dorsum of the hand. Sterile technique is critical, especially in cases where implants will be used.

MONITORING

Cardiovascular

A precordial stethoscope (or esophageal stethoscope in patients receiving endotracheal general anesthesia) is a useful monitor of cardiac rate and rhythm, but it may be difficult to hear during cases when laminar flow is used. An electrocardioscope is essential. The leads should be positioned well away from the surgical field. In patients with coronary artery disease, a V_5 lead is helpful for early detection of ischemic changes. A conventional sphygmomanometer or automatic noninvasive blood pressure monitor is usually satisfactory. An arterial line is seldom necessary but should be considered under a number of circumstances. These include gross obesity where a cuff does not give accurate information, severe hypertension or myocardial ischemia, expected rapid and extensive blood loss, severe pulmonary disease, and risk of malignant hyperpyrexia. A central venous catheter or pulmonary artery catheter should be considered in patients with severe cardiac or pulmonary disease or when a large blood loss is expected.[13]

Respiratory

In addition to the basic precordial or esophageal stethoscope, expired carbon dioxide can be sampled from patients receiving general or regional anesthesia and displayed on an apnea monitor, capnograph, or mass spectrometer if these devices are available.

Supplemental oxygen, 2 to 4 liters per minute, should be administered by nasal cannula or oxygen mask to patients receiving regional anesthesia. Transcutaneous oxygen saturation (SaO_2) can be measured continuously. To permit frequent arterial blood gas analysis, an arterial line should be considered for patients with severe pulmonary disease.

Other

When general anesthesia is used, the usual monitors and alarm systems associated with modern anesthesia machines should be used. These are well known to qualified anesthesiologists. A neuromuscular blockade monitor will permit titration of muscle relaxants to produce optimal conditions during surgery and to confirm reversal of the action of these drugs at the end of the case. Monitoring of patient temperature during general anesthesia is routine.

POSITIONING

The majority of surgical procedures on the shoulder can conveniently be carried out in the sitting or semi-sitting position. This position has the advantage of lowering local venous pressure which in turn reduces bleeding. Exceptions include arthroscopy and arthroscopic surgery. These may be more easily performed in the lateral position. Posterior repairs and many scapular procedures require the patient to be prone. Rolls under the chest and pelvis in this position will reduce pressure on the abdomen and make breathing easier. Whichever position is chosen, care and attention to detail in positioning is important. In patients with arthritis, the operating table should be especially well padded. It should be adjusted to minimize stress on each joint. Additional padding should be placed to protect vulnerable nerves, as well as over bony prominences. In the lateral position, an axillary roll should be used and adequate peripheral pulses confirmed after final positioning. During surgery in any position, the patient's face may need protection from retractors and other instruments; for example, during reaming of the humeral canal. Surgeons may need to be reminded of the proximity of the face (covered by drapes) to the incision. An unobstructed upper airway at all times is essential.

Choice of Anesthetics—Regional Versus General

Although each patient should be considered individually, after 10 years' experience administering anesthetics to patients undergoing shoulder surgery, I have concluded that under most circumstances regional anesthesia has significant advantages. Regional techniques provide optimal operating conditions without disturbance to the function of major organ systems. This is particularly important in patients with serious underlying medical conditions which, in combination with general anesthesia, may represent a major risk. Recovery time after regional anesthesia is short, and nausea, vomiting, and urinary retention are uncommon. With the appropriate choice of local anesthetic agents, duration of a neuronal block may be varied between one hour (for short procedures in ambulatory patients) and 12 to 24 or more hours. The choice of long-acting local anesthetics permits analgesia for many hours following painful shoulder procedures in hospitalized patients. This is particularly useful when early mobilization is indicated, such as after release of contractures and adhesions.

A number of studies have demonstrated reduced intraoperative blood loss during hip replacement using regional blocks.[14–19] The same is true during major chest wall surgery.[20] These benefits are thought to result from reduced local venous pressure secondary to sympathetic block and the absence of positive airway pressures that can cause venous distention during general anesthesia if mechanical ventilation is used. If these observations apply to shoulder procedures, the risks associated with blood transfusions would be reduced by using regional anesthesia.

Emergency surgery on the shoulder is not common but is occasionally necessary. Regional anesthesia minimizes the risk of aspiration of gastric contents in these circumstances. Other complications unique to general anesthesia are also eliminated.

It has been argued that regional anesthesia takes more time to initiate than general anesthesia. With care in scheduling cases, optimal utilization of manpower and space resources, and technically skilled anesthesiologists, these time differences can be reduced or eliminated. An "induction area" equipped to permit the safe placement of regional blocks before patients enter the operating room is a valuable resource. Also, by using extra anesthesia personnel qualified to monitor patients once surgery has started, thus freeing the anesthesiologist to place the next block, it may be possible to eliminate any anesthetic-related delays between cases. Each anesthesiologist has a responsibility to use regional anesthesia efficiently. However, when medical considerations make regional anesthesia a safer choice for a particular patient, surgeons should be tolerant of additional anesthetic induction time, if necessary, to provide the best anesthetic for that patient.

Some patients express a fear of needles or a wish not to be aware that surgery is being performed. With modern techniques, patients can be offered the advantages of regional anesthesia and also have these concerns addressed. Appropriate sedation during block placement and during surgery is the answer for these patients. A number of drugs alone or in combination may be used. These include nitrous oxide, incremental doses of a benzodiazepine (diazepam, midazolam), or an infusion of a dilute solution of methohexital titrated to produce lack of awareness.

Surgery involving the lower scapula (below the spine) represents special challenges for the use of regional anesthetic techniques. Complete anesthesia requires block of the brachial plexus plus the upper chest wall (T2–T7). The need to perform multiple nerve blocks, combined with the use of the prone position and attendant need for airway control, leads to the recommendation for general anesthesia for these cases unless contraindications exist.

Patients occasionally express a strong preference for general anesthesia. In the absence of strong medical contraindications, this preference should be respected. A number of techniques well known to qualified anesthesiologists may be appropriate, depending on underlying medical conditions. Special caution is needed in the presence of suspected difficult airways. Options for management in these situations include inhalation induction of the spontaneously breathing patient with a potent anesthetic agent followed by laryngoscopy to assess airway access; awake nasal intubation preceded by topical anesthesia to the upper airway; and awake passage of an endotracheal tube over a fiberoptic bronchoscope. Experienced anesthesiologists vary in their preferences. Once inserted and checked for correct placement, the endotracheal tube should be taped securely on the side opposite to the site of surgery. Surgical exposure may be improved by moderate neck extension and rotation of the head away from the surgical site. Following surgery, extubation should be considered only when full airway control has returned.

Techniques for Regional Anesthesia

A number of regional anesthetic techniques can be used for shoulder surgery. These include supraclavicular block,[21] subclavian perivascular block,[22, 23] and interscalene brachial plexus block.[23, 24] For completeness, cervicothoracic epidural block should also be included in this list.

SUPRACLAVICULAR BLOCK

Supraclavicular block is performed by inserting the block needle above the midpoint of the clavicle just lateral to the clavicular head of the sternocleidomastoid muscle. It is advanced toward the trunks of the brachial plexus where they lie posterior to the subclavian artery on the first rib. When a paresthesia is elicited, 30 to 50 ml of local anesthetic is injected. For shoulder surgery, the superficial cervical plexus, intercostobrachial nerve, and medial brachial cutaneous nerve must also be blocked.

SUBCLAVIAN PERIVASCULAR BLOCK

The subclavian perivascular approach is similar to the supraclavicular technique. In this case the important surface landmark is the palpable groove between the anterior and middle scalene muscles. The block needle is inserted into the most inferior palpable portion of this groove and advanced in a direct caudal direction toward the trunks of the brachial plexus. When a paresthesia below the shoulder is elicited, 30 to 50 ml of local anesthetic is injected. As with supraclavicular block, the superficial cervical plexus, intercostobrachial nerve, and medial brachial cutaneous nerve must be blocked separately if surgery extends to areas they innervate.

INTERSCALENE BLOCK

Since I and other writers have found the interscalene brachial plexus block to be nearly ideal for shoulder surgery,[25, 26, 27] it will be described in considerable detail. As an alternative to eliciting sensory paresthesia in performing this block, I use a peripheral nerve stimulator and electrically insulated block needle to produce muscle twitch. The characteristics of a stimulator suitable for this purpose are listed in Table 7–1.[28]

The technique is as follows: Well before the time of surgery, the patient is transported from the ward to an induction area near the operating room. An intravenous cannula is inserted on the forearm of the normal upper extremity. An electrocardioscope and automatic blood pressure measuring device are attached, as well as a grounding skin electrode just below the clavicle on the operative side. It is confirmed that equipment and drugs (thiopental, succinyl choline, atropine, ephedrine) are available to permit immediate airway suctioning, positive pressure ventilation with 100 per cent oxygen, insertion of an endotracheal tube, and

Table 7–1. CHARACTERISTICS OF A NERVE STIMULATOR SUITABLE FOR BRACHIAL PLEXUS OR PERIPHERAL NERVE BLOCK

1. The pulse current should be variable over a range of 0 to at least 3 mA. and be independent of load resistance variations between 200 and 2000 ohms. The current dial should have ample spread over the range of 0.1 to 1.0 mA.
2. The delivered current should be displayed on a meter or calibrated dial.
3. The pulse repetition rate should be about 2 per second.
4. The pulse duration should be between 0.1 and 1.0 millisecond (with preference for the shorter duration since it improves ability to discriminate varying distances between the needle and the nerve).
5. The polarity of the output terminals should be clearly marked.
6. There should be a battery condition indicator and lead fault indicator.

maintenance of heart rate and systemic blood pressure in the event a complication requires these measures. The setup, including block equipment, local anesthetic solution, and peripheral nerve stimulator, is illustrated in Figure 7–1. Intravenous premedication is titrated to produce the desired effect. This typically includes 50 to 100 μg of fentanyl and 1 to 5 mg of midazolam. Additional sedation can be provided as needed with a 0.2 per cent methohexital drip. The endpoint, depending on patient preference, varies between relaxed but alert to total lack of awareness. Heavy sedation may add to the risk of nerve injury unless electrical stimulation is used to aid needle placement.

With the patient supine, the pillow removed, and the head turned to the opposite side, the shoulder is lowered as far as possible. The groove between the anterior and middle scalene muscles is identified by palpation at the C6 level using the surface landmarks described by Winnie.[23] The skin is cleaned with tincture of benzoin swabs, and drapes are applied in a manner that permits visualization of the entire extremity. Local infiltration of skin and subcutaneous tissue over the injection site is performed using 0.5 ml of dilute local anesthetic solution (0.5 per cent lidocaine or mepivacaine or 0.125 per cent bupivacaine). More concentrated solutions may interfere with subsequent electrostimulation. A 1½-inch short bevel, electrically insulated needle attached to the negative output terminal of a nerve stimulator set to deliver one milliamp is inserted into the groove (Fig. 7–2). Its direction is perpendicular to the skin in all planes, with a definite slightly caudal direction. Correct needle orientation will make it difficult for the needle to pass between the cervical transverse processes to enter the vertebral artery or a cervical nerve root dural cuff. Current is reduced as the needle approaches the trunks of the brachial plexus. Correct needle placement is indicated by a twitch of the forearm flexors with a stimulating current of 0.5 milliamps or less. Typically, this is 1 to 2 cm deep to the skin. The needle is immobilized and 30 to 50 ml of local anesthetic solution (depending on the patient's age and physical status) is injected. Twitching of other muscles (pectoralis, deltoid) is often seen. If injection is carried out under these circumstances, satisfactory anesthesia can result but is less certain. Repositioning of the needle to cause a twitch in the forearm flexors is recommended. Suggested agents, their concentrations, and expected duration of action are listed in Table 7–2. An additional 5 to 10 ml of the local anesthetic solution is injected along the midportion of the posterior border of the sternocleidomastoid muscle to block the superficial fibers of the cervical plexus and speed onset of sensory block over the shoulder.

Surgical analgesia is usually present in 15 to 20 minutes. Onset of sensory block is characteristically from proximal to distal. Motor block of the shoulder abductors is almost immediate, followed rapidly by weakness in the forearm flexors. Triceps weakness usually takes longer to develop, while hand and finger

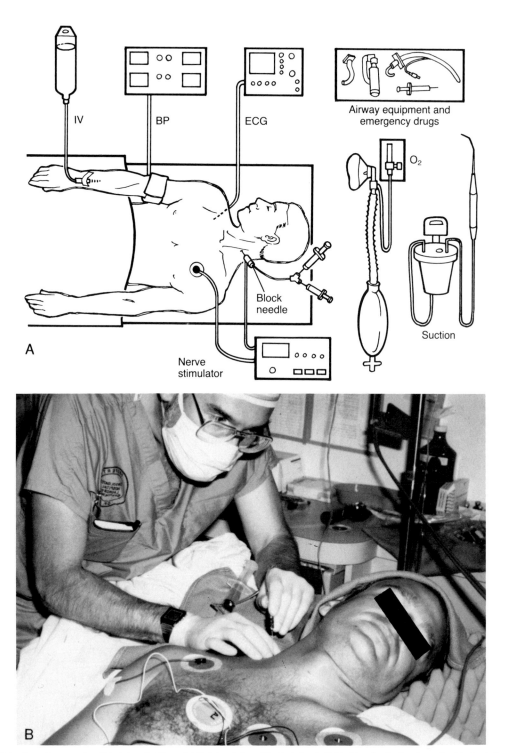

Figure 7–1. *A,* Setup to perform a regional block (see text for a detailed description of the technique). *B,* Position of patient and anesthesiologist during interscalene block.

Table 7–2. LOCAL ANESTHETIC DRUGS SUITABLE FOR INTERSCALENE BRACHIAL PLEXUS BLOCK*

Generic Name (Brand Name)	Concentration	Volume† (ml)	Onset of Surgical Analgesia (Minutes)	Duration of Surgical Analgesia (Hours)
Chloroprocaine (Nesacaine)	2%	25–50	10–25	0.75–1
Lidocaine (Xylocaine)	0.7–1%	25–50	10–25	1.5–3
Mepivacaine (Carbocaine, Polocaine)	0.7–1%	25–50	10–25	2–4
Bupivacaine (Marcaine, Sensorcaine)	0.25–0.5%	25–50	15–25	8–24+

*Doses stated are for adults. See text for additional details.
†All solutions contain epinephrine 1:200,000 (0.05 ml of 1:1000 epinephrine added to each 10 ml of local anesthetic solution).

movements may not be completely lost. In a successful block, serial examinations every five minutes should show progressive sensory and motor loss. Failure to see this progressive change suggests a likely incomplete final block. This determination can be made within 15 minutes after injection. Supplemental injection of 10 to 20 ml of local anesthetic solution superficially in the interscalene groove (without seeking paresthesias) will usually correct the deficit.

Interscalene block can be performed without a nerve stimulator by seeking a sensory paresthesia that radiates to the hand or fingers. Using this method, patients must remain alert enough to report the paresthesia promptly and accurately.

Figure 7–3 shows the extent of sensory block with the technique described. (It is very similar to using a subclavian perivascular or supraclavicular block.) This is satisfactory for most shoulder surgery including total joint replacement. It should be noted that the skin of

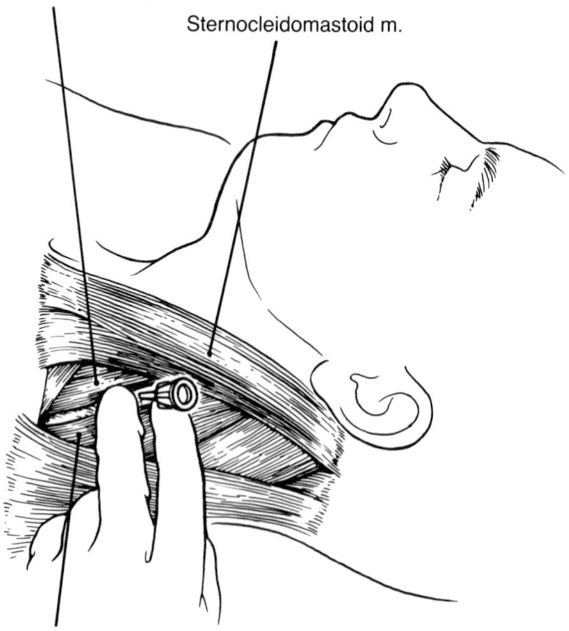

Figure 7–2. Block needle correctly positioned to perform interscalene brachial plexus block.

the axilla below the anterior axillary line and on the medial side of the arm (intercostobrachial nerve and medial brachial cutaneous nerve) is not anesthetized. If a low anterior incision is planned, it is necessary to infiltrate this area subcutaneously with 5 to 10 ml of local anesthetic solution before incision. Since this area is in the surgical field, it is blocked by the surgeon after surgical skin prep and draping are completed. As discussed earlier, this anesthetic technique alone is not adequate for surgery below the spine of the scapula.

Figure 7–4 shows a typical operating room setup for shoulder surgery. Note that the patient's head and airway remain accessible to the anesthesiologist. Before incision, sedation should be tailored to meet individual patients' needs.

Interscalene brachial plexus block has proved safe and effective for shoulder surgery over 10 years of use. Serious complications are rare, but when they occur, they must be recognized and treated promptly to avoid morbidity.

Horner's syndrome and recurrent laryngeal nerve block are common and are of no consequence as long as patients are warned of their possible occurrence.[29]

The phrenic nerve lies on the anterior surface of the anterior scalene muscle at the level the block needle is inserted. It is blocked in 35 to 40 per cent of patients who receive brachial plexus anesthesia using above-the-clavicle approaches, including interscalene block.[30] Figure 7–5 shows postoperative elevation of the right hemidiaphragm in a patient following ipsilateral interscalene block. This change may produce subjective dyspnea in occasional patients. Treatment consists of reassurance and monitoring the adequacy of ventilation.

Pneumothorax must be considered in the differential diagnosis but does not occur if the technique is used correctly. It is more likely with the supraclavicular and subclavian perivascular techniques. An upright chest x-ray should be obtained in any patient with distressing dyspnea after a block. Figure 7–6 shows a pneumothorax following an interscalene block attempted lower in the neck than the recommended level.

A number of blood vessels are present near the injection area. A small volume of local anesthetic injected into the vertebral artery will cause a convulsion.[31] This complication is rare and can be prevented

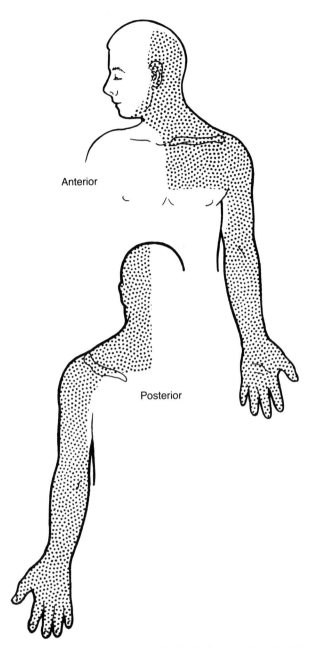

Figure 7–3. Distribution of cutaneous analgesia following interscalene brachial plexus block. (Superficial cervical plexus block is included.)

Damage to nerves is a rare event with any form of regional anesthesia. The etiology may be difficult to determine because of the multiple factors that might be involved. Overt or latent neurological disease (such as diabetic neuropathy) predating surgery should be considered. Whether such conditions contraindicate a block depends on the status of individual patients and the risks to them associated with the administration of a general anesthetic.

Intraoperative factors include nerve damage owing to the surgical procedure and the trauma it causes; chemical injury from local anesthetics; injury caused by intraoperative position of an anesthetized extremity; and trauma caused by the block needle, either directly with nerve injury or indirectly by causing local bleeding and subsequent nerve compression. Contaminants such as soap or sterilizing solutions remaining on block equipment can be neurotoxic. Single-use, disposable equipment eliminates this risk. The use of block needles with short bevels or noncutting "pencil point" tips may reduce direct or indirect needle trauma.[36]

A possible mechanism for nerve injury during interscalene block is needle trauma to the fifth or sixth cervical nerve roots where they lie cradled in the bony troughs of their respective cervical transverse processes. The risk can be minimized by seeking correct needle placement superficially and by the use of a nerve stimulator which will cause muscle twitching before a nerve is contacted. Great care is needed if the needle position is changed after injection of a portion of the local anesthetic. Sensory paresthesias and muscle twitches, otherwise indicative of proximity of the needle to a nerve, may be attenuated or absent.

Another mechanism for nerve injury is intraneural injection of local anesthetic. This produces high intraneural pressure, ischemia, and severe pain. It should be suspected and the injection stopped any time that severe pain is associated with injection of local anesthetic solution.

The risks of nerve injury caused by regional anesthesia may be minimized by placing the blocks in alert or lightly sedated patients, using disposable needles designed for nerve blocks, gentle technique, and possibly electrical stimulation.

Dhuner reviewed a series of cases of "postanesthetic brachial plexus palsy" following surgical procedures.[37] He found that neural injury was far more common after general than regional anesthesia and that the most common cause was improper position of the extremity during surgery.

Most brachial plexus injuries that occur in the perioperative period are reversible over a few days, although rarely, full return to normal may take several months. Careful, serial neurological examinations will help to demonstrate the extent of the injury and the recovery process. Electromyographic examination can help pinpoint the site of injury. There is no specific therapy. Maintenance of a normal range of motion across involved joints should be undertaken while recovery progresses. Patients should be instructed to

in most cases by seeking correct needle placement superficially in the interscalene groove, careful aspiration before injection, and injection of local anesthetic in small increments rather than as a single large bolus.

Rarely, the block needle may enter a cervical nerve root dural sleeve leading to cervical epidural[32, 33] or spinal block.[34, 35] This can be prevented by use of correct needle orientation and injection superficially into the interscalene space. Should the complication occur, support of ventilation, blood pressure, and heart rate may be necessary. Equipment and drugs to provide this care must always be close at hand.

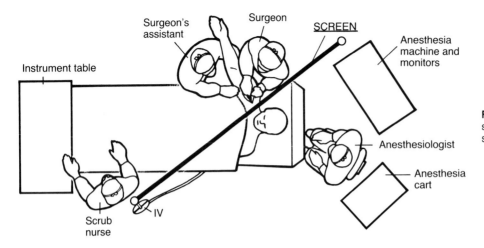

Figure 7–4. Arrangement of operating room for surgery on the right shoulder. The setup for left shoulder surgery is a mirror image.

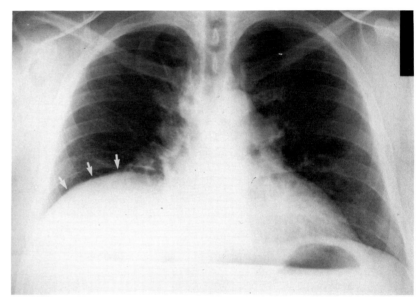

Figure 7–5. Postoperative elevation of the right hemidiaphragm *(arrows)* with block of the phrenic nerve after ipsilateral interscalene brachial plexus block.

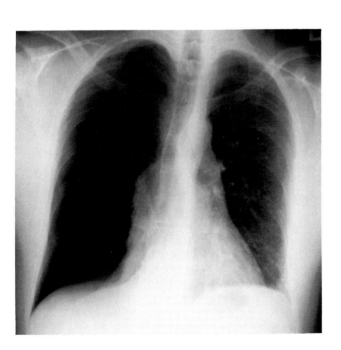

Figure 7–6. Pneumothorax following an interscalene block attempted at a site in the neck below the recommended level. The x-ray shows nearly complete collapse of the right lung and a shift of the mediastinum and heart into the left chest consistent with tension.

protect partially denervated extremities from further injury. Analgesics are appropriate for residual pain. Reassurance and support should be offered by the anesthesiologist and surgeon. A rare patient who suffers persistent pain may benefit from referral to a facility experienced in treating chronic pain. A number of empirical regimens (such as the combination of a phenothiazine and a tricyclic antidepressant) may offer relief, while avoiding the problems associated with long-term narcotics use.

CERVICOTHORACIC EPIDURAL BLOCK

Cervicothoracic epidural block can produce bilateral anesthesia suitable for surgical procedures on the shoulder. It may rarely have application when bilateral surgery under regional anesthesia is indicated or when technical problems contraindicate brachial plexus block. This technique should be used only by very experienced practitioners of epidural anesthesia.

Special Considerations

ACRYLIC BONE CEMENT

Shoulder joint replacement is facilitated by the use of the acrylic cement methylmethacrylate to hold the prosthetic components in place. The cement consists of granular methylmethacrylate to which a liquid monomer is added just before use. A number of problems have been reported in the period immediately following cement application.

Charnley reported hypotension after inserting acrylic cement into the femur.[38] Cardiac arrest has also been reported.[39] In a subsequent study,[40] it was found that intravenous infusions of an acrylic powder suspension into dogs did not alter blood pressure, but an infusion of the liquid monomer produced hypotension and tachycardia. It was proposed that absorbed monomer produced a reduction in peripheral vascular resistance which in turn led to the changes observed. More recent research indicates that respiratory and circulatory changes with monomer infusion occur only at concentrations many times those used clinically.[41]

A factor that may play an important role in causing cardiopulmonary changes is embolization of fat and bone marrow to the lungs.[42] High intermedullary pressures generated with insertion of a prosthesis have been demonstrated.[43] These and the resultant risk of embolization can be reduced by venting the medullary cavity during prosthesis insertion.[44] Oxygen desaturation following cement application has been demonstrated[44, 45] and further suggests pulmonary embolization.

It is not known whether the findings of these studies involving hip surgery also apply to the use of bone cement in shoulder surgery. However, since there is a possibility that cement application can lead to occasional life-threatening changes, it is prudent to minimize risks in every way possible. This should include maintenance of normal volume status and blood pressure prior to cement application, supplemental oxygen by mask or nasal cannula in awake patients, or high inspired oxygen concentrations in patients receiving general anesthesia. Good communication between the surgeon and anesthesiologist is necessary to ensure correct timing of these measures. Monitoring of oxygen saturation is desirable. Meticulous lavage to eliminate reamed intermedullary contents and venting of the medullary cavity during prosthesis insertion may be helpful.[46]

BONE GRAFTS

Corrective shoulder surgery will on some occasions require the use of a fresh bone graft harvested from a site distant from the shoulder. The need for a graft will sometimes be unknown or uncertain at the beginning of surgery but must be considered in a regional anesthetic management plan. The most common site for obtaining a graft is the iliac crest. In thin patients, small grafts can be removed comfortably with prior local anesthetic infiltration by the surgeon. For a larger graft or a graft in an obese patient, segmental epidural anesthesia may be used. In such cases, a regional block to produce shoulder anesthesia is administered in the usual fashion. Then a lumbar epidural catheter is placed, tested, and fixed in position. If during surgery it is determined that an iliac crest bone graft will be needed, sufficient local anesthetic is injected into the catheter to produce dense segmental sensory anesthesia over the donor site. In most cases, 5 to 10 ml of 2 per cent lidocaine or 2 per cent mepivacaine would be satisfactory choices.

Postoperative Anesthetic Care

At least one postoperative visit by the anesthesiologist is necessary. At that time it should be determined and documented whether any anesthetic complications have occurred. If so, it should be determined that adequate evaluation and treatment are being provided. In the case of regional anesthesia, return of normal neurological function should be confirmed. Questions or concerns about the anesthetic experience should be addressed. Only through careful postoperative follow-up can anesthesiologists learn what aspects of the care they provide help or distress their patients. Modifications in future practice based on this information lead to the evolution of better care.

Postoperative Pain Management

It has been shown in a number of studies that postoperative pain is frequently inadequately treated.[47-52] Anesthesiologists may be able to have a positive impact in this area. The choice of long-acting local anesthetics for regional blocks permits patients to remain comfortable for 12 to 24 hours following shoulder surgery. When these techniques are used, it is important to recognize that the blocks may recede rapidly. In such patients, analgesics should be started at the earliest sign of pain. Waiting longer may result in severe incisional pain that is then difficult to control. The administration of a long-acting narcotic (like methadone) intravenously at the end of a general anesthetic can improve comfort for many hours.

New techniques for postoperative analgesia may have application. Patient-controlled analgesia (PCA) permits patients to self-administer small boluses of intravenous narcotic to obtain immediate relief when pain becomes distressing. A microprocessor-controlled device developed for the purpose ensures that only safe doses are delivered. It has been shown that better analgesia using less narcotic is provided with these devices compared with traditional intramuscular injections given on an as needed basis. Patient satisfaction with pain control is high while using PCA. With all routes of narcotic administration, a surgical population will show wide variability in effective analgesic doses. There are no short cuts to careful, ongoing assessment and adjustment of dose to ensure the comfort and safety of each individual patient.

Under special circumstances, continuous or intermittent local anesthetic administration to maintain sensory anesthesia for the shoulder may be indicated. These should be used only by those experienced in the techniques and in hospital locations where appropriate monitoring and immediate treatment of complications can be provided. It should be noted that after a large bone graft, the donor site may cause more discomfort than the shoulder incision.

Summary

Anesthesia for patients undergoing surgical procedures on the shoulder has been considered in this chapter. For optimal care, anesthetic management should be planned before surgery by a qualified anesthesiologist who considers the individual needs, medical condition, and preferences of each patient. Adequate evaluation and optimal treatment of medical conditions should precede the administration of an anesthetic. Anesthetic techniques that do not alter the function of major organ systems, in particular regional anesthetic techniques, should be considered. Special problems that can occur during shoulder procedures, including their prevention and treatment, should be

well understood. Careful follow-up of patients after an anesthetic is mandatory.

Optimal perioperative care requires good communication between the anesthesiologist and surgeon. This includes, for each, a thorough understanding of the concerns and problems faced by the other in undertaking to care for each patient. A mutually supportive team concept coupled with modern anesthetic practice makes possible the administration of a safe anesthetic to most patients who require shoulder surgery.

References

1. Adam S: The Genuine Works of Hippocrates, Volume II. (Translated from the Greek.) New York: William Wood and Company, 1886, p 94.
2. Halsted WS: Surgical Papers. (Burket WC, ed). Baltimore: Johns Hopkins Press, 1925, pp 167–176.
3. Hirschel G: Anesthesia of the brachial plexus for operations on the upper extremity. Munchen Med Wochenschr 58:1555–1556, 1911.
4. Kulenkampff D: Anesthesia of the brachial plexus. Zentralbl Chir 38:1337–1350, 1911.
5. Gardiner DL, and Holmes F: Anaesthetic and postoperative hazards in rheumatoid arthritis. Br J Anaesth 33:258, 1961.
6. Edelist G: Principles of anesthetic management in rheumatoid arthritic patients. Anesth Analg 43:227, 1964.
7. Jenkins LC, and McGraw RW: Anaesthetic management of the patient with rheumatoid arthritis. Can Anaesth Soc J 16:407, 1969.
8. Cathcart ES, and Spodick DH: Rheumatoid heart disease: a study of the incidence and nature of cardiac lesions in rheumatoid arthritis. N Engl J Med 266:959, 1962.
9. Lee FI, and Brain AT: Chronic diffuse interstitial pulmonary fibrosis and rheumatoid arthritis. Lancet 2:693, 1962.
10. Cooper T: High blood pressure—scope of the problem. In Wolf GL, and Eliot RS (eds): Practical Management of Hypertension. Mount Kisco, New York: Futura Publishing Company Inc., 1975.
11. Edelist G: Extreme obesity. Anesthesiology 29:846, 1968.
12. Lamberth IE: Obesity and anesthesia. Clin Anesth 3:56, 1968.
13. Sprung CL, and Jacobs LJ: Indications for pulmonary artery catheterization. In (Sprung CL, ed): The Pulmonary Artery Catheter. Baltimore: University Park Press, 1983, pp 7–19.
14. Keith I: Anaesthesia and blood loss in total hip replacement. Anaesthesia 32:444, 1977.
15. Hole A, Terjesen T, and Breivik H: Epidural versus general anaesthesia for total hip arthroplasty in elderly patients. Acta Anaesthesiol Scand 24:279, 1980.
16. Modig J, Hjelmstedt A, Sahlstedt B, and Maripuu E: Comparative influences of epidural and general anaesthesia on deep vein thrombosis and pulmonary embolism after total hip replacement. Acta Chir Scand 147:125, 1981.
17. Chin SP, Abou-Madi MN, Eurin B, et al: Blood loss in total hip replacement: extradural v. phenoperidine analgesia. Br J Anaesth 54:491, 1982.
18. Hole A, Unsgaard G, and Breivik H: Monocyte functions are depressed during and after surgery under general anaesthesia but not under epidural anaesthesia. Acta Anaesthesiol Scand 26:301, 1982.
19. Modig J, Borg T, Karlstrom G, et al: Thromboembolism after total hip replacement: role of epidural and general anesthesia. Anesth Analg 62:174, 1983.
20. Takeshima R, and Dohi S: Cervical epidural anesthesia and surgical blood loss in radical mastectomy. Reg Anaesth 11:171–175, 1986.
21. Moore DC: Regional Block, 4th ed. Springfield, IL: Charles C Thomas, 1965, pp 221–242.
22. Winnie AP, and Collins VJ: The subclavian perivascular tech-

nique of brachial plexus anesthesia. Anesthesiology 25:353–363, 1964.

23. Winnie AP: Perivascular Techniques of Brachial Plexus Block. Philadelphia: WB Saunders, 1983.

24. Winnie AP: Interscalene brachial plexus block. Anesth Analg 49:455–466, 1970.

25. Dekrey JA, and Balas GI: Regional anaesthesia for surgery on the shoulder. A review of 1500 cases. Reg Anaesth 4:46–48, 1981.

26. Peterson DO: Shoulder block anesthesia for shoulder reconstruction surgery. Anesth Analg 64:373–375, 1985.

27. Mitchell EI, Murphy FL, Wyche MQ, and Torg JS: Interscalene brachial plexus block anesthesia for the modified Bristow procedure. Am J Sports Med 10:79–82, 1982.

28. Bashein G: Electrical nerve location for peripheral nerve blocks. Proceedings of the Washington State Society of Anesthesiologists Annual Meeting, 1986.

29. Seltzer JL: Hoarseness and Horner's syndrome after interscalene brachial plexus block. Anesth Analg 56:585–586, 1977.

30. Farrar MD, Scheybani M, and Nolte H: Upper extremity block. Effectiveness and complications. Reg Anaesth 6:133–134, 1981.

31. Kozody R, Ready LB, Barsa JE, and Murphy TM: Dose requirement of local anesthetic to produce grand mal seizure during stellate ganglion block. Can Anaesth Soc J 29:489–91, 1982.

32. Kumar A, Battit GE, Froese AB, and Long MC: Bilateral cervical and thoracic epidural blockade complicating interscalene brachial plexus block: report of two cases. Anesthesiology 35:650–652, 1971.

33. Scammell SJ: Inadvertent epidural anaesthesia as a complication of interscalene brachial plexus block. Anaesth Intensive Care 7:56–57, 1979.

34. Ross S, and Scarborough CD: Total spinal anesthesia following brachial plexus block. Anesthesiology 39:458, 1973.

35. Edde RR, and Deutsch S: Cardiac arrest after interscalene brachial plexus block. Anesth Analg 56:446–447, 1977.

36. Galindo A, and Galindo A: A special needle for nerve blocks. Reg Anaesth 5:12–13, 1980.

37. Dhuner, KG: Nerve injuries following operations: a survey of cases occurring during a six-year period. Anesthesiology 11:289–293, 1950.

38. Charnley J: Acrylic Cement in Orthopaedic Surgery. Baltimore: Williams & Wilkins, 1970.

39. Powell JN, McGrath PJ, Lahiri SK, et al: Cardiac arrest associated with bone cement. Br J Med 3:326, 1970.

40. Peebles DJ, Ellis RH, Stride SD, et al: Cardiovascular effects of methylmethacrylate cement Br J Med 1:349, 1972.

41. Modig J, Busch C, and Waernbaum G: Effects of graded infusions of monomethylmethacrylate on coagulation, blood lipids, respiration, and circulation. Clin Orthop 113:187, 1975.

42. Modig J, Busch C, Olerud S, et al: Arterial hypotension and hypoxemia during total hip replacement: the importance of thromboplastic products, fat embolism, and acrylic monomers. Acta Anaesth Scand 19:28, 1975.

43. Kallos T, et al: Bone marrow embolism during hip prosthesis. Proceedings of the Annual Meeting of the American Society of Anesthesiologists, San Francisco, California, 1973.

44. Kallos T: Impaired arterial oxygenation associated with use of bone cement in the femoral shaft. Anesthesiology 42:210, 1975.

45. Park WY, Balingit P, Kenmore PI, et al: Changes in arterial oxygen tension during total hip replacement. Anesthesiology 39:642, 1973.

46. Orsini EC, Byrick RJ, Mullen JBM, et al: Cardiopulmonary function during arthroplasty using cemented or non-cemented components. J Bone Joint Surg 69A:822–832, 1987.

47. Nageman J: Measurement and control of postoperative pain. Ann R Coll Surg Engl 61:419–426, 1979.

47a. Bonica JJ: Current status of postoperative pain therapy. In Yokota T, Dubner R. (eds): Current Topics in Pain Research and Therapy. Amsterdam: Excerpta Medica, 1983, pp 169–189.

48. Cronin M, Redfern PA, and Utting JE: Psychometry and postoperative pain complaints in surgical patients. Br J Anaesth 45:879–886, 1973.

49. Cohn FL: Postsurgical pain relief: status and nurses' medication choices. Pain 9:265–272, 1980.

50. Donovan BD: Patient attitudes to postoperative pain relief. Anaesth Intensive Care 11:125–129, 1983.

51. Sriwatanakul K, Weiss OF, Alloza JL, et al: Analysis of narcotic usage in the treatment of postoperative pain. JAMA 250:926–929, 1983.

52. Weis OF, Sriwatanakul K, Alloya JL, et al: Attitudes of patients, house staff, and nurses toward postoperative analgesic care. Anesth Analg 62:70–74, 1983.

Shoulder Arthroscopy

David W. Altchek, M.D.
Russell F. Warren, M.D.
Michael J. Skyhar, M.D.

In the past decade, shoulder arthroscopy has become a relatively common procedure. This has occurred despite the fact that its usefulness and indications in the diagnosis and treatment of disorders of the shoulder are yet evolving. As with arthroscopy of the knee in its earlier stages, the most common uses of shoulder arthroscopy today are to confirm the diagnosis, establish the specific details of the pathology, and formulate the plan for subsequent management. In recent years, arthroscopic techniques have been adapted to the shoulder as a treatment modality, thereby reducing the morbidity associated with the more traditional approaches to intra-articular and subacromial pathology. Although these surgical approaches are yet controversial in many situations, they are gaining increased acceptance in the management of disorders of the shoulder.

History

The first arthroscopic examination of the shoulder is credited to Burman who in 1931 examined, with a primitive arthroscope, multiple joints in a cadaver.[10] Published data on this subject did not reappear until Wantabe in 1950 developed the No. 21 arthroscope, with which most arthroscopies of the 1970s were performed.[49] This instrument, with a tungsten bulb in a fragile carrier, provided inconsistent illumination and a high risk of breakage within the joint. With the development of the rigid telescope and fiberoptic illumination in the 1970s, arthroscopy became a safer and more dependable procedure.

Arthroscopy of the shoulder has evolved at a much slower pace than that of the knee. The first clinical reports of shoulder arthroscopy were by Andren and

colleagues in 1965,[3] Conti in 1979,[13] and Wiley in 1980,[52] who investigated, arthroscopically, patients with "frozen shoulders" and other problems. Wantabe and colleagues[47] clearly described the anterior and posterior portals. Wantabe was also the first to publish reports of arthroscopy of the shoulder to diagnose osteochondral fractures, identify loose bodies, evaluate the extent of rheumatoid arthritis, and identify lesions of the biceps brachii and glenoid labrum.[47, 48] Since 1980 there has been a proliferation of publications dealing with shoulder arthroscopy and a rapid advance in its use. Several small series with short follow-ups have been published to propose arthroscopic management of acromial arch decompression, debridement of rotator cuff tears and labral lesions, as well as shoulder stabilization procedures using both suturing and stapling techniques. These represent exciting new areas of clinical research that could usher in a new era of shoulder surgery.

Arthroscopic Anatomy of the Glenohumeral Joint and Subacromial Space

Possibly the greatest contribution of shoulder arthroscopy has been to better delineate intra-articular and subacromial anatomy, both normal and pathological. Unlike conventional operative exposures, whether performed on patients or cadaver specimens, arthroscopic evaluation can be performed without distorting the joint structure for access. Via magnification, arthroscopic inspection provides a more extensive visualization of the joint than can be achieved during open surgery.

Intra-articular Anatomy

BICEPS TENDON

The tendon of the biceps brachii is the structure that should be visualized first when the arthroscope is inserted from the primary puncture segment. Several authors have noted that the intracapsular segment of the tendon is in continuity with the superior portion of the glenoid labrum as it passes from its origin on the supraglenoid tubercle (Fig. 8–1).[6] As the tendon is followed laterally out of the sleeve, it can be seen to extend past the transverse humeral ligament. Intra-articular lesions of the biceps tendon, including degenerative fraying, most often seen in conjunction with chronic impingement syndrome, and tenosynovitis, are all clearly evident. At times the tendon may exist as two or three bands, but this should not be interpreted as abnormal.

GLENOID LABRUM

The glenoid labrum has been likened to the knee meniscus in both structure and function. Moseley and Overgaard, in their elegant dissection and histological study, demonstrated that the labrum is composed primarily of fibrous tissue, unlike the fibrocartilaginous meniscus of the knee.[31] According to Moseley, an area of fibrocartilaginous tissue is present within the labrum but is confined to a small transition zone where the labrum attaches to the glenoid rim.[31] They concluded that the glenoid labrum is a redundant fold of capsular

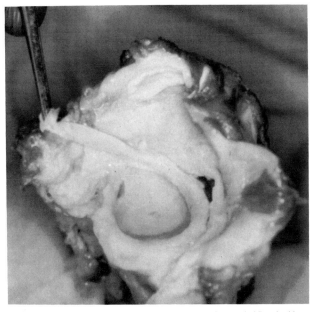

Figure 8–2. Photograph of a cadaveric specimen with forceps holding the biceps tendon, again seen in continuity with the labrum, which can be followed circumferentially along the glenoid.

tissue that changes shape with different states of rotation of the humeral head (Fig. 8–2).

The exact function of the labrum remains somewhat in debate. It clearly has a significant role in the stability of the glenohumeral joint. The glenoid labrum, through its wedge shape, increases both the depth and conformity of the glenoid and serves as the site of attachment of the glenohumeral ligament capsule to the scapula.[2] It is generally accepted that a disruption

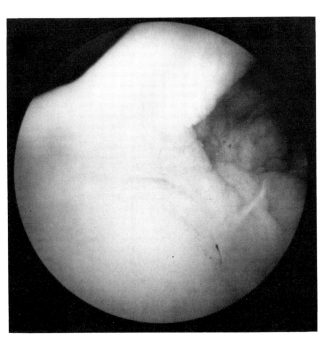

Figure 8–1. An arthroscopic photograph demonstrating the biceps tendon (seen at 12 o'clock) in continuity with the superior glenoid labrum.

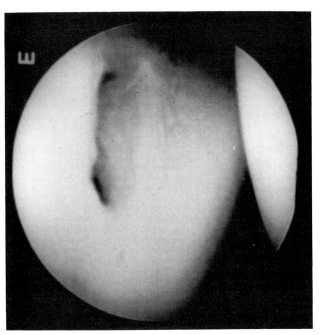

Figure 8–3. An arthroscopic photograph demonstrating the labral sulcus. The humeral head is seen to the right and the glenoid to the left. The labrum is seen well attached above and below.

of the glenoid labrum is the most common lesion noted in a shoulder with instability.[28, 29, 38, 42] This disruption may range from fraying to a tear in its substance, or it may be a separation of the labrum from its attachment to the glenoid margin. Detrisac and Johnson, in anatomical dissections, have documented the presence of a labral sulcus as a normal variant in approximately 20 per cent of individuals.[17] This sulcus is present anteriorly, superior to the equator of the glenoid, and can be differentiated from a detachment by its smooth and well-rounded borders (Fig. 8–3).

There is a large amount of individual variation in the normal labrum. Commonly, the labrum is thin superiorly and thick inferiorly. The labrum ranges in width from 5 mm to a barely discernible fold of 1 mm. In cross-section, the labrum is wedge shaped and in the thicker portion can be meniscoid in appearance (Fig. 8–4).

The glenoid is oval in shape and covered by articular cartilage. Frequently the normal glenoid has evidence of a central bare area devoid of articular cartilage. At the waist of the glenoid a notch is present anteriorly and can be confused with bony abnormalities seen on the anterior glenoid in patients with anterior instability.

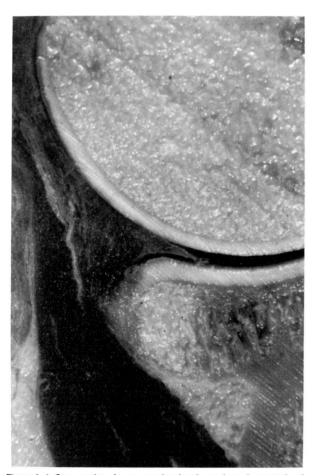

Figure 8–4. Cross-section of a preserved cadaveric specimen demonstrating the labrum interposed as a wedge between the humeral and glenoid articular surfaces. (Courtesy of Steven P. Arnoczky, DVM.)

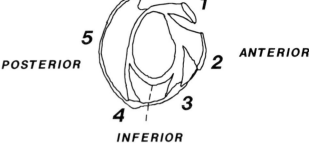

Figure 8–5. Drawing demonstrating the glenohumeral ligament system: (1) the biceps tendon, (2) the middle glenohumeral ligament, (3) the superior band of the inferior glenohumeral ligament, (4) the posterior band of the inferior glenohumeral ligament, and (5) the posterior capsule.

CAPSULAR LIGAMENTS AND SUBSCAPULARIS TENDON

When viewed from its exterior surface in open surgery, the shoulder joint capsule appears to have a relatively uniform appearance. It is only on close examination of the intra-articular surface, as is provided by the arthroscope, that discrete capsular ligaments become evident. As Schlemm described in 1853, the capsule has three areas of distinct thickening which he named as glenohumeral ligaments, superior, middle, and inferior (Fig. 8–5).[43] The superior glenohumeral ligament has been consistently described as originating from the supraglenoid tubercle. The adjacent labrum, together with the tendon of the long head of the biceps, attaches to the humerus in a small fovea, the fovea capitis, proximal to the lesser tuberosity.

The middle glenohumeral ligament is described as having two alternative sites of glenoid origin. The first and most common is from the supraglenoid tubercle and superior labrum just below the superior glenohumeral ligament. Alternatively, it is found to arise not from the labrum but the scapular neck. The insertion site is at the junction of the lesser tuberosity and anatomical neck of the humerus. This variability in origin site can have important functional implications as a scapular, rather than labral, origin creates a large anterior pouch that could theoretically contribute to anterior instability.[31, 46]

The inferior glenohumeral ligament is the most well defined and substantial of the three glenohumeral ligaments. Originating from the anteroinferior and posterior margins of the glenoid labrum below the equator of the glenoid, it inserts on the inferior aspect of the neck of the humerus. Turkel and coworkers were able to define two discrete parts of the inferior glenohumeral ligament: the thickened anterosuperior edge, which they named the superior band of the inferior glenohumeral ligament (Fig. 8–6), and the diffuse thickening of the anteroinferior part of the capsule, which they named the axillary pouch of the inferior glenohumeral ligament (Fig. 8–7).[45] Recent

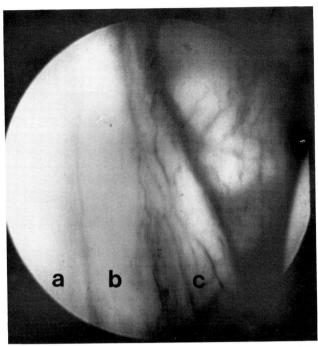

Figure 8–6. The inferior glenohumeral ligament seen attaching to the inferior glenoid labrum. Left to right: (a) glenoid, (b) labrum, and (c) inferior glenohumeral ligament.

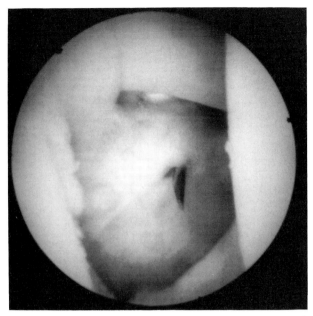

Figure 8–8. The spinal needle is seen piercing the intra-articular anterior triangle. The glenoid is to the left, the humeral head to the right, the biceps tendon above, and the subscapularis below. The middle glenohumeral ligament is draped over the subscapularis below.

work performed at the Hospital for Special Surgery has focused attention on the posterior portion of the inferior glenohumeral ligament (IGHL). The postero-superior portion of the IGHL is similar to its anterior counterpart, presenting as a distinctly thickened band. As will be described below, this posterior portion acts in concert with the anterior segment to stabilize the glenohumeral joint against both anteriorly as well as

posteriorly directed forces.[44] This posterior portion of the IGHL is seen most directly with the arthroscope in an anterior portal.

The tendon of the subscapularis is seen anteriorly in the shoulder joint, intimately related to the glenohumeral ligaments (Fig. 8–8). Mosely and colleagues studied the synovial recesses of the anterior capsular mechanism and found that the tendon of the subscapularis enters the joint most commonly via the subscapularis bursae, situated between the superior and middle glenohumeral ligaments.[31] Arthroscopically, it is clearly evident in this position as a discrete, tendinous structure.

The capsular mechanism, including the subscapularis and glenohumeral ligaments and glenoid labrum, as well as their contribution to normal joint stability can be demonstrated on arthroscopic examination. Under direct vision using the arthroscope, the subscapularis tendon can be seen to tighten during both external rotation and abduction of the glenohumeral joint, while during internal rotation the tendon becomes lax. As abduction progressively increases, the subscapularis tendon can be seen to move to a superior position, leaving the inferior portion of the humeral head uncovered anteriorly. Turkel and colleagues, in their selective cutting studies, were able to analyze the contribution of the glenohumeral ligaments and subscapularis tendon to anterior stability at different arm positions. They concluded that the subscapularis is not an effective check or block to anterior dislocation at the higher degrees of abduction.[45]

The superior glenohumeral ligament, which becomes lax with progressive arm abduction, takes up tension only with the arm at the side. Therefore it does not

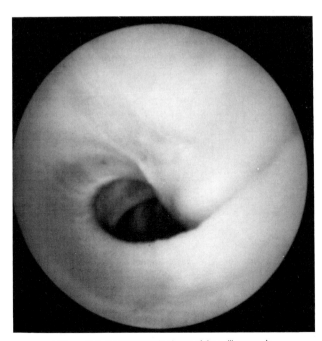

Figure 8–7. An arthroscopic picture of the axillary pouch.

function in the resisting of anterior translation of the humerus on the glenoid but possibly functions more as a stabilizer against inferior subluxation or dislocation.

The middle glenohumeral ligament, similar to the subscapularis tendon, can be seen to become taut with external rotation, lax with internal rotation, and move progressively higher in relation to the humeral head with abduction. Cutting of the middle glenohumeral ligament demonstrated it to be effective in limiting external rotation below 45 degrees of abduction only.

The inferior glenohumeral ligament when assessed arthroscopically from a posterior portal is seen clearly to have two parts as described by Turkel and colleagues.[45] The anterosuperior tendon of the glenohumeral ligament becomes taut with progressive external rotation with the arm in the adducted position. In adduction and neutral rotation, the axillary pouch portion of the ligament is lax; in progressive abduction and external rotation the axillary pouch disappears as these fibers of the ligament become taut. At maximal external rotation and 90 degrees of abduction, the anterior and inferior aspects of the humeral head are covered by a continuous taut ligamentous structure. These anatomical findings correlate with the results of Turkel's cutting studies, which demonstrated that with division of the anterosuperior band, external rotation with the arm adducted allowed dislocation; however, with abduction, cutting of this band alone did not produce instability.[45] When in addition the inferior portion of the axillary pouch was sectioned, external rotation caused frank dislocation in 45 or 90 degrees of abduction.

Posterior stability studies were performed by Schwartz and coworkers at the Hospital for Special Surgery and demonstrated that increased posterior translation of the humeral head occurred with sectioning of the posterior component of the inferior glenohumeral ligament but that dislocation did not occur routinely until the anterosuperior structures were sectioned as well.[44]

HUMERAL HEAD

Arthroscopic examination of the humeral head includes evaluation of the cartilage and subchondral plate as well as the insertion of the joint capsule and rotator cuff.

Examination of the entire humeral head is possible by rotating the arthroscope anteriorly and posteriorly as well as rotating the humeral head internally and externally. Posteriorly, a normal sulcus, as recognized by DePalma, is present between the insertion of the posterior capsule and overlying synovial membrane and the edge of the articular surface.[16] DePalma found a variability in the size of this bare area that was directly proportional to age. No such area is seen in young patients. He postulated that the capsule and synovium retract beginning in the third decade, producing this "sulcus" of bare bone. This bare area is identified by punctate vessel penetration and is located lateral to the area of a Hill-Sachs lesion.

ROTATOR CUFF AND SUBACROMIAL SPACE

The intra-articular portion of the rotator cuff can be viewed arthroscopically as it courses to its insertion on the humeral head. Any violation in its integrity can be demonstrated through examination by probing both the tendon and its insertion for evidence of fraying or avulsion.

Visualization of the subacromial space with the arthroscope affords a complete view of the coracoacromial arch, including the acromioclavicular joint as well as the superficial surface of the rotator cuff and subacromial bursae. The space in a normal subject should demonstrate a thin layer of bursal tissue covering an intact rotator cuff that can be followed laterally to its insertion on the humeral head. The coracoacromial arch should be smooth in contour and covered by a layer of fibrous tissue and periosteum without evidence of spurring.

The acromioclavicular joint, seen in the medialmost aspect of the space, is evident by its glistening white joint capsule. Inspection of the anterior wall of the subacromial space reveals the coracoacromial ligament with its thick fibers coursing in an oblique fashion from the anterior aspect of the acromion to its insertion on the coracoid.

Indications

As with any relatively new procedure the indications for shoulder arthroscopy are still in an evolutionary stage. At the present time, shoulder arthroscopy has been performed more often as a diagnostic procedure. Final surgical management for most shoulder pathology is still carried out by open surgery. Recent advances in technique and instrumentation have made surgical arthroscopic shoulder procedures more accessible and easier to perform.

We will discuss the indications for shoulder arthroscopy as they pertain to particular pathological conditions.

SHOULDER INSTABILITY

The cornerstone of the diagnosis and treatment of patients with shoulder instability is accurate history and physical examination. There exists, however, a subset of patients, particularly those with subluxation, in whom complex symptoms and office examination cannot prove instability to be the sole source of the problem. This is not uncommon in athletes involved in overhead sports, in whom instability can be the result of the high intrinsic forces directed both ante-riorly and posteriorly, depending on arm position.[47] Translation of the humeral head is prevented by a competent labral ligamentous complex and by decel-eration forces generated by the rotator cuff and biceps tendon. Failure or dysfunction of any part of the restraint system, whether it be rotator cuff, biceps tendon, or labrum-ligament complex, leads to in-creased load being borne by the other portions of the system, accounting for the possible coexistence of instability and impingement in the throwing athlete. These patients often present with pain as their only complaint. Accurate assessment of the amount and direction of glenohumeral translation is often difficult, and differentiation between apprehension and pain is at times impossible.

Examination under anesthesia alone in this group of patients is often not enough to confirm the instability pattern. Owing to the previously described mechanism, translation may be increased symmetrically in both anterior and posterior directions. Arthroscopy of the glenohumeral joint can aid in solving the diagnostic puzzle. A violation of the integrity of the glenoid labrum, depending on the site, either with frank de-tachment or tearing within its substance, can document the presence and direction of the instability. The location of the labral lesion is of crucial importance because the majority of labral lesions, whether anterior or posterior, when occurring below the equator of the glenoid, are felt to be secondary to instability whereas superior lesions are not. Other findings, such as a Hill-Sachs defect, loose bodies, or glenohumeral ligament detachment or deficiency, would be important factors supportive of a diagnosis of instability. In addition, arthroscopic inspection of the intra-articular surface of the rotator cuff and the subacromial space should be carried out since rotator cuff disease frequently accom-panies labral damage above the equator of the glenoid.

We should emphasize that in the majority of situa-tions arthroscopy does not play a major role in the diagnosis of instability. In experienced hands, arthro-scopic stabilization for patients with traumatic unidi-rectional (anterior) glenohumeral instability is an op-tion. The technique will be discussed in detail in a following section.

IMPINGEMENT

Impingement syndrome, a term coined by Neer, is the most common cause for anterior shoulder pain.[35] This situation is caused by microtrauma to the rotator cuff mechanism as tuberosities of the humerus glide under the coracoacromial arch during arm elevation (Fig. 8–9). Over time there results a thickening of the subacromial bursae and progressive degeneration of rotator cuff and biceps tendon. By affording visuali-zation of both the intra-articular and subacromial spaces, shoulder arthroscopy can help document the presence and extent of a rotator cuff tear, the degree

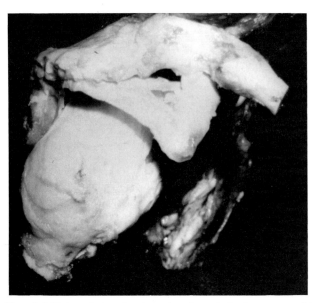

Figure 8–9. Photograph of a cadaveric specimen demonstrating the coracoacromial arch with the underlying rotator cuff.

of inflammatory changes present in the subacromial bursae, and the condition of the undersurface of the coracoacromial arch and acromioclavicular joint. In the circumstance where the diagnosis is unclear, intra-articular examination with the arthroscope will provide additional information. This is most important in the patient with coexistent instability, in whom preopera-tive examination may be misleading.

Preliminary results indicate that shoulder arthros-copy may have a role in the treatment of these lesions as well as in their diagnosis. The most well-accepted surgical treatment for the impingement syndrome is the anterior acromioplasty by Neer.[35] In the traditional open approach, this is achieved by releasing a portion of the anterior deltoid to allow exposure of the anterior acromion and subacromial space. With the arthroscope the anterior acromioplasty can be performed without violating the deltoid sleeve. Concerns about the tech-nical feasibility of performing a complete acromioplasty arthroscopically are answered by the study of Gartsman and colleagues.[19] In cadaver specimens, open acro-mioplasty was compared with arthroscopic acromio-plasty. They concluded that the arthroscopic procedure was as effective as the open procedure both in loca-tion and amount of acromial removal as well as cor-acoacromial ligament excision. Preliminary results in clinical studies are encouraging, demonstrating an earlier return to full activity than with the open ap-proach.[1, 18, 39]

The therapeutic role of shoulder arthroscopy in the presence of a documented rotator cuff tear is less well defined. Andrews and coworkers have performed a limited intra-articular debridement of partial (incom-plete) tears of the rotator cuff in a population of throwing athletes, resulting in a favorable clinical out-come.[4] Our results with this form of treatment show some deterioration of clinical result over time, indicating that simple arthroscopic debridement is not the final solution for these patients. At present, in young, active patients with partial tears demonstrated by arthrograms, we pursue an initial conservative program of spring or elastic exercises to develop the cuff, followed by arthroscopy only if the pain persists. If indicated, a partial-thickness tear would be treated with arthroscopic cuff debridement and subacromial decompression. A frank full-thickness tear, if present, would be treated by open cuff repair combined with acromioplasty.

In older patients with moderate to large full-thickness tears of the rotator cuff, arthroscopic subacromial decompression without repair has proved unpredictable in outcome. In a small review of patients at the Hospital for Special Surgery with a minimum of one-year follow-up, approximately 75 per cent had good to excellent results and the rest fair with incomplete relief of symptoms.[1] It has been our observation that patients who preoperatively demonstrate significant rotator cuff weakness, as evidenced by shoulder shrugging during arm elevation, respond less well to decompression alone and should be considered for cuff repair.

INFLAMMATORY AND DEGENERATIVE DISEASES OF THE SHOULDER

Inflammatory disease such as rheumatoid arthritis (RA) not uncommonly causes a synovitis of the glenohumeral joint. As in the knee and elbow, synovectomy for the patient who has not had significant loss of articular cartilage has proved to be of benefit. Arthroscopic synovectomy of the shoulder for RA, gout, pigmented villonodular synovitis, and synovial chondromatosis has been performed with relatively good short-term results.

In cases of symptomatic degenerative arthritis in the young patient who is not a candidate for joint replacement or the older patient in whom a limited surgical approach is more appropriate, arthroscopy can offer diagnostic, therapeutic, and prognostic advantages. More so than by x-ray, a precise evaluation of the location and amount of remaining articular cartilage can be performed, aiding future management plans.[10, 52] In the short term, careful debridement of loose flaps of tissue combined with a wash-out procedure can provide symptomatic relief.[12]

ADHESIVE CAPSULITIS

As described by Neviaser in 1945, adhesive capsulitis represents an inflammatory reaction in the capsule and synovium that leads to the formation of adhesions in the axillary recess.[33] Using the arthroscope Neviaser has established a four-stage pathological sequence for adhesive capsulitis.[32, 34] Beginning with a fibrous synovial reaction (Stage I), there is a progressive increase in synovitis and adhesion formation. In the final stage (Stage IV), there are mature adhesions and loss of the axillary recess. Contrary to this, Johnson contends that adhesive capsulitis does not result in intra-articular adhesions. Johnson believes that an inflammatory process begins in the synovium in the region of the subscapularis bursa and progresses to a circumferential thickening and tightening of the entire capsule.[21]

Many of the earliest published studies on shoulder arthroscopy dealt with its use in adhesive capsulitis.[3, 5, 12, 20] Distention of the joint combined with intra-articular capsular release and manipulation has produced mixed results. At present, most authors agree that the arthroscope has little indication in treating adhesive capsulitis. An arthrogram demonstrating obliteration of the inferior pouch is the simplest diagnostic modality. Treatment is generally conservative with manipulation under anesthesia performed only if a several-month course of rehabilitation fails to improve motion.

SEPSIS

As in the knee, arthroscopic debridement and lavage coupled with the establishment of continuous drainage and appropriate intravenous antibiotics have been used successfully in the treatment of the septic glenohumeral joint.[11, 37] Special attention must be given to the sheath of the biceps tendon, which is a site of potential extra-articular tracking of infection. Its presence would require a separate open incision and drainage of the biceps sheath.

Technique

OPERATING ROOM SET-UP

Choice of the operating table depends on lateral or beach chair positioning. For the lateral position, we employ a fracture table with well-padded kidney rests. A shoulder-holding device is positioned at the foot of the table on the contralateral side to allow abduction and flexion of the operated shoulder. Traction is placed through a suspended pulley system using 5 to 15 pounds, depending on the size of the patient. Alternatively, the beach chair position uses a regular operating room table that allows for hip and knee flexion. A well-padded support is placed at the foot of the table. No traction device is used.

The television monitor and video equipment are placed contralateral to the shoulder being operated upon. The arthroscopic irrigating solution, light source, and shaver source are placed on the same side as the monitor. We used normal saline for the majority of arthroscopic procedures. However, for use of the electrocautery, a nonconductive solution such as sterile water (as opposed to an electrolyte solution) is needed. Our inflow tubing allows for four separate solution bags. For shoulder arthroscopy we use three bags of saline and one of sterile water. In this way, the sterile water may be used in isolation and only when the electrocautery is in use.

Necessary equipment for shoulder arthroscopy includes

1. A 30-degree 4.5-mm arthroscope.
2. A video camera and monitor.
3. A suction shaving system with varying sizes of full radius resectors and arthroplasty burs.
4. An interchangeable cannula system that allows for inflow, sealed probe, and shaver insertion.
5. A complete set of basic arthroscopy hand instruments.

ANESTHESIA AND POSITIONING

Unlike arthroscopy of the knee, local anesthesia is rarely used in the shoulder. The thick covering layers of subcutaneous tissue and muscle make the shoulder more difficult to anesthetize properly for complete arthroscopic examination.

Although general anesthesia with endotracheal intubation is the most widely used, we have performed most of our arthroscopic procedures on the shoulder under scalene block.

After induction of anesthesia the shoulder is examined. The passive range of motion is recorded. If an adhesive capsulitis is present and a manipulation is planned, we usually wait until the completion of the arthroscopic procedure. The lysis of adhesions via manipulation will cause acute hemorrhage, making arthroscopic visualization difficult.

Glenohumeral stability in the anterior, posterior, and inferior direction should be assessed in all patients regardless of preoperative diagnosis. For example, impingement syndrome may be secondary to instability that is often subtle and difficult to detect in the awake patient. In addition, patients with known instability may have other components (directions) to their instability that may be identified only by examination under anesthesia.

We initially performed the procedure in the lateral position with the arm suspended by a traction device. Although we have had no complications directly related to the position, transient neuropraxia, presumably due to excessive strain on the brachial plexus, has been reported by several authors.[23] Paulos and colleagues reported a 30 per cent incidence of transient neuropraxia following shoulder arthroscopy using traction.[39]

Beginning in 1986 we began positioning the patient in the upright seated position with the arm free at the side. We have performed more than 75 shoulder arthroscopic procedures since that time including diagnostic arthroscopy, subacromial decompression, and arthroscopic stabilization. There are several advantages to this position. Patient positioning is easier regardless of anesthetic technique. The upright position facilitates management of the airway. When scalene block anesthesia is used, the awake, upright patient may observe

the procedure on an overhead monitor. Under scalene block, tolerance of the lateral position is poor, whereas the seated position is usually comfortable. There is no need to prepare and drape the patient again if an anterior arthrotomy needs to be performed following the arthroscopy. The capsular anatomy within the glenohumeral joint is not placed in the nonanatomical, stretched-out attitude, which occurs with arm traction. This assumes importance when performing arthroscopic stabilization because an accurate assessment of glenohumeral ligament laxity must be obtained, in addition to the necessity of reapproximating tissues under minimal tension. There is more mobility of the arm using the beach chair position, enabling the assistant to manipulate the arm and affording a very complete view of the intra-articular and subacromial spaces. Exact arm positioning becomes crucial during arthroscopic rotator cuff repair and stabilization. In addition, with the vertical position of the joint and the arm at the side the external anatomy is easier to visualize and palpate.

The only disadvantage to this position is fogging of the camera. The beach chair position places the arthroscope in a dependent position during certain procedures, most notably subacromial decompression. This problem can be helped by minimizing the outflow of effluent onto the arthroscope and solved by newer fog-free equipment. The rubber diaphragm from the Acufex disposable cannula, when placed over the arthroscopic sheath, will decrease the flow of effluent down the cannula onto the camera (Fig. 8–10).

Description of Beach Chair Position

After the table is adjusted so that the patient is sitting upright with the torso placed at 70 degrees to the horizontal, a pad is placed under the medial border

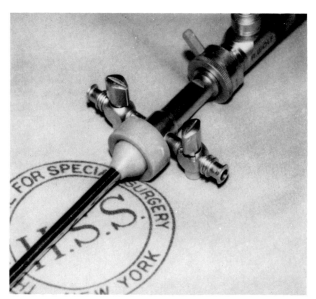

Figure 8–10. The arthroscopic cannula with the Acufex diaphragm in place.

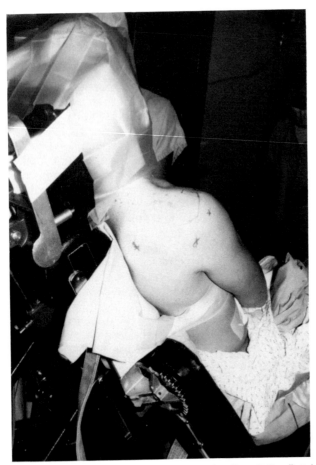

Figure 8–11. Posterior view of a patient in the seated position with the affected scapula lying free over the edge of the table.

placing the fingers anteriorly and the thumb posteriorly and by moving the humeral head in an anteroposterior direction on the glenoid. The *posterior portal site* can be localized by a soft spot and can be palpated posteriorly by the thumb; this point is 3 cm inferior and 2 cm medial to the posterolateral tip of the acromion (Fig. 8–12). Anatomically, this portal passes through the lower border of the infraspinatus near the interval between it and the teres minor. The closest major neurovascular structure is the axillary nerve, which is well inferior, exiting posteriorly beneath the teres minor. The final localization of the joint is performed by placing a finger on the coracoid, which demonstrates the plane of the glenoid articular surface. The skin overlying this posterior portal site is then infiltrated with a 1:300,000 epinephrine solution and incised. The subacromial space is then entered through this portal using a No. 18 spinal needle and filled with 30 ml of this solution. The spinal needle is then withdrawn to the skin and placed in the shoulder joint, directing the tip of the needle toward the coracoid process. The tip of the spinal needle can be felt to pop through the posterior capsule. The joint is then distended using 60 ml of the epinephrine solution. The arthroscopic sleeve with the blunt trocar is then introduced into the shoulder joint following the same path as the spinal needle. The newly distended capsule provides an easier target. As with the spinal needle, a distinct pop will be felt as the cannula passes through both intervals between the infraspinatus and teres minor and the capsule. The trocar is removed, and the arthroscope with light source is inserted through the cannula into the joint.

of the scapula, and the patient is placed with shoulder free over the edge of the table (Fig. 8–11). If an arthroscopic stabilization is to be attempted with the suture technique, the entire scapula should be accessible. This is achieved by placing a 10-pound sandbag under the ipsilateral hip to facilitate rotation of the upper torso away from the edge of the table. The arm is allowed to hang free at the side. An arm board is used at the side of the table at the bend of the elbow. The shoulder and axilla are scrubbed with a sterile soap, then prepared and draped using adhesive sterile drapes at the borders.

Arthroscopic Technique

DIAGNOSTIC ARTHROSCOPY

Portal Placement and Portal Anatomy

The first step in accurate portal placement is identification of the external anatomical landmarks. The acromial borders, acromioclavicular joint, clavicle, and coracoid should be clearly marked out. Next, the humeral head and glenohumeral joint are palpated by

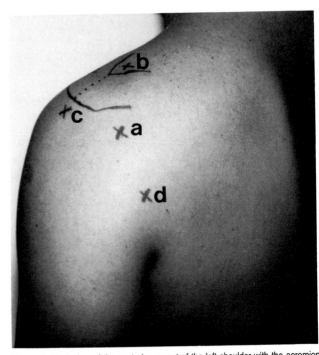

Figure 8–12. A view of the posterior aspect of the left shoulder with the acromion and posterior clavicular borders outlined. The X's represent the potential portal sites: the primary posterior portal *(a),* the Neviaser or supraspinatus portal *(b),* the lateral subacromial portal *(c),* and the posterior axillary portal *(d).*

Inflow is established through the arthroscopic cannula, and the joint is visualized.

We orient the joint on the monitor in anatomical or vertical position. The most consistent landmark is the biceps tendon in its intra-articular course. It should be followed from its lateral exit, from the joint above the humeral head, to its medial insertion on the superiormost aspect of the glenoid where it blends with the glenoid labrum.

Prior to carrying out our primary examination of the joint, we establish an anterior portal for use both as an inflow and instrumentation portal. We use a disposable cannula with a side port for inflow (or outflow) and a diaphragm covering its exterior to prevent water leakage. It should be emphasized that maintenance of a clearly established inflow portal is crucial. Without the benefit of a tourniquet, as in knee arthroscopy, bleeding is prevented only by the presence of constant intra-articular hydrostatic pressure.

After localization of the biceps tendon and orientation of the glenohumeral joint into the vertical axis, the triangular space for the *anterior portal* can be localized. This intra-articular space is bordered superiorly by the biceps tendon, inferiorly by the subscapularis tendon, and medially by the anterosuperior portion of the glenoid (see Fig. 8–8). The subscapularis tendon is recognized as a rounded, discrete, tendinous structure in the area of the anterior capsule. The exterior site of entrance is then created in the anterior aspect of the shoulder. The spot chosen should be

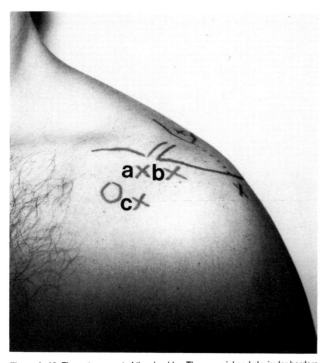

Figure 8–13. The outer aspect of the shoulder. The acromial and clavicular borders and the coracoid are outlined. The three X's seen anteriorly represent potential anterior portal sites: the most common site of the anterior portal *(a)*, and additional potential portal sites *(b* and *c)*.

lateral and superior to the coracoid. This avoids potential injury to the neurovascular structures in this area. Anatomical studies of the anterior portal performed by Matthews and colleagues have demonstrated that the region medial to the coracoid contains the brachial plexus and axillary artery and vein. In the lateral inferior region, the musculocutaneous and subscapularis nerves are at risk.[27] With these exterior and intra-articular landmarks clearly established, a spinal needle is placed into the joint from a point lateral to the coracoid piercing the intra-articular triangle (Fig. 8–13). With this as a guide, the cannula with a removable trocar is inserted into the joint along the same path as the spinal needle. The inflow tubing is now switched to this anterior cannula, and a joint examination is performed.

Primary Joint Examination

We begin by following the biceps tendon throughout its intra-articular course from its lateral sleeve, where it passes out into the bicipital groove, to its insertion into the supraglenoid tubercle where it blends with the superior glenoid labrum. Any evidence of flattening or fraying should be noted. Using the biceps tendon as our guide, we follow the labrum around the glenoid face. The labrum must be carefully probed for evidence of detachment or tearing (the probe now inserted through the anterior cannula). At the same time an evaluation of the integrity of the glenoid articular surface is performed. Attention is then directed laterally to the humeral head. With a sequence of internal rotation to assess the anterior aspect, external rotation to assess the posterior aspect, and abduction to examine superiorly, the entire articular surface of the humeral head can be visualized through the posterior portal. Particular attention should be paid to the posterolateral portion of the humeral head for the presence of a Hill-Sachs compression fracture while remembering that with advancing age a bare area is commonly seen in this region.

From the posterior portal we next view the anterior and inferior capsular mechanism. The most distinct structure seen anteriorly is the subscapularis tendon. It is seen entering into the joint via the subscapularis recess between the superior and middle glenohumeral ligament. The superior glenohumeral ligament is rarely distinct, and it is often obscured from view by the biceps tendon. The middle glenohumeral ligament is seen draped over the subscapularis tendon and becomes taut with external rotation. The division between the inferior glenohumeral ligament and the middle glenohumeral ligament is demarcated by the superior band of the inferior glenohumeral ligament, which is often a distinct structure seen directly attaching to the labrum in the inferior portion of the anterior wall (see Fig. 8–6). During external rotation and abduction, this can be seen to tighten. The inferior glenohumeral ligament can be followed inferiorly as it becomes the axillary pouch (see Fig. 8–7). During external rotation, the capsule in this region will twist and tighten, diminishing considerably the volume of the axillary pouch.

The axillary pouch should be thoroughly examined for evidence of loose bodies, and the area of insertion of the inferior capsule into the humeral neck should be free of adhesions, as seen in adhesive capsulitis.

The rotator cuff is evaluated by viewing superiorly, following the tendon laterally to its insertion site into the tuberosity, which can be seen with arm abducted. This should be carefully probed for avulsion or fraying as evidence of rotator cuff disease.

For a more complete view of the posterior labrum, the arthroscope may be switched to the anterior portal and the probe and inflow to the posterior portal. This will provide an improved view of the posterior component of the inferior ligament and the posterior labrum.

Additional Portals

Superior Portal

The superior portal, or supraspinatus inflow portal (Neviaser), is sometimes valuable as an inflow or viewing portal for visualization of the anterior glenoid in stabilization procedures (discussed later in this chapter). The point of entry is the supraspinatus fossa, bounded anteriorly by the clavicle, laterally by the medial border of the acromion, and inferiorly by the scapular spine (see Fig. 8–12). The portal is identified by a spinal needle passed through this spot, directed 20 degrees laterally and 15 degrees anteriorly. The needle tip is identified in the joint above the supero-posterior junction of the glenoid neck. A cannula is then inserted along the same path. Anatomical dissections have shown the cannula to pass through the trapezius muscle and the muscle belly portion of the supraspinatus. The suprascapular nerve and artery lie 3 cm medial to this portal site, well out of range of possible injury.[32]

Lateral (Subacromial) Portal

This portal is useful as an instrument or viewing portal for work in the subacromial space. Located 2 cm below the midlateral acromion, it has several advantages (see Fig. 8–12). First, it allows for triangulation in the subacromial space. Second, because of the shape of the acromion (hooked anteriorly), it is easier to pass instruments beneath the acromion laterally than it is anteriorly or posteriorly. Third, its position parallel to the coracoacromial ligament allows easy resection. Fourth, it is perpendicular to the acromioclavicular joint allowing resection. Finally, its position is well suited to grasping and stapling of rotator cuff tears.

The portal passes through the deltoid and deltoid fascia directly into the subacromial bursa. The axillary nerve lies well distal, approximately 5 cm from the lateral acromial border.

Anterosuperior Portal

As will be detailed in a later section of this chapter, additional anterior portals (all lateral and superior to the coracoid) can be added to allow simultaneous visualization and instrumentation of the anterior glenoid (see Fig. 8–13). The exact location of each portal should be localized by a spinal needle passed percutaneously into the joint under direct vision. In the region of the coracoacromial ligament the thoracoarcromial artery is at risk.

Posterior Portal

A posterior axillary portal is useful for inflow, removing loose bodies, or releasing adhesions in the axillary pouch. The portal position is identified using a spinal needle placed directly into the axillary pouch. It is placed slightly inferior (1 to 2 cm) to the original posterior portal (see Fig. 8–12). One must be clearly aware of the proximity of this portal to the axillary nerve. The cannula should be placed strictly along the needle tract, taking care not to stray distal to the inferior capsular recess.

Arthroscopic Procedures for the Shoulder

IMPINGEMENT SYNDROME

The appropriate operating room setup and arthroscopic equipment for shoulder arthroscopy have been outlined in an earlier portion of this chapter. A few salient features should be reviewed. The patient may be positioned in the lateral or seated position, depending on the surgeon's preference and familiarity. Besides the usual arthroscopic equipment, a commercially available electocautery device, motorized bur, and full radius resector are necessary. As well, sterile water will be needed as inflow when the electrocautery is in use.

After examination under anesthesia and prior to arthroscopic insertion, the subacromial space is entered using the 18-gauge spinal needle and distended with 30 to 40 ml of a 1:300,000 epinephrine solution. Complete arthroscopic examination of the glenohumeral joint is then performed as previously described. We use the initial posterior portal to redirect the arthroscopic cannula, with the blunt trocar in place, into the subacromial space. The cannula is swept from a medial to lateral direction within the subacromial space to break up adhesions in the bursa. The trocar is then withdrawn, and a long blunt rod is passed through the cannula into the bursa and directed toward the previously described anterior portal site. A large-bore anterior inflow is then established by the retrograde technique. As the arthroscope is withdrawn posteriorly, visualization of the anterior cannula should be possible. Often there is a great deal of inflammation present, and visualization at this stage in the procedure is difficult. At this time the lateral acromial portal is established, approximately 2 cm below the lateral tip of the acromion. A cannula with a shaver adapter is then introduced through this portal, and the full radius resector is introduced. Visualization improves as inflammatory bursal tissue is removed from the rotator cuff below and the acromion above.

After completion of the bursectomy, examination of the subacromial space is performed. The probe is used again through the lateral portal to (1) identify the anterior and lateral bony margins of the acromion, (2) palpate for spurs on the undersurface of the acromion, (3) evaluate the integrity of the rotator cuff, and (4) establish the position and condition of the acromioclavicular joint and identify the coracoacromial (CA) ligament. On occasion we have noted, in young patients, an unusually thick layer (up to 1 cm) of ligamentous tissue on the undersurface of the acromion. Debridement of this with resection of the CA ligament

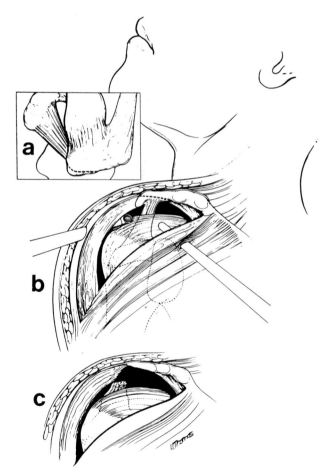

Figure 8–14. *a,* A schematic drawing of the superior view of the acromion with the distal clavicular and coracoid represented as well. The *dotted line* represents the proposed resection of the anterolateral acromion, which would include the site of attachment of the coracoacromial ligament. *b,* A schematic drawing of a posterior view of a left shoulder. The arthroscope has been inserted posteriorly and the bur is entered laterally. *c,* After completion of acromioplasty, the anterior acromial lip has been excised and the coracoacromial ligament detached.

has, in this select group of patients, provided adequate decompression. In all other patients we proceed with a formal bony acromioplasty. The 5.5-mm arthroplasty bur is introduced through the lateral portal, and a centering hole is made in the clearly visible midanterior acromion to the depth of the bur (Fig. 8–14). Beginning posteriorly and laterally the acromion is then thinned to this depth. At this point burring does not extend to the most anterior or medial acromion since these areas are more prone to incur bleeding. Once thinning is complete, the bur is used to continue the acromial removal anteriorly until the leading anterior edge of the acromion is clearly identifiable. The anterior acromion is then recessed with the bur, and an attempt is made to leave the deep fascia of the deltoid muscle intact. If perforation of the fascia occurs and bleeding is encountered, the electrocautery is used to achieve hemostasis. The classic acromioplasty of Neer describes a wedge of bone measuring 0.9 cm in anterior thickness and extending 2 cm posteriorly to be removed from the undersurface of the acromion. We achieve this by removing anterior acromion from the acromioclavicular joint medially to the lateral deltoid insertion until the leading acromion edge is recessed posterior to the clavicle. With this amount of acromial removal, the coracoacromial ligament should be totally detached from its acromial insertion (Fig. 8–14*a*). If deemed necessary, the acromioclavicular joint is now approached. Any osteophytes on the deep surface are removed, and, if symptoms warrant, a distal clavicular excision can be performed. In some instances it is easier to gain access to the acromioclavicular joint by switching the arthroscope to the lateral portal and the bur to the anterior portal. As well, from this position the remaining undersurface of the acromion can be re-evaluated for the presence of missed spurs or irregularity.

ROTATOR CUFF LESIONS

If a bursal side partial-thickness tear is seen arthroscopically, we proceed with the acromioplasty and perform a limited debridement of the tear. If a full-thickness tear is found, its location, size, and mobility must be assessed. If the cuff tear is essentially a peripheral leak, we would possibly treat this by decompressing the subacromial space. Only tears that are 1 to 3 cm in size with good tissue that is not retracted may allow for an arthroscopic repair. However, if difficulty is encountered, a mini-incision may facilitate this repair. Large tears in a patient with rehabilitation capability require open repairs, particularly when dealing with retracted tissue. Massive tears in patients with poor rehabilitation potential are treated by acromioplasty and debridement. Mobility is gauged by grasping the edge of the torn rotator cuff through the lateral portal. If the cuff can be reduced easily to a position lateral to the articular margin of the humerus and if the tear is limited to the supraspinatus, we would consider arthroscopic stapling, using an absorbable tack. At present, we rarely attempt arthroscopic rotator cuff repair. It is indicated only when the patient refuses open surgery or in the setting of acute avulsion of the rotator cuff. An additional lateral portal will usually be necessary. If the existing lateral portal is good for grasping and reducing the cuff, the second lateral portal should be created to prepare the humeral bed and insert the tack. The exact location is best found by using an 18-gauge spinal needle; the site in general is more anterior than the previous midlateral portal. As with open cuff repair, a raw bony surface should be prepared with the shaver and bur at the proposed site of cuff reattachment. With the grasper reducing the cuff (usually through the midlateral portal) to the trough, the humerus should be positioned to minimize the tension on the repair. The tack is placed through the other lateral portal, transfixing the cuff to the humeral bed. If possible, a second tack is then placed to provide additional fixation. The arm is then carefully adducted while the repair is probed to determine a safe zone of abduction for postoperative immobilization.

Large retracted rotator cuff tears are managed either by acromioplasty from above or by open reconstruction, depending on patient demands, desires, and the exact nature of the tear.

Postoperative Regimen

Postoperatively, patients who have undergone arthroscopic acromioplasty are initially placed in a sling. They are instructed to begin Codman exercises on the first postoperative day, progressing from passive range of motion exercises to active range of motion exercises by the first week to 10 days. Sling use is diminished daily and should be eliminated by five days postoperatively. Gentle resistance exercises emphasizing internal and external rotation with the arm in adduction can begin as early as two weeks postoperatively. Return to overhead sports is delayed until at least four to six weeks postoperatively.

Results of Arthroscopic Acromioplasty

We analyzed, in a prospective fashion, an initial group of 43 patients who underwent arthroscopic acromioplasty.[2] Included were those patients with both Stage II impingement and rotator cuff tears. In this group of patients with an average age of 42 years, 86 per cent were regularly active in sports and disabled because of shoulder pain. At an average of 18 months follow-up, there were good to excellent results in 84 per cent and fair to poor results in 16 per cent. Of those active in sports, 83 per cent had a full return. Return to work averaged nine days; return to sports averaged 2.4 months; and total recovery averaged 3.8 months. Of the seven unsatisfactory results, four were only slightly symptomatically improved or never achieved an adequate level of function postoperatively

to be satisfactory, and three required reoperation. Of the three reoperations, one was a technical failure: inadequate removal of anterior acromion successfully managed by subsequent open acromioplasty. The second had postoperative acromioclavicular pain requiring subsequent arthroscopic decompression of the acromioclavicular joint. The third was a failure to provide symptomatic relief by acromioplasty alone in a 40-year-old semiprofessional softball pitcher with a full-thickness rotator cuff tear. Subsequent open cuff repair was performed with a fair result.

When the results were analyzed to determine outcome based on the presence or absence of rotator cuff tears, we found the following: Patients with full-thickness rotator cuff tear (n = 10) achieved lower functional levels but had similar pain relief and satisfaction when compared with patients with impingement alone; patients with partial-thickness rotator cuff tears (n = 6) achieved nearly identical results to those with intact rotator cuffs.[1] In particular, patients with large, seemingly irreparable rotator cuff tears had a favorable outcome. This finding of symptomatic relief provided by decompression alone in patients with massive rotator cuff tears supports the results by Rockwood. In a group of patients with large rotator cuff tears, he performed open acromioplasty without cuff repair and found a high percentage to have excellent symptomatic relief at follow-up.

SHOULDER INSTABILITY

Diagnosis

The arthroscope can be useful both in the diagnosis and treatment of the unstable shoulder. As stated in the section on indications, we rarely use the arthroscope as a primary diagnostic modality. The history and physical examination dictate our treatment plan in the majority of cases.

Pathological Anatomy

Labrum and Glenoid

The labrum plays a significant role in the prevention of shoulder instability. Through its wedge shape it increases both the depth and conformity of the glenoid and serves as the site of attachment of the glenohumeral ligaments of the scapula. It appears that the inferior half of the labrum, in the area of attachment of the inferior glenohumeral ligament, is the important component in stabilizing the glenohumeral joint.

Inferior labral lesions felt to occur secondary to increased humeral head translation take one of two forms: detachment from the scapular neck (Bankart lesions) (Fig. 8–15) or tearing of its substance (Figs. 8–16 and 8–17), similar to a knee meniscus. Associated erosion or fracture of the glenoid margin may be found in the area of labral detachment.

Superior labral lesions are frequently degenerative,

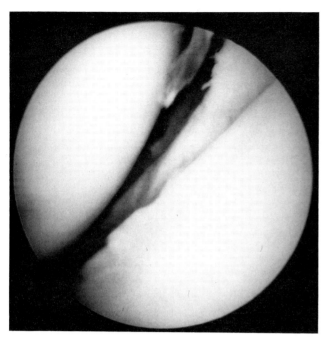

Figure 8–15. An arthroscopic photograph from a posterior portal viewing the anterior labrum. The humeral head is to the left; the glenoid is to the right. The labrum is seen detached from the glenoid margin.

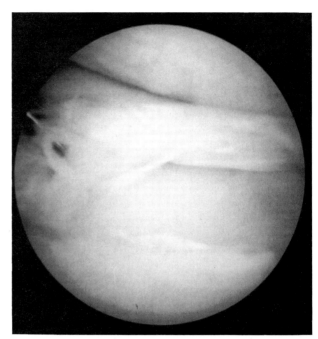

Figure 8–17. An arthroscopic photograph from a posterior portal viewing the posterior glenoid labrum. The humeral head is seen superiorly. A displaced bucket-handle tear of the posterior labrum is seen; a spinal needle (left) is interposed between the fragments.

resulting in tearing of the labrum. Overhead athletes, particularly throwers, will often demonstrate superior labral pathology. Andrews and colleagues have demonstrated that tension in the biceps muscle is transmitted to the anterosuperior portion of the labrum. They hypothesize that with repetitive throwing, tearing of

the labrum will occur in this region.[5] Detrisac and Johnson have noted a labral "sulcus" appears at the 2 o'clock position as a normal variant in approximately 20 per cent of individuals. This is not a detachment and is recognized by its smooth borders (see Fig. 8–3).[17]

Glenohumeral Ligaments

As stated previously, the inferior glenohumeral ligaments (IGHL) are the prime stabilizers of the joint. The ligament is effective only when firmly attached to the glenoid rim. Since the labrum serves as the site of attachment, a detached inferior labrum represents a nonfunctional inferior glenohumeral ligament. Less frequently, the ligament may be avulsed from the labrum, torn within its substance, or congenitally poorly formed or absent. When a multidirectional component is present, the anterior and axillary pouch will appear more capacious than usual and often the labrum will appear intact and firmly attached. The anterosuperior band, if present, will not become taut during external rotation, and the axillary portion of the IGHL will not wind up in its usual fashion. If, in the presence of anterior instability, the labrum is well attached and yet the ligaments are loose, the site of ligamentous attachment laterally to the humeral head should be inspected.[7]

Humeral Head

In cases of recurrent anterior dislocation, greater than 80 per cent of the patients will have a Hill-Sachs lesion.[50] This is found at the posterolateral margin of

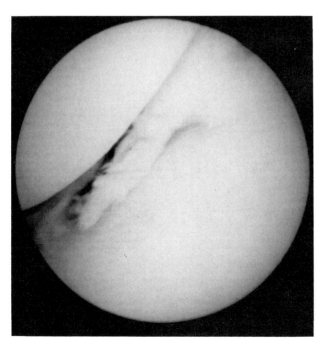

Figure 8–16. An arthroscopic photograph from a posterior portal viewing the anterior labrum. The humeral head is to the left; the glenoid is to the right. A flap tear of the anterior glenoid labrum is seen interposed between the humeral head and the glenoid.

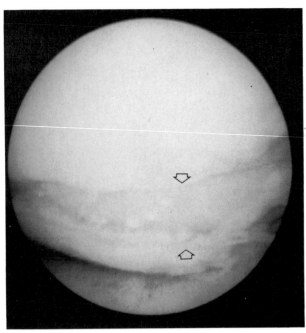

Figure 8–18. An arthroscopic photograph from the posterior portal viewing the posterior lateral head. A compression fracture is seen interposed between two areas of cartilage *(between arrows),* indicating the presence of a Hill-Sachs lesion.

the humeral articular surface. The location of the Hill-Sachs lesion is just medial to the normal bare area or "sulcus" previously described. The Hill-Sachs lesion will have articular cartilage lateral to it and a raw, cancellous surface, whereas the normal sulcus will be smooth with vascular channels (Fig. 8–18). Minor

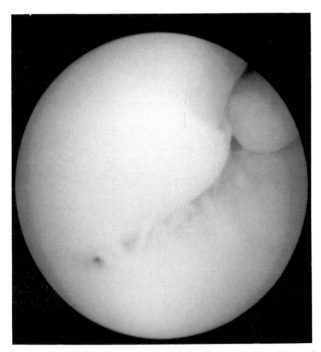

Figure 8–19. An arthroscopic photograph viewing the posterior lateral humeral head and axillary pouch from a posterior portal. A well-rounded loose body is seen at the 2 o'clock position.

variants of the Hill-Sachs lesion may be observed in subluxating shoulders.

Loose Bodies

Loose bodies formed secondary to the repetitive trauma of instability are present in about 10 per cent of unstable shoulders and should be specifically looked for, particularly in the axillary recess where they often collect (Fig. 8–19). When loose bodies are found in the shoulders of a patient undergoing arthroscopy for any reason, the patient's history and physical examination should be carefully re-evaluated for evidence of instability.

Treatment

Labral Debridement

The majority of lesions of the glenoid labrum will occur in association with glenohumeral instability. The instability may be clinically evident in patients with recurrent dislocation or subluxation in whom the labrum will frequently be detached in the direction of primary instability. Conversely, the instability may be subtle as in the overhead athlete in whom increased anteroposterior translation of the humeral head on the glenoid can occur, leading to increased shear stresses on the labrum with resulting labral tears. Pappas pointed out that the torn labrum can, as in the meniscus of the knee, became intermittently interposed between the articular surfaces, causing symptoms of "functional instability." If the labrum margin remains attached, the torn fragment can be removed, resulting in relief of symptoms. Pappas reported on 19 athletes with functional instability who underwent open excision of labral tears without stabilization, with good results at 1.5- to 14-year follow-up.[38]

Labral tears can result from degenerative processes. Kohn, in his examination of autopsy specimens, noted fissuring and fibrillation in 76 per cent of labrums in specimens averaging 84 years of age.[24]

Andrews has reported superior labral tears at the biceps insertion that occur in throwers presumably because of overpull of the biceps during the throwing motion.[5]

The diagnosis of labral pathology can be difficult. If associated with instability, it is diagnosed by history and physical examination, and labral pathology is confirmed at the time of surgical treatment. Labral lesions occurring secondary to "functional instability" or degenerative or traumatic causes do not often produce specific findings on physical examination.[24, 28, 38] Arthrography, CT arthrography, and arthrotomography have all been used to diagnose labral lesions.[25, 29] We have not found these radiographic studies to be sensitive or specific enough to guide our patient management. If clinical suspicion of labral pathology is high, we would proceed with arthroscopic examination.

Technique of Labral Debridement. The operating room setup and positioning have been previously described. Before arthroscope insertion we perform a thorough examination to rule out instability as the underlying problem. Once the joint has been visualized and a second portal (usually anterior) established, the labrum is identified and probed. The surgeon should identify if the labrum is torn or detached and the precise location of the lesion. A detached labrum (particularly in the inferior half of the glenoid) usually indicates instability. Other signs, such as a Hill-Sachs lesion or loose body, should be looked for to provide supporting evidence. Resection of labral tissue in these cases will provide no benefit and may cause a patient to develop frank instability.

Tears in the labrum may be longitudinal, producing a bucket handle fragment (see Fig. 8–17), or radial with a longitudinal component, producing a flap (see Fig. 8–16). Torn labral fragments may be resected if the glenohumeral ligaments and labral rim remain firmly attached. Debridement technique is similar to partial meniscectomy in the knee. Using hand or motorized shaving instruments, the torn labrum is resected back to a stable rim, and the leading edges are contoured to achieve a smooth transition. Excessive removal of labral tissue should be avoided since it may make the ligament system nonfunctional.

Postoperatively, the patient is placed in a sling for comfort and begins range-of-motion exercises on the second postoperative day. Light resistance exercises for the rotator cuff are begun within the first week. Return to sports is delayed for three to four weeks.

Results

Andrews, in his review of 73 throwing athletes who had tears of the anterosuperior labrum (42.5 per cent had partial-thickness rotator cuff tears in addition), reported good to excellent results in 88 per cent at 13.5-month follow-up.[4, 5] At The Hospital for Special Surgery we have a group of 23 athletic patients who underwent glenoid labral debridement for complaints of shoulder pain. The diagnosis of instability was suspected, but not documented, in all.[1] Of these patients, 13 had lesions which were anteroinferior. Of these lesions, 12 were tears and one a detachment. Six had anterosuperior labral tears. The remaining four were posterior lesions of which one was a detachment and three were tears. At an average 31-month follow-up, we found good to excellent results in 70 per cent. Both patients with labral detachments required subsequent open stabilization procedures. The best results were achieved in the subset with anteroinferior tears.

STABILIZATION

The common denominator underlying all arthroscopic shoulder stabilization procedures for anterior instability is re-establishment of a functional inferior glenohumeral ligament. This is achieved by reattaching the avulsed labrum with ligament in continuity or reattaching the ligament directly to the glenoid neck.

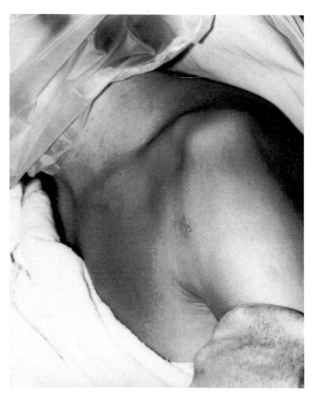

Figure 8–20. This photograph demonstrates the sulcus produced between the acromion and the humeral head when traction is placed on the arm of a patient with multidirectional instability of the shoulder.

We have performed the procedure successfully on patients with acute/recurrent or traumatic anterior subluxation or dislocation, avoiding those with inferior or multidirectional components (Fig. 8–20). These patients have marked redundancy of capsular tissue, making appropriate tensioning difficult to achieve with an arthroscopic procedure.

Many methods of fixation have been advocated: metallic implants such as staples and screws, sutures, and recently biodegradable tacks. In addition, Caspari has developed a technique of inferior glenohumeral ligament reconstruction using a section of allograft iliotibial band similar to a Galli procedure. The allograft is affixed to the humerus by a screw with ligament washer and to the scapula through a drill hole. It functions as a sling which tightens during abduction and external rotation of the arm. Caspari has reported 100 cases thus far with no recurrent instability and excellent preservation of motion.[11]

At the Hospital for Special Surgery we are in agreement with Matsen and Zuckerman who reported on the unacceptably high rate of significant complications related to the use of metal screws and staples placed in and around the shoulder.[53] The most commonly used arthroscopic metallic device is the dual-pronged staple by Instrument Makar. Johnson has reported the largest series, with a 20 per cent redislocation rate in the early group. With experience and the implementation of three weeks of immobilization and discontinuance of contact sports, the short-term redislocation rate was reduced to 3 per cent.[22] Besides redislocation, problems

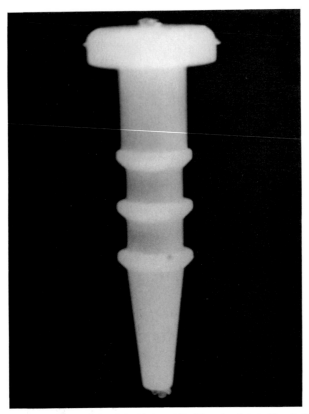

Figure 8–21. Magnified view of a biodegradable (Maxon) tack (actual length 15 mm).

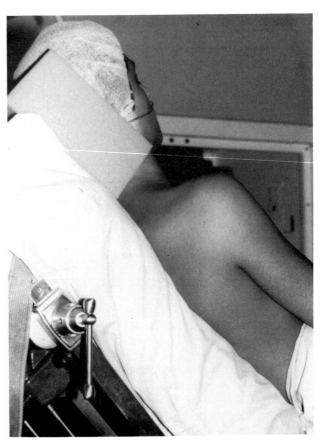

Figure 8–22. This photograph demonstrates the upright position of a patient prepared for arthroscopic stabilization of the shoulder. Only the medial border of the scapula rests on the edge of the table.

such as impingement of the staple and loosening occur and are felt to be related to initial positioning. The staple must be implanted with both prongs in bone and must be placed superior to the equator of the glenoid. Wiley has reported a small series of arthroscopic stabilizations performed with a metal rivet that is removed at six weeks postoperatively.[51] The redislocation and complication rates are low, but follow-up is short.

Since 1983 we have used a suture technique in which knotted PDS sutures transfix the tissue and are passed through transglenoid drill holes. More recently, we have used a biodegradable (Maxon) tack that is placed in a predrilled hole for stabilization of anterior dislocation or subluxation (Fig. 8–21).

Techniques

Suture Technique

Besides the standard operating equipment and setup previously described for shoulder arthroscopy, we use pins, 30 cm × 2 mm, with two eyelets and a sharp point to drill the suture through the bone. A power drill should be available for insertion. The suture material used is absorbable 0 PDS.

After induction of anesthesia and after examination confirms that the instability pattern is anterior, we proceed with placing the patient into the upright sitting position with the arm free at the side (Fig. 8–22). The

arthroscope is inserted through the posterior portal as previously described; the standard anterior portal is established with a cannula; and a complete diagnostic arthroscopy is carried out. In particular, the labrum is probed for site of detachment, continuity with ligamentous structures, and overall tissue quality. If a detached labrum is present, it is grasped by an instrument placed through the anterior cannula. As tension is placed on the labrum, the inferior glenohumeral ligament is viewed. A functional labrum should transmit the tension, and tightening of the ligament should occur. If the labrum is absent, nonfunctional, or of poor quality, a discrete superior band of IGHL should be identified. This is grasped and pulled up to the 3 o'clock position on the anterior glenoid rim. As this is done, the anterior pouch should disappear, and tension should be seen in the anterior ligamentous structures. If neither a functional labrum nor a discrete ligamentous band is present, the arthroscopic procedure should be aborted and open stabilization performed.

To proceed with the arthroscopic stabilization, a careful but complete debridement of the anterior glenoid rim and scapular neck is performed to achieve a raw bony surface (Fig. 8–23a). Localization of the drill holes is then performed. We use two drill holes: superior (1 o'clock) and inferior (3 o'clock), each with two sutures. The pins should enter 2 to 3 mm medial

Figure 8–23. *A*, A superior transaxial view of the glenohumeral joint. A Bankart lesion is present anteriorly with separation of the glenoid labrum. The arthroscope has been introduced posteriorly and the bur from an anterior portal. The bur is used to freshen the anterior margin. *B*, The Beath pin drilled from anterior to posterior across the glenoid at an oblique angle to avoid possible injury to the suprascapular nerve and artery. *C*, Passage of the suture through the anterior cannula using the eyelet of the Beath pin.

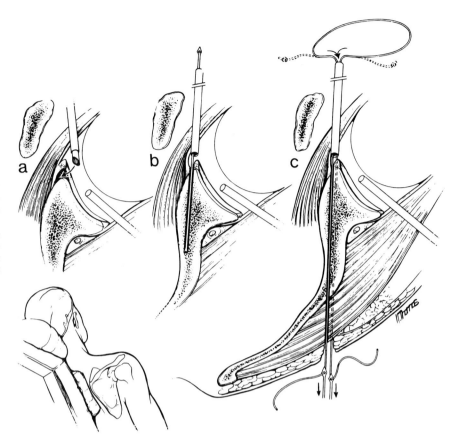

to the edge of the glenoid rim and travel posteriorly, diverging from the articular surface of the glenoid. Excessive lateral exit of the pin posteriorly must be avoided to prevent injury to the suprascapular nerve (Fig. 8–23*b*). If the original anterior portal is adequate for pin placement, a second, more superoanterior portal is created to allow for grasping and tensioning of the labral or ligamentous tissue. Localization of this portal is performed using a percutaneous spinal needle, and the portal is established using a cannula.

The tissue is grasped through the superior portal and reduced under tension to the anterior glenoid rim. With humeral rotation set at neutral, the pin is placed through the drilling portal, and the sharp end is used to spear a robust section of the tissue. The point is then placed at the superior drill hole, and the pin is then drilled by power from anterior to posterior, diverging medial to the glenoid surface. The pin is drilled through the posterior cortex and to the skin posteriorly at which point a 5-mm skin portal is created. The drill is then placed on the extruding pin posteriorly, and the two 0 PDS sutures are threaded through the eyelets. The pin is then drilled completely through posteriorly, while one end of the suture is retained anteriorly (Fig. 8–23*c*). The anterior sutures are then grasped intra-articularly through the superior portal and pulled up through this portal. This frees the suture from the drilling portal. A second set of sutures is then passed in a similar fashion at the 4 to 5 o'clock position.

The posterior tails from the second set of sutures are transferred subcutaneously to the first posterior skin portal. One anterior suture from each set of two is tied to a suture from the other set, using a bulky knot. The

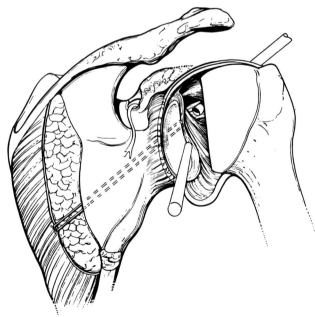

Figure 8–24. The suture placed under tension and tied posteriorly over the thick fascia of the infraspinatus, reducing the anterior glenoid labrum with the attached inferior glenohumeral ligament.

knots are then pulled through the anterior cannula by posterior tension. Under direct vision, the knots should oppose the labral or ligamentous tissue to the glenoid rim under tension. Because this tightens the entire anterior recess, visualization of the anterior rim may become more difficult at this point. The tissue should be probed to be sure that the knots have not cut through. If satisfactory, the sutures are tied to themselves subcutaneously in the posterior portal over the thick fascia of the infraspinatus (Fig. 8–24). The skin is closed meticulously over the sutures with no dermal pouching. The arthroscope is removed, and the patient is placed in a shoulder immobilizer in complete internal rotation. The patient is transferred to the recovery room and may be discharged if conditions are appropriate.

Postoperative Regimen

The shoulder is maintained in an internal rotation attitude in an immobilizer for a full five-week period. We use an immobilizer that allows elbow flexion and extension exercises to be performed without changing the position of the humerus. At six weeks, the immobilizer is removed and range of motion exercises are begun. Once a complete range of motion is established through passive and active assisted exercise, resistance exercises for deltoid and rotator cuff are initiated. At four months, motion is usually complete and strength sufficient to allow return to light throwing or racquet sports. Contact sports and unrestricted activity begin at six months.

Technique Using Biodegradable Tack

The equipment for this procedure is still in an evolutionary stage. At present, we use a cannulated tack made of biodegradable material. A cannula system that allows for drilling and tack insertion is used.

The initial setup, examination under anesthesia, and diagnostic arthroscopy are performed as previously described. The same criteria for tissue laxity, quality, and location are used to decide whether the procedure can be successfully carried out.

If conditions are appropriate, again, the glenoid rim is prepared, and a second superoanterior portal is created. The tissue (labrum or ligament) is reduced with appropriate tension to the glenoid rim. The tissue is then speared with a pointed guidewire and positioned on the glenoid far enough superior to allow fixation of the tissue with tension. The wire is impacted into the glenoid rim 2 to 3 mm medial to the articular surface. A cannulated drill is passed over the wire and drilled to the depth of the staple. The staple is impacted under direct vision, and the tissue and staple are probed to ensure that the staple has not cut through and is well fixed. Postoperative management is identical to the suture procedure.

Results

We have performed 17 stabilizations using the suture technique with follow-up at a maximum of five years. Thus far, we have had no recurrences and one complication. Our index patient developed a synovial cyst that emanated from a glenoid drill hole. The patient was aware of a posterior mass and underwent excisional biopsy with excellent results. Morgan and Bodenstab have reported a series of arthroscopic stabilizations performed using a modification of the suture technique. Over a short follow-up period, 25 patients who underwent the procedure had no episodes of recurrence and had excellent shoulder function.[30]

The biodegradable tack has been in use since the fall of 1987. Twenty patients have undergone the procedure, and at the time of this writing, there have been no recurrences and no complications. The patients' range of motion both with the hand at the side and at 90 degrees of abduction has been excellent, with essentially no loss noted if the inferior glenohumeral ligament was reattached. In one patient with poor quality ligament, the superior edge of the subscapularis tendon was incorporated with the capsule, resulting in a 20-degree loss of external rotation.

The role of the arthroscope in managing patients with shoulder instability is still evolving. At present, we are developing techniques that have some advantages in managing instability if it is anterior-unidirectional with good ligament tissues available that allow for reattachment. The basic goal is to pull the inferior glenohumeral ligament superiorly to place tension on it. The advantages include less injury to the deltoid and no reattachment of the subscapularis. Shortening of the capsule should be lessened, resulting in improved range of motion at follow-up. Present systems, though, require healing to occur before stressing the repair. Thus, postoperative protection for three to five weeks is important.

We have (in contrast to Johnson) allowed our athletes to go back to contact sports and, in particular, sports requiring overhead activity. In essence, the surgical approach, whether open or arthroscopic, is similar and is simply a matter of technical ability rather than philosophy. It is our impression, based on 43 stabilizations performed arthroscopically (with only one recurrence), that the results are predictable in the short term. The best methods to be used are still to be determined, but it is our impression that absorbable materials will play an increasing role in this area. The future for arthroscopic approaches to the shoulder is bright, and it will continue to provide an improved understanding of the pathophysiology of shoulder disease. In addition to skill and improved techniques, arthroscopy should allow surgeons further options in treatment and decrease patient morbidity.

References

1. Altchek DW, Ortiz G, Warren RF, and Skyhar MJ: Arthroscopic labral debridement: a retrospective analysis abstract. Unpublished data.

2. Altchek DW, Skyhar MJ, Warren RF, and Schwartz E: Arthroscopic acromioplasty: a prospective study. Unpublished data presented to Arthroscopy Association of North America, March 1988, Washington, D.C.

3. Andren L, and Lundberg BJ: Treatment of rigid shoulders by joint distention during arthroscopy. Acta Orthop Scand 36:45–53, 1965.

4. Andrews JR, and Carson WG: The arthroscopic treatment of glenoid labrum tears in the throwing athlete. Orthop Trans 8(1):44, 1984.

5. Andrews JR, Carson WG, and McLeod WD: Glenoid labrum tears related to the long head of the biceps. Am J Sports Med 13(5):337–341, 1985.

6. Andrews JR, Carson WG, and Ortega U: Arthroscopy of the shoulder: technique and normal anatomy. Sports Med 12(1):1–7, 1984.

7. Bach BR, Warren RF, and Fronek J: Disruption of the lateral capsule of the shoulder. A cause of recurrent dislocation. J Bone Joint Surg 70B(2):274–276, 1988.

8. Bankart ASB: The pathology and treatment of recurrent dislocation of the shoulder. Br J Surg 26:23–29, 1938.

9. Blazina E, and Saltzman JS: Recurrent anterior subluxation of the shoulder in athletes: a distinct entity. J Bone Joint Surg 51A:1037–1038, 1969.

10. Burman MS: Arthroscopy on the direct visualization of joints: an experimental cadaver study. J Bone Joint Surg 8:669, 1931.

11. Caspari RB: Arthroscopic evaluation and reconstruction for shoulder instability. Unpublished data presented to Arthroscopy Association of North America, February 7, 1988, Atlanta, GA.

12. Cofield RH: Arthroscopy of the shoulder. Mayo Clin Proc 58:501–508, 1983.

13. Conti V: Arthroscopy in rehabilitation. Orthop Clin North Am 10(3):709, 1979.

14. DePalma AF: Degenerative lesions of the shoulder joint at various age groups which are compatible with good function. American Academy of Orthopaedic Surgeons Instr Course Lect 7:168–180, 1950.

15. DePalma AF: Surgery of the Shoulder. Philadelphia: JB Lippincott, 1973.

16. DePalma AF, Callery G, and Bennett GA: Variational anatomy and degenerative lesions of the shoulder joint. American Academy of Orthopaedic Surgeons Instr Course Lect 6:255–280, 1949.

17. Detrisac DA, and Johnson LL: Arthroscopic Shoulder Anatomy. Pathologic and Surgical Implication. Thorofare, NJ: Slack, Inc., 1986.

18. Ellman H: Arthroscopic subacromial decompression: 1–3 year follow-up study. Instr Course Lect, American Academy of Orthopaedic Surgeons, Atlanta, GA, February 1988.

19. Gartsman GM, Blair ME, Noble MS, Bennett JB, et al.: Arthroscopic subacromial decompression. An anatomical study. Am J Sports Med 16(1):48–50, 1988.

20. Ha'en GB, and Maitland A: Arthroscopic findings in the frozen shoulder. J Rheumatol 8:149–152, 1981.

21. Johnson LL: Arthroscopic staple capsulorrhaphy. A preliminary report. Unpublished data presented at The American Shoulder and Elbow Surgeons Meeting, February 7, 1988, Atlanta, GA.

22. Johnson LL: The shoulder joint: an arthroscopist's perspective of anatomy and pathology. Clin Orthop 223:113–125, 1987.

23. Klein AH, France JC, Mutschler TA, and Fu FH: Measurement of brachial plexus strain in arthroscopy of the shoulder. Arthroscopy 3(1):45–52, 1987.

24. Kohn D: The clinical relevance of glenoid labrum lesions. Arthroscopy 3(4):223–230, 1987.

25. Kummel BM: Arthrography in anterior capsular derangements of the shoulder. Clin Orthop 83:170–176, 1982.

26. Kummel BM: Spectrum of lesions of the anterior capsular mechanism of the shoulder. Am J Sports Med 7:111, 1979.

27. Matthews LS, Zarins B, Michael RH, and Helfet DL: Anterior portal selection for shoulder arthroscopy. Arthroscopy 1(1):33–39, 1985.

28. McGlynn FJ, and Caspari RB: Arthroscopic findings in the subluxating shoulder. Clin Orthop 183:173–178, 1984.

29. McGlynn FJ, El-Khoury G, and Albright JP: Arthrotomography of the glenoid labrum in shoulder instability. J Bone Joint Surg 64A:506, 1982.

30. Morgan CD, and Bodenstab AB: Arthroscopic Bankart suture repair: technique and early results. Arthroscopy 3(2):111–122, 1987.

31. Moseley HF, and Overgaard B: The anterior capsular mechanism in recurrent anterior dislocation of the shoulder. J Bone Joint Surg 44B(4):913–927, 1962.

32. Neviaser TJ: Arthroscopy of the shoulder. Orthop Clin North Am 18(5):361–386, 1987.

33. Neviaser JS: Adhesive capsulitis of the shoulder: study of pathological findings in periarthritis of the shoulder. J Bone Joint Surg 27A:219, 1945.

34. Neviaser RJ, and Neviaser TJ: The frozen shoulder: diagnosis and management. Clin Orthop 223:59–64, 1987.

35. Neer CS: Anterior acromioplasty for chronic impingement syndrome in the shoulder. J Bone Joint Surg 54A(1):41–50, 1972.

36. Neer CS, and Foster CR: Inferior capsular shift for involuntary inferior and multidirectional instability of the shoulder. J Bone Joint Surg 62A(6):897–908, 1980.

37. Olgilvie-Harris DJ, and Wiley AM: Arthroscopic surgery of the shoulder: a general appraisal. J Bone Joint Surg 68B(2):201–207, 1986.

38. Pappas AM, Goss TP, and Kleinman PK: Symptomatic shoulder instability due to lesions of the glenoid labrum. Am J Sports Med 11(5):279–288, 1983.

39. Paulos L: Arthroscopic subacromial decompression; technique and preliminary results. Unpublished data presented to Arthroscopy Association of North America, April, 1985.

40. Rathbun JB, and Macnab I: The microvascular pattern of the rotator cuff. J Bone Joint Surg 52B(3):540–553, 1970.

41. Rowe CR, Patel D, and Southmayd WM: The Bankart procedure. J Bone Joint Surg 60A(1):1–16, 1978.

42. Rowe CR, and Zarins B: Recurrent transient subluxation of the shoulder. J Bone Joint Surg 63A(6):863–872, 1981.

43. Schlemm F: Über die Verstarklingsbänder am Schultergelenk. Arch Anat 1853, pp 45–48.

44. Schwartz R, O'Brien SJ, and Warren RF: Posterior stability of the shoulder. Presented to American Shoulder and Elbow Surgeons Meeting, Atlanta, GA, February 1988.

45. Turkel SJ, Panio MN, Marshall JL, and Girgis FG: Stabilizing mechanisms preventing anterior dislocation of the glenohumeral joint. J Bone Joint Surg 63A(8):1208–1217, 1986.

46. Uthoff HU: Anterior capsular redundancy of the shoulder: congenital or traumatic. J Bone Joint Surg 67B:363–366, 1985.

47. Wantabe M, Takeda S, and Ikeuchi H: Atlas of Arthroscopy, 3rd ed. New York: Igaku-Shoin, 1978.

48. Wantabe M: Arthroscopy: the present state. Orthop Clin North Am 10:505–522, 1979.

49. Wantabe M: The development and present status of the arthroscope. J Jpn Med Inst 25:11, 1954.

50. Warren RF: Subluxation of the shoulder in athletes. Clin Sports Med 2(2):339–354, 1983.

51. Wiley AM: Arthroscopy for shoulder instability and a technique for arthroscopic repair. Arthroscopy 4(1):25–30, 1988.

52. Wiley AM, and Older MB: Shoulder arthroscopy: investigation with a fiberoptic instrument. Am J Sports Med 8:18–31, 1980.

53. Zuckerman JD, and Matsen FA III: Complications about the glenohumeral joint related to the use of screws and staples. J Bone Joint Surg 66A(2):175–180, 1984.

Fractures of the Proximal Humerus

Louis U. Bigliani, M.D.

The diagnosis and treatment of the proximal humerus fracture is a challenging and difficult problem. A great deal of information has been published in recent decades as new techniques have been developed[116] and old ones have been rediscovered. Hippocrates is credited with documenting the first fracture of the proximal humerus in 460 B.C. and describing a method of weight traction which aided in bone healing. However, little was written concerning this subject until the latter part of the 19th century.[26, 50, 102, 154, 157] These reports discussed treatment of most fractures by immobilization in a sling followed by range of motion exercises. This treatment was adequate for undisplaced fractures. However, the more complex fractures were not appreciated or understood, and the results of treatment in these cases were quite poor.

In 1896 Kocher[135] developed an anatomical classification in an attempt to improve diagnosis and treatment, but this simplified scheme was not thorough enough and lacked consistency. Other early attempts at overly simple classifications were confusing and incomplete.[56, 120, 126, 129, 222, 234] Lack of consensus concerning fracture description and classification made it difficult to evaluate treatment adequately.

In 1934, Codman[45] made a significant contribution when he divided proximal humeral fractures into four basic parts. These parts were divided along the epiphyseal lines and consisted of the head, greater tuberosity, lesser tuberosity, and shaft. The subsequent four-part classification reported by Neer[190] in 1970 is based on this anatomical classification. This classification is a comprehensive system that integrates fracture, anatomy, biomechanics, and displacement allowing for consistent diagnosis and treatment. It is the most useful and commonly used classification system.

In the early part of the 20th century methods of closed reduction,[3, 234] traction,[129] casting,[81, 94] and abduction splints[13, 240, 274] were developed to achieve and maintain accurate anatomical alignment of displaced fractures. Often, however, these closed techniques were not sufficient to allow an adequate anatomical reduction. In 1932, Roberts[222] reported that elaborate apparatus and prolonged immobilization were not as beneficial as simpler forms of fixation and early motion. Other authors also stressed the importance of early motion and avoiding the abduction position.[31, 81, 120, 128, 132, 276] Howard and Eloesser[120] developed a complex theoretical shoulder model that simulated muscle forces and demonstrated that the abduction splint was not beneficial for reduction and control of muscle forces.

Open reduction of severely displaced fracture dislocations gained popularity during the same period in an effort to provide better anatomical alignment.[18, 43, 56, 217, 234, 245, 257] Roberts[222] and Meyerding[173] suggested the use of open reduction early to improve alignment and avoid malunions that would limit motion. Also, in some instances, internal fixation was performed. Suture material, wire, and screws were types of early fixation. The first report of intramedullary nailing of a transcervical fracture was by Widen[281] in 1949, and he credits Palmer with the development of the technique. In 1955, Rush[230] described his method of intramedullary nailing for the treatment of displaced fractures, which became quite popular. In the early 1970s the Association for Study of Internal Fixation (ASIF) group popularized the use of the Study Group for the Problem of Osteosynthesis (AO) plates and screws for displaced fractures. However, recent reports have stressed a high incidence of complications when this technique is used in more displaced fractures with osteoporotic bone.[138, 205, 254] Recently refined techniques of internal fixation with wire and nonabsorbable sutures have been successful and have a low complication rate.[104, 188, 191]

In the early 1950s, interest developed in the use of a humeral head prosthesis for the treatment of severely displaced fracture dislocations of the proximal humerus.[8, 70, 196, 210, 220] Closed reduction, open reduction and internal fixation, arthrodesis, and humeral head excision proved generally unsuccessful in the treatment of this problem.[191] In 1955, Neer[195] reported good results with the use of a metal humeral head prosthesis in 27 patients with fracture dislocations. In 1973, the prosthesis was redesigned to a more conforming head, and recent technical improvements have led to better results.[186] Currently, there are several different types of proximal humeral replacements; the Neer prosthesis is the most common.

Complications of treatment of proximal humeral fractures are not uncommon and have a wide range, including avascular necrosis, malunion, nonunion, infection, and neurovascular injury. In this chapter, I will outline a comprehensive approach to proximal humeral fractures which will aid in diagnosis and treatment.

Anatomy

It is important to understand the complex anatomy of the shoulder since optimum function of the glenohumeral joint is dependent on proper alignment and interaction of its anatomical structures. Malunion and nonunion of fractures will disrupt the balance of forces across the shoulder, interfering with smooth scapular-humeral rhythm and causing impingement beneath the subacromial arch.

The shoulder has an almost global range of motion, more than any other major joint in the body. This occurs because the glenoid cavity is a shallow socket approximately one-third to one-fourth the size of the humeral head.[231] Therefore, it depends on capsule, ligaments, and muscle rather than bone for stability. The capsule is quite loose and approximately double the size of the humeral head, allowing for a great deal of motion. The subdeltoid bursa lies on top of the rotator cuff and greatly facilitates movement of the cuff beneath the coracoacromial arch.

THE PROXIMAL HUMERUS

The proximal humerus consists of the humeral head, the lesser tuberosity, the greater tuberosity, the bicipital groove, and the proximal humeral shaft (Fig. 9–1). It is important to differentiate between the anatomical neck, which is at the junction of the head and the tuberosities, and the surgical neck, which is at the area below the greater and lesser tuberosities. The boundaries of the latter are somewhat variable without a distinct line. Anatomical neck fractures are quite rare and have a poor prognosis since the blood supply to the head is completely disrupted (Fig. 9–2), whereas surgical neck fractures are quite common and the blood supply to the head is preserved. The lesser tuberosity, the area of attachment for the subscapularis muscle,

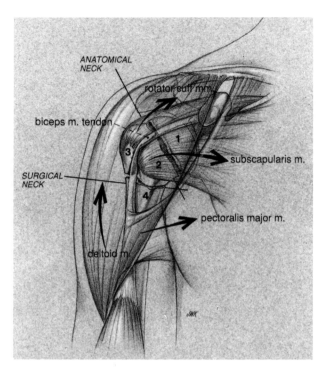

Figure 9–1. The anatomy of the shoulder is complex and depends on proper alignment and interaction of anatomical structures. Displacement of a fracture fragment is due to the pull of muscles attaching to the various bony components. The four anatomical components of the proximal humerus are the head (1), the lesser tuberosity (2), the greater tuberosity (3), and the shaft (4). The anatomical neck is at the junction of the head and tuberosities, and the surgical neck is below the area of the greater and lesser tuberosities. The subscapularis inserts on the lesser tuberosity, causing medial displacement; the supraspinatus and infraspinatus insert on the greater tuberosity and can cause superior and posterior displacement. The pectoralis major inserts on the humeral shaft and displaces it medially.

lies on the anterior aspect of the humerus and is smaller than the greater tuberosity. The bicipital or intertubercular groove lies between the greater and the lesser tuberosities and is on the anterior aspect of the proximal humerus. There are considerable variations in both the height and depth of the groove.[58, 117, 118] The biceps tendon lies in the bicipital groove and is covered by the transverse humeral ligament. The greater tuberosity lies posterior and superior on the humeral shaft and provides attachment for the supraspinatus, infraspinatus, and teres minor muscles. The greater tuberosity does not protrude above the humeral head. The glenoid is a shallow, concave structure with the shape of an inverted comma,[58] approximately one-third to one-fourth the surface area of the humeral head. It articulates with the humeral head and also provides attachment at its rim for the glenoid labrum and capsule.

THE ACROMION

The acromion protects the superior aspect of the glenohumeral joint and provides origin and mechanical leverage for the deltoid muscle, which is a prime mover of the shoulder. It also forms the lateral component of the acromioclavicular joint. The acromion together

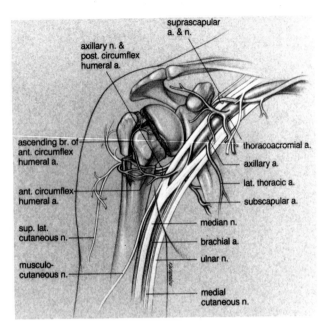

Figure 9–2. The acromion together with the coracoacromial ligament and the coracoid process form the coracoacromial arch. The brachial plexus and axillary artery are medial to the coracoid process and can be injured with fractures of the proximal humerus. The major blood supply to the humeral head is through the ascending branch of the anterior humeral circumflex artery, which penetrates the head at the superior aspect of the bicipital groove and becomes the arcuate artery. The three important nerves around the shoulder are the axillary, the suprascapular, and the musculocutaneous.

with the coracoacromial ligament and the coracoid process forms the coracoacromial arch (see Fig. 9–2). This is a rather rigid structure under which the proximal humerus, rotator cuff, and subacromial bursa must pass. Displaced fractures may disrupt the smooth flow of these structures below the coracoacromial arch, which may result in impingement and prevent normal glenohumeral motion. The subacromial (subdeltoid) bursa is a large synovial membrane. The roof is adherent to the under surface of the coracoacromial ligament, acromion, and deltoid muscle laterally, while the floor is closely adherent to the rotator cuff and greater tuberosity.[118] It also extends anteriorly and posteriorly around the humerus, creating a gliding mechanism that facilitates the movement of the proximal humerus under the coracoacromial arch. This structure may become injured even in undisplaced fractures, resulting in fibrotic thickening and loss of glenohumeral motion. Early institution of range of motion exercises following a fracture will limit the formation of bursal adhesions.

THE ROTATOR CUFF AND MUSCLES

The dynamic interplay of the rotator cuff and deltoid muscles is essential for glenohumeral function. The stability of the humeral head in the glenoid created by these muscles allows the deltoid muscle to function optimally. The rotator cuff consists of four muscles: the subscapularis, supraspinatus, infraspinatus, and teres minor. The long head of the biceps tendon is also an important component of this complex (see Fig. 9–1). The subscapularis is an internal rotator, while the supraspinatus is a head depressor and, in certain positions, an internal rotator. The infraspinatus and the teres minor are external rotators. These muscles work as a unit, rather than individually, to maintain dynamic glenohumeral stability.

Since the rotator cuff muscles are attached to the tuberosities, it is important to understand the direction of pull of their fibers as this will facilitate the understanding of displacement of bone fragments. For example, in a fracture of the greater tuberosity, the fragment will be pulled superiorly and posteriorly because of the supraspinatus and teres minor muscles, whereas in a fracture of the lesser tuberosity, the fragment will be pulled anteriorly and medially by the subscapularis muscle. The long head of the biceps attaches to the supraglenoid tubercle of the glenoid and has a stabilizing and depressing action on the humeral head. It is a significant structure to consider in closed reductions as it can act as a tether and block closed reduction. Also, during operative procedures, it is a useful landmark from which the rotator interval can be identified so that bone fragments are properly identified and the rotator cuff muscles are preserved.

Two other important muscles must be considered in relation to the proximal humerus: the deltoid and the pectoralis major. The deltoid is a prime mover in the shoulder and takes origin from the lateral one-third of the clavicle, the acromion, and spine of the scapula. It inserts at the deltoid tuberosity on the lateral shaft of the humerus, and it can cause displacement of fractures of the proximal humeral shaft. The pectoralis major is a large fan-shaped muscle that has a broad origin from the clavicle, the upper ribs, and sternocostal area. It inserts on the lower portion of the lateral lip of the bicipital groove, and it can displace the proximal shaft of the humerus medially as is usually seen in surgical neck fractures.

BLOOD SUPPLY

It is important to consider the blood supply to the proximal humerus since avascular necrosis is not uncommon following displaced fractures. The major blood supply to the humeral head is from the anterior humeral circumflex artery[142, 181, 215, 227] (see Fig. 9–2). Laing[142] was the first to describe the arcuate artery, which is a continuation of the ascending branch of the anterior humeral circumflex as it penetrates the bone. This tortuous artery supplies blood to a large portion of the humeral head. It routinely enters the bone in the area of the intertubercular groove and gives branches to the lesser and greater tuberosities. Also, a small contribution to the humeral head blood supply comes from branches of the posterior circumflex and from the vascular rotator cuff through tendinous osseous anastomosis.

Rothman[227] has outlined the blood supply to the rotator cuff as routinely derived from six arteries: the anterior humeral circumflex, the posterior humeral circumflex, the suprascapular, the thoracoacromial, the suprahumeral, and the subscapular. The anterior humeral circumflex is the major supplier to the anterior cuff and the long head of the biceps, while the posterior humeral circumflex and suprascapular anastomosis supply the posterior cuff. The thoracoacromial artery supplies the supraspinatus, while the suprahumeral and subscapular arteries supply the anteroinferior aspect of the cuff.

NERVE SUPPLY

Injury to the nerves about the shoulder can occur with fractures. The brachial plexus and axillary artery are medial to the coracoid process and can be injured with anterior fracture dislocations and violent trauma to the proximal humerus (see Fig. 9–2). Isolated injuries to the major nerves innervating the muscles around the shoulder—the axillary, suprascapular, and musculocutaneous—can also occur.

The most commonly injured nerve is the axillary nerve. In most cases, the axillary nerve is composed of fibers from the fifth and sixth cervical roots and takes its origin from the posterior cord at the level of the axilla. Then it crosses the anterior surface of the subscapularis muscle and dips back posteriorly under its inferior border. It passes along the inferior border of the capsule of the glenohumeral joint and then through the quadrangular space (see Fig. 9–2). After emerging from the quadrangular space, it gives off a branch to the teres minor and divides into anterior and posterior branches. The posterior branch supplies the posterior deltoid and gives off the superior lateral brachial cutaneous nerve. The anterior branch supplies the middle and anterior deltoid muscles as the axillary nerve winds around the inner surface. Owing to its relative fixation at the posterior cord and the deltoid, any abnormal downward motion of the proximal humerus can result in traction and injury to this nerve. Also, its close relationship to the inferior capsule makes it susceptible to injury from anterior dislocation and during open repairs for anterior fracture dislocations.

The suprascapular nerve may also be injured, but this is much less common. It is made up of fibers from the fifth and sixth cervical roots and originates from the upper trunk of the brachial plexus. It runs laterally deep to the omohyoid and trapezius, passing through the suprascapular notch (see Fig. 9–2). After giving off two branches to the supraspinatus, it passes around the lateral border of the scapular spine to the infraspinatus. The two points of fixation of the nerve are at its origin from the upper trunk and at the suprascapular notch, where it passes beneath the transverse scapular ligament making it susceptible to traction injuries.

Injury to the musculocutaneous nerve is rare but does occur. Composed of fibers from C5 to C6 with the occasional addition of C7 fibers, it originates from the lateral cord at the level of the pectoralis minor and passes obliquely distally through the coracobrachialis and between the biceps and brachialis (see Fig. 9–2). In the 93 cadaver shoulders I have dissected, the distance from the coracoid to the point of entrance into the coracobrachialis muscle has been between 3.1 and 8.2 cm, with a mean of 5.6 cm.[76] More important, 29 per cent entered less than 5 cm from the coracoid. The frequently cited safe zone of 5 to 8 cm is inaccurate. The nerve terminates as the lateral antebrachial cutaneous nerve as it exits the deep fascia at the level of the elbow. Injury to the musculocutaneous nerve can result from blunt trauma as well as traction injuries.

Classification

A workable classification system for fractures of the proximal humerus is necessary for proper management. A classification system must be comprehensive enough to encompass all factors, yet specific enough to allow accurate diagnosis and treatment. Also, it must be flexible enough to accommodate variations and allow logical deductions for treatment. The majority of proximal humeral fractures are undisplaced and must be differentiated from the more displaced fractures as the treatment is significantly different. Inadequate diagnosis of complex fractures will only create confusion and lead to improper management.

It is important to emphasize that the first steps in any classification system are a thorough knowledge of the anatomy and accurate radiographic views to outline the anatomical structures. The most logical and commonly used classification is the four-part fracture classification developed by Neer[190] in 1970.

THE NEER CLASSIFICATION

Prior to the Neer classification, various other methods had been proposed including anatomical level or location of injury,[31, 45, 125, 129, 135] mechanism of injury,[57, 252, 274] amount of contact by the fracture fragments,[68] degree of displacement,[133] and vascular status of the articular segment.[8, 124] Furthermore, others have devised classifications using combinations of the above criteria, resulting in confusion concerning the diagnosis and treatment of these complex fractures.[20, 57, 59, 69, 71, 111, 133, 216, 222]

In 1896, Kocher was the first to devise a classification of proximal humeral fractures.[135] His classification was based on different anatomical levels for fractures—anatomical neck, epiphyseal region, and surgical neck (Fig. 9–3). The problem with this type of classification is that it does not allow for multiple fractures at two different sites, nor does it differentiate between displaced and undisplaced fractures, which causes confusion since they require different treatment. Classification according to the mechanism of injury can also be misleading, as in the Watson-Jones classification of an

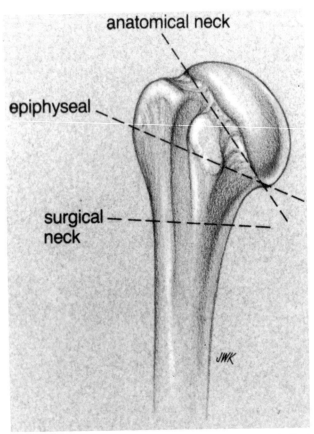

Figure 9–3. The Kocher classification is based on three different anatomical levels for fractures: anatomical neck, epiphyseal region, and surgical neck. This classification does not allow for differentiation of multiple fractures at two different sites, nor does it differentiate between displaced and undisplaced fractures. (Adapted from Kocher T: Beitrage zur Kenntnis einiger praktisch wichtiger Fracturenformen. Basel: Carl Sallman Verlag, 1896.)

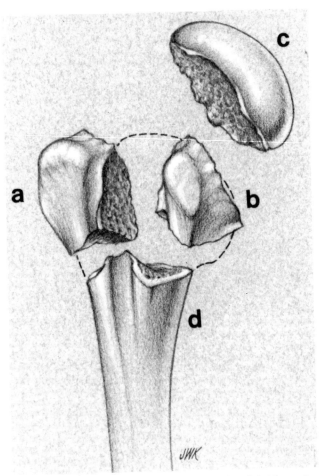

Figure 9–4. Codman divided the proximal humerus into four distinct fragments, which roughly occur along anatomical lines of epiphyseal union. He differentiated the four major fragments as the greater tuberosity (a), lesser tuberosity (b), head (c), and shaft (d). (Redrawn with permission from Codman EA: The Shoulder; Rupture of the Supraspinatus Tendon and Other Lesions in or About the Subacromial Bursa. Malabar, FL: Robert E. Krieger Publishing Company, 1984.)

abduction or adduction type of fracture.[274] It has since been pointed out that the deformity in these fractures is anterior angulation and, with internal or external rotation of the arm, the fracture can become either an abduction or an adduction fracture.[190, 283]

In 1934, Codman[45] made a significant contribution to the understanding of proximal humeral fractures by proposing that fractures be separated into four distinct fragments, occurring roughly along the anatomical line of epiphyseal union (Fig. 9–4). He was able to differentiate four major fragments: the anatomical head, the greater tuberosity, the lesser tuberosity, and the shaft. Codman's conclusion was that all fractures were some combination of these different fracture fragments. Furthermore, the musculotendinous cuff attaches to the more proximal fragments and can hold the fractured fragments together.

This was the cornerstone on which Neer,[190] in 1970, based his four-part classification (Fig. 9–5). This was the first truly comprehensive system: It considered anatomy, biomechanical forces, and the resultant amount of displacement of fracture fragments and related these to diagnosis and treatment. It is a commonly used classification for proximal humeral frac-

tures and will be used extensively in this chapter to identify fracture patterns.

The Neer classification of fractures of the proximal humerus is a system based on the accurate identification of the four major fragments and their relationship to each other. There is nothing to memorize, but an adequate knowledge of the anatomy and the insertions of the tendons of the rotator cuff is essential to use it properly (Fig. 9–5). The identification of fragments can be accomplished only with proper x-rays including the trauma series, which consists of anteroposterior and lateral views in the scapular plane as well as an axillary view. This fracture system is a concept rather than a numerical classification and sets forth guidelines that are arbitrary and designed to be helpful in recognizing displaced fractures. Emphasis is placed on determining the adequacy of vascular supply to the humeral head since avascular necrosis is a common complication of displaced fractures.

The majority of fractures are minimally displaced (more than 80 per cent),[188] although Rose[224] and

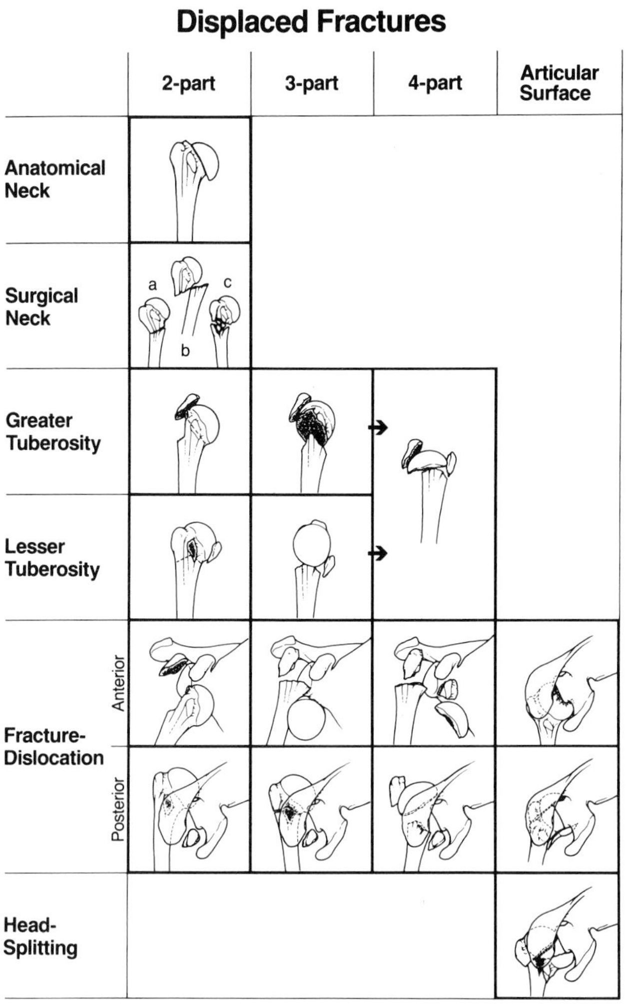

Displaced Fractures

	2-part	3-part	4-part	Articular Surface
Anatomical Neck				
Surgical Neck	a c / b			
Greater Tuberosity				
Lesser Tuberosity				
Fracture-Dislocation (Anterior)				
Fracture-Dislocation (Posterior)				
Head-Splitting				

Figure 9–5. The most commonly used classification is the Neer four-part classification, a comprehensive system that encompasses anatomy and biomechanical forces that result in the displacement of fracture fragments. It is based on accurate identification of the four major fragments and their relationships with one another. A displaced fracture is either two-part, three-part, or four-part. In addition, fracture dislocations can either be two-part, three-part, or four-part. Fissure lines or hairline fractures are not considered displaced fragments. A fragment is considered displaced when there is over 1 cm of separation or when a fragment is angulated more than 45 degrees from the other fragments. Impression fractures of the articular surface also occur and are usually associated with an anterior or posterior dislocation. Head splitting fractures are usually associated with fractures of the tuberosities or surgical neck. (Adapted from Neer CS: Displaced proximal humeral fractures. Part I. Classification and evaluation. J Bone Joint Surg 52A:1077–1089, 1970.)

Horak[119] have reported lower incidences—78 and 61 per cent, respectively. (Minimally displaced fractures must be accurately identified so that they may be differentiated from the more serious displaced fractures.) In the Neer four-part classification, the four parts are the same as those described by Codman: the articular segment or the head, the greater tuberosity, the lesser tuberosity, and the shaft (see Fig. 9–5). When any of the four major segments is displaced over 1 cm or angulated more than 45 degrees, the fracture is considered to be displaced. Fissure lines or hairline fractures are not to be considered displaced fragments. A fragment may have several undisplaced components; these should not be considered separate fragments

since they are in continuity and they are held together by soft tissue. If the above criteria are not met and there is no displacement of fragments, then the fracture should be considered minimally displaced and only one part. A two-part fracture is one in which one fragment is displaced in reference to the other three fragments. A three-part fracture is one in which two fragments are displaced in relationship to each other and the other two are undisplaced fragments, but the head remains in contact with the glenoid. A four-part fracture is one in which all four fracture fragments are displaced; the head is out of contact with the glenoid and angulated either laterally, anteriorly, posteriorly, inferiorly, or superiorly. Furthermore, it is detached from both tuberosities and therefore from its blood supply. The central focus of this fracture classification is the status of the blood supply to the humeral head and the relationship of the humeral head to the displaced parts and the glenoid.

Neer[190] has also emphasized the term fracture dislocation and the accurate diagnosis of this problem (see Fig. 9–5). A fracture dislocation exists when the head is displaced outside the joint space rather than subluxated or rotated and there is, in addition, a fracture. Fracture dislocations can be classified according to direction, usually anterior or posterior, as well as according to the number of fracture fragments, that is, two part, three part, or four part. Head splitting fractures and impression fractures of the articular surface are special fractures (see Fig. 9–5). Impression fractures of the articular surface are graded according to the percentage of the articular surface involved. The general guidelines that have been adopted for these are less than 20 per cent, between 20 and 45 per cent, and greater than 45 per cent of the articular head.[103] Head splitting fractures can also be graded in a similar fashion but are generally involved with other fractures of the proximal humerus and, in many instances, are the result of violent trauma.

THE AO CLASSIFICATION

Recently, based on a review of 730 fractures, Jakob[124] and the AO group have modified Neer's classification and have emphasized the vascular supply to the articular segment. The vascular supply to the articular segment plays a pivotal role in the prognosis of a proximal humeral fracture since avascular necrosis is such a common complication. The system is divided into three categories according to the severity of the injury. The least severe is the Type A fracture in which vascular isolation of the articular segment is not present and avascular necrosis is unlikely. It is extracapsular and involves two of the four primary segments. A Type B fracture is more severe, and there is partial isolation of the articular segment and a low risk of avascular necrosis. It is partially intracapsular, and three of the four primary segments are involved. In a Type C fracture, the most severe, total vascular isolation of the articular segment occurs with a high risk of avascular necrosis. It is intracapsular, and all four primary segments are involved. In addition, each alphabetical group is subgrouped numerically, and higher numbers generally reflect greater severity. This more complicated system is supposed to create a framework for more detailed therapeutic and prognostic guidelines; however, long-term results regarding treatment of various fractures have never been presented.

RATING SYSTEM

It is important to have a consistent method for evaluating results. Unless results from different series are reported in a uniform manner, it will be very difficult to draw valid comparisons. When Hagg[98] reported his series of fractures, he had 52 per cent satisfactory results using Santee's criteria[234] and 35 per cent satisfactory results using Neer's criteria.[191] Confusion persists because authors continue to use their own criteria for evaluation. The most commonly used rating system for fracture has been the one devised by Neer, based on 100 units. There are 35 units for pain, 30 units for function, 25 units for range of motion, and 10 units for anatomy. Pain is the most significant factor. An excellent result is over 89 units, satisfactory over 80 units, unsatisfactory over 70 units, and failure under 70 units.

In an effort to standardize results, the American Society of Shoulder and Elbow Surgeons has recently developed a rating system that is useful for evaluation.[16] The assessment form has five categories: pain, range of motion, strength, stability, and function. It also considers the patient's subjective response to a surgical procedure. Pain is graded from zero to five, with a score of zero signifying constant pain and five no pain. Both active and passive range of motion are tested in forward flexion, external rotation, and internal rotation. Also, motion should be checked with the patient both sitting and supine. Strength is scored from zero to five, from paralysis to normal function. The deltoid, trapezius, biceps, triceps, external rotators, and internal rotators should all be tested. Stability is graded from zero to five, from fixed dislocation to a stable joint.

Function is graded from zero to four, unable to function to unrestricted activity. Activities of daily living, such as cooking and combing hair, as well as throwing and lifting are tested. Finally, the patient's response is recorded from zero to five, worse than before to much improved. It is hoped that this method of evaluation will shortly be widely adopted.

Incidence

Fractures of the proximal humerus are not that uncommon, especially in older age groups. They have previously been reported to account for approximately 4 to 5 per cent of all fractures, but this figure may be low.[190, 253] A recent epidemiological study reported by Bengner[24] from Malmo, Sweden of over 2125 fractures showed a steady and significant increase in the incidence of proximal humeral fractures. In two other recent, comprehensive studies, one from Rochester, Minnesota,[224] and another also from Malmo, Sweden,[119] the age-adjusted incidence rates of proximal humeral fractures among adult residents were practically identical: 105 and 104 per 100,000 person years, respectively. Furthermore, it was correlated in the Minnesota study that proximal humeral fractures occur at nearly 70 per cent of the reported rate of proximal femur fractures, all ages considered. A comparison was made with a previous study concerning proximal femur fractures in the same population.[82] Based on the epidemiological data available, it was concluded that a majority of proximal humeral fractures are primarily osteoporosis related and an important source of morbidity among the elderly population. Brehr and Cooke[34] also noted a strong similarity in the incidence and pattern of these two fractures.

Proximal humeral fractures were the most common humeral fractures (45 per cent) in Rose's study concerning the epidemiological features of humeral fractures in Rochester, Minnesota.[224] When considering adults over 40 years of age, the incidence of proximal humeral fractures increases to 76 per cent. The major reason for this increase is the osteoporosis factor, since the amount of trauma responsible for the fracture was significantly less in the older age group. Shaft and distal humeral fractures are more common in the younger age groups where more violent trauma is usually associated with the injury. Also, a higher incidence in proximal humeral fractures was noted in women than in men, by a rate of approximately two to one. Horak[119] has also reported increased incidence with age and in females and the same frequency as fractures of the proximal end of the femur. The patients with proximal humeral fractures had an increased incidence of alcoholism and prior gastric resection. Furthermore, prevalence of other fractures was about doubled in patients who have had a proximal humeral fracture. Both Rose[224] and Horak[119] concluded that osteoporosis was a significant factor in these fractures.

Mechanism of Injury

The most common mechanism of injury for proximal humeral fracture is a fall on outstretched hands from standing height or less. In most instances, severe trauma does not play a significant role. Rather, the trauma need only be minor to moderate in degree because osteoporosis is usually present. The position of the arm and hand during the fall and obesity have also been suggested as factors in these trivial falls. Severe trauma may play a role in younger individuals, and the resulting fracture is often more serious. These patients usually have fracture dislocations with significant soft tissue disruption and multiple trauma. In dealing with multiple trauma, the proximal humeral fracture is commonly initially ignored, as attention is focused on more life-threatening problems. However, as the patient regains consciousness or awareness, complaints of pain in the shoulder may prove to be secondary to a fracture. Another mechanism of injury, first mentioned by Codman, is excessive rotation of the arm especially in the abducted position. The humerus locks against the acromion in a pivotal position and a fracture can occur, especially in older patients with osteoporotic bone. Another mechanism of injury is a direct blow to the side of the shoulder. This usually occurs in the lateral position and may result in a greater tuberosity fracture.

An often ignored etiology for fracture dislocations of the proximal humerus is electrical shock or a convulsive episode.[65, 103, 218, 233, 242, 284] The fracture dislocation may be anterior or posterior and is often overlooked. Metastatic disease may significantly weaken the bone so that a pathological fracture may occur with just trivial activity. Whenever a trivial event causes a fracture of the proximal humerus, a pathological etiology should be considered.

Clinical Presentation

The majority of fractures of the proximal humerus present acutely, and therefore, the most common symptoms are pain, swelling, and tenderness about the shoulder, especially in the area of the greater tuberosity. Palpation of the bony contour of the shoulder may be difficult since the soft tissue covering of the shoulder is generous. Crepitus may be present upon motion of the fracture fragments if they are in contact. However, diagnosis of a fracture of the shoulder is made radiographically, and the history and physical signs only corroborate radiographic findings. Ecchymosis generally occurs within 24 to 48 hours of the injury and may spread to the chest wall and flank and distally down the extremity. It is important to warn the patient that this development may occur since it may alarm a patient and he or she may think that further internal damage has occurred after the initial fracture. In most instances, patients find it difficult to initiate active motion, and the arm is held closely against the chest wall. However, history and physical examination are only suggestive of a fracture; the definitive diagnosis is made with the proper x-rays.

A detailed neurovascular evaluation is essential in all fractures of the proximal humerus. The brachial plexus and axillary artery are just medial to the coracoid process, and injury to these structures are not uncommon. They can occur even in undisplaced fractures.[106, 247] It is important to test the peripheral pulses and question the patient concerning paresthesias and loss of sensations in the distal extremity. The easiest way to make a diagnosis of a neurovascular complication is to suspect the injury and test for it at the initial examination. The most common nerve injury seen with fractures about the shoulder is injury to the axillary nerve. Sensation should be tested over the deltoid muscle, since testing for deltoid activity or weakness may be very difficult because of pain. Occasionally, in the immediate postfracture or postoperative period, there may be inferior subluxation of the humerus. In the majority of instances this is secondary to deltoid fatigue or atony rather than to an injury to the axillary nerve.[53, 57, 74, 259, 273, 282] The arm should be supported in a sling, and gentle isometric exercises will help recover deltoid tone. If the situation is severe and persists for more than four weeks, it must be differentiated from a true axillary nerve palsy.

Examination of the chest should not be ignored as complications involving the thoracic cavity have been reported following fractures of the proximal humerus. Although rare, they do occur, and several authors have reported intrathoracic penetration by the humeral head associated with fractures.[87, 101, 208, 278] Also, a pneumothorax may occur, especially with patients who have multiple trauma.

Fracture dislocations of the proximal humerus are difficult to diagnose and often are missed by the initial examiner.[103, 105, 115, 167, 268, 269] This is especially true of posterior fracture dislocations where it is estimated that more than 50 per cent of these injuries are missed by the initial treating physician.[10, 103, 188] In a fracture dislocation, there is loss of contour of the shoulder. With an anterior fracture dislocation, there is an anterior bulge, and the posterior aspect of the joint is flattened or hollow. The reverse is true with a posterior fracture dislocation, where the anterior aspect of the shoulder is flattened, the coracoid is more prominent, and there is a posterior bulge with the axis of the humerus pointing posteriorly. There will always be a loss of external rotation and abduction secondary to pain. However, if there is a surgical neck fracture component to the fracture, rotation and abduction can occur. This diagnosis must be confirmed by proper x-rays, i.e., a lateral view in the scapular plane, axillary view (Fig. 9–6B), or CT scan.

When a patient has a convulsive episode or a history of an electrical shock accident, and there is pain and swelling about the shoulder, the patient must first be evaluated for a posterior dislocation or fracture dislocation as well as an anterior displacement.[11, 103, 131, 242] Although this seems obvious, there was a recent case reported of bilateral posterior fracture dislocations which were undiagnosed for 14 days following injury.[152] The patient had significant swelling and ecchymosis, as well as a fixed internal rotation contracture. The ecchymosis was attributed to a drug reaction by the initial physician. It cannot be overemphasized that a fixed posterior fracture dislocation is commonly missed and to avoid this there must be a high degree of suspicion by the examining physician so that appropriate radiographs can be ordered.

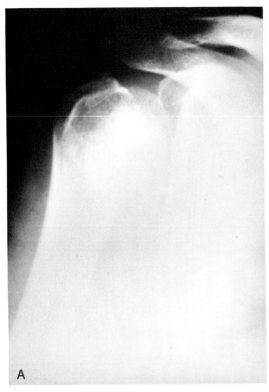
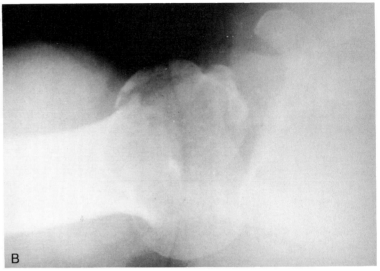

Figure 9–6. *A,* An anteroposterior radiograph of an obese female, taken in the emergency room and initially read as a minimally displaced fracture. This poor quality radiograph was the only view taken. The patient was started on early range of motion exercises but after four weeks had −30 degrees of external rotation, forward elevation to 70 degrees, and no abduction. *B,* An axillary radiograph taken after four weeks revealed a missed posterior fracture dislocation. An axillary radiograph is essential for diagnosis of posterior fracture dislocations.

Differential Diagnosis

In the majority of instances, the diagnosis of a fracture is readily made when proper and accurate x-rays of the shoulder are available. However, the patient may have acute pain following a traumatic incident, and radiographs may be negative for a fracture. The differential diagnosis of proximal humeral fractures includes any abnormality which will cause acute pain, swelling, and loss of active motion. Acute hemorrhagic bursitis, a traumatic rotator cuff tear, a simple dislocation, an acromioclavicular separation, and calcific tendinitis may all present clinically with these symptoms. A fall on an outstretched hand may injure the soft tissues about the shoulder causing hemorrhage into the subacromial space, leading to inflammation and scarring of the subacromial bursa. If this condition does not resolve several weeks after injury, one must consider the possibility of a full thickness rotator cuff tear, especially in an older individual or in cases where there was a previous anterior dislocation. Tenderness of the greater tuberosity, weakness of forward elevation and external rotation, an arc of pain, and a positive impingement sign are generally present in these patients. If there is a high degree of suspicion, ultrasonography or an arthrogram may be indicated. Calcific

tendinitis may have been a pre-existing problem that was activated by trauma. Patients with an acromioclavicular separation have direct tenderness over the acromioclavicular joint, and in more severe cases, the distal clavicle is displaced superiorly. A careful history, in addition to radiographs, will help differentiate a spontaneously reduced dislocation.

Another, more important factor to consider is the possibility of an underlying problem which may have contributed to the fracture. Treatment of a pathological fracture is more complicated, and bone healing is usually compromised. One should be suspicious that a pathological fracture may have occurred when a trivial incident is the cause. Metastatic carcinoma, metabolic bone disease, rheumatoid arthritis, osteonecrosis, and osteoporosis are some of the more common processes that may weaken bone and result in a pathological fracture.

Radiographic Evaluation

Accurate radiographic evaluation of fractures of the proximal humerus is essential for diagnosis and treatment. Incorrect or oblique x-rays will only misrepresent the fracture and create confusion.

TRAUMA SERIES

The trauma series is still the best initial method for diagnosing proximal humeral fractures.[190] This consists of anteroposterior and lateral radiographs in the scap-ular plane and, if motion and pain permit, an axillary view (Fig. 9–7). The lateral view in the scapular plane is also called the tangential, or Y view, of the scapula. This series allows evaluation of the fracture in three separate perpendicular planes so that accurate assess-ment of fracture displacement may be achieved. The

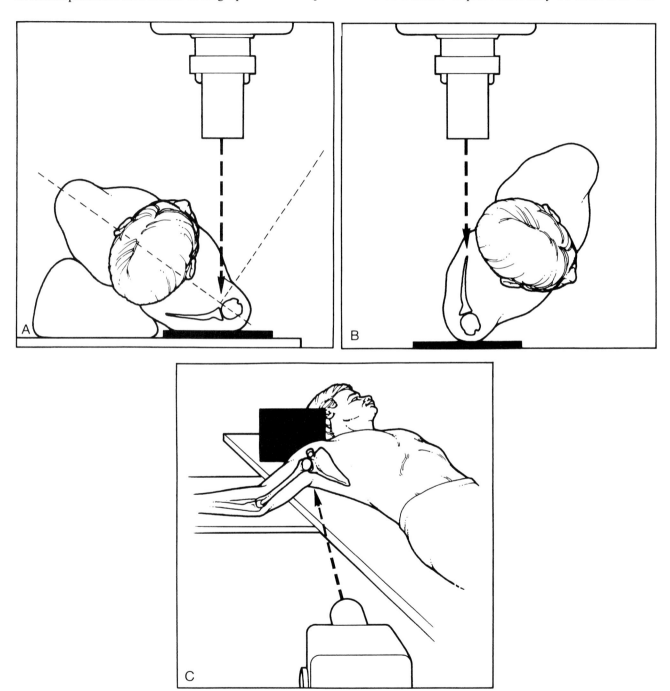

Figure 9–7. The trauma series consists of anteroposterior *(A)* and lateral *(B)* views in the scapular plane as well as an axillary view *(C)*. These views may be done sitting, standing, or prone. The lateral is called the tangential or Y view of the scapula. This series permits evaluation of the fracture in three perpendicular planes to allow accurate assessment of the fracture displacement. The scapula sits obliquely on the chest wall, and the glenoid surface is tilted approximately 35 to 40 degrees anteriorly. Therefore, the glenohumeral joint is not in the sagittal or the coronal plane. For the anteroposterior view in the scapular plane, the posterior aspect of the affected shoulder is placed up against the x-ray plate and the opposite shoulder is rotated out approximately 40 degrees. For the lateral view in the scapular plane, the anterior aspect of the affected shoulder is placed against the x-ray plate and the other shoulder is rotated out approximately 40 degrees. The x-ray tube is then placed posteriorly along the scapular spine. The axillary view is performed with the patient supine and the arm supported in abduction. The patient is usually placed on a cushion or foam pad so that the fracture is not obstructed by the table.

scapula sits obliquely on the chest wall, and the glenoid surface is tilted approximately 35 to 40 degrees anteriorly. Therefore, the glenohumeral joint does not lie in either the sagittal or coronal plane. The anteroposterior and lateral x-rays in this scapular plane can be taken without removing the patient from the sling. They can be done in either a sitting, standing, or prone position. For the anteroposterior view in the scapular plane, the posterior aspect of the affected shoulder is placed up against the x-ray plate, and the opposite shoulder is rotated out approximately 40 degrees. This will give a true anteroposterior view of the shoulder joint and will avoid any superimposition of other tissues which will obscure bony detail. The lateral view in the scapular plane is accomplished by placing the anterior aspect of the affected shoulder against the x-ray plate and rotating the other shoulder out approximately 40 degrees. The x-ray tube is then placed posteriorly along the scapular spine, and this will provide a true lateral view of the shoulder.

The axillary view allows for evaluation in the axial plane and is essential for evaluating the glenoid articular surface and the relationship of anterior and posterior fracture dislocations (see Figs. 9–6B and 9–7C). This view is often ignored despite the fact that its importance has been stressed for years by several authors.[81, 173, 191, 222, 280] An axillary view may also be obtained in either the standing, sitting, or prone position. If possible, the supine position is preferable. The arm can be held in abduction by a knowledgeable person so that further displacement of the fracture does not occur. The x-ray plate is placed above the patient's shoulder, and the arm is gently abducted to 30 degrees. The x-ray tube is placed slightly below the patient, and the beam goes from inferior to superior. It is helpful in these cases to rest the patient's shoulder on a soft cushion so that it is elevated off the table and bony pathology is not obscured. The Velpeau axillary view has also been described in which the arm is not removed from the sling.[28] The patient is seated and tilted obliquely backward 45 degrees. The plate is below and the x-ray tube above.

In attempting to judge the amount of angular displacement at the surgical neck level, it is important to consider the neck shaft angle of the humerus in both the anteroposterior and lateral planes. On the anteroposterior projections, the neck shaft angle is the angle created at the intersection of lines that are perpendicular to the anatomical neck and parallel to the shaft of the humerus. On the lateral radiograph, the neck shaft angle is the angle formed at the intersection of the lines parallel to the anatomical neck and parallel to the shaft of the humerus. Keene[130] has demonstrated that the neck shaft angle can vary with humeral rotation. Therefore, it is important to consider the position of the arm when evaluating radiographs and comparing them with the unaffected side if necessary. In Keene's studies of 25 control patients, the average neck shaft angle in the anteroposterior projection was 143 degrees, with a range of 134 to 166 degrees. This angle

was less with external rotation and greater with internal rotation. Therefore, it can vary as much as 30 degrees with rotation of the arm. The posterior angulation, which was measured on the lateral x-ray, averaged approximately 25 degrees, with a range of −9 to 59 degrees. Supplemental radiographic views, such as a transthoracic and various rotational views, may at times be useful to estimate the amount of displacement of specific segments. These may also be useful in malunions, especially with greater tuberosity fractures.

OTHER X-RAY TECHNIQUES

Several other diagnostic tests are also helpful including tomograms and computed tomography (CT). Tomograms may be useful in evaluating a proximal humeral fracture for a nonunion or the amount of articular surface (glenoid and humeral head) involvement (Fig. 9–8). However, in most instances, CT has replaced tomography as the initial procedure of choice. Morris has recently reported a series of patients in which CT was helpful in judging the amount of displacement of greater tuberosity fractures.[180a] CT is also

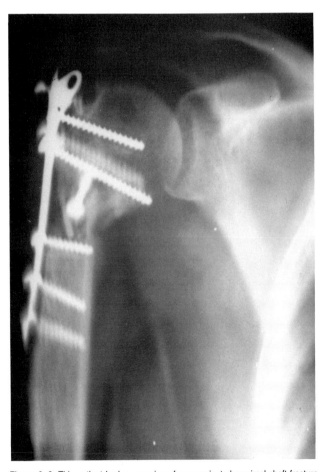

Figure 9–8. This patient had a nonunion of a comminuted proximal shaft fracture following buttress plate fixation. A tomogram was helpful in establishing a nonunion. Note that the plate is placed extremely high and is impinging on the acromion. Also, the plate is distracting the fracture.

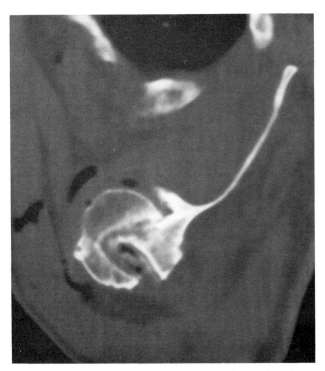

Figure 9–9. This 64-year-old male had a chronic anterior fracture dislocation that was missed for approximately one year. This CT scan was helpful in evaluating the amount of head and glenoid involvement.

extremely helpful in evaluating the amount of articular involvement with a head splitting fracture, impression fractures, chronic fracture dislocations (Fig. 9–9), and glenoid rim fractures. Magnetic resonance imaging, a relatively new procedure, may hold some promise for evaluating displacement of proximal humeral fractures.

Complications

Complications following fractures of the proximal humerus encompass a rather large spectrum and are not uncommon. Some of these include a frozen shoulder, pneumothorax or pneumohemothorax, nonunion, malunion, avascular necrosis, myositis ossificans, and neurovascular injuries. Adhesions of the subacromial bursa, rotator cuff tendons, and glenohumeral joint capsule may occur and can significantly limit rotation and function.[36, 83, 222] Therefore, it is important to institute a well-supervised and well-organized rehabilitation program in the immediate postinjury period. This should be started when there is sufficient clinical stability so that the fracture moves as a unit. With impacted and stable fractures, this is generally within 10 days of injury.

NONUNION

Nonunion has generally been associated with displaced two-part unimpacted surgical neck fractures, but it can occur with all types of proximal humeral

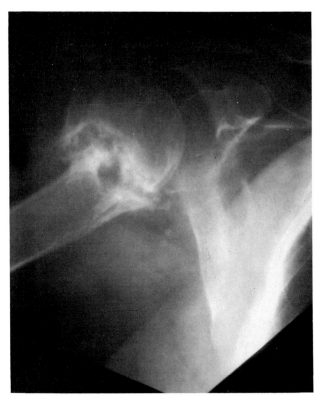

Figure 9–10. This minimally displaced surgical neck fracture went on to a nonunion. Note the sclerotic margins of the fracture. This patient was started on overly aggressive physiotherapy and was not sufficiently supervised.

fractures, even those that are minimally displaced (Fig. 9–10).[54, 68, 144, 163, 223, 249] The cause of a nonunion can be an unstable closed reduction, interposition of soft tissue (capsule, muscle, long head of biceps), a hanging cast, insufficient immobilization, an uncooperative patient, overaggressive physiotherapy, or poor bone quality. As a result, it is extremely important to closely monitor the physiotherapy program so that it will coincide with fracture healing and stability.

MALUNION

Malunion from insufficient treatment of displaced fractures can be an especially disabling problem. Excessive anterior angulation (greater than 45 degrees) of a surgical neck fracture will restrict forward elevation. Also, retraction of the tuberosities beneath the acromion can significantly limit rotation and elevation. In a greater tuberosity malunion, the supraspinatus and infraspinatus will pull the fragment both superiorly and posteriorly, resulting in subacromial impingement (Fig. 9–11). In three- and four-part fractures, the deformity is more severe and includes displacement of the head and shaft. These are formidable lesions to reconstruct, as there is fixed retraction of the tuberosities, scarring of the soft tissue, and loss of bone. At the same time, nerve deficits and joint incongruity may be present. It is much easier to deal with an acute injury.

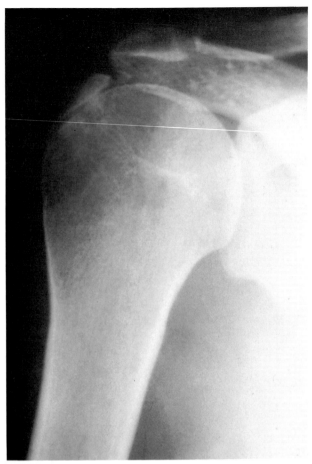

Figure 9–11. This greater tuberosity malunion resulted from the unopposed pull of the supraspinatus and infraspinatus muscles, which displaced the fragment superiorly and posteriorly. Subacromial impingement resulted, with pain on forward elevation and external rotation and a restricted range of motion.

AVASCULAR NECROSIS

Avascular necrosis can also occur after proximal humeral fractures.* It more commonly occurs after four-part fractures but can also occur following three- and two-part fractures. In reviewing several large series, Hagg[98] has recently reported an avascular necrosis rate between 3 and 14 per cent following closed reduction of displaced three-part fractures. In addition to the avascular necrosis, malunion and glenohumeral arthritis may be present, resulting in significant pain and loss of glenohumeral motion. The example, seen in Figure 9–12, is that of an active 72-year-old female who had a painful stiff shoulder secondary to avascular necrosis and a malunion of a four-part fracture, treated by closed reduction and early motion. Degenerative arthritis of the glenohumeral joint developed, and a total shoulder replacement was required for pain relief and improved function. This was an especially difficult procedure to perform since there was joint incongruity and capsular, bursal, and tendon scarring with contracture and loss of bone.

*See references 20, 85, 98, 124, 133, 138, 190, 205, 237, 254.

VASCULAR INJURY

Vascular complications following proximal humeral fractures are infrequent but do occur and can have profound consequences.† Injury to the axillary artery accounts for approximately 6 per cent of all arterial trauma secondary to fractures of the proximal humerus and is the most common vascular injury. In a series of 81 fractures, Stableforth[250] reported a 4.9 per cent incidence of arterial damage in displaced fractures. The injury is usually associated with penetrating or violent blunt trauma, resulting in a displaced fracture. However, it has also been reported with minimally displaced fractures. In addition, the risk is increased in older patients with arterial sclerosis because the vessel walls have lost elasticity and cannot stretch in response to the trauma. Therefore, in the elderly, a trivial accident may result in an arterial injury.

The most common site of injury to the axillary artery is proximal to the take-off of the anterior circumflex artery. Recent reports have stressed the need to suspect vascular injury whenever there is a fracture near a major vessel because the key to successful treatment is early diagnosis and repair.[106, 237, 292] The physical examination of the axillary artery may be difficult when pain and muscle spasm prevent abduction. It is important to check the radial pulse in the injured extremity; however, the presence of peripheral pulses may be secondary to collateral circulation. Therefore, an intact radial pulse is not a guarantee that significant arterial injury has not occurred. Doppler ultrasonography can be helpful in detecting a pulse but can also be misleading because collateral circulation can create a pulse detectable by Doppler examination. Other signs include an expanding hematoma, pallor, and paresthesias. Paresthesias are probably the most reliable sign of inadequate distal circulation and should raise suspicion of a vascular injury.

If an arterial injury is not recognized, the complications could be catastrophic and include gas gangrene, amputation, and compressive neuropathies of the brachial plexus leading to permanent deficits unless there is early evacuation of the hematoma. Angiography should be performed to confirm the diagnosis and to establish the exact location and nature of the injury. Arterial repair should be performed without delay and if necessary coordinated with appropriate orthopedic fracture repair.

BRACHIAL PLEXUS INJURY

Brachial plexus injuries also occur following fractures of the proximal humerus. Stableforth[250] reported an incidence of 6.1 per cent following proximal humeral fractures. Any or all components of the brachial plexus may be involved. Isolated injury to the axillary nerve is not uncommon and has been reported.[27] This is especially true concerning anterior fracture dislocations

†See references 106, 110, 137, 153, 191, 221, 237, 247, 250, 258, 292.

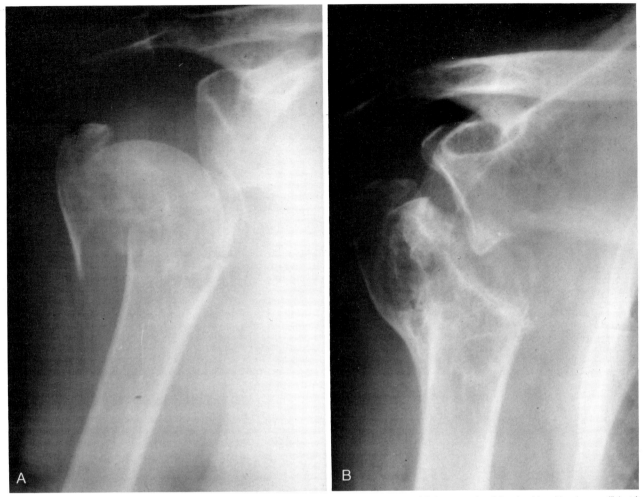

Figure 9–12. *A,* An anteroposterior radiograph of a four-part fracture in an active 72-year-old female. It was felt that congruity of the glenoid and head was sufficient for early motion to be started, and that the patient was too old for an operative procedure. *B,* Ten months after the fracture, the patient had avascular necrosis and degenerative arthritis. There was significant pain and disability and inability to use the upper extremity for even simple activities of daily living. The patient required a total shoulder replacement for pain relief and improved function.

as the nerve courses on the inferior surface of the capsule and is susceptible to injury. Injury to the suprascapular and musculocutaneous nerves is less common. It is important to establish, at the time of initial evaluation, if there are any nerve injuries. This can be done clinically by testing skin sensation and motor power. If nerve injury is suspected, this should be explained to the patient and should be carefully followed. Electromyogram and nerve conduction studies should be used to follow the progress of the injury. In complete axillary nerve injuries that do not show any signs of improvement within two to three months of injury, early exploration may be indicated.

CHEST INJURY

Injury to the thorax can also occur following fractures of the proximal humerus.[190, 250] There have been several reports of intrathoracic dislocation of the head

with surgical neck fractures of the humerus.[87, 101, 208] In addition, a pneumothorax or a pneumohemothorax can occur after fractures of the proximal humerus.

MYOSITIS OSSIFICANS

Myositis ossificans, especially after fracture dislocations, has been reported by several authors.[59, 191, 211] It is unusual for this to occur with uncomplicated fractures, but it can be present, especially when there is a chronic unreduced fracture dislocation.

Methods of Treatment

Many methods of treatment of proximal humeral fractures have been proposed through the years, creating a great deal of controversy and, at times, confusion. Fortunately, the majority of proximal humeral fractures are minimally displaced and can be satisfactorily treated with a sling and early range of motion exercises. Controversy exists when the fractures are significantly displaced. Needless to say, it is imperative to make the appropriate diagnosis initially. Precise x-rays and a reproducible classification system are essential to achieve consistent treatment of displaced fractures. Through the years, various treatment methods have been proposed including closed reduction, casts, splints, percutaneous pinning, open reduction and internal fixation, and the use of a humeral head prosthesis. It is important to realize that one method does not fit all cases and that we must use sound judgment as to what is the appropriate treatment for each specific fracture.

INITIAL IMMOBILIZATION AND EARLY MOTION

Initial immobilization and early motion have been continually described as having a high degree of success because the majority of proximal humeral fractures are minimally displaced.[22, 71, 83, 180, 222, 228, 276] The shoulder has a large capsule allowing a wide range of motion which can compensate for even moderate amounts of displacement. The arm is supported by a sling at the side or in the Velpeau position. A swath may be needed in the immediate postfracture period to enhance immobilization and comfort. An axillary pad may also be useful. Gentle range-of-motion exercises can be started by 7 to 10 days following a fracture when the pain has diminished and the patient is less apprehensive. It is important to establish that the fracture is clinically stable and moves as a unit before starting exercises. Overly aggressive exercises may distract a minimally displaced fracture and result in a malunion or nonunion (see Fig. 9–10). Intermittent x-rays in two perpendicular planes (an anteroposterior and a lateral in the scapular plane) are essential to determine if there has been any fracture displacement. Bertoft[25] has reported that the greatest amount of improvement in range of movement occurs between three to eight weeks following injury. Therefore, it is very important to have an organized and supervised physiotherapy program in place during this period. The exercises can be performed by the patient at home, but supervision by a physical therapist is beneficial in most instances. The exercises should be performed at least three to four times a day. The results of this treatment with complex displaced fractures are not as successful.

CLOSED REDUCTION

For years, closed reduction has been a popular method of treatment for all types of displaced proximal humeral fractures.[85, 94, 129, 175, 222, 274, 290] However, it is important to differentiate between which fractures are suited to closed reduction and which are not. Repeated and forceable attempts at closed reduction may complicate a fracture by causing further displacement, fragmentation, or neurovascular injury. Various other types of reduction maneuvers have been used with mixed results.[94, 129, 175, 240, 274]

Before performing a closed reduction, it is important to understand the type of deformity and the forces involved in fracture. Without recognition of pathophysiology of a particular fracture, it is almost impossible to perform an adequate closed reduction. Watson-Jones[273] described a classic technique of hyperabduction and traction to achieve a closed reduction. This technique was thought to be necessary because in the surgical neck "abduction type fracture" the proximal fragment was pulled into abduction. However, the deformity is anterior angulation and not hyperabduction; therefore, this type of reduction is not necessary. Also, in the displaced two-part surgical neck fracture, the deforming force is created by the pectoralis major muscle and other internal rotators pulling the shaft medially. This force must be neutralized before an adequate reduction can be performed. To perform a closed reduction, adequate relaxation is necessary. The patient is usually more comfortable supine. An intravenous catheter should be in place in the contralateral arm. A muscle relaxant and narcotic should be given intravenously after a small test dose. Whenever possible, fluoroscopic C-arm visualization should be employed to enhance visualization of the reduction and precise location of the fracture fragments. Also, the stability of the fracture reduction can be tested in different positions. If a fracture after reduction is unstable, further operative stabilization may be necessary.

Two-Part Anatomical Neck Fractures

Displaced anatomical neck fractures are difficult to treat by closed reduction. The thickness of the head is quite small and may be rotated or angulated in the joint capsule, not allowing adequate head and neck alignment. However, several other types of two-part fractures and fracture dislocations are very amenable to closed reduction.

Two-Part Surgical Neck Fractures

In the displaced two-part surgical neck fracture, both tuberosities are attached to the head so that it remains in a neutral position. The shaft is usually displaced medially by the pull of the pectoralis major. The hyperabduction overhead technique is not required nor is significant traction with weight needed. Gentle traction with flexion and some adduction is usually all that is required to get the arm to the pivotal portion so that it can be impacted under the head. If a reduction is not possible, there may be interposition of soft tissue—muscle, capsule, or long head of the biceps. Often, the long head of the biceps is caught in the fracture site and creates a tether which will distract the fracture with repeated attempts at reduction (Fig. 9–13).

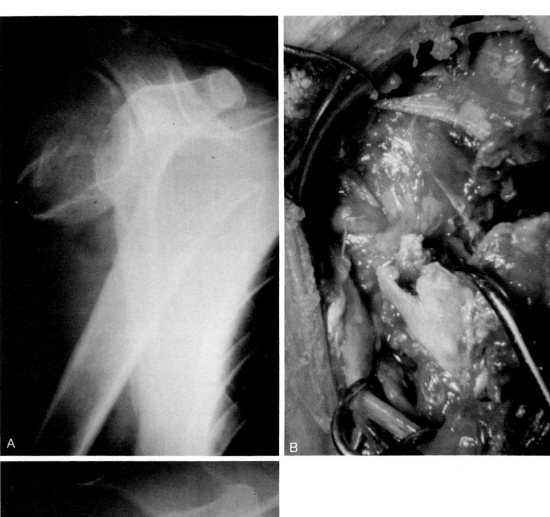

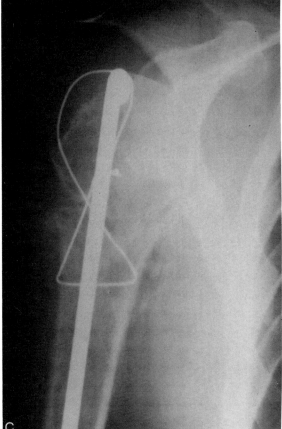

Figure 9–13. *A,* An anteroposterior radiograph of a displaced two-part surgical neck fracture. The shaft is displaced medially by the pull of the pectoralis major muscle. Several attempts at closed reduction were performed, both in the emergency room and in the operating room under general anesthesia with the use of an image intensifier. However, the fracture could not be reduced. *B,* A photograph at the time of surgery shows interposition of the biceps tendon between the proximal fragment and the shaft. The loop retractor is in the biceps tendon, which was tethering the head and wedged between the shaft and the head, preventing reduction. *C,* A six-week postoperative radiograph reveals early healing of the fracture, which was fixed with a figure-of-eight wire; in this instance a Rush rod was used for longitudinal support because of comminution. The Rush rod was removed to avoid impingement with forward elevation. (Courtesy of Dr. Charles S. Neer II.)

This situation requires open reduction and internal fixation. An impacted but angulated two-part surgical neck fracture may also be improved with a closed reduction. If the anterior angulation is more than 45 degrees, this will limit forward elevation. The head should be disimpacted from the shaft. Then the shaft is reduced and placed underneath the head with less anterior angulation. A minimally displaced and stable comminuted fracture can be treated without the need for surgery, but displaced and unstable fractures require open reduction and internal fixation to properly align the fragments.[44, 46, 191, 250, 255, 290]

Two-Part Greater Tuberosity Fractures

Greater tuberosity fractures are usually retracted posteriorly and superiorly, and closed reduction is difficult. However, if this fracture is associated with an anterior dislocation, a closed reduction of the glenohumeral dislocation may successfully reduce the greater tuberosity fracture (Fig. 9–14). If the fracture heals in an adequate alignment, the chance of recurrent dislocation is low. However, there is a tendency for the greater tuberosity fragment to displace superiorly and posteriorly after a reduction (Fig. 9–15).[166] Oni[203] reported a case where the greater tuberosity fracture blocked reduction of the anterior glenohumeral dislocation. The literature reports isolated greater tuberosity fractures associated with an anterior dislocation

in 5 to 8 per cent of cases.[90, 222, 238] However, higher rates of between 10 and 15 per cent have also been reported.[173, 175, 188, 276]

Two-Part Lesser Tuberosity Fractures

If the fragment is small and does not block medial rotation, successful treatment by closed reduction of the rare two-part lesser tuberosity fracture has been reported.[124, 188] Usually this injury is associated with a posterior dislocation and may also be treated by closed reduction if the articular involvement is minimal and the injury occurred within two to three weeks (Fig. 9–16). The arm should be immobilized in neutral or slight external rotation.

Three-Part Fractures

Three-part fractures are quite unstable and difficult to treat by closed reduction. There is a tuberosity fragment as well as a surgical neck fragment. In three-part lesser tuberosity fractures, the greater tuberosity is attached to the head, pulling it into external rotation, i.e., the articular surface faces anteriorly. In a greater tuberosity three-part fracture, the lesser tuberosity remains attached to the head, pulling it into internal rotation, i.e., the articular surface faces posteriorly. In addition, the shaft is pulled medially by the pectoralis major, adding another component to be considered

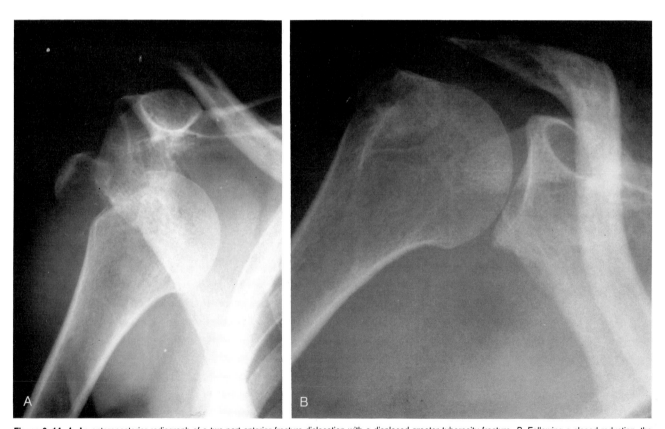

Figure 9–14. *A,* An anteroposterior radiograph of a two-part anterior fracture dislocation with a displaced greater tuberosity fracture. *B,* Following a closed reduction, the greater tuberosity fracture reduced and healed without further displacement. The patient achieved a normal range of motion without any further anterior dislocations.

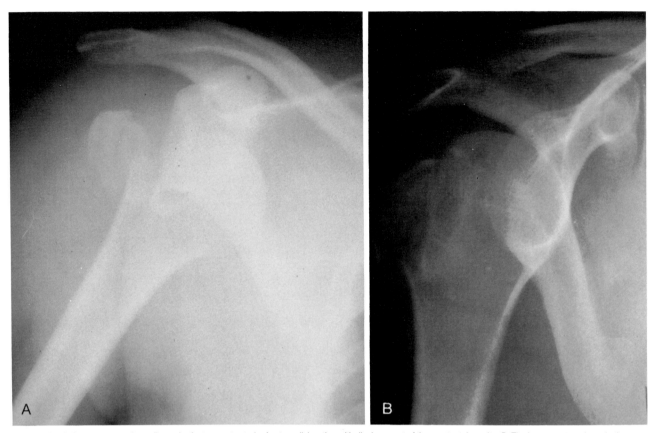

Figure 9–15. *A,* An anteroposterior radiograph of a two-part anterior fracture dislocation with displacement of the greater tuberosity. *B,* The large greater tuberosity fragment remained displaced and required open reduction internal fixation with nonabsorbable sutures.

during the closed reduction. These deforming forces must be considered when attempting a closed reduction. The long head of the biceps tendon may also be caught between the fragments obstructing the reduction. Repeated attempts at a closed reduction in these

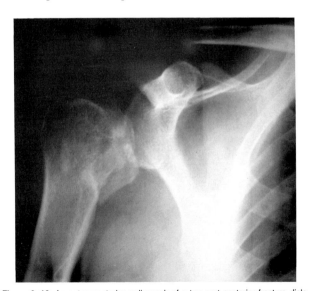

Figure 9–16. An anteroposterior radiograph of a two-part posterior fracture dislocation after reduction. The lesser tuberosity fragment was minimally displaced and did not block medial rotation. This injury was treated closed, with excellent return of function.

fractures should not be done because most of them are in elderly people with osteoporotic bone. However, several authors have reported good results with closed reduction of three-part fractures.[71, 150, 178, 290] The better results were in older, sedentary individuals with limited goals. Pain relief was adequate, but functional activity was limited. Dingley[66] has described a modified closed technique for fracture dislocations using a percutaneous pin in the dislocated head to facilitate reduction and then removing the pin. Other literature has reported poor results with closed reduction, a high incidence of pain, malunion, and avascular necrosis.[44, 85, 98, 133, 216, 255]

Four-Part Fractures

Closed reduction of four-part fractures of the proximal humerus generally produce poor results. In various series, there have been extremely high incidences of avascular necrosis—between 13 and 34 per cent.[85, 98, 133, 191, 209, 237, 250, 255] Malunion and degenerative arthritis also occur. Lee[146] has reported the only series of satisfactory results with closed reduction.

Impression Fractures

If a missed dislocation with an impression fracture is diagnosed within two to three weeks, and the impression fracture of the head is less than 20 per cent, an attempt at a closed reduction may be worthwhile. It is important to assess accurately the degree of the head impression fracture with a CT or axillary view to judge whether the reduction will be stable. An adequate result may be obtained with a closed reduction in some displaced fractures because the shoulder has a great capacity to compensate within a restricted range of motion. Many functional activities involving the shoulder can be done with a restricted range of motion. However, it must be emphasized that an anatomical reduction should be the goal in the treatment of the majority of displaced fractures of the proximal humerus. In older sedentary individuals who do not place great demand on their arms, one may accept a less than perfect closed reduction, especially in the nondominant extremity.

PERCUTANEOUS PINS

Percutaneous pinning may be used following a closed reduction if it is unstable. This technique is very useful in the treatment of unimpacted two-part surgical neck fractures. Jacob[124] has nicely outlined the technique and reported satisfactory results in 35 of 40 cases. Two distal 2.5 AO threaded tip pins are placed in the proximal shaft just above the deltoid insertion and then air drilled into the head fragment using a C-arm image intensifier to visualize the fracture. A pin from the tuberosity into the shaft may enhance fixation. This procedure can be technically difficult, and a power drill is usually required to penetrate the shaft. The pins are removed when there is adequate stability of the fracture and range of motion can progress without fear of displacement. Percutaneous pin technique has also been reported for three- and four-part fractures and comminuted fractures of the proximal humerus; however, it is a much more difficult procedure for these fractures with less than ideal results.

PLASTER SPLINTS AND CASTS

Many types of splints and casts have been proposed through the years, with varying success, for the treatment of displaced fractures.* At present, a sling and swathe or a Velpeau sling is the most commonly used method of immobilization for proximal humeral fractures, and more elaborate devices are generally not required. However, a plaster slab along the humeral shaft and superior aspect of the shoulder can be used for extra support and comfort.

Older literature suggests that reduction in an abducted and flexed position was essential for proper alignment. Milch[175, 176] and others[240, 274] felt that the abducted and overhead position better neutralized the muscle forces about the shoulder than the anatomical position of Kocher, with the arm at the side. The

shoulder spica casts and braces needed to maintain this position were extremely cumbersome and uncomfortable for the patient. These devices began to lose popularity in the 1920s.[222] However, a shoulder spica cast with some degree of abduction (20 to 30 degrees) may be needed to provide extra stability for a severely comminuted fracture of the proximal humerus. Jakob[124] recommends the use of an abduction splint for the treatment of selected greater tuberosity fractures.

Good results have been reported with the hanging cast, especially with humeral shaft fractures.† However, a significant amount of patient cooperation is required, and frequent supervision is necessary to avoid angulation and distraction. The weight of a heavy cast may cause distraction of the fracture fragments. This is especially true of comminuted proximal shaft fractures where there is inferior subluxation.[259] Stewart[252] recommended supplementing a hanging cast with an abduction brace for extra support and comfort in the immediate postfracture period. If traction is needed, the weight of the arm should provide sufficient distraction. In general, the use of hanging casts for fractures of the proximal humerus should be avoided as there is a tendency for distraction of the fracture fragments, leading to nonunion or malunion. The hanging cast technique probably has more application in the treatment of humeral shaft fractures.

SKELETAL TRACTION

The use of traction is not commonly indicated but may be helpful in management of a comminuted fracture.[132, 188, 189, 197] Traction can be difficult to maintain and restricts patient mobility, especially if the patient has multiple injuries and requires other diagnostic and treatment procedures. However, it can provide temporary benefit until a more definitive procedure can be performed.

The arm should be held flexed and slightly adducted to relax the pectoralis major, which is the most important deforming force. The abducted position should be avoided. The shoulder is flexed to 90 degrees, and the elbow is also flexed to 90 degrees. A threaded Kirschner wire, Steinmann pin, or an AO screw should be placed in the ulna, and the forearm and wrist should be suspended in a sling. This will allow some hand and elbow motion to avoid stiffness. The goal is to try to hold the shoulder in a neutral position, since in this fracture both tuberosities are attached to the head and the head is essentially in a neutral position. When there is sufficient callus formation, the traction may be discontinued, and the patient may be placed in a sling or spica cast.

OPEN REDUCTION AND INTERNAL FIXATION

Open reduction of displaced fractures gained popularity in the early part of the 20th century.[18, 45, 90, 222, 234, 257]

---

*See references 3, 13, 71, 94, 123, 197, 234, 240, 274, 276, 279, 280, 286.

†See references 37, 38, 39, 93, 121, 123, 141, 214, 280, 286.

In many instances, closed reduction and external fixation was unable to correct deformity and maintain reduction sufficiently. Various techniques and devices have been proposed to treat fractures. The choice of technique and devices depends on several factors including the type of fracture, the quality of the bone and soft tissue, and the age and reliability of the patient. The goal of internal fixation should be a stable reduction allowing for early motion of the fracture. The current trend is toward limited dissection of the soft tissue about the fracture fragments and the minimal amount of hardware required for stable fixation.[46]

Two-Part Anatomical Neck Fractures

Anatomical neck fractures are extremely rare, and very few cases are reported in the literature on which to base a discussion concerning treatment. The prognosis for survival of the head is poor since it has been completely separated from its blood supply. However, several authors recommend an attempt at open reduction and internal fixation, especially if the patient is young.[59, 124, 188] If the small head cannot be secured to the proximal humerus, a prosthesis is indicated.

Two-Part Surgical Neck Fractures

Two-part displaced surgical neck fractures often require an open reduction and internal fixation either because interposition of soft tissue prevents a closed reduction or the reduction is not stable. Various devices have been proposed for fixation, including intramedullary nails or rods, plates and screws, staples, wire, nonabsorbable suture material, multiple pins, and combinations of the above.

The Rush rod technique can be performed through a very limited incision and split in the deltoid and the rotator cuff. It has been a very popular device with several authors reporting good results.[149, 230, 259, 277, 283] However, the relative lack of fixation of this device to control rotation may be inadequate for some displaced surgical neck fractures. Furthermore, a second procedure may be required to remove the device since it can impinge against the anterior or inferior acromion during forward elevation and rotation. This technique may be useful in older debilitated patients where minimal surgery is indicated and the functional goals are limited. The use of an AO buttress plate and screw has been associated with good results, especially with two-part surgical neck fractures, but the soft tissue dissection should be limited and the bone quality must be adequate for screw fixation (Fig. 9–17). Yamano[288] has reported a high success rate with a hooked plate. A figure-of-eight tension band technique with wire or nonabsorbable sutures is also useful and in most instances provides adequate fixation (Fig. 9–18; see also Fig. 9–13). Furthermore, if the quality of the bone is poor, the wires can be passed through the rotator cuff for proximal fixation as it may be stronger than the bone. In cases where there is comminution, intramedullary fixation with either a Rush rod or Enders nails will improve fixation and maintain length (Fig. 9–19).

Two-Part Greater Tuberosity Fractures

Greater tuberosity fractures displaced more than one centimeter may require open reduction internal fixation, because the posterior and superior displacement will cause impingement beneath the acromion[59, 166, 191] (Fig. 9–20). Screws, wire, and suture material have all been proposed as types of fixation of the greater tuberosity. The rent in the rotator cuff that occurs with displaced greater tuberosity fractures must also be repaired. Screws may not provide adequate fixation in osteoporotic bone (Fig. 9–21). Nonabsorbable sutures are probably a better choice of fixation.

Two-Part Lesser Tuberosity Fractures

Displaced isolated fractures of the lesser tuberosity are rare injuries and may require internal fixation with nonabsorbable sutures, especially if the fragment is quite large and blocks medial rotation.[7, 96, 124, 140, 165, 188, 243, 283] Stangl[251] has described removal of the bone fragment and suture of the subscapularis tendon to the cortical edge of the fracture site. When the fragment is large, it may involve part of the articular surface.

Three-Part Fractures

Open reduction and internal fixation is the treatment of choice for displaced three-part fractures of the proximal humerus.[98, 104, 205, 225, 235] It is important to avoid extensive exposure and soft tissue dissection of the fragments which may compromise blood supply. Hagg[98] has reported a high rate of avascular necrosis, between 12 and 25 per cent, in a review of several series of open reduction and internal fixation of three-part fractures.

Regardless of the type of fixation used, it must secure the displaced tuberosity to both the head and shaft. The use of intramedullary nails or rods is usually not adequate fixation to neutralize the deforming forces in this type of fracture and could result in a malunion (Fig. 9–22). Mouradian[182] developed an intramedullary nail with screw fixation for the head and tuberosities. However, the incidence of avascular necrosis was high, and follow-up was short. The AO buttress plate technique has been a popular procedure for this fracture, but recent reports from several authors have reflected poor results with the AO plate for both three- and four-part fractures.[138, 205, 254] The complications include avascular necrosis, secondary to extensive soft tissue dissection; superior placement of the plate, leading to impingement; loss of plate fixation with screw loosening; malunion; and infection. Paavolainen[205] reported that the most common technical errors were placing the plate too high on the tuberosity, which restricted motion, and reducing the fracture into a varus position (see Fig. 9–8). Kristiansen[138] reported 55 per cent unsatisfactory results in a series of 20 patients with two-, three-, and four-part fractures that were managed with plate and screws. Sturzenegger[254] has reported a high incidence (34 per cent) of avascular necrosis.

Text continued on page 303

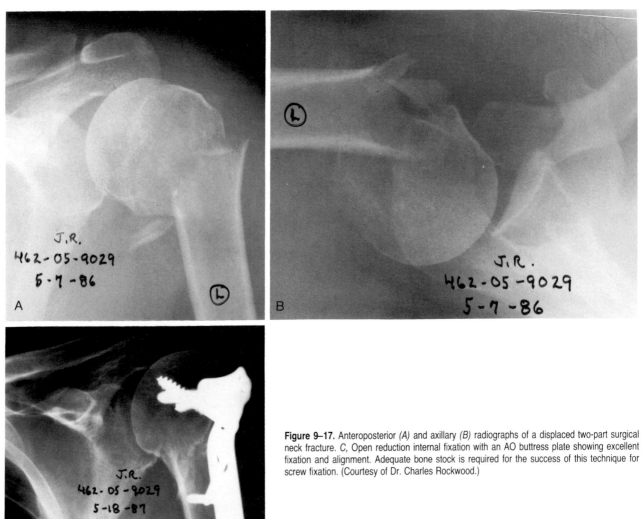

Figure 9–17. Anteroposterior *(A)* and axillary *(B)* radiographs of a displaced two-part surgical neck fracture. *C,* Open reduction internal fixation with an AO buttress plate showing excellent fixation and alignment. Adequate bone stock is required for the success of this technique for screw fixation. (Courtesy of Dr. Charles Rockwood.)

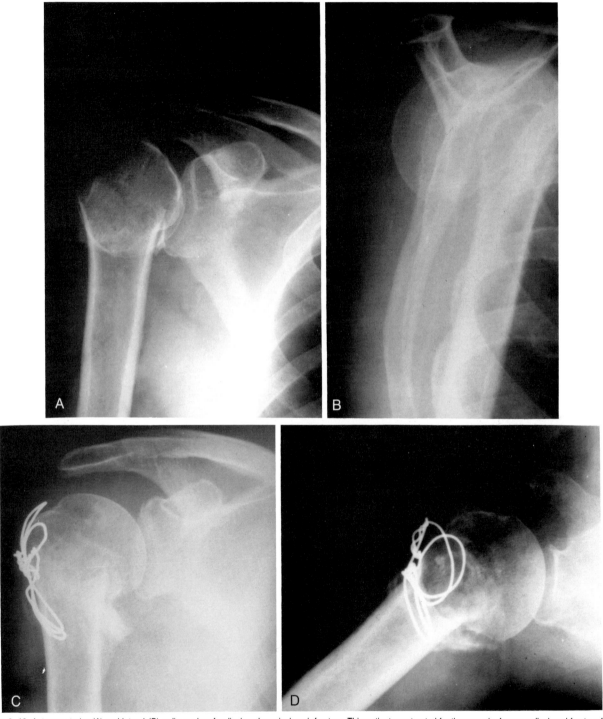

Figure 9–18. Anteroposterior *(A)* and lateral *(B)* radiographs of a displaced surgical neck fracture. This patient was treated for three weeks for an undisplaced fracture from only the anteroposterior radiograph. The follow-up lateral x-ray in the scapula plane revealed a significant anterior shaft displacement. Anteroposterior *(C)* and axillary lateral *(D)* radiographs were taken following open reduction internal fixation with two figure-eight wires. The wires are placed through both the cuff and the tuberosities, as well as the proximal shaft.

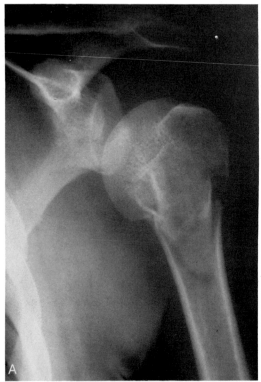

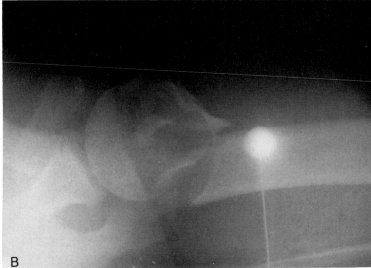

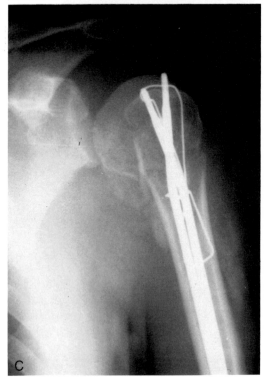

Figure 9–19. *A,* An anteroposterior radiograph of a comminuted surgical neck fracture. *B,* An axillary x-ray that shows displacement of the head. This fracture was extremely unstable, with excessive motion at the fracture site. *C,* Open reduction internal fixation with two Enders nails as well as a figure-eight wire providing rigid fixation. (Courtesy of Dr. Evan L. Flatow.)

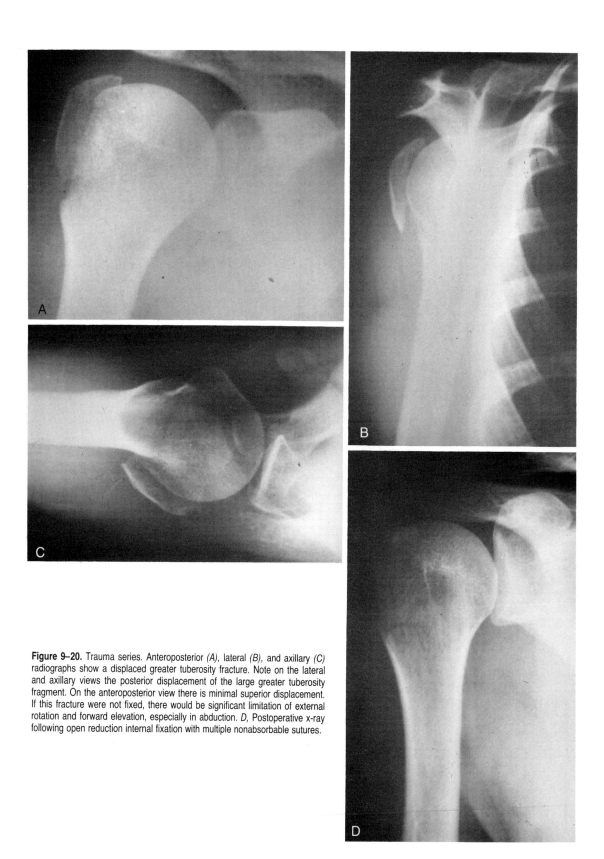

Figure 9–20. Trauma series. Anteroposterior *(A)*, lateral *(B)*, and axillary *(C)* radiographs show a displaced greater tuberosity fracture. Note on the lateral and axillary views the posterior displacement of the large greater tuberosity fragment. On the anteroposterior view there is minimal superior displacement. If this fracture were not fixed, there would be significant limitation of external rotation and forward elevation, especially in abduction. *D,* Postoperative x-ray following open reduction internal fixation with multiple nonabsorbable sutures.

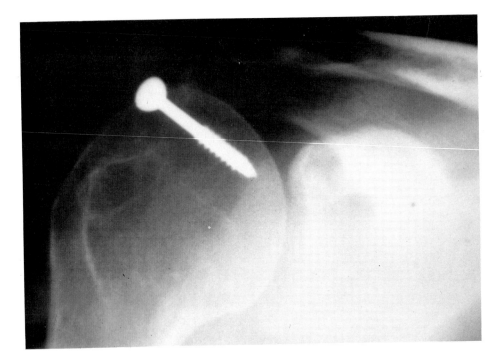

Figure 9–21. Anteroposterior radiograph of an AO screw that had migrated superiorly with the greater tuberosity fragment. This led to significant impingement and loss of motion. There was loss of fixation of the screw since it was placed in the soft cancellous bone of the humeral head.

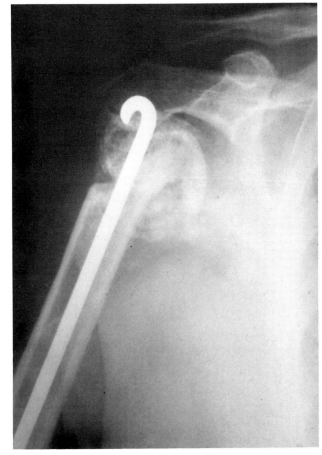

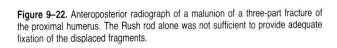

Figure 9–22. Anteroposterior radiograph of a malunion of a three-part fracture of the proximal humerus. The Rush rod alone was not sufficient to provide adequate fixation of the displaced fragments.

Neer[191] reported good results with internal fixation of three-part fractures if the displaced tuberosity is reattached to the shaft and head with wire or, more recently, nonabsorbable sutures. The poor results in his series were due to tuberosity displacement from failure of vertical fixation devices (Rush rods, Kirschner wires, splints) to hold the tuberosities in position. In 1986, Hawkins[104] reported, in a series of 15 patients, that good results were obtained in 14 patients with the use of a figure-of-eight wire for three-part fractures of the proximal humerus. The only early failure in his series was a patient who had a buttress plate and screws for fixation. Two patients developed avascular necrosis, and one of these required a humeral head prosthesis. In osteoporotic bone, the soft tissues of the rotator cuff are stronger than the bone, and these can be used with this technique. The wire is passed through the rotator cuff as well as the bone of the tuberosity and then attached to the shaft below. This method usually supplies sufficient stability to begin early motion.

Four-Part Fractures

Open reduction and internal fixation of four-part fractures generally yields unsatisfactory results, as confirmed by numerous reports.[98, 138, 191, 205, 250, 254–256] The complications are essentially the same as with three-part fractures, just more severe and with a higher percentage of avascular necrosis and malunion.

A significant number of four-part fractures occur in the elderly in whom osteoporosis and poor bone quality are more common. This is not the ideal setting for internal fixation with pins, rods, or plate and screws. Jakob[124] has recently reported that open reduction and internal fixation with multiple pins (minimal fixation techniques) of a subgroup of four-part fractures may be indicated (Fig. 9–23). In this subgroup, the head is impacted on the shaft, and the tuberosities are split but in close proximity to the head and shaft. The head is not dislocated or displaced laterally, and some contact with the glenoid is maintained. However, this type of fracture is not a true four-part displacement, according to the Neer classification. The head is elevated and the tuberosities are placed beneath it. Multiple pins are used to provide fixation and left under the skin. The pins are removed between the fourth and sixth week when there is early healing and some stability. Acceptable function and pain relief may be achieved despite avascular necrosis because of the reasonable position of the head with respect to the glenoid, allowing adequate glenohumeral congruity. However, long-term follow-up of cases was not reported. As a rule, the results of internal fixation of four-part fractures are generally poor.

Replacement Prosthesis

The use of the humeral head prosthesis for fractures of the proximal humerus was first published in the early 1950s. Several authors reported on different designs that were being developed for use in displaced fracture dislocations of the proximal humerus.[8, 70, 75, 139, 196, 210, 220, 266, 267] The design that has become the most commonly used is the one developed by Neer. In 1953, Neer[196] reported the first use of this prosthesis for complex fracture dislocation of the proximal humerus.

At that time, alternative treatment of this fracture included closed reduction,[81] open reduction and internal fixation,[196, 222, 234] arthrodesis,[196] and humeral head excision.[126, 127] The results of all these treatments were usually unsatisfactory. However, several authors earlier in this century reported satisfactory results with humeral head excision.[174, 264] The use of this procedure yields a weakened, short, and painful extremity. In 1955 and 1970, Neer[191, 194] reported on a series of patients successfully treated with the proximal humeral prosthesis. The original prosthesis (Fig. 9–24) was revised by Neer in 1973 to a more conforming surface design (Fig. 9–25).

The prosthesis has two head sizes, 15 and 22 mm in thickness. The larger gives better leverage and mechanical advantage for forward elevation, but the smaller may be required for coverage by the rotator cuff. There are three stem sizes, 7, 9.5, and 12 mm, and two stem lengths, 125 and 150 mm (see Fig. 9–24). Longer stem lengths are available on special order if needed to bridge a shaft fracture.

The surgical technique has evolved over the past 30 years, and it is a reliable procedure for four-part fractures and fracture dislocations of the proximal humerus. Most recently, Neer[186] has reported better results secondary to technical considerations concerning the anatomical approach, the surgical technique, and rehabilitation. Of the 61 patients in his series, 51 were rated excellent, 9 were rated satisfactory, and only 1 was rated unsatisfactory. The technical considerations will be outlined in the next section in the description of the technique. Several other series have reported good results using this prosthesis, including adequate pain relief and function.[60, 61, 256, 263] Others have reported adequate pain relief but a higher incidence of unsatisfactory results secondary to postoperative stiffness and limitation of function.[69, 137, 162, 178, 285]

It is important to remember that the surgical approach, care of the soft tissue, and postoperative rehabilitation are equally as important as the insertion of the prosthesis. A humeral head prosthesis may be required for an anatomical neck fracture if internal fixation is not feasible. Also, in certain selected comminuted osteoporotic three-part fractures in older individuals, a primary humeral head prosthesis may be a better choice than internal fixation, because internal fixation does not achieve a stable reduction allowing early motion.[46, 188, 256] A humeral head prosthesis will allow secure tuberosity fixation so that rehabilitation can be started earlier and a more functional result can be achieved. A prosthesis is indicated in head splitting fractures and also in impression fractures in which more than 45 per cent of the articular surface is involved. The results from use of a prosthesis in acute fractures are generally better than the results seen with

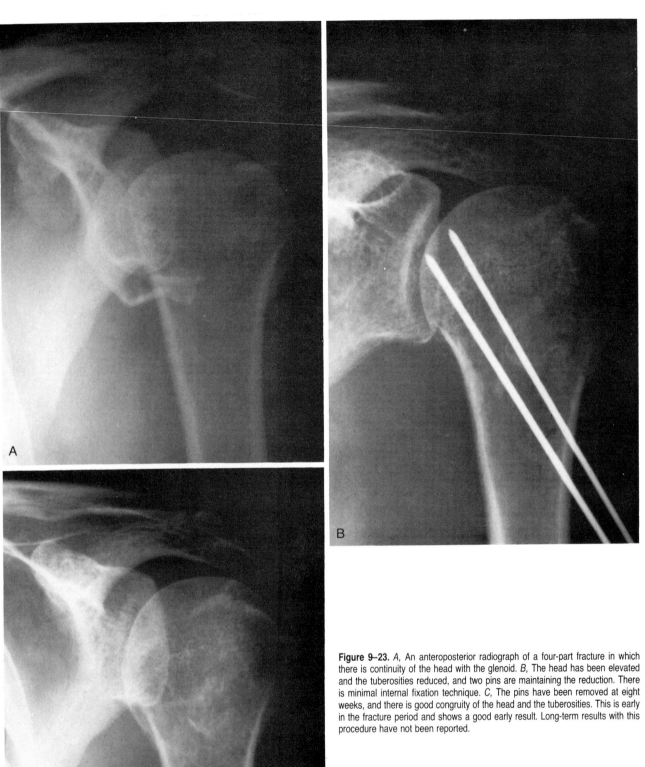

Figure 9–23. *A,* An anteroposterior radiograph of a four-part fracture in which there is continuity of the head with the glenoid. *B,* The head has been elevated and the tuberosities reduced, and two pins are maintaining the reduction. There is minimal internal fixation technique. *C,* The pins have been removed at eight weeks, and there is good congruity of the head and the tuberosities. This is early in the fracture period and shows a good early result. Long-term results with this procedure have not been reported.

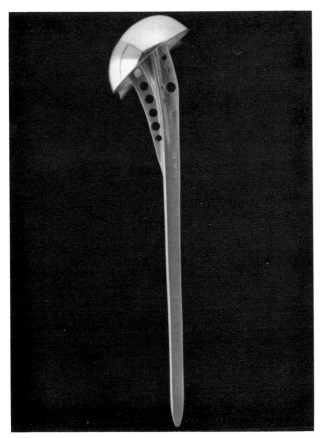

Figure 9-24. The original Neer I prosthesis, which was designed in 1951.

use in chronic fractures or in revisions of failed internal fixation because of malunion, scar tissue, and muscle contractures.

Fracture Dislocation

Two- and three-part fracture dislocations are readily treated by open reduction and internal fixation. In these fracture dislocations, the vascular supply to the head is maintained by the soft tissue attachments to the intact tuberosity, and therefore, adequate fixation should be attained by the procedures that have been previously outlined. Redislocation is rare following adequate fracture healing. In two-part fracture dislocations, a closed reduction may have adequately treated the glenohumeral dislocation. However, if there is a persistent tuberosity displacement, this will require open reduction and internal fixation. The results from internal fixation of four-part fracture dislocations have been poor, and a prosthesis is generally indicated in this type of lesion (Fig. 9–26).

Surgical Approaches

There are two basic surgical approaches for treatment of proximal humeral fractures. The first is the superior deltoid approach (Fig. 9–27A).[188] The skin in-

cision is made in Langer's lines, just lateral to the anterior lateral aspect of the acromion. Through this approach, the deltoid can be split from the edge of the acromion distally for approximately 4 to 5 cm (Fig. 9–27B). The deltoid origin is not removed, allowing exposure of the superior aspect of the proximal humerus. It is useful for internal fixation of greater tuberosity fractures and is also helpful for the insertion of a proximal intramedullary rod. Rotation, flexion, or extension of the humerus greatly enhances exposure of the underlying structures.

The second approach is a long deltopectoral approach (Fig. 9–28A).[187] In this approach, both the deltoid origin and insertion are preserved. The skin incision is started just inferior to the clavicle and extends across the coracoid process and down to the area of insertion of the deltoid. The cephalic vein should be preserved and retracted either laterally or medially, depending on which is the easiest direction. The deltopectoral interval is dissected proximally and distally (Fig. 9–28B). If more exposure is needed, the insertion of the deltoid can be partially elevated, and the superior part of the pectoralis major tendon insertion can be divided.

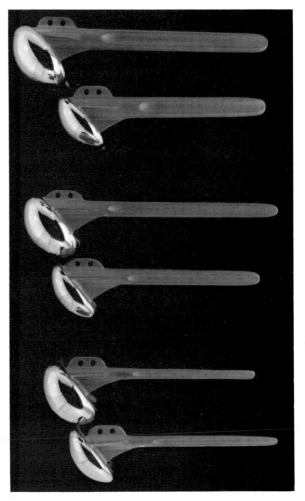

Figure 9-25. The Neer II prosthesis, which was redesigned in 1973. There are two head sizes (15 and 22 mm) as well as six different stem sizes.

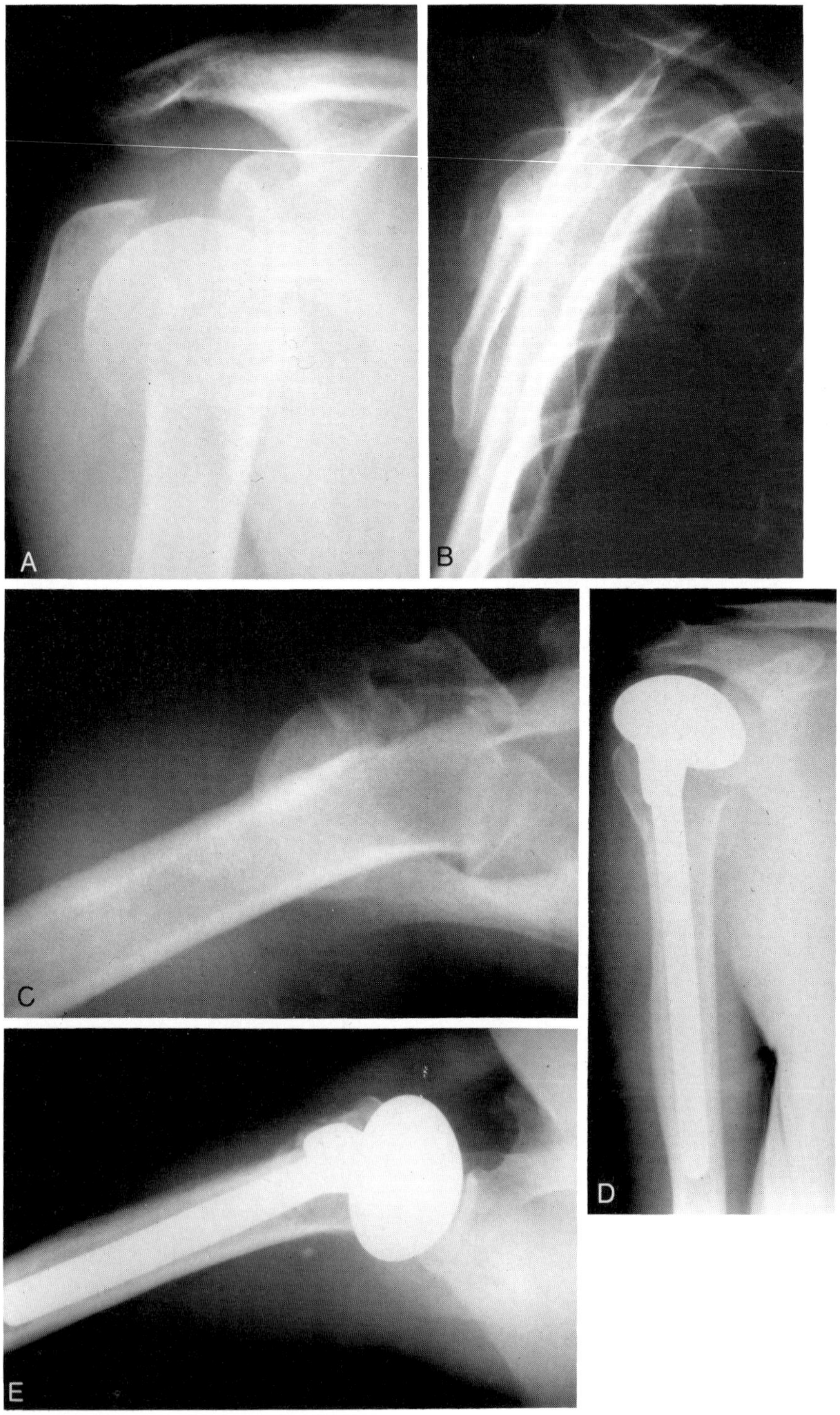

Figure 9–26. *A,* An anteroposterior radiograph in the scapular plane reveals a four-part fracture with the head displaced laterally, the greater tuberosity displaced superiorly, and the lesser tuberosity displaced medially. *B,* A lateral radiograph in the scapular plane reveals the posterior displacement of the greater tuberosity, with the head in the center and the lesser tuberosity medially below the coracoid. *C,* The axillary view shows the lateral displacement of the head as well as the displacement of the lesser and greater tuberosities. Anteroposterior *(D)* and axillary *(E)* radiographs show a large humeral head prosthesis in place. In this instance a press fit was obtained; in most instances cement is needed to support the prosthesis. Three years after operation the patient has essentially a normal range of motion and activity.

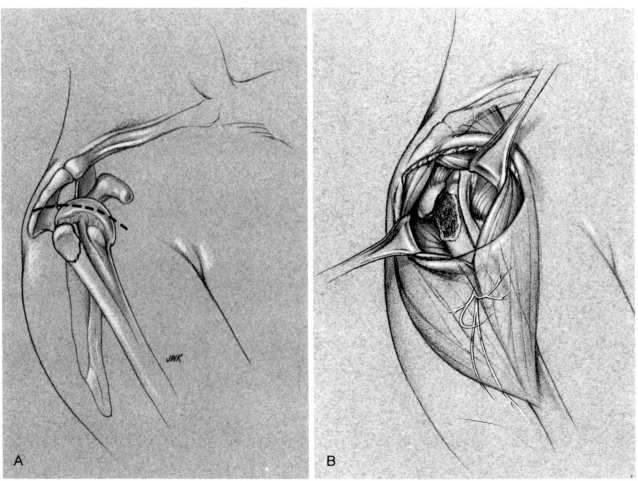

Figure 9–27. *A*, The skin incision for the superior-anterior approach to the shoulder consists of an oblique incision in Langer's lines beginning on the anterolateral aspect of the acromion and extending obliquely down for approximately 8 to 9 cm. *B*, Two Richardson retractors are placed in the deltoid as it is split approximately 4 to 5 cm from the tip of the acromion. This gives adequate exposure for greater tuberosity fractures. Great care is taken not to extend the slit below 6 cm as there may be injury to the axillary nerve. Rotation of the humerus allows for improved exposure of the different parts of the proximal humerus.

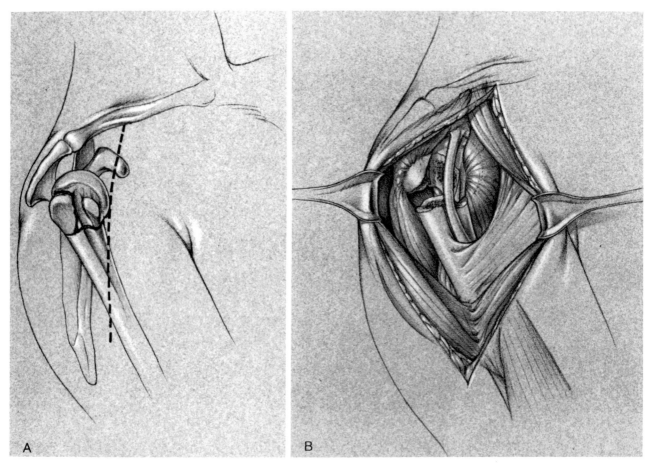

Figure 9–28. *A,* A long deltopectoral approach is useful for two-, three-, and four-part fractures. The incision is made from the clavicle medially over the coracoid and extended down to the shaft of the humerus near the deltoid insertion. *B* shows the exposure that can be achieved. The insertion of the pectoralis major may also be released to improve exposure. Care is taken never to remove the deltoid origin from the clavicle; if more exposure is needed, the deltoid insertion may be elevated.

Procedures that split or remove the lateral part of the acromion are unnecessary and may lead to complications. Furthermore, splitting the middle deltoid beyond 5 cm from the edge of the acromion has a high risk of injury to the axillary nerve. Both of these approaches are extremely worthwhile because they preserve deltoid function, which allows a more rapid rehabilitation in the postoperative period. Removal of the deltoid origin is unnecessary because it will seriously affect the function of this important muscle and slow down the postoperative rehabilitation program. Splitting the middle deltoid beyond 2 inches from the edge of the acromion presents a high risk of injury to the axillary nerve.

Author's Preferred Method of Treatment

MINIMALLY DISPLACED FRACTURES

Minimally displaced fractures are treated with a sling and swathe for comfort. The swathe can usually be removed after a few days. On rare occasions, if there is significant swelling and discomfort, I may use a plaster slab on the shaft of the humerus and the superior aspect of the shoulder.

If the fracture is stable, range of motion exercises can be started early—within 10 days when the pain is tolerable. The physician must evaluate the fracture for clinical stability by standing on the side of the patient and supporting the elbow and forearm with one hand and placing the other hand over the proximal humerus. Then the physician gently rotates the elbow and forearm. If the fracture appears to move as a unit, it is stable and gentle, and passive range of motion exercises may be started. Elbow supination, pronation, and flexion may be started while the patient is in the sling. The complete physical therapy regimen is outlined in the rehabilitation section. Frequent radiographic evaluation is needed to check for displacement of fracture fragments.

TWO-PART ANATOMICAL NECK FRACTURES

Anatomical neck fractures, as has been noted, are extremely rare, and there are very few reports of treatment.[59, 124, 191] Certainly, no surgeon has treated large numbers of this type of fracture. In young patients, I recommend an attempt at open reduction and internal fixation. If there is some soft tissue attachment to the head, and if the quality of the bone is good, it may be possible to achieve fixation to the tuberosities and shaft. In older patients, a primary prosthesis is a better choice, allowing early motion and a more rapid recovery.

TWO-PART SURGICAL NECK FRACTURES

Displaced two-part surgical neck fractures are divided into three distinct types: unimpacted, angulated impacted, and comminuted. The majority of these may be initially treated by closed reduction. The exception is the severely comminuted surgical neck fracture where there is little chance of improvement of alignment and stability is not possible.

In the displaced surgical neck fracture, the shaft is displaced medially by the pectoralis major and is in close proximity to the brachial plexus and axillary artery. The head remains within the glenohumeral joint in a neutral position since both tuberosities are attached. To achieve a closed reduction, gentle traction should be placed on the arm as it is brought out to the side and then gently flexed. Traction should be maintained, and flexion is increased as the arm is gradually adducted to gain reduction of the shaft beneath the head (Fig. 9–29). The adduction will neutralize the pull of the pectoralis major and other internal rotators, which are creating the deformity. Counterpressure by an assistant may be needed beneath the armpit, or digital pressure on the proximal fragment may be necessary to achieve stabilization. An attempt is made to hook the proximal shaft beneath the humeral head, and then the arm is slightly abducted and the shaft is impacted beneath the head. To adequately perform this procedure it is important to have good relaxation. This may not be possible in an emergency room situation with only intramuscular or intravenous analgesics and muscle relaxants. Multiple attempts at closed reduction in the emergency room without adequate relaxation are ill advised.

If the first attempt of closed reduction is unsuccessful, I prefer to perform the next closed reduction in the operating room under adequate anesthesia and image intensifier control. This monitoring will allow precise visualization of the fracture fragments. If a satisfactory reduction is achieved and it is stable, the arm is immobilized in a sling and swathe. However, if the reduction is unstable, percutaneous pinning should be performed. The patient should be prepared and draped, and IV antibiotics should be given. The arm is then reduced and held in a stable position. Two pins are directed proximally starting above the deltoid insertion through the shaft fragment and into the head and tuberosity fragment (Fig. 9–30). These pins should be 2.5-mm terminally threaded AO pins. It is important to use a power drill as it may be very difficult to pierce the cortex of the proximal humerus. Each pin should be individually checked with the image intensifier in two perpendicular planes. A third pin is started proximally from above into the greater tuberosity and then into the distal shaft. An additional fourth pin from distal to proximal through the anterior shaft into the head will achieve extra stability if required. Care must be taken not to enter the articular surface of the head. Following this, the arm is rotated and stability is

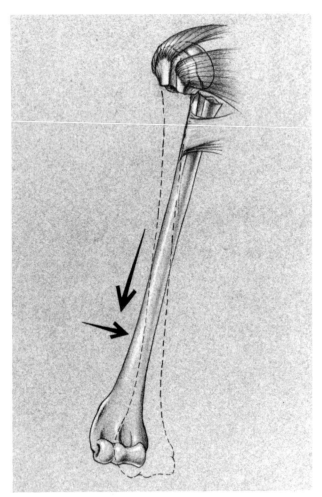

Figure 9–29. To achieve a closed reduction of a surgical neck fracture, general traction should be placed on the arm as it is brought out to the side and gently flexed. Traction should be maintained and flexion is increased as the arm is gradually adducted to gain reduction of the shaft beneath the head. Adduction will neutralize the pull of the pectoralis major and other internal rotators, which is creating the deformity. Counterpressure by the assistant may be needed beneath the armpit, or digital pressure on the proximal fragment may be necessary to achieve stabilization. The shaft should be impacted beneath the head for a stable reduction.

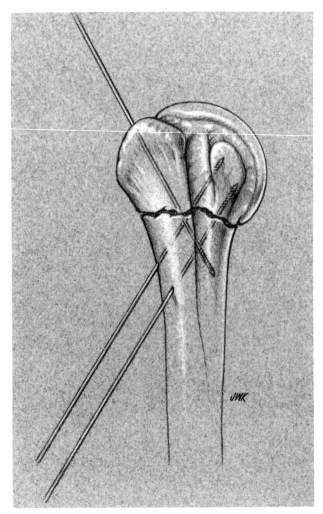

Figure 9–30. Technique of percutaneous pinning of surgical neck fractures. The arm is reduced and held in a stable position. Two pins are then directed proximally, starting above the deltoid insertion, through the proximal fragment and into the head and tuberosity fragment. These pins should be 2.5-mm terminally threaded AO pins. It is important to use a power drill as it may be difficult to pierce the cortex. The third pin is started proximally from above into the greater tuberosity and then into the shaft.

assessed. The pins are cut short beneath the skin and not removed until there is radiographic evidence of fracture stability, usually between four and six weeks.

If closed reduction is not possible and the percutaneous pinning is unsuccessful, open reduction and internal fixation is required. There may be soft tissue interposition. The long head of the biceps can act as a tether between the fracture fragments and actually prevent reduction by causing distraction (see Fig. 9–13B).

The surgical exposure is a long deltopectoral approach in which the origin and insertion of the deltoid are preserved. It provides adequate exposure without injuring the deltoid muscle or axillary nerve. Care should be taken to avoid extensive dissection of soft tissue from the fracture fragments. I prefer to treat these fractures with a figure-of-eight wire (18 gauge)

technique or No. 5 nonabsorbable nylon suture. Wire provides greater stability but may be an irritant in the subacromial space. It may also break or migrate. Therefore, if possible, nonabsorbable sutures are preferable. The suture or wires should be passed through and under the rotator cuff as well as through the tuberosity. In many instances, the cuff may be better quality tissue than the bone in the proximal humerus. A large 14- or 16-gauge spinal needle or plastic angiocath is helpful in passing suture or wire through the cuff. A drill hole is made in the shaft of the humerus approximately 1 inch below the fracture site, and the wire or nonabsorbable sutures can be passed through the hole and then looped back in a figure-of-eight manner. Two separate sutures or wires are used, one through the greater tuberosity and the other through the lesser tuberosity. Then both sutures or wires are placed through the same drill hole in the proximal

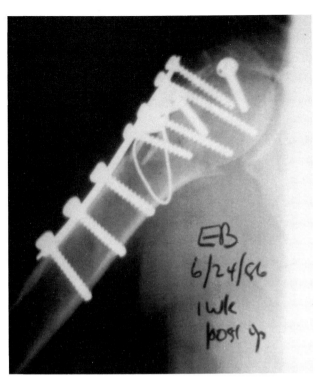

Figure 9–31. An anteroposterior radiograph of an open reduction internal fixation with a plate and screws of a comminuted fracture of the proximal humerus. Excellent fixation was achieved; the patient had excellent union and achieved a good functional result. (Courtesy of Dr. Howard Rosen.)

humerus. Excellent stability can be achieved, allowing for early range of motion exercises. If the longitudinal stability is not sufficient, secondary to comminution or poor bone quality, intramedullary fixation is necessary to supplement the wire or suture (see Figs. 9–13 and 9–19). The intramedullary fixation should be removed at six weeks to avoid subacromial impingement.

Impacted surgical neck fractures angulated greater than 45 degrees should be reduced. The deformity is usually in the anterior plane, and malunion will limit forward elevation. Multiple rotational radiographic views, as well as comparison radiographs of the normal shoulder, are important to fully judge the amount of angulation. The reduction maneuver includes abduction and flexion to the pivotal position. This usually distracts the fracture fragments and frees the shaft from under the head, allowing correction of the deformity. A hyperabduction maneuver is not indicated in this fracture, as it is not the deformity. The head may be reimpacted so that stability can be achieved and early motion started. The arm is immobilized at the side in a sling and swathe.

Initially, comminuted proximal humeral fractures without significant displacement should be treated with a sling and swathe and a plaster splint applied along the shaft of the humerus and onto the top of the shoulder. Occasionally, a shoulder spica cast is helpful. Traction is difficult to maintain and tolerate and is a problem in patients with multiple injuries. If closed reduction is not successful, open reduction and internal fixation, with a plate and screws and multiple sutures or wire, if necessary, is indicated (Fig. 9–31). Although

this fixation may not always be rigid enough to allow early motion, it will be adequate to maintain alignment until there is early healing and motion can be started. Addition of a shoulder spica cast can be helpful to enchance fixation.

TWO-PART GREATER TUBEROSITY FRACTURES

Two-part greater tuberosity fractures displaced greater than one centimeter require open reduction and internal fixation. It is very difficult to achieve a closed reduction because there is a tear in the rotator cuff and the fragment is pulled posteriorly and superiorly. If left in this position, impingement will develop, and the patient will lose motion of the shoulder (see Fig. 9–11). The surgical approach for this type of fracture is a superior approach in Langer's lines (see Fig. 9–27). The deltoid is split a short distance from the acromion for 3 to 4 cm. I prefer to stabilize the bone fragment with multiple nonabsorbable nylon sutures (Fig. 9–32). The rotator cuff must also be repaired. Repairing the rent in the cuff first offers stability and takes tension off the fracture repair. The greater tuberosity is anatomically replaced using several No. 2 Tevdek nylon sutures placed through drill

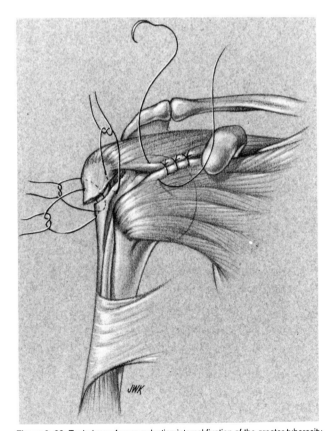

Figure 9–32. Technique of open reduction internal fixation of the greater tuberosity fracture. The ideal method of fixation for greater tuberosity fractures is the use of multiple nonabsorbable nylon sutures. The cuff must also be repaired. It is advisable to repair the cuff first as this reduces tension from the bony sutures and stabilizes the fracture fragment. Several drill holes are placed in the proximal shaft and through the greater tuberosity and then secured.

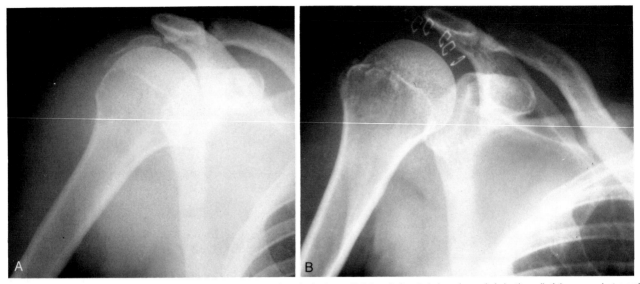

Figure 9–33. *A,* An anteroposterior radiograph of the displaced greater tuberosity fracture, which is pulled posteriorly and superiorly by the pull of the supraspinatus and the infraspinatus. *B,* Postoperative x-ray showing stabilization of the fracture with multiple nonabsorbable sutures.

holes in the tuberosity and shaft (Fig. 9–33). Bone fragments and hematoma may need to be removed from the fracture surface of the greater tuberosity to improve the reduction. Exercises are started early, on the second or third postoperative day.

TWO-PART LESSER TUBEROSITY FRACTURES

Displaced isolated fractures of the lesser tuberosity are also extremely rare. If the fragment is small and rotation is not affected, the arm can be supported in a sling and the patient is given instructions in range of motion exercises. If the fragment is large and blocks medial rotation, open reduction and internal fixation with nonabsorbable sutures is needed. The fracture fragment may also be removed and the tendon of the subscapularis repaired back to the proximal humerus.

THREE-PART FRACTURES

Most three-part fractures are quite unstable, and closed reduction is very difficult. In general, open reduction and internal fixation is the treatment of choice in active patients since a stable reduction can usually be achieved, allowing early motion. Closed reduction is an option only in debilitated patients or patients for whom surgery is contraindicated. The surgical approach to this procedure is also a deltopectoral approach.

Great care must be taken not to denude the fracture fragments of their blood supply, which may lead to avascular necrosis. In the majority of cases, I prefer to use internal fixation of the fragments with No. 5 nonabsorbable sutures or 18-gauge figure-of-eight wires. The technique is similar to that previously described for two-part surgical neck fractures (Fig. 9–34). The displaced tuberosity should be attached to the head and remaining tuberosity fragment as well as the shaft below (Fig. 9–35). Multiple sutures are necessary for stability. In selected cases, when there is significant osteoporosis and the quality of the bone is poor, therefore not allowing internal fixation, a primary humeral head prosthesis is indicated. This will allow earlier mobilization of the shoulder. The patient is usually an older female.

FOUR-PART FRACTURES

The treatment of choice for four-part fractures of the proximal humerus is a humeral head prosthesis, as other methods of treatment are associated with poor results. Occasionally, in patients under 40 years of age without a dislocation, if the head is still in continuity with the glenoid and there appears to be some soft tissue attachment, an open reduction may be attempted. Fixation of the head fragment is difficult and best achieved with multiple Kirschner wires that are removed after adequate healing. However, it must be emphasized that this type of fracture has a high incidence of avascular necrosis.

My preference is use of the Neer humeral head prosthesis. It is available in various sizes. The surgical approach is very important because the deltoid must be preserved to allow optimum postoperative shoulder function. It should not be detached from its origin as this will weaken it. A long deltopectoral approach (deltoid on) avoids detachment of the deltoid origin but still allows adequate exposure (see Fig. 9–28). If more exposure is needed, the deltoid insertion should be slightly elevated. Another important aspect is to restore proper length to the humerus with the pros-

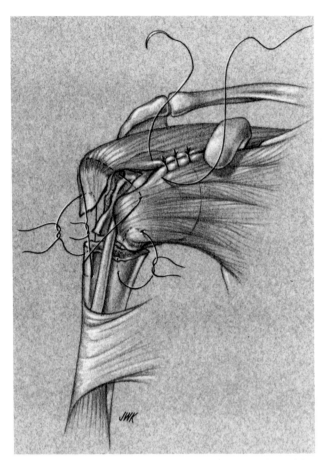

Figure 9–34. Technique of internal fixation of a three-part fracture. This technique may be done with either absorbable sutures or 18-gauge wire. It is important to secure the displaced tuberosity (in this case the greater tuberosity) to both the head and the lesser tuberosity, as well as to the shaft below. The lesser tuberosity and head fragment should also be secured to the shaft below with several sutures. Generally this gives very stable fixation, allowing for early motion.

thesis, preserving proper tension in the myofascial sleeve. The tendency is to set the prosthesis against the remaining humeral shaft, which significantly shortens the humerus, thereby creating an unstable situation leading to inferior subluxation and inability to elevate the extremity. In this situation, the deltoid is shortened and its function is significantly compromised (Fig. 9–36). The addition of cement enhances stability when there is inadequate bony support for the stem and allows for adjustment of the prosthesis to the proper length. The prosthesis has to be set at the proper degree of retroversion, which is generally between 30 to 40 degrees (Fig. 9–37). The distal humeral condyles must be palpated to aid in estimating the amount of humeral head retroversion. This is performed with the elbow flexed and the prosthesis in position so that anterior and posterior stability can be assessed. A sponge may be placed into the shaft of the humerus, which will allow sufficient support of the prosthesis so that stability can be checked. If part of the biceps groove is intact, this can be a useful landmark. The lateral fin with holes in it for the prosthesis should sit just at the posterior aspect of the bicipital groove (Fig. 9–38).

Secure fixation of the tuberosities is essential to allow early postoperative motion of the shoulder. The tuberosities should be sutured with nonabsorbable suture to each other and to the shaft of the humerus through the fin of the prosthesis (Fig. 9–39). Two or three sutures should be placed from the greater tuberosity to the shaft, and two sutures should be placed from the greater tuberosity through the holes in the fin of the prosthesis to the lesser tuberosity. It is important to close the rent in the rotator cuff. One or two sutures are also passed from the lesser tuberosity to the shaft of the humerus. If possible, preserve the long head of the biceps by retracting it anteriorly or posteriorly and then replace it into its groove in the humerus. The head of the prosthesis should be positioned above the greater tuberosity to avoid impingement of the greater tuberosity against the acromion (Fig. 9–26*E*).

If there is a humeral shaft fracture, it should be stabilized before cementing the prosthesis. This may be done with a cerclage wire and multiple nonabsorbable nylon sutures. The wound is irrigated with saline, and two closed suction irrigation tubes are placed deep in the deltoid muscle. The deltoid is closed with chromic sutures, and if the insertion has been elevated, this should be reattached. The skin is closed with a subcuticular dexon or nylon suture. Prophylactic antibiotics are given preoperatively, intraoperatively, and postoperatively for 48 hours. The operating physician may start range-of-motion exercises within 48 hours and gently rotate and elevate the arm. Passive-assistive range-of-motion exercises are started on the third postoperative day, and resistive exercises are not performed until there is healing of the tuberosities, generally by six weeks. After six weeks, the resistance in active exercising is gradually increased, and stretching exercises are continued.

FRACTURE DISLOCATIONS

Two-Part Fracture Dislocations

Two-part fracture dislocations should initially be treated by a closed reduction. The head is attached to the shaft and it is hoped that in most instances, the displaced tuberosity fragment will be reduced to an acceptable position (see Fig. 9–14). Anterior two-part fracture dislocations are immobilized at the side with a sling and swathe. Posterior fracture dislocations are immobilized in neutral or slight external rotation with the arm in a cast or brace. There is a tendency for redisplacement of the tuberosity fragment, especially with greater tuberosity fractures. Therefore, frequent follow-up x-rays are essential in the postreduction period. If the tuberosities are displaced, these should be treated the same as two-part fractures.

Usually with repair of the tuberosity, further glenohumeral dislocations do not occur. Two-part fracture dislocations involving the anatomical or surgical neck are extremely rare. If an anatomical head fragment is dislocated, I would use a humeral head prosthesis. For

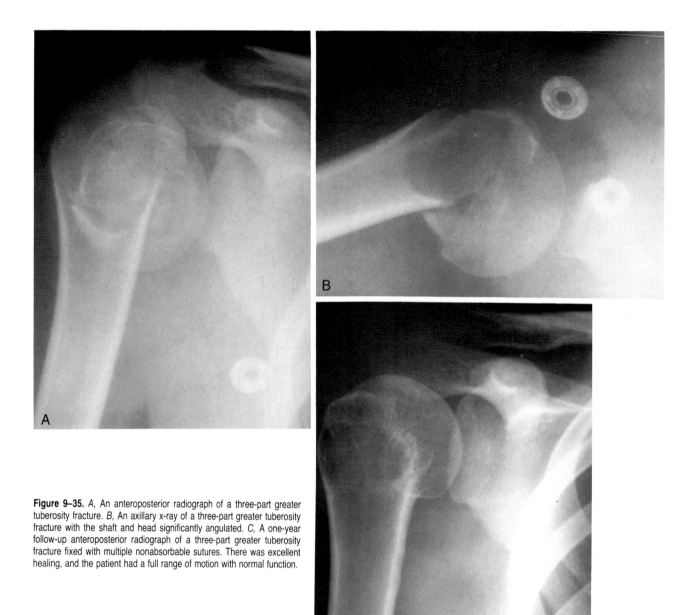

Figure 9-35. *A,* An anteroposterior radiograph of a three-part greater tuberosity fracture. *B,* An axillary x-ray of a three-part greater tuberosity fracture with the shaft and head significantly angulated. *C,* A one-year follow-up anteroposterior radiograph of a three-part greater tuberosity fracture fixed with multiple nonabsorbable sutures. There was excellent healing, and the patient had a full range of motion with normal function.

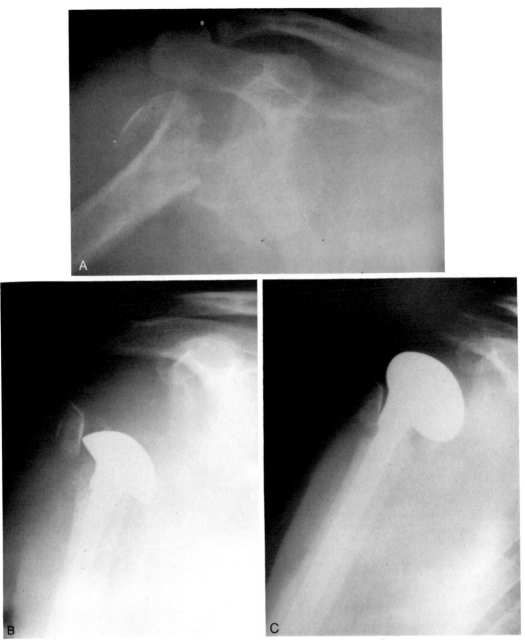

Figure 9–36. *A,* An anterior four-part fracture dislocation with the head displaced beneath the coracoid. *B,* A failed Neer I prosthesis in which the prosthesis was placed up against the proximal shaft, creating an unstable situation leading to inferior subluxation. In addition, both tuberosities became detached owing to inadequate fixation. *C,* Revision of the prosthesis in which cement was used to elevate the prosthesis approximately 4 cm. This was enough to impart stability. There was enough bone left on the greater tuberosity to place it beneath the head. This patient in addition had a partial axillary nerve palsy. However, he did achieve a pain-free shoulder with approximately 80 degrees of forward elevation and 30 degrees of external rotation.

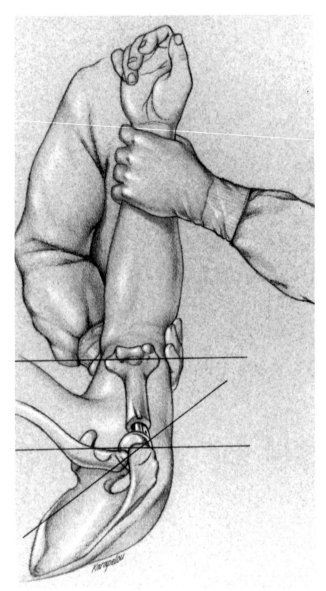

Figure 9–37. The humeral head prosthesis should be placed in 30 to 40 degrees of retroversion. This can be accomplished by palpating the distal humeral condyles with the elbow flexed and estimating the amount of humeral head retroversion. Anterior and posterior stability should be assessed with the prosthesis in the shaft. A sponge may be stuffed in the shaft of the humerus to allow sufficient support of the prosthesis. If part of the biceps groove is intact, this can be used as a landmark. The lateral fin of the prosthesis should sit at the posterior aspect of the bicipital groove.

fracture dislocation involving the surgical neck, I prefer open reduction and internal fixation.

Three-Part Fracture Dislocations

I prefer open reduction and internal fixation of these fractures. I might attempt one closed reduction. In anterior fracture dislocation, it must be remembered that the head is very close to the brachial plexus and axillary artery. Therefore, great care must be taken in an open reduction of an anterior three-part fracture

dislocation to gently reduce the head to avoid injury to the neurovascular structures. The glenoid surface should also be inspected for impression fractures. Open reduction and internal fixation using sutures is performed with the same technique as that described for the three-part fractures.

Four-Part Fracture Dislocations

Four-part fracture dislocations are treated with a humeral prosthesis. The head is devoid of any soft tissue attachment with fracture dislocations and usually is a free-floating fragment. Once again great caution should be exercised when trying to remove the head in an anterior fracture dislocation (Fig. 9–40), especially if surgery has been delayed for several weeks, since adhesions are usually present. With a posterior fracture dislocation, there may be excessive posterior instability, and less retroversion may be required for the prosthesis. If the prosthesis is unstable posteriorly, retroversion may be decreased by 10 to 15 degrees, and this will usually create stability.

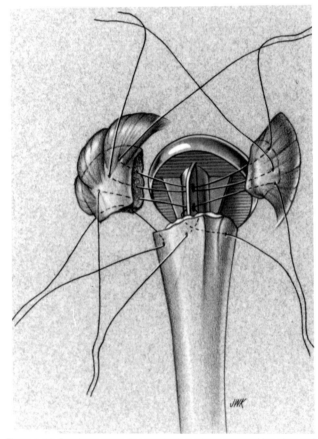

Figure 9–38. Prosthesis repair. The prosthesis has been cemented into place and is elevated off the shaft. Both tuberosities should be able to fit below the head. The tuberosities should not be repaired superior to the head. Drill holes should be placed through both tuberosities, and the shaft and the tuberosities should be attached to each other through the fin of the prosthesis as well as to the shaft below.

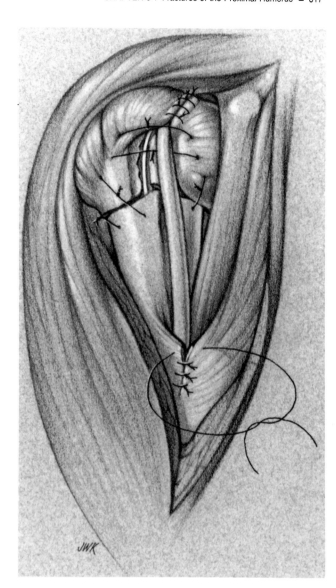

Figure 9–39. The completed repair of the tuberosities with the rotator cuff interval closed and the biceps preserved. In general, nonabsorbable sutures provide a firm repair that allows for early motion.

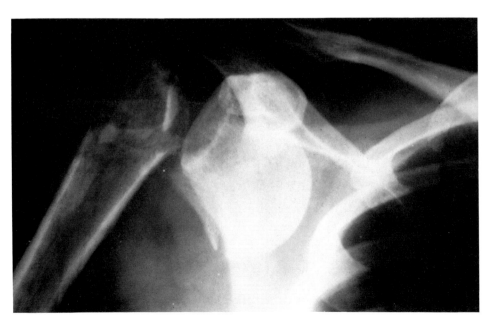

Figure 9–40. An anteroposterior radiograph of a four-part fracture dislocation. The head is displaced below the coracoid and is adjacent to the neurovascular bundle.

IMPRESSION AND HEAD SPLITTING FRACTURES

Treatment of impression fractures of the articular surface differs with the size of the defect and the time of the diagnosis. If there is less than 20 per cent head involvement and the treatment is within two to three weeks after injury, closed reduction may be adequate. The arm should be immobilized in external rotation after reduction if the dislocation is posterior. For defects involving 20 to 45 per cent of the anterior head associated with a posterior dislocation, I prefer to use a modification of the McLaughlin procedure as reported by Neer.[188] Using an anterior approach, the lesser tuberosity, as with the tendon of the subscapularis, is transferred into the defect in the head and fixed with a screw. For head defects greater than 45 per cent, I prefer to use a prosthesis. If the glenoid is fractured, eroded, or worn, it may also require replacement. Generally, impression fractures occur with posterior fracture dislocations.

Head splitting fractures also require a prosthesis. These are usually associated with fractures of either tuberosities or the surgical neck (Fig. 9–41). In a younger patient, if there is adequate bone stock, open reduction and internal fixation may be attempted, but in my experience, this is usually a very difficult procedure and is associated with a high incidence of failure.

REHABILITATION

Rehabilitation of proximal humeral fractures is essential because adequate motion is needed for optimum function. If a fracture or fracture repair is stable, therapy should be started early. The most useful rehabilitation protocol is the three-phase system that has been devised by Neer[122] (Fig. 9–42). The first phase consists of passive-assistive exercises. In the second phase, active and early resistive exercises, as well as stretching exercises, are started. The third phase is a maintenance program aimed at advanced stretching and strengthening exercises.

Application of this system is variable and depends on the type of fracture, the stability of the fracture or fracture repair, and the ability of the patient to comprehend the exercise program. The exercises are performed three to four times per day for 20 to 30 minutes. A hot pack applied 20 minutes before the exercise session begins is beneficial. Early in the program, an analgesic may be needed to control pain, allowing sufficient stretching. In many instances, it is advisable to involve a physical therapist for guidance and management of the exercise program.

Phase I exercises are started early in the postfracture or postoperative period. If a fracture is minimally displaced or has been treated by closed reduction and is stable, exercises are generally started between the seventh and tenth day following fracture. The first exercise is usually a pendulum exercise (Codman) in which the arm is rotated both outwardly and inwardly in small circles (Fig. 9–42A, B). The second exercise is supine external rotation with a stick (Fig. 9–42C). It is important to support the elbow and the distal humerus with either a folded towel or sheet as this will create a sense of security for the patient. A slight amount of abduction, approximately 15 to 20 degrees, may also aid in performing this exercise.

Three weeks after fracture, assisted forward elevation (Fig. 9–42D) as well as pulley exercises (Fig. 9–42E) may be added. Extension can also be added a little later. Isometric exercises are generally started at four weeks (Fig. 9–42F, G). Following a secure surgical repair, the exercises may be started by the physician within 24 to 48 hours. The physician should start with elbow flexion and extension and then gently assist the patient with pendulum exercises. Supine external rotation and assisted forward elevation, either supine or sitting, are also performed. Between three and five days postoperatively, formal exercises with the therapist are started. These consist of pendulum, pulley supine, external rotation with a stick, supine forward flexion, and extension with a stick. Isometrics may be started after three weeks.

Phase II exercises involve early active, resistive, and stretching exercises. The first exercise is supine active forward elevation as gravity is partially eliminated, making elevation easier (Fig. 9–42H, I, J). The forward elevation can then progress to the erect position, with a stick in the unaffected arm assisting the involved arm in forward elevation (Fig. 9–42K, L, M). As the arm gains strength, active erect elevation can be performed unassisted, but it is important to keep the elbow bent and the arm close to the midline. Strips of rubber sheeting of various strengths (Therabands) are used to strengthen the internal rotators, the external rotators, and the anterior, middle, and posterior deltoids (Fig. 9–42N, O). Three sets of 10 to 15 repetitions are recommended at each exercise session. Stretching for forward elevation on the top of the door or wall is started (Fig. 9–42T), as well as stretching in the door jam for external rotation. Also, the arm is raised over the head with hands clasped, and then the hands are placed behind the head and the arms are externally rotated and abducted (Fig. 9–42P, Q, R). This exercise is extremely important to achieve abduction and external rotation. Wall climbing is generally not performed as this does not promote stretching. Internal rotation is helped by using the normal arm to pull the involved arm into internal rotation (Fig. 9–42S).

Phase III exercises are generally started at three months. Rubber tubing is substituted for the rubber strips to increase resistance. The arm is stretched higher on the wall by leaning the torso into the wall. Also, stretching on the end of the door and prone stretching for forward elevation are extremely useful. A hot shower prior to stretching will promote relaxation. Light weights could be used after three months and should be started at 1 pound and increased at 1-pound increments, with the limit being 5 pounds. If

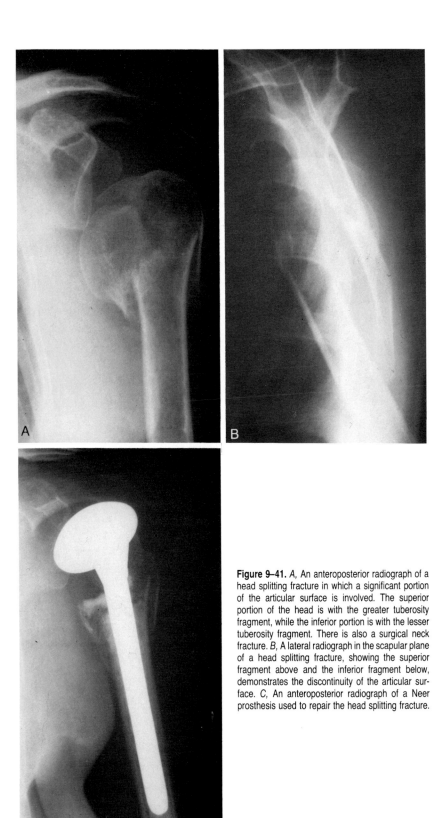

Figure 9–41. *A,* An anteroposterior radiograph of a head splitting fracture in which a significant portion of the articular surface is involved. The superior portion of the head is with the greater tuberosity fragment, while the inferior portion is with the lesser tuberosity fragment. There is also a surgical neck fracture. *B,* A lateral radiograph in the scapular plane of a head splitting fracture, showing the superior fragment above and the inferior fragment below, demonstrates the discontinuity of the articular surface. *C,* An anteroposterior radiograph of a Neer prosthesis used to repair the head splitting fracture.

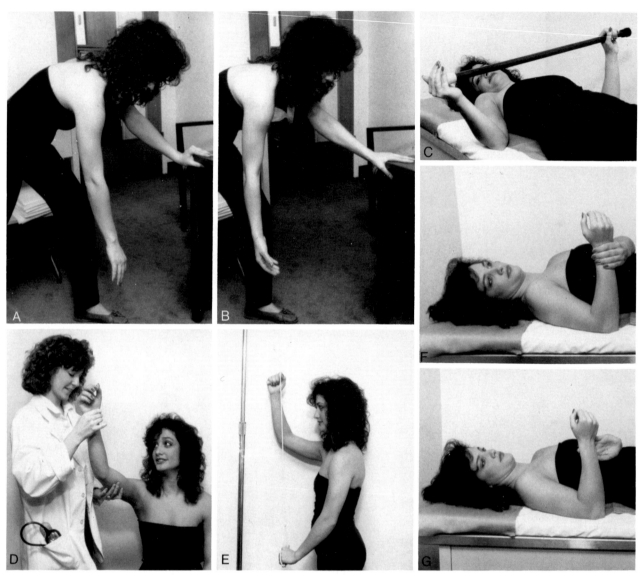

Figure 9–42. Exercises should be done at least three to four times a day. It is best to warm up first with a hot shower, heating pad, or hot water bottle. The exercise regimen should take between 15 and 20 minutes. *A, B,* Pendulum exercises are performed standing and bent over at the waist. Large circles are made with the entire arm with the palm forward and backward. *C,* External rotation with a stick should be performed supine with the elbow abducted slightly from the side. The noninvolved arm pushes the involved arm out, supplying the power. *D,* Assisted forward elevation is done by the therapist, either erect or supine. *E,* Pulley exercises are performed with the uninvolved arm supplying the power for elevation of the involved arm. *F, G,* Isometric exercises to strengthen both the external and internal rotators are started with the patient supine.

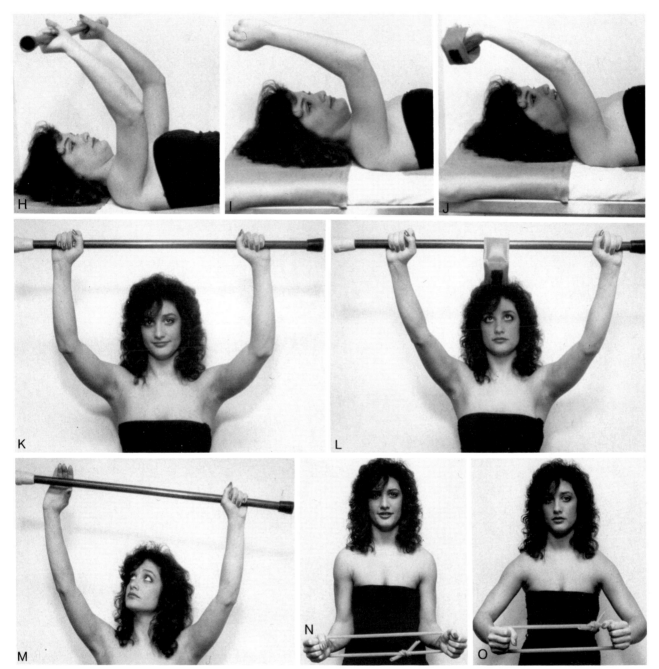

Figure 9–42 *Continued. H, I, J,* Active forward elevation with a stick is started supine with the elbow bent. As strength permits, it may be done with the arm unassisted. Later, a 1- or 2-pound weight may be added for strengthening. *K, L, M,* Erect forward elevation may also be performed with a stick, using the uninvolved arm to assist the involved arm. As the patient gets stronger, an attempt should be made to release the stick from the involved hand and to lower the arm on its own. Weights may be added for strengthening. *N,* Strips of rubber sheeting of various strengths or rubber tubing can be used to strengthen the external rotators by placing the tubing around the wrist, keeping the elbows at the side and externally rotating. *O,* This can also be used to strengthen the deltoid by abducting the shoulders. In addition, by attaching the rubber tubing to a doorknob, the anterior and posterior deltoids may also be strengthened.

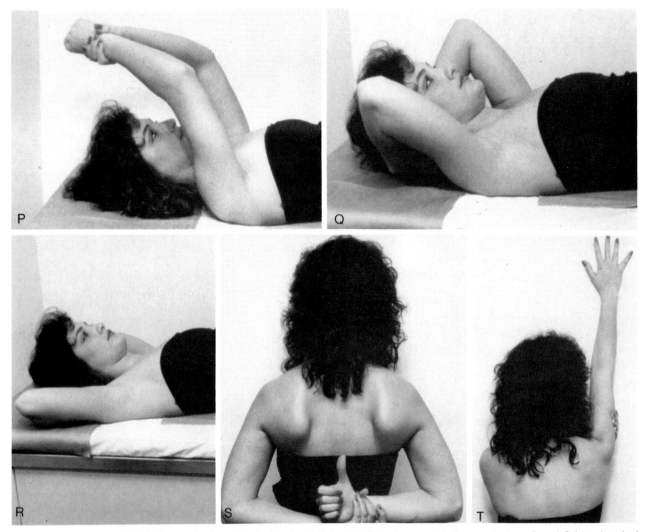

Figure 9–42 *Continued. P, Q, R,* As healing permits, the arm is raised overhead with the help of the other arm; abduction may also be performed. *S,* Internal rotation is done with the aid of the uninvolved arm or a towel over the shoulder. *T,* Stretching for a forward elevation may be done against the wall or the end of a door. It is important to try to lean the weight of the body into the wall so as to stretch the shoulder in forward elevation.

there is persistent pain after exercises with weights, weights should be decreased or eliminated. Strength can be achieved with functional activity. A well-supervised rehabilitation regimen is essential for successful fracture treatment. Even the most perfect fracture reduction or surgical repair will not achieve a good result without proper exercises.

COMPLICATIONS

Displaced fractures of the proximal humerus are difficult to manage, and many complications have been reported following both closed and open treatment. The more common complications include avascular necrosis, nonunion, malunion, hardware failure, frozen shoulder, infection, and neurovascular injury.

Avascular Necrosis

Avascular necrosis is not uncommon following both three- and four-part fractures and has also been reported following some two-part fractures.* The result is usually a stiff, painful joint. However, some reports have described adequate function if there is reasonable congruity of the glenohumeral joint.[146, 182] Besides the severity of the fracture, extensive exposure of soft tissue has been identified as a major contributing factor. Sturzenegger[254] reported a 34 per cent incidence of avascular necrosis in a series of 17 patients treated with an AO buttress T plate. The extensive soft tissue exposure needed for plate fixation was thought to be a factor in this series (Fig. 9–43). The treatment of choice for avascular necrosis is a humeral head prosthesis or total shoulder replacement if the glenoid is involved.

Nonunion

Nonunions of the proximal humerus are not that common.[54, 144, 191, 236, 249] Unfortunately, treatment may be difficult because they often occur in older, debilitated patients with soft, osteoporotic bone. Also, loss of bone stock may occur. The literature concerning this subject is scarce. In 1964, Sorensen[249] reported on only seven cases, five found in the literature and two of his own. Neer[190, 191] reported 16 cases of nonunions in his paper concerning displaced proximal humeral fractures in 1970. Eight of the nonunions were secondary to a hanging cast or excessive overhead traction. Other causes following closed treatment include severe displacement; comminution; soft tissue interposition such as capsule, deltoid muscle, or the long head of biceps; systemic disease; a pre-existing stiff glenohumeral joint; an uncooperative patient; and overly aggressive physiotherapy. Nonunion may also occur after open treatment secondary to poor bone quality, inadequate fixation, or infection (Fig. 9–44).

Neer[188] has described a pathological condition in

nonunion of surgical neck fractures in which there is significant resorption of bone beneath the head and a characteristic cavitation of the head fragment which is produced by the upper end of the shaft (Fig. 9–45). In this situation, there is constant motion because of the unopposed pull of the pectoralis major muscle. A pseudarthrosis with a synovial lining occurs because of the communication with the joint and the flow of joint fluid into this area. Internal fixation with heavy metal, such as screw and plate fixation, is impossible in this situation because of the poor quality of the remaining humeral head.

The indications for surgical treatment are pain, loss of function, and deformity. Pain may not be that severe if the arm is not being used. Open reduction and internal fixation with the addition of an autogenous iliac crest bone graft is the preferred treatment. However, a humeral head prosthesis may be necessary if there is articular damage or inadequate bone in the humeral head. Humeral head excision and arthrodesis should be avoided and are strictly salvage procedures. Conservative treatment may be an option in older patients who are pain free, especially if the nondominant extremity is involved.

The choice of hardware should be either Enders rods and figure-of-eight wire or suture or a plate and screws. Rods and wire are preferred in surgical neck nonunions and when the bone is soft. A plate is more suited for proximal shaft nonunions with good bone stock so that the screws can hold the cortex. In most cases, a spica cast is necessary for six to eight weeks because of poor bone quality. Electrical stimulation may be a helpful adjunct to promoting healing. After the cast is removed, range-of-motion exercises are started and progressed if healing is sufficient. A second procedure may be needed to release adhesions and remove hardware, especially a prominent rod.

Malunion

Malunion occurs following inadequate closed reduction or a failed open reduction and internal fixation. This problem is especially difficult to treat because there is excessive scar tissue with retraction of the tuberosities or displacement of the shaft. In addition, neurological and soft tissue deficits may compromise surgical repair. Greater tuberosity malunions will lead to impingement against the acromion[259] (see Fig. 9–11). They are best managed through a superior approach in which the fragment is completely mobilized and all of the scar tissue is lysed. It is important also to mobilize the rotator cuff and bring this tissue out to length. These are generally treated the same as acute greater tuberosity fractures. If there is excessive scarring and there seems to be residual impingement, an anterior acromioplasty and removal of coracoacromial ligament may be helpful.

Malunions of three-part fractures are more difficult since there are more components involved. If avascular necrosis or post-traumatic degenerative arthritis are not present, an attempt at osteotomy of the displaced

*See references 77, 85, 98, 133, 138, 146, 182, 205, 254, 255.

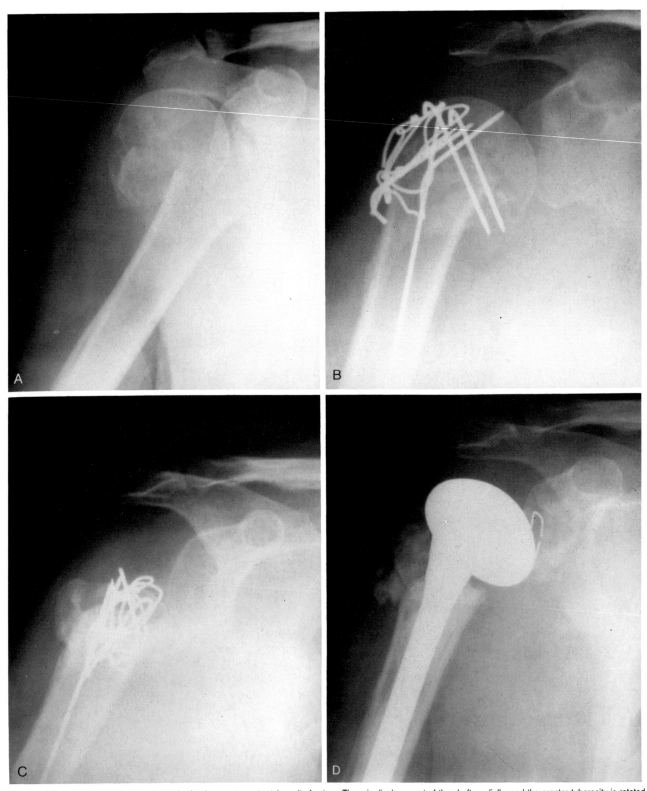

Figure 9–43. *A,* An anteroposterior radiograph of a three-part greater tuberosity fracture. There is displacement of the shaft medially, and the greater tuberosity is rotated and separated from the head. *B,* Open reduction internal fixation was achieved with numerous pins and wires. Extensive soft tissue dissection was needed for this repair. *C,* Eight months postoperatively the head has disappeared, as there is significant avascular necrosis. *D,* This failed fracture repair was salvaged with a total shoulder replacement, since the glenoid was also involved with degenerative disease.

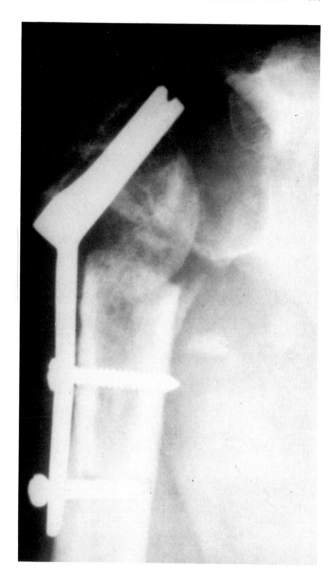

Figure 9–44. This patient had an open reduction internal fixation of a four-part fracture with a baby Jewett nail. This hip device was not appropriate for the shoulder, and the patient went on to have a nonunion as well as an infection after this procedure.

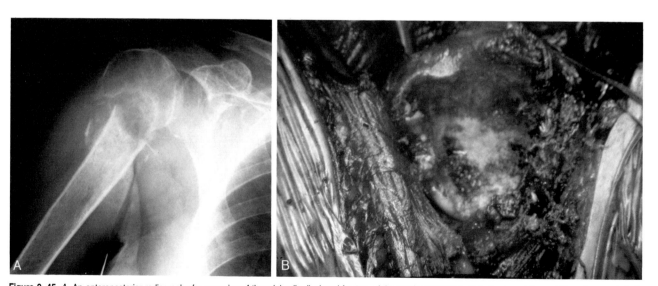

Figure 9–45. *A,* An anteroposterior radiograph of a nonunion of the minimally displaced fracture of the proximal humerus. Note the lucent line and the osteoporosis in the subtuberous region. *B,* An operative photograph showing the cavitation beneath the head with significant loss of bone stock.

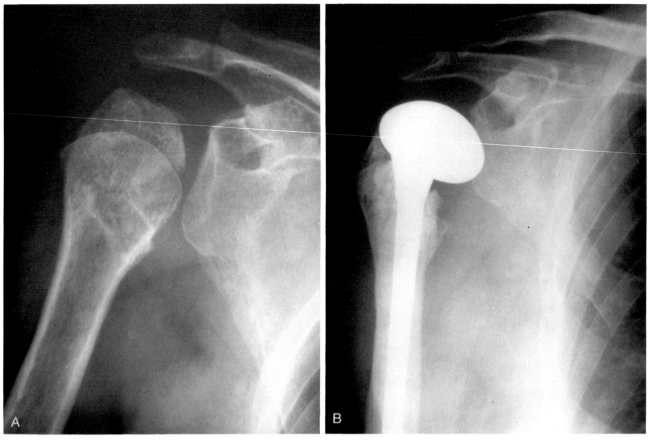

Figure 9–46. *A,* An anteroposterior radiograph of a malunion of a four-part fracture in which the greater tuberosity has healed above the head. The patient's surgery was delayed for eight months because of neurological complications. *B,* A prosthesis was eventually inserted; the repair was quite difficult because of the malunion and scarring of the soft tissues. The patient eventually achieved 130 degrees of forward elevation with 30 degrees of external rotation. There was some discomfort and weather ache, but the patient did have a functional shoulder.

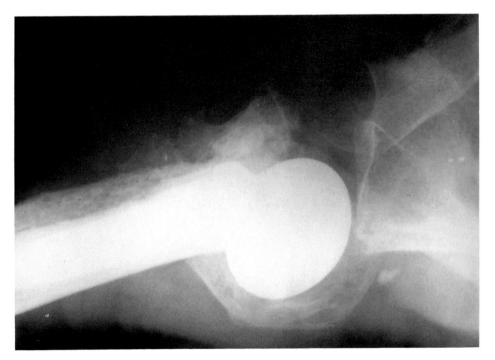

Figure 9–47. This patient had a posterior fracture dislocation that was treated with a Neer prosthesis, which also dislocated posteriorly. There was extensive myositis ossificans in the soft tissues.

fracture components and internal fixation should be attempted. A prosthesis is generally indicated for avascular necrosis and joint incongruity. A glenoid component may be required if there is arthritis of the glenoid surface. Dissection is quite difficult, and it is important to always be aware of the position of the axillary, suprascapular, and musculocutaneous nerves. A malunion of a surgical neck fracture with increased anterior angulation will limit forward elevation. Surgical treatment involves osteotomy to correct the anterior angulation and the rotational deformities.[248]

Malunion and avascular necrosis of a four-part fracture require a prosthesis. The head is usually quite distorted, and often there is significant displacement of the tuberosities (Fig. 9–46A, B). A tuberosity osteotomy must often be performed to allow adequate

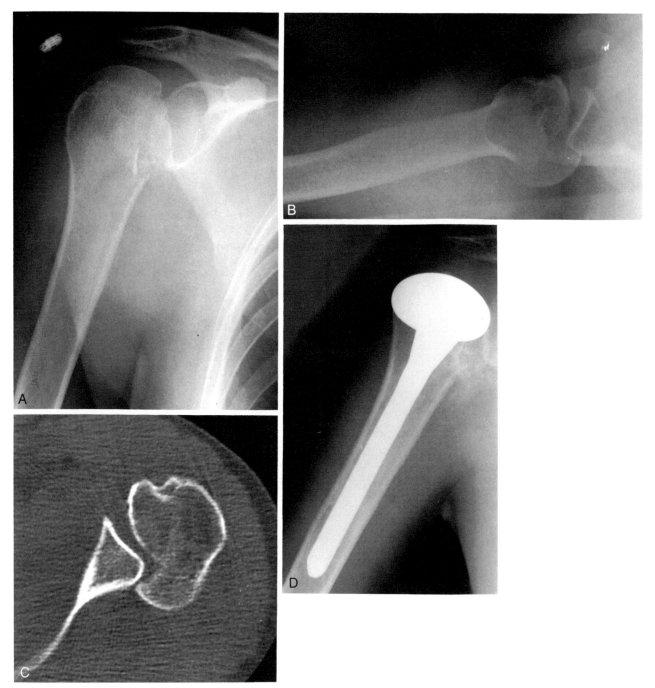

Figure 9–48. *A,* An anteroposterior radiograph shows a posterior fracture dislocation with involvement of the lesser tuberosity as well as a component of the articular surface. *B,* An axillary x-ray shows significant involvement of the humeral head with a fracture of the lesser tuberosity. *C,* A CT scan of the head shows a greater than 50 per cent involvement of the articular surface of the head. *D,* A humeral head prosthesis was put in excessive retroversion and dislocated posteriorly. The patient experienced significant pain for approximately eight months following surgery and had a fixed internal rotation contraction of approximately 30 degrees.

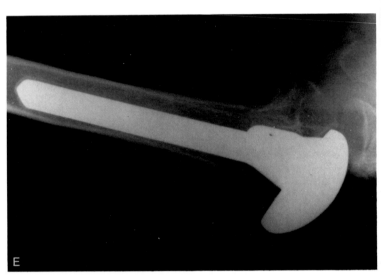
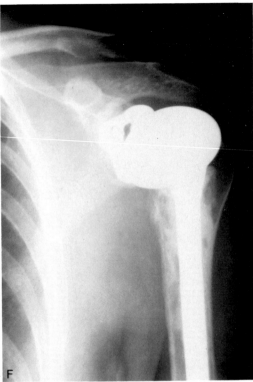

Figure 9–48 *Continued. E,* An axillary radiograph shows the prosthesis dislocated posteriorly. *F,* An anteroposterior radiograph shows a total shoulder replacement, which was used to revise the failed humeral head prosthesis. The glenoid was also significantly degenerated. The humeral head was placed in less retroversion (approximately 20 degrees); this achieved satisfactory stability. In the postoperative period the patient was held in a neutral position for approximately two weeks, and forward elevation was done in the neutral position.

placement of the humeral head prosthesis. Unless the head is centered and proper length of the humerus is maintained, function will be impaired. The results of these procedures are not as good as a primary prosthesis, since the scarring and retraction of the tuberosities and soft tissues often limit the range of motion and restrict overhead function. However, the pain relief is usually satisfactory.

Malunion of a fracture dislocation is extremely difficult to treat because the head component may be totally out of the glenohumeral joint area and wedged up against the anterior or posterior aspect of the glenoid. Mobilizing the head from the anterior subcoracoid area is especially dangerous as the neurovascular bundle may be attached to the scar tissue surrounding the head. A very careful dissection should be performed. Furthermore, there is an increased incidence of myositis ossificans with fracture dislocations (Fig. 9–47).

Revision of Failed Prosthesis

Revision of a failed prosthesis is especially difficult. There may be associated soft tissue deficits and bone loss as well as nerve paralysis, which may complicate revision surgery. An electromyogram is helpful in the evaluation before any reconstruction. The purpose of a revision of a prosthesis should be pain relief, since

it may be difficult to significantly improve function because of nerve and muscle damage (Fig. 9–48).

Adhesive Capsulitis

Adhesive capsulitis may result if there is inadequate rehabilitation following a fracture or operative repair. It is essential to have a well-organized and monitored physiotherapy program. In general, the first step with a stiff shoulder is to start the patient on a progressive exercise program. In cases of minimally displaced fracture where there is adequate anatomical congruity, the next step may be a manipulation under anesthesia and arthroscopic debridement of both the joint and subacromial space. The arthroscopic examination creates a brisement and distention of the joint space as well as the subacromial space. Scar tissue and adhesions may also be resected using the arthroscope. If there is painful hardware or impingement of hardware and the patient does have a union, an open release and removal of hardware may be required.

References

1. Ahlgren O, and Appel H: Proximal humeral fractures. Acta Orthop Scand *44:*124–125, 1973.
2. Aitken AP: End results of fractures of the proximal humeral epiphysis. J Bone Joint Surg *18:*1036–1041, 1936.

3. Albee FH: Juxta-epiphyseal fracture of the upper end of the humerus. Med Rec *81:*847, 1912.
4. Albee FH: Restoration of shoulder function in cases of loss of head and upper portion of the humerus. Surgery *32:*1–19, 1921.
5. Alberts KA, and Engstrom CF: Fractures of the proximal humerus. Opuscula Medica *24*(4), 1979.
6. Aldredge RH, and Knight MP: Fractures of the upper end of the humerus treated by early relaxed motion and massage. New Orleans Med Surg J *92:*519–524, 1940.
7. Andreasen AT: Avulsion fracture of the lesser tuberosity of the humerus. Lancet *1:*750, 1941.
8. de Anquin CL, and de Anquin A: Prosthetic replacement in the treatment of serious fractures of the proximal humerus. *In* Bayley I, and Kessel L (eds): Shoulder Surgery. New York: Springer-Verlag, 1965.
9. Ansorge D: Fracture dislocation as a result of a high voltage current accident. Zentralbl Chir *107:*465, 1980.
10. Arndt JH, and Sears AD: Posterior dislocation of the shoulder. Am J Roentgenol *94:*639–645, 1965.
11. Aufranc OE, Jones WN, and Turner RH: Bilateral shoulder fracture-dislocations. JAMA *195:*1140–1143, 1966.
12. Aufranc OE: Nonunion of humerus. JAMA *175:*1092–1095, 1961.
13. Austin MD: Fractures hazards, reporting 3 uncommon fracture cases, with use of original crucifixion splint in fracture of surgical neck of humerus. J Indiana Med Assoc *16:*129, 1923.
14. Autin A: Traitement des fractures de l'ESH. These Medecine no 840. Paris, 1960.
15. Baker DM, and Leach RE: Fracture-dislocation of the shoulder. Report of three unusual cases with rotator cuff avulsion. J Trauma *5:*659–664, 1965.
16. Bandi W: Zur operativen Therapie der Humeruskopf-und-halsfrakturen. Unfallheilkunde *196:*38–45, 1976.
17. Bandmann F: Beitrag für Behandlung der Oberarmkopffrakturen. Zentralbl Chir, *76:*97, 1951.
18. Bardenheuer FH, cited by Hans Lorenz, Deut Zeit Chir *58:*593, 1900–1901, 1949.
19. Barrett WP, Franklin JL, Jackins SE, Wyss CR, et al.: Total shoulder arthroplasty. J Bone Joint Surg *69A:*865–872, 1987.
20. Baudin P: Intramedullary nailing of fractures of the proximal humerus. These Medecine Bordeaux, 1977.
21. Baxter MP, and Wiley JJ: Fractures of the proximal humeral epiphysis. Their influence on humeral growth. J Bone Joint Surg *68B:*570–573, 1986.
22. Bechtol CO: See Hitchcock reference (117).
23. Bell HM: Posterior fracture-dislocation of the shoulder. A method of closed reduction. A case report. J Bone Joint Surg *47A:*1521–1524, 1965.
24. Bengner U: Changes in the incidence of fracture of the upper end of the humerus during a 3-year period. A study of 2125 fractures. Clin Orthop *231:*179–182, 1988.
25. Bertoft ES, Lundh I, and Ringqvist I: Physiotherapy after fracture of the proximal end of the humerus. Scand J Rehab Med *16:*11–16, 1984.
26. Bigelow HJ: A Memoir of Henry Jacob Bigelow. Boston: Little, Brown, 1900.
27. Blom S, and Dahlback LO: Nerve injuries in dislocations of the shoulder joint and fractures of the neck of the humerus. A clinical and electromyographical study. Acta Chir Scand *136:*461–466, 1970.
28. Bloom MH, and Obata W: Diagnosis of posterior dislocation of the shoulder with use of Velpeau axillary and angle-up roentgenographic views. J Bone Joint Surg *49A:*943–949, 1967.
29. Boehler J: Les fractures recentes de l'epaule. Acta Orthop Belg *30:*235–242, 1964.
30. Bohler L: The Treatment of Fractures, 5th ed. New York: Grune & Stratton, 1956.
31. Bohler L: The Treatment of Fractures, 4th English ed. Baltimore: Williams Wood & Co., 1935.
32. Bohler L: Die Behandlung von Verrenkungsbruchen der Schulter. Dtsch Z Chir *219:*238–245, 1929.
33. Bosworth DM: Blade plate fixation. JAMA *141:*1111, 1949.
34. Brehr AJ, and Cooke AM: Fracture patterns. Lancet *1:*531–536, 1959.
35. Brighton CT, Friedenberg ZD, Zemsky LM, and Pollis, RR: Direct-current stimulation on non-union and congenital pseud-arthrosis. J Bone Joint Surg *57A:*368–377, 1975.
36. Brostrom F: Early mobilization of fractures of the upper end of the humerus. Arch Surg *46:*614, 1943.
37. Caldwell GA: The treatment of fractures of the upper end of the humerus. Rocky Mountain Med J *40:*33, 1943.
38. Caldwell JA: Treatment of fractures in the Cincinnati General Hospital. Ann Surg *97:*174–177, 1933.
39. Caldwell JA, and Smith J: Treatment of unimpacted fractures of the surgical neck of humerus. Am J Surg *31:*141–144, 1936.
40. Callahan DJ: Anatomic considerations. Closed reduction of proximal humeral fractures. Orthop Rev *13*(3):79–85, 1984.
41. Carew-McColl M: Bilateral shoulder dislocations caused by electric shock. Br J Clin Pract *34:*251, 1980.
42. Cathcart CW: Movements of the shoulder girdle involved in those of the arm on the trunk. J Anat Physiol *18:*211–218, 1884.
43. Chalier A: Fracture de l'epaule avec luxation de la tete humerale et avec section tendineuse du long biceps. Repo Lyon Chir *29:*226, 1932.
44. Clifford PC: Fractures of the neck of the humerus. A review of the late results. Injury *12:*91–95, 1980.
45. Codman EA: The Shoulder; Rupture of the Supraspinatus Tendon and Other Lesions in or About the Subacromial Bursa. Boston: Thomas Todd, 1934.
46. Cofield RH: Comminuted fractures of the proximal humerus. Clin Orthop *230:*49–57, 1988.
47. Collin I: Brug og misbrug af massage hos ulykkesforsikrede patienter. *In* Kiaer S (ed): Ulykkesforsikringsbogen. Copenhagen: Nordisk Forlag 1931.
48. Conforty B: The results of the Boytchev procedure for treatment of recurrent dislocation of the shoulder. Int Orthop *4:*127–132, 1980.
49. Conforty B: Boytchev's procedure for recurrent dislocation of the shoulder. J Bone Joint Surg *56B:*386, 1974.
50. Cooper A: A Treatise in Dislocations and Fractures of the Joints. Philadelphia: HC Carey & L Lea, 1825.
51. Cooper A: On the dislocation of the os humeri upon the dorsum scapulae and upon fractures near the shoulder joint. Guy Hosp Rep *4:*265–284, 1839.
52. Cotton FJ: Dislocations and Joint Fractures. Philadelphia: WB Saunders, 1910.
53. Cotton FJ: Subluxation of the shoulder downward. Boston Med Surg J *185:*405–407, 1921.
54. Coventry MB, and Laurnen EL: Ununited fractures of the middle and upper humerus. Special problems in treatment. Clin Orthop *69:*192–198, 1970.
55. Dameron TB: Complications of treatment of injuries to the shoulder. *In* Epps CH (ed): Complications in Orthopaedic Surgery, 2nd ed. Philadelphia: JB Lippincott, 1986.
56. DeBernardi L: Sul trattamento della dussazione con frattura dell' estremita superiore dell' omero. Boll Mem Soc Piemontese Chir *11:*193, 1932.
57. Dehne E: Fractures at the upper end of the humerus. Surg Clin North Am *25:*28–47, 1945.
58. DePalma AF: Surgery of the Shoulder, 3rd ed. Philadelphia: JB Lippincott, 1983.
59. DePalma AF, and Cautilli RA: Fractures of the upper end of the humerus. Clin Orthop *20:*73–93, 1961.
60. Des Marchais JE, and Morais G: Treatment of complex fractures of the proximal humerus by Neer hemiarthroplasty. *In* Bateman JE, and Welsh RP (eds): Surgery of the Shoulder. Philadelphia: BC Decker, 1984.
61. Des Marchais JE, and Benazet JP: Evaluation de l'hemi-arthroplastie de Neer dans le traitement des fractures de l'humerus. Can J Surg *26:*469–471, 1983.
62. Destree C, and Safary A: Le traitement des fractures hyumerales, col et diaphyse, par l'enclouage fascicule de Hackethal. Acta Orthop Belg *45:*666, 1979.
63. Dewar FP, and Yabsley RH: Fracture-dislocation of the shoulder. Report of a case. J Bone Joint Surg *49B:*540–543, 1967.
64. Dimon JH: Posterior dislocation and posterior fracture dislo-

cation of the shoulder. A report of 25 cases. South Med J 60:661, 1967.

65. Din KM, and Meggitt BF: Bilateral four-part fractures with posterior dislocation of the shoulder. A case report. J Bone Joint Surg 65B:176–178, 1983.

66. Dingley A, and Denham R: Fracture-dislocation of the humeral head. A method of reduction. J Bone Joint Surg 55A:1299–1300, 1973.

67. Drapanas T, Hewitt RL, Weichert RF, et al.: Civilian vascular injuries. A critical appraisal of three decades of management. Ann Surg 172:351–360, 1970.

68. Drapanas T, McDonald J, and Hale HW: A rational approach to classification and treatment of fractures of the surgical neck of the humerus. Am J Surg 99:617–624, 1960.

69. Duparc J, and Largier A: Les luxations-fractures de l'extremitie superieure de l'humerus. Rev Chir Orthop 62:91–110, 1976.

70. Edelman G: Immediate therapy of complex fractures of the upper end of the humerus by means of acrylic prosthesis. Presse Med 59:1777–1778, 1951.

71. Einarsson F: Fracture of the upper end of the humerus. Acta Orthop Scand [Suppl] 3:10–209, 1958.

72. Ekstrom T, Lagergren C, and von Schreeb T: Procaine injections and early mobilisation for fractures of the neck of the humerus. Acta Chir Scand 130:18–24, 1965.

73. Elliot JA: Acute arterial occlusion. An unusual cause. Surgery 39:825–826, 1956.

74. Fairbank TJ: Fracture-subluxations of the shoulder. J Bone Joint Surg 30B:454–460, 1948.

75. Fellander M: Fracture-dislocations of the shoulder joint. Acta Chir Scand 107:138–145, 1954.

76. Flatow EL, Bigliani LU, and April EW: An anatomic study of the musculocutaneous nerve and its relationship to the coracoid process. Clin Orthop 244:166–171, 1989.

77. Fourrier P, and Martini M: Post-traumatic avascular necrosis of the humeral head. Int Orthop 1:187–190, 1977.

78. Frankau C: A manipulative method for the reduction of fractures of the surgical neck of the humerus. Lancet 2:755, 1933.

79. Freg EK: Zur operation der bruche am oberen ende des oberarmes. Zentralbl Chir 61:851, 1934.

80. Frey F: Die knöcherne Heilung von Schienbeinschaftbrüchen. Arch Orthop Unfallchir 46:482–484, 1954.

81. Funsten RV, and Kinser P: Fractures and dislocations about the shoulder. J Bone Joint Surg 18:191–198, 1936.

82. Gallagher JC, Melton LJ, Riggs BL, and Bergstrath E: Epidemiology of fractures of the proximal femur in Rochester, Minnesota. Clin Orthop 150:163–171, 1980.

83. Garceau GJ, and Cogland S: Early physical therapy in the treatment of fractures of the surgical neck of the humerus. J Indiana Med Assoc 34:293–295, 1941.

84. Garraway WM, Stauffer RN, Kurland LT, and O'Fallon WM: Limb fractures in a defined population. I. Frequency and distribution. Mayo Clin Proc 54:701, 1979.

85. Geneste R, et al.: Closed treatment of fracture-dislocations of the shoulder joint. Rev Chir Orthop 66:383–386, 1980.

86. Gerard-Marchant P: Diagnostic et traitement des luxations de l'epaule compliquees de fracture de l'humerus. J Chir 31:659, 1928.

87. Glessner JR: Intrathoracic dislocation of the humeral head. J Bone Joint Surg 43A:428–430, 1961.

88. Gold AM: Fractured neck of the humerus with separation and dislocation of the humeral head. Bull Hosp Jt Dis 32:87–99, 1971.

89. Graham J, and Wood S: Aseptic necrosis of bone following trauma. In Davidson JK (ed): Aseptic Necrosis of Bone. Amsterdam: Excerpta Medica, 1976, pp 113–117, 136–137.

90. Greeley PW, and Magnuson PB: Dislocation of the shoulder accompanied by fracture of the greater tuberosity and complicated by spinatus tendon injury. JAMA 102:1835–1838, 1934.

91. Greenhill BJ: Persistent posterior shoulder dislocation. Its diagnosis and its treatment by posterior Putti-Platt repair. J Bone Joint Surg 54B:763, 1972.

92. Grimes DW: The use of Rush pin fixation in unstable upper humeral fracture. A method of blind insertion. Orthop Rev 9(4):75–79, 1980.

93. Griswold RA, Hucherson DC, and Strode EC: Fractures of the humerus treated with hanging cast. South Med J 34:777–778, 1941.

94. Gurd FB: A simple effective method for the treatment of fractures of the upper part of the humerus. Am J Surg 47:433–453, 1940.

95. Haas K: Displaced proximal humeral fractures operated by Rush pin technique. Opuscula Medica 23(4), 1978.

96. Haas SL: Fracture of the lesser tuberosity of the humerus. Am J Surg 63:252, 1944.

97. Hackethal KH: Die Bundelnagelung. Berlin: Springer-Verlag, 1961.

98. Hagg O, and Lundberg B: Aspects of prognostic factors in comminuted and dislocated proximal humeral fractures. In Bateman JE, and Welsh RP (eds): Surgery of the Shoulder. Philadelphia: BC Decker, 1984.

99. Hall MC, and Rosser M: The structure of the upper end of the humerus, with reference to osteoporotic changes in senescence leading to fractures. Can Med Assoc J 88:290–294, 1963.

100. Hall RH, Isaac F, and Booth CR: Dislocations of the shoulder with special reference to accompanying small fractures. J Bone Joint Surg 41A:489–494, 1959.

101. Hardcastle PH, and Fisher TR: Intrathoracic displacement of the humeral head with fracture of the surgical neck. Injury 12:313–315, 1981.

102. Hartigan JW: Separation of the lesser tuberosity of the head of the humerus. NY Med J 61:276, 1895.

103. Hawkins RJ, Neer CS, Pianta RM, and Mendoza FX: Locked posterior dislocation of the shoulder. J Bone Joint Surg 69A:9–18, 1987.

104. Hawkins RJ, Bell RH, and Gurr K: The three-part fracture of the proximal part of the humerus. Operative treatment. J Bone Joint Surg 68A:1410–1414, 1986.

105. Hawkins RJ: Unrecognized dislocations of the shoulder. Instr Course Lect 34:258–263, 1985.

106. Hayes MJ, and Van Winkle N: Axillary artery injury with minimally displaced fracture of the neck of the humerus. J Trauma 23:431–433, 1983.

107. Hendenach JCR: Recurrent posterior dislocation of the shoulder. J Bone Joint Surg 29:582–586, 1947.

108. Henderson MS: The massive bone graft in ununited fractures. JAMA 107:1104, 1936.

109. Henderson RS: Fracture-dislocation of the shoulder with interposition of long head of the biceps. Report of a case. J Bone Joint Surg 34B:240–241, 1952.

110. Henson GF: Vascular complications of shoulder injuries. A report of two cases. J Bone Joint Surg 38B:528, 1956.

111. Heppenstall RB: Fractures of the proximal humerus. Orthop Clin North Am 6(2):467–475, 1975.

112. Herbert JJ, and Paillot J: Treatment of complicated fractures of the upper end of the humerus. Epiphysio-diaphysial pegging. Rev Chir Orthop 46:739–747, 1960.

113. Hermann OJ: Fractures of the shoulder joint with special reference to correction of defects. Instr Course Lect 2:359–370, 1944.

114. Heuget L, et al.: Bone cement in the treatment of certain fractures of the proximal humerus. Ann Chir 27:311–313, 1973.

115. Hill NA, and McLaughlin HL: Locked posterior dislocation simulating a 'frozen shoulder.' J Trauma 3:225–234, 1963.

116. Hippocrates: The Genuine Works of Hippocrates. Baltimore: Williams & Wilkins, 1939.

117. Hitchcock HH, and Bechtol CO: Painful shoulder. Observations on the role of the tendon of the long head of the biceps brachii in its causation. J Bone Joint Surg 30A:263–273, 1948.

118. Hollinshead WH: Anatomy for Surgeons, Volume 3. The Back and Limbs, 3rd ed. Philadelphia: Harper & Row, 1982.

119. Horak J, and Nilsson B: Epidemiology of fractures of the upper end of the humerus. Clin Orthop 112:250–253, 1975.

120. Howard NJ, and Eloesser L: Treatment of the fractures of the upper end of the humerus. An experimental and clinical study. J Bone Joint Surg 16:1–29, 1934.

121. Hudson RT: The use of the hanging cast in treatment of fractures of the humerus. South Surgeon 10:132–134, 1941.

122. Hughes M, and Neer CS: Glenohumeral joint replacement and postoperative rehabilitation. Phys Ther 55:850–858, 1975.

123. Hundley JM, and Stewart MJ: Fractures of the humerus. A

comparative study in methods of treatment. J Bone Joint Surg *37A*:681–692, 1955.

124. Jakob RP, Kristiansen T, Mayo K, Ganz R, et al.: Classification and aspects of treatment of fractures of the proximal humerus. *In* Bateman JE, and Welsh RP (eds): Surgery of the Shoulder. Philadelphia: BC Decker, 1984.

125. Johansson O: Complications and failures of surgery in various fractures of the humerus. Acta Chir Scand *120*:469–478, 1961.

126. Jones L: Reconstructive operation for non-reducible fractures of the head of the humerus. Ann Surg *97*:217–225, 1933.

127. Jones L: The shoulder joint. Observations on the anatomy and physiology with analysis of reconstructive operation following extensive injury. Surg Gynecol Obstet *75*:433–444, 1942.

128. Jones R: On certain fractures about the shoulder. Irish J Med Sci *78*:282–291, 1932.

129. Jones R: Certain injuries commonly associated with displacement of the head of the humerus. Br Med J *1*:1385–1386, 1906.

130. Keene JS, Huizenga RE, Engber WD, and Rogers SC: Proximal humeral fractures. A correction of residual deformity with long-term function. Orthopedics *6*:173–178, 1983.

131. Kelly JP: Fractures complicating electroconvulsive therapy and chronic epilepsy. J Bone Joint Surg *36B*:70–79, 1954.

132. Key JA, and Conwell HE: Fractures, Dislocations, and Sprains, 5th ed. St. Louis: CV Mosby, 1951.

133. Knight RA, and Mayne JA: Comminuted fractures and fracture-dislocations involving the articular surface of the humeral head. J Bone Joint Surg *39A*:1343–1355, 1957.

134. Knowelden J, Buhr AJ, and Dunbar O: Incidence of fractures in persons over 35 years of age. A report to the M.R.C. Working Party on fractures in the elderly. Br J Prev Soc Med *18*:130, 1964.

135. Kocher T: Beitrage zur Kenntnis einiger praktisch wichtiger Fracturenformen. Basel: Carl Sallman Verlag, 1896.

136. Krakovic M, et al.: Indications and results of operation in proximal humeral fractures. Mschr Unfallheilk *78*:326–332, 1975.

137. Kraulis J, and Hunter G: The results of prosthetic replacement in fracture-dislocations of the upper end of the humerus. Injury *8*:129–131, 1976.

138. Kristiansen B, and Christensen SW: Plate fixation of proximal humeral fractures. Acta Orthop Scand *57*:320–323, 1986.

139. Krueger FT: Vitallium replica arthroplasty of shoulder. Care of aseptic necrosis of proximal end of humerus. Surgery *30*:1005–1011, 1951.

140. LaBriola JH, and Mohaghegh HA: Isolated avulsion fracture of the lesser tuberosity of the humerus. A case report and review of the literature. J Bone Joint Surg *57A*:1011, 1975.

141. LaFerte AD, and Nutter PD: The treatment of fractures of the humerus by means of hanging plaster cast. "Hanging cast." Ann Surg *114*:919–930, 1955.

142. Laing PG: The arterial supply of the adult humerus. J Bone Joint Surg *38A*:1105–1116, 1956.

143. Lane LB, Villacin A, and Bullough PG: The vascularity and remodelling of subchondral bone and calcified cartilage in adult human femoral and humeral heads. An age- and stress-related phenomenon. J Bone Joint Surg *59B*:272–278, 1977.

144. Leach RE, and Premer RF: Nonunion of the surgical neck of the humerus. Method of internal fixation. Minnesota Med *48*:318–322, 1965.

145. LeBorgne J, LeNeel JC, and Mitland D: Les lesions de l'artere axillaire et de ses branches consecutives a un traumatisme ferme de l'epaule. Ann Chir (Paris) *27*:587, 1973.

146. Lee CK, and Hansen HR: Post-traumatic avascular necrosis of the humeral head in displaced proximal humeral fractures. J Trauma *21*:788–791, 1981.

147. Lee CK, Hansen HT, and Weiss AB: Surgical treatment of the difficult humeral neck fracture. Acromial shortening anterolateral approach. J Trauma *20*:67–70, 1980.

148. Leikkonen O: Osteosynthesis with special modified plate in fractures of the proximal end of the humerus. Ann Clin Gynaec Fenn *49*:309–314, 1960.

149. Lentz W, and Meuser P: The treatment of fractures of the proximal humerus. Arch Orthop Trauma Surg *96*:283–285, 1980.

150. Leyshon RL: Closed treatment of fractures of the proximal humerus. Acta Orthop Scand *55*:48–51, 1984.

151. Lim TE, Ochsner PE, Marti RK, and Holscher AA: The results of treatment of comminuted fractures and fracture dislocations of the proximal humerus. Neth J Surg *35*:139–143, 1983.

152. Lindholm TS, and Elmstedt E: Bilateral posterior dislocation of the shoulder combined with fracture of the proximal humerus. A case report. Acta Orthop Scand *51*:485–488, 1980.

153. Linson MA: Axillary artery thrombosis after fracture of the humerus. A case report. J Bone Joint Surg *62A*:1214–1215, 1980.

154. Lorenz H: Die isolirte Fractur des Tuberculum minus humeri. Dtsch Zeitschr Chir *58*:593, 1900–1901.

155. Lorenzo FT: Osteosynthesis with Blount staples in fracture of the proximal end of the humerus. A preliminary report. J Bone Joint Surg *37A*:45–48, 1955.

156. Lovett RW: The diagnosis and treatment of some common injuries of the shoulder joint. Surg Gynecol Obstet *34*:437, 1922.

157. Lucas-Championniere J: Traitement des fractures par le massage et la mobilisation. Paris: Rueff, 1895.

158. Lundberg BJ, Svenungson-Hartwig E, and Vikmark R: Independent exercises versus physiotherapy in non-displaced proximal humeral fractures. Scand J Rehabil Med *11*:133, 1979.

159. Luppino D, Santangelo G, Vicenzi G, Innao V et al.: Le fratture dell'estremita prossimale dell'omero di interesse chirurgico (studio di 40 casi). Chir Organi Mov *67*:373–381, 1982.

160. MacDonald FR: Intra-articular fractures in recurrent dislocations of the shoulder. Surg Clin North Am *43*:1635–1645, 1963.

161. Machmull G, and Weeder SD: Bilateral fracture of the humeral heads. Cases with bilateral fracture of the anatomical and surgical necks of the humeri due to convulsion. Radiology *55*:735–739, 1950.

162. Marotte JH, Lord G, and Bancel P: L'arthroplastie de Neer dans les fractures et fractures-luxations complexes de l'epaule. A propos de 12 cas. Chirurgie *104*:816–821, 1978.

163. Mauclaire M: Bull Mem Soc Chir Paris *46*:572, 1920.

164. McBurney C, and Dowd CN: Dislocation of the humerus complicated by fracture at or near the surgical neck with a new method of reduction. Ann Surg *19*:399, 1894.

165. McGuinness JP: Isolated avulsion fracture of the lesser tuberosity of the humerus. Lancet *1*:508, 1939.

166. McLaughlin HL: Dislocation of the shoulder with tuberosity fracture. Surg Clin North Am *43*:1615–1620, 1963.

167. McLaughlin HL: Locked posterior subluxation of the shoulder. Diagnosis and treatment. Surg Clin North Am *43*:1621–1622, 1963.

168. McLaughlin HL: Posterior dislocation of the shoulder. J Bone Joint Surg *34A*:584–590, 1952.

169. McLaughlin HL: Treatment of shoulder injuries. *In* American Academy of Orthopaedic Surgeons: Regional Orthopedic Surgery and Fundamental Orthopedic Problems. Ann Arbor, MI: Edwards, 1947.

170. McQuillan WM, and Nolan B: Ischemia complicating injury. A report of thirty-seven cases. J Bone Joint Surg *50B*:482–492, 1968.

171. Mazet R: Intramedullary fixation in the arm and the forearm. Clin Orthop *2*:75–92, 1953.

172. Mestdagh H, Butruille Y, Tillie B, and Bocquet F: Resultats du traitement des fractures de l'extremite superieure de l'humerus par embrochage percutane. A propos de cent quarante-deux cas. Ann Chir *38*:5–13, 1984.

173. Meyerding HW: Fracture-dislocation of the shoulder. Minn Med *20*:717–726, 1937.

174. Michaelis LS: Comminuted fracture-dislocation of the shoulder. J Bone Joint Surg *26*:363–365, 1944.

175. Milch H: The treatment of recent dislocations and fracture-dislocations of the shoulder. J Bone Joint Surg *31A*:173–180, 1949.

176. Milch H: Treatment of dislocation of the shoulder. Surgery 3:732–740, 1938.
177. Miller SR: Practical points in the diagnosis and treatment of fractures of the upper fourth of the humerus. Indust Med 9:458–460, 1940.
178. Mills KLG: Severe injuries of the upper end of the humerus. Injury 6:13–21, 1974.
179. Mills KLG: Simultaneous bilateral posterior fracture-dislocation of the shoulder. Injury 6:39, 1974.
180. Moriber LA, and Patterson RL: Fractures of the proximal end of the humerus. J Bone Joint Surg 49A:1018, 1967.
180a. Morris MF, Kilcoyne RF, and Shuman W: Humeral tuberosity fractures: Evaluation by CT scan and management of malunion. Orthop Trans 11:242, 1987.
181. Moseley HF: The arterial pattern of the rotator cuff of the shoulder. J Bone Joint Surg 45B:780–789, 1963.
182. Mouradian WH: Displaced proximal humeral fractures. Seven years' experience with a modified Zickel supracondylar device. Clin Orthop 212:209–218, 1986.
183. de Mourgues G, et al.: Fracture-dislocations of the shoulder joint. Rev Chir Orthop 51:151, 1965.
184. Murphy JB: Nailing of fracture of surgical neck of humerus after an unsuccessful attempt to secure union by bone transplantation. Surg Clin Chicago 3:531, 1914.
185. Neer CS, McCann PD, Macfarlane EA, and Padilla N: Earlier passive motion following shoulder arthroplasty and rotator cuff repair. A prospective study. Orthop Trans 11:231, 1987.
186. Neer CS, and McIlveen SJ: Recent results and technique of prosthetic replacement for 4-part proximal humeral fractures. Orthop Trans 10:475, 1986.
187. Neer CS, Watson KC, and Stanton FJ: Recent experience in total shoulder replacement. J Bone Joint Surg 64A:319–337, 1982.
188. Neer CS, and Rockwood CA: Fractures and dislocations of the shoulder. In Rockwood CA, and Green DP (eds): Fractures, 2nd ed. Philadelphia: JB Lippincott, 1984.
189. Neer CS: Four-segment classification of displaced proximal humeral fractures. Instr Course Lect 24:160–168, 1975.
190. Neer CS: Displaced proximal humeral fractures. Part I. Classification and evaluation. J Bone Joint Surg 52A:1077–1089, 1970.
191. Neer CS: Displaced proximal humeral fractures. Part II. Treatment of three-part and four-part displacement. J Bone Joint Surg 52A:1090–1103, 1970.
192. Neer CS: Prosthetic replacement of the humeral head. Indications and operative technique. Surg Clin North Am 43:1581–1597, 1963.
193. Neer CS: Degenerative lesions of the proximal humeral articular surface. Clin Orthop 20:116–124, 1961.
194. Neer CS: Indications for replacement of the proximal humeral articulation. Am J Surg 89:901–907, 1955.
195. Neer CS: Articular replacement for the humeral head. J Bone Joint Surg 37A:215–228, 1955.
196. Neer CS, Brown TH, and McLaughlin HL: Fracture of the neck of the humerus with dislocation of the head fragment. Am J Surg 85:252–258, 1953.
197. Neviaser JS: Complicated fractures and dislocations about the shoulder joint. J Bone Joint Surg 44A:984–998, 1962.
198. Newton-John HF, and Morgan DB: The loss of bone with age, osteoporosis, and fractures. Clin Orthop 71:229, 1970.
199. Nicola FG, Ellman H, Eckardt J, and Finerman G: Bilateral posterior fracture-dislocation of the shoulder treated with a modification of the McLaughlin procedure. J Bone Joint Surg 63A:1175–1177, 1981.
200. Nissen-Lie HS: Pseudarthroses of humerus. Acta Orthop Scand 21:22–30, 1951.
201. North JP: The conservative treatment of fractures of the humerus. Surg Clin North Am 20:1633–1643, 1940.
202. O'Flanagan PH: Fracture due to shock from domestic electricity supply. Injury 6:244–245, 1975.
203. Oni OO: Irreducible acute anterior dislocation of the shoulder due to a loose fragment from an associated fracture of the greater tuberosity. Injury 15:138, 1984.
204. Ostapowicz G, and Rahn-Myrach A: The functional treatment of fractures of the head of the humerus. Bruns' Butr Klin Chir 202:96–114, 1961.
205. Paavolainen P, Bjorkenheim J-M, Slatis P, and Paukku P: Operative treatment of severe proximal humeral fractures. Acta Orthop Scand 54:374–379, 1983.
206. Palmer IA: A dualistic method of treating pseudoarthrosis. Acta Chir Scand 107:261, 1954.
207. Palmer I: On the complications and technical problems of medullary nailing. Acta Chir Scand 101:491–492, 1951.
208. Patel MR, Pardee ML, and Singerman RC: Intrathoracic dislocation of the head of the humerus. J Bone Joint Surg 45A:1712–1714, 1963.
209. Pilgaard S, Och Oster A: Four-segment fractures of the humeral neck. Acta Orthop Scand 44:124, 1973.
210. Poilleux F, and Courtois-Suffit M: Des fractures du col chirurgical de l'humerus. Rev Chir 133–158, 1954.
211. Post M: Fractures of the upper humerus. Orthop Clin North Am 11(2):239–252, 1980.
212. Prillaman HA, and Thompson RC: Bilateral posterior fracture-dislocation of the shoulder. A case report. J Bone Joint Surg 51A:1627–1630, 1969.
213. Proximal humeral fractures. What price history? Editorial. Injury 12:89–90, 1981.
214. Raney RB: The treatment of fractures of the humerus with the hanging cast. North Carolina Med J 6:88–92, 1945.
215. Rathbun JB, and Macnab I: The microvascular pattern of the rotator cuff. J Bone Joint Surg 52B:540–553, 1970.
216. Razemon JP, and Baux S: Fractures and fracture-dislocations of the proximal humerus. Rev Chir Orthop 55:387–396, 1965.
217. Rechtman AM: Open reduction of fracture dislocation of the humerus. JAMA 94:1656, 1934.
218. Reckling FW: Posterior fracture-dislocation of the shoulder treated by a Neer hemiarthroplasty with a posterior surgical approach. Clin Orthop 207:133–137, 1986.
219. Rendlich RA, and Poppel MH: Roentgen diagnosis of posterior dislocation of the shoulder. Radiology 36:42–45, 1941.
220. Richard A, Judet R, and Rene L: Reconstruction prothetique acrylique de l'extremite superieure de l'humerus specialement au cours des fratures-luxations. J Chir 68:537–547, 1952.
221. Rob CG, and Standeven A: Closed traumatic lesions of the axillary and brachial arteries. Lancet 1:597–599, 1956.
222. Roberts SM: Fractures of the upper end of the humerus. An end-result study which shows the advantage of early active motion. JAMA 98:367–373, 1932.
223. Rooney PJ, and Cockshott WP: Pseudarthrosis following proximal humeral fractures. A possible mechanism. Skeletal Radiol 15:21–24, 1986.
224. Rose SH, Melton LJ, Morrey BF, Ilstrup DM, et al.: Epidemiologic features of humeral fractures. Clin Orthop 168:24–30, 1982.
225. Rosen H: Tension band wiring for fracture dislocation of the shoulder. Proceedings of the 12th Congress of the International Society of Orthopaedic Surgery and Traumatologie. Tel Aviv, October 9–12, 1972, pp 939–941.
226. Rothman RH, Marvel JP, and Heppenstall RB: Anatomic considerations in the glenohumeral joint. Orthop Clin North Am 6(2):341–352, 1975.
227. Rothman RH, and Parke WW: The vascular anatomy of the rotator cuff. Clin Orthop 41:176–186, 1965.
228. Rowe CR, and Colville M: The glenohumeral joint. In Rowe CR (ed): The Shoulder. New York: Churchill Livingstone, 1988.
229. Rowe CR, and Marble H: Shoulder girdle injuries. In Cave EF (ed): Fractures and Other Injuries. Chicago: Year Book Medical Publishers, 1958.
230. Rush LV: Atlas of Rush Pin Techniques. Meridian, MI: Beviron Co., 1959.
231. Saha AK: The zero position of the glenohumeral joint: Its

recognition and clinical importance. Ann R Coll Surg Engl 22:223, 1958.

232. Sakai K, Hattori S, Kawai S, Saiki K, et al.: One case of the fracture at the attachment of the subscapularis muscle. The Shoulder Joint 7:58, 1981.

233. Salem MI: Bilateral anterior fracture-dislocation of the shoulder joints due to severe electric shock. Injury 14:361–363, 1983.

234. Santee HE: Fractures about the upper end of the humerus. Ann Surg 80:103–114, 1924.

235. Savoie FH, Geissler WB, and Vander Griend RA: Open reduction and internal fixation of three-part fractures of the proximal humerus. Orthopedics 12:65–70, 1989.

236. Scheck M: Surgical treatment of nonunions of the surgical neck of the humerus. Clin Orthop 167:255–259, 1982.

237. Schuhl JF: Fracture-dislocations of the proximal humerus. These medicine, Lyon, 1973.

238. Schweiger G, and Ludolph E: Fractures of the shoulder joint. Unfallchir 6, 1980.

239. Scudder CL: The Treatment of Fractures, 11th ed. Philadelphia: WB Saunders, 1939.

240. Sever JW: Fracture of the head of the humerus. Treatment and results. N Engl J Med 216:1100–1107, 1937.

241. Sever JW: Nonunion in fracture of the shaft of the humerus. Report of five cases. JAMA 104:382–386, 1935.

242. Shaw JL: Bilateral posterior fracture-dislocation of the shoulder and other trauma caused by convulsive seizures. J Bone Joint Surg 53A:1437–1440, 1971.

243. Shibuya S, and Ogawa K: Isolated avulsion fracture of the lesser tuberosity of the humerus. A case report. Clin Orthop 211:215–218, 1986.

244. Shuck JM, Omer GE, and Lewis CE: Arterial obstruction due to intimal disruption in extremity fractures. J Trauma 12:481–489, 1972.

245. Silfverskiold N: On the treatment of fracture-dislocations of the shoulder-joint. With special reference to the capability of the head-fragment, disconnected from capsule and periosteum to enter into bony union. Acta Chir Scand 64:227–293, 1928.

246. Sjovall H: A case of spontaneous backward subluxation of the shoulder treated by the Clairmont-Ehrlich operation. Nord Med (Hygeia) 21:474–476, 1944.

247. Smyth EHJ: Major arterial injury in closed fracture of the neck of the humerus. Report of a case. J Bone Joint Surg 51B:508–510, 1969.

248. Solonen KA, and Vastamaki M: Osteotomy of the neck of the humerus for traumatic varus deformity. Acta Orthop Scand 56:79–80, 1985.

249. Sorensen KH: Pseudarthrosis of the surgical neck of the humerus. Two cases. One bilateral. Acta Orthop Scand 34:132–138, 1964.

250. Stableforth PG: Four-part fractures of the neck of the humerus. J Bone Joint Surg 66B:104–108, 1984.

251. Stangl FH: Isolated fracture of the lesser tuberosity of the humerus. Minn Med 16:435–437, 1933.

252. Stewart MJ, and Hundley JM: Fractures of the humerus. A comparative study in methods of treatment. J Bone Joint Surg 37A:681–692, 1955.

253. Stimson BB: A Manual of Fractures and Dislocations, 2nd ed. Philadelphia: Lea & Febiger, 1947.

254. Sturzenegger M, Fornaro E, and Jakob RP: Results of surgical treatment of multifragmented fractures of the humeral head. Arch Orthop Trauma Surg 100:249–259, 1982.

255. Sven-Hansen H: Displaced proximal humeral fractures. A review of 49 patients. Acta Orthop Scand 45:359–364, 1974.

256. Tanner MW, and Cofield RH: Prosthetic arthroplasty for fractures and fracture-dislocation of the proximal humerus. Clin Orthop 179:116–128, 1983.

257. Tanton J: Fractures de l'extremite superiere de l'humerus. In LeDentu A, and Delbet P (eds): Noveau Traite de Chirurgie, Fasc 4. Paris: Bailliere et Fils, 1915.

258. Theodorides T, and Dekeizer G: Injuries of the axillary artery caused by fractures of the neck of the humerus. Injury 8:120, 1976.

259. Thompson FE, and Winant EM: Comminuted fracture of the humeral head with subluxation. Clin Orthop 20:94–97, 1961.

260. Thompson FR, and Winant EM: Unusual fracture subluxations of the shoulder joint. J Bone Joint Surg 32A:575–582, 1950.

261. Thompson JE: Anatomical methods of approach in operations on the long bones of the extremities. Ann Surg 68:309–329, 1918.

262. Tondeur G: Les fractures recentes de l'epaule. Acta Orthop Belg 30:1–144, 1964.

263. Tonino AJ, and van de Werf GJIM: Hemi arthroplasty of the shoulder. Acta Orthop Belg 51:625–631, 1985.

264. Trotter E: Apropos d'un cas de resection de la tete de l'humerus. J l'Hotel-dieu Montreal 11:368, 1933.

265. Vainio S: Observation on serious fractures of the proximal end of the humerus. Ann Clin Gynaec Fenn 49:302–308, 1960.

266. Valls J: Acrylic prosthesis in a case with fracture of the head of the humerus. Bal Soc Orthop Trauma 17:61, 1952.

267. Vander-Ghirst M, and Houssa R: Acrylic prosthesis in fractures of the head of the humerus. Acta Chir Belg 50:31, 1951.

268. Vastamaki M, and Solonen KA: Posterior dislocation and fracture-dislocation of the shoulder. Acta Orthop Scand 51:479–484, 1980.

269. Vastamaki M, and Solonen KA: Posterior dislocation and posterior fracture-dislocation of the shoulder. Acta Orthop Scand 50:124, 1979.

270. Vesely DG: Use of the split diamond nail for fractures of the humerus. 1958–1964. Clin Orthop 41:145–156, 1965.

271. Vichard PH, and Bellanger P: Ascending bipolar nailing using elastic nails in the treatment of fractures of the upper end of the humerus. Nouv Presse Med 7:4041–4043, 1978.

272. Wallace WA: The dynamic study of shoulder movement. In Bayley I, and Kessel L (eds): Shoulder Surgery. New York: Springer-Verlag, 1982.

273. Watson-Jones R: Fractures and Joint Injuries, 4th ed. Baltimore: Williams & Wilkins, 1955, pp 473–476.

274. Watson-Jones R: Fractures and Joint Injuries, 3rd ed. Baltimore: Williams & Wilkins, 1943, pp 460–461.

275. Weise K, Meeder PJ, and Wentzensen A: Indications and operative technique in osteosynthesis of fracture-dislocations of the shoulder joint in adults. Langenbecks Arch Chir 351:91–98, 1980.

276. Wentworth ET: Fractures involving the shoulder joint. NY State J Med 40:1282–1288, 1940.

277. Weseley MS, Barenfeld PA, and Eisenstein AL: Rush pin intramedullary fixation for fractures of the proximal humerus. J Trauma 17:29–37, 1977.

278. West EF: Intrathoracic dislocation of the humerus. J Bone Joint Surg 31B:61, 1949.

279. Whitman R: A treatment of epiphyseal displacements and fractures of the upper extremity of the humerus designed to assure definite adjustment and fixation of fragments. Ann Surg 47:706, 1908.

280. Whitson TB: Fractures of the surgical neck of the humerus. A study in reduction. J Bone Joint Surg 36B:423–427, 1954.

281. Widen A: Fractures of the upper end of humerus with great displacement treated by marrow nailing. Acta Chir Scand 97:439–441, 1949.

282. Wilson GE: Fractures and Their Complications. New York: Macmillan, 1931.

283. Wilson JN (ed): Watson-Jones Fractures and Joint Injuries, 6th ed. New York: Churchill Livingstone, 1982.

284. Wilson JC, and McKeever FM: Traumatic posterior (retroglenoid) dislocation of the humerus. J Bone Joint Surg 31A:160–172; 180, 1949.

285. Willems WJ, and Lim TEA: Neer arthroplasty for humeral fracture. Acta Orthop Scand 56:394–395, 1985.

286. Winfield JM, Miller H, and LaFerte AD: Evaluation of the "hanging cast" as a method of treating fractures of the humerus. Am J Surg 55:228–249, 1942.

287. Wood JP: Posterior dislocation of the head of the humerus and diagnostic value of lateral and vertical views. US Naval Med Bull 39:532–535, 1941.

288. Yamano Y: Comminuted fractures of the proximal humerus treated with hook plate. Arch Orthop Trauma Surg *105:*359–363, 1986.
289. Yano S, Takamura S, and Kobayshi I: Use of the spiral pin for fractures of the humeral neck. J Jpn Orthop Assn *55:*1607, 1981.
290. Young TB: Conservative treatment of fractures and fracture-dislocations of the upper end of the humerus. J Bone Joint Surg *67B:*373–377, 1985.

291. Zadik FR: Recurrent posterior dislocation of the shoulder. J Bone Joint Surg *30B:*531–532, 1948.
292. Zuckerman JD, Flugstad DL, Teitz CC, and King HA: Axillary artery injury as a complication of proximal humeral fractures. Two case reports and a review of the literature. Clin Orthop *189:*234–237, 1984.

CHAPTER
10

The Scapula

Kenneth P. Butters, M.D.

The scapula has an important role in arm function. It sits congruently against the ribs and serves to stabilize the upper extremity against the thorax. It is also the link between the upper extremity and the axial skeleton through the glenoid, acromioclavicular, clavicular, and sternoclavicular joints. The scapula is subject to indirect injury through axial loading on the outstretched arm (scapular neck), through direct trauma, often high energy, from a blow or fall (body), and through direct trauma to the point of the shoulder (acromion, coracoid). Shoulder dislocation may cause glenoid fracture. Traction by muscles or ligaments may also occur. Scapular fracture patterns have been identified and will be discussed.

Fracture of the scapula occurs infrequently,[69] the incidence being 3 to 5 per cent of shoulder girdle injuries[39, 103] and 0.4 to 1 per cent of all fractures.[85, 121] This may be due to its thickened edges, its great mobility with recoil, and its position between layers of muscle. The mean age of patients with scapula fractures is 35 to 45.[3, 67, 118]

Associated injuries to other points in the shoulder girdle, the thoracic cage, and soft tissues are common and may lead to a delay in diagnosis of the scapular fracture. Such problems as cervical spine fracture or vascular injury often require immediate attention. Operative surgical indications for scapular fracture are rare. Significant trauma is required to fracture the scapula, as is evidenced by the cause of injury—motor vehicle accidents in about 50 per cent of cases[48, 67] and motorcycle accidents in 11 to 25 per cent.

Anatomy

The practice of orthopedics is applied anatomy. Bony contour, muscle attachments, and the location of adjacent neurovascular structures should be understood in evaluating scapular fractures and certainly should be studied prior to undertaking surgery.

The anterior scapular surface is covered with the attachment of the subscapularis muscle with the serratus anterior muscle attaching to the anterior medial border of the scapula (Figs. 10–1 and 10–3). The posterior scapula has on its surface the supraspinatus and infraspinatus muscles, with the trapezius muscle overlying the supraspinatus and attaching to the spine and clavicle (Fig. 10–2). The deltoid overlies a portion of the infraspinatus posteriorly and the lateral subscapularis anteriorly; its origin is from the scapular spine, acromion, and anterior clavicle. Many other muscles attach to the scapular margin—the levator scapulae and rhomboids to the medial border, the teres minor and teres major from the lateral border, and an inconsistent latissimus attachment to the inferior tip of the scapula. The pectoralis minor, the short head of the

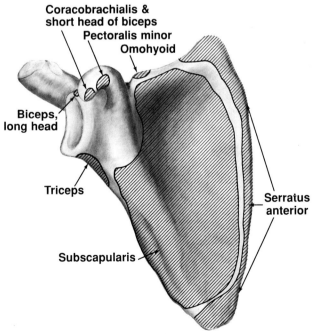

Figure 10–1. The muscle attachments to the anterior surface of the scapula.

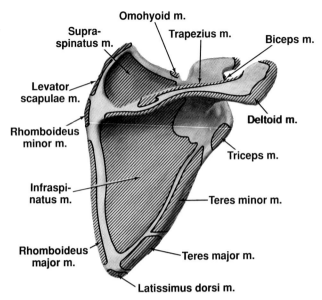

Figure 10–2. The muscle attachments to the posterior surface of the scapula.

biceps, and the coracobrachialis attach to the coracoid; the long head of the biceps attaches to the superior glenoid; and the triceps attaches to the inferior glenoid (Figs. 10–1 and 10–4).

The coracoid process projects upward, forward, and lateral from the superior border of the scapula. The brachial plexus and axillary artery run posterior to the pectoralis minor tendon, which inserts on the medial aspect of the base of the coracoid. Just medial to the coracoid base is the scapular notch, bridged by the transverse scapular ligament. The suprascapular nerve passes through the notch under the ligament, and the suprascapular artery passes over the ligament. The acromion continues laterally from the spine; a gap between it and the neck of the scapula constitutes the spinoglenoid notch transmitting the suprascapular nerve and vessels to the infraspinatus. Figure 10–4B shows this relationship and the proximity of the axillary and suprascapular nerves and the brachial plexus to the scapula.

The dorsal scapular and accessory nerves travel with the deep and superficial branches of the transverse cervical artery, respectively, parallel to and medial to the vertebral border of the scapula.

Most shoulder function involves simultaneous humeral and scapular movements with a definite rhythm. The scapula is a platform for the upper extremity. It rotates into abduction to assist the arm with forward elevation and undergoes adduction, elevation, or depression to help position the extremity. With all these movements, the scapula is in its bed against the chest wall. Scapular fracture malunion, soft tissue scarring, and muscle and nerve injury can all affect rhythm and limit scapular excursion, decreasing shoulder motion.

Classification of Fractures of the Scapula

Certain fracture patterns are seen in the scapula. They will be described by anatomical area for ease of discussion (i.e., body and spine, glenoid neck, intraarticular, glenoid, coracoid, and acromion). Several areas of the scapula are often involved but the neck (10 to 60 per cent) and body (49 to 89 per cent) are most common.[3, 48, 67, 120] Zdravkovic[124] divided scapular fractures into three types: I—fractures of the body; II—fractures of the apophysis, including the coracoid and acromion; and III—fractures of the superior lateral angle, including the neck and glenoid. This classification was devised to separate the Type III fracture, which is generally considered the most difficult to deal with. Displaced or comminuted Type III (neck and glenoid) fractures constituted only 6 per cent of this entire series of scapular fractures.

Thompson and colleagues[118] in their trauma center series of wide-impact blunt trauma, classified scapular fractures into Class I—the coracoid and acromion and small fractures of the body; Class II—the glenoid and neck; and Class III—major scapular body fractures.

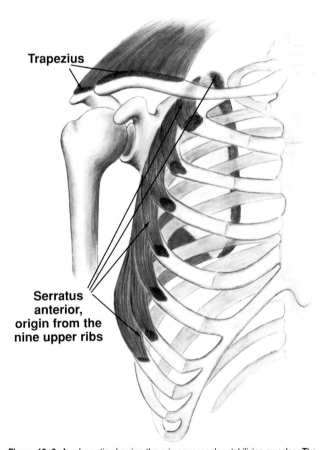

Figure 10–3. A schematic showing the primary scapular stabilizing muscles. The serratus anterior passes deep to the scapula, attaching to the medial border holding the scapula against the chest wall.

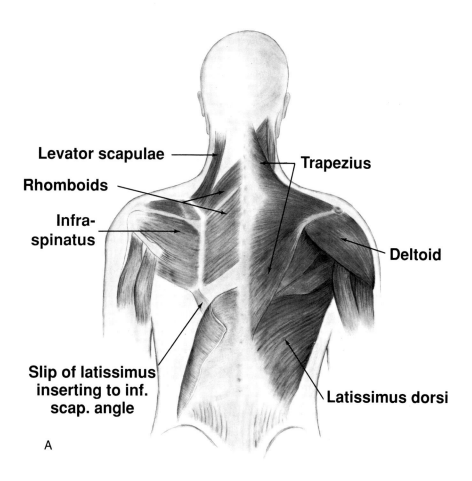

Levator scapulae

Trapezius

Rhomboids

Infra-
spinatus

Deltoid

Slip of latissimus
inserting to inf.
scap. angle

Latissimus dorsi

A

Figure 10–4. *A,* The posterior torso musculature, superficial *(right)* and deep *(left).* *B,* A schematic diagram showing the positions of the major nerves relative to the scapula.

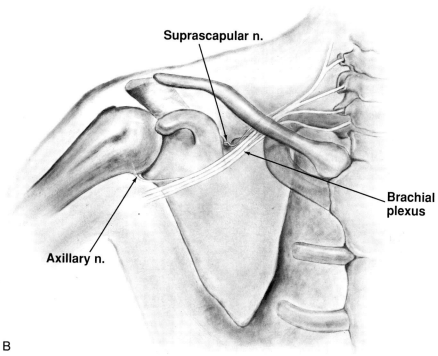

Suprascapular n.

Brachial
plexus

Axillary n.

B

Class II and III fractures were much more likely to have associated injuries. Ideberg[47] has proposed a classification of five types of intra-articular glenoid fractures (described later in this chapter).

Clinical Presentation

Throughout the literature, a classic clinical description of scapular fracture, that of scapular glenoid neck, is noted. According to Hitzrot and Bolling,[44] Sir Astley Cooper described flattening of the shoulder and prominence of the acromion. When the deformity was reduced by supporting the elbow, the movement was associated with bony crepitus. Interestingly, two of his three cases proved to be humeral neck fractures. Some authors have tried to make a clinical diagnosis by measuring arm length or midline-to-coracoid distance[44] without finding that this offers consistent, accurate help in diagnosis.

The typical presentation is that the arm is held adducted and protected from all movements, with abduction especially painful. Local tenderness is present. The shoulder may appear flattened with a displaced neck or acromion fracture. Ecchymosis is less than expected from the degree of bony injury present, as opposed to fracture of the upper humerus. Pain with deep inspiration may be present with coracoid fracture (pectoralis minor) or body fracture (serratus anterior). One should always be aware of the possibility of associated pneumothorax, either immediate or delayed. With body fractures especially, deep swelling may be quite painful, producing "pseudorupture of the rotator cuff."[84] Neviaser[84] described the syndrome of weak cuff function and loss of active arm elevation, which is probably only inhibition of muscle contractions from intramuscular hemorrhage and which usually resolves within a few weeks. This can be differentiated from rotator cuff tear, as the fracture is seen on x-ray and the swelling present with fracture and pseudorupture syndrome exceeds that normally seen with a cuff tear. It is important to re-emphasize that a scapular fracture often presents with associated injuries needing more urgent treatment.

Associated Injuries and Complications

Significant associated injuries occur in 35 to 98 per cent of scapular fractures, the higher incidence coming from serious trauma unit admission.[3, 30, 48, 67, 118, 120] This reflects the degree of trauma necessary to fracture the scapula.

Fischer[30] and Thompson[118] have stated that direct scapular trauma and resultant scapular body fracture from wide-impact trauma have a particularly high incidence of associated ipsilateral upper torso injuries, so these fractures should be regarded as warnings.

Similarly, the diagnosis of scapular fracture is often delayed as more urgent care is provided.[3]

Pneumothorax was found in 16 of 30 patients in a prospective study of fractured scapulae.[70] Interestingly, 10 of the 16 pneumothoraces were delayed in onset from one to three days. A follow-up chest x-ray, an examination, and blood gases determinations should then be considered in scapular fracture patients. Other series have reported a lower overall incidence of pneumothorax (11 to 38 per cent).[3, 30, 118]

Ipsilateral fractured ribs are present in 27 to 54 per cent of cases.[118] Correlation with pneumothorax is probably strong enough to warrant a prophylactic chest tube before early surgery is done for other injuries.[30] Armstrong found a fracture of the scapula with an underlying first rib fracture a particularly severe injury.[3]

Pulmonary contusion can be a life-threatening associated injury and is present in 11 to 54 per cent of scapular fractures.[30, 118] This may result in marked oxygen desaturation requiring tracheal intubation and positive end-expiratory pressure ventilation. Figure 10–5 illustrates several of the common associated injuries. Fracture of the clavicle frequently (23 to 39 per cent) is associated with a fracture of the glenoid or glenoid neck. This may represent a continuation of an impaction force. Brachial plexus injury (5 to 13 per cent) is usually a supraclavicular type with a poor prognosis.[3, 30, 48, 67, 118] In his series, McGahan noted the association of brachial plexus injury with injuries about the acromion. He postulated that this may be due to depression of the shoulder and contralateral neck flexion as a mechanism of injury.[67, 82] However, in Fischer and coworkers' series of badly injured trauma unit patients, 70 per cent of the brachial plexus injuries seen occurred with major body fracture caused by wide, blunt trauma. Also, 57 per cent of those patients with scapular fracture and a brachial plexus injury also had ipsilateral upper torso arterial injury. A scapular fracture alone had an 11 per cent incidence of arterial injury.[30] Case reports in the literature of nerve and arterial injuries[67, 88, 113] with scapular fracture supplement the trauma studies and reinforce the importance of a complete neurovascular examination. Skull fractures, which occur in 24 per cent of scapular fracture patients, and closed head injuries, which occur in 20 per cent, generate concern, especially with a history of loss of consciousness.[67]

Distal extremity and spinal injury, blunt abdominal trauma, and pelvic fracture are all reported to increase in occurrence with major scapular body fracture.

Associated injuries were responsible for the 15 per cent mortality with scapular fracture in the patients reported by Fischer and colleagues[30] and in 10 per cent of the patients reported by Armstrong.[3] Half of these deaths were from pulmonary contusion with sepsis.

In summary, then, the presence of scapular fracture on initial anteroposterior chest x-ray is an indication for a good work-up for additional torso and extremity trauma on the injured side. In McGahan's and Armstrong's series, 50 per cent of the fractures had grave

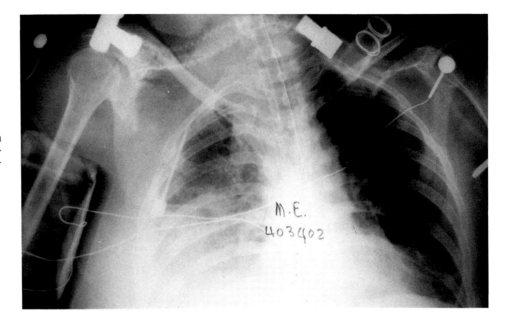

Figure 10–5. X-ray of a multiple trauma patient with a fractured neck of the scapula and associated upper extremity fractures and pulmonary contusion.

associated injuries and no scapular surgery could even be carried out, indicating simple immobilization treatment followed by range of motion exercises.[3, 67]

Differential Diagnosis

X-RAY EVALUATION

Fracture of the scapula is an x-ray diagnosis, but visualization is not always easy. Superimposition of the thorax may cloud the structural details of the scapula; however, most scapular fractures can be adequately evaluated by multiple plane views. A single view cannot provide all the information. A true anteroposterior view of the shoulder and an axillary or true scapular lateral (Trauma Series) are basic views showing glenoid neck (Fig. 10–6), body (Fig. 10–7), and acromion (Fig. 10–8) fractures. The axillary lateral view is helpful for acromial and glenoid rim fractures, and the cephalic tilt or Stryker notch view is useful for coracoid fractures (Fig. 10–9). Tomograms have not been very helpful in the overall evaluation of scapular

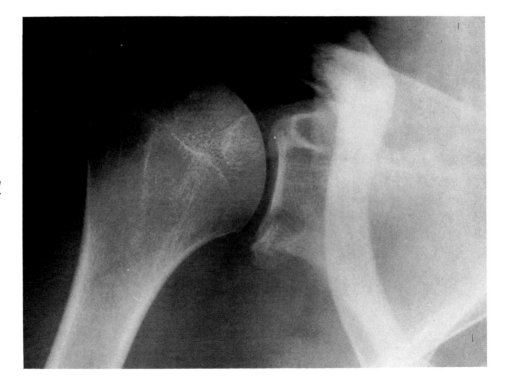

Figure 10–6. A true anteroposterior view of the glenoid showing an anterior-inferior glenoid fracture.

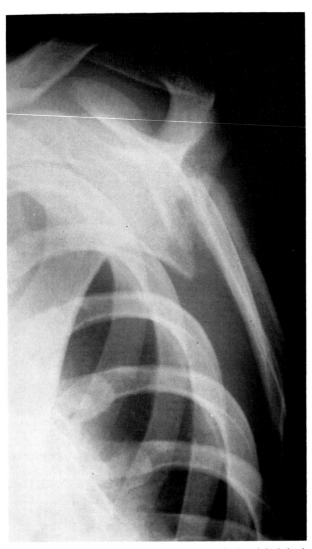

Figure 10-7. A tangential scapular lateral view (trauma series lateral view) showing a displaced scapular body fracture with a bayonet position.

fractures; they can be used in carefully chosen planes to evaluate union or displacement of the fracture.

The oblique position of the scapula on the chest wall and its narrow width make tomographic evaluation difficult to interpret. A computed tomography (CT) scan in the standard transverse plane again may not allow a three-dimensional concept of the fracture. The CT scan can be used in evaluating a glenoid fracture to confirm the reduced position of the humeral head. A three-dimensional reconstruction can be used to evaluate the shoulder girdle complex.[86]

EPIPHYSEAL LINES

Most important in the discussion of differential diagnosis is understanding the development of the scapula and its ossification pattern.[68, 89, 116] At birth the body and spine form one ossified mass, with the coracoid, acromion, glenoid, and inferior angle all being cartilaginous. At 3 to 18 months a center of ossification,

which may be bipolar, appears at the midcoracoid. At 7 to 10 years the coracoid base, including the upper third of the glenoid, appears. Sometimes called a subcoracoid bone, it joins the rest of the coracoid at 14 to 16 years (adolescence). An ossification center at the tip and a shell-like center at the medial apex of the coracoid may appear at the same time and go on to fusion at age 18 to 25 (Figs. 10–10 and 10–11).

Two or three acromial centers form at age 14 to 16, coalesce at age 19, and fuse to the spine at age 20 to 25. Failure of this to occur, with persistence of one ossification center past age 25, is known as *os acromiale*.

The glenoid fossa ossifies from four sources: (1) the coracoid base (including the upper third of the glenoid), (2) the deep portion of the coracoid process, (3) the body, and (4) the lower pole (joining the body at age 20 to 25 and deepening the glenoid cavity). At age 8 to 13 the glenoid border may be dentate from irregular ossification.[53]

At the inferior angle of the scapula, an ossification center appears at age 15 and fuses at age 20; the vertebral border center appears at age 16 to 18 and fuses by the 25th year. The ossification centers may be asymmetrical, and comparison films may not be helpful.

OS ACROMIALE

Clinically, os acromiale is the best known separate bone (resulting from failure of coalescence of the adjacent ossification centers) simulating acromial frac-

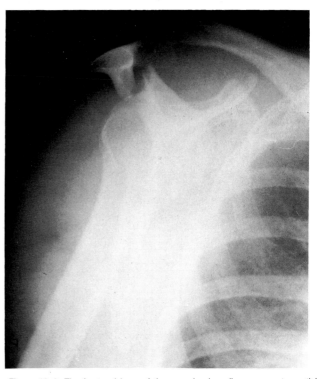

Figure 10-8. The fractured base of the acromion is well seen on a tangential scapular lateral view.

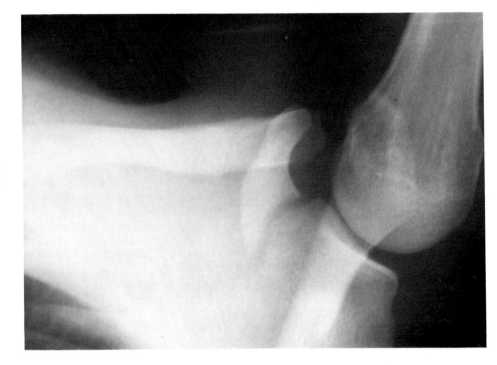

Figure 10–9. A fracture of the base of the coracoid, seen best on a Stryker notch view.

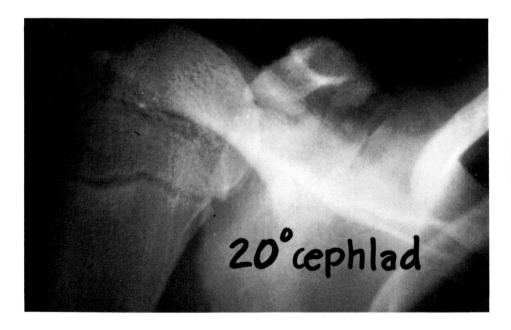

Figure 10–10. A normal ossification pattern at the base of the coracoid. A crescent-shaped center is seen at the apex of the coracoid.

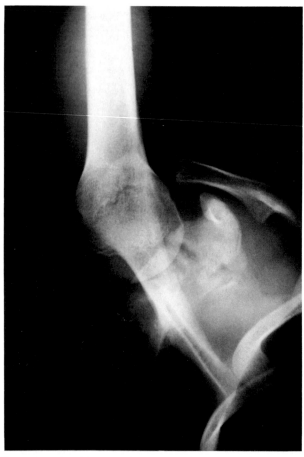

Figure 10–11. An epiphyseal line is seen across the upper third of the glenoid as this portion of the glenoid ossifies in common with the base of the coracoid. This may be confused with a fracture and is the precise location of most Type III glenoid fractures.

ture. The open epiphyseal line occurs at the level of the acromioclavicular joint (Fig. 10–12).[9] (Interestingly, Liberson's classic 1937 study was stimulated by a worker's compensation claim.[60]) The unfused apophysis is present in 2.7 per cent of random patients and when present is bilateral in 60 per cent.[60] Four ossification centers are present in the acromion, as seen in Figure 10–13. The most common site of nonunion is between the meso-acromion and the meta-acromion at the mid-acromioclavicular joint. An axillary lateral x-ray is essential for an accurate description. Factors favoring the diagnosis of os acromiale over fracture are bilaterally rounded borders with uniform space and the position of the bony ossification center even with or above the posterior acromion on the anteroposterior view. Norris[87] has reported that the unfused physis has been mistaken for fracture and that there is an association between os acromiale and rotator cuff tear. Fracture separation, or at least some movement at this site, has been seen during acromioplasty, and surgical fixation with pins or screws at the time of cuff repair has been necessary.[81, 82]

GLENOID DYSPLASIA

Scapular neck dysplasia (hypoplasia of the glenoid) resembling an impaction of the glenoid may have an associated acromial or humeral head abnormality. It usually has a benign course; many are found inadvertently, first being evaluated in the sixth or seventh decade.[94, 98] Rockwood has seen glenoid dysplasia present in college age and become symptomatic with increased athletic use of the shoulder.[99] One might suspect an increased incidence of impingement with

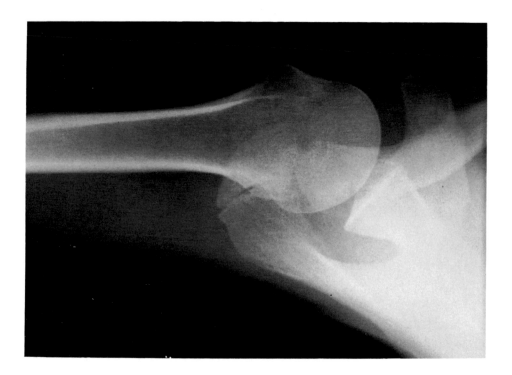

Figure 10–12. Os acromiale.

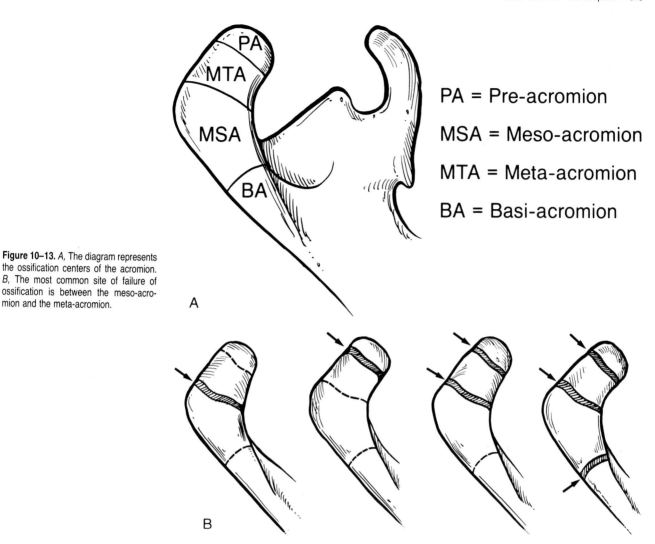

PA = Pre-acromion

MSA = Meso-acromion

MTA = Meta-acromion

BA = Basi-acromion

Figure 10–13. *A,* The diagram represents the ossification centers of the acromion. *B,* The most common site of failure of ossification is between the meso-acromion and the meta-acromion.

A

B

medial head position and less rotator cuff lever arm. Figure 10–14 is a radiograph of a 60-year-old with mild shoulder pain and stiffness.

NORMAL SCAPULAR FORAMINA

Scapular foramina[98] from disrupted ossification of the body and neck are common. They are benign appearing and well circumscribed.

Types of Fractures and Methods of Treatment

GLENOID NECK (EXTRA-ARTICULAR) FRACTURE

The literature in the early 20th century interestingly parallels that of today. A fractured scapula was thought to be produced by trauma, usually of great violence, with associated injuries. The treatment was usually conservative. The published work focused on displaced scapular neck fractures. Scudder[111] felt that traction with abduction of the arm was helpful. Cotton and Brickley[18] in 1921 described a closed reduction, using an axillary pad and three weeks in bed with "hypnotics" and with a pillow placed between the scapulae. Hitzrot and Bolling[44] in 1916 believed that manipulation and traction had no effect, and even with displaced fractures the results were satisfactory enough that reduction attempts were unnecessary. The posterior approach was used if surgery was done on intra-articular fractures. Findlay[29] in 1931 kept even his scapular body fracture patients flat in bed for 10 days. Most authors agreed that "early motion" was important.

A fracture of the neck of the scapula is probably the second most common scapular fracture, occurring from direct trauma, a fall on the point of the shoulder, or a fall on the outstretched arm from impaction. True anteroposterior, tangential scapular lateral, axillary lateral x-rays, and often CT are necessary to confirm

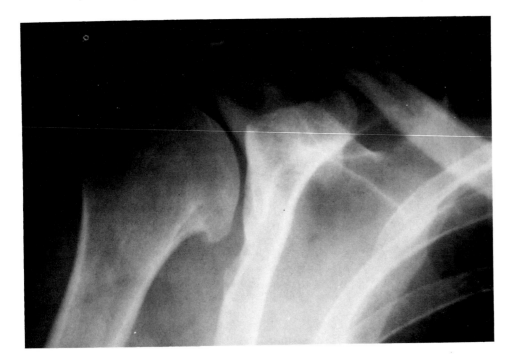

Figure 10–14. Scapular dysplasia.

the extra-articular nature of the fracture and the reduced position of the humeral head.

With neck fracture, the glenoid articular surface is intact and the fracture pattern extends from the suprascapular notch area across the neck to the lateral border of the scapula. The glenoid and coracoid may be comminuted or remain as an intact unit. The glenoid neck fracture is often displaced, but an intact clavicle and acromioclavicular joint will limit this displacement and enhance stability as opposed to the clavicle fracture seen in Figure 10–15.

Reduction of the scapular neck fracture and restoration of the glenoid to its anatomical position is not necessary. Sling immobilization for comfort is probably enough. Further displacement is rare. In a study of neck and body fractures, Lindblom and Leven found that, if untreated, all healed in the position displayed at the time of the primary examination.[61]

For displaced fracture, DePalma[21] recommends closed reduction and olecranon pin traction for three weeks, followed by use of a sling. Bateman[6] favored closed reduction in a shoulder spica for six to eight weeks in those cases where ''shortening of the neck is sufficient to favor subluxation or interfere with abduction.'' McLaughlin[69] felt that most neck fractures were impacted, making attempts at correction difficult.

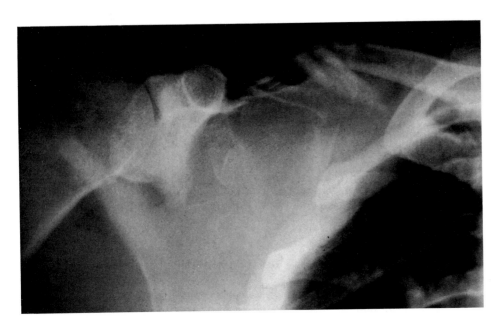

Figure 10–15. A scapular neck fracture with an associated body and clavicle fracture.

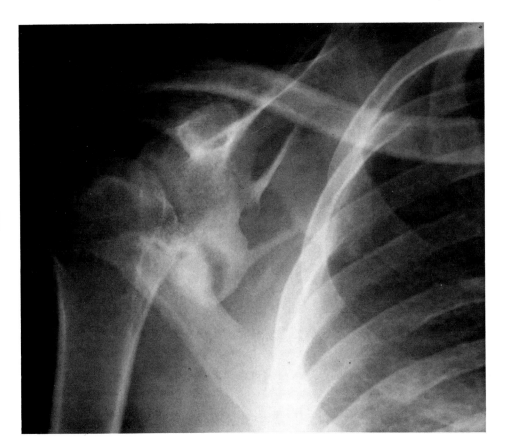

Figure 10–16. A healed glenoid neck fracture with marked medial displacement and full range of motion.

Most series report good range of motion and function in follow-up of neck and body fractures (Fig. 10–16).[47, 61, 120] Armstrong[3] reported that some residual stiffness was present in six of seven neck fractures, but there was no functional disability in his patients. Zdravkovic[124] came to the same conclusion in a study with an average follow-up of nine years. Gagney and colleagues,[34] in a French article, found a good result in only one of 12 displaced fractures. They felt that the injury would "disorganize the coracoacromial arch" and recommended open reduction. A fractured glenoid neck may be significantly displaced. Hardegger and coworkers believed that the amount of displacement and stability is dependent upon the presence of an associated fracture of the clavicle or a coracoclavicular ligament tear. The altered glenohumeral-acromial relationship results in "functional imbalance."[39] They recommended open reduction and scapular fixation of this fracture. Figure 10–17 is an x-ray of such a scapular neck fracture with an associated fractured clavicle, and Figure 10–18 shows the importance of an intact clavicle in glenoid fracture stability.

GLENOID (INTRA-ARTICULAR) FRACTURE

Intra-articular glenoid fractures may lure the orthopedist into choosing surgical treatment. True anteroposterior, axillary lateral, and West Point views

and often CT scans are needed to assess these fractures. A direct force on the lateral shoulder or indirect axial compression of the extremity may cause a stellate glenoid fracture. Most of these require no reduction as the head remains centered (Figs. 10–19 and 10–20).

Ideberg[46, 47] classified glenoid fractures into five types (Fig. 10–21), based on 300 cases: Type I—avulsion of the anterior margin; Type II—transverse fracture through the glenoid fossa, with an inferior triangular fragment displaced with the humeral head; Type III—oblique fracture through the glenoid exiting at the midsuperior border of the scapula, often associated with acromioclavicular fracture or acromioclavicular dislocation; Type IV—horizontal, exiting through the medial border of the blade; and Type V—combines Type IV with a fracture separating the inferior half of the glenoid.

Type I

This is an anterior avulsion fracture occurring most probably from dislocations and subluxations, but in some cases from direct injury. These fractures, if displaced, may predispose to instability. There is usually maintenance of continuity between the capsule, labrum, and fracture fragment. Interestingly, however, a history of recurrent dislocation may precede the episode, causing a fracture of the anterior glenoid

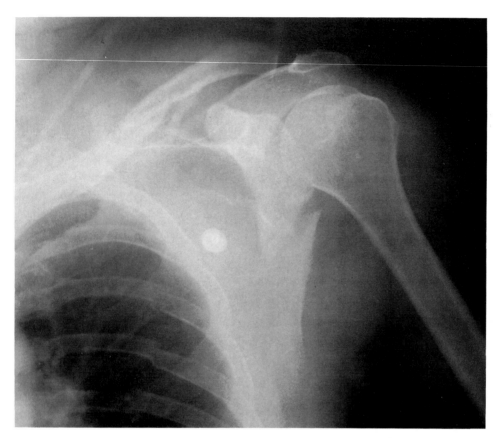

Figure 10–17. Surgical stabilization is helpful for this unstable glenoid neck fracture. With a fractured clavicle Hardegger recommends a scapular plate; the author has used clavicular plate fixation.

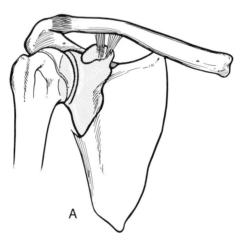 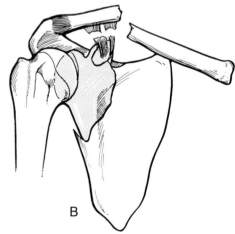

Figure 10–18. This diagram shows the distinction between stable (A) and unstable (B) scapular neck fractures. The injury in B shows clavicular fracture or coracoclavicular ligament disruption.

A

B

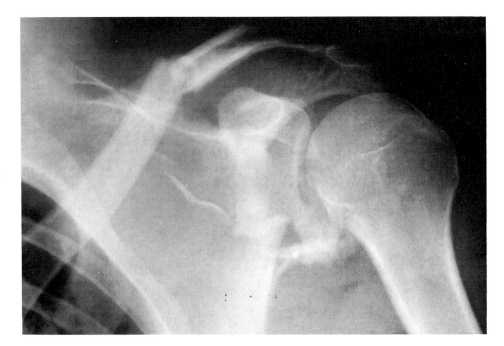

Figure 10–19. A comminuted glenoid articular surface fracture with satisfactory position.

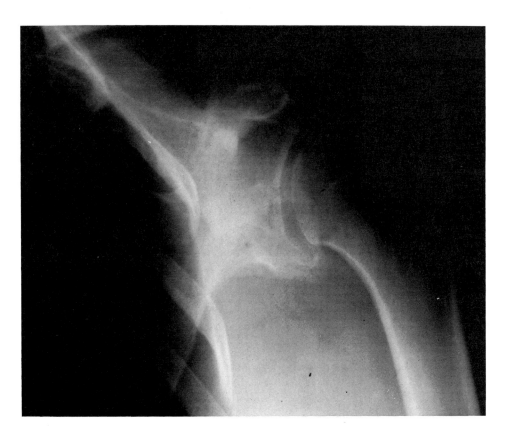

Figure 10–20. This fracture healed well without problems and with good preservation of the joint surface.

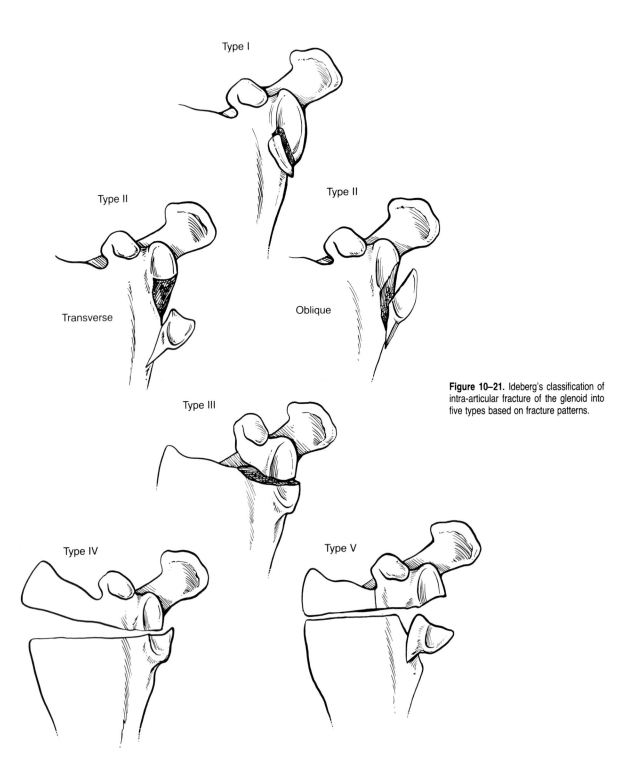

Figure 10–21. Ideberg's classification of intra-articular fracture of the glenoid into five types based on fracture patterns.

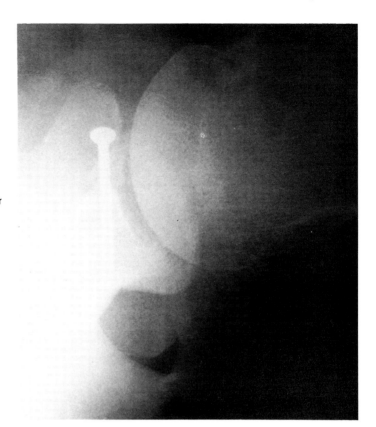

Figure 10–22. An anterior glenoid fracture seen on an axillary view after open reduction internal fixation.

margin. Figure 10–22 shows such a fracture repaired with open reduction and AO screw fixation.

Ideberg believed that the size of the fragment is not prognostic for further instability. DePalma thought that displacements greater than 10 mm, particularly if the size of the fragment is one-fourth of the glenoid, would indicate an open reduction.[21] Late open reduction of the displaced fragment or reconstruction of the anterior glenoid is difficult, often requiring a bone graft or coracoid bone block. In his Bankart study, Rowe found that those fractures involving one-fourth or even one-third of the glenoid had equal success with repair compared with those in which one-sixth or less of the glenoid was involved.[106]

Rockwood recommended that a fracture involving one-fourth of the glenoid fossa that is associated with shoulder instability is an indication for open reduction of the fragment with screw fixation.[99] A CT scan is helpful in determining fragment size and humeral head position (Fig. 10–23).

Ideberg's indication for operation is persisting subluxation or an unstable reduction (recurrent instability soon after reduction). No details were given, but 125 to 130 cases of glenoid avulsion in Ideberg's report had a satisfactory outcome. Of the 68 with associated dislocations, 11 had surgery, 5 with satisfactory results.

A distinction must be made between a glenoid avulsion fracture and a small glenoid rim or labrum avulsion fracture, which is commonly seen with trau-

matic anterior shoulder instability. These lesions are evidence of injury from traumatic anterior instability, not an indication for acute repair or reconstruction. Posterior rim fractures are much less common and similar judgment is applied.

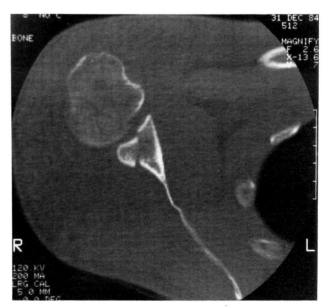

Figure 10–23. A CT scan showing a large glenoid fracture with residual humeral head subluxation.

When the decision is made to treat a large anterior glenoid fracture nonsurgically, follow-up x-rays must be taken and an examination done. A chronic dislocation may occur, especially in older patients, and postreduction resubluxation may go unnoticed.[56]

Type II

A Type II fracture involves a transverse or oblique fracture through the glenoid with the inferior glenoid as a free fragment. The humeral head may sublux inferiorly, with the fragment leading the surgeon to consider open reduction (Figs. 10–24, 10–25, and 10–26).

Type III

A Type III fracture involves the upper third of the glenoid and includes the coracoid; it may occur along the old epiphyseal line separating ossification centers. This fracture is often accompanied by a fractured acromion or clavicle or by acromioclavicular separation (Figs. 10–27, 10–28, and 10–29).

Intact glenohumeral ligaments may keep the incongruity slight, and early motion may spontaneously improve fracture position. Open reduction is difficult, as it is in Type II. One technique uses an anterior arthrotomy (deltopectoral approach) as used for anterior reconstruction, plus superior exposure for a superior-to-inferior glenoid screw. Partial-thickness clavicle removal or even resection of the distal clavicle may need to be done to clear a path for the screw. Five of Ideberg's 17 cases in Type III had a poor result, usually with associated injuries. Only one of the 17 had open reduction.

Type IV

A Type IV fracture is a horizontal glenoid fracture extending all the way through the body to the axillary border. Four of Ideberg's 23 patients had poor results from an extra-articular origin, and three of the 23 from glenoid irregularity. Again, open reduction was difficult.

Type V

Type V combines Types II and IV. Direct violent trauma was the cause in most cases, often delaying scapular treatment and probably influencing the results. Interestingly, of the seven patients out of 20 who had poor results, all 7 had surgery, whereas only 1 of 13 good results had open reduction (Figs. 10–30 and 10–31).

Ideberg's experiences with Types II through V, which represent 40 per cent of the total series, are summarized as follows. Closed reduction under anesthesia was always unsuccessful in improving fracture

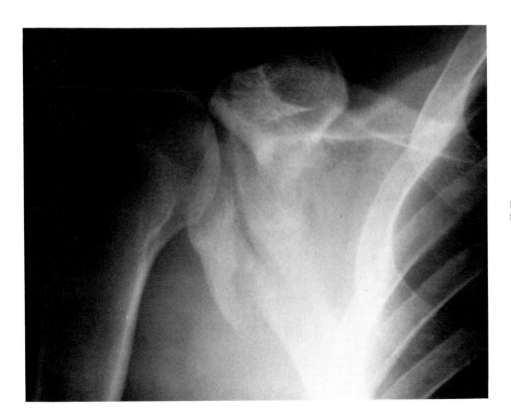

Figure 10–24. A Type II (oblique) glenoid fracture treated with early rehabilitation.

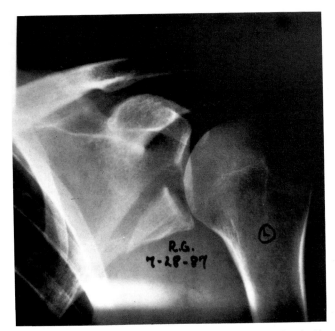

Figure 10–25. An anterior glenoid fracture associated with anterior shoulder instability.

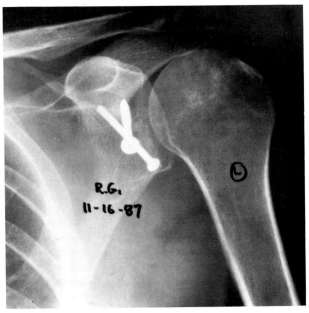

Figure 10–26. Anterior glenoid rim fracture fixed with open reduction and fixation with two screws.

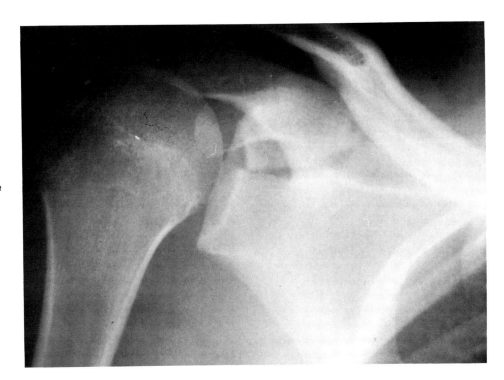

Figure 10–27. A Type III glenoid fracture along an old epiphyseal line.

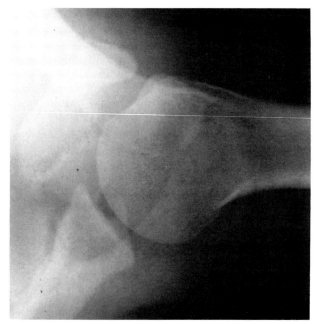

Figure 10–28. A Type III glenoid fracture including the base of the coracoid and the upper third of the glenoid, seen on an axillary view.

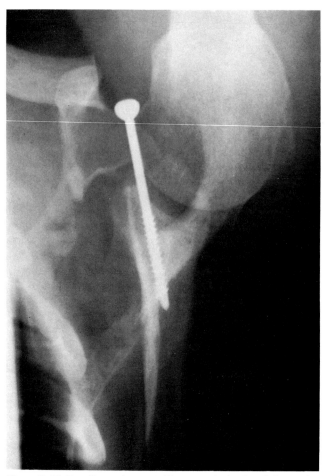

Figure 10–29. Type III nonunion, treated by open reduction through the anterior and superior approaches with resection of the distal clavicle.

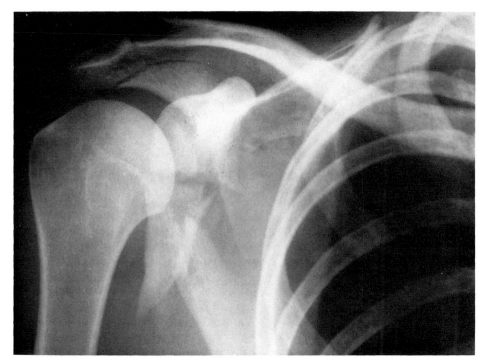

Figure 10–30. Type V glenoid fracture.

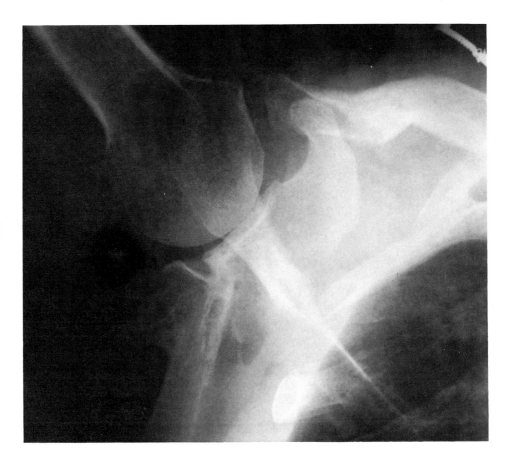

Figure 10–31. Type V glenoid fracture, well healed, with good functional motion without pain.

position at the time, but some late improvement in displacement was seen in most of the conservatively treated fractures. This improvement in fracture position may come from molding by muscle forces across the joint. A good result occurred in 75 per cent of the cases of Types II to V and was obtained mainly by early mobilization. Open reduction, however, can also produce a good result. Associated problems, such as other fractures about the shoulder, nerve, or muscle lesions, may worsen the outcome.

Some European literature suggests a more aggressive surgical indication to scapular fracture treatment. Basing their evaluation on true anteroposterior, tangential scapular lateral, and axillary lateral x-rays, Hardegger and coworkers[39] described eight varieties of fracture with some surgical indication: (1) fracture of the body with a lateral spike entering the joint; (2) fracture of the glenoid rim with instability after reduction of dislocation; (3) fracture of the glenoid fossa, displaced; (4) extra-articular fracture of the glenoid neck with lateral and distal displacement; (5) similar displaced neck fractures with a displaced clavicle fracture or coracoclavicular ligament rupture (they felt that these extra-articular fractures resulted in functional imbalance and altered the glenohumeral-acromial relationship); (6) fracture of the acromion (if significant displacement is present, nonunion may develop or the deltoid may tilt the acromion fragment inferiorly, in-

terfering with rotator cuff function); (7) fracture of the coracoid, displaced with neurovascular compression or with coracoclavicular ligament rupture; and (8) avulsion of the coracoid tip in an athlete.

The surgical approach is anterior for anterior glenoid rim and coracoid fractures. The posterior approach is employed for neck and glenoid fossa fractures, detaching the infraspinatus and using a lag screw or inferior buttress plate fixation.

SCAPULAR BODY FRACTURE

Direct violence and sudden contraction of divergent muscles may cause fractures of the body of the scapula. Other reported causes include electrical shock treatments and accidental electrical shock causing seizures.[10, 42a, 64, 117] Of all scapular fractures, body fractures have the highest incidence of associated injury. Scapular fractures may be quite comminuted and displaced. True anteroposterior and trauma lateral (tangential scapular lateral) x-rays of the shoulder will show the scapular body fracture (Figs. 10–32 and 10–33). Axillary and cephalic tilt views may also be helpful in looking for other fractures, as injury often is not isolated to the body. CT is not usually helpful in treatment (Fig. 10–34). In the immediate treatment of these fractures, no reduction is attempted. The patient

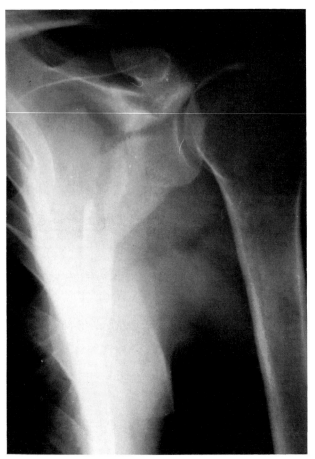

Figure 10–32. A comminuted fracture of the body of the scapula.

ACROMION FRACTURE

The acromion commonly absorbs direct superior blows, with acromioclavicular separation being a much more common sequela than acromion fracture. Most acromial fractures have very little displacement. Commonly the fracture line is lateral to the acromioclavicular joint, causing confusion with os acromiale. In addition to the standard views, x-ray evaluation must include axillary and 30-degree caudal tilt views. A supraspinatus outlet view may be helpful, as well as x-rays of the contralateral shoulder to look for os acromiale (bilateral in 60 per cent of patients) and to compare acromial configuration.

Another mechanism of acromial fracture is traumatic or superior displacement of the humeral head. This often causes an associated extensive rotator cuff tear. If the humeral head is displaced upward in the subacromial space (acromiohumeral distance is reduced), a rotator cuff tear should be suspected and an arthrogram obtained. A stress fracture can occur in association with the superior migration of the humeral head as is seen with long-standing cuff disease (Fig. 10–35). Cuff repair and open reduction of the end of the acromion probably should be done. Acromionectomy should, as always, be avoided. An acromial avulsion by deltoid force has been reported.[57]

is given local ice and immobilization for comfort. Cross-strapping with adhesive moleskin to immobilize the scapula in a nonambulatory patient was described by Neer and Bateman.[6] Such immobilization may produce a stiff shoulder.[69] Pendulum exercises, use of overhead pulleys, and a further passive or active assisted range-of-motion program are begun within a week after injury. Multiple muscle attachments form an excellent environment for healing, and nonunion is very rare. Pain may persist until the fracture is solid, but a full range of motion should be the goal in rehabilitation to mobilize the scapula, and progressive-resistance exercises to the rotator cuff and deltoid are essential.

Normal bony anatomy is not necessary for good function in a healed scapular body fracture. Perceived malunion with scapulothoracic irritation rarely restricts shoulder function, although when accompanied by associated scarring, it may impair scapular motion.

There is mention in the literature of operative treatments of body fractures. These include an acute excision of a displaced inferolateral fragment[40] and an open reduction for body fracture, which "interferes in unity of the scapula in performing function as adjunct to arm elevation."[31]

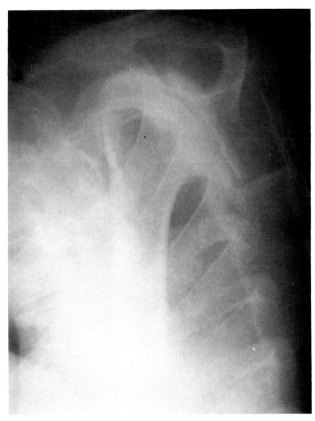

Figure 10–33. A tangential scapulolateral view showing a comminuted body fracture.

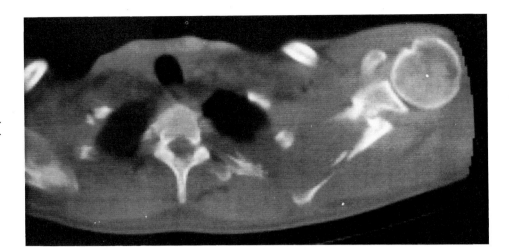

Figure 10–34. A CT scan showing fracture of the body with an intact glenohumeral joint.

A nondisplaced fracture of the acromion should respond well to initial symptomatic treatment and the use of a sling for three weeks. Rehabilitation is begun immediately with range-of-motion exercises—passive initially—progressing to isometrics and an active program of rotator cuff and deltoid progressive-resistance exercises after fracture healing.

Results of simple acromial fracture treatment are generally good. Loss of motion, however, was noted by Wilbur and Evans,[120] who recommended cast im-

mobilization in 60 degrees of abduction, 25 degrees of forward flexion, and 25 degrees of external rotation for six weeks. Displaced fractures occasionally require elevation and Kirschner wire or screw fixation to eliminate impingement or to reduce the acromioclavicular joint (Fig. 10–36).[82] Acromial nonunion is reported in isolated cases. Darrach[20] recommended open reduction, fixation, and immobilization. Ruther[109] used a bone graft and cast. Wong-Pack and associates used a plate across the clavicle to the acromion.[123] Mick and

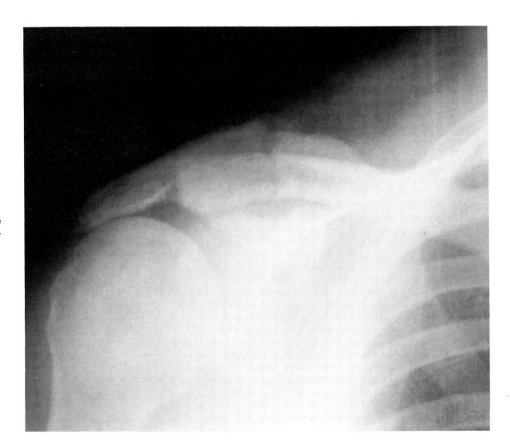

Figure 10–35. A stress fracture of the acromion in a patient with cuff arthropathy.

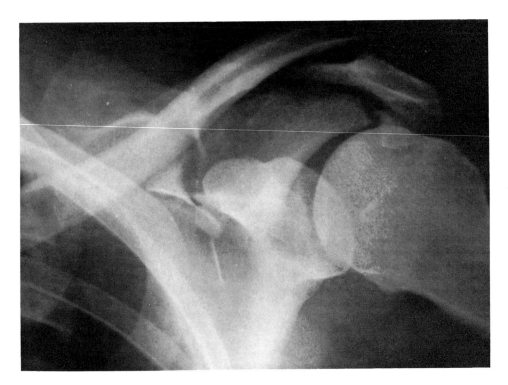

Figure 10–36. A displaced acromion fracture, a reasonable candidate for open reduction.

Weiland employed a lag screw and plate along the scapular spine.[74] Neer reminds us that no more than a small fragment of acromion should ever be excised.[82]

A fracture of the base of the acromion near the spine, if displaced, may progress to nonunion, and acute open reduction fixation is a good option (Figs. 10–37, 10–38, and 10–39). As always, when contemplating early surgery for the scapular fracture, the clinical picture, age, and occupation of the patient must be carefully considered. With the small cross-section of contact area in acromion fractures, postoperative protection is necessary.

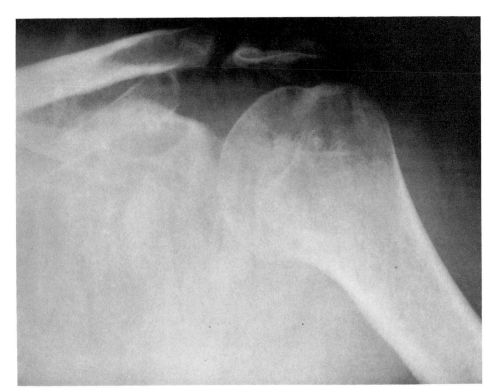

Figure 10–37. Nonunion of the acromion.

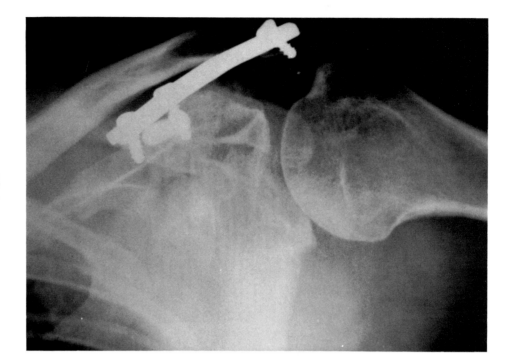

Figure 10–38. Nonunion of the acromion, fixed with an intercalary graft and AO plate anchored along the spine of the scapula.

CORACOID FRACTURE

The coracoid is an important part of the attachment of the limb flexion muscles and ligaments, especially those stabilizing the clavicle. The coracoid is not readily visualized by an anteroposterior x-ray; an axillary view and an anteroposterior cephalic tilt view of 35 to 60 degrees are needed (Fig. 10–40). A Stryker notch view[123] and Goldberg[37] posterior oblique 20-degree cephalic tilt views are also helpful. Weight-hanging films may also be helpful if an associated acromioclavicular separation is present. Fractures of the coracoid may be isolated, occurring from a direct blow to the coracoid or to the point of the shoulder. Coracoid fracture may also occur along with acromioclavicular dislocation, with the coracoclavicular ligaments remaining intact.[9, 49, 125] This occurs with traction exerted on the intact ligaments, avulsing the coracoid at its base or through an epiphyseal line. A radiographic clue to diagnosis is a normal and symmetrical coracoclavicular distance with x-ray and clinical evidence of third-degree acromioclavicular separation with a high-riding clavicle (Fig. 10–41). A cephalic tilt view, especially taken to evaluate the clavicle, may reveal the fracture. I believe the best view is the Stryker notch view. This coracoid fracture may be overlooked when attention is restricted to the obvious acromioclavicular separation. The coracoid tip may be avulsed by muscle pull of the biceps and coracobrachialis[102] or from direct contact from a dislocating humeral head.[35, 69] Garcia-Elias and Salo pointed out that this association is easily missed and that follow-up postreduction axillary lateral x-ray is necessary if pain continues in the shoulder (Fig. 10–42).[35] Fatigue fractures, such as trapshooter's

shoulder,[11] have been reported. There are case reports of coracoid fractures with complications from surgical use of the coracoclavicular tape fixation[78] and from medial humeral head migration from cuff arthropathy (Fig. 10–43).

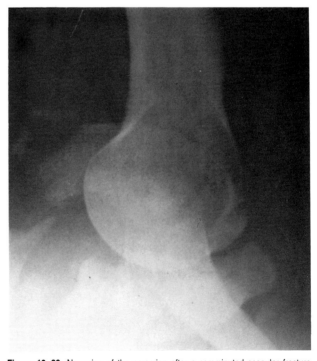

Figure 10–39. Nonunion of the acromion after a comminuted scapular fracture, well seen on an axillary view.

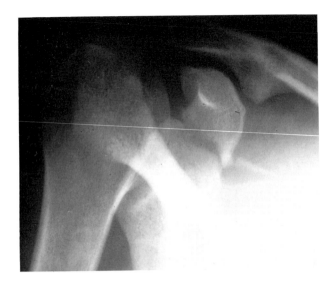

Figure 10–40. A 35-degree cephalic tilt view showing a fracture of the base of the coracoid.

The fracture occurs most commonly through the base and is minimally displaced unless significant acromioclavicular separation occurs. A fracture line may extend across the suprascapular notch to the superior surface of the scapula or into the upper third of the glenoid. Confusion may exist with a normal accessory ossification center; such a center may be present at the ligament insertion at the site of an avulsion. (See the section on epiphyseal lines.)

In the coracoid fracture with acromioclavicular separation, surgical and nonsurgical treatment appear to offer equally favorable results. The literature is not clear about the time required for union, but no nonunions are reported. Some authors believe that open reduction is indicated, but only for treatment of the acromioclavicular separation. Stability of the fractured coracoid is supplied by the coracoacromial and coracoclavicular ligaments superiorly and by the pectoralis

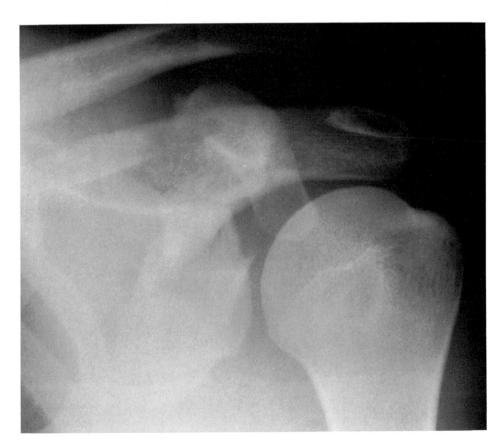

Figure 10–41. A third-degree acromioclavicular separation with fractured base of the coracoid and a comminuted glenoid fracture. Note the normal coracoclavicular distance, indicating intact ligaments.

minor and conjoined tendon inferiorly. For the isolated coracoid fracture, therefore, most authors feel that no specific treatment is needed since an anatomical alignment is not essential for adequate function or healing. For a displaced fracture, especially with associated acromioclavicular separation, Bateman recommended shoulder spica or acromioclavicular fixation (Fig. 10–44).[6] Other authors' indications for surgery include "marked displacement,"[105] associated acromioclavicular separation,[58, 63, 82, 112, 120] and compression of the brachial plexus.[82] Neer also described suprascapular nerve paralysis with fracture in the area of the suprascapular notch. Electromyography is essential in the diagnosis, and early exploration is usually indicated.[82]

McLaughlin felt that fibrous union is not uncommon but is rarely symptomatic.[69] Garcia-Elias and Salo reported a case of a painful coracoid nonunion discovered late after shoulder dislocation, which did well after excision of the fragment.[35] Both Steindler[114] and Benton and Nelson[8] have reported that the tip of the corocoid can be excised and the conjoined tendons reattached to the remaining corocoid process.

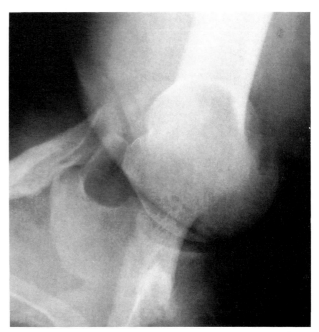

Figure 10–42. Fracture of the coracoid tip from a direct blow, seen on Stryker notch, cephalic tilt view.

AVULSION FRACTURES OF THE SCAPULA

Some of these injuries have been discussed within the anatomical groups, but they will be mentioned here for completeness owing to a common mechanism. Scapular fracture due to avulsion of its many muscular and ligament attachments is uncommon. Four mechanisms may be involved:[43] (1) uncoordinated muscle contraction due to electrical shock, electroconvulsive therapy, or seizures; (2) muscle pull as the result of trauma or unusual exertion; (3) ligamentous avulsion; and (4) stress fracture near a muscle attachment.

A coracoid fracture may occur by a coracoclavicular ligament avulsion associated with acromioclavicular separation,[49, 82, 112] by resisted muscle force (coracobrachialis, short head of the biceps) with direct blow,[22, 102] and by stress fracture of the tip.[8, 11] An electroshock treatment caused an avulsion fracture.[51, 96] A superior scapular border avulsion is seen as an extension of the fractured coracoid, created by the coracoclavicular ligament or possibly by avulsion of the omohyoid muscle.[49] Deltoid avulsion of the acromion is seen in case reports[43, 57, 97] and can be easily confused with os acromiale.

Results of Treatment

Results of scapular fracture treatment have been reported generally across the spectrum of injuries, with satisfactory functional results with conservative treatment. McGahan and coworkers,[67] Lindblom and Leven,[61] McLaughlin,[69] Zdravkovic and Damholt,[124]

and Armstrong[3] all had series of patients with fractures of the scapula treated nonsurgically. Few patients had long-term disability of the shoulder. Steindler[114] in 1946 reported insignificant disability associated with nonsurgical treatment and found occasional limitation of abduction in neck fractures with grating and limitation of motion due to surrounding scar in body fractures. He thought that intra-articular glenoid fracture, however, could lead to painful post-traumatic arthritis. Armstrong[3] found 6 of 11 extra-articular neck fractures

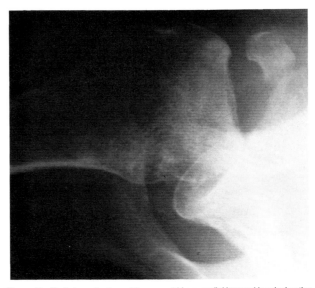

Figure 10–43. A stress fracture of the coracoid from medial humeral head migration in cuff arthropathy.

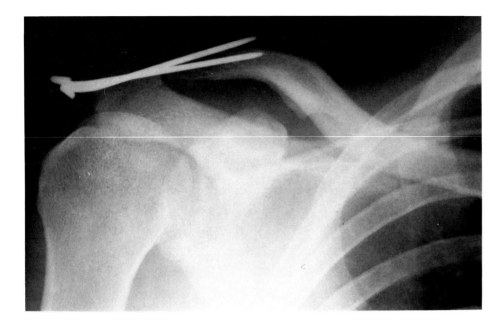

Figure 10–44. Open reduction of the acromioclavicular joint with transacromion clavicular joint pins.

to have residual stiffness but no functional disability. Three of his six patients with glenoid fractures, however, had restricted painful movement in follow-up. Wilbur and Evans[120] grouped their acromion, glenoid, and coracoid fractures and found 10 of 11 to have a decreased range of motion, with poor results in only 2. Zdravkovic and Damholt[124] found 23 of 28 patients to have moderately severe deformity by x-ray in follow-up, but only two had restricted elevation (both were intra-articular glenoid fractures). Only two patients changed occupation, and only one had severe osteoarthritis after nine years. Again, published results support conservative management of most scapular fractures.

Author's Preferred Method of Treatment

GLENOID NECK FRACTURE

Reduction of displaced extra-articular scapular neck fractures is not necessary to obtain a good clinical result. Early experience with traction does not improve the fracture position and necessitates prolonged recumbency and hospital stay. Symptomatic local care, followed in a few days by passive exercises, allows satisfactory motion and does not interfere with fracture healing. When a displaced clavicle fracture accompanies a medially displaced glenoid neck fracture, an unstable segment that includes the glenoid, acromion, and lateral clavicle is created. Stabilization by plate fixation of the clavicle allows for much faster rehabilitation.

BODY AND SPINE

Patients are examined for associated injuries, which are very common with body fractures. Symptomatic treatment is indicated, with ice and sling immobilization followed by stretching exercises and later, after fracture healing, by scapular mobilization and shoulder girdle strengthening.

GLENOID

X-ray evaluation is important. Axillary and West Point views as well as CT are used to diagnose significant glenoid fractures involving 25 per cent or more of the joint surface. One must separate these from a small avulsion fracture. If these larger fragments are displaced, open reduction and small AO screw fixation is indicated, possibly using the new AO small cannulated screws. The chance for continued instability if left untreated, especially in the younger age group, approaches 100 per cent. The operative approach, although difficult, is easier than in later reconstruction with fragment fixation, iliac bone graft, coracoid bone block, or Bankart repair. I start gentle motion at seven days in these patients.

The other types of glenoid fractures described by Ideberg (Types II through V), have less clear indications for operative treatment. If the humeral head is centered on the major portion of the glenoid and the shoulder joint is stable, then nonsurgical treatment is indicated as the head remains intracapsular. When the humeral head appears to be subluxed along with a major fragment, surgical treatment with capsular repair is indicated. Again, a work-up with carefully positioned tomograms and CT gives the surgeon a three-dimensional view of the fracture. I usually prefer the anterior approach to reduce the fracture, combined with superior visualization to pass the screw. The path of the screw is cleared by partial-thickness clavicle removal or even by resection of the distal clavicle. It is critical to understand the obliquity of the fracture before this can be planned. This surgery is most difficult and the fixation often is not pleasing.

ACROMION

As stated earlier, most fractures of the acromion are without significant displacement. They should be protected in a supervised passive and active assisted exercise program with no resisted deltoid function until union occurs. If there has been upward movement of the humeral head, fracturing the acromion, then the rotator cuff must be investigated and repaired. It is important to remember the presence of os acromiale as part of the differential diagnosis for fracture; its presence alone is associated with an increased incidence of cuff disease.[82] The use of a dorsal tension band wire is a good technique for acromial fracture fixation.

CORACOID

The Stryker notch or the 35-degree cephalic tilt view provides the information needed to assess the displacement of the coracoid fracture. Complete third-degree acromioclavicular separation combined with the significantly displaced coracoid fracture is an indication for open reduction of both injuries with trans-acromioclavicular Steinmann pin fixation (see Fig. 10–44). I have experience with two late explorations of suprascapular nerve injury in association with coracoid and body fractures and agree with Neer, who favors early exploration of the nerve.

Other Disorders

DISLOCATION OF THE SCAPULA

Dislocation of the scapula between the ribs and into the thoracic cage is very rare. Ainscow describes one type with little violence and a pre-existing factor such as generalized laxity or locking osteochondroma.[1] The medial border is lodged between the third and fourth ribs or in the fourth to fifth intercostal space.[83] A second type is associated with more violent trauma with chest injury. This is a rare variation of the injury and usually causes fracture of the scapula and ribs. The rhomboid muscles must be stretched or torn.[52] The diagnosis is suspected by upper extremity exami

nation and inspection of the posterior chest wall, but may be missed owing to associated injuries or not appreciated on anteroposterior views of the chest.

Nettrour and colleagues' series had a case where the displaced scapula was felt to be a chest wall hematoma on plain chest films.[83] The Nettrour anterior oblique or tangential scapular lateral (trauma lateral) views or CT scan will confirm the diagnosis. Reduction under general anesthesia is accomplished by hyperabducting the arm and manually manipulating the axillary border, rotating the scapula forward and at the same time pushing it back, as described by DePalma.[21] Acute reduction is usually stable, but adhesive strapping plus collar and cuff is recommended by Key and Conwell.[52] Late discovery may require open reduction and soft tissue reattachment to maintain reduction.[83]

SCAPULOTHORACIC DISSOCIATION

A new term, *scapulothoracic dissociation,* describes violent lateral displacement of the scapula with clavicle disruption and severe soft tissue injury (i.e., to the brachial plexus and with or without vascular disruption) with intact skin.[24, 25] It has been described by Ebraheim and coworkers[25] as "closed, traumatic forequarter amputation" and has been infrequently reported, as most patients have died. Soft tissue injury includes complete or partial tears of the deltoid, pectoralis, and posterior scapular muscles. Vascular disruption occurs most frequently at the level of the subclavian artery. Most often there is complete avulsion of the brachial plexus, but incomplete neuropraxia is possible. Bony injury may appear as acromioclavicular or sternoclavicular separation or clavicle fracture. Ipsilateral upper extremity fractures are often also present. Associated injuries are usually discovered early, without full appreciation of the magnitude of the injury. The diagnosis is made when a nonrotated chest x-ray shows significant lateral displacement of the scapula as measured by the distance from the sternal notch to the coracoid, glenoid margin, or medial scapular border. Kelbel and associates[50] found the ratio of the medial border to spine distances to be 1.5 or greater. Figure 10–45 shows this measurement.

The primary mode of injury is direct trauma occurring, for example, during a motorcycle, millwheel, haybaler, or motor vehicle accident.[90] Extremities are flail and pulseless, but swelling from dissecting hematoma may be the only external signs. A more distal vascular injury may divert attention from the more severe proximal injury. Following resuscitation of the patient, the chest x-ray should be carefully inspected and arteriography performed to delineate the vascular lesion. Exploration to restore vascular integrity and diagnose the level and severity of the brachial plexus injury is next. Based on this information and on assessment of scapular muscle damage, early above-elbow amputation and shoulder fusion is considered.[24, 25] Rorabeck found no advantage to shoulder arthrodesis

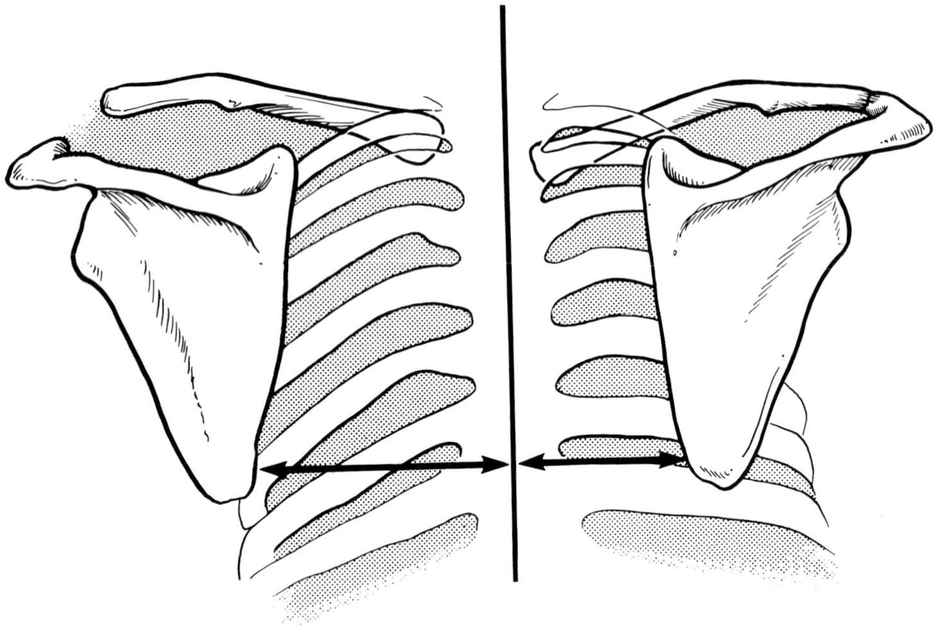

Figure 10–45. A diagram of scapulothoracic dissociation, demonstrating a lateral displacement of the scapula on the injured side *(left)* compared with the normal side *(right)* on a nonrotated chest x-ray.

in this setting.[101] If parts of the brachial plexus remain intact, vascular and neurological repair for limb salvage is indicated.

SNAPPING SCAPULA

Scapulothoracic crepitus (snapping scapula) should not always be considered a pathological symptom, nor is it an entity often with a clear cause. Scapulothoracic pain often is related to disease of the glenohumeral joint, subacromial bursa, or cervical spine. Such pain may also be part of the syndrome of multiple trigger points termed fibrositis.

A localized anatomical diagnosis for the snapping scapula is rarely made. This fact leads the surgeon to a conservative approach to treatment. The convex chest wall normally is congruent and allows smooth, gliding motion to the convex deep surface of the scapula and interposed muscles. The inferior, medial, and superior borders are not as well cushioned. Clinically, according to Milch,[76] the snapping scapula was first described by Boinet in 1867. In the same year, DeMarquay presented a postmortem examination with exostosis on the deep surface of the scapula. The recent literature on snapping scapula is scant and is mostly provided by Milch.[75, 76, 77] Scapular sounds have been described by Milch[75, 76, 77] and attributed to Boinet and Mauclaire. *Froissement* is a general friction sound, the consequence of normal muscle action, and is considered physiological and usually asymptomatic. *Froittement* is somewhat louder and may be a grating or snapping sound, possibly pathological. *Craquemont* is a loud, snapping sound, often associated with pain and functional complaints. The intensity of the sound,

however, does not parallel the severity of symptoms, nor does it indicate the presence of a diagnosable anatomical entity. Scapular sounds have been found in 8 to 70 per cent of the normal population in older studies cited by Milch.[75] "Abnormally loud sounds," however, are quite rare.

There are anatomical causes for snapping scapula. Changes in the bony structure of the deep surface of the scapula or in the opposing surface of the ribs are the most easily understood. Osteochondroma is the most common scapular tumor and may present as a mass on the deep surface projecting into the scapulothoracic space. A rib exostosis could do the same and cause snapping. These lesions are often difficult to see on anteroposterior x-ray, and a tangential scapulolateral view or CT scan is needed (Figs. 10–46 and 10–47).

Osteochondromata are usually sessile[79] and will grow until overall growth plate closure occurs. Milch[76] described a three-year-old girl with subscapular exostosis causing thumping sounds. Complete relief followed excision. Parsons[92] had four similar patients who responded well to excision of the mass. Exostoses with adventitious bursae have been described.[71, 92]

The symptoms range from the shoulder "jumping out of place" to "winging" (posterior scapular prominence) and slight crepitation. Cooley and Torg[17] described a case of "pseudowinging" with the scapula pushed posteriorly by deep surface osteochondroma. This patient also had mild compression of the long thoracic nerve. There was no residual deformity 10 weeks after tumor removal. A palpable mass, scapular grating, prominence at rest, and the presence of normal scapulohumeral rhythm are important in the differential diagnosis favoring pseudowinging or a scapular

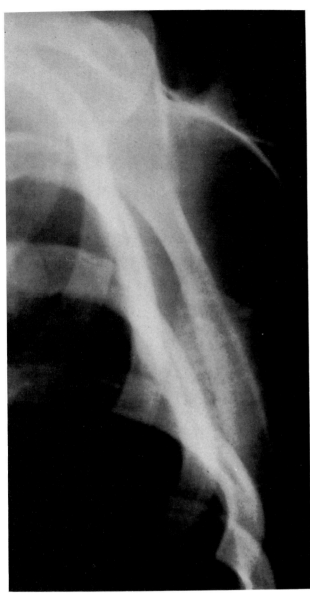

Figure 10–46. A slightly oblique tangential scapulolateral view showing a large, deep scapular surface osteochondroma.

prominence forced out by a deep surface mass. Electrical studies, of course, are important in the diagnosis of neurological causes of true winging.

Serratus anterior function, holding the scapula against the chest wall, is thought to be necessary for the snapping to occur. Other bony projections described in the past include Luschka's tubercle, referring to an exostosis with bony enlargement of the superiomedial scapula. Also described is a so-called scapular hook with the superior angle of the scapula being unusually long or having increased curvature. Both of these entities are considered to be causes of snapping scapula, but clinical data (after resection) are not available. It is important to stress that their presence may not cause symptoms nor their removal result in improvement. Snapping may occur with Sprengel's

deformity, possibly from the omovertebral bone or from the abnormal scapular shape. Milch believes that a bony mass at the site of a healing rib fracture can also cause the snapping.[75, 76]

A scapular fracture malunion causing snapping, however, was not seen in Rockwood's scapular fracture cases. The concave anterior surface of the scapula is usually maintained with fracture healing. Scapular grating was mentioned in a description of follow-up results of scapular fracture by Steindler.[114]

Soft tissue causes of snapping scapula are less well understood. Milch in 1961 described interstitial scar changes in the muscle (attributed to Volkmann in 1922) or anatomical variation in muscle (Testut).[75] Bateman[6] described the lesion as periosteal microtears with scars and spur formation in the medial muscle attachment. Strizak and Cowen in 1982 documented such a case, with part of the levator scapulae insertion being successfully excised.[115] Rockwood has seen a rhomboid muscle avulsion flap excised with elimination of snapping and pain.[100]

The subscapular bursae are described in 19th-century literature.[75] One is at the superomedial angle between the serratus anterior and the subscapularis; a second is between the serratus anterior and the lateral chest wall; a third may be present at the inferior angle of the scapula. Steroid injections are often given in the posterior scapula, ostensibly for "subscapular bursitis." How often such bursae or adventitious bursae occur is unknown. Loss of muscle bulk from muscle atrophy or after shoulder fusion or weight loss reduces the cushion and may be a cause of the scapular sounds. Clinically the patient describes an audible and palpable snapping in the scapulothoracic area with shoulder girdle movements. It is usually voluntarily produced, may be painful, and often is bilateral.

Differential Diagnosis

A differential diagnosis of painful snapping scapula includes all causes of posterior scapular pain, ignoring the snapping symptom. Such posterior pain may have its origin as referred pain from the glenohumeral joint or subacromial bursa or from cervical root compression, joint disease, or neck muscle strain. Thoracic outlet compression is part of the differential diagnosis. "Thoracic disc" with root compression is rare and difficult to diagnose but usually includes unilateral pain in a dermatomal distribution.

Treatment

A work-up usually fails to turn up either an obvious cause (e.g., an osteochondroma) or a possible surgical solution. Palliative treatment includes local care with heat and scapular adduction and postural shoulder shrug exercises. Local injection of bupivacaine hydrochloride (Marcaine) and a steroid into the tender area or into the subscapular region can be helpful; care must be taken to stay in the proper plane, as the author

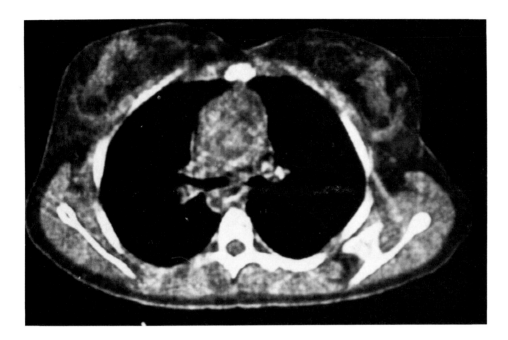

Figure 10–47. A CT scan of the body showing the same large osteochondroma on the deep surface of the scapula, causing posterior prominence of the scapula and snapping scapula symptoms.

has had experience with pneumothorax with such a deep injection.

Surgical treatment that has been described includes removal of the documented bony intrusion into the scapulothoracic space from the scapula or ribs. Resection of the medial border, especially the superomedial border of the scapula, without definite bony deformity has been indicated by Milch in the past after careful localization of the sounds.[75] Mauclaire also has described the creation of a muscle flap of the trapezius or rhomboids sewn onto the deep surface of the scapula.

The scapular deep surface can be exposed readily by subperiosteal detachment of muscles. The superomedial angle can be dissected through an approach that opens the trapezius fascia and splits the fibers, exposing the levator scapulae, subscapularis, and rhomboids. Subperiosteal dissection is done, staying medial to the suprascapular notch and lateral to the dorsal scapular nerves, which lie medial to the vertebral border of the scapula.

Author's Preferred Treatment

Unless an exostosis is clearly seen in the scapulothoracic space, off the scapula or ribs, or unless rib deformity is present, I believe that the best course of treatment is one of rehabilitation. If one feels that there is a clear soft tissue abnormality of the scapular border, exploration under local anesthesia may be tried with the patient able to demonstrate the snapping. I have excised the superomedial angle of the scapula in several patients, blaming it for painful snapping. These cases of normal-appearing x-ray studies with positive injection tests had mixed results. One should beware of patients who can grind, pop, or snap the scapula,

particularly in cases of litigation, after minor trauma, or in worker's compensation cases. Often these patients have a similar sound on the contralateral side. A complete history, physical examination, plain x-ray, or bone scan will suggest an unusual cause, such as a neoplasm or an infection or intrathoracic or abdominal disease. Fibrositis remains a common differential, especially when multiple trigger points are also present elsewhere, away from the posterior scapula.

References

1. Ainscow DA: Dislocation of the scapula. J Coll Surg Edinb *27:*56–57, 1982.
2. Anderson LD: Fractures. *In* Crenshaw AH (ed): Campbell's Operative Orthopaedics, 5th ed. St. Louis: CV Mosby, 1971.
3. Armstrong CP, and Vanderspuy J: The fractured scapula: importance in management based on a series of 62 patients. Injury *15:*324–329, 1984.
4. Aston JW, and Gregory CF: Dislocation of the shoulder with significant fracture of the glenoid. J Bone Joint Surg *55A:*1531–1533, 1973.
5. Banerjee AK, and Field S: An unusual scapular fracture caused by a water skiing accident. Br J Radiol *58:*465–467, 1985.
6. Bateman JE: The Shoulder and Neck, 2nd ed. Philadelphia: WB Saunders, 1978.
7. Benchetrit E, and Friedman B: Fracture of the coracoid process associated with subglenoid dislocation of the shoulder. J Bone and Joint Surg *61A:*295, 1979.
8. Benton J, and Nelson C: Avulsion of the coracoid process in an athlete. J Bone Joint Surg *53A:*356–358, 1971.
9. Bernard TN, Brunet ME, and Haddad RJ Jr: Fractured coracoid process in acromioclavicular dislocations. Clin Orthop *175:*227–231, 1983.
10. Beswick DR, Morse SD, and Barnes AU: Bilateral scapular fractures from low voltage electrical injury—a case report. Ann Emerg Med *11:*12–13, 1982.
11. Boyer DW: Trap shooter's shoulder: stress fracture of the coracoid process. J Bone and Joint Surg *57A:*862, 1975.
12. Caffey J (ed): Pediatric X-ray Diagnosis, 7th ed. Chicago: Year Book Medical Publishers, 1978, pp 320–321.

13. Cameron HU: Snapping scapula: a report of three cases. Eur J Rheumatol Inflamm 7:66–67, 1984.
14. Charlton MR: Fracture, neck of the scapula. NW Med 37:18–21, 1938.
15. Cigtay OS, and Mascatello VJ: Scapular defects: a normal variation. AJR 132:239–241, 1979.
16. Cockshott WP: The coracoclavicular joint. Radiology 132:313–316, Feb. 1979.
17. Cooley LH, and Torg JS: "Pseudo-winging" of the scapula secondary to subscapular osteochondroma. Clin Orthop 162:119–124, 1982.
18. Cotton FJ, and Brickley WJ: Treatment of fracture at the neck of the scapula. Boston Med Surg J 185:326–329, 1921.
19. Coues WP: Fracture of the coracoid process of the scapula. N Engl J Med 212:727–728, 1935.
20. Darrach W: Fractures of the acromion process of the scapula. Ann Surg 54:455, 1914.
21. DePalma AF: Surgery of the Shoulder, 3rd Ed. Philadelphia; JB Lippincott, 1983, pp 366–367.
22. De Rosa GP, and Kettelkamp DB: Fracture of the coracoid process of the scapula: a case report. J Bone and Joint Surg 59A:696–697, 1977.
23. Dzioba RB, and Quinlan WJ: Avascular necrosis of the glenoid. J Trauma 24:448–451, 1984.
24. Ebraheim NA, An S, Jackson WT, et al: Scapulothoracic dissociation. J Bone Joint Surg 70A:428–432, 1988.
25. Ebraheim NA, Pearlstein SR, Savolaine ER, et al: Scapulo-thoracic dissociation (avulsion of the scapula, subclavian artery, and brachial plexus): an early recognized variant, a new clas-sification, and a review of the literature and treatment options. J Orthop Trauma 1:18–23, 1987.
26. Edeland HG, and Zachrisson HE: Fracture of the scapular notch associated with lesion of the suprascapular nerve. Acta Orthop Scand 46:758–763, 1975.
27. Fery A, and Sommelet J: Fractures de l'apophyse coracoide. Rev Chir Orthop 65:403–407, 1979.
28. Findlay RT: Fractures of the scapula and ribs. Am J Surg 38:489–494, 1937.
29. Findlay RT: Fractures of the scapula. Ann Surg 93:1001–1008, 1931.
30. Fischer RP, Flynn TC, Miller PW, and Thompson DA: Scap-ular fractures and associated major ipsilateral upper-torso in-juries. Curr Concepts Trauma Care 1:14–16, 1985.
31. Fischer WR: Fracture of the scapula requiring open reduction: report of a case. J Bone Joint Surg 21:459–461, 1939.
32. Friedrich B, and Winter G: Zur Operativen Therapie von Frakturen der Scapula. Chirurg 44:37–39, 1973.
33. Froimson AI: Fracture of the coracoid process of the scapula. J Bone Joint Surg 60A:710, 1978.
34. Gagney O, Carey JP, and Mazas F: Les fractures recentes de l'omoplate a propos de 43 cas. Rev Chir Orthop 70:443–447, 1984.
35. Garcia-Elias M, and Salo JM: Nonunion of a fractured coracoid process after dislocation of the shoulder. J Bone Joint Surg 67B:722–723, 1985.
36. Gleich JJ: The fractured scapula, a significance in prognosis. Missouri Med 77:24–26, 1980.
37. Goldberg RP, and Vicks B: Oblique angle to view for coracoid fractures. Skeletal Radiol 9:195–197, 1983.
38. Halpern AA, Joseph R, Page J, and Nagel DA: Subclavian artery injury and fracture of the scapula. J Am Coll Emerg Physicians 8:19–20, 1979.
39. Hardegger FH, Simpson LA, and Weber BG: The operative treatment of scapular fractures. J Bone Joint Surg 66B:725–731, 1984.
40. Harmon PH, and Baker DR: Fracture of the scapula with displacement. J Bone Joint Surg 25:834–838, 1943.
41. Hayes J, and Zehr D: Traumatic muscle avulsion causing winging of the scapula. J Bone Joint Surg 68A:495, 1981.
42. Heatly MD, Breck LW, and Higinbotham NL: Bilateral frac-ture of the scapula. Am J Surg 71:256–259, 1946.
42a. Henneking K, Hofmann D, and Kunze K: Skapulafrakturen nach electronunfall. Unfallchirurgie 10:149–151, 1984.

43. Heyse-Moore GH, and Stoker DJ: Avulsion fractures of the scapula. Skeletal Radiol 9:27–32, 1982.
44. Hitzrot T, and Bolling RW: Fracture of the neck of the scapula. Ann Surg 63:215–234, 1916.
45. Hollinshead R, and James KW: Scapulothoracic dislocation (locked scapula). J Bone Joint Surg 61A:1102–1103, 1979.
46. Ideberg R: Unusual glenoid fractures: a report on 92 cases. Acta Orthop Scand 58:191–192, 1987.
47. Ideberg R: Fractures of the scapula involving the glenoid fossa. In Bateman JE, and Welsh RP: Surgery of the Shoulder. BC Decker, 1984, pp 63–66.
48. Imatani RJ: Fractures of the scapula. A review of 53 fractures. J Trauma 15:473–478, 1975.
49. Ishizuki M, Yamaura I, Isobe Y, et al: Avulsion fracture of the superior border of the scapula. A report of five cases. J Bone Joint Surg 63A:820–822, 1981.
50. Kelbel JM, Hardon OM, and Huurman WW: Scapulothoracic dissociation—a case report. Clin Orthop 209:210–214, 1986.
51. Kelly JP: Fractures complicating electroconvulsive therapy in chronic epilepsy. J Bone Joint Surg 36B:70–79, 1954.
52. Key JA, and Conwell HE: The Management of Fractures, Dislocations and Sprains. St. Louis: CV Mosby, 1964.
53. Kohler A, and Zimmer EA: Borderlands of the Normal and Early Pathologic Skeletal Roentgenogram. New York: Grune & Stratton, 1968.
54. Kopecky KK, Bies JR, and Ellis JH: CT diagnosis of fracture of the coracoid process of the scapula. Comput Radiol 8:325–327, 1984.
55. Kozlowski K, Colavita N, Morris L, and Little KET: Bilateral glenoid dysplasia (report of eight cases). Aust Radiol 29:174–177, 1985.
56. Kummel BM: Fractures of the glenoid causing chronic dislo-cation of the shoulder. Clin Orthop 69:189–191, 1970.
57. Laing R, and Dee R: Fracture symposium. Orthop Rev 13:717–720, 1984.
58. Lasda NA, and Murray DG: Fracture separation of the cora-coid process associated with acromioclavicular dislocation. Clin Orthop 134:222–224, 1978.
59. Leffmann R: A case of "rattling shoulder blade." Acta Med Orientalia 6:292–295, 1947.
60. Liberson F: Os acromiale—a contested anomaly. J Bone Joint Surg 19:683–689, 1937.
61. Lindblom A, and Leven H: Prognosis in fractures of the body and neck of the scapula. Acta Chir Scand 140:33, 1974.
62. Longabaugh RI: Fracture simple, right scapula. US Naval Med Bull 27:341–343, 1924.
63. Mariani PP: Isolated fracture of the coracoid process in an athlete. Am J Sports Med 8:129–130, 1980.
64. Mathews RE, Cocke TB, and D'Ambrosia RD: Scapular fractures secondary to seizures in patients without osteodystro-phy. J Bone Joint Surg 65:850–853, 1983.
65. McCally WC, and Kelly DA: Treatment of fractures of the clavicle, ribs and scapula. Am J Surg 50:558–562, 1940.
66. McGahan JP, and Rab GT: Fracture of the acromion associated with axillary nerve deficit. Clin Orthop 147:216–218, 1980.
67. McGahan JP, Rab GT, and Dublin A: Fractures of the scapula. J Trauma 20:880–883, 1980.
68. McClure JG, and Raney RB: Anomalies of the scapula. Clin Orthop 110:22–31, 1975.
69. McLaughlin HL: Trauma. Philadelphia: WB Saunders, 1959.
70. McLennen JG, and Ungersma J: Pneumothorax complicating fractures of the scapula. J Bone Joint Surg 64A:598–599, 1982.
71. McWilliams CA: Subscapular exostosis with adventitious bursa. JAMA 63:1473–1474, 1914.
72. Mencke JB: The frequency and significance of injuries to the acromion process. Ann Surg 59:233–238, 1914.
73. Michele AA, and Davies JJ: Scapulocostal syndrome (fatigue-postural paradox). NY State J Med 50:1353–1356, 1950.
74. Mick CA, and Weiland AJ: Pseudo-arthrosis of a fracture of the acromion. J Trauma 23:248–249, 1983.
75. Milch H: Snapping scapula. Clin Orthop 20:139–150, 1961.
76. Milch H: Partial scapulectomy for snapping in the scapula. J Bone Joint Surg 32A:561–566, 1950.

77. Milch H, and Burman MS: Snapping scapula and humerus varus. Arch Surg 26:570–588, 1933.
78. Moneim MS, and Balduini FC: Coracoid fractures—a complication of surgical treatment by coraclavicular tape fixation. A case report. Clin Orthop 168:133–135, 1982.
79. Montgomery SP, and Loyd RD: Avulsion fracture of the coracoid epiphysis with acromioclavicular separation. J Bone Joint Surg 59:963, 1977.
80. Moseley HF: Shoulder Lesions, 2nd ed. New York: Paul Hoeber, 1953, pp 171–175.
81. Mudge MK, Wood VE, and Frykman GK: Rotator cuff tears associated with os acromiale. J Bone Joint Surg 66A:427–429, 1984.
82. Neer CS II: Fractures about the shoulder. In Rockwood CA, and Green DP (eds): Fractures. Philadelphia: JB Lippincott, 1984, pp 713–721.
83. Nettrour LF, Krufty LE, Mueller RE, and Raycroft JF: Locked scapula: intrathoracic dislocation of the inferior angle. J Bone Joint Surg 54A:413–416, 1972.
84. Neviaser J: Traumatic lesions: injuries in and about the shoulder joint. Am Acad Orthop Surg Instructional Course Lectures 13:187–216, 1956.
85. Newell ED: Review of over 2,000 fractures in the past seven years. South Med J 20:644–648, 1927.
86. Norris T: Fractures and dislocations of the glenohumeral complex. In Chapman M (ed): Operative Orthopedics. Philadelphia: JB Lippincott, 1984, pp 205–210.
87. Norris TR: Unfused epiphysis mistaken for acromion fracture. Orthopedics Today 3(10):12–13, 1983.
88. Nunley RL, and Bedini SJ: Paralysis of the shoulder subsequent to comminuted fracture of the scapula: rationale and treatment methods. Phys Ther Rev 40:442–447, 1960.
89. Ogden JA, and Phillips SB: Radiology of postnatal skeletal development. Skeletal Radiol 9:157–169, 1983.
90. Oreck SL, Burgess A, and Levine AM: Traumatic lateral displacement of the scapula: a radiologic sign of neurovascular disruption. J Bone Joint Surg 66A:758–763, 1984.
91. Orthopedic Knowledge Update, 1985, Scapular Fractures.
92. Parsons TA: The snapping scapula and subscapularis exostosis. J Bone Joint Surg 55B:345–349, 1973.
93. Pate D, Kursunoglu S, Resnick D, and Resnick, CS: Scapula foramina. Skeletal Radiol 14:270–275, 1985.
94. Pettersson H: Bilateral dysplasia of the neck of the scapula and associated anomalies. Acta Radiol [Diagn] 22:81–84, 1981.
95. Protiss JJ, Stampfli FW, and Osmer JC: Coracoid process fracture diagnosis in acromioclavicular separation. Radiology 116:61–64, 1975.
96. Ramin JE, and Veit H: Fracture of the scapula during electroshock therapy. Am J Psychiatry 110:153–154, 1953.
97. Rask MR, and Steinberg LH: Fracture of the acromion caused by muscle forces. J Bone Joint Surg 60A:1146–1147, 1978.
98. Resnick D, Walter RD, and Crudale AS: Bilateral dysplasia of the scapular neck. AJR 139:387–390, 1982.
99. Rockwood CA: Personal communication, 1989.
100. Rockwood CA: Management of fractures of the scapula. J Bone Joint Surg 10:219, 1986.
101. Rorabeck CH: The management of the flail upper extremity in brachial plexus injuries. J Trauma 20:491–493, 1980.
102. Rounds RC: Isolated fracture of the coracoid process. J Bone Joint Surg 31A:662–663, 1949.
103. Rowe CR: Fractures of the scapula. Surg Clin North Am 43:1565–1571, 1963.
104. Rowe CR: The Bankart procedure. A study of late results. J Bone Joint Surg Proceedings 59B:22, 1977.
105. Rowe CR: The Shoulder. New York: Churchill Livingstone, 1987, pp 373–381.
106. Rowe CR, Patel D, and Southmayd WW: The Bankart procedure—a long-term end-result study. J Bone Joint Surg 60A:1–16, 1978.
107. Rubenstein JD, Abraheim NA, and Kellam JF: Traumatic scapulothoracic dissociation. Radiology 157:297–298, 1985.
108. Rush LV: Fracture of the coracoid process of the scapula. Ann Surg 90:1113, 1929.
109. Ruther H: Therapy of pseudoarthroses of the scaphoid, internal malleollus, and acromion. Ztschr Orthop 79:485–499, 1950.
110. Sandrock AR: Another sports fatigue fracture: stress fracture of the coracoid process of the scapula. Radiology 117:274, 1975.
111. Scudder CL (ed): The Treatment of Fractures, 4th Ed. Philadelphia: WB Saunders, 1904, p 201.
112. Smith DM: Coracoid fracture associated with acromioclavicular dislocation. A case report. Clin Orthop 108:165–167, 1975.
113. Stein RE, Bono J, Korn J, and Wolff WI: Axillary artery injury in closed fracture of the neck of the scapula—a case report. J Trauma 11:528, 1971.
114. Steindler A: Traumatic Deformities and Disabilities of the Upper Extremity. Springfield, IL: Charles C Thomas, 1946, pp 112–118.
115. Strizak AM, and Cowen MH: The snapping scapula syndrome. J Bone Joint Surg 64A:941–942, 1982.
116. Tachdjian MO: Pediatric Orthopedics. Philadelphia; WB Saunders, 1972, pp 1553–1555.
117. Tarquinio T, Weinstein ME, and Virgilio RW: Bilateral scapular fractures from accidental electric shock. J Trauma 19:132–133, 1979.
118. Thompson DA, Flynn TC, Miller PW, and Fischer RP: The significance of scapular fractures. J Trauma 25:974–977, 1985.
119. Varriale PL, and Adler ML: Occult fracture of the glenoid without dislocation. J Bone Joint Surg 65A:688–689, 1983.
120. Wilbur MC, and Evans EB: Fractures of the scapula—an analysis of forty cases and review of literature. J Bone Joint Surg 59A:358–362, 1977.
121. Wilson PD: Experience in the Management of Fractures and Dislocations (Based on an Analysis of 4390 Cases) by the Staff of the Fracture Service MGH, Boston. Philadelphia: JB Lippincott, 1938.
122. Wolfe AW, Shoji H, and Chuinard RG: Unusual fracture of the coracoid process. Case report and review of the literature. J Bone Joint Surg 58A:423–424, 1976.
123. Wong-Pack WK, Bobechko PE, and Becker EJ: Fractured coracoid with anterior shoulder dislocation. J Can Assoc Radiol 31:228, 1980.
124. Zdravkovic D, and Damholt VV: Comminuted and severely displaced fractures of the scapula. Acta Orthop Scand 45:60–65, 1974.
125. Zettas JP, and Muchnic PD: Fracture of the coracoid process base and acute acromioclavicular separation. Orthop Rev 5:77–79, 1976.
126. Zilberman Z, and Rejovitzky R: Fracture of the coracoid process of the scapula. Injury 13:203–206, 1982.

Fractures of the Clavicle

Edward V. Craig, M.D.

Fractures of the clavicle are usually not difficult to recognize and typically unite uneventfully with many different treatment methods. Nevertheless, the frequency with which this injury is seen and the difficulty in managing the early and late complications of this fracture attest to its importance. Its clinical relevance is underscored when one considers that the clavicle is the most common fracture site in childhood,[39, 229] that it has been estimated that 1 out of 20 fractures involves the clavicle,[153] and that fractures of the clavicle may constitute as much as 44 per cent of shoulder girdle injuries.[200]

Historical Review

The clavicle is entirely subcutaneous and thus easily accessible to inspection and palpation. This may account for its inclusion in some of the earliest descriptions of injuries of the human skeleton and their treatment. As early as 400 B.C., Hippocrates recorded a number of observations about clavicular fractures: (1) With a fractured clavicle, the distal fragment and arm sag while the proximal fragment, held securely by the sternoclavicular joint attachments, points upward. (2) It is difficult to reduce the fracture and maintain the reduction: ". . . They act imprudently who think to depress the projecting end of the bone. But it is clear that the underpart ought to be brought to the upper, for the former is the moveable part, and that which has been displaced from its natural position." (3) Union is usual, rapid, and produces prominent callus, and despite the deformity healing usually proceeds uneventfully.

A fractured clavicle like all other spongy bone, gets speedily united; for all such bone forms callus in a short time. When, then, a fracture has recently taken place, the patients attach much importance to it, as supposing the mischief greater than it really is. . . ; but, in a little time, the patients having no pain, nor finding any impediment to their walking or eating, become negligent, and the physician, finding they cannot make the parts look well, take themselves off, and are not sorry at the neglect of the patients, and in the mean time the callus is quickly formed.[2]

The Edwin Smith papyrus provides what is probably the earliest description of the accepted method of fracture reduction, indicating that an unknown Egyptian surgeon in 3000 B.C. recommended treating fractures of the clavicle thus: "Thou shouldst place him prostrate on his back with something folded between his shoulder-blades, thou shouldst spread out with his two shoulders in order to stretch apart his collar-bone until that break falls into place."[39, 66, 153]

Paul of Aegina, a 17th-century Byzantine, reported that all that could ever be written about fractures of the clavicle had been written, and that treatment included the supine position and the application of potions of olive oil, pigeon dung, snake oil, and other essences.[153]

Some of the earliest documented cases resulted from reports of riding accidents. William III in 1702 died from a fracture of the clavicle three days after falling when his horse shied at a molehill. Sir Benjamin Brodie described a "diffuse false venous aneurysm" complicating a fracture of the clavicle in Sir Robert Peel, who fell from his horse in 1850 on the way to Parliament. As he lapsed into unconsciousness, a pulsatile swelling rapidly developed behind the fracture and his arm was paralyzed. The *Lancet* defended the physician's handling of the case, as many skeptics doubted that death could occur from a clavicular fracture.[45, 117, 254]

Dupuytren, a keen though controversial anatomist and observer, noted in 1839 that the cumbersome devices of his day used to hold the reduction were often unnecessary; he advocated simply placing the arm on a pillow until union occurred. A number of the devices of the time often appeared to aggravate the difficulty created by the fracture or to create new problems. He described a case on which he consulted in which bleeding could not be arrested: "When I was summoned I merely removed the apparatus (the pressure of which was the cause of the mischief) and placed the arm on a pillow. The bleeding immediately ceased."[48, 254] He railed against cumbersome and painful treatment methods. In the late 1860s the present-day ambulatory treatment (early mobilization of the patient) was described by Lucas-Championniere, who advocated a figure-of-eight dressing and suggested that recumbency, a popular treatment method of his day, be abandoned.[73] In 1871 Sayre, recognizing the difficulty of maintaining the reduction, advocated a method of ambulatory treatment employing a rigid dressing to maintain the reduction and support the extremity, a method that was echoed and taught in the textbooks of his time and still has many advocates.[207]

Malgaigne, however, concluded in 1859

. . . but while for a century and a half we see the most celebrated surgeons striving to prefer, or perhaps more strictly to complicate, the contrivances for treating fractured clavicle we may follow parallel to them another series of no less estimable surgeons, who disbelieving in these so-called improvements, return to the simplest means, as to Hippocrates before them. If now we seek to judge of all these contrivances by their results we see that most of them are extolled as producing cures without deformity; but we see also that subsequent experience has always falsified these promises, I therefore, regard the thing (absence of deformity) as not impossible, although for my own part I have never seen such an instance.[133]

This well summarizes the results of most conservative methods of treatment of the fractured clavicle—that is, most of them unite uneventfully by a variety of treatment methods, many of the patients end up with residual deformity, some shortening, and a lump, yet interference with function, cosmesis, activity level, and satisfaction appears to be minimal.

Ambulatory treatment of clavicular fractures with support of the arm while maintaining satisfactory and acceptable alignment of the fracture fragments remains the mainstay of care today.

Anatomy

The embryology of the clavicle is unique in that it is the first bone in the body to ossify (fifth week of fetal life) and is the only long bone to ossify by intramembranous ossification, without going through a cartilaginous stage.[69, 146, 147] The ossification center begins in the central portion of the clavicle; it is this area that is responsible for growth of the clavicle up to about age five.[39, 61] Epiphyseal growth plates develop at both the medial and lateral ends of the clavicle, but only the

sternal ossification center is present radiographically.[39, 235] This medial growth plate of the clavicle is responsible for the majority of its longitudinal growth, probably contributing as much as 80 per cent of the length of the clavicle.[166] The appearance and fusion of the sternal ossification center occurs relatively late in life, with ossification occurring between ages 12 and 19 and fusion to the clavicle occurring from ages 22 to 25.[98, 237] Thus many of the so-called sternoclavicular dislocations in young adults are, in fact, epiphyseal fractures and are a potential source of confusion unless the late sternoclavicular epiphyseal closure is remembered.

Since the clavicle is subcutaneous along its entire length, the only structures that cross it are the supraclavicular nerves.[11] In most individuals it is possible to grasp the bone and manipulate it, which can be helpful in producing crepitus if an acute fracture is suspected or movement in the case of suspected nonunion.

The clavicle is the sole bony strut connecting the trunk to the shoulder girdle and arm, and it is the only bone of the shoulder girdle forming a synovial joint with the trunk.[125] Its name is derived from the Latin word *clavis* (key), the diminutive of which is clavicula, referring to the musical symbol of similar shape.[146]

The shape and configuration of the clavicle not only is important for its function but also provides an explanation for the pattern of fractures encountered in this bone. Although it appears nearly straight when viewed from the front, when viewed from above the clavicle appears as an S-shaped double curve, concave ventrally on its outer half and convex ventrally on its medial half (Fig. 11–1). Although some reports have noted differences in the shape and size of the clavicle from male to female and from dominant to nondomi-

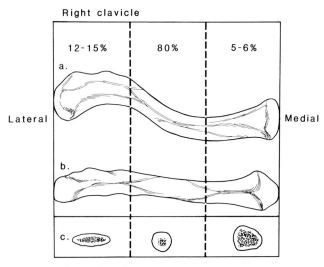

Figure 11–1. The clavicle appears as an S-shaped double curve when viewed from above (*a*); it appears nearly straight when viewed from in front (*b*). The outer end of the clavicle is flat in cross-section but becomes more tubular in the medial aspect (*c*).

nant arm, others have not found this to be so or have discounted its clinical significance.[40, 62, 125, 166] DePalma found that the outer third of the clavicle exhibited varying degrees of anterior torsion and suggested that changes in torsion might be responsible for altered stresses that lead to changes of primary degenerative disease in the acromioclavicular joint.[40] The cross-section of the clavicle differs in shape along its length, varying from flat along its outer third to prismatic along its inner third. The exact curvature of the clavicle and its thickness, to a high degree, vary according to the attachments of the muscles and the ligaments.[125] The flat outer third is most compatible with pull from muscles and ligaments, whereas the tubular medial third is a shape consistent with axial pressure or pull. The junction between the two cross-sections varies as to its precise location in the middle third of the clavicle. This junction is a weak spot, particularly to axial loading.[125] This may be one of the several reasons that fractures occur so commonly at the middle third. Another may be that it is an area not reinforced by muscles and ligaments and that it is just distal to the subclavius insertion.[88, 93, 153] It is curious that nature has strengthened, through ligaments or muscular reinforcement, every part of the clavicle except the end of the outer part of the middle third, which is the thinnest part of the bone.[16]

The clavicle articulates with the sternum through the sternoclavicular joint, which has little actual articular contact but suprisingly strong ligamentous attachments. The medial end of the clavicle is moored firmly against the first rib by the intra-articular sternoclavicular joint cartilage (which functions as a ligament), the oblique fibers of the costoclavicular ligaments, and, to a lesser degree, the subclavius muscle.[40] The scapula and clavicle are bound securely through both the acromioclavicular and coracoclavicular ligaments, the mechanism and function of which have been extensively reported and which contribute in a significant way to the movement and stability of the entire upper extremity (Fig. 11–2).[67, 239] The clavicle in the adult is dense, honeycombed, and lacks a well-defined medullary cavity. The bone of the clavicle has been described as "thick compacta,"[68] and its main nutrient vessel enters just medial to the attachment of the coracoclavicular ligaments.[166]

The tubular one-third of the clavicle, which is thicker in cross-section, offers protection for the neurovascular structures of great importance that pass beneath the medial one-third of the clavicle. The intimate relationship between these structures and the clavicle assumes great importance both in acute fractures, in which direct injury may occur, and in the unusual fracture sequelae of malunion, nonunion, or production of excessive callus, in which compression of these structures may lead to late symptoms. The brachial plexus, at the level where it crosses beneath the clavicle, comprises three main branches (see Fig. 11–2). Of these, two are anterior. One (lateral) originates from the fifth, sixth, and seventh cervical roots and forms

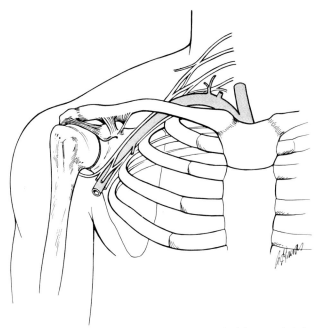

Figure 11–2. The clavicle is bound securely by ligaments at both the sternoclavicular and acromioclavicular joints. It is the only bony strut from the torso to the extremity. In addition, the brachial plexus and greater vessels are seen posterior to the medial third of the clavicle between the clavicle and first rib.

the musculocutaneous nerve and a branch of the median nerve; the other (medial) originates from the eighth cervical and first thoracic roots and forms another branch of the median nerve, the entire ulnar nerve, and the medial cutaneous nerve. The posterior branch of the plexus forms the axillary and radial nerves. The cord of the brachial plexus, which contains the first components of the ulnar nerve, crosses the first rib directly under the medial third of the clavicle. The other two cords are farther to the lateral side and posterior. Therefore, the ulnar nerve is more frequently involved in complications arising from fractures of the medial third of the clavicle.

The space between the clavicle and the first rib has been called the costoclavicular space. This space has been measured in gross anatomical studies and often appears quite adequate. However, it is not as large in the living subject as in the cadaver, possibly because in the living subject the vessels are distended and the dimensions of the cords of the brachial plexus are larger than in the cadaver. In addition, in the living subject the space is diminished as the first rib elevates owing to contraction of the scalenus anticus. Hence, when the inner end of the outer fragment of the fractured clavicle is depressed, there is much less space between the first rib and the clavicle; the result is that the vessels (especially the subclavian and axillary vessels) and nerves (especially the ulnar) are potentially subject to injury, pressure, or irritation.[16] The internal jugular, which is adjacent to the sternoclavicular joint (see Fig. 11–2), is usually not injured with middle third fractures but has the potential for injury in more medial trauma involving the sternum and sternoclavicular joint.

SURGICAL ANATOMY

The surgical anatomy relative to the fascial arrangements about the clavicle has been extensively detailed by Abbott and Lucas.[1] Knowledge of these will lessen the risk of damage to the neurovascular structures during surgical dissection.[198] It is useful to divide them into the areas above, below, and behind the clavicle.

1. Above the clavicle—at the sternal notch a layer of cervical fascia splits into two layers, a superficial layer attached to the front and a deep layer attached to the back of the manubrium. The space between these layers contains lymphatics and a communicating vessel between the two anterior jugular veins. The two layers of fascia proceed laterally to enclose the sternocleidomastoid muscle before passing down to the clavicle. For an inch above the clavicle, they are separated by loose fat. The superficial layer is ill defined and is continuous with the fascia covering the undersurface of the trapezius muscle. A prolongation from the deep layer forms an inverted sling for the posterior belly of the omohyoid muscle, and it continues below to blend with the fascia enclosing the subclavius muscle. Medially, the omohyoid fascia covers the sternohyoid muscle.

2. Below the clavicle—two layers consisting of muscle and fascia form the anterior wall of the axilla. The pectoralis major and pectoral fascia form the superficial layer; the pectoralis minor and clavipectoral fascia form the deep layer. The pectoral fascia closely envelops the pectoralis major. Above, it is attached to the clavicle, and laterally it forms the roof of the superficial infraclavicular triangle (formed by the pectoralis major, a portion of the anterior deltoid, and the clavicle). The deep layer—the clavipectoral fascia—extends from the clavicle above to the axillary fascia below. At the point where it attaches to the clavicle, it consists of two layers that enclose the subclavius muscle. The subclavius muscle arises from the manubrium and first rib and inserts into the inferior surface of the clavicle. At the lower border of the subclavius, the two fascial layers join to form the costocoracoid membrane. This membrane fills a space between the subclavius above and the pectoralis minor below, and is attached medially to the first costal cartilage and laterally to the coracoid process. Below, it splits into two layers, which ensheathe the pectoralis minor. The costocoracoid membrane is pierced by the cephalic vein, the lateral pectoral nerve, and the thoracoacromial artery and vein.[1]

3. Behind the clavicle—a continuous myofascial layer, which has not been commonly appreciated in surgical anatomy, lies in front of the large vessels and nerves as they pass from the root of the neck to the axilla. From above to below, this layer consists of (1) the omohyoid fascia enclosing the omohyoid muscle and (2) the clavipectoral fascia enclosing the pectoralis minor and subclavius muscles.[1] Behind the medial clavicle and the sternoclavicular joint, the internal jugular and subclavian veins join to form the innominate vein. These veins are covered by the omohyoid fascia and by its extension medially over the sternohyoid and sternothyroid muscles. Behind the clavicle, at the junction between the middle and medial thirds, the junction of the subclavian and axillary veins lies very close to the clavicle and is also protected by this myofascial layer.

Between the omohyoid fascia posteriorly and the investing layer of cervical fascia anteriorly is a space, described by Grant, in which the external jugular vein usually joins the subclavian vein at its confluence with the internal jugular vein.[76] Before this junction, the external jugular is joined on its lateral aspect by the transverse cervical and scapular veins and on its medial aspect by the anterior jugular vein. This anastomosis usually lies just behind the fascial envelope and the angle formed by the posterior border of the sternocleidomastoid muscle and clavicle.[1]

Function of the Clavicle

The function of the clavicle may be inferred, in part, by some study of comparative anatomy. Codman has stated that

We are proud that our brains are more developed than the animals: we might also boast of our clavicles. It seems to me that the clavicle is one of man's greatest skeletal inheritances, for he depends to a greater extent than most animals except the apes and monkeys on the use of his hands and arms.[31]

Mammals that depend on swimming, running, or grazing have no clavicles, whereas those species with clavicles appear to be predominantly fliers or climbers. Codman theorized that animals with strong clavicles needed to use their arms more in adduction and abduction. The long clavicle may facilitate the placement of the shoulder in a more lateral position so that the hand can be more effectively positioned to deal with the three-dimensional environment.[170] The teleological role of the clavicle has been disputed, however, as there have been reports following complete excision of the clavicle of entirely normal function of the upper limb.[36, 83, 91] These reports, combined with observations in patients with congenital absence of the clavicle (cleidocranial dysostosis) who appear not to show any impairment of limb function, probably are responsible for the often stated belief that this bone is a surplus part that can be excised without disturbance of function. However, others have noted drooping of the shoulder, weakness, and loss of motion following clavicular excision and have used these observations to attribute to the clavicle its important role in normal extremity function (Figs. 11–3 and 11–4).[196, 216]

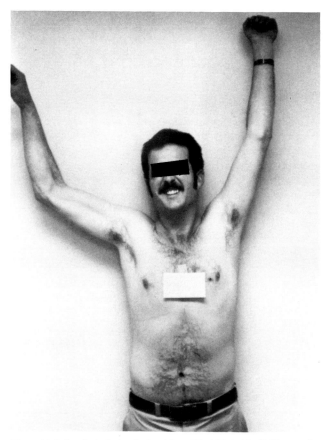

Figure 11–3. A patient who has had excision of his right clavicle. Eight years after right clavicle resection, the patient has a painful and limited range of motion of his shoulder.

The clavicle does have several important functions, each of which would be expected to be altered not only by excision of the bone but also by fracture, nonunion, or malunion.

POWER AND STABILITY OF THE ARM

The clavicle, by serving as a bony link from the thorax to the shoulder girdle, provides a stable linkage of the arm-trunk mechanism and contributes significantly to power and stability of the arm and shoulder girdle, especially in movement above the shoulder level.[147] It transmits the support and force of the trapezius muscle to the scapula and arm via the coracoclavicular ligaments.

Although patients with cleidocranial dysostosis and absence of the clavicle do not appear to have a significantly decreased range of motion and, in fact, may have an increase in protraction and retraction of the scapula (due to absence of the clavicle), they may exhibit some weakness in supporting a load overhead; this further suggests that the clavicle adds stability to the extremity under load in extreme ranges of motion.[91]

The clavicle is predominantly supported and stabilized by passive structures,[125] particularly the sternoclavicular ligaments.[13, 14] Although it has been reported

that there is electromyographic evidence of trapezius muscle activity at rest, suggesting a role for that muscle in support of the clavicle,[1] other authors have not been able to demonstrate that muscle activity plays any role in clavicular support.

MOTION OF THE SHOULDER GIRDLE

When the arm is elevated 180 degrees, the clavicle angles upward 30 degrees and backward 35 degrees at the sternoclavicular joint. It also rotates upward on its longitudinal axis approximately 50 degrees. During combined glenohumeral, acromioclavicular, and sternoclavicular movement, the humerus moves approximately 120 degrees at the glenohumeral joint and the scapula moves along the chest wall approximately 60 degrees. These complex and combined simultaneous movements of the joints and their articulating bony structures (scapula, humerus, and clavicle) seem to imply an important role for the clavicle in range of motion of the arm. There is some debate about this, however. It has been observed by some that loss of the clavicle does not in fact impair abduction of the arm at all,[1, 253] and that excision of the clavicle may permit range of motion just as well. However, Rockwood has observed loss of the clavicle to result in disabling loss of function, weakness, drooping of the

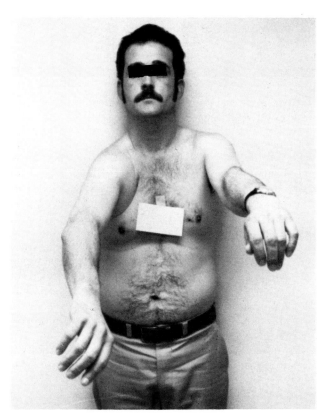

Figure 11–4. During flexion the shoulder collapses medially. The patient has no strength in abduction or flexion. He has significant drooping of the upper extremity with symptoms of brachial plexitis.

arm, and pain secondary to brachial plexus irritation (see Figs. 11–3 and 11–4).[196]

It has been stated that contribution to motion may be the most important function of the clavicle and that this is related to its curvature, especially its lateral curvature. The 50-degree rotation of the clavicle on its axis appears to be important for free elevation of the extremity. In fact, a direct relationship has been found between the line of attachment of the coracoclavicular ligaments, the amount of clavicular rotation, the extent and relative lengthening of the ligaments, and scapula rotation itself. Of the total of 60 degrees of scapular rotation, the first 30 degrees is due to elevation of the clavicle as a whole by movement of the sternoclavicular joint, and the second 30 degrees is permitted through the acromioclavicular joint by clavicular rotation and elongation of the coracoclavicular ligaments. Thus the lateral curvature of the clavicle permits it to act as a crankshaft, effectively allowing half of scapular movement.[124]

The smooth, rhythmic movement of the shoulder girdle is a complex interaction of muscle groups acting on joints and both subacromial and scapulothoracic spaces. Although it is difficult to break down all of the contributions of the clavicle to the total motion, it appears that its geometrical and kinematic design, by permitting rotation, maximizes the stability of the upper limb against the trunk while permitting mobility, particularly of the scapula along the chest wall. The practical result of this is that the glenoid fossa continually moves, facing and contacting the humeral head as the arm is used overhead.[91]

MUSCLE ATTACHMENTS

The clavicle also acts as a bony framework for muscle origin and insertion. The upper third of the trapezius inserts on the superior surface of the outer third of the clavicle, opposite the site of origin of the clavicular head of the deltoid along its anterior edge. The clavicular head of the sternocleidomastoid muscle arises from the posterior edge of the inner third of the clavicle. The clavicular head of the pectoralis major muscle arises from the anterior edge of the clavicle. During active elevation of the arm, these muscles contract simultaneously. It has been suggested that, in theory, those muscles above the clavicle could be directly attached to those muscles below the clavicle as a continuous muscular layer without an interposed bony attachment,[1] but the stable bony framework clearly provides the advantage of a solid foundation for muscle attachment. The other muscle that inserts on the clavicle is the subclavius. After it arises from the first rib anteriorly at the costochondral junction, it proceeds obliquely and posteriorly into a groove on the undersurface of the clavicle. This muscle appears to aid in depressing the middle third of the clavicle. Fractures of the clavicle often occur at the distal portion of its insertion. In midclavicular fractures, this muscle may

offer some protection to the neurovascular structures beneath.

PROTECTION OF THE NEUROVASCULAR STRUCTURES

The clavicle also acts as a skeletal protection for adjacent neurovascular structures and for the superior aspect of the lung. The subclavian and axillary vessels, the brachial plexus, and the lung are directly behind the medial third of the clavicle. As noted earlier, the tubular cross-section of the medial third of the clavicle increases its strength and adds to its protective function at this level. The anterior curve of the medial two-thirds of the clavicle provides a rigid arch beneath which the great vessels pass as they move from the mediastinum and thoracic outlet to the axilla. It has been shown that during elevation of the arm the clavicle, as it rotates upward, also moves backward, with the curvature providing increased clearance for the vessels.[233] Loss of the clavicle eliminates this bony barrier against external trauma.[1]

RESPIRATORY FUNCTION

Elevation of the lateral part of the clavicle results in increased pull on the costoclavicular ligament and subclavius muscle. Owing to the connection between the clavicle and the first rib and between the first rib and the sternum, elevation of the shoulder girdle brings about a cephalad motion of the thorax, corresponding to an inspiration. This relationship is utilized in some breathing exercises and in some forms of artificial respiration.[1]

COSMESIS

By providing a graceful curve to the base of the neck, a cosmetic function is served by the smooth, subcutaneous bony clavicle. After surgical excision, in some patients the upper limb may fall downward and forward, giving a foreshortened appearance to this area. In addition, the cosmetic function of the clavicle is noted by many concerned patients after excessive formation of callus following clavicular fracture or deformity caused by clavicular malunion.[1]

Classification of Clavicular Fractures

Although clavicular fractures have been classified by fracture configuration (greenstick, oblique, transverse, and comminuted),[231] the usual classification is by location of the fracture since this appears to better compartmentalize our understanding of fracture anatomy, mechanism of injury, clinical presentation, and alternative methods of treatment.[5, 51, 59, 155, 173]

A useful classification is as follows:

Group I—fracture of the middle third

Group II—fracture of the distal third

    Type I—minimal displacement (interligamentous)

    Type II—displaced secondary to a fracture medial to the coracoclavicular ligaments

        A. Conoid and trapezoid attached

        B. Conoid torn, trapezoid attached

    Type III—fractures of the articular surface

    Type IV—ligaments intact to the periosteum (children), with displacement of the proximal fragment

    Type V—comminuted, with ligaments attached neither proximally nor distally, but to an inferior, comminuted fragment

Group III—fracture of the proximal third

    Type I—minimal displacement

    Type II—displaced (ligaments ruptured)

    Type III—intra-articular

    Type IV—epiphyseal separation (children and young adults)

    Type V—comminuted

Group I fractures, or fractures of the middle third, are the commonest fractures seen in adults and children. They occur at the point at which the clavicle changes to a flattened cross-section from a prismatic cross-section. The force of the traumatic impact follows the curve of the clavicle and disperses upon reaching the lateral curve.[160-162, 219] In addition, the proximal and distal segments of the clavicle are mechanically secured by ligamentous structures and muscular attachments, whereas the central segment is relatively free. This fracture accounts for 80 per cent of clavicular fractures (Figs. 11–5, 11–6, and 11–7).[153, 200]

Group II fractures account for 12 to 15 per cent of all clavicular fractures and are subclassified according to the location of the coracoclavicular ligaments relative to the fracture fragments.[86] Neer first pointed out the importance of this fracture while subdividing it into three types. Type I fractures are the most common by a ratio of four to one. In this fracture the ligaments remain intact to hold the fragments together and

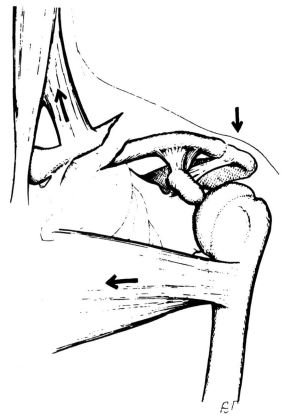

Figure 11–6. When displacement occurs, the proximal fragment is pulled superiorly and posteriorly by the pull of the sternocleidomastoid, while the distal segment droops forward by the weight of gravity and the pull of the pectoralis. (Reproduced with permission from Rockwood CA, and Green DP (eds): Fractures (3 vols), 2nd ed. Philadelphia: JB Lippincott, 1984.)

prevent rotation, tilting, or significant displacement. This is an interligamentous fracture occurring between the conoid and trapezoid or between the coracoclavic-

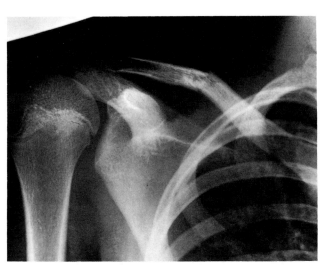

Figure 11–5. Typical location for a Group I fracture of the clavicle, nondisplaced.

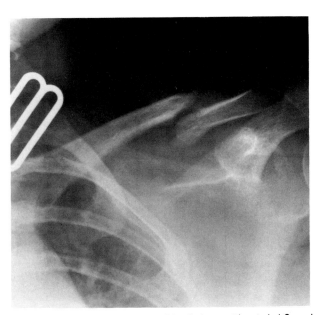

Figure 11–7. Radiographic appearance of the displacement in a typical Group I fracture of the clavicle.

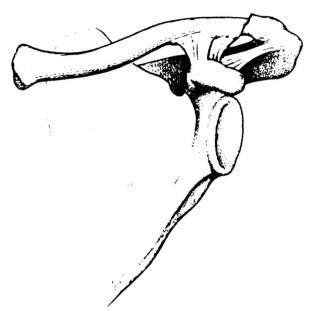

Figure 11-8. A Type I fracture of the distal clavicle (Group II). The intact ligaments hold the fragments in place. (Reproduced with permission from Rockwood CA, and Green DP (eds): Fractures (3 vols), 2nd ed. Philadelphia: JB Lippincott, 1984.)

ular and acromioclavicular ligaments (Figs. 11-8 and 11-9).[156] In Type II distal clavicular fractures, the coracoclavicular ligaments are detached from the medial segment. Both the conoid and trapezoid may be on the distal fragment (IIA) (Fig. 11-10), or the conoid ligament may be ruptured while the trapezoid ligament remains attached to the distal segment (IIB) (Fig. 11-11).[39] Four forces act on this fracture that may impair healing and may be contributing factors to the reported high incidence of nonunion: (1) when the patient is erect, the outer fragment, retaining the attachment of the trapezoid ligament to the scapula through the intact acromioclavicular ligaments, is pulled downward and forward by the weight of the arm; (2) the pectoralis

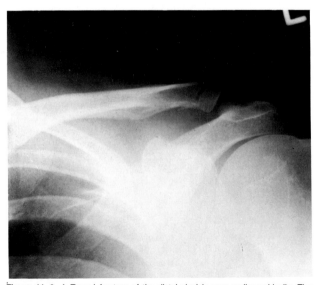

Figure 11-9. A Type I fracture of the distal clavicle seen radiographically. The fragments are held in place securely by the intact coracoclavicular and acromioclavicular ligaments.

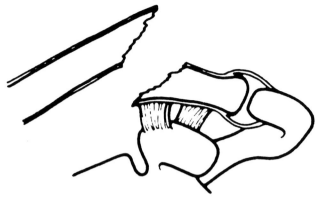

Figure 11-10. A Type II distal clavicle fracture. In Type IIA, both conoid and trapezoid ligaments are on the distal segment, while the proximal segment, without ligamentous attachments, is displaced. (Reproduced with permission from Rockwood CA, and Green DP (eds): Fractures (3 vols), 2nd ed. Philadelphia: JB Lippincott, 1984.)

major, pectoralis minor, and latissimus dorsi draw the distal segment downward and medially, causing overriding; (3) the scapula may rotate the distal segment as the arm is moved; and (4) the trapezius muscle attaches upon the entire outer two-thirds of the clavicle while the sternocleidomastoid attaches to the medial third, and these muscles act to draw the clavicular segment superior and posterior, often into the substance of the trapezius muscle.[155] Type III distal clavicular fractures involve the articular surface of the acromioclavicular joint alone (Fig. 11-12). Although Type II fractures may have intra-articular extension (Fig. 11-13), in Type III fractures there is a break in the articular surface without a ligamentous injury. The Type III injury may be subtle, may be confused with a first-degree acromioclavicular separation, and may require special views to visualize. It may, in fact, present as late degenerative joint arthrosis of the acromioclavicular joint. In addition, it has been suggested that "weightlifter's clavicle," resorption of the distal end of the clavicle, may occur from increased vascularity secondary to microtrauma or microfractures that lead to this resorption.[26, 153, 188]

It appears logical to add a fourth and fifth type of distal clavicular fracture, as there is a series of fractures

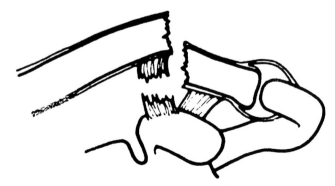

Figure 11-11. A Type IIB fracture of the distal clavicle. The conoid ligament is ruptured while the trapezoid ligament remains attached to the distal segment. The proximal fragment is displaced. (Reproduced with permission from Rockwood CA, and Green DP (eds): Fractures (3 vols), 2nd ed. Philadelphia: JB Lippincott, 1984.)

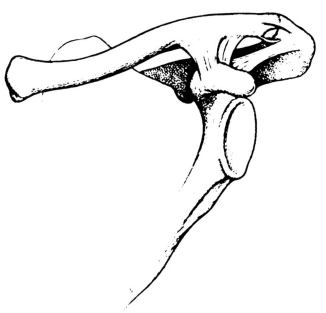

Figure 11–12. A Type III distal clavicle fracture, involving the articular surface of the acromioclavicular joint alone. There is no ligamentous disruption or displacement. These fractures present as late degenerative changes of the joint. (Reproduced with permission from Rockwood CA, and Green DP (eds): Fractures (3 vols), 2nd ed. Philadelphia: JB Lippincott, 1984.)

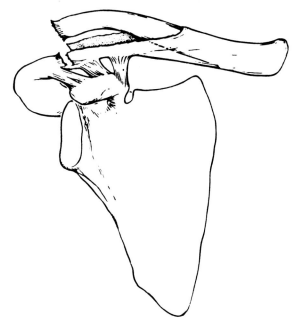

Figure 11–14. A Type IV fracture occurring in children, which has been called a "pseudodislocation" of the acromioclavicular joint. The coracoclavicular ligaments remain attached to the bone or the periosteum, while the proximal fragment ruptures through the thin superior periosteum and may be displaced upward by muscle forces. (Reproduced with permission from Rockwood CA, and Green DP (eds): Fractures (3 vols), 2nd ed. Philadelphia: JB Lippincott, 1984.)

in which bone displacement occurs because of deforming muscle forces, yet the coracoclavicular ligaments remain attached to bone or periosteum. Type IV fractures occur in children and may be confused with a complete acromioclavicular separation (Fig. 11–14). Called *pseudodislocation* of the acromioclavicular joint, they typically occur in children under the age of 16.[198] There is a fracture of the distal clavicle, and the acromioclavicular joint remains intact. In children and young adults, the attachment between bone and periosteum is relatively loose. The proximal fragment ruptures through the thin periosteum and may be

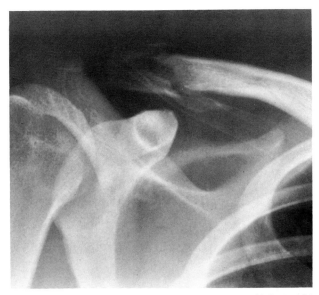

Figure 11–13. Although there is an intra-articular component to this fracture, it is not a Type III fracture but a Type II with intra-articular extension.

displaced upward by muscular forces. The coracoclavicular ligaments remain attached to the periosteum or may be avulsed with a small piece of bone.[51, 59, 198] Clinically and radiographically it may be impossible to distinguish between Grade III acromioclavicular separations, Type II fractures of the distal clavicle, and Type IV fractures involving rupture of the periosteum.[153, 155, 156] In Type V fractures occurring in adults, neither of the main fracture fragments have functional coracoclavicular ligaments. These fracture fragments are displaced by the deforming muscles as in Type I distal clavicular fractures, but the coracoclavicular ligaments are intact and remain attached to a small, third comminuted intermediary segment.[173] This fracture is thought to be more unstable than Type II distal clavicular fractures.

Group III fractures, or fractures of the inner one-third of the clavicle, constitute 5 to 6 per cent of clavicular fractures. As with distal clavicle fractures, they can be subdivided according to the integrity of the ligamentous structures. If the costoclavicular ligaments remain intact and attached to the outer fragment, there is little or no displacement.[5, 109] When these lesions occur in children, they are usually epiphyseal fractures.[39] In adults, articular surface injuries can also lead to degenerative changes.[153, 252]

Finally, the panclavicular dislocation or the traumatic floating clavicle is neither a clavicular fracture nor an isolated sternoclavicular or acromioclavicular separation.[15, 70, 96, 181] In this injury, both sternoclavicular ligaments and coracoclavicular and the acromioclavicular ligamentous structures are disrupted.

Mechanism of Injury

Since the clavicle is the bone that is most frequently fractured, a great many causes of clavicular fracture, both traumatic and nontraumatic, have been reported.[52]

TRAUMA IN CHILDREN

Fractures of the clavicle in children share many of the same mechanisms of injury as in adults and may occur either by a direct blow to the clavicle or the point of the shoulder or by an indirect blow, such as a fall on the outstretched hand. However, other features are unusual and unique to children, including the obstetrical clavicular fracture and the plastic bowing injury.

Birth Fractures

In 15,000 deliveries from 1954 to 1959, Rubin found that clavicular fractures were the most common birth injury.[201] Although it has been stated that intrapartum traumatic injuries are decreasing owing to improvement in obstetrical care,[77, 240] the incidence of clavicular fracture remains quite high, and, in infants, may actually be increasing.[8] Moir and Myerscough found an incidence of clavicular fractures of 5 per 1000 vertex births, increasing to 160 per 1000 if there was a breech presentation.[144] The mechanism of injury in the full-term newborn infant delivered vaginally, when the baby is in a cephalic presentation, is compression of the leading clavicle against the maternal symphysis pubis.[131, 230] In a breech delivery, direct traction may occur as the obstetrician, trying to depress the shoulders and free the arm in the delivery of the head, may produce the same bony injury.[105, 228]

The overall incidence of clavicular fracture during birth is approximately 2.8 to 7.2 per 1000 births. In addition to the presentation of the infant, a number of factors appear to be involved: (1) Birth weight clearly plays a role, since the incidence of clavicular fractures increases with increasing birth weight and in larger children.[29, 75] Children weighing 3800 to 4000 gm or measuring 52 cm or longer seem to be at higher risk for fracture. (2) The experience of the physician is probably also related. Cohen and Otto reported an increased incidence of clavicular fractures when babies were delivered by less experienced residents, with a decrease in incidence for each year of obstetrical experience.[30] This certainly is a statistic that merits consideration in obstetrical house staff training. (3) The method of delivery also is important, as there is an increase in the risk of fracture with mid forceps deliveries, calling into question the wisdom of this obstetrical maneuver. On the other hand, Balata and coworkers noted no fracture in babies delivered by cesarean section.[8]

There seems to be no relationship between clavicular fractures and the type of anesthesia, length of active labor, length of second stage labor, Apgar score, or parity of the mother. The exact anatomy of fractures that occur during delivery varies, with incomplete, greenstick, and bicortical disruption with or without displacement having all been reported.[229] In one study, males were more commonly affected than females and the right clavicle was more frequently fractured than the left.[8]

Injuries in Infancy and Childhood

Fractures of the clavicle are particularly common in childhood, with nearly half occurring before the age of seven.[11] Fractures commonly result from a fall on the point of the shoulder or on an outstretched hand. In younger children this not uncommonly is from a high-chair, bed, or a changing table. The fracture occasionally may be due to a direct violent force applied from the front of the clavicle; like other fractures of long bones, clavicular fractures may be one of several signs of trauma in the physically abused child.

Unlike in the adult, direct and indirect trauma to the child's clavicle may result in incomplete or greenstick fractures rather than displaced fractures.[160] In addition, trauma to the child's clavicle may result in plastic bowing alone without evident cortical disruption. Despite presenting only with bowing, on later examination these fractures usually present evidence of gross healing of complete fractures with obvious callus visible on x-rays.[20, 218]

TRAUMA IN ADULTS

The incidence of clavicular fractures in adults appears to be increasing owing to a number of factors, including the occurrence of many more high-velocity vehicular injuries and the increase in popularity of contact sports.[40] The mechanism of injury of clavicular fractures in adults has been widely reported to consist of either direct or indirect forces. It has generally been assumed that the most common mechanism of adult fractures is a fall onto the outstretched hand.[40] Allman, in dividing clavicular fractures into three groups, proposed different mechanisms of injuries for each group.[5] He felt that in Group I, fractures of the middle third, the most common mechanism of injury is a fall onto an outstretched hand, with the force being transmitted up the arm and across the glenohumeral joint, dispersing along the clavicle. Group II fractures, those distal to the coracoclavicular ligaments, occur from a fall on the lateral shoulder, driving the shoulder and scapular downward. Group III fractures, proximal clavicular fractures, usually are due to direct violence caused by a force applied from the lateral side.

Fowler, in 1962,[64] pointed out that all clavicular

injuries nearly always follow a fall or a blow on the point of the shoulder whereas a blow on the bone itself is rarely a cause, although direct blow has certainly been recognized in athletics, particularly in stick sports such as lacrosse and hockey.[211] In a large series of clavicular fractures (342 patients) studied by Sankarankutty and Turner, 91 per cent sustained a fall or blow to the point of the shoulder whereas only 1 per cent had a fall onto the outstretched hand.[206]

More recently, Stanley and colleagues studied a consecutive series of 150 patients with clavicular fractures, with 81 per cent of the patients presenting detailed information about the mechanism of injury.[220] They found that 94 per cent had fractured the clavicle from a direct blow on the shoulder, whereas only 6 per cent had fallen onto an outstretched hand. Further biomechanical analysis by this group of the forces involved in clavicular fracture revealed that direct injury produced a critical buckling load, which is exceeded at a compression force equivalent to the body weight, resulting in fracture of the bone. When the force is applied along the axis of the arm, the buckling force is rarely reached in the clavicle. These investigators recorded fractures at every site along the clavicle with a direct injury to the point of the shoulder and found little support for Allman's concept that fractures at different anatomical sites have different mechanisms of injury. In addition, they theorized that a direct blow on the shoulder might even be the mechanism of injury in those who described a fall on the outstretched hand: as the hand makes contact with the ground, the patient's body weight and falling velocity are such that the fall continues, with the shoulder becoming the upper limb's next point of contact with the ground.

Another indirect mechanism of clavicular fractures is a direct force applied to the top of the shoulder, which forces the clavicle against the first rib and often produces a spiral fracture of the middle third.[40]

NONTRAUMATIC FRACTURES

It is well recognized that the clavicle can be the site of neoplastic or infectious destruction of bone, and fracture may occur from relatively minor trauma (Fig. 11–15). Certainly, lack of a traumatic episode should lead the clinician to focus on the possibility that long bone fracture may have occurred in pathological bone. In addition to both malignant and benign lesions producing pathological clavicular fractures,[17] pathological fracture has also been described in association with arteriovenous malformation, an entity that may mimic neoplasm.[143]

Atraumatic stress fracture has also been reported in the clavicle.[108] In addition, spontaneous fracture of the medial end of the clavicle has been reported as a "pseudotumor" following radical neck dissection.[38, 63, 167, 227]

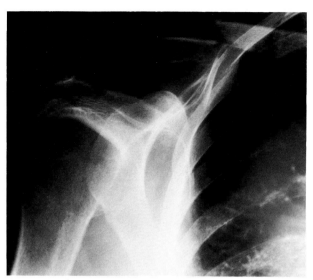

Figure 11–15. A pathological fracture of the clavicle from metastatic thyroid carcinoma. The patient presented without a traumatic episode.

Clinical Presentation

BIRTH FRACTURES

Two clinical presentations of birth fractures appear to predominate:

1. Clinically inapparent—there may be great difficulty in diagnosing these, as there are few clinical symptoms. A crack heard during the delivery may be the only clue to the clavicular fracture.[11] Whether in this group of fractures the lesion is truly asymptomatic and is overlooked in the neonatal examination is uncertain, but Farkas and Levine emphasized that many of these initially are not diagnosed. Of the five cases of clavicular fractures in 300 newborns in their series, none were suspected following routine physical examination in the delivery room and newborn nursery.[60] On re-examination, however, crepitus could usually be demonstrated at the fracture site (Fig. 11–16). Thus it appears that fractures may be easily overlooked. However, as they are usually unilateral, close examination may reveal asymmetry of clavicular contour or shortening of the neck line. Often the fracture is first recognized after the swelling caused by fracture callus, which typically appears 7 to 11 days after the fracture, is recognized by the mother.[37]

2. Clinically apparent (pseudoparalysis) (Fig. 11–17)—there is a disinclination or unwillingness of the infant to use the extremity, with a unilateral lack of movement of the whole upper limb either spontaneously or during elicitation of Moro's reflex.[65, 205] Again, because these are often complete fractures, local swelling, tenderness, and crepitus may suggest the diagnosis. This injury must be distinguished from other conditions that may make the infant disinclined or unable to use the extremity, such as birth brachial

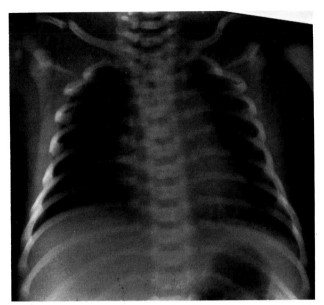

Figure 11–16. An obstetrical fracture in a day-old infant. The fracture is complete and presented with crepitus demonstrable at the fracture site.

plexus injury, separation of the proximal humeral epiphysis, and acute osteomyelitis of the clavicle or proximal humerus. It is important to remember that a fractured clavicle and a brachial plexus injury may coexist.[229]

FRACTURES IN CHILDREN

More than one-half of clavicular fractures in children occur in those under the age of seven. Because in these young children the fracture may be incomplete or of the greenstick variety, it may not be obvious and thus may be overlooked. The mother of the infant may notice that the baby cries after being picked up and appears to be hurt.[11] The baby does not seem to use the arm naturally and cries when the arm is used for any activities or moved during dressing. On palpation, a tender, uneven upper border of the clavicle may be felt, which is asymmetrical when compared with the contralateral side. As with a newborn, the mother may take the baby to the pediatrician because of the "sudden" appearance of a lump (Figs. 11–18, 11–19, and 11–20).[39]

However, if the fracture is complete in children who are ambulatory and verbal, the diagnosis is usually obvious. In addition to the child's complaints of pain localized to the clavicle, when these fractures are displaced there is a typical deformity caused by muscle displacement of the fracture fragments. The shoulder on the affected side may appear lower and droop forward and inward. The child splints the involved extremity against the body and supports the affected elbow with the contralateral hand. Because of the pull of the sternocleidomastoid muscle on the proximal fragment, the child tilts the head toward and the chin away from the side of the fracture in an effort to relax the pull of this muscle (Fig. 11–21).[229] Physical examination reveals tenderness, crepitus, and swelling typical for this fracture at any age.

It must be remembered that complete acromioclavicular separations are very unusual in children under the age of 16. What may present clinically as a high-riding clavicle above the acromioclavicular joint and an apparent acromioclavicular separation is often either a transperiosteal distal clavicular fracture or, more commonly, a rupture through the periosteum with a distal clavicular fracture, the coracoclavicular ligaments remaining behind attached to the periosteum. This lesion is often not recognized in the child under 16 years of age.[51]

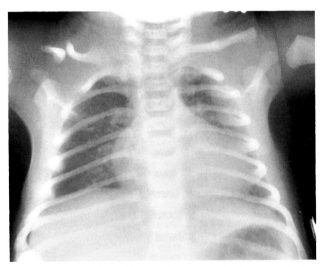

Figure 11–17. In a newborn with multiple fractures at birth, this clavicular fracture was overlooked until it became evident that the infant had a disinclination to use the extremity. This "pseudoparalysis" is typical of the clinically apparent type of birth fracture.

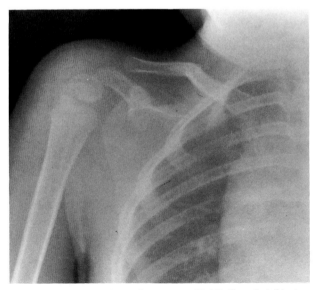

Figure 11–18. A clavicular fracture in a two-year-old child. The patient did not use the arm and cried whenever the arm was elevated.

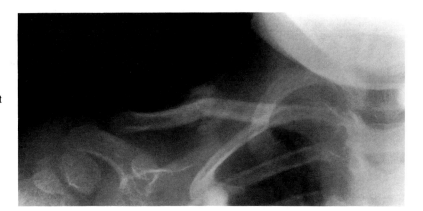

Figure 11–19. Two and a half weeks later there is prominent callus formation, manifested clinically as a bump.

Similarly, since the sternal epiphysis is the last epiphysis of the long bones to fuse with the metaphysis (this usually occurs from ages 22 to 25), the joint may be subject to the usual types of epiphyseal injuries. Many misdiagnosed sternoclavicular dislocations are, in fact, separations through the medial clavicular epiphysis. Occasionally, sternoclavicular separations may occur with adjacent clavicular fractures in children.[23, 119]

FRACTURES IN ADULTS

Because of the characteristic clinical presentation in adults, displaced fractures of the clavicle present little difficulty with diagnosis if the patient is seen soon after injury. There is usually a clear history of some form of either direct or indirect injury to the shoulder. Clinical deformity is obvious and may be out of proportion to the amount of discomfort that the patient experiences.[11] The proximal fragment is displaced upward and backward and may be tenting the skin.

Compounding of this fracture is unusual but may occur (Fig. 11–22).[191] The patient usually presents splinting the involved extremity at the side, since any movement elicits pain. The involved arm droops forward and down (Fig. 11–23). Although the initial deformity may be obvious later, with acute swelling of soft tissue and hemorrhage it may be obscured. In a fracture near the

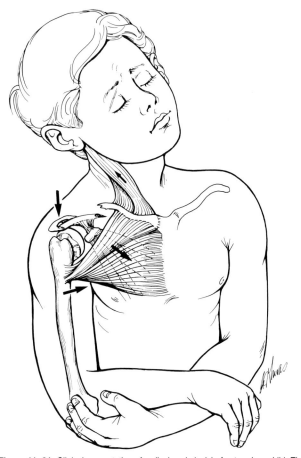

Figure 11–21. Clinical presentation of a displaced clavicle fracture in a child. The shoulder on the affected side appears lower and droops forward and inward. The child splints the involved extremity against the body, supports the affected elbow with the contralateral hand, and tilts the head forward and the chin away from the site of the fracture in order to relax the pull of the sternocleidomastoid.

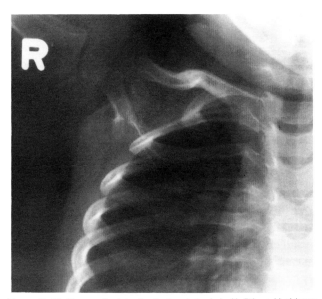

Figure 11–20. Five months later the fracture is healed with little residual bump evident.

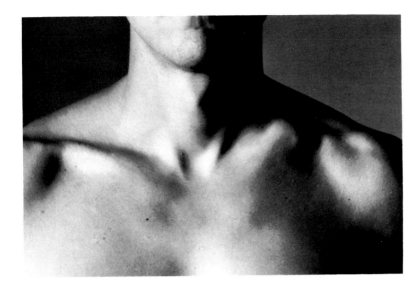

Figure 11–22. An adult clavicle fracture showing prominence of the proximal fragment, which is displaced upward and backward. This may tent the skin, although compounding is unusual.

ligamentous structures (acromioclavicular and sterno-clavicular joints), the deformity may mimic a purely ligamentous injury.

Examination of the patient reveals tenderness directly over the fracture site, and any movement of the arm is painful. There may be ecchymosis over the

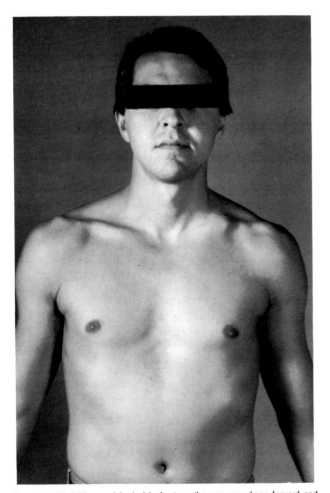

Figure 11–23. With an adult clavicle fracture, the arm may droop forward and downward to varying degrees.

fracture site, especially if severe displacement of the bony fragments has produced associated tearing of soft tissue. The patient may angle his or her head toward the injury, attempting to relax the pull of the trapezius on the fragment. As in children, the patient may be more comfortable with the chin tilted to the opposite side. Gentle palpation and manipulation will usually produce crepitus and motion, and the site of the fracture is easily palpable owing to the subcutaneous position of the bone. The skin over the clavicle, the scapula, or the chest wall may give a clue to the mechanism of injury and may indicate other areas to be evaluated for associated injuries. The lungs must be examined for the presence of symmetrical breath sounds, and the whole extremity must be carefully examined.

Undisplaced fractures or isolated fractures of the articular surfaces may not cause deformity and may be overlooked unless they are specifically sought for radiographically. If the diagnosis is in doubt, special x-rays or a repeat x-ray of the clavicle in 7 to 10 days may be indicated.

The panclavicular dislocation is typically produced by extreme and forceful protraction of the shoulder. This injury is usually the result of a major traumatic episode such as a high-speed motor vehicle accident, a fall from a height, or a very heavy object falling on the shoulder,[70] although it has been reported following a minor fall at home.[96] Clinically, there is usually bruising over the spine of the scapula, swelling, and tenderness at both ends of the clavicle. This injury is associated with anterosuperior sternoclavicular dislocation and either posterosuperior or subjacent displacement of the clavicle. The whole clavicle may be freely mobile and may feel as if it is floating. X-rays usually confirm this injury.

ASSOCIATED INJURIES

In 1830 Gross reported that "fractures of the clavicle usually assume a mild aspect, being seldom accom-

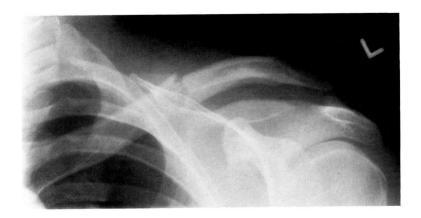

Figure 11–24. An unusual case of a clavicular fracture associated with a complete acromioclavicular separation. The associated clavicular fracture makes treatment of the ligamentous injury very difficult.

panied by any serious accident."[78] Although statistically most clavicular fractures are relatively innocuous injuries, serious associated injuries may occur, delay in treatment of which may be potentially life threatening.[47] Therefore, in a patient with a clavicular fracture it is critical that a careful examination of the entire upper extremity be performed with particular emphasis on the neurovascular status, and, as mentioned previously, a careful examination of the lungs.[47]

Associated injuries accompanying acute fractures of the clavicle may be divided into (1) associated skeletal injuries, (2) injuries to the lung and pleura, (3) vascular injuries, and (4) brachial plexus injuries.

Associated skeletal injuries may include sternoclavicular or acromioclavicular separations or fracture dislocations through these joints (Fig. 11–24).[25, 102, 119] As might be anticipated with ipsilateral sternoclavicular or acromioclavicular joint injuries, closed reduction of the ligamentous injury is usually impossible because of the accompanying clavicular fracture.[102]

Head and neck injuries may be present,[251] especially with displaced distal clavicular fractures. In one series, 10 per cent of patients were comatose.[156]

Fractures of the first rib are not infrequent and are easily overlooked.[3, 248] These rib fractures may be directly responsible for accompanying lung, brachial plexus, or subclavian vein injury. Under-recognition of this associated injury may be due to the fact that they are not easily seen on standard chest x-rays. Weiner and O'Dell recommended either an anteroposterior view of the cervical spine or an anteroposterior view of the thoracic spine associated with a lateral view of the thoracic spine to decrease the likelihood that this injury would be overlooked.[248] The location of a first rib fracture may be either the ipsilateral or contralateral rib to the clavicle fracture. Weiner and O'Dell have outlined how a number of these rib fractures occur. The scalenus anticus muscle attaches on a tubercle of the first rib. On either side of this tubercle lies a groove for the subclavian vein anteriorly

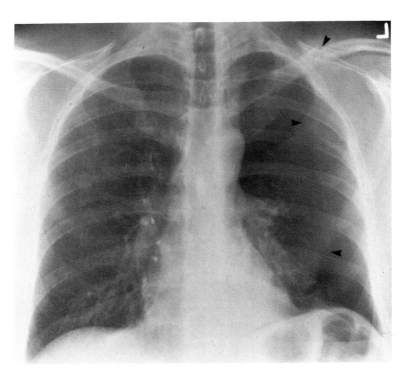

Figure 11–25. A fracture of the left clavicle associated with a left pneumothorax. The lung markings are absent on the left side. In this patient there is also a fracture of the second rib.

and the subclavian artery posteriorly. Posterior to the groove for the subclavian artery lies a roughened area for the attachment of the scalene medius muscle. These two muscles elevate the rib during inspiration. The serratus anterior arises from the outer surfaces of the upper eight ribs and fixes the rib posteriorly during inspiration. These structures may interact to contribute to the occurrence of fractures of the first rib as the clavicle is fractured. Three basic mechanisms have been theorized to be responsible for this combination of injuries: (1) indirect forces transmitted via the manubrium; (2) an avulsion fracture at the weakest portion of the rib by the scalene anticus; and (3) injury to the lateral clavicle that causes an acromioclavicular separation, leading to indirect force from the subclavius muscle to the costal cartilage and the anterior aspect of the first rib.[182, 248]

A number of authors have commented on the potentially serious complication of associated pneumothorax or hemothorax with fractures of the clavicle, since the apical pleura and upper lung lobes lie adjacent to this bone (Fig. 11–25). Rowe reported a 3 per cent incidence of pneumothorax in a series of 690 clavicular fractures, although he did not comment on how many had associated rib or scapular fractures.[200] Although it is easy to see how a severely displaced fracture may puncture the pleura with a sharp shard of bone to produce this lesion, the x-ray appearance may be misleadingly benign, with little evidence to suggest what might have been significant fragment displacement at the time of injury.[47] It is essential that careful physical examination of the lung be undertaken at the time of the initial presentation, searching for presence and symmetry of breath sounds. In addition, an upright chest film appears to be important in the assessment of all patients with clavicular fractures who have de-creased breath sounds or other physical findings suggestive of a pneumothorax, with particularly close attention being paid to the lung outline.[132] This is especially true in the multiply traumatized or unconscious patient who has neither obvious blunt chest trauma nor any external signs of trauma to the chest that might yield a clue to potential lung or pleural complications.[47, 94, 132, 221, 224, 254]

Although nerve injuries with clavicular fractures are rare, acute injuries to the brachial plexus do occur. The neurovascular bundle emerges from the thoracic outlet under the clavicle on top of the first rib.[192] As it passes under the clavicle it is protected to a certain extent by the thick, medial clavicular bone; considerable trauma is usually necessary to damage the brachial plexus and break the clavicle at the same time. When the force is severe enough to break the clavicle and injure the brachial plexus, a subclavian vascular injury often occurs concomitantly (Fig. 11–26). The force resulting in nerve injury usually comes in a direction from above downward or from in front downward. As the force is applied the nerves may be stretched, with the fulcrum of maximum tension being the transverse process of the cervical vertebra. The roots can also be torn above the clavicle, or they may be avulsed from their attachment to the spinal cord.[12] Although the posterior periosteum, subclavius muscles, and bone offer some protection to the underlying plexus, the plexus may be injured directly by the fragments of bone. This is especially worthy of emphasis; manipulation of clavicular fragments should not be done without adequate x-ray studies of the position of these fracture fragments.[241]

Direct injury to the brachial plexus usually involves the ulnar nerve, as this is the portion of the plexus lying adjacent to the middle third of the clavicle.

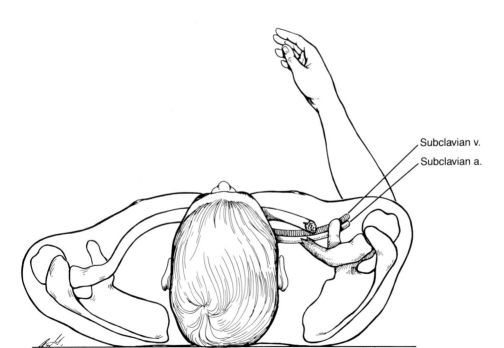

Subclavian v.

Subclavian a.

Figure 11–26. As the clavicle fractures and displaces, the subclavian vessels immediately posterior to the clavicle may be injured by sharp shards of bone.

Acute vascular injuries are unusual owing to many of the same local anatomical factors that protect the nerves from direct injury. The subclavius muscle and the thick, deep cervical fascia also act as barriers against direct injury to the vessels. If the initial displacement of the fracture fragment has not injured the adjacent vessels, they are unlikely to be injured further, since the distal fragment is pulled downward and forward by the weight of the limb and the proximal fragment is pulled upward and backward by the trapezius. Thus, as with acute nerve injury, a major injury is usually required to produce acute vascular insult.[175] Nevertheless, injury has been reported even with a greenstick fracture.[142] In addition, acute vascular compression resulting from fracture angulation has been described.[42]

When they occur, vascular injuries include laceration, occlusion, spasm, or acute compression; the vessels most commonly injured are the subclavian artery, subclavian vein, or the internal jugular vein.[97, 113, 123, 137] The subclavian vein is particularly vulnerable to tearing since it is fixed to the clavicle by a fascial aponeurosis.[82, 223] Injuries to the suprascapular and axillary arteries have also been reported.[92, 238] Laceration may result in life-threatening hemorrhage, whereas arterial thrombus and occlusion may lead to distal ischemia. Damage to the arterial wall, in addition, may lead to aneurysm formation and late embolic phenomena. Venous thrombosis may be problematic as well in that, although its clinical presentation is not typically life- or limb-threatening, there is a potential for pulmonary embolism, which certainly may be.[213] Clinical recognition of an acute vascular injury may be difficult, particularly in the unconscious patient or the patient presenting in shock. Although a complete laceration certainly may present with a life-threatening hemorrhage or an extremity that is cold, pulseless, and pale, a partial laceration is more likely to present with uncontrolled bleeding and life-threatening blood loss. The color and temperature of the extremity may be normal, but the absence of a pulse, the presence of a bruit, or a pulsatile hematoma (as the hematoma is walled off or produces a false aneurysm) should make the clinician strongly suspicious of a major vascular injury.[238] If there is a significant obstruction to blood flow, the injured limb is usually colder than the uninjured limb; there may also be a difference in blood pressure between the two.[254] Vascular contusion or spasm may result in thrombotic and, later, thromboembolic phenomena.[247] It is sometimes difficult to recognize the difference between arterial spasm and interruption or occlusion, and it may be reasonable to consider a sympathetic block to help distinguish spasm from more serious injury.

If major injury to a vessel is suspected, an arteriogram should be performed.[254] In the rare event of a tear of a large vessel, surgical exploration is mandatory. To gain adequate exposure, as much of the clavicle should be excised as is needed to isolate and repair the injured major vessel. Although in some instances the vessel may be ligated, ligation of a major vessel in the elderly patient may well be dangerous because of inadequate remaining circulation to the extremity. In any event, a surgeon skilled in the decision making and in techniques regarding vascular repair is essential if a major injury has occurred.

X-ray Evaluation

FRACTURES OF THE SHAFT

In most instances of clavicular shaft fractures, the diagnosis is not in doubt because of the clinical deformity and confirmatory x-rays. Nevertheless, to obtain an accurate evaluation of the fragment position two projections of the clavicle are typically used, an anteroposterior and a 45-degree cephalic tilt view. In the former, the proximal fragment is typically displaced upward and the distal fragment downward (Fig. 11–27). In the latter, the tube is directed from below upward and more accurately assesses the anteroposterior relationship of the two fragments (Figs. 11–28 and 11–29).[249] Quesana recommended two views at right angles to each other, a 45-degree angle superiorly and a 45-degree angle inferiorly, to assess the extent and displacement of clavicular fractures.[185]

Rowe has suggested that with an anteroposterior x-ray the film should include the upper third of the humerus, the shoulder girdle, and the upper lung fields, so that other shoulder girdle fractures and pneumothorax can be identified more speedily.[200] The configuration of the fracture is also important to assess, as it may give a clue to the presence of associated injuries. The usual clavicular shaft fracture in the adult is slightly oblique; if it is more comminuted, and especially if the middle spike is projecting from superior to inferior, this usually results from a greater force and may alert the surgeon to the potential for associated neurovascular or pulmonary injuries.

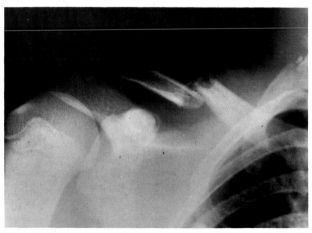

Figure 11–27. An anteroposterior view of a right clavicle fracture, showing the typical deformity with a proximal fragment displaced superiorly.

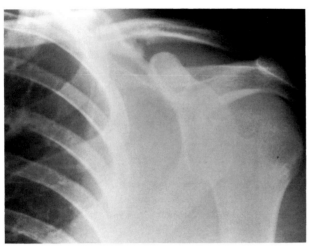

Figure 11–28. An anteroposterior view of this left comminuted clavicular fracture poorly defines and identifies the fracture fragments owing to overlying bone in the area of the fracture fragments.

Children's fractures may be greenstick, nondisplaced, or present only as bony bowing, and thus the diagnosis of shaft fractures may be more difficult (Fig. 11–30). This is especially true in newborns or infants, in whom the clinical presentation may be difficult to assess. Movement by the child or bony overlap may obscure radiographic detail, and an incomplete fracture may not be noted. However, the surrounding soft tissues of the clavicle are normally and frequently displayed as parallel shadows above the body of the clavicle. Although this "accompanying shadow" may not be seen along the proximal one-third of the clavicle medial to the crossing of the first rib, it is invariably present on most x-rays. Suspicion for clavicular fractures should be aroused by loss of the accompanying shadow unilaterally.[218] If there is any doubt about the presence of a fracture in the child, a repeat x-ray taken 5 to 10 days after the injury will usually reveal callus formation.

Recently, the technique of ultrasonography has been described for evaluation of clavicular birth fractures.[105]

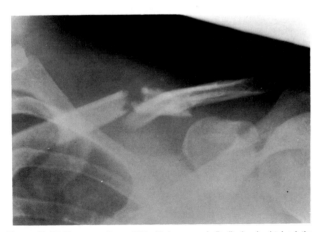

Figure 11–29. However, when a 20 to 45 degree cephalic tilt view is obtained, the fracture anatomy is more clearly delineated.

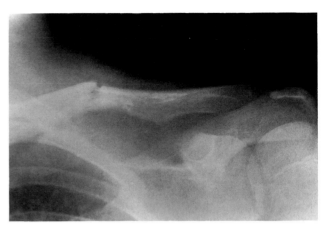

Figure 11–30. A greenstick fracture of the left clavicle in a 14-year-old patient. In these patients the diagnosis may be more difficult.

These birth fractures may easily be overlooked and may be confused clinically with birth palsy. In their study, Katz and associates noted no difference in diagnostic accuracy between ultrasonography and plain x-ray.[105] In addition, a medial clavicular fracture not seen on plain film was picked up with ultrasonography. In fact, the authors noted that the individual fracture fragments were seen to move up and down with respiration.

With either plain x-ray or ultrasonography, it may be difficult to differentiate congenital pseudarthrosis from an acute fracture. However, the radiographic features, the lack of trauma, and the absence of callus usually help to distinguish an atraumatic condition such as this from a birth fracture.

FRACTURES OF THE DISTAL ONE-THIRD

In both children and adults, the usual radiographic views obtained for shaft fractures are inadequate to completely assess distal clavicular fractures. The standard exposure for evaluation of shoulder or shaft fractures overexposes the distal clavicle. The usual exposure for the distal clavicle should be approximately one-third that used for the shoulder joint. This is especially true if it is important to determine articular surface involvement.

Type II distal clavicular fractures may be particularly difficult to diagnose, as the usual anteroposterior and 40-degree cephalic tilt views typically do not reveal the extent of the injury.[156] If the exposure is appropriate, this distal clavicular fracture may be identified on the anteroposterior and lateral views of the trauma series (Figs. 11–31 and 11–32), but to accurately assess the extent of the injury and the presence or absence of associated ligamentous damage, Neer has recommended three views: (1) The anteroposterior view includes both shoulders on one plate with the patient erect and with 10 pounds of weight strapped to each wrist (Figs. 11–33 and 11–34). If the distance between the coracoid and the medial fragment is increased when

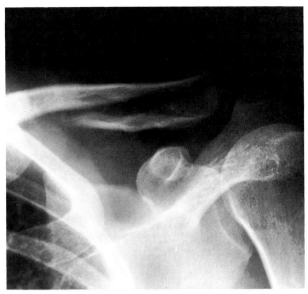

Figure 11–31. An anteroposterior view of a distal clavicle fracture. This is a cephalic tilt view of approximately 15 degrees which brings the clavicle and acromioclavicular joint away from the overlying bony anatomy.

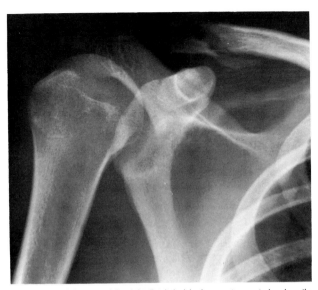

Figure 11–33. A fracture of the right distal clavicle. In an anteroposterior view, the fracture location is suggestive of ligamentous involvement, with the ligaments attached to the distal fragment.

compared with the normal side, ligamentous detachment from the medial fragment can be assumed to be present. However, since much of the displacement of the fracture is in the anteroposterior plane, two additional views were suggested. (2) An anterior 45-degree oblique view, with the patient erect and the injured shoulder against the plate, gives a lateral view of the scapula and shows the medial fragment posteriorly with the outer fragment displaced anteriorly. (3) A posterior 45-degree oblique view, with the patient erect

and the injured shoulder against the plate, also demonstrates the extent of separation of the two fragments.

Articular surface fractures of the distal clavicle are easily overlooked unless high-quality x-rays are obtained. If the fracture is not seen on a plain x-ray view and the clinical suspicion is strong, tomography or a CT scan may reveal the presence and extent of the articular surface injury (Fig. 11–35).

FRACTURES OF THE MEDIAL ONE-THIRD

These may be particularly difficult to detect by routine x-rays owing to the overlap of ribs, vertebrae,

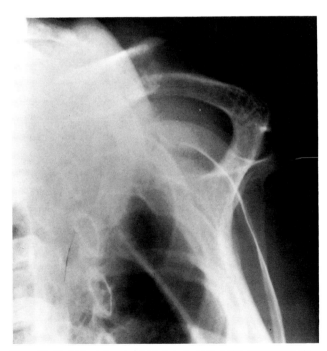

Figure 11–32. A lateral view of a distal clavicular fracture. The displacement of the proximal segment is identified, but the fracture detail may be obscured by bony and soft tissue anatomy.

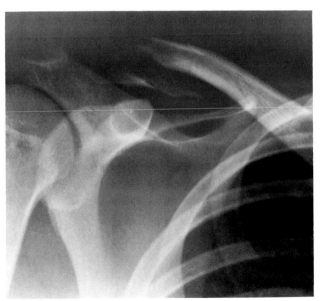

Figure 11–34. The extent of ligamentous involvement is confirmed on a weighted view, where there is a separation of the coracoclavicular distance. The coracoclavicular ligaments are attached to the distal clavicular segment.

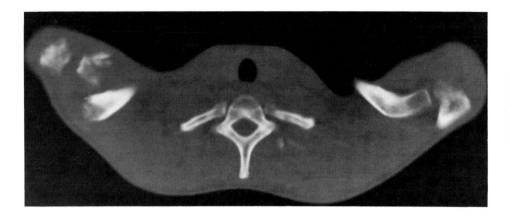

Figure 11–35. CT scan of a right clavicular fracture. Not only does it confirm the site of the clavicular fracture as the distal clavicle, but it also identifies a previously unsuspected intra-articular extension of the distal clavicle fracture.

and mediastinal shadows. However, a cephalic tilt view of 40 to 45 degrees often reveals the fracture, whether in a child or an adult. In children particularly, fractures of the medial end of the clavicle are often misdiagnosed as sternoclavicular dislocations, when in fact they are usually epiphyseal injuries. As with the distal clavicular injuries, tomography or a CT scan may be useful in demonstrating the intra-articular or epiphyseal nature of the injury in this location.

Differential Diagnosis

In adults, fractures of the shaft of the clavicle are usually not confused with any other diagnosis, although pathological fractures are occasionally difficult to recognize as such. However, fractures of the distal or medial end of the clavicle may clinically appear to be complete acromioclavicular or sternoclavicular separations, although these rarely cause confusion once proper radiographic studies are performed.

In children, it may be easy to confuse injuries to the clavicle with other entities, including congenital disorders and other traumatic conditions:

Congenital Pseudarthrosis. When recognized at birth or shortly thereafter, congenital pseudarthrosis may be confused with either cleidocranial dysostosis or a birth fracture, especially if there is a history of some trauma associated with the delivery. However, birth fractures unite rapidly and leave no disability. The deformity of congenital pseudarthrosis may become more conspicuous as the child grows.[74] Clinically the lump is painless; there is usually no history of injury, pain, or disability with this lesion.[112, 187] It is invariably in the lateral portion of the middle third of the clavicle, and usually affects the right clavicle unless there is dextrocardia, when it may occur on the left side.[126, 243] Bilateral congenital pseudarthrosis has been reported, particularly in the presence of bilateral cervical ribs.[39]

The cause of this entity is unclear. Although a family history is not typical, in some reported cases there has been a familial incidence, raising the question of genetic transmission.[74]

Although there may be a history of trauma with the birth, this is probably incidental; most investigators now agree that congenital pseudarthrosis is not a nonunion of normal bone following trauma.[169] It is probable that abnormal intrauterine development plays the primary role in its appearance, and it has been suggested that pressure from the subclavian artery as it arches over the first rib and under the clavicle may be a primary factor in its development.[126, 127] The cervical ribs may also displace the subclavian artery and cause pressure in the same area of the clavicle.[39]

Radiographically there are characteristic changes. The sternal fragment, consisting of the medial one-third of the clavicle, is larger and protrudes forward and upward, while the lateral one-half is situated below, pointing upward and backward and ending in a bulbous mass at the pseudarthrosis site. Other identifying features are an increase in the deformity with age, the proximity of the bone ends to one another, and a large lump palpable clinically. This contrasts quite markedly with cleidocranial dysostosis.

Cleidocranial Dysostosis. Cleidocranial dysostosis is a hereditary abnormality of membranous bone, with the clavicle most frequently involved. The abnormality varies from a central defect of the clavicle to complete absence of the clavicle; the most common presentation is absence of the distal portion of the clavicle.[39, 135] Radiographically, it is distinguished from congenital pseudoarthrosis by the larger gap between the bone ends and by the tapered ends of the clavicle rather than the larger bulbous ends.[74] It is more clearly aplastic bone. In addition, multiple membranous bones are involved, and these may each have their own clinical manifestations. Some children suffer from bossing or other skull defects, smallness of facial bones, scoliosis, abnormal epiphyses of hands or feet, and deficiencies of the pelvic ring. Usually there is a familial history of bone disorders.[4, 57]

Sternoclavicular Dislocation. Epiphyseal fractures of the medial end of the clavicle may mimic sternoclavicular separations in children, owing to the late closure of the sternal epiphysis. If it is important to distinguish between these two entities, tomography or CT scanning may be indicated.

Acromioclavicular Separation. Fracture of the lateral clavicle in children may also be identical with a complete acromioclavicular separation, clinically and radiographically. If plain radiography does not identify the small fracture fragment, tomography or CT scanning may. However, as the coracoclavicular ligaments remain attached to the periosteal tube in children and healing is uneventful, it is difficult to justify these more elaborate diagnostic modalities in children with this injury.[198, 215]

Complications

NONUNION

Despite the frequency of clavicular fractures, nonunion of unoperated shaft fractures is rare, with a reported incidence of 0.9 to 4.0 per cent.* There is some debate in the literature as to the definition, but most authors consider a clavicular nonunion to be defined as failure to show clinical or radiographic progression of healing at four to six months,[100, 124, 184, 203, 250] although there is some temporal difference between atrophic and hypertrophic nonunions. Manske and Szabo reported that tapered, sclerotic, atrophic bone ends at 16 weeks were unlikely to unite, while they classified other fractures as delayed unions at the 16-week period as long as there is some potential for healing.[134] Bilateral post-traumatic pseudarthrosis has been reported in an adult.[85]

Although nonunion of the clavicle is predominantly a problem following fracture in adults, it has been described in children.[164] However, when nonunion is seen in a child, it is likely to be a congenital pseudarthrosis. There appear to be several factors predisposing to nonunion of the clavicle: (1) inadequate immobilization, (2) severity of trauma, (3) refracture, (4) location of fracture (outer third), (5) degree of displacement (marked displacement), and (6) primary open reduction.

Inadequate Immobilization. It has long been recognized that the clavicle is one of the most difficult bones to immobilize properly and completely following fracture, while providing the patient with the simplicity and comfort that is ideal and practical in fracture treatment. Immobilization, by whatever means employed, should be continued until union is complete, although it may be difficult to determine this time with certainty. Rowe has provided some guidelines for the usual healing period of fractures of the middle third of the clavicle: infants—two weeks; children—three weeks; young adults—four to six weeks; adults—six weeks or longer.[200] It has been recognized, moreover, that radiographic union may progress more slowly than clinical union, with x-ray evidence of union not appearing for 12 weeks or longer.[163] When in doubt,

immobilization should probably be continued. It has been suggested that once clinical union has occurred with absence of motion or tenderness at the fracture site, a gradual increase in activity may safely be permitted, even if radiographic union is incomplete.[163]

Severity of Trauma. Up to one-half of fractures resulting in nonunion follow severe trauma.[101] In their series, Wilkins and Johnston reviewed 33 ununited clavicular fractures.[250] Many of their patients had severe trauma, manifested by the degree of displacement of the fracture fragments, the amount of soft tissue damage, and associated injuries such as multiple long bone, spine, pelvic, and rib fractures. They pointed out the similarities between the clavicle and another subcutaneous long bone, the tibia, which is also prone to nonunion, and emphasized that the subcutaneous position of the clavicle predisposes it to more severe trauma, more severe soft tissue damage, and thus to nonunion. As with other bones, open fractures have been implicated as a factor in nonunion of the clavicle.[124] Late perforation of the skin with a free compounding fragment has also been reported.[191]

It may be that most factors associated in some series with clavicular nonunion, such as the degree of displacement, compounding, operative management, poor immobilization, and soft tissue interposition, may simply reflect the cases that have been associated with more severe trauma to the clavicle. The independent statistical importance of some of these associations with nonunion may be questioned.

Refracture. A number of studies have identified refracture of a previously healed clavicular fracture as a factor contributing to the development of nonunion.[101, 136] In Wilkins and Johnston's series, 7 out of 31 nonunions were in such patients.[250] There appears to be no relationship between the length of time between injuries, the age of the patient, the duration of immobilization of the original fracture, or the severity of the initial or subsequent traumatic injuries and the complication of nonunion following refracture. It has been theorized that since the vascular anatomy of fractured bone remains altered for a long period even after fracture union,[193] reinjury might in some way prevent this altered blood supply from reacting to the new fracture.[250]

Location of Fracture. Approximately 85 per cent of nonunions of the clavicle occur in the middle third of the bone.[189] Despite this, it appears that fractures of the distal one-third of the clavicle are much more prone to nonunion than shaft fractures (see Fig. 11–49). In his series on clavicular nonunions, Neer noted that distal clavicular fractures accounted for over one-half of ununited clavicles following closed treatment.[154] He found the reasons for this increased incidence of nonunion to be multifactorial: (1) The fracture is very unstable, and the muscle forces and weight of the arm tend to displace the fracture fragments.[217] (2) Since these distal clavicular injuries are often the result of severe trauma, there is extensive local soft tissue injury, and there may be associated injuries that may affect generalized biological and specific fracture heal-

---

*See references 7, 55, 99, 114, 136, 154, 200, 208, 232, 242.

ing.[156] (3) There may be difficulty in securing adequate external immobilization.

Even in those fractures in which union may occur with closed methods, the union time for distal clavicular fractures is often delayed; this long healing time, combined with the associated degree of soft tissue trauma, may lead to stiffness and prolonged disability from disuse. For these reasons, Neer advocated early open reduction and internal fixation for this injury.[155, 156]

Degree of Displacement. In a large series reported by Jupiter and Leffert, the degree of displacement was the most significant factor in nonunion.[101] However, in many clavicular fractures, marked displacement is often associated with other factors that delay fracture healing, such as severe trauma, soft tissue damage, open fractures, and soft tissue interposition. Manske and Szabo felt that soft tissue interposition alone was a major contributing factor in fractures that failed to heal, and at surgery they frequently found a fracture fragment impaled in the trapezius muscle.[134] They particularly implicated soft tissue interposition in the development of atrophic nonunions. However, others have reported that muscle interposition is uncommon.[101]

Primary Open Reduction. A number of authors have associated primary open reduction of acute clavicular shaft fractures with an increase in incidence of nonunion.[214] Rowe reported an incidence of 0.8 per cent nonunion in fractures treated nonoperatively, which rose to 3.7 per cent in those treated operatively.[200] Neer had a similar experience, with a nonunion rate of 0.1 per cent in those fractures treated nonoperatively rising to 4.6 per cent when the initial fracture was treated surgically (Fig. 11–36).[154] Schwartz and Leixnering reported a nonunion rate of 13 per cent in

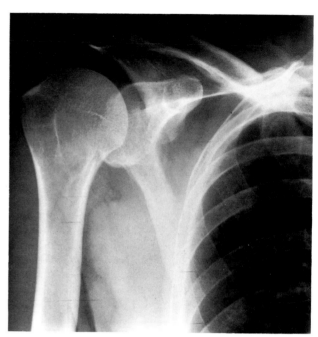

Figure 11–37. An anteroposterior view of a right shoulder in a patient who has had a clavicular fracture and now has a painful right shoulder. The area of the fracture is poorly seen.

patients with primary open reduction of clavicular fractures, although they suggested that inadequate internal fixation may have played a prominent role in this high incidence.[214] Poigenfurst and coworkers reported a complication rate of 10 per cent, with 4 nonunions in 60 fresh clavicular fractures that were plated.[179]

Poor internal fixation rather than the surgery itself may play the primary role in the increased incidence of nonunion in those patients treated with primary surgery. Zenni and associates reported a series of 25 acute clavicular fractures treated with primary open reduction, utilizing open intramedullary pin or cerclage suture and bone grafting, all of which healed without complications.[257] In some series reporting an increased incidence of nonunions with open reduction, it is probable that the operative fractures also included many of the more difficult fractures, such as those with more severe trauma, soft tissue damage, and associated injuries, thus contributing to the poor results. Nevertheless, the excellent results of nonoperative treatment are undeniable, and primary open reduction of clavicular fractures is rarely indicated.

X-ray Evaluation

Although nonunion often may be demonstrated clinically by motion at the fracture site, radiographic confirmation is obtained by anteroposterior and 45-degree cephalic tilt views. The radiographic signs of nonunion may not always be clear. If there is minimal displacement of the fracture fragments and if there is no gross motion, tomography or even bone scan may be useful in demonstrating the presence of a nonunion in a symptomatic patient (Figs. 11–37 to 11–41). As

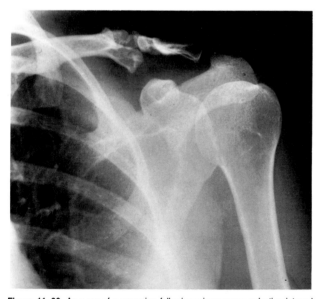

Figure 11–36. An x-ray of a nonunion following primary open reduction internal fixation of a clavicular fracture using an intramedullary pin. Inadequate internal fixation, rather than the fixation itself, may be a contributing factor in nonunion of surgically treated acute fractures.

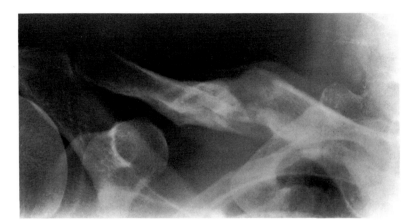

Figure 11–38. A 45-degree cephalic tilt view shows the clavicle much more clearly, but it is still uncertain whether there is clear bridging of the fracture site.

with other fractures, nonunions of the clavicle may present with hypertrophic or atrophic bone ends. There may be real or apparent bone loss, particularly if there has been comminution. It is particularly helpful in evaluating nonunions to obtain an anteroposterior view of both clavicles on a single large cassette. In this way the distance from the sternum to the acromion can be measured on the normal side and compared with the symptomatic side. This may help in deciding whether primary osteosynthesis with bone grafting will be adequate or whether an intercalary segment of bone will be needed to span the area of segmental bone loss.

Symptoms

Approximately 75 per cent of patients with an ununited clavicular fracture are symptomatic with moderate to severe pain.[101, 134] However, there is some evidence that patients with atrophic nonunions, although symptomatic initially, may become less so with time.[250] Pain from nonunion may radiate to the neck,

down into the forearm, or even into the hand, especially if there is nerve irritation.[203] The patient may complain of grating or crepitation, which is often palpable. The shoulder may appear to sag forward, inward, and medial, and the apex of the medial fragment may be observed angling upward underneath the trapezius. Twenty-five per cent or more of patients may be affected by neurological symptoms, often due to compromise of the brachial plexus by overabundant callus.[101, 203] Similarly, chronic vascular symptoms may be present owing to pressure on the subclavian vein producing symptoms of thoracic outlet syndrome.[9, 33, 101, 177]

When considering a nonunion as the cause of the patient's painful symptoms, it must be emphasized that nonunion may be an incidental finding. A careful history and physical examination must be obtained, as many soft tissue and bony abnormalities around the shoulder, including post-traumatic arthrosis of either

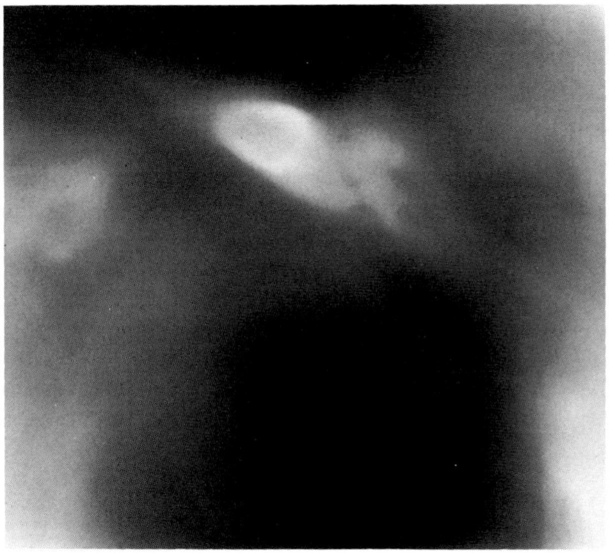

Figure 11–39. With tomography, there is a suggestion of a lucent line in the area of the fracture, which occurred four years previously.

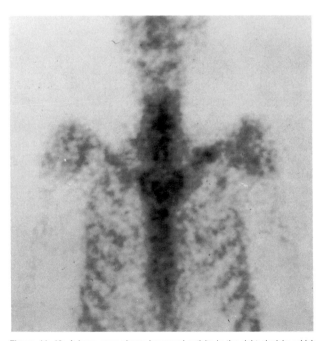

Figure 11–40. A bone scan shows increased activity in the right clavicle, which confirmed the presence of a clavicular nonunion.

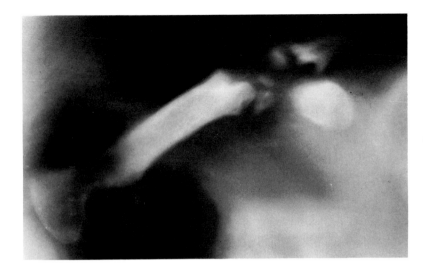

Figure 11–41. A tomogram showing bone fragmentation in a clear-cut, established nonunion of the clavicle.

the sternoclavicular or acromioclavicular joint, may mimic the symptoms of a nonunion. These degenerative changes in the joint may appear several years after the injury.[250]

Physical Examination

Physical examination may reveal motion as the clavicle is manipulated or pain upon pressure at a nonunion site. Prominent bone of comminuted fragments may be palpable. Occasionally there may be limited range of motion at the shoulder joint, but this often is associated with soft tissue, subacromial, or glenohumeral joint disease rather than a direct result of the clavicular nonunion. If there are neurological symptoms, often these are referred to the ulnar nerve distribution, and intrinsic weakness may occur.[72, 203]

MALUNION

In children with clavicular fractures, foreshortening is frequent but has not been reported to be a problem, and the angular deformity will often remodel. In adults, however, there is no remodeling potential and shortening or angulation may occur. This has been described by some authors as a purely cosmetic deformity with little interference with function.[11] However, Eskola and associates reported that patients with shortening of the clavicular segments of more than 15 mm at follow-up examination had significantly more pain than those without these findings, and they recommended taking care to avoid the acceptance of a shortened clavicle.[54]

If the malunited fracture is a significant cosmetic or functional problem, simply shaving down the bone may be inadequate[153]; several authors have recommended osteotomy, internal fixation, and bone graft.[11] The patient must be made aware, however, that nonunion may be a sequela, and that the cosmetic appearance of the surgical scar may be more troublesome than the bump from the malunited bone.

NEUROVASCULAR SEQUELAE

Despite the large amount of callus that follows healing of the fracture in children, the callus mass rarely causes any compression of the costoclavicular space and usually decreases with time.[39] In adults, however, late neurovascular sequelae can follow both united and ununited fractures.[71, 148, 215, 226, 235]

Normally the sternoclavicular angle and anterior bow of the clavicle provide abundant room for the brachial plexus and subclavian vessels in the costoclavicular space. Although there is some normal variability in the width and space between the clavicle and first rib, this room is usually adequate.[90] Occasionally a congenital anomaly, such as a bifid clavicle or a straight clavicle with no medial or anterior angulation (Fig. 11–42), may narrow the costoclavicular space and cause neu-

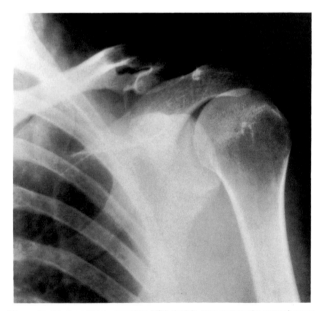

Figure 11–42. A partial or complete bifid clavicle may narrow the normal space between the clavicle and the first rib, leading to neurovascular compression syndromes.

rovascular compression.[199] Thus it is not surprising that abundant callus or significant fracture deformity in some patients may narrow this space sufficiently to cause symptoms, which most frequently involve the subclavian vessels, the carotid artery, or the brachial plexus.[104] These compression phenomena, although infrequent, are important since their clinical presentation may be confusing to the clinician and problematic for the patient until definitive treatment is instituted. The vascular structures that have been reported to be involved in compression syndromes include the following:

1. Carotid artery—obstruction of this artery may lead to symptoms of syncope. If present, this obstruction would be expected to be associated with fracture deformity or callus at the medial end of the clavicle.

2. Subclavian vein—compression of the subclavian vein between the clavicle and first rib, with subsequent obstruction, is probably the most common late vascular complication and may be accompanied by plexus and subclavian artery involvement. The point of this obstruction has been shown by Lusskin and coworkers to be the site where the vein crosses the first rib and passes beneath the subclavius muscle and costoclavicular ligament.[130] A number of authors have emphasized the role of the subclavius muscle and the condensation of the clavipectoral fascia known as the costocoracoid ligament in producing venous obstruction and subsequent thrombosis.[130] The syndrome is characterized by dilatation of the veins of the upper extremity and anterior chest on the affected side, produced by congestion of the collateral venous network. This compression is relieved by a downward thrust of the shoulder.[58, 128, 204, 225] Lusskin and associates reported that this costoclavicular syndrome could be distinguished from the typical anterior scalene, cervical rib, and thoracic outlet compression syndromes, which may also produce arterial and neurological symptoms but which typically are reproduced by Adson's maneuver. The other syndromes are not typically accentuated by shoulder girdle extension.[42, 81, 90, 210]

The treatment described by a number of authors has depended on the offending structure. If it is overabundant callus, addressing the surgery to the clavicle may be indicated. If the clavicle is more normal, however, it might make more sense to resect the first rib.

3. Subclavian artery—subclavian artery compression was reported by Guilfoil and Christiansen, who described a case of thrombosis secondary to a clavicular nonunion.[81] Although injury to this artery is recognized to occur with acute clavicular injuries,[79, 151] it is unusual as a late complication secondary to clavicular callus overabundance or nonunion. However, Yates and Guest recorded a case of death from embolus to the basilar artery that originated from a thrombosis in the subclavian artery following ununited clavicular fracture.[255]

4. Aneurysm—both traumatic aneurysm[28, 44, 157] and pseudoaneurysm[209] have been reported following clavicular fractures. These may present as pulsatile masses or soft tissue densities in the area of the clavicular fracture or nonunion and may also be the source of thrombi.

5. Brachial plexus—a number of neurological symptoms have been described relating to late complications of clavicular fractures.[80] As the onset of symptoms may be variable between fracture and the establishment of nonunion, the late sequelae can be confused with nerve injuries occurring at the time of acute injury. Thus it is particularly important to perform a careful neurological examination of the patient with an acute fracture. Whereas an early nerve injury is usually a traction neuropraxia, involves the lateral cord, and has a guarded prognosis, late compression neuropathies typically affect the medial cord, produce ulnar nerve symptoms, and have a more benign prognosis. In this complication, which typically is associated with middle third fractures, the proximal tip of the distal nonunion fragment is pulled downward and posterior, bringing it into contact with the neurovascular bundle, which is squeezed by the nonunion site above and the first and second ribs below. As one would expect, this is more commonly a problem with hypertrophic rather than atrophic nonunions.

The diagnosis of late compression syndrome is usually made by a careful history, physical examination, and electrical studies such as electromyography and nerve conduction velocities.*

POST-TRAUMATIC ARTHRITIS

Post-traumatic arthritis of the joint may follow intra-articular injuries of both the sternoclavicular and acromioclavicular joints, although degenerative disease of the distal clavicle is much more common. Often, this is the result of an intra-articular fracture that has gone unrecognized (Type III distal clavicle). The patient may present with symptoms specifically related to pain at the acromioclavicular joint or with symptoms of impingement due to an inferior protruding osteophyte of the acromioclavicular joint, causing extrinsic pressure on the subacromial bursa and rotator cuff.[152] Radiographically there may be cystic changes, spur formation, or narrowing of the acromioclavicular joint, or resorption of the distal clavicle may be found. Further radiologic studies may be needed to define the lesion, especially in the area of the sternoclavicular joint, and additional tomograms or a CT scan may be indicated. The patient will often be symptomatically improved following a diagnostic injection of 1 per cent lidocaine (Xylocaine) into the affected joint. If appropriate nonoperative treatment, including administration of nonsteroidal medications or a steroid injection, does not provide lasting relief, surgical excision of the joint may be indicated. If the outer clavicle is to be resected, the distal 2 cm of bone are removed, lateral to the coracoclavicular ligaments, and the deltoid is

*See references 16, 53, 90, 107, 130, 141, 162, 203.

repaired to the trapezius fascia. If resection of the sternoclavicular joint is indicated, the clavicular head of the sternocleidomastoid muscle may be used to fill in the area of resection.[153]

Treatment

As early as the late 1920s, more than 200 different treatment methods had already been described for fractures of the clavicle (Fig. 11–43).[115, 121] In general, excellent results have been reported with nonoperative treatment of these fractures.

The exact method of treatment of the fractured clavicle depends on several factors, including the age and medical condition of the patient, the location of the fracture, and associated injuries.

CHILDREN

Because of their excellent healing potential and the tremendous remodeling that accompanies growth, there is little role for any form of treatment other than nonoperative in children; in fact, it has been stated that operative treatment is contraindicated in chil-

dren.[229] Occasionally, however—such as for debridement of an open fracture, for neurovascular compromise that does not resolve with closed reduction, or for severe irreducible displacement of the fragments—operative management may be indicated.[19, 93, 122, 142] Although it is generally agreed that closed treatment methods are usually successful, the exact method may vary since children may differ in their comprehension or ability to cooperate with nonoperative treatment regimens.

In the newborn with a birth fracture, little treatment is needed other than measures to keep the baby comfortable. Healing is usually rapid, occurring within the first two weeks with no untoward effects. However, both the nurse and the mother must be instructed in methods of careful, safe, and gentle turning of the infant to minimize discomfort. The arm may be gently bound to the child for a few days to increase the comfort level.[39] Direct pressure over the clavicle while dressing the child is avoided.

In children with a greenstick or nondisplaced fracture, treatment often consists of the use of a sling until the symptoms have subsided.[194] In displaced fractures or those requiring reduction, most treatment methods have entailed using some form of a figure-of-eight bandage or splint, either alone or reinforced with plaster, to hold the shoulder upward and backward in

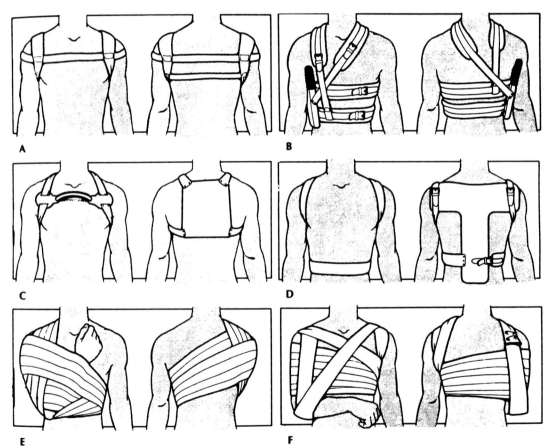

Figure 11–43. A variety of closed treatment methods have been utilized for fractures of the clavicle. A number of these are illustrated: A, Parham support; B, Bohler brace; C, Taylor clavicle support; D, unidentified support; E, Velpeau wrap; F, modified Velpeau wrap. (Reproduced with permission from Rockwood CA, and Green DP (eds): Fractures (3 vols), 2nd ed. Philadelphia: JB Lippincott, 1984.)

an attempt to reduce the degree of displacement. Fortunately, in children these fractures heal rapidly without much morbidity (Figs. 11–44 and 11–45).[180] Treatment of older children and teenagers may be more troublesome and more frequently requires plaster reinforcement because of their high level of activity.

Frequent adjustment is often needed by the physician or parent in attempting to treat these young patients with figure-of-eight methods, which can prove frustrating for both patients and surgeons. There is a real question as to whether there is any significant long-term advantage to aggressive attempts at maintaining the reduction with these treatment methods.

ADULTS

In adults with clavicular fractures, the goal of treatment (as with other fractures) is to achieve healing of bone with minimal morbidity, loss of function, and residual deformity. If this is kept in mind, re-evaluation of some of the traditional, cumbersome methods of immobilization of clavicular fractures might be considered. The main principles of nonoperative treatment historically have included the following points: (1) to brace the shoulder girdle to raise the outer fragment upward, outward, and backward; (2) to depress the inner fragment; (3) to maintain its reduction; and (4) to enable the ipsilateral elbow and hand to be used so that associated problems with immobilization can be avoided.

An extensive review of the literature generally leads one to conclude that immobilization is nearly impossible to achieve, that deformity and shortening are usual, and that even if some shortening occurs it generally does not interfere with function. The literature is replete with methods of various complexity to immobilize the clavicle, and treatment has been described ranging from long-term recumbency

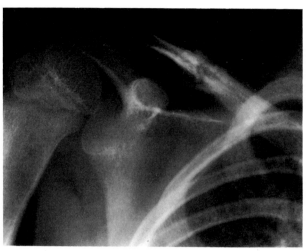

Figure 11–45. Same patient as in Figure 11–44. Fourteen days later there is clinical absence of pain and significant callus formation.

alone,[11, 186] various forms of ambulatory treatment,[34] and, finally, various internal fixation methods.*

In general, the methods of treatment of clavicular fractures can be broadly grouped into the following:

1. Simple support of the arm (Fig. 11–46). Whether by sling alone, a sling-and-swathe, a Sayre bandage, or a Velpeau bandage,[121] no attempt is made to maintain a clavicular reduction, provided that satisfactory positioning of the bone appears to be present so that union is anticipated.[178] Although sling treatment is certainly the simplest way to treat the fractured clavicular shaft, it is often unsettling to the orthopedic surgeon who wishes to effect realignment of the fracture fragments; this probably explains the popularity of the many methods of effecting and maintaining a closed reduction.

2. Reduction. This is followed by the attempt to maintain and hold reduction by bringing the distal fragment up and back. This may be done by a bandage alone (including the figure-of-eight),[18, 186] with plaster reinforcement,[35, 256] or by full immobilization of the shoulder in various forms of spica cast (Figs. 11–47 and 11–48).[111, 153, 171, 200, 237] A variety of materials have

---

*See references 21, 93, 106, 118, 120, 145, 150, 158, 172, 176, 202, 257.

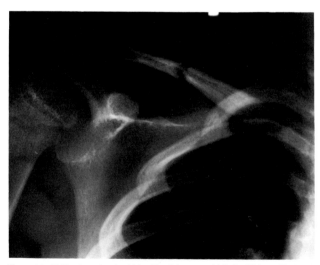

Figure 11–44. Fractures heal quickly with minimum morbidity in children with simple immobilization. An x-ray of a clavicular fracture in a five-year-old is illustrated.

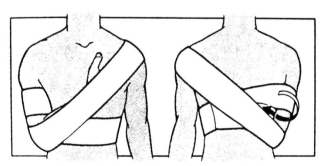

Figure 11–46. Modification of a Sayre bandage, which is intended not to reduce the fracture but to simply support the arm. (Reproduced with permission from Rockwood CA, and Green DP (eds): Fractures (3 vols), 2nd ed. Philadelphia: JB Lippincott, 1984.)

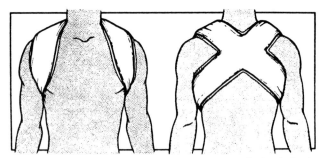

Figure 11–47. A Billington yoke, a method of attempting to maintain reduction by plaster reinforcement of a figure-of-eight–type immobilization. (Reproduced with permission from Rockwood CA, and Green DP (eds): Fractures (3 vols), 2nd ed. Philadelphia: JB Lippincott, 1984.)

been described to maintain the closed reduction, including metal, leather, plastic, plaster, and muslin.[153] The position required to reduce the fracture and maintain the reduction (upward, lateral, and backward) is difficult to achieve, may often be uncomfortable for the patient, and occasionally has been reported to cause symptoms of either neurovascular compression or displacement of the fragment[200] if careful attention is not paid to placing the external immobilization precisely. Few studies have attempted in a controlled

fashion to evaluate whether a vigorous attempt to effect and maintain a reduction provides a greater chance for a better outcome than simple arm support for comfort. In two studies directly comparing a figure-of-eight dressing with sling support, it was noted that figure-of-eight dressings were time consuming, required frequent adjustments, might contribute to other problems, and had more complications than a simple sling treatment. The authors concluded that functional and cosmetic sequelae of the two methods of treatment were identical and that alignment of the healed fracture was unchanged from the initial displacement.[6, 140]

3. Open or closed reduction with internal fixation. A number of techniques have been described for treatment of clavicular fractures with internal fixation.[84, 168, 212] These techniques have included cerclage sutures,[237] intramedullary devices (Steinmann pin, K-wire, Knowles, Perry, or Rush pins),* or plate fixation.[110, 149]

4. In rare instances, primary excision of both ends of the fracture with skin closure and intentional formation of a pseudarthrosis has been advocated.[174]

---

*See references 21, 120, 145, 150, 158, 172, 176, 202, 257.

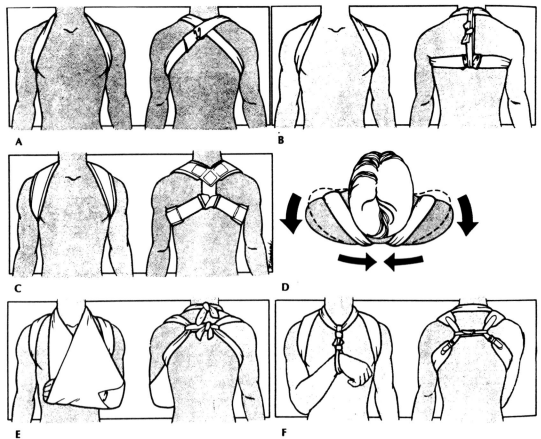

Figure 11–48. Various types of figure-of-eight bandages. The figure-of-eight method is intended to maintain a reduction that has been achieved by closed means. *A,* Stockinette that has been padded with three layers of sheet wadding and held in place with safety pins. *B,* Padded stockinette that is not crossed in the back. The upper and lower borders are tied to each other and tightened daily, increasing the tension to maintain the reduction. *C,* A commercial figure-of-eight support. *D,* Superior view of the patient, showing how the figure-of-eight support pulls the shoulder up and backward. *E,* A modified figure-of-eight bandage with a sling. *F,* A figure-of-eight support used with a collar and cuff. (Reproduced with permission from Rockwood CA, and Green DP (eds): Fractures (3 vols), 2nd ed. Philadelphia: JB Lippincott, 1984.)

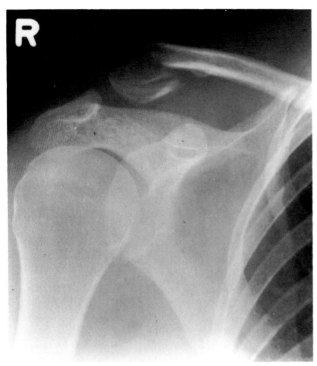

Figure 11–49. A distal clavicular fracture. The ligaments are attached to the distal clavicular piece, and there is high riding and instability of the proximal fragment. Open reduction internal fixation was elected as the treatment method because of the potential for nonunion in this fracture.

Although distal clavicular fractures may heal quite well without surgical treatment[197, 198] because of the deforming forces and high incidence of nonunion, many authors continue to recommend primary open reduction and internal fixation,[56] either with an intramedullary pin[155, 156] or with some method of dynamic fixation to bring the proximal clavicular segment to the distal (Figs. 11–49 to 11–53).[106] Complications have been reported with each of these methods, including

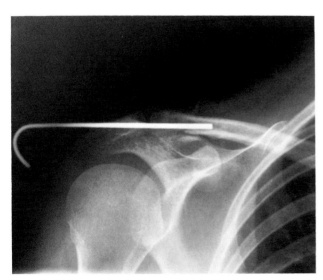

Figure 11–50. Intramedullary fixation was elected with a heavy Kirschner wire, bent to prevent migration.

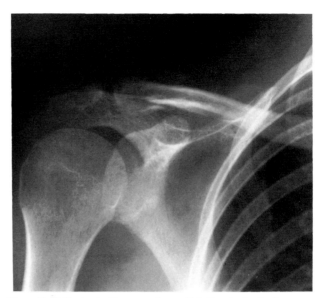

Figure 11–51. Fracture healing occurred uneventfully. Once fracture healing occurs, the shoulder and clavicle are stable because the ligaments are attached to the distal fragment.

migration of intramedullary wires. In addition, musculocutaneous nerve injuries have been reported with the use of the coracoid process transferred to the proximal clavicular segment in this fracture.[28] Plate fixation is often impractical because of the small distal segment. It appears that some type of intramedullary device not prone to migration might offer the safest method of treatment for distal clavicular fractures.

NONUNION

Asymptomatic clavicular nonunions need not be treated. In addition, nonunions in the elderly should probably be considered for nonoperative treatment. Although nonoperative methods to obtain union have been reported—particularly the use of electrical stim-

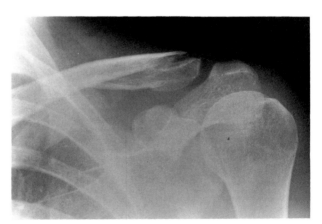

Figure 11–52. Distal clavicular fractures may heal quite well without surgical treatment in some instances, as evidenced by this x-ray. This adult had an oblique distal clavicular fracture treated nonoperatively. Clinical and radiographic union has occurred.

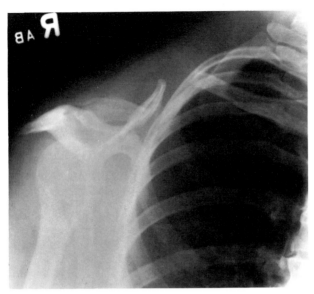

Figure 11-53. Radiographic appearance of a 26-year-old woman who had fractured her clavicle five years previously. A painful nonunion was present, with an intermediate gap and atrophic ends.

ulation—there have been only a few documented cases of healing of clavicular nonunions by pulsed electromagnetic fields.[22, 43] Most authors share the view that there is little role for electrical stimulation in the treatment of clavicular nonunions, especially since operative methods have shown such a high degree of success.[10, 32]

Indications for surgical treatment include: (1) pain or aching clearly attributable to the nonunion; (2) shoulder girdle dysfunction, weakness, or fatigue; and (3) neurovascular compromise.[172] Although bone drilling has been suggested as a means of stimulating a delayed union to progress,[183] there is little role for this in established nonunion. Alternatively, some authors have advocated resection of the nonunion.

Partial claviculectomy, with excision of the nonunion site, has been reported by some as a means of treating ununited clavicular fracture. Certainly, in the short term this may alleviate the crepitus and often will eliminate the pain.[134] However, many patients treated in this way may remain mildly to moderately symptomatic,[101, 250] the stabilizing function of the clavicle is lost, and neurogenic symptoms may be a problem.[124, 250] However, resection of the nonunion and filling of the defect with cancellous bone chips may stimulate regeneration of the clavicle and, in addition, may decompress the neurovascular structures if nonunion is accompanied by symptoms of thoracic outlet syndrome.[33] Surgical treatment most commonly consists of an attempt to gain union through some means of internal fixation with bone grafting. The techniques for surgical treatment of nonunions have evolved, as have internal fixation techniques for other long bone fractures and nonunions.

A number of open treatment methods have been detailed. Some authors have used *wire sutures* through the ends of either clavicular fragment and through an iliac crest graft.[11, 72, 154] Sutures of other materials including catgut, braided suture, and even loops of kangaroo tendon have been utilized in the past.[153] Simple *intrafragmentary screw fixation* has been advocated, with fixation of the iliac bone as an onlay graft and cancellous bone grafting at either junction.[138, 203] However, because of the amount of movement in multiple planes that the clavicle exhibits and because these methods control rotation poorly, neither suture nor screw fixation is secure enough to be reliable when used independently of additional protection. External cast or brace support is necessary to prevent screw or wire breakage and possible wire fragment migration which can produce disastrous results.[116, 139, 165]

Open reduction internal fixation with intramedullary fixation has been a popular means of internal fixation, either with the use of K-wires (with or without screws),* Steinmann pins,[110, 155, 200] Knowles pins,[158] or modified Hagie pins.[195] Although reports have been encouraging with these methods and they can be successful, rotation is poorly controlled under most circumstances, the intramedullary fixation can be difficult to insert if there are atrophic bone ends (especially with the flat, curved clavicle), and often external plaster support is required. In addition, distraction of the fracture at the nonunion site with threaded pins may occur.[110] The intramedullary device may bend or break, and a number of complications have been reported with pin migration.[116, 139, 165] Despite reports of success,[234] the complication rate can be high with intramedullary fixation—as high as 75 per cent in one series.[250]

The application of rigid internal fixation in acute fractures has aided management in the treatment of many traditionally difficult fractures, and this concept of rigidly immobilizing fragment ends has had its natural application in the treatment of nonunions as well. Although rigid internal fixation techniques utilizing AO plates without bone grafting have been reported to be successful in clavicular nonunions as in nonunions of other long bones,[87, 184] the addition of supplemental bone graft to rigid plating has been the most popular treatment of clavicular nonunions (Fig. 11–54). With this method of treatment, reports in the literature have approached 100 per cent union rate.† Manske and Szabo reported an incidence of 100 per cent union by 10 weeks postoperatively without complications, using open reduction and internal fixation with compression plating and bone grafting.[134] Jupiter and Leffert reported on 23 clavicular nonunions, including 2 resulting from clavicular osteotomies for surgical access, with an overall success rate of 89 per cent in achieving union. However, 93.7 per cent of those treated with grafting and dynamic compression plating achieved union.[101] Eskola and colleagues reported 20 to 22 clavicular nonunions healing with rigid plate fixation and bone grafting, but they warned

---

*See references 136, 153, 163, 214, 232, 236, 244.

†See references 49, 50, 103, 184, 190, 234, 246.

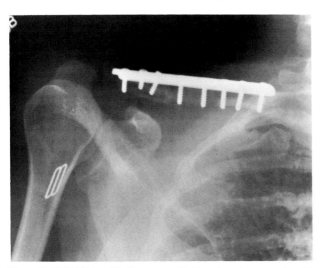

Figure 11–54. Rigid internal fixation was provided by a dynamic compression plate with an intercalary bone graft. Clinical and radiographic union has occurred.

against shortening of the clavicle to achieve union.[55] For this reason, if resection of the sclerotic edges of the atrophic margin in order to achieve primary osteosynthesis would result in significant clavicular shortening, many authors recommend intercalary bone grafting along with plate fixation.[16, 124] Plate fixation and bone grafting is reliable, safe, has few complications, and has the added benefit that rigid internal fixation usually is secure enough so that no postoperative external cast immobilization is needed—use of a sling alone is usually adequate. The plate does have the disadvantage of requiring a second operation to remove the hardware if its prominent position irritates the skin. In addition, the screw holes weaken the bone and protection is needed after hardware removal.

However, there is one instance in which intramedullary fixation is probably the treatment of choice. In nonunion of the distal third of the clavicle, particularly the Type II distal clavicular fracture, the distal fragment is usually too small for adequate plate and screw fixation, and there has been excellent success using intramedullary fixation with bone grafting for this specific nonunion.[156]

NEUROVASCULAR COMPLICATIONS

In general, the treatment for late neurovascular lesions has depended on the cause of the compromised structure.

1. If there is neurovascular compromise by massive callus formation and callus debulking is risky, if internal fixation with bone grafting of pseudarthrosis is impractical because of comminution, or if there is a malunion with a severe deformity and realignment osteotomy cannot be achieved, then *resection* of the middle third of the clavicle may be the best choice if the lesion is in this portion. Abbott and Lucas have outlined the various areas of the clavicle that can be resected without untoward sequelae and those areas

that do less well with resection.[1] Although some authors have advocated a total claviculectomy, it is probably wiser to do careful subtotal resections when possible.

2. If there is excessive callus buildup or malunion of the clavicle and the lesion is amenable to bone grafting and plate fixation, then removal of the hypertrophic callus buildup and realignment osteotomy with or without segmental interposition of bone graft and cancellous bone grafting will often relieve the neurovascular symptoms.

3. If the clavicle has a satisfactory appearance and is stable, enlargement of the costoclavicular space—and thus, neurovascular decompression—can be accomplished by first rib resection with partial excision of the scalene or subclavius muscle.[42, 215]

Postoperative Care

In the operating room following operative treatment of the nonunion or an acute fracture, the patient is placed in a sling and swathe. A postoperative x-ray is reviewed; it should include not only the fracture site and the internal fixation, to determine the fracture alignment and hardware placement, but also enough of the lung to ensure that no injury has occurred during the surgical procedure. When comfortable, the patient is discharged and wound care is the same as for any surgical procedure on the shoulder.

If the glenohumeral joint and the subacromial bursa have not been surgically violated and are otherwise not diseased, there appears to be no need for institution of early range-of-motion exercises, as shoulder range of motion, if normal preoperatively, will usually remain so. Thus the patient may be kept safely supported in a sling or immobilizer until radiographic signs of union occur, without fear of producing a frozen shoulder.

Early in the postoperative period, isometric exercises for the rotator cuff may be begun, although isometric strengthening of the trapezius and deltoid are delayed until their suture junction is healed securely (three to four weeks). Range of motion following surgery is not permitted past 45 degrees of flexion in the plane of the scapula until there are clinical signs of union, usually at four to six weeks.

When clinical or radiographic union is present, the patient may begin full range of motion, particularly in forward elevation (utilizing an overhead pulley); external rotation (with the use of a cane or stick), and hyperextension–internal rotation are then added. Resistive exercises of the deltoid, trapezius, cuff, and scapula muscles are also added. When radiographic union is present, full active use of the arm is permitted.

The patient is not permitted to return to full, strenuous work or athletic activities until there is a nearly full range of motion of the shoulder, strength has returned to near normal, and bone healing is presumed solid. In adults this is usually four to six months postoperatively.

Author's Preferred Method of Treatment

NEWBORNS AND INFANTS

Despite some information that this fracture in the newborn may be asymptomatic, I prefer to ensure comfort by treating clavicular birth fractures for a few days. The newborn is supine for many hours in the day; one who is not particularly active may be treated simply by avoiding pressure on the clavicle when dressing the infant and taking care to handle him or her gently, avoiding movement of the affected arm during feeding, diapering, and dressing change. When the newborn is prone, soft padding may be placed under the anterior aspect of the shoulder, using the weight of the body to help keep the lateral clavicle back. Avoiding handling a newborn is neither practical nor desirable. If "pseudoparalysis" is present in which the infant avoids using the arm because of pain, I prefer to place a cotton abdominal pad under the infant's arm, flex the elbow fully to 90 degrees, and gently strap the arm to the chest with a padded elastic bandage, Kling, or Kerlix bandage. A sling is difficult to apply and maintain and is not necessary. The parents may be taught to reapply the bandage for skin care and after bathing. Usually within 7 to 10 days the patient is asymptomatic, and healing is usually complete by two weeks. The infant will use the arm normally once symptoms subside. Unrestricted use of the arm is permitted once the wrap is off, and the parents may be reassured that deformity and exuberant callus will remodel in time. After adequate healing, the infant is retested with Moro's reflex to make certain that the disinclination to move the arm was, in fact, a pseudoparalysis rather than inability to move the arm secondary to an injury to the brachial plexus.[229]

CHILDREN

Ages 2 to 12

Young children are treated symptomatically. Under age six no attempt is made to reduce the fracture, as the fracture will remodel and the large lump will be gone in six to nine months.[229] The child is made more comfortable with some type of applied figure-of-eight bandage. Commercial figure-of-eight bandages are usually too large; the simplest way to construct one out of materials is to use 2-inch stockinette filled with cotton wadding, cast padding, or felt. The child is seated and the dressing is applied as follows: the surgeon, standing behind the patient, passes the stockinette across the front of the uninjured clavicle, through the uninjured axilla and across the back, through the axilla on the fracture site, across the front of the anterior shoulder and clavicle on the fracture site, and across the back behind the neck. To help keep the shoulder up and back, tension is placed on the stockinette and a safety pin binds both ends of the stockinette together as the tension is maintained. An elastic bandage or 2-inch tape securing the bandage can be placed from one posterior strap to the other, maintaining the tension and securing the position. Alternatively, the figure-of-eight stockinette may be crisscrossed behind the patient before being applied to the fracture side and subsequently pinned and tightened. If the 2-inch stockinette appears to be an irritation to the skin, an abdominal cotton pad can be placed beneath the anterior straps. Parents should be instructed on how to tighten the figure-of-eight bandage to maintain this tension by reapplying the anchoring safety pin. This should be done *in situ* without taking the stockinette off. The stockinette may have a tendency to loosen quickly; it should be retightened two or three days after the initial application and then weekly thereafter. I prefer to see the child weekly to assure that the bandage is secure and that there are no skin problems, neurovascular irritation, or any other problems with treatment. Parents should be made aware of potential circulatory difficulties or skin problems if the bandage is too tight, and I ask them to practice tightening the bandage with my supervision to minimize the anxiety of having to bear the responsibility for handling the bandage adjustment themselves. In young children three weeks is usually adequate immobilization, but in the older ambulatory child clinical signs of union, such as absence of tenderness to pressure over the fracture site or movement of the arm, are good signs that can help the physician decide when immobilization may be discontinued. Although union typically occurs in three to six weeks, symptoms are often dramatically diminished within the first two to three weeks (Figs. 11–55 and 11–56).

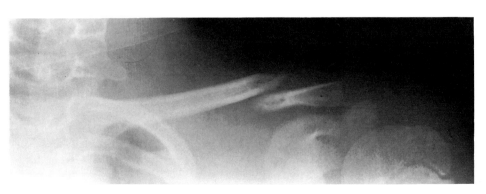

Figure 11–55. A nine-year-old boy with a fracture of the lateral portion of the middle third of the clavicle.

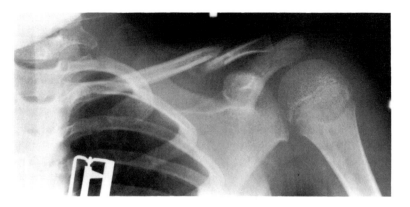

Figure 11–56. Two and a half weeks postoperatively, periosteal reaction and early callus formation are seen. The patient was clinically nontender. Union progresses rapidly in childhood fractures of the clavicle, and little attempt is made to produce and maintain a reduction.

Nondisplaced fractures, incomplete fractures, or plastic bone bowing need not be treated with the figure-of-eight bandage, as the position is unlikely to change with ambulatory treatment if activity can be curtailed and reinjury avoided. A simple sling for comfort until clinical union takes place is sufficient.

It should be suggested that the child avoid unusually vigorous activities such as gym class until the bone is solid, typically at about three months.

Repeat x-ray evaluation is not necessary at each return visit. I typically order an x-ray of the involved shoulder with the immobilization in place, another x-ray to check the progress of healing and the amount of callus, and one final x-ray when union is definite (between 6 to 12 weeks). An additional x-ray showing healing is helpful; in the event of reinjury, x-ray interpretation can be confusing if there is no x-ray showing radiographic union after the first injury.

Ages 12 to 16

This group may be difficult to treat because their activity level often frustrates the most aggressive attempts to maintain reduction and immobilization. Whereas in very young children little or no attempt is made to reduce the fracture, the teenage population has limited remodeling potential and an attempt is made to reduce the fracture before applying the immobilization. Teenagers are often self-conscious about the deformity and bump that may remain after the fracture is healed, and this is another reason to attempt closed reduction. With meticulously sterile technique and careful preparation of the area, the hematoma is infiltrated with 6 to 10 ml of 1 per cent lidocaine (Xylocaine) or bupivacaine hydrochloride (Marcaine); the resulting anesthesia usually permits reduction and molding of the fracture into satisfactory position (Fig. 11–57). With the fracture reduced, a 4-inch stockinette with cast padding may be passed in the figure-of-eight fashion as with young children. To reduce the fracture, the knee is placed in the midback between both scapulae as the teenager is sitting on a stool, both shoulders are brought upward and backward, and the fracture may be molded into place. In more active children a plaster yoke should be considered, fashioned in the

same way as the figure-of-eight bandage. However, caution should be taken that the skin is well padded with cast padding, felt, or cotton wadding in stockinette and that the soft padding under the plaster extends out past the sharp edges of the plaster. The cast may be trimmed where the edges are sharp. Treatment for six weeks is usually adequate in the older child and adolescent. In cooperative older children and young adults, a commercial figure-of-eight clavicular splint—usually an elastic bandage with well-padded areas for the axilla—may be applied. The commercial splint has several advantages including easy removal for bathing and more resistance to "stretching out" over time than the fashioned stockinette. This figure-of-eight bandage does not serve to reduce or rigidly immobilize the

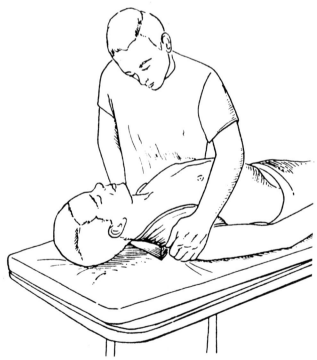

Figure 11–57. Recumbency has been prescribed as one of the treatment methods for clavicular fractures. This may be useful in the multiply traumatized patient. A bump or pillow is placed between the scapulae, allowing the weight of the arm to reduce the fracture. However, in a multiply traumatized patient, consideration should be given to open reduction and rigid internal fixation. (Reproduced with permission from De Palma A: Surgery of the Shoulder, 3rd ed. Philadelphia: JB Lippincott, 1983.)

fracture, but it may serve as a reminder to hold the shoulders "back" when the child wants to slump forward.[39]

Despite reports that there may not be any long-term difference between the use of the sling and the figure-of-eight bandage, I still prefer the latter after an attempt is made to reduce the fracture, maintaining alignment of the clavicle. The figure-of-eight bandage has one advantage that the sling lacks—it leaves both hands and elbows free for use in activities of daily living. In addition, the sling in its usual position holds the arm forward and inward, and the distal clavicular segment is not in position to be lined up with the proximal.

In the older children, fractures usually heal within six weeks. However, I usually maintain the clavicular immobilizer for another four weeks after healing to serve as a reminder to restrict activities. Vigorous athletic activities should be avoided until union is solid, which in the teenager should be after 12 to 16 weeks.[39, 42]

In the multiply traumatized child the clavicular fracture can be treated by recumbency if a small pillow is placed between the scapulae, allowing the weight of the arm to reduce the fracture. If recumbent treatment is to be instituted, the use of a sling may make the arm more comfortable.

Medial and Distal Fractures in Children

I prefer to treat both medial and distal clavicular fractures in children with a sling for support and an elastic (Ace) wrap for comfort. Medial clavicular fractures are rare problems and rarely produce significant displacement. Lateral clavicular fractures, although clinically dramatic (appearing to be a high-grade acromioclavicular separation), are stable since the coracoclavicular ligaments and acromioclavicular ligaments remain attached to the periosteal tube and both sides of the joint, respectively. Despite the degree of displacement, the bone will remodel in time (Fig. 11–58). For lateral clavicular fractures, I find a figure-of-eight bandage difficult to maintain over the most lateral aspect of the shoulder; the sling-and-swathe is more practical and quite comfortable, and the healing potential in children negates the need for precise maintenance of reduction.

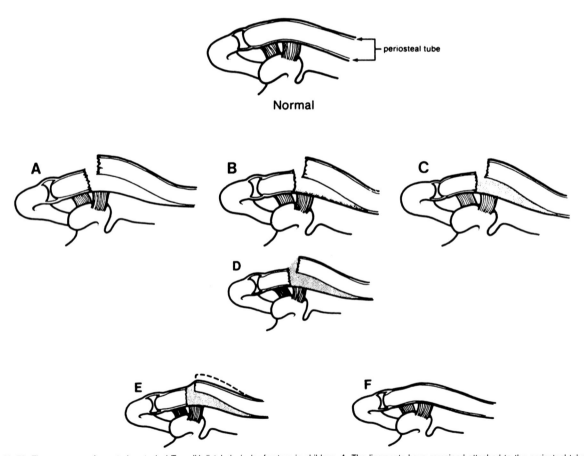

Figure 11–58. The sequence of events in a typical Type IV distal clavicular fracture in children. *A*, The ligaments have remained attached to the periosteal tube as the medial clavicular fragment ruptures through the superior thin periosteum. This may mimic an acromioclavicular separation. *B*, Early filling of the area between the periosteum and the bone is seen. *C*, Further filling in of the bone is seen. *D*, Bridging callus is seen to reach the top of the medial clavicular segment. *E*, Early remodeling has begun to occur with further consolidation of the fracture. *F*, Remodeling has occurred with complete union. This fracture is best treated nonoperatively, and excellent results can be expected. (Reproduced with permission from Rockwood CA, and Green DP (eds): Fractures (3 vols), 2nd ed. Philadelphia: JB Lippincott, 1984.)

ADULTS

Fractures of the adult clavicle are much more difficult to treat, since the quality of the bone and periosteum is different from that in children and associated soft tissue or bony injury is often greater. In addition, the potential for healing is less in adults.

Fractures of the Shaft

Despite the broad range of treatment methods for clavicular shaft fractures in adults, I prefer a commercially available figure-of-eight splint following closed reduction. To reduce the clavicle, the patient is seated on a stool with the surgeon behind; after meticulous preparation, the area of fracture and fracture hematoma is infiltrated with 8 to 12 ml of 1 per cent Xylocaine. The knee is placed between the scapulae, the outer edges of the shoulders are held securely, and the shoulders are pulled upward, outward, and backward (Fig. 11–59). The fracture may then be manipulated into place. The commercially available figure-of-eight bandage (usually supplemented with an abdominal pad in the area of the axilla) is preferred because it is more comfortable, less cumbersome, and more attractive than (for example) a plaster spica cast,

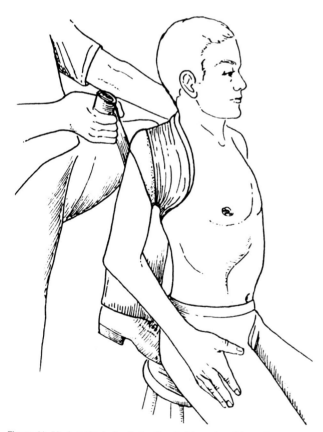

Figure 11–59. A method of reducing the clavicle and applying a figure-of-eight bandage. The knee is placed between the scapulae, both outer edges of the shoulder are held securely, and the shoulders are pulled upward, outward, and backward. (Reproduced with permission from De Palma A: Surgery of the Shoulder, 3rd ed. Philadelphia: JB Lippincott, 1983.)

and immobilization of the fracture is as adequately achieved as with more drastic and bulky forms of external fixation. The figure-of-eight bandage has the added advantage of leaving both hands and elbows free. A sling may be added to the figure-of-eight to provide additional support for the arm and to make sleeping more comfortable. Because adults usually have more trouble healing the fracture than children, immobilization must be maintained for six to eight weeks. Although I permit rotation of the arm at the side in any direction and to any extent, I limit the active use of the arm until clinical union takes place. If refracture occurs during the treatment period, continued immobilization by this means is appropriate. Athletics are not permitted until at least six weeks after clinical and radiographic union. At six to eight weeks, the patient is taken out of the figure-of-eight and placed in the sling for an additional three to four weeks for added protection, while gentle isometric and mobilization exercises are begun at this time.

Indications for Primary Open Fixation

My indications for operative treatment of acute clavicular fractures include the following:

1. Neurovascular injury or compromise that is progressive or that fails to reverse with closed reduction of the fracture.

2. Severe displacement caused by comminution with resulting angulation and tenting of the skin severe enough to threaten its integrity, and which fails to respond to a closed reduction.

3. An open fracture that will require operative debridement.

4. Multiple trauma, when mobility of the patient is desirable and closed methods of immobilization are impractical or impossible.

5. Type II distal clavicular fractures (see below).

6. Factors that render the patient unable to tolerate closed immobilization, such as the neurological problems of parkinsonism, seizure disorders, or other neurovascular disorders.[257]

7. The very rare patient for whom the cosmetic lump over the healed clavicle is intolerable and who is willing to exchange this for a potentially equally noncosmetic surgical scar and the possibility of a nonunion.

Although there are numerous relative or absolute indications for surgery, it must be emphasized that very few fractures of the shaft need to be treated with primary surgical open reduction and internal fixation.[153, 162]

If surgery for a fractured clavicle is to be undertaken, historically the choices have tended to be between plate fixation (AO) and intramedullary fixation.[139, 148] I prefer intramedullary fixation for acute fractures for the following reasons: (1) there is less exposure of the fracture and therefore a smaller skin incision; (2) little periosteal stripping is needed and therefore there is less interference with the healing potential of the fracture; (3) removal of hardware is less problematic and can usually be done with a local anesthetic; and (4) no screw holes remain to act as potential areas of weakness of the bone.

Although the use of a threaded Steinmann pin bent at the lateral end to avoid migration is a well-described technique, my preference is a Knowles pin, a method described by Neviaser.[158] The Knowles pin has a hub that is large enough to prevent pin migration and is easily palpable beneath the skin when removal is desired. The threaded distal end of the pin also helps to prevent migration. To insert this pin, the patient is placed in a "beach chair" position; a small horizontal incision is made at the level of the fracture, which is then exposed. The fracture is reduced and held with towel clips. The Knowles pin is drilled from lateral to medial, entering the clavicle at the posterolateral aspect of the acromion, avoiding the acromioclavicular joint if possible. It is then directed toward the medial fragment of the clavicle and down the intramedullary portion of the fragment.

Alternatively, a 4-mm Steinmann pin may be drilled retrograde from medial to lateral after the fracture is exposed, entering the lateral fragment at the fracture site and emerging at the posterolateral aspect of the acromion. At the point of egress of the pin, a Knowles pin is drilled antegrade through the acromion, following the Steinmann pin as the latter is withdrawn. At the fracture site, the fracture is reduced and held with towel clips and the Knowles pin is drilled into the medullary canal. If the Knowles pin penetrates the anterior cortex and the tip of the pin is excessively prominent, it may be cut even with the anterior edge of the clavicle to avoid prominence under the skin. In addition, the subacromial space must be palpated to ensure that the intramedullary pin is not in the subacromial space but is in fact transacromial.

I also prefer to add bone graft acutely along with

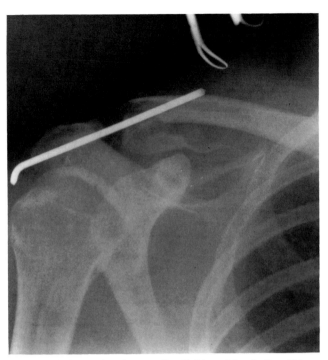

Figure 11–61. It was elected to treat this with intramedullary fixation utilizing a heavy Kirschner wire.

internal fixation when any acute shaft fracture is treated with open reduction and internal fixation.

Fractures of the Distal Clavicle

In Type I distal clavicular fracture the ligaments are intact, displacement is minimal, and the patient may be treated with a sling for comfort, early isometric exercises, and discontinuation of the immobilization as symptoms permit.

Type II distal clavicular fractures, as has been discussed previously, are difficult to treat nonoperatively. Immobilization is difficult, the fragments are distracted by muscle forces and the weight of the arm, the proximal fragment is unstable and has no ligamentous attachment, and nonunion is an all-too-frequent sequela. The usual sling does not reduce the deformity, and the use of a figure-of-eight bandage can actually increase the deformity by holding the proximal fragment posteriorly. Although closed treatment has been successful,[198] union often is delayed and shoulder stiffness may add morbidity to the treatment. Patients with this fracture are probably best treated with open reduction and internal fixation acutely (Figs. 11–60 to 11–63). The operative treatment of this fracture depends on the size of the lateral fragment and the position and integrity of the coracoclavicular ligaments relative to the fragments.

Although a variety of encircling wires,[160, 162] pins, and sutures[156] binding the proximal fragment to the coracoid process have been described, I prefer open intramedullary fixation utilizing the Knowles pin (Fig. 11–64). It must be remembered that because of the fracture anatomy, the coracoclavicular ligaments are usually

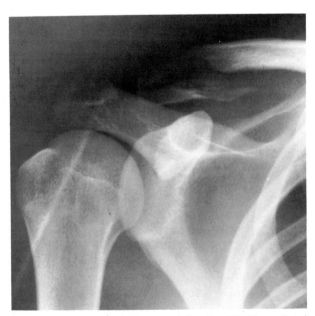

Figure 11–60. A distal clavicular fracture, probably a Type V that is comminuted.

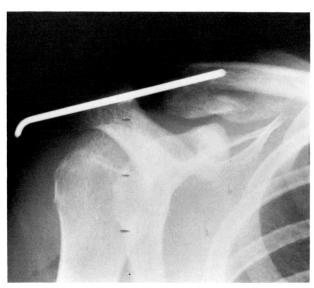

Figure 11–62. Early healing is seen.

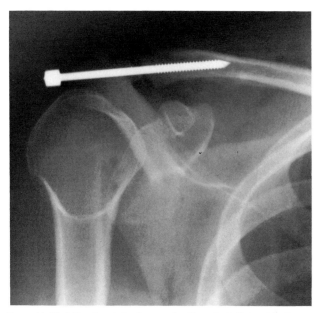

Figure 11–64. A Knowles pin is often a preferable method of internal fixation, as the hub prevents migration and is easily palpable for later removal. It can be buried underneath the skin.

attached to the distal fragment, with the proximal fragment pulled upward by the contraction of the trapezius muscle. Therefore, if fracture union can be achieved, the acromioclavicular joint and clavicle are stable.

With the patient in the "beach chair" position and the head turned away from the side of the fracture, a small vertical incision is made at the fracture site. The deltoid–trapezius interval is split horizontally and the fracture site exposed. I often place a very heavy nonabsorbable suture or a piece of Mersilene tape around the coracoid process and proximal clavicular segment to aid in security of the reduction. This is passed prior to reduction of the fracture. In addition,

prior to reduction of the fracture a Knowles pin is drilled from the posterolateral aspect of the acromion, emerging from the medullary canal of the distal clavicular segment. Once the pin is seen and the subacromial space is palpated to make certain that the pin has not violated it, the fracture is reduced; reduction may be maintained with towel clips, and the Knowles pin is advanced through the intramedullary canal of the proximal clavicular fragment. It is usually not a problem if the pin penetrates the anterior cortex; any excessive length can be cut flush with the anterior clavicle. The nonabsorbable suture or tape from the coracoid to the clavicle is then securely tied for added fixation. Although both the conoid and trapezoid ligaments may be attached to the distal clavicular segment, not infrequently the conoid ligament is torn with the trapezoid alone attached to the distal segment. If this is the case, the conoid ligament may be sutured into the clavicular periosteum or into the clavicular insertion of the trapezoid ligament. With adequate internal fixation of an acute fracture of the lateral clavicle, I typically do not perform bone graft for these fractures since union usually ensues, but bone graft may be added if desirable acutely. The patient is then placed in a sling and swathe postoperatively, and isometric exercises are begun in the early postoperative period. The Knowles pin is removed after radiographic signs of early fracture healing (six weeks) since the coracoclavicular sutures contribute to added security, early healing has generally occurred by this time, and the hub of the Knowles pin may be irritating to the skin.

Type III fractures of the distal clavicle are not often recognized acutely. When they are seen acutely, if they are unstable, or when they appear to be an extension of a Type II injury into the joint they should be treated

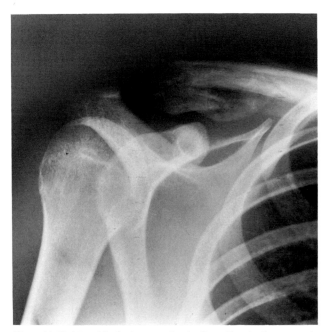

Figure 11–63. Internal fixation is removed and radiographic union has occurred.

as a Type II injury. If they lead to symptomatic late degeneration of the acromioclavicular joint, the distal 2 cm of clavicle may be excised with little morbidity and excellent results. If treated surgically, the distal fragment should be retained because of its attachment to the coracoclavicular ligaments unless there is hopeless damage of the articular surface or severe comminution. In extremely rare instances, if it is necessary to excise the distal segment, the proximal clavicular segment must be stabilized, usually with an intramedullary pin, and the ligaments transferred from the distal fragment to the proximal fragment. Occasionally the coracoacromial ligament may be secured to the proximal fragment acutely.[245]

Fractures of the Medial Clavicle

Fractures of the medial clavicle require symptomatic support only unless there is severe neurovascular compromise or injury. If this occurs and the fracture must be operated upon, open reduction should be considered. However, even if this fracture is openly reduced, I prefer to avoid intramedullary fixation of the clavicle because of the difficulty of securing and positioning the fragment and the danger of pin migration with its potentially catastrophic results.

Nonunion

Fortunately, clavicular nonunions are rare. When they occur, 75 per cent are in the shaft (30 per cent atrophic, 70 per cent hypertrophic) and 25 per cent are in the distal third.[101, 134] A nonunion that is asymptomatic need not be treated.

My preference for treatment of a symptomatic clavicular shaft nonunion is to use a compression plate and bone graft, ideally utilizing a six- or seven-hole

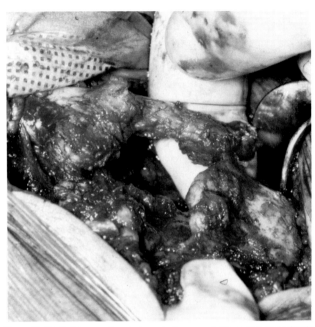

Figure 11–66. An intraoperative photograph shows small, thin, and tapered sclerotic edges of the nonunion.

dynamic compression plate (3.5 mm) with at least six cortices secured on each clavicular segment (Figs. 11–65 to 11–68; see also Fig. 11–54). I prefer a dynamic compression plate to the semitubular plate because the former uses small fragment screws as compared with the 4.5 mm screws with the latter. In addition, compression appears to be less difficult to achieve.

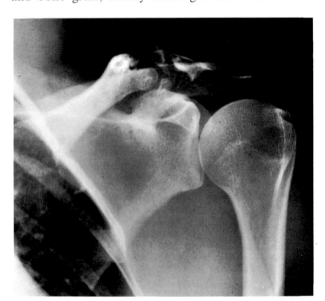

Figure 11–65. Three years after clavicular fracture, this patient has a symptomatic left clavicular nonunion. The ideal treatment for this is bone grafting and rigid internal fixation, preferably with a dynamic compression plate.

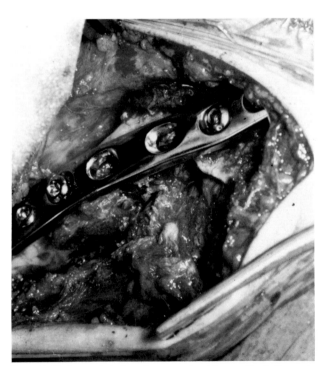

Figure 11–67. A seven-hole dynamic compression plate was utilized with massive cortical cancellous grafting. Because the lateral segment was small, only two screws could be placed in it.

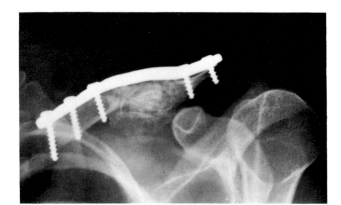

Figure 11-68. Healing of the nonunion has occurred. A disadvantage of plate fixation for nonunion is that the plate may need to be removed if it is irritating and subcutaneous.

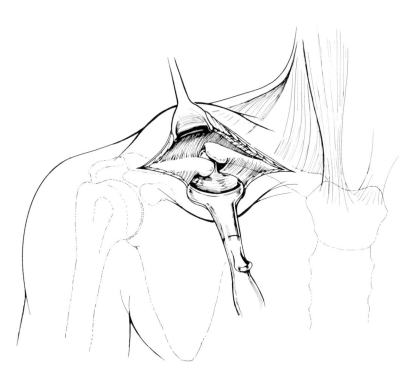

Figure 11-69. Operative approach for a surgical treatment of symptomatic nonunion. A horizontal incision is made. The trapezius and deltoid muscles are elevated off the clavicle and the nonunion is exposed. Blunt retractors protect the retroclavicular vital structures.

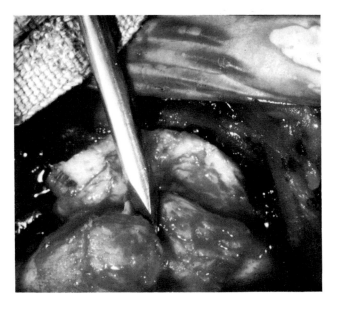

Figure 11-70. The nonunion is exposed. Sclerotic edges are trimmed and fibrous tissue is removed. Usually the fragments are large enough to be able to take six cortices on either side of the fracture.

The surgical technique requires the patient to be in a semiseated or "beach chair" position with the head turned to the opposite shoulder. A horizontal incision is made paralleling the medial clavicular segment along its superior border. The interval between the deltoid and trapezius is found, and a horizontal incision is made in this interval. The ends of the clavicle are exposed subperiosteally and any interposed soft tissue is removed (Figs. 11–69 to 11–71). In a hypertrophic nonunion, the excessive callus buildup and excessively hypertrophic bone may be shaved down to a more normal clavicular size for ease of fitting of the plate. With an atrophic nonunion, if the sclerotic ends need to be resected, an intercalary segment of iliac crest graft is fashioned to fit between the two clavicular segments. If it is anticipated in an atrophic nonunion that an intercalary bone graft will be needed, it is useful to be able to palpate the distance from the acromial tip to the midsternum on both the injured and uninjured side (Figs. 11–72 and 11–73). In addition, the distance between the acromion and sternum on each side can be measured preoperatively on an x-ray taken on a large cassette, in an effort to judge how much clavicular length will need to be made up by the intercalary graft.

Blunt retractors (Darrach, Bennett) are used to protect the infraclavicular structures during drilling of the holes for plate fixation. I prefer to place the plate superiorly and have not found this to be cosmetically or symptomatically a problem. The 3.5-mm plate (DCP Synthes, Wayne PA) is used; I attempt to place three

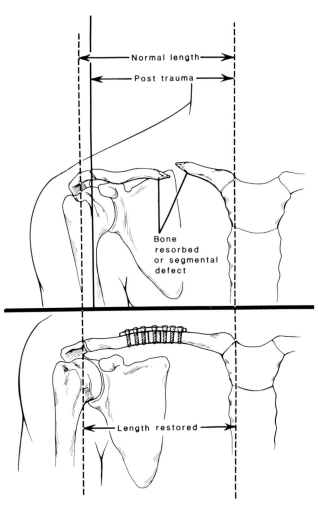

Figure 11–72. In an atrophic nonunion there are often tapered sclerotic edges, and an intercalary bone graft may be needed between the two ends of the clavicular nonunion. The normal manubrial acromial length is seen; the post-traumatic manubrial acromial length is decreased owing to bone resorption or a segmental defect. To restore the normal length of the clavicle, an intercalary bone graft can be placed between the two sides of the nonunion. It is often helpful to internally fix the intercalary segment (fibula or iliac crest) with a cortical screw.

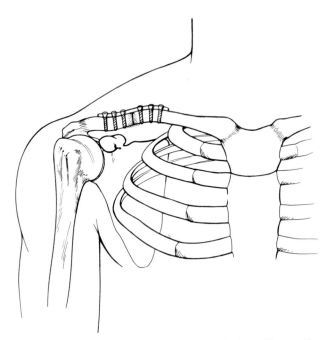

Figure 11–71. Diagrammatic representation of internal fixation and bone grafting of an nonunited middle third clavicle fracture. An attempt is made to incorporate at least six cortices on the dynamic compression plate. Care must be taken that the screws do not project too far inferiorly. The bone graft should be packed in the nonunion site and inferiorly, but packing of the retroclavicular space with bone graft should be avoided.

screws in each clavicular segment as bicortical fixation, and I use a six- or seven-hole plate depending on fracture configuration. Occasionally an interfragmentary screw can be used if the bony anatomy warrants it and the nonunion anatomy is oblique enough. The plate is contoured to the clavicle and secured to the bone. If an intercalary iliac crest segment is to be used, the middle hole of a seven-hole plate may be used to place a screw from the plate into the intercalary segment directly. Following secure plate fixation, iliac crest bone is then placed at the fracture site along the superior and inferior clavicular borders. An excessive amount of bone is avoided posteriorly and inferiorly so as to avoid late irritation or crowding of the neurovascular structures. The trapezius and deltoid fascia are repaired and the patient is placed in a sling and swathe postoperatively.

For lateral clavicular nonunions, I prefer the same method of internal fixation as with acute fractures, that

Figure 11-73. Operative photograph of an intercalary bone graft segment placed between two sides of a nonunion.

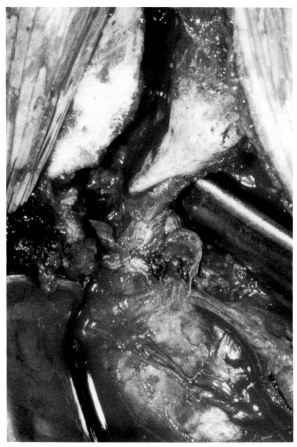

Figure 11-74. Two years after a Type II distal clavicle fracture, a painful nonunion has occurred.

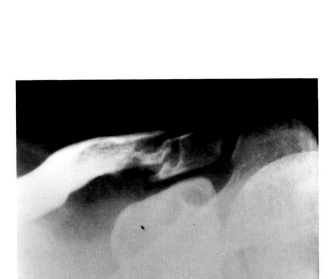

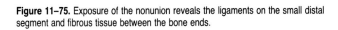

Figure 11-75. Exposure of the nonunion reveals the ligaments on the small distal segment and fibrous tissue between the bone ends.

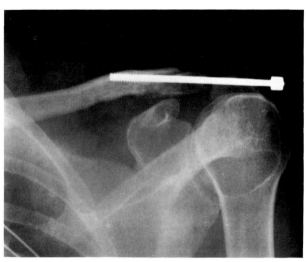

Figure 11-76. Internal fixation utilizing a Knowles pin (which was cut off when it protruded past the anterior cortex) and bone grafting of the nonunion site was performed. Ligament reconstruction ordinarily is not needed, as the ligaments remain attached to the distal fragment.

is, use of a Knowles pin. However, iliac crest graft is always added (Figs. 11–74 to 11–77). In addition I usually add, as with an acute fracture, a piece of Mersilene tape or heavy nonabsorbable suture from the coracoid around the proximal fragment of clavicle for added fixation. In this type of procedure, the fracture site is exposed as with an acute fracture and the Knowles pin is passed from the posterolateral corner of the acromion, across the acromioclavicular joint and small distal segment of the clavicle; after the nonunion edges are trimmed to satisfactory bone, the Knowles pin is advanced across the nonunion site. Coracoclavicular fixation is then tightened and bone graft is added. As with an acute fracture, the Knowles pin is taken out in approximately six to eight weeks.

It must be remembered that the healing time for a nonunion of the adult clavicle is longer than for an acute fracture. It may often be a period of three to six months; the patient should be protected until radio-

graphic signs of union are present. A sling usually provides enough immobilization for at least six to eight weeks, and gentle range of motion may be begun after immobilization is discontinued. Removal of the plate is optional after healing of the fracture, and the intramedullary Knowles pin is removed in approximately six weeks.

In the rare instance when the surgeon is confronted with a previously excised lateral clavicular segment and an unstable proximal segment following a Type II distal clavicular fracture, I prefer using Mersilene tape around the proximal segment to secure the segment to the coracoid, transfixing the proximal segment with an intramedullary pin (Knowles) after reduction, and transferring the coracoacromial ligament into the end of the clavicle.[159, 245]

References

1. Abbott LC, and Lucas DB: The function of the clavicle. Its surgical significance. Ann Surg 140:583–599, 1954.
2. Adams CF: The Genuine Works of Hippocrates. Baltimore: Williams & Wilkins, 1939.
3. Aitken AD, and Lincoln RE: Fractures of the first rib due to muscle pull. Report of a case. N Engl J Med 220:1063–1064, 1939.
4. Alldred AJ: Congenital pseudoarthrosis of the clavicle. J Bone Joint Surg 45B:312–319, 1963.
5. Allman FL: Fractures and ligamentous injuries of the clavicle and its articulation. J Bone Joint Surg 49A:774–784, 1967.
6. Anderson K, Jensen P and Lauritzen J: Treatment of clavicular fractures. Figure-of-eight bandage vs. a simple sling. Acta Orthop Scand 57:71–74, 1987.
7. Apeli L, and Burch HB: Study on the pseudoarthrosis of the clavicle. In Chapchal G (ed): Pseudoarthroses and Their Treatment. Eighth International Symposium on Topical Problems in Orthopaedic Surgery. Stuttgart: Thieme, 1979, pp 188–189.
8. Balata A, Olzai MG, Porcu A, et al: Fractures of the clavicle in the newborn. Riv Ital Ped.
9. Bargar WL, Marcus RE, and Ittleman FP: Late thoracic outlet syndrome secondary to pseudoarthrosis of the clavicle. J Trauma 24(9):857–859, 1984.
10. Basom WC, Breck LW, and Herz JR: Dual grafts for nonunion of the clavicle. South Med J 40:898–899, 1987.
11. Bateman JE: The Shoulder and Neck. Philadelphia: WB Saunders, 1978.
12. Bateman JE: Nerve injuries about the shoulder in sports. J Bone Joint Surg 49A:785–792, 1967.
13. Bearn JG: An electromyographic study of the trapezius, deltoid, pectoralis major, biceps, triceps muscles during static loading of the upper limb. J Anat 140:103–108, 1961.
14. Bearn JG: Direct observation in the function of the capsule to the sternoclavicular joint in clavicular support. J Anat 10:159–170, 1967.
15. Beckman T: A case of simultaneous luxation of both ends of the clavicle. Acta Chir Scand 56:156–163, 1923.
16. Berkheiser EJ: Old ununited clavicular fractures in the adult. Surg Gynecol Obstet 64:1064–1072, 1937.
17. Bernard TN, and Haddad RJ: Enchondroma of the proximal clavicle. An unusual cause of pathologic fracture dislocation of the sternoclavicular joint. Clin Orthop 167:239–241, 1982.
18. Billington RW: A new (plaster yoke) dressing for fracture of the clavicle. South Med J 24:667, 1931.
19. Bonnett J: Fracture of the clavicle. Arch Chir Neerl 27:143–151, 1975.
20. Bowen AD: Plastic bowing of the clavicle in children: a report of two cases. J Bone Joint Surg 65A:403–405, 1983.
21. Breck L: Partially threaded round pins with oversized threads for intramedullary fixation of the clavicle and the forearm bones. Clin Orthop 11:227–229, 1958.

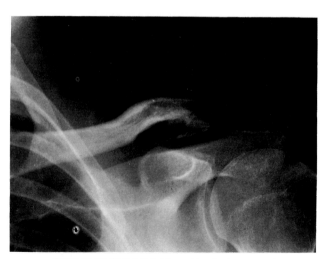

Figure 11-77. Clinical and radiographic union has occurred.

22. Brighton CT, and Pollick SR: Treatment of recalcitrant non-union with a capacitively coupled electrical field. A preliminary report. J Bone Joint Surg 67A:577–585, 1985.

23. Brooks AL, and Henning GD: Injuries to the proximal clavicular epiphysis. J Bone Joint Surg 54A:1347, 1972.

24. Bronz G, Heim D, and Posterla C: Die stabile Clavicula Osteosynthese. Unfallheilkunde 84:319–325, 1981.

25. Butterworth RD, and Kirk AA: Fracture dislocation sternoclavicular joint: case report. Virginia Med Month, 79:98–100, 1952.

26. Cahill BR: Osteolysis of the distal part of the clavicle in male athletes. J Bone Joint Surg 64A:1053–1058, 1982.

27. Campbell E, Howard WB, and Breklund CW: Delayed brachial plexus palsy due to ununited fracture of the clavicle. JAMA 139:91–92, 1949.

28. Caspi I, Ezra E, Nerubay J, et al: Musculocutaneous nerve injury after coracoid process transfer for clavicle instability. Acta Orthop Scand 58:294–295, 1987.

29. Cayford EH, and Tees FJ: Traumatic aneurysm of the subclavian artery as a late complication of fractured clavicle. Can Med Assoc J 25:450–452, 1931.

30. Cohen AW, and Otto SR: Obstetric clavicular fractures. J Reprod Med 25:119–122, 1980.

31. Codman EA: The Shoulder: Rupture of the Supraspinatus Tendon and Other Lesions in or about the Subacromial Bursa. Boston: Thomas Todd, 1934.

32. Connolly JF: Electrical treatment of nonunion. Its use and abuse in 100 consecutive fractures. Orthop Clin North Am 15:89–106, 1984.

33. Connolly JF, and Dehne R: Delayed thoracic outlet syndrome from clavicular non-union: management by morseling. Nebr Med J 71(8):303–306, 1986.

34. Conwell HE: Fractures of the clavicle. JAMA 90:838–839, 1928.

35. Cook T: Reduction and external fixation of fractures of the clavicle in recumbency. J Bone Joint Surg 36A:878–880, 1954.

36. Copeland SM: Total resection of the clavicle. Am J Surg 72:280–281, 1946.

37. Cumming WA: Neonatal skeletal fractures. Birth trauma, or child abuse? J Can Assoc Radiol 30:30–33, 1979.

38. Cummings CW, and First R: Stress fracture of the clavicle after a radical neck dissection. Case report. Plast Reconstr Surg 55(3):366 n367, 1975.

39. Dameron TB Jr, and Rockwood CA Jr: Fractures of the shaft of the clavicle. In Rockwood CA, Wilkins KE, and King RE (eds): Fractures in Children. Philadelphia: JB Lippincott, 1984, pp 608–624.

40. DePalma A: Surgery of the Shoulder, 3rd ed. Philadelphia: JB Lippincott, 1983.

41. Das NK, and Deb HK: Synovioma of the clavicle. Report of a case. J Internat Coll Surg 35:776–780, 1961.

42. Dash UN, and Handler D: A case of compression of subclavian vessels by a fractured clavicle treated by excision of the first rib. J Bone Joint Surg 42A:798–801, 1960.

43. Day L: Electrical stimulation in the treatment of ununited fractures. Clin Orthop 161:54–57, 1981.

44. De Bakey E, Beall C Jr, and Ukkasch DC: Recent developments in vascular surgery with particular reference to orthopaedics. Am J Surg 109:134–142, 1965.

45. Dickson JW: Death following fractured clavicle. Br Med J 2:666, 1952.

46. Dolin M: The operative treatment of midshaft clavicular non-unions (letter). J Bone Joint Surg 68A:634, 1986.

47. Dugdale TW, and Fulkerson JB: Pneumothorax complicating a closed fracture of the clavicle. A case report. Clin Orthop 221:212–214, 1987.

48. Dupuytren, Le Baron: On the Injuries and Diseases of Bone. (Trans Legros Clark.) London: Sydenham Society, 1847.

49. Echtermeyer V, Zwipp H, and Oestern HJ: Fehler und Gefahren in der Behandlung der Fracturen und Pseudarthrosen des Schlusselbeins. Langenbecks Arch Chir 364:351–354, 1984.

50. Edvardsen P, and Odegard O: Treatment of posttraumatic clavicular pseudoarthrosis. Acta Orthop Scand 48:456–457, 1977.

51. Eidman DK, Siff SJ, and Tullos HS: Acromioclavicular lesions in children. Am J Sports Med 9(3):150–154, 1981.

52. Elliott AC: Tripartite injury of the clavicle. A case report. S Afr Med J 70(2):115, 1986.

53. Enker SH, and Murthy KK: Brachial plexus compression by excessive callus formation secondary to a fractured clavicle. A case report. Mt Sinai J Med (NY) 37(6):678–682, 1970.

54. Eskola A, Vainionpaa S, Myllynen P, et al: Outcome of clavicular fracture in 89 patients. Arch Orthop Trauma Surg 105:337–338, 1986.

55. Eskola A, Vainionpaa S, and Myllynen P: Surgery for ununited clavicular fracture. Acta Orthop Scand 57:366–367, 1986.

56. Eskola A, Vainionpaa S, Patiala H, et al: Outcome of operative treatment in fresh lateral clavicle fracture. Ann Chir Gynaecol 76(3):167–168, 1987.

57. Fairbank H: Cranio-cleido-dystostosis. J Bone Joint Surg 31B:608, 1949.

58. Falconer MA, and Weddell G: Costoclavicular compression of the subclavian artery and vein. Lancet 2:539, 1943.

59. Falstie-Jensen S: Psuedodislocation of the acromioclavicular joint. J Bone Joint Surg 64B:368–369, 1982.

60. Farkas R, and Levine S: X-ray incidents of fractured clavicle in vertex presentation. Am J Obstet Gynecol 59:204–206, 1950.

61. Fawcett J: The development and ossification of the human clavicle. J Anat 47:225–234, 1913.

62. Fich R: Handbuch der Anatomie und Mechanic der Galanke. In Bvdeleben V: Handbuch der Anatomie des Menschen, Vol 2, Section 1. Jena: Gustava Discher, 1910, pp 163–187.

63. Fini-Storchi O, LoRusso D, and Agostini V: "Pseudotumors" of the clavicle subsequent to radical neck dissection. J Laryngol Otol 99(1):73–83, 1985.

64. Fowler AW: Fractures of the clavicle. J Bone Joint Surg 44B:440, 1962.

65. Freedman M, Gamble J, and Lewis C: Intrauterine fracture simulating a unilateral clavicular pseudarthrosis. J Assoc Radiol 33(1):37–38, 1982.

66. Fry J: [Photo of the "Edwin Smith Surgical Papyrus."] In Rockwood CA, Wilkins KE, and King RE (eds): Fractures in Children. Philadelphia: JB Lippincott, 1984, p 679.

67. Fukuda K, Craig EV, An KN, et al: Biomechanical study of the ligamentous system of the acromioclavicular joint. J Bone Joint Surg 68A:434–440, 1986.

68. Gardner ED, Grey DJ, and Orahilly R: Anatomy. Philadelphia: WB Saunders, 1960.

69. Gardner E: The embryology of the clavicle. Clin Orthop 58:9–16, 1968.

70. Gearen PF, and Petty W: Panclavicular dislocation: report of a case. J Bone Joint Surg 64A454–455, 1982.

71. Gebuhr P: Brachial plexus involvement after fractures of the clavicle. Ugeskr Laeger 150(2):105–106, 1988.

72. Ghormley RK, Black JR, and Cherry JH: Ununited fractures of the clavicle. Am J Surg 51:343–349, 1941.

73. Gibbon JH: Lucas-Championniere and mobilization in the treatment of fractures. Surg Gynecol Obstet 43:271–278, 1926.

74. Gibson DA, and Carroll N: Congenital pseudoarthrosis of the clavicle. J Bone Joint Surg 52B:629–643, 1970.

75. Gitsch VG, and Schatten C: Frequenz und potentielle Faktoren in der Genese der geburtstraumatisch bedingten Klavicula fraktur. Zentralbl Gynakol 109:909–912, 1987.

76. Grant JCB: A Method of Anatomy, 5th ed. Baltimore: Williams & Wilkins, 1952.

77. Gresham EL: Birth trauma. Pediatr Clin North Am 22:317, 1975.

78. Gross SD: The Anatomy, Physiology, and Diseases of the Bones and Joints. Philadelphia: John Grigg, 1830.

79. Gryska PF: Major vascular injuries. N Engl J Med 266:381–385, 1982.

80. Guattieri G, and Frassi G: Late truncal paralysis of the brachial plexis in sequella of fracture of the clavicle. Arch di Ortopedia 74:840–848, 1961.

81. Guilfoil PH, and Christiansen T: An unusual vascular complication of fractured clavicle. JAMA 200:72–73, 1967.
82. Guillemin A: Dechrune de la vein sous-claviere par fracture fermie de la clavicule. Bull et Mem Soc Nat Chir 56:302–304, 1930.
83. Gurd FB: The treatment of complete dislocation of the outer end of clavicle: a hitherto undescribed operation. Ann Surg 113:1094–1097, 1941.
84. Hackstock H, and Hackstock, H.: Surgical treatment of clavicular fracture. Unfallchirurg 91(2):64–69, 1988.
85. Hargan B, and Macafee AL: Bilateral pseudoarthrosis of the clavicles. Injury 12(4):316–318, 1981.
86. Heppenstall RB: Fractures and dislocations of the distal clavicle. Orthop Clin North Am 6(2):477–486, 1975.
87. Hicks JH: Rigid fixation as a treatment for hypertrophic nonunion. Injury 8:199–205, 1976.
88. Hoyer HE, Kindt R, and Lippert H: Zur Biomechanik der menschlichen Clavicula. Z Orthop 118:915–922, 1980.
89. Houston HE: An unusual complication of clavicular fracture. J Ky Med Assoc 75(4):170–171, 1977.
90. Howard FM, and Schafer SJ: Injuries to the clavicle with neurovascular complications. A study of fourteen cases. J Bone Joint Surg 47A:1335–1346, 1965.
91. Inman VT, and Saunders JB: Observation in the function of the clavicle. Calif Med 65:158–165, 1946.
92. Iqbal O: Axillary artery thrombosis associated with fracture of the clavicle. Med J Malaysia 26:68–70, 1971.
93. Jablon M, Sutker A, and Post M: Irreducible fractures of the middle third of the clavicle. J Bone Joint Surg 61A:296–298, 1979.
94. Jackson WJ: Clavicle fractures. Therapy is dictated by the patient's age. Consultant 177, 1982.
95. Jacobs P: Posttraumatic osteologies of the outer end of the clavicle. J Bone Joint Surg 46B:705–707, 1964.
96. Jain AS: Traumatic floating clavicle. A case report. J Bone Joint Surg 66B:560–561, 1984.
97. Javid H: Vascular injuries of the neck. Clin Orthop 28:70–78, 1963.
98. Jit I, and Kulkrani M: Times of appearance and fusion of epiphysis at the medial end of the clavicle. Indian J Med Res 64(5):773–792, 1976.
99. Johnson EW Jr, and Collins HR: Nonunion of the clavicle. Arch Surg 87:963–966, 1963.
100. Joukainen J, and Karaharju E: Pseudoarthrosis of the clavicle. Acta Orthop Scand 48:550, 1977.
101. Jupiter JB, and Leffert RD: Nonunion of the clavicle. J Bone Joint Surg 69A:753–760, 1987.
102. Kanoksikarin S, and Wearne WN: Fracture and retrosternal dislocation of the clavicle. Aust NZ J Surg 48:95–96, 1978.
103. Kabaharjve E, Joukainen J, and Peltonen J: Treatment of pseudoarthrosis of the clavicle. Injury 13(5):400–403, 1982.
104. Karwasz RR, Kutzner M, and Krammer WG: Late brachial plexus lesion following clavicular fracture. Unfallchirurg 91(1):45–47, 1988.
105. Katz R, Landman J, Dulitzky F, et al: Fracture of the clavicle in the newborn. An ultrasound diagnosis. J Ultrasound Med 7(1):21–23, 1988.
106. Katznelson A, Nerubay JN, and Oliver S: Dynamic fixation of the avulsed clavicle. J Trauma 16(10):841–844, 1976.
107. Kay SP, and Eckardt JJ: Brachial plexus palsy secondary to clavicular nonunion. A case report and literature survey. Clin Orthop 206:219–222, 1986.
108. Kaye JJ, Nance EP Jr, and Green NE: Fatigue fracture of the medial aspect of the clavicle. An academic rather than athletic injury. Radiology 144(1):89–90, 1982.
109. Key JA, and Conwell EH: The Management of Fractures, Dislocations, and Sprains, 2nd ed. St. Louis: CV Mosby, 1937, p 437.
110. Khan MAA, and Lucas HK: Plating of fractures of the middle third of the clavicle. Injury 9:263–267, 1978.
111. Kini MG: A simple method of ambulatory treatment of fractures of the clavicle. J Bone Joint Surg 23:795–798, 1941.
112. Kite JH: Congenital pseudoarthrosis of the clavicle. South Med J 761:703–710, 1968.
113. Klier I, and Mayor PB: Laceration of the innominate internal jugular venous junction. Rare complication of fracture of the clavicle. Orthop Rev 10:81–82, 1981.
114. Koch F, Papadimitriou G, and Groher W: Die Clavicula pseudoarthroseihse Entstehung und Bahandlung. Unfallheilkunde 74:330–337, 1971.
115. Kreisinger V: Sur le traitement des fractures de le clavicule. Rev Chir Paris 43:376, 1927.
116. Kremens V, and Glauser F: Unusual sequelae following pinning of medial clavicular fracture. Am J Roentgenol 74:1066–1069, 1956.
117. Lancet editorial: Sir Robert Peel's death. Lancet 2:19, 1850.
118. Lee HG: Treatment of fracture of the clavicle by internal nail fixation. N Engl J Med 234:222–224, 1946.
119. Lemire L, and Rosman M: Sternoclavicular epiphyseal separation with adjacent clavicular fracture. J Pediatr Orthop 4:118–120, 1984.
120. Lengua F, Nuss J, Lechner R, et al: The treatment of fracture of the clavicle by closed-medio-lateral pinning. Rev Chir Orthop 73:377–380, 1987.
121. Lester CW: The treatment of fractures of the clavicle. Ann Surg 89:600–606, 1929.
122. Liechtl R: Fracture of the clavicle and scapula. In Webber BG, Brunner C, and Freuler F (eds): Treatment of Fractures in Children and Adolescents. New York: Springer-Verlag, 1988, pp 88–95.
123. Lim E, and Day LJ: Subclavian vein thrombosis following fracture of the clavicle. A case report. Orthopedics 10(2):349–351, 1987.
124. Lipton HA, and Jupiter JB: Nonunion of clavicular fractures: characteristics and surgical management. Surg Rounds Orthop, 1988.
125. Ljunggren AE: Clavicular function. Acta Orthop Scand 50:261–268, 1979.
126. Lloyd-Roberts GC, Apley AG, and Owen R: Reflections upon the etiology of congenital pseudoarthrosis of the clavicle. J Bone Joint Surg 57B:24–29, 1975.
127. Lombard JJ: Pseudoarthrosis of the clavicle. A case report. S Afr Med J 66(4):151–153, 1984.
128. Lord JW, and Rosati JM: Neurovascular compression syndromes of the upper extremity. CIBA Clin Symposia 10(2), 1958.
129. Lukin AV, and Grishken VA: Two cases of successful treatment of fracture dislocation of the clavicle. Ortop Travmatol Protez 11:35, 1987.
130. Lusskin R, Weiss CA, and Winer J: The role of the subclavius muscle in the subclavian vein syndrome (costoclavicular syndrome) following fracture of the clavicle. Clin Orthop 54:75–84, 1967.
131. Madsen ET: Fractures of the extremities in the newborn. Acta Obstet Gynecol Scand 34:41–74, 1955.
132. Malcolm BW, Ameli FN, and Simmons EH: Pneumothorax complicating a fracture of the clavicle. Can J Surg 22(1):84, 1979.
133. Malgaigne JF: A Treatise on Fractures (Translated by Packard JH). Philadelphia: JB Lippincott, 1859, pp 374–401.
134. Manske DJ, and Szabo RM: The operative treatment of midshaft clavicular non-unions. J Bone Joint Surg 67A:1367–1371, 1985.
135. Marie P, and Sainton P: On hereditary cleidocranial dysostosis. Clin Orthop 58:5–7, 1968.
136. Marsh HO, and Hazarian E: Pseudoarthrosis of the clavicle. In Proceedings of the American, British, Canadian, Australia, New Zealand, and South African Orthopaedic Associations. J Bone Joint Surg 52B:793–794, 1970.
137. Matry C: Fracture de la clavicule gauche au tiers interne. Blessure de la vein sous-claviere. Osteosynthese Bull Mem Soc Nat Chir 58:75–78, 1932.
138. Mayer JH: Nonunion of fractured clavicle. Proc Roy Soc Med 58:182, 1965.

139. Mazet R: Migration of a Kirschner wire from the shoulder region into the lung. Report of two cases. J Bone Joint Surg 25:477–483, 1943.

140. McCandless DN, and Mowbray M: Treatment of displaced fractures of the clavicle. Sling vs. figure-of-eight bandage. Practitioner 223:266–267, 1979.

141. Miller DS, and Boswick JA: Lesions of the brachial plexus associated with fractures of the clavicle. Clin Orthop 64:144–149, 1969.

142. Mital MA, and Aufranc OE: Venous occlusion following greenstick fracture clavicle. JAMA 206:1301–1302, 1968.

143. Mnaymneh W, Vargas A, and Kaplan J: Fractures of the clavicle caused by arteriovenous malformation. Clin Orthop 148:256–258, 1980.

144. Moir JC, and Myerscough PR: Operative Obstetrics, 7th ed. Baltimore: Williams & Wilkins, 1964.

145. Moore TO: Internal pin fixation for fracture of the clavicle. Am Surg 17:580–583, 1951.

146. Moseley HF: The clavicle. Its anatomy and function. Clin Orthop 58:17–27, 1968.

147. Moseley HF: Shoulder Lesions. Edinburgh: Churchill Livingstone, 1972, pp 207–235.

148. Mulder DS, Greenwood FA, and Brooks CE: Post-traumatic thoracic outlet syndrome. J Trauma 13:706–713, 1973.

149. Mueller ME, Allgower N, and Willenegger H: Manual of Internal Fixation. New York: Springer-Verlag, 1970.

150. Murray G: A method of fixation for fracture of the clavicle. J Bone Joint Surg 22:616–620, 1940.

151. Natali J, Maraval M, Kieffer E, et al: Fractures of the clavicle and injuries of the subclavian artery. Report of 10 cases. J Cardiovasc Surg 16(5):541–547, 1975.

152. Neer CS II: Impingement lesions. Clin Orthop 173:70–77, 1983.

153. Neer CS II: Fractures of the clavicle. In Rockwood CA and Green DP (eds): Fractures in Adults. Philadelphia: JB Lippincott, 1984, pp 707–713.

154. Neer CS II: Nonunion of the clavicle. JAMA 172:1006–1011, 1960.

155. Neer CS II: Fractures of the distal third of the clavicle. Clin Orthop 58:43–50, 1968.

156. Neer CS II: Fracture of the distal clavicle with detachment of coracoclavicular ligaments in adults. J Trauma 3:99–110, 1963.

157. Nelson HP: Subclavian aneurysm following fracture of the clavicle. St. Bartholomew's Hospital Report 65:219–229, 1932.

158. Neviaser RJ, Neviaser JS, Neviaser TJ, et al: A simple technique for internal fixation of the clavicle. Clin Orthop 109:103–107, 1975.

159. Neviaser JS: Acromioclavicular dislocations treated by transference of the coracoacromial ligament. Bull Hosp Joint Dis 12:46–54, 1951.

160. Neviaser JS: Injuries of the clavicle and its articulations. Orthop Clin North Am 11(2):233–237, 1980.

161. Neviaser JS: Injuries in and about the shoulder joint. Instr Course Lect 13:187–216, 1956.

162. Neviaser JS: The treatment of fractures of the clavicle. Surg Clin North Am 43:1555–1563, 1963.

163. Nevaiser RJ: Injuries to the clavicle and acromioclavicular joint. Orthop Clin North Am 18:433–438, 1987.

164. Nogi J, et al: Nonunion of the clavicle in the child. A case report. Clin Orthop 110:19–21, 1975.

165. Norell H, and Llewellyn RC: Migration of a threaded Steinmann pin from an acromioclavicular joint into the spinal canal. A case report. J Bone Joint Surg 47A:1024, 1965.

166. Ogden JA, Conologue GJ, and Bronson NL: Radiology of postnatal skeletal development, Volume 3. The clavicle. Skeletal Radiol 4:196–203, 1979.

167. Ord RA, and Langon JD: Stress fracture of the clavicle. A rare late complication of radical neck dissection. J Maxillofac Surg 14(5):281–284, 1986.

168. O'Rourke IC, and Middleton RW: The place and efficacy of operative management of fractured clavicle. Injury 6(3):236–240, 1975.

169. Owen R: Congenital pseudoarthrosis of the clavicle. J Bone Joint Surg 52B:642–652, 1970.

170. Oxnard CE: The architecture of the shoulder in some mammals. J Morphol 126:249–290, 1968.

171. Packer BD: Conservative treatment of fracture of the clavicle. J Bone Joint Surg 26:770–774, 1944.

172. Paffen PJ, and Jansen EW: Surgical treatment of clavicular fractures with Kirshner wires. A comparative study. Arch Chir Neerl 30:43–53, 1978.

173. Parkes JC, and Deland JD: A three-part distal clavicle fracture. J Trauma 23(5):437–438, 1983.

174. Patel CV, and Audenwalla HS: Treatment of fractured clavicle by immediate partial subperiosteal resection. J Postgrad Med 18:32–34, 1972.

175. Penn I: The vascular complications of fractures of the clavicle. J Trauma V 4:819–831, 1964.

176. Perry B: An improved clavicular pin. Am J Surg 112:142–144, 1966.

177. Pipkin G: Tardy shoulder hand syndrome following ununited fracture of clavicle. A case report. J Missouri Med Assoc 48:643–646, 1951.

178. Piterman L: "The fractured clavicle." Aust Fam Phys 11(8):614, 1982.

179. Poigenfurst J, Reiler T, and Fischer W: Plating of fresh clavicular fractures. Experience with 60 operations. Unfallchirurg 14(1):26–37, 1988.

180. Pollen AG: Fractures and Dislocations in Children. Baltimore: Williams & Wilkins, 1973.

181. Porral A: Observation d'une double luxation de la clavicule dorite. Juniva Hibd Med Chir Part 2:78–82, 1931.

182. Post M: Injury to the shoulder girdle. In Post M (ed): The Shoulder: Surgical and Non-Surgical Management. Philadelphia: Lea and Febiger, 1988.

183. Pusitz ME, and Davis EV: Bone-drilling in delayed union of fractures. J Bone Joint Surg 26A:560–565, 1944.

184. Pyper JB: Nonunion of fractures of the clavicle. Injury 9(4):268–270, 1978.

185. Quesana F: Technique for the roentgen. Diagnosis of fractures of the clavicle. Surg Gynecol Obstet 42:4261–4281, 1926.

186. Quigley TB: The management of simple fracture of the clavicle in adults. N Engl J Med 243:286–290, 1950.

187. Quinlan WR, Brady PG, and Regan BF: Congenital pseudoarthrosis of the clavicle. Acta Orthop Scand 51:489–492, 1980.

188. Quinn SF, and Glass TA: Post-traumatic osteolysis of the clavicle. South Med J 76:307–308, 1983.

189. Rabenseifner L: Zur Atiologie und Therapie bei Schlusselbeinpseudarthosen. Aktuel Traumatol 11:130–132, 1981.

190. Raymakers E, and Marti R: Nonunion of the clavicle. In Pseudarthroses and Their Treatment. Eighth International Symposium on Topical Problems in Orthopaedic Surgery. Thieme, 1979.

191. Redmond AD: A complication of fracture of the clavicle (letter). Injury 13(4):352, 1982.

192. Reid J, and Kenned J: Direct fracture of the clavicle with symptoms simulating a cervical rib. Br Med J 2:608–609, 1925.

193. Rhinelander FW: Tibial blood supply in relation to fracture healing. Clin Orthop 105:34–81, 1974.

194. Ring M: Clavicle. In Children's Fractures, 2nd ed. Philadelphia: JB Lippincott, 1983.

195. Rockwood CA: Fractures of the outer clavicle in children and adults. J Bone Joint Surg 64B:642, 1982.

196. Rockwood CA: Personal communications, 1989.

197. Rockwood CA: Management of fracture of the clavicle and injuries of the SC joints. Orthop Trans 6:422, 1982.

198. Rockwood CA: Treatment of the outer clavicle in children and adults. Orthop Trans 6:472, 1982.

199. Rosati LM, and Lord JW Jr: Neurovascular Compression Syndromes of the Shoulder Girdle. New York: Grune and Stratton, 1961.

200. Rowe CR: An atlas of anatomy and treatment of mid-clavicular fractures. Clin Orthop 58:29–42, 1968.

201. Rubin A: Birth injuries: incidents, mechanisms and end result. Obstet Gynecol 23:218–221, 1964.

202. Rush LV, and Rush HL: Technique of longitudinal pin fixation in fractures of the clavicle and jaw. Mississippi Doctor 27:332, 1949.

203. Sakellarides H: Pseudoarthrosis of the clavicle. J Bone Joint Surg 43A:130–138, 1961.

204. Sampson JJ, Saunders JB, and Capp CS: Compression of the subclavian vein by the first rib and clavicle with reference to prominence of the chest veins as a sign of collaterals. Am Heart J 19:292–315, 1940.

205. Sandford HN: The Moro reflex as a diagnostic aid in fracture of the clavicle in the newborn infant. Am J Dis Child 41:1304–1306, 1931.

206. Sankarankutty M, and Turner BW: Fractures of the clavicle. Injury 7(2):101–106, 1975.

207. Sayre L: A simple dressing for fractures of the clavicle. Am Practitioner 4:1, 1871.

208. Schewior T: Die Durckpallenostesynthese bei Schlusselpein pseudarthrosen. Acta Traumatol 4:113–125, 1974.

209. Shih J, Chao E, and Chang C: Subclavian pseudoaneurysm after clavicle fracture. A case report. J Formosan Med Assoc 82:332–335, 1983.

210. Siffrey and Aulong: Thrombose post-traumatique de l'artere sous-claviere gauche. Lyon Chir 51:479–481, 1956.

211. Silloway KA, Mclaughlin RE, Edlichy RC, et al: Clavicular fractures and acromioclavicular joint injuries in lacrosse: preventable injuries. J Emerg Med 3:117–121, 1985.

212. Simpson LA, and Kellam J: Surgical management of fractures of the clavicle, scapula, and proximal humerus. Orthop Update Series 4(4):1–8, 1985.

213. Scarpa FJ, and Levy RM: Pulmonary embolism complicating clavicle fracture. Conn Med 43(12):771–773, 1979.

214. Schwartz N, and Leixnering M: Technik und Ergebienisse der Klavikula-markdrahtung. Zentralbl Chir 111(11):640–647, 1986.

215. Shauffer IA, and Collins WV: The deep clavicular rhomboid fossa. JAMA 195:778–779, 1966.

216. Spar I: Total claviculectomy for pathological fractures. Clin Orthop 129:236–237, 1977.

217. Smith RW: A Treatise on Fractures in the Vicinity of Joints. Dublin: Hodges & Smith, 1847, pp 209–224.

218. Snyder LA: Loss of the accompaning soft tissue shadow of clavicle with occult fracture. South Med J 72:243, 1979.

219. Sorrells RB: Fracture of the clavicle. J Arkansas Med Soc 71(8):253–256, 1975.

220. Stanley D, Trowbridge EA, and Norris SH: The mechanism of clavicular fracture. J Bone Joint Surg 70B:461–464, 1988.

221. Steenburg RW, and Ravitch MM: Cervico-thoracic approach for subclavian vessel injury from compound fracture of the clavicle: considerations of subclavian axillary exposures. Ann Surg 1(57):839, 1963.

222. Steffelaar H, and Heim V: Sekundare Plattenosteosynthesen an der Clavicula. Arch Orthop Unfallchir 79:75, 1974.

223. Steinberg I: Subclavian vein thrombosis associated with fractures of the clavicle. Report of two cases. N Engl J Med 264:686–688, 1961.

224. Stimson LA: A Treatise on Fractures. Philadelphia: Henry A. Lea's Son and Co, 1883, p 332.

225. Stone PW, and Lord JW: The clavicle and its relation to trauma to the subclavian artery and vein. Am J Surg 98:834–839, 1955.

226. Storen H: Old clavicular pseudoarthrosis with late appearing neuralgias and vasomotor disturbances cured by operation. Acta Chir Scand 94:187, 1946.

227. Strauss M, Bushey MJ, Chung C, and Baum S: Fractures of the clavicle following radical neck dissection or postoperative radiotherapy. A case report and review of the literature. Laryngoscope 92(11):1304–1307, 1982.

228. Swischuk LE: Radiology of Newborn and Young Infants, 2nd ed. Baltimore: Williams & Wilkins, 1981, p 630.

229. Tachdjian MO: Pediatric Orthopaedics. Philadelphia: WB Saunders, 1972.

230. Tanchev S, Kolishev K, Tanches P, et al: Etiology of a clavicle fracture due to the birth process. Akush Ginekol 24(2):39–43, 1985.

231. Taylor AR: Nonunion of fractures of the clavicle. A review of 31 cases. Proceedings of the British Orthopaedic Association. J Bone Joint Surg 51B:568–569, 1969.

232. Taylor AR: Some observations on fractures of the clavicle. Proc Roy Soc Med 62(10):1037–1038, 1969.

233. Telford ED, and Mottershead S: Pressure at the cervico-brachial junction: an operative and an anatomical study. J Bone Joint Surg 30B:249, 1948.

234. Thompson AG, and Batten RC: The application of rigid internal fixation to the treatment of nonunion and delayed union using AO technique. Injury 8:88, 1977.

235. Todd TW, and D'errico J Jr: The clavicular epiphysis. Am J Anat 41:25–50, 1928.

236. Tregonning G, and Macnab I: Post-traumatic pseudoarthrosis of the clavicle. Proceedings of the New Zealand Orthopaedic Association. J Bone Joint Surg 58B:264, 1976.

237. Tyrnin AH: The Bohler clavicular splint in the treatment of clavicular injuries. J Bone Joint Surg 19:417–424, 1937.

238. Tse DHW, Slabaugh PB, and Carlson PA: Injury to the axillary artery by a closed fracture of the clavicle. J Bone Joint Surg 62A:1372–1373, 1980.

239. Urist MR: Complete dislocation of the acromioclavicular joint. J Bone Joint Surg 28:813–837, 1946.

240. Valdes-dopena MA, and Arey JB: The causes of neonatal mortality: an analysis of 501 autopsies on new born infants. J Pediatr 77:366, 1970.

241. Van Vlack HG: Comminuted fracture of the clavicle with pressure on brachial plexus. Report of case. J Bone Joint Surg 22A:446–447, 1940.

242. Wachsmudh W: Allgemeine und Specielle Operationslettie. Berlin: Martin Kirschner, Springer-Verlag, 1956, p 375.

243. Wall JJ: Congenital pseudoarthrosis of the clavicle. J Bone Joint Surg 52A:1003–1009, 1970.

244. Watson-Jones R: Fractures and Other Bone and Joint Injuries. Edinburgh: E. & S. Livingstone, 1940, pp 90–91.

245. Weaver JK, and Dunn HK: Treatment of acromioclavicular injuries, especially acromioclavicular separation. J Bone Joint Surg 54A:1187–1198, 1972.

246. Weber BG: Pseudoarthrosis of the clavicle. In Pseudoarthrosis: Pathophysiology, Biomechanics, Therapy, Results. New York: Grune and Stratton, 1976, pp 104–107.

247. Weh L, and Torklus DZ: Fracture of the clavicle with consecutive costoclavicular compression syndrome. Z Orthop 118(1):140–142, 1980.

248. Weiner DS, and O'Dell HW: Fractures of the first rib associated with injuries to the clavicle. J Trauma 9(5):412–422, 1969.

249. Widner LA, and Riddewold HO: The value of the lordotic view in diagnosis of fractured clavicle. Rev Int Radiol 5:69–70, 1980.

250. Wilkins RM, and Johnston RM: Ununited fractures of the clavicle. J Bone Joint Surg 65A:773–778, 1983.

251. Wilkes JA, and Hoffer M: Clavicle fractures in head-injured children. J Orthop Trauma 1(1):55–58, 1987.

252. Worcester JN, and Green DP: Osteoarthritis of the acromioclavicular joint. Clin Orthop 58:69–73, 1968.

253. Wood VE: The results of total claviculectomy. Clin Orthop 207:186–190, 1986.

254. Yates DW: Complications of fractures of the clavicle. Injury 7(3):189–193, 1976.

255. Yates AG, and Guest D: Cerebral embolus due to ununited fracture of the clavicle and subclavian thrombosis. Lancet 2:225–226, 1928.

256. Young CS: The mechanics of ambulatory treatment of fractures of the clavicle. J Bone Joint Surg 13:299–310, 1931.

257. Zenni EJ Jr, Krieg JK, and Rosen MJ: Open reduction and internal fixation of clavicular fractures. J Bone Joint Surg 63A(1):147–151, 1981.

Disorders of the Acromioclavicular Joint

Charles A. Rockwood, Jr., M.D.
D. Christopher Young, M.D.

Historical Review

Dislocation of the acromioclavicular joint, and particularly the treatment of the injuries, has been a subject of controversy from the earliest medical writings. Hippocrates[2] (460 to 377 B.C.) wrote, "Physicians are particularly liable to be deceived in this accident (for as the separated bone protrudes, the top of the shoulder appears low and hollow), so that they may prepare as if for dislocation of the shoulder; for I have known many physicians otherwise not expert at the art who have done much mischief by attempting to reduce shoulders, thus supposing it as a case of dislocation." Galen[2] (129 to 199 A.D.) obviously had paid close attention to Hippocrates, because he diagnosed his own acromioclavicular dislocation received from wrestling in the palestra. It is appropriate that one of the earliest reported cases in the literature was related to sports, as certainly today sports participation is one of the most common causes of acromioclavicular dislocations. This famous physician of the Graeco-Roman period treated himself in the manner of Hippocrates, i.e., tight bandages to hold the projecting clavicle down while keeping the arm elevated. Galen reported that this type of treatment was so uncomfortable that he discontinued it after just a few days.

From these earliest of publications on through the time of Paul of Aegina (seventh century), the acromioclavicular joint became better recognized, but the treatment remained essentially unchanged.

Hippocrates[2] stated that no impediment, small or great, will result from such an injury. However, he went on to write that there would be a "tumefaction" or deformity, "for the bone cannot be properly restored to its natural situation." I suppose that this statement was, has been, and will be received by the orthopedic world as a challenge, since there is probably not another joint in the body that has been treated in so many different ways as the acromioclavicular joint in attempts to "properly restore" it to "its natural situation."

Surgical Anatomy

The acromioclavicular joint is classified as a diarthrodial joint, and the articular surfaces are covered with fibrocartilage. Tyurina[409] has reported that the articular cartilage of the acromial end of the clavicle is hyaline cartilage until age 17, by which time it acquires the structure of fibrocartilage. The articular surface of the clavicular surface of the acromion changes more slowly and does not become fibrocartilage until age 23 or 24. The joint exists between the lateral end of the clavicle and the medial margin of the acromion process of the scapula (Fig. 12–1). Bosworth[65] stated that the average size of the adult acromioclavicular joint is 9.0 mm by 19.0 mm. Codman[89] related that the acromioclavicular joint is only slightly movable, that it might swing a little, rock a little, twist a little, slide a little, and act like a hinge. DePalma[111] has shown that there is marked variability in the plane of the joint. Viewed from the front, the inclination of the joint may be almost vertical, or it may be inclined downward medially, with the clavicle overriding the acromion by as much as an angle of 50 degrees (Fig. 12–2). Moseley[272] stated that there may be an underriding type of inclination with the clavicle facet under the acromion process. In his experience, the vertical and underriding type of facets appear to be most prone to prolonged

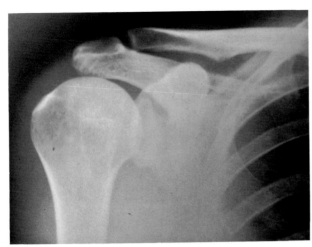

Figure 12–1. Anteroposterior x-ray of the normal shoulder. Note the acromioclavicular joint, the coracoid process, and the coracoclavicular interspace. (Reproduced with permission from Rockwood CA, and Green DP (eds): Fractures (3 vols), 2nd ed. Philadelphia: JB Lippincott, 1984.)

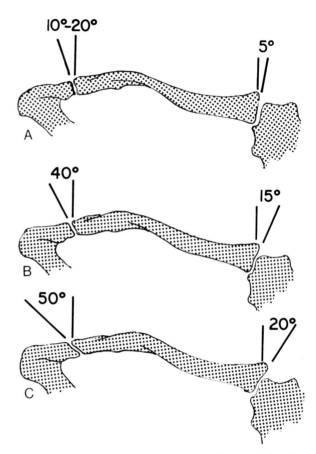

Figure 12–2. Variations in the shape and inclination of the acromioclavicular and sternoclavicular joints. (Redrawn from DePalma AF: Surgery of the Shoulder, 3rd ed. Philadelphia: JB Lippincott, 1983.)

disability after injury. Urist[411] has shown that in 100 random x-rays of the shoulder, the articular surface of the clavicle overrides the articular surface of the acromion approximately 50 per cent of the time.

There may be two types of the fibrocartilaginous interarticular discs—complete and partial (meniscoid). The disc has great variation in its size and shape. DePalma[113] has demonstrated that with age, the meniscus undergoes rapid degeneration until it is essentially no longer functional beyond the fourth decade. These findings have been further substantiated by work by Petersson[310] and by Salter and colleagues.[356] The nerve supply to the acromioclavicular joint is from branches of the axillary, suprascapular, and lateral pectoral nerves.

ACROMIOCLAVICULAR LIGAMENTS

The joint is surrounded by a thin capsule that is reinforced above and below by the superior and inferior acromioclavicular ligaments and by the anterior and posterior acromioclavicular ligaments (Fig. 12–3). The fibers of the superior acromioclavicular ligament blend with the fibers of the deltoid and trapezius muscles, which are attached to the superior aspect of the clavicle and the acromion process. These muscle attachments are important in that they strengthen the acromioclavicular ligaments and add stability to the acromioclavicular joint.

MOTION OF THE ACROMIOCLAVICULAR JOINT

The article in 1944 by Inman and colleagues[196] suggested that the total range of motion of the acromioclavicular joint is 20 degrees. They reported that the motion occurs in the first 30 degrees of abduction of

the arm and after 135 degrees of elevation of the arm. They also demonstrated that with full elevation of the arm, the clavicle rotates upward 40 to 50 degrees. This was measured by drilling a pin into the clavicle and observing the rotation upward during overhead elevation of the arm. When they manually held the pin, which prevented clavicular rotation, overhead elevation of the arm was restricted to 110 degrees. Inman and colleagues concluded that the clavicular rotation was a fundamental feature of shoulder motion. Furthermore, they concluded that a coracoclavicular screw between the clavicle and the coracoid or an arthrodesis of the acromioclavicular joint would limit clavicular rotation and, hence, severely limit abduction of the arm. Since 1944, most authors have condemned the use of the coracoclavicular screw, because it would produce an extra-articular acromioclavicular arthrodesis, which would prevent the normal clavicular rotation, the end result of which would be limitation of elevation or abduction of the arm.

Significant differences of opinion have been reported by Caldwell,[83] Kennedy and Cameron,[209, 210] and Rockwood.[340, 341] Caldwell[83] reported two cases of acromioclavicular dislocation treated by arthrodesis of the acromioclavicular joint. One patient gained a full free

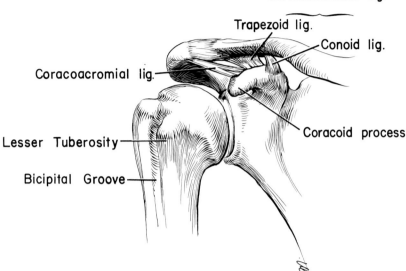

Figure 12–3. Normal anatomy of the acromioclavicular joint. (Reproduced with permission from Rockwood CA, and Green DP (eds): Fractures (3 vols), 2nd ed. Philadelphia: JB Lippincott, 1984.)

range of motion of the shoulder and the other had abduction to 165 degrees. Kennedy and Cameron[209, 210] have demonstrated that patients who have a coracoclavicular screw in place and have an arthrodesis between the clavicle and the coracoid are capable of almost full overhead motion. They drilled pins into the clavicle and into the spine of the scapula in patients who had a coracoclavicular lag screw in place and noted normal clavicular rotation during overhead elevation of the arm. In further studies of motion of the clavicle and the scapula, Kennedy and Cameron[209] demonstrated that with the coracoclavicular screw in place, the degree of elevation of the clavicular pins corresponds to the degree of depression of pins drilled into the scapular spine. In their operative procedure, the clavicle is depressed down to and in contact with the coracoid by the screw, and the screw is left permanently in place, with the hope that a coracoclavicular arthrodesis will be obtained.

The authors have seen patients who had developed a solid bar of bone between the clavicle and the coracoid following acromioclavicular operations. Despite this arthrodesis of the clavicle to the scapula, the patients have had essentially a full range of motion (Fig. 12–4). There is no anatomical difference between an arthrodesis of the coracoclavicular area and an arthrodesis of the acromioclavicular area.

The senior author has drilled Kirschner wires into both clavicles of patients who have a coracoclavicular lag screw in place in one of the shoulders (Fig. 12–5). The degree of upward rotation of each pin during 180 degrees of shoulder abduction and forward flexion was essentially the same—45 degrees. This is in complete agreement with the work of Kennedy and Cameron,[209] who concluded that with the screw in place the clavicle rotates normally. As the clavicle rotates upward, the scapula rotates downward, i.e., the so-called "synchronous scapuloclavicular rotation" (see Fig. 12–52).

Studies of the motion that occurs in the normal acromioclavicular joint in young adults have been conducted. Kirschner wires were drilled into the superolateral edge of the acromion and into the distal superior aspect of the clavicle. These two pins were placed parallel to each other and were within ½ inch of the acromioclavicular joint (Fig. 12–6). These pins were then observed during range of motion of the upper extremity (i.e., flexion, abduction, rotation, etc.). No matter where or how much the arm was actively moved or rotated by the patient, only 5 to 8 degrees of motion could be detected in the acromioclavicular joint. This indication of the small amount of motion in the acromioclavicular joint explains why a coracoclavicular lag screw or coracoclavicular arthrodesis does not significantly limit shoulder motion—and even why Caldwell's[83] patients who had an arthrodesis of the acromioclavicular joint had such a surprisingly good range of motion. We completely concur that the clavicle and scapula rotate in a "synchronous scapuloclavicular" motion, as described originally by Codman,[89] and more recently by Kennedy and Cameron.[209]

CORACOCLAVICULAR LIGAMENT

The coracoclavicular ligament is a very strong, heavy ligament whose fibers run from the outer inferior surface of the clavicle to the base of the coracoid process of the scapula (Fig. 12–7). The coracoclavicular ligament has two parts: the conoid and the trapezoid ligaments. A bursa may separate these two parts of the ligament.

The conoid ligament[202] is cone shaped, with the apex of the cone attaching on the posteromedial side of the base of the coracoid process. The base of the cone attaches onto the conoid tubercle on the posterior undersurface of the clavicle. The conoid tubercle is

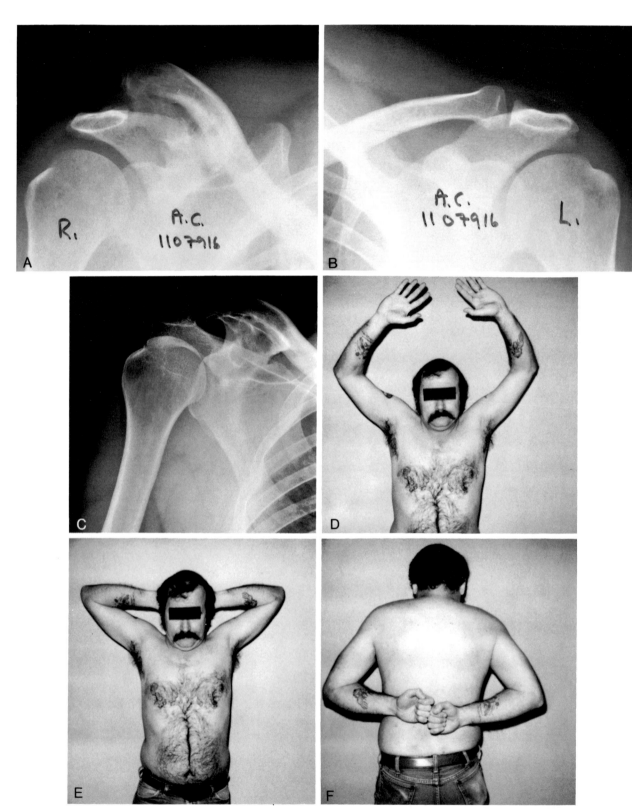

Figure 12–4. *A,* Chronic Type III dislocation with massive new bone formation between the coracoid and the clavicle of the right shoulder. *B,* The patient's normal left shoulder. Despite the mass of bone, the patient had essentially a normal range of motion. *C,* Solid bar of bone between the upper scapula and coracoid and the distal clavicle. *D–F,* Despite the fusion of the clavicle to the scapula, the patient had essentially a full range of motion with little or no discomfort in the right shoulder.

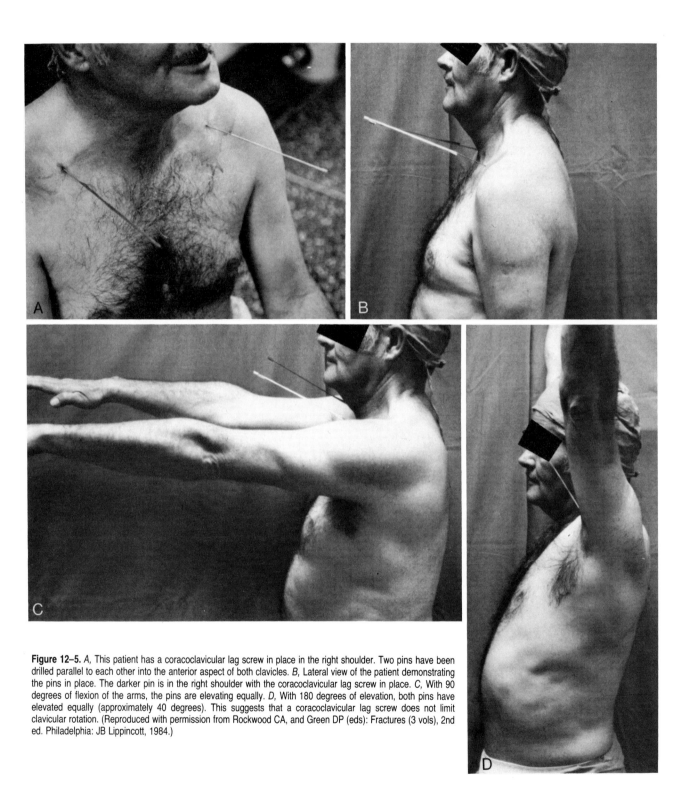

Figure 12–5. *A,* This patient has a coracoclavicular lag screw in place in the right shoulder. Two pins have been drilled parallel to each other into the anterior aspect of both clavicles. *B,* Lateral view of the patient demonstrating the pins in place. The darker pin is in the right shoulder with the coracoclavicular lag screw in place. *C,* With 90 degrees of flexion of the arms, the pins are elevating equally. *D,* With 180 degrees of elevation, both pins have elevated equally (approximately 40 degrees). This suggests that a coracoclavicular lag screw does not limit clavicular rotation. (Reproduced with permission from Rockwood CA, and Green DP (eds): Fractures (3 vols), 2nd ed. Philadelphia: JB Lippincott, 1984.)

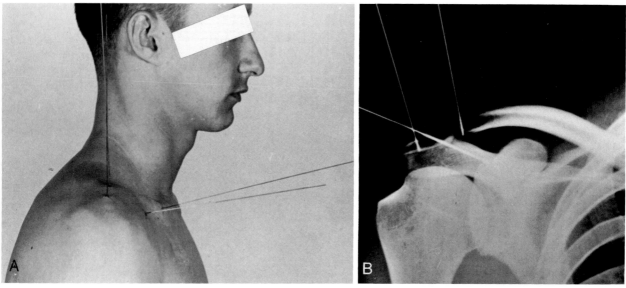

Figure 12–6. *A,* Lateral view of a "volunteer" with normal shoulders. Pins have been drilled into the coracoid and clavicle and into the acromion process. *B,* X-ray with pins in place. When the patient puts the shoulder through a full range of motion, the maximum amount of motion that occurred in the acromioclavicular joint, as determined by deviation of the pins in the clavicle and in the acromion, was 8 degrees. (Reproduced with permission from Rockwood CA, and Green DP (eds): Fractures (3 vols), 2nd ed. Philadelphia: JB Lippincott, 1984.)

located at the apex of the posteroclavicular curve, which is at the junction of the lateral third of the flattened clavicle with the medial two-thirds of the triangular-shaped shaft.

The trapezoid[202] arises anterior and lateral to the conoid ligament on the coracoid process and just behind the attaching pectoralis minor tendon. It extends superiorly to a rough line on the undersurface of the clavicle, which extends anteriorly and laterally from the conoid tubercle.

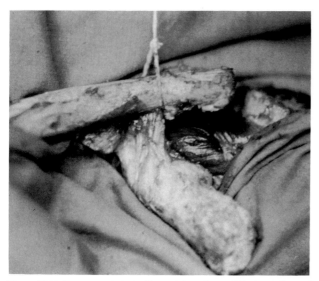

Figure 12–7. The coracoclavicular ligament is a dense, thick, heavy ligament running from the base of the coracoid up to the inferior surface of the clavicle. In this view, the trapezoid component, which is distal to the conoid ligament, has been resected. The normal trapezoid ligament extends out to the distal end of the clavicle. Despite the trapezoid removal, the conoid ligament is quite strong. (Reproduced with permission from Rockwood CA, and Green DP (eds): Fractures (3 vols), 2nd ed. Philadelphia: JB Lippincott, 1984.)

Function of the Coracoclavicular Ligament

Most authors agree that the coracoclavicular ligaments are the primary support ligaments of the acromioclavicular articulation.* They are the primary ligaments between the distal clavicle and the scapula. The only connection of the upper extremity with the axial skeleton is through the clavicular articulations at the acromioclavicular and sternoclavicular joints.

Bearn[40] has demonstrated that the sternoclavicular ligaments are the most important anatomical structures to hold the distal end of the clavicles up (i.e., the shoulder) in their normal position. Hence, in the erect position, it is not the shoulder muscles which hold the shoulders in their anatomical position. The normal poise of the shoulder (i.e., normal anatomical position of the shoulder) is then primarily through the strength of the sternoclavicular ligaments. The clavicles are then supported out, away from the body like the wings off the body of an airplane. Furthermore, just like the jet engines are suspended from the underside of the wings of an airplane, the upper extremities are suspended from the distal ends of the clavicles. Thus, the coracoclavicular ligament becomes the prime suspensory ligament of the upper extremity. However, it is important to remember that when the trapezius muscle is paralyzed, as is seen following an injury to the spinal accessory nerve, the entire shoulder complex does droop downward and forward. This presumably would have to occur secondary to the stretching out of the sternoclavicular ligaments. The attachment of the coracoclavicular ligament on the apex of the posterior

---

*See references 1, 13, 36, 39, 43, 62, 81, 135, 189, 192, 201, 210, 272, 297, 348, 353, 403.

curve of the clavicle aids in clavicular rotation with abduction and elevation of the arm.

According to Bosworth,[65] the average space between the clavicle and the coracoid process is 1.3 cm, and Bearden and co-workers[39] have found variations from 1.1 to 1.3 cm. Salter and colleagues[356] measured the coracoclavicular ligaments in 20 cadaver joints. They found the trapezoid to vary from 0.80 cm to 2.50 cm in length and 0.80 cm to 2.50 cm in width. The conoid varied from 0.70 cm to 2.45 cm in length and 0.40 cm to 0.95 cm in width.

Cadenat,[81] in 1917, very carefully studied the importance of the coracoclavicular ligament in stabilizing the acromioclavicular joint. He concluded that a moderate blow to the acromion process would rupture the acromioclavicular ligament and produce an incomplete acromioclavicular dislocation and that a heavier blow would rupture the acromioclavicular ligament and then the coracoclavicular ligament and produce a complete dislocation of the acromioclavicular joint. He agrees with the studies of Poirier and Rieffel,[319] done in 1891, and of Delbet[81] and Mocquot,[81] which confirm that both the trapezoid and conoid portions of the coracoclavicular ligament must be divided to produce a complete dislocation of the acromioclavicular joint. He further pointed out that before the functional and clinical end results of a given injury can be evaluated, the physician must determine whether the dislocation was incomplete (a mild sprain to the joint) or complete (a complete dislocation of the joint).

Experimental Studies by Urist

Urist,[411] after a series of experiments, concluded that *complete dislocation* of the acromioclavicular joint can

occur without rupture of the coracoclavicular ligament. In a cadaver shoulder with the coracoclavicular ligament intact, he divided the superior acromioclavicular ligament and the entire joint capsule and detached the deltoid and trapezius muscles from the region of the acromioclavicular joint. He then demonstrated that under these conditions, the distal clavicle could be completely dislocated anteriorly and posteriorly away from the acromion process (i.e., in a horizontal plane). Since the coracoclavicular ligament was intact, upward displacement or subluxation of the acromioclavicular joint was minimal. Only after the coracoclavicular ligament was transected did a complete upward or vertical dislocation of the acromioclavicular joint occur.

I have repeated some of the cadaver studies of Urist[411] and agree with his anatomical findings, but I disagree with his terminology. Indeed, with the muscles and acromioclavicular ligaments detached, the clavicle can be dislocated away from the acromion, but only in a horizontal direction (Fig. 12–8A). However, the clavicle cannot be dislocated in a vertical plane (see Fig. 12–7). Only when the conoid and trapezoid ligaments have been divided can the clavicle be vertically dislocated from the acromion process (Fig. 12–8B). These experiments have led me to the following conclusions:

1. The horizontal stability is controlled by the acromioclavicular ligament.

2. The vertical stability is controlled by the coracoclavicular ligaments.

In keeping with the world literature in discussing dislocations of the acromioclavicular joint, I suggest that we refer to an injury where *both* the acromiocla-

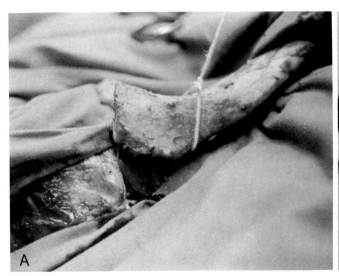 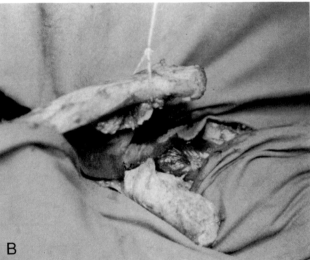

Figure 12–8. The importance of the acromioclavicular and coracoclavicular ligaments for stability of the acromioclavicular joint in a fresh cadaver. *A,* With the muscles and the acromioclavicular ligaments resected, and with the coracoclavicular ligaments intact, the clavicle can be displaced anteriorly (as shown) or posteriorly from the articular surface of the acromion. However, since the conoid component of the coracoclavicular ligaments is intact, the clavicle cannot be significantly displaced upward (see Fig. 12–7). *B,* Following the transection of the conoid ligament, the clavicle can be easily displaced above the acromion. This suggests that the horizontal stability of the acromioclavicular joint is accomplished through the acromioclavicular ligaments, and vertical stability is obtained through the coracoclavicular ligaments. (Reproduced with permission from Rockwood CA, and Green DP (eds): Fractures (3 vols), 2nd ed. Philadelphia: JB Lippincott, 1984.)

vicular *and* the coracoclavicular ligaments are disrupted.*

Fukuda and colleagues[135] recently studied the individual ligament contributions to acromioclavicular stability by performing load-displacement tests with a fixed displacement and sequential ligament section. The contribution of the acromioclavicular, trapezoid, and conoid ligaments was determined at small and large displacements. At small displacements, the acromioclavicular ligaments were the primary restraint to both posterior (89 per cent) and superior (68 per cent) translation of the clavicle—the most common failure patterns clinically. At large displacements, the conoid ligament provided the primary restraint (62 per cent) to superior translation, while the acromioclavicular ligaments remained the primary restraint (90 per cent) to posterior translation. The primary role of the trapezoid was serving as the primary restraint to the acromioclavicular joint compression at both large and small displacements.

Coracoclavicular Articulation

The existence of a joint between the clavicle and the coracoid process is rare. Gradoyevitch[160] reported, in 1939, that only 15 cases were known to medical science. Ten had been proven anatomically, and five were demonstrated by radiography. He reported one instance of a patient with bilateral coracoclavicular joints. The patient's shoulders were asymptomatic and symmetrical, and he had a normal range of motion. There were no abnormal findings of either the acromioclavicular or the sternoclavicular joints.

X-ray Appearance

X-rays reveal a bony outgrowth from the undersurface of the clavicle. The outgrowth is triangular, with the base of the triangle on the inferior surface of the clavicle, and the lateral border of the triangle forming the articular surface with the tubercle of the dorsomedial surface of the coracoid process (Fig. 12–9). Not only does it look like a typical joint on the x-ray, but Gradoyevitch[160] dissected the specimens and found a diarthrodial joint (i.e., articular surfaces, a true capsule, and an intra-articular synovial membrane).

Incidence

In an attempt to determine the frequency of the coracoclavicular joint, Nutter[294] reviewed 1000 x-rays of adult shoulders at random and found 12 cases, an incidence of 1.2 per cent. Six of the 12 cases were bilateral, and 11 of the 12 were in men. Liberson[234] reported an incidence of 9 patients in 1800 shoulders studied; 5 had bilateral coracoclavicular joints. According to Wertheimer,[437] Poirier found 1 case in 2300

---

*See references 5, 10, 16, 20, 39, 62, 65, 81, 85, 111, 112, 189, 195, 210, 234, 248, 257, 271, 272, 275, 277, 330, 354.

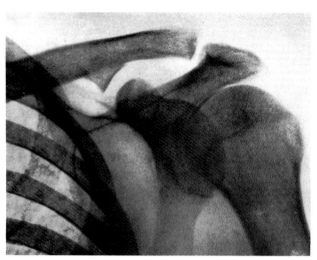

Figure 12–9. Coracoclavicular articulation. This x-ray demonstrates the triangular bony outgrowth from the inferior surface of the clavicle with the dorsal medial aspect of the coracoid process. (Reproduced with permission from Rockwood CA, and Green DP (eds): Fractures (3 vols), 2nd ed. Philadelphia: JB Lippincott, 1984.)

shoulders. Frassetto[437] believes that a coracoclavicular articulation predisposes to fracture of the neck of the humerus. His reasoning is that a fall on an outstretched hand is normally buffered somewhat by the rotation of the scapula about the thorax, and this is not possible when there is an extra articulation between the coracoid process of the scapula and the clavicle. Wertheimer[437] excised the coracoclavicular joint in a manual laborer because of pain.

I have seen this anatomical variation on many x-rays of the shoulder and believe that it is an incidental x-ray finding that has little clinical significance.

Mechanism of Injury

DIRECT FORCE

Injury by direct force is produced by the patient falling on the point of the shoulder with the arm at the side in the adducted position (Fig. 12–10). This is the most common cause of acromioclavicular injuries. The force drives the acromion downward. Bearn[40] has shown that the downward displacement of the clavicle is primarily resisted through an interlocking of the sternoclavicular ligaments. The result, then, of a downward force being applied to the superior aspect of the acromion is that either the acromioclavicular and coracoclavicular ligaments give way or a fracture of the clavicle occurs.

If a fracture of the clavicle does not occur, the force is transmitted first to the acromioclavicular ligaments (a mild sprain), then tears the acromioclavicular ligaments (a moderate sprain), then stresses the coracoclavicular ligament, and finally—if the downward force continues—tears the deltoid and trapezius muscle attachments from the clavicle and ruptures the coraco-

through the acromioclavicular ligament and by the surrounding musculature. Therefore, when a severe downward force is applied to the point of the shoulder and the sternoclavicular ligaments do not rupture and the clavicle does not fracture, the coracoclavicular ligaments rupture and the suspension system of the scapula, from the clavicle with its attaching upper extremity, is lost and the arm droops downward (Fig. 12–11). Since the weight of the arm is no longer suspended from the clavicle, there may be a slight upward pull by the trapezius muscle. However, the major deformity seen in a complete acromioclavicular dislocation is a downward displacement of the shoulder.

Bearn[40] has stressed the importance of the sternoclavicular ligaments in supporting the distal end of the clavicle. Through anatomical dissections and selective division of the sternoclavicular ligaments, he has demonstrated how these ligaments prevent the downward displacement of the distal end of the clavicle. However, there must be an important interplay between the trapezius muscle and the sternoclavicular ligaments, because we have all seen patients who have downward droop of the entire shoulder complex, including the clavicle, following an injury to the spinal accessory nerve supplying the trapezius muscle.

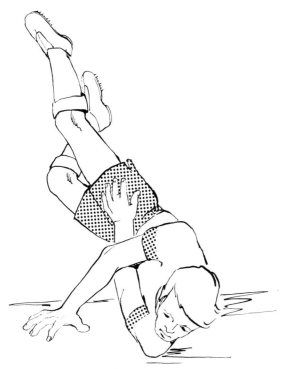

Figure 12–10. The most common mechanism for injury of the acromioclavicular joint is a direct force that occurs from a fall on the point of the shoulder. (Reproduced with permission from Rockwood CA, and Green DP (eds): Fractures (3 vols), 2nd ed. Philadelphia: JB Lippincott, 1984.)

clavicular ligament (a severe acromioclavicular sprain, which completes the dislocation). At this point, the upper extremity has lost its ligament support from the distal end of the clavicle and droops downward.

The mechanism for the inferior dislocation of the clavicle under the coracoid, Type VI, is thought to be a very severe direct force onto the superior surface of the distal clavicle, along with abduction of the arm and retraction of the scapula.[254, 306]

Complete Acromioclavicular Dislocation (Type III, IV, or V): Clavicle Up or Shoulder Down?

Classically, the literature indicates that it is the upward displacement of the clavicle that is diagnostic of a complete acromioclavicular dislocation. Although there may be a slight upward displacement of the clavicle by the upward pull of the trapezius muscle, the true anatomical feature is the downward sag of the shoulder and arm. The framework of the shoulder in the upright position is maintained in its normal anatomical position through a linkage system formed by two mechanisms. First, and probably most important, is the interlocking of the sternoclavicular ligaments, which are quite strong and which resist any significant downward displacement of the distal end of the clavicle.[443] The second mechanism is by the upward support of the trapezius muscle. The scapula and attached upper extremity are suspended from the clavicle primarily by the coracoclavicular ligament and secondarily

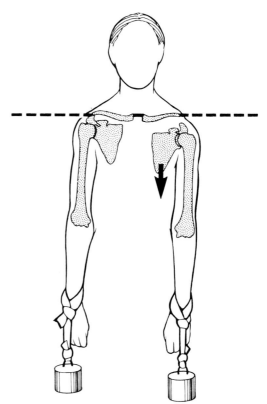

Figure 12–11. A schematic drawing of a patient with a complete Grade III acromioclavicular dislocation. The deformity in the acromioclavicular joint is caused by a downward displacement of the upper extremity, not from an upward elevation of the clavicle.

INDIRECT FORCE

Upward Indirect Force by the Upper Extremity

A force from a fall on the outstretched hand is transmitted up the arm through the humeral head into the acromion process. The strain is referred only to the acromioclavicular ligaments and not to the coracoclavicular ligaments, since the coracoclavicular space is actually decreased (Fig. 12–12). This indirect force then can produce mild, moderate, or severe acromioclavicular joint injury. If the force were severe enough, it could fracture the acromion and cause a superior dislocation of the glenohumeral joint and disrupt the acromioclavicular ligament. This is indeed a very rare mechanism of injury.

Downward Indirect Force Through the Upper Extremity

Forces can be applied directly to the acromioclavicular joint by a pull through the upper extremity. Liberson[234] reported a case in which the scapula was forcibly drawn downward and anteriorly by a sudden change in the position of a heavy burden being carried. Again, this is a very rare mechanism of injury to the acromioclavicular joint.

Classification of Injury

Injuries to the acromioclavicular joint are best classified according to the amount of damage that is done

by a given force. The differential diagnosis of injury to the acromioclavicular joint is based on the amount of injury to the ligament of the joint and on the amount of damage that has been done to the extra-articular ligaments (i.e., the coracoclavicular ligaments) and to adjacent supporting muscles (i.e., the deltoid and trapezius muscles). Therefore, injuries to the acromioclavicular joint are usually graded on the amount of injury to the acromioclavicular and coracoclavicular ligaments. Anatomically, injuries of the acromioclavicular joint should really be referred to as scapuloclavicular injuries. Zaricznyj[448] discusses this terminology in his report. However, because of tradition, subject indexing, and commonly used nomenclature, we will refer to the injuries in this anatomical area as injuries to the acromioclavicular joint.

Classically, injuries of the acromioclavicular joint have been referred to as either Type I, II, or III, and each injury is classified depending on the type of ligament disruption to the acromioclavicular and the coracoclavicular ligaments (Fig. 12–13).[13, 403] However, over the past 15 years, the senior author has recognized and treated three other types of injuries that are added to the classification. In a Type IV injury, the clavicle is grossly displaced posteriorly, back into or through the trapezius muscle. In a Type V injury, the vertical separation of the clavicle from the scapula is greatly exaggerated over a Type III. In a Type VI injury, the clavicle is dislocated inferiorly under the coracoid process.[254, 306, 354] This injury has been described by Patterson,[306] McPhee,[254] and Sage.[354] In 1987, Gerber and Rockwood[145] reported on three cases of inferior dislocation of the distal clavicle under the coracoid—one case in a child and two cases in adults. Thus,

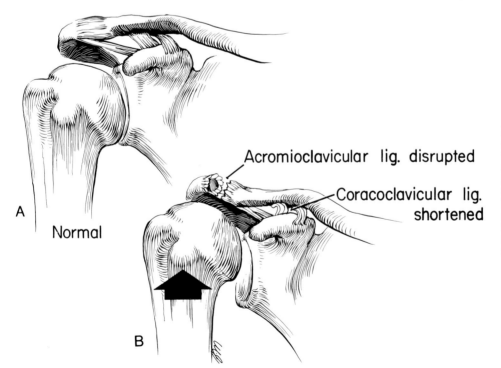

Acromioclavicular lig. disrupted

Coracoclavicular lig. shortened

A Normal

B

Figure 12–12. An indirect force applied up through the upper extremity that might occur from a fall on the outstretched hand can superiorly displace the acromion up from the clavicle, producing an injury to the acromioclavicular ligaments but leaving the coracoclavicular ligaments intact. (Reproduced with permission from Rockwood CA, and Green DP (eds): Fractures (3 vols), 2nd ed. Philadelphia: JB Lippincott, 1984.)

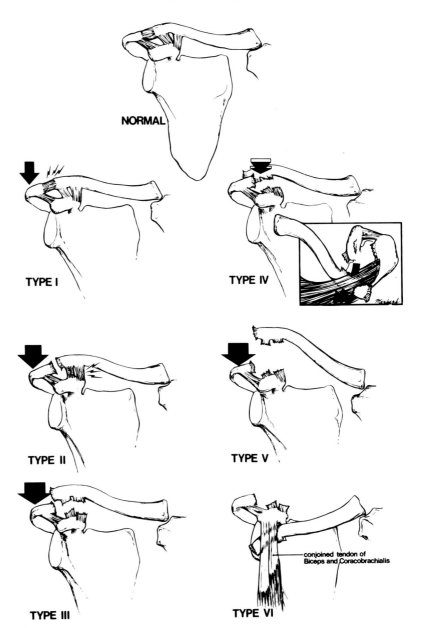

Figure 12–13. Schematic drawings of the classification of ligamentous injuries that can occur to the acromioclavicular ligament. Type I: A mild force applied to the point of the shoulder does not disrupt either the acromioclavicular or the coracoclavicular ligaments. Type II: A moderate to heavy force applied to the point of the shoulder will disrupt the acromioclavicular ligaments, but the coracoclavicular ligaments remain intact. Type III: When a severe force is applied to the point of the shoulder, both the acromioclavicular and coracoclavicular ligaments are disrupted. Type IV: In this major injury, not only are the acromioclavicular and coracoclavicular ligaments disrupted, but the distal end of the clavicle is displaced posteriorly into or through the trapezius muscle. Type V: A violent force has been applied to the point of the shoulder that not only ruptures the acromioclavicular and coracoclavicular ligaments but also disrupts the deltoid and trapezius muscle attachments and creates a major separation between the clavicle and the acromion. Type VI: Another major injury is an inferior dislocation of the distal end of the clavicle to the subcoracoid position. The acromioclavicular and coracoclavicular ligaments are disrupted.

for completion of the usual classification of Type I, II, and III injuries, Types IV, V, and VI were added. Knowing that there is extreme controversy concerning the treatment of Type III injuries, i.e., operative versus nonoperative, and knowing that most surgeons would opt to treat Types IV, V, and VI with surgery, it seems reasonable and practical to remove them from the all-inclusive Type III category and create the new classification.[341] The modified classification is as follows:

TYPE I
 Sprain of acromioclavicular ligament
 Acromioclavicular joint intact
 Coracoclavicular ligaments intact
 Deltoid and trapezius muscles intact
TYPE II
 Acromioclavicular joint is disrupted
 Acromioclavicular joint wider; may be a slight vertical separation when compared with the normal shoulder

 Sprain of the coracoclavicular ligaments
 Coracoclavicular interspace might be slightly increased
 Deltoid and trapezius muscles intact
TYPE III
 Acromioclavicular ligaments disrupted
 Acromioclavicular joint dislocated and the shoulder complex displaced inferiorly
 Coracoclavicular ligaments disrupted
 Coracoclavicular interspace greater than the normal shoulder (i.e., 25 to 100 per cent greater than in the normal shoulder)
 Deltoid and trapezius muscles usually detached from the distal end of the clavicle
 In children, a pseudodislocation of the acromioclavicular joint occurs. The coracoclavicular ligaments remain intact to the intact periosteal tube, and the clavicle is displaced out of the periosteal tube.

TYPE IV
    Acromioclavicular ligaments disrupted
    Acromioclavicular joint dislocated and clavicle ana-
        tomically displaced posteriorly into or through the
        trapezius muscle
    Coracoclavicular ligaments completely disrupted
    Coracoclavicular space may be displaced, *but* may
        appear to be same as the normal shoulder
    Deltoid and trapezius muscles detached from the
        distal clavicle
TYPE V
    Acromioclavicular ligaments disrupted
    Coracoclavicular ligaments disrupted
    Acromioclavicular joint dislocated and gross dispar-
        ity between the clavicle and the scapula (i.e., 100
        to 300 per cent greater than the normal shoulder)
    Deltoid and trapezius muscles detached from the
        distal half of the clavicle
TYPE VI
    Acromioclavicular ligaments disrupted
    Coracoclavicular ligaments disrupted
    Acromioclavicular joint dislocated and clavicle dis-
        placed inferior to the acromion or the coracoid
        process
    Coracoclavicular interspace reversed with the clavi-
        cle being inferior to the acromion or the coracoid
    Deltoid and trapezius muscles are detached from the
        distal clavicle

TYPE I

A mild force to the point of the shoulder produces
a minor strain to the fibers of the acromioclavicular
ligaments. The ligaments remain intact, and the acromioclavicular joint remains stable (see Fig. 12–13).

TYPE II

A moderate force to the point of the shoulder is
severe enough to rupture the ligaments of the acromioclavicular joint (see Fig. 12–13). The distal end of
the clavicle is unstable, because now the scapula has
attachments only to the clavicle through the coracoclavicular ligament. The scapula may rotate medially,
producing a widening of the acromioclavicular joint.
There may be a slight downward displacement of the
scapula from the distal end of the clavicle, secondary
to a minor stretching of the coracoclavicular ligament.

TYPE III

When a severe force is applied to the point of the
shoulder, the acromioclavicular and the coracoclavicular ligaments are disrupted (see Fig. 12–13). Occasionally, the coracoclavicular ligaments remain intact,
and this is associated with an avulsion fracture of part
or all of the coracoid process.
Another possible mechanism of vertical displace-

ment between the acromion and the clavicle is when
the acromioclavicular and coracoclavicular ligaments
remain intact to the periosteal tube of the clavicle and
the clavicle is displaced out of the periosteal tube,
secondary to a longitudinal split in the periosteal
sleeve. This injury occurs in children, but has been
reported in adults by Falstie-Jensen and Mikkelsen[131]
and by Katznelson and associates.[207]
In the complete dislocation of the acromioclavicular
joint, the distal end of the clavicle appears, on x-ray
and clinically, to be displaced above the acromion
process. However, as previously described, the actual
deformity is an inferior displacement of the scapula
and entire upper extremity from the clavicle. The
deltoid and trapezius muscles are disrupted from the
distal end of the clavicle, or the periosteal sleeve with
muscle attachments may be separated from the outer
clavicle.

TYPE IV

The mechanism of injury and the pathology of this
injury is similar to that of a Type III problem, except
that the distal end of the clavicle is displaced posteriorly
into and occasionally through and locked within the
fibers of the trapezius muscle (see Fig. 12–13). The
posterior displacement of the clavicle may be so
marked that it may tent the skin on the posterior aspect
of the shoulder. Hastings and Horne[176] and Nieminen
and Aho[290] have reported on this type of injury and
refer to them as anterior dislocations of the scapula.
Malcapi and colleagues[244] and Sondergard-Petersen
and Mikkelsen[352] have reported cases and referred to
them as posterior acromioclavicular dislocations.
In describing dislocations of joints, we realize that
the customary terminology used for the reference point
is the proximal part, i.e., in anterior dislocation of the
hip, the pelvis is the proximal part and the head is
dislocated anteriorly. The pelvis is also the most stable
component of the hip joint. The same is true for
dislocation of the shoulder joint. When the head of
the humerus is dislocated anterior to the scapula, it is
referred to as an anterior dislocation of the shoulder—again, the scapula is the proximal and the stable
part of the joint. It is because the scapula is the stable
component of the acromioclavicular joint that we have
termed a posterior displacement of the clavicle from
the acromion a posterior dislocation. In a Type IV
injury, the acromion process of the scapula remains in
its usual anatomical position, and the clavicle is indeed
dislocated posteriorly back into the trapezius muscle.
Similarly, in a Type VI injury, the clavicle is anatomically displaced inferiorly under the coracoid—not a
superiorly displaced scapula over the clavicle.

TYPE V

Type V injury is a very severe Type III injury. In
addition to the rupture of the supporting acromiocla-

vicular and coracoclavicular ligaments and detachment of the deltoid and trapezius muscles from the distal third of the clavicle, the entire upper extremity droops inferiorly, making the clavicle appear quite prominent (see Fig. 12–13). Sometimes, through muscle spasm, the clavicle may be displaced superiorly upward toward the base of the neck. The combination of the superiorly displaced clavicle and a downward droop of the shoulder produces a grotesque disfiguration of the shoulder.

TYPE VI

This injury is usually secondary to a significant traumatic abduction force to the upper extremity. The distal end of the clavicle is dislocated under the coracoid process and posterior to the conjoined tendons (see Fig. 12–13). This has been reported by Patterson,[306] McPhee,[254] and Gerber and Rockwood.[145] Sage[354] reported a case of recurring inferior dislocation, and Nauman[279] reported a case of spontaneous habitual inferior dislocation of the clavicle under the acromion.

Incidence of Injury

Cave has shown, from a review of 394 dislocations about the shoulder, that 85 per cent of the dislocations occurred to the glenohumeral joint, 12 per cent to the acromioclavicular joint, and 3 per cent to the sternoclavicular joint. Most authors report that the incidence of injury to the acromioclavicular joint occurs more often in males in a ratio of 5 to 1. In some series, the ratio is 10 to 1. Most authors also agree that incomplete injuries are twice as common as complete dislocations of the acromioclavicular joint.

Signs and Symptoms of Injury

When an acromioclavicular joint injury is suspected, the patient should be examined in the standing or sitting position whenever possible. The weight of the arm pulling downward stresses the acromioclavicular joint and will make a deformity more apparent.

TYPE I INJURY

There is minimal to moderate joint tenderness and swelling over the acromioclavicular joint without palpable displacement of the joint. Usually, there is only minimal pain with arm movements. Pain is not present in the coracoclavicular interspace.

TYPE II INJURY

With subluxation of the acromioclavicular joint, moderate to severe pain is noted at the joint. If the patient is seen soon after the injury, the outer end of the clavicle may be noted to be slightly superior to the acromion. Motion of the shoulder produces pain in the acromioclavicular joint. With gentle palpation, the outer end of the clavicle may appear to be unstable and free floating. When the midclavicle is grasped and the shoulder stabilized, a to-and-fro motion of the clavicle in the horizontal plane can be detected. Pain is also noted with palpation of the coracoclavicular interspace.

TYPE III INJURY

The patient with Type III injury, a complete dislocation of the acromioclavicular joint, characteristically presents with the upper extremity adducted close to his body and held upward by the other arm to relieve the discomfort in the acromioclavicular joint. The entire upper extremity is depressed when compared with the normal shoulder, and the distal end of the clavicle may be prominent enough to tent the skin (Fig. 12–14). Moderate pain is the rule, and any motion of the arm, particularly abduction, increases the pain.

With palpation, pain is noted in the acromioclavicular joint, the coracoclavicular interspace, and along the superior aspect of the lateral one-fourth of the clavicle. The lateral clavicle is quite unstable and seems to be floating free. Delbet[81] has stated that the distal end of the clavicle may be so prominent that it can be depressed like a piano key.

Cooper,[93] in 1832, described a technique that could be used even by a blind man to detect the complete acromioclavicular dislocation: "The easiest mode of detecting this accident is to place the finger upon the

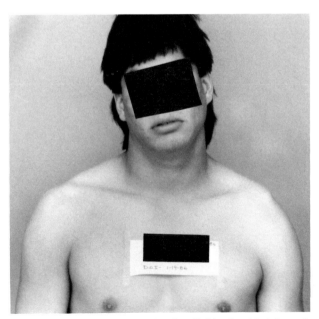

Figure 12–14. This patient has a complete Type III dislocation of the left acromioclavicular joint. The left shoulder is drooping and there is prominence of the left distal clavicle.

spine of the scapula and to trace this portion of the bone forward to the acromion in which it ends; the finger is stopped by the projection of the clavicle, and so, as the shoulders are drawn back, the point of the clavicle sinks into place, but it reappears when the shoulders let go."

TYPE IV INJURY

The patient has essentially all the clinical findings as those described with a Type III injury, plus the striking feature that the patient has much more pain than with a Type III injury, and the distal end of the clavicle is posteriorly displaced away from the acromion and into and occasionally through the trapezius muscle. The physician standing above and behind the seated patient will observe that the outline of the involved clavicle will have a definite posterior inclination when compared with the normal shoulder (Fig. 12–15). On occasion, the clavicle is displaced completely through the trapezius muscle, locked between the fibers of the muscle, and the clavicle can be tenting the skin of the posterior shoulder. The patient experiences much more pain with shoulder movements with a Type IV injury than with a Type III injury.

TYPE V INJURY

The Type V injury is an exacerbation of the Type III injury in which the upper extremity is grossly drooping lower than the normal extremity. The clavicle

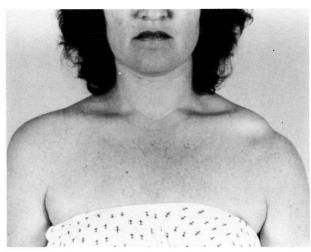

Figure 12–16. This patient has a Type V acromioclavicular dislocation of the left shoulder. The entire left upper extremity is displaced inferiorly. The left clavicle is prominent, but it is not superiorly displaced compared with the normal right clavicle.

is usually not superiorly displaced; the upper extremity is inferiorly displaced (Fig. 12–16). However, in some acute cases, there may be spasm of the trapezius muscle, which may displace the clavicle upward (Fig. 12–17). This upward displacement, along with the downward displacement of the shoulder, presents a gross disfigurement to the shoulder. The patient has more pain than with a Type III injury, and pain is noted over the distal half of the clavicle, secondary to the extensive muscle and soft tissue disruption from the clavicle.

TYPE VI INJURY

The superior aspect of the shoulder has a flat appearance, as opposed to the rounded contour of the normal shoulder. With palpation, the acromion is prominent, and there is a definite inferior step-down to the superior surface of the coracoid process. Because of the amount of trauma that is required to produce a subcoracoid dislocation of the clavicle, there may be associated fractures of the clavicle, upper ribs, or injury to the upper roots of the brachial plexus. These associated injuries may produce so much swelling of the shoulder that the disruption of the acromioclavicular joint may not initially be recognized. Vascular injuries that were secondary to the dislocation were not present in the patients presented by Patterson,[306] McPhee,[254] and Gerber and Rockwood.[145] However, all of the adult cases reported by Patterson,[306] McPhee,[254] and Gerber and Rockwood[145] had transient paresthesias prior to reduction of the dislocation. Following reduction, the neurological deficits cleared.

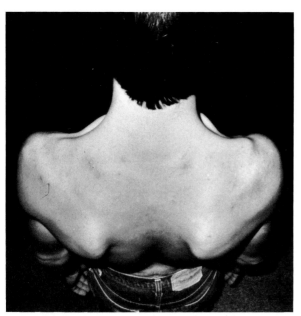

Figure 12–15. Superior view of a seated patient who has a Type IV acromioclavicular joint injury of the right shoulder. The right clavicle has more posterior inclination than the normal left clavicle. There is a prominent "bump" on the dorsal posterior aspect of the right shoulder secondary to the clavicle's prominence into the trapezius muscle. (Reproduced with permission from Rockwood CA, and Green DP (eds): Fractures (3 vols), 2nd ed. Philadelphia: JB Lippincott, 1984.)

X-ray Evaluation

In most instances, x-rays of the acromioclavicular joint are taken by the technician using the same x-ray

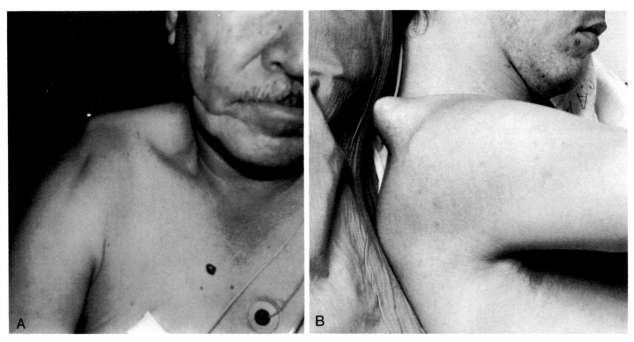

Figure 12–17. Clinical photographs of patients with Type V acromioclavicular dislocations. *A,* The clavicle is quite prominent secondary to the downward displacement of the right upper extremity. *B,* Severe prominence of the right clavicle.

exposure settings used for penetrating the heavier and thicker glenohumeral joint. This produces a very dark, overpenetrated film of the acromioclavicular joint that is impossible to interpret (Fig. 12–18*A*). Therefore, many times the technician must be requested to take x-rays specifically of the "acromioclavicular joint," and not just x-rays of the "shoulder." Quality films of the acromioclavicular joint require about one-half the x-ray intensity that is required for a quality x-ray of the glenohumeral joint (Fig. 12–18*B,C*).

ANTEROPOSTERIOR VIEWS

Even good quality anteroposterior films of the acromioclavicular joint are not always sufficient to diagnose the injuries. Zanca[445] recommended that a 10- to 15-degree cephalic tilt view of the acromioclavicular joint be routine (Fig. 12–19). Unless there is a slight superior tilt to the x-ray beam, the acromioclavicular joint will be superimposed on the spine of the scapula, and small fractures will be missed (Fig. 12–20).

LATERAL VIEWS

In addition to having clear anteroposterior x-rays of the acromioclavicular joint, an axillary view of the shoulder should also be taken. This will indicate any posterior displacement of the clavicle and may reveal small fractures that cannot be seen on the anteroposterior view. The scapular lateral x-ray is another technique to study the acromioclavicular joint. This view was described by Alexander,[7] and he called it the

shoulder forward view and used it to demonstrate dislocations of the acromioclavicular joint (Fig. 12–21). This view is recommended by Waldrop and co-workers[424] for the routine evaluation of all injuries to the acromioclavicular joint.

Technique of Alexander Scapular Lateral View

In the Alexander view, the patient is positioned as if a true scapulolateral x-ray is to be taken, as described in Chapter 5. The patient is asked to thrust both shoulders forward, and then an x-ray is made of the normal shoulder, as well as the injured shoulder. The acromioclavicular joint in the normal shoulder will maintain its integrity, whereas in an acromioclavicular dislocation, the joint will be disrupted, and the acromion is displaced anteriorly and inferiorly under the distal end of the clavicle (see Fig. 12–21).

STRESS X-RAYS

Patients who clinically present with the obvious prominent clavicle and drooping shoulder will have the characteristic x-ray findings of a Type III, IV, or V injury. However, it is impossible to clinically differentiate all cases of Type II subluxations from a Type III complete dislocation. Therefore, stress films of both shoulders, which test the integrity of the coracoclavicular ligaments, should be made routinely when an injury of the acromioclavicular joint is suspected.

The patient should be standing or sitting with his or her arms hanging free and his back against a cassette

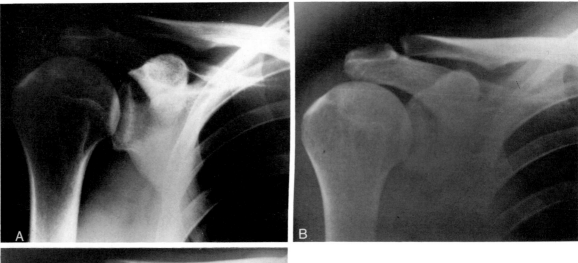

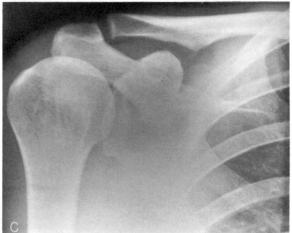

Figure 12–18. Explanation of why the acromioclavicular joint is poorly visualized on routine x-rays of the shoulder. *A,* A routine anteroposterior view of the shoulder demonstrates the glenohumeral joint well. However, the acromioclavicular joint is too dark to interpret because it has been overpenetrated by the x-ray technique. *B,* When the exposure is decreased by about 50 per cent, the acromioclavicular joint is better visualized. However, the inferior corner of the joint is superimposed on the spine of the scapula. *C,* Using the Zanca view with a 10- to 15-degree upward tilt of the x-ray beam affords a clear view of the acromioclavicular joint. (Reproduced with permission from Rockwood CA, and Green DP (eds): Fractures (3 vols), 2nd ed. Philadelphia: JB Lippincott, 1984.)

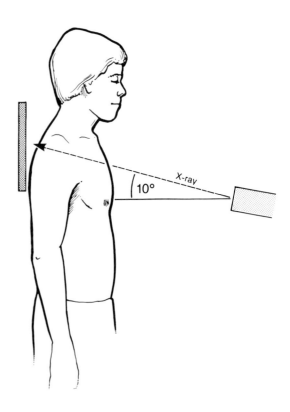

Figure 12–19. Position of the patient for the Zanca view—a 10- to 15-degree cephalic tilt of the x-ray of the acromioclavicular joint.

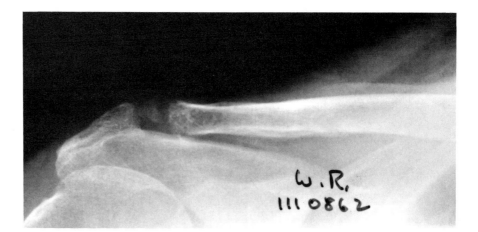

Figure 12–20. The Zanca x-ray view demonstrates a loose body in the acromioclavicular joint.

large enough to visualize both shoulders (Fig. 12–22A). If the patient is large and has broad heavy shoulders, it is better to take two separate 10-inch × 12-inch x-rays of each shoulder rather than having to rotate the 14-inch × 17-inch cassette so that both shoulders can be seen on the same x-ray film. Ten to 15 pounds of weight—not held in the hand but suspended by a loop of webbing around the wrists—allows for total relaxation of the muscles of the upper extremity and prevents any muscle forces from lifting the arm upward, which could alter the amount of coracoclavicular separation. The average distance between the superior aspect of the coracoid process and the inferior aspect of the clavicle varies from 1.1 cm to 1.3 cm.[39, 65] However, the coracoclavicular distance will vary in normal subjects depending on how far the patient is from the cassette, the distance the tube is from the patient or cassette, and so on. The most important detail is not the distance in the coracoclavicular interspace of the injured shoulder but the comparison of the coracoclavicular space between the injured shoulder and the normal one (Fig. 12–22B). According to Bearden and colleagues,[39] an increase of the coracoclavicular distance of the injured shoulder over the normal shoulder by 40 to 50 per cent can be considered a complete coracoclavicular ligament disruption. The senior author has documented that a difference of 25 per cent has been diagnostic of a complete disruption of the coracoclavicular ligaments.

The routine use of stress films in doubtful cases prevents the patient from holding up the injured arm while the x-ray is being taken. We have seen normal x-rays of the acromioclavicular joint in patients who have total dislocations, because instead of using weights strapped about the wrists, the patient was allowed to hold the injured shoulder up, which reduced the joint injury and produced a near normal x-ray (Fig. 12–23).

Bossart and colleagues[61] reviewed the stress x-rays of 82 patients who did not have an obvious Type III injury of the acromioclavicular joint. Their study unmasked five cases with Type III injuries. Because of this low percentage yield, they did not believe that stress x-rays of the acromioclavicular joint were justi-

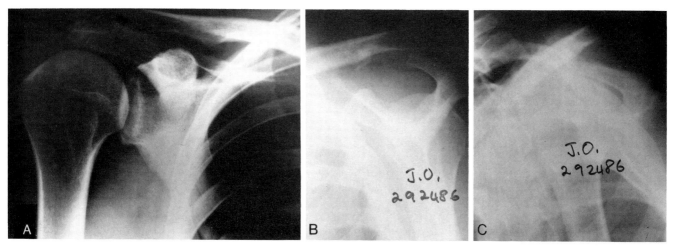

Figure 12–21. Technique of obtaining the Alexander view or modified scapulolateral view to evaluate injuries of the acromioclavicular joint. *A,* Anteroposterior x-ray of a patient with a suspected injury to the acromioclavicular joint. *B,* Alexander view taken with the shoulder in the relaxed position. Note that the acromioclavicular joint is only minimally displaced. *C,* With the shoulders thrust forward there is gross displacement of the acromioclavicular joint, with the clavicle displaced posteriorly and superiorly over the acromion. (Reproduced with permission from Rockwood CA, and Green DP (eds): Fractures (3 vols), 2nd ed. Philadelphia: JB Lippincott, 1984.)

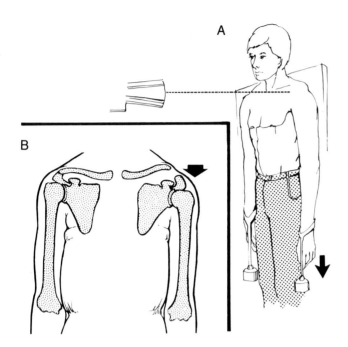

Figure 12–22. Technique of obtaining stress x-rays of the acromioclavicular joint. *A,* Anteroposterior x-rays are made of both acromioclavicular joints with 10 to 15 pounds of weight hanging from the wrists. *B,* The distance between the superior aspect of the coracoid process and the undersurface of the clavicle is measured to determine whether or not the coracoclavicular ligaments have been disrupted.

Figure 12–23. Importance of obtaining stress x-rays of the acromioclavicular joint. *A,* The patient may present with only a mild deformity in the vicinity of the acromioclavicular joint. *B,* With weight added to the wrist of the upper extremity, the deformity is obvious. However, if the x-ray is taken while the patient holds the arm upward to reduce the pain, it will show minimal, if any, displacement of the acromioclavicular joint. (Reproduced with permission from Rockwood CA, and Green DP (eds): Fractures (3 vols), 2nd ed. Philadelphia: JB Lippincott, 1984.)

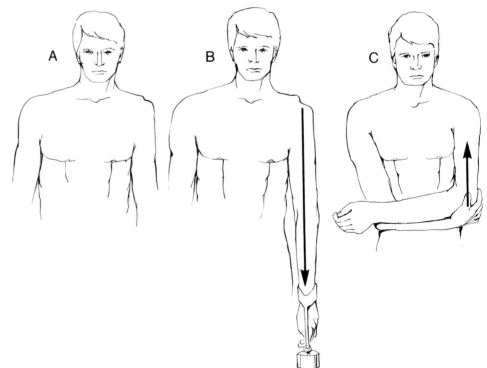

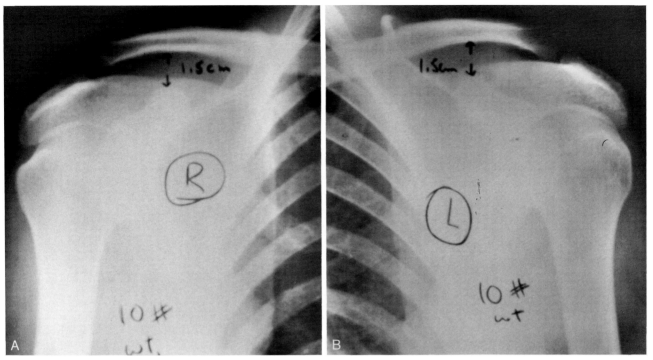

Figure 12–24. X-ray appearance of a Type II injury to the right shoulder. With stress x-rays the coracoclavicular distance in both shoulders measures 1.5 cm. However, the injured right shoulder has a widened acromioclavicular joint compared to the normal left shoulder.

fied. If the physician believes that Type III or greater injury needs surgery, or if the physician wants to make a correct diagnosis as to the degree of ligament injury, stress x-rays of the acromioclavicular joint are justified, just as they are for evaluation of ankle, knee, and spine injuries.

X-RAY FINDINGS IN TYPE I INJURY

In a Type I injury, the x-rays of the acromioclavicular joint are essentially normal as compared with those of

the normal shoulder. There is no widening, no separation, and no deformity.

X-RAY FINDINGS IN TYPE II INJURY

In a Type II injury, the lateral end of the clavicle may be slightly elevated, and the acromioclavicular joint, when compared with the normal side, may appear to be widened. The widening probably is the result of a slight medial rotation of the scapula and a slight posterior displacement of the clavicle by the pull

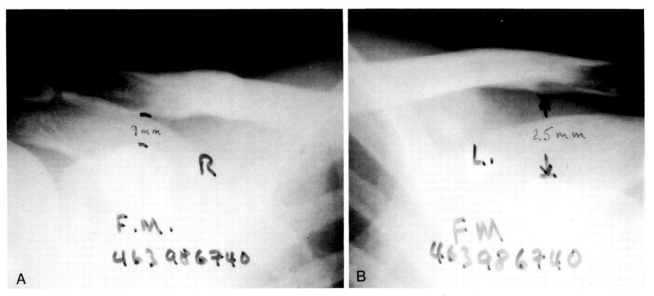

Figure 12–25. X-ray appearance of a Type III injury in the left shoulder. Stress x-rays indicate a 25.0-mm gap in the coracoclavicular space on the left compared with a 9.0-mm gap in the right shoulder.

of the trapezius muscle. Stress films of both shoulders to test the integrity of the coracoclavicular ligaments reveal that the coracoclavicular space of the injured shoulder is essentially the same as that of the normal shoulder (Fig. 12–24).

X-RAY FINDINGS IN TYPE III INJURY

In obvious cases of complete acromioclavicular dislocations, the joint is totally displaced. The lateral end of the clavicle is above the superior border of the acromion, and the coracoclavicular interspace is signif-

icantly greater than in the normal shoulder (Fig. 12–25). When the injury is questionable, which it usually is in most instances, stress films comparing the injured and normal shoulders will reveal a major discrepancy in the coracoclavicular distances. Fractures of the distal clavicle, the acromion, or the coracoid process may be noted.

Rarely, instead of the coracoclavicular ligaments disrupting, there may be a fracture of the coracoid process (Fig. 12–26). In this instance, the distal clavicle is clearly superiorly displaced from the acromion, but the coracoclavicular interspace is the same as in the normal shoulder. The fracture of the coracoid is hard to

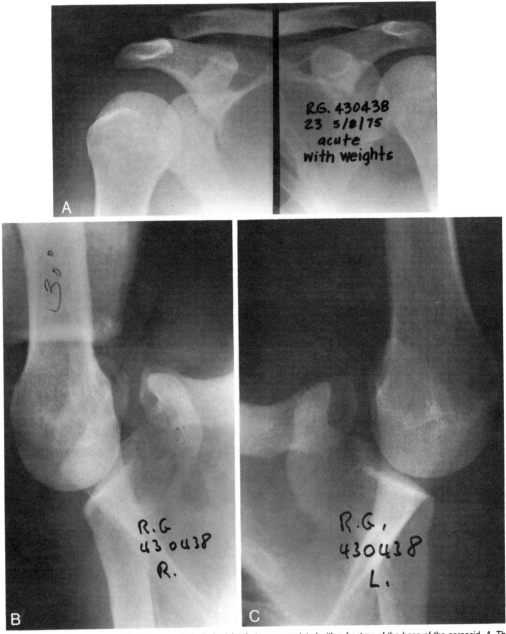

Figure 12–26. X-rays of an adult with an injury to the right acromioclavicular joint that was associated with a fracture of the base of the coracoid. *A,* The distal end of the right clavicle is displaced from the acromion as compared with the normal shoulder. However, the coracoclavicular interspace is the same in both shoulders. This would suggest a fracture through the coracoid. *B,* The Stryker notch view demonstrates the fracture through the base of the coracoid. *C,* A Stryker notch view of the normal left shoulder demonstrates the normal appearance of the base of the coracoid. (Reproduced with permission from Rockwood CA, and Green DP (eds): Fractures (3 vols), 2nd ed. Philadelphia: JB Lippincott, 1984.)

visualize on routine x-rays. The best "special view" to visualize this fracture is the Stryker notch view (Fig. 12–27). This technique is described in detail in Chapter 5.

X-RAY FINDINGS IN TYPE IV INJURY

Although the patient with a Type IV injury may have x-ray findings of an increase in the acromioclavicular joint and an increase in the coracoclavicular interspace, the most striking feature is the posterior displacement of the distal clavicle as seen on the axillary lateral x-ray (Fig. 12–28A,B). In patients with heavy, thick shoulders or in patients with multiple injuries in whom an axillary lateral view of the shoulder or a scapular lateral x-ray cannot be taken, a CT scan can be of great value in helping to confirm clinical suspicions of a posteriorly dislocated acromioclavicular joint (Fig. 12–28C,D).

X-RAY FINDINGS IN TYPE V INJURY

The characteristic x-ray feature in Type V injuries is a gross inferior displacement of the scapula from the

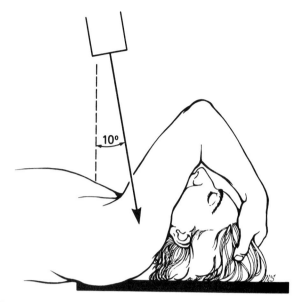

Figure 12–27. Technique for taking the Stryker notch view to demonstrate fractures of the base of the coracoid. The patient is supine with a cassette placed posterior to the shoulder. The humerus is flexed approximately 120 degrees so that the patient's hand can be placed on top of the head. The x-ray beam is directed 10 degrees superior.

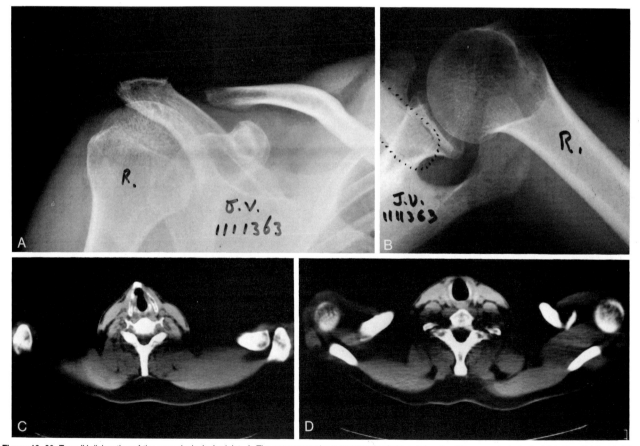

Figure 12–28. Type IV dislocation of the acromioclavicular joint. *A,* The anteroposterior x-ray reveals obvious deformity of the acromioclavicular joint. The distal end of the clavicle appears to be inferior to that of the acromion. *B,* The axillary view confirms that the clavicle is displaced posteriorly away from the acromion process. *C,* CT scans reveal that the left clavicle is in its normal position adjacent to the acromion. Note that the right clavicle is completely absent. *D,* A lower CT cut demonstrates the posterior displacement and also confirms the fact that the clavicle is inferior to the acromion.

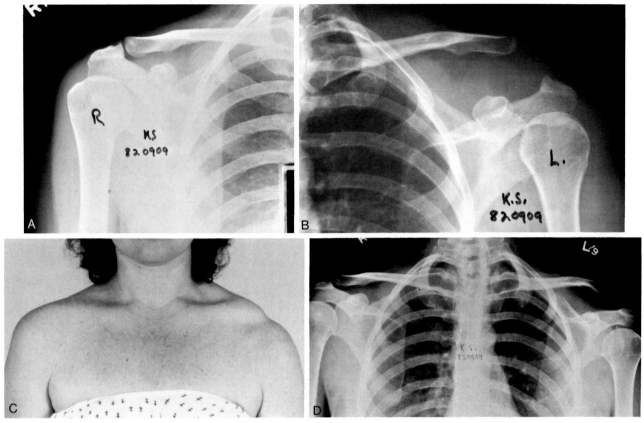

Figure 12–29. X-rays of a patient with a Type V injury. *A,* The normal right shoulder. *B,* The injured left shoulder. Note the gross disparity in the coracoclavicular space interval. *C* and *D,* Comparison of the patient's clinical deformity with the x-ray deformity. Note that a line drawn through both clavicles would indicate that they are essentially at the same level. The deformity is due to the inferior displacement of the upper extremity, which is secondary to the loss of the coracoclavicular suspensory ligaments.

clavicle. On a horizontal 14-inch × 17-inch x-ray cassette showing both shoulders, it will be noted that both clavicles are at the same horizontal level. This again demonstrates that the clavicle of the injured shoulder is not up—the injured shoulder is down (Fig. 12–29). The coracoclavicular interspace may be two to three times that of the normal shoulder.

X-RAY FINDINGS IN TYPE VI INJURY

There are two types of inferior dislocation: subacromial and subcoracoid. In the subacromial type of injury, the distal end of the clavicle is inferiorly displaced and located under the acromion. In the subcoracoid injury, the distal end of the clavicle is completely inferior to the coracoid process (Fig. 12–30). There may well be associated fractures of the clavicle and ribs.

Treatment of Injuries

One of the interesting things revealed in a review of acromioclavicular joint injuries is that about half of

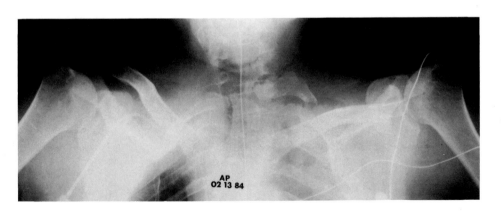

Figure 12–30. Type VI acromioclavicular dislocation of the left shoulder. Note that the distal end of the left clavicle is inferior to the coracoid process. (See Fig. 12–55.)

more than 300 articles have contributed a new technique or a new twist to an old technique on how to manage dislocations of the acromioclavicular joint. There are three basic and fundamentally different schools of thought in the management of the acute, complete Type III acromioclavicular dislocation: (1) those whose approach is conservative, or no-operation-is-necessary school; (2) those who recommend surgical repair in all patients; and (3) those who recommend surgical repairs for selected patients. Each group thinks the others are radical.

Some authors tend to lump mild injuries, subluxations, and dislocations together under one form of treatment and quote the end results for all the cases combined. Only when the injuries to the acromioclavicular joint are graded according to severity and the final results are also graded according to severity can readers evaluate the adequacy of a given form of treatment.

Most authors agree on conservative management of acute Type I and Type II sprains. The treatment of the acute Type III acromioclavicular joint dislocation is extremely controversial.

TREATMENT OF TYPE I INJURY

In Type I injury, the acromioclavicular and coracoclavicular ligaments are intact, but the acromioclavicular ligaments have been strained. Usually, after 7 to 10 days of rest, the symptoms subside. The application of ice bags will help to ease the discomfort. However, the shoulder should be protected from further injury until there is a painless full range of motion.

TREATMENT OF TYPE II INJURY

The damage in a Type II sprain is localized primarily to the acromioclavicular joint, with coracoclavicular ligaments remaining intact. There may be some associated partial detachment of the deltoid and trapezius muscles from the distal clavicle, which increases the pain and discomfort.

Closed Treatment

Most authors agree that nonsurgical measures are indicated to treat this injury. However, a report by Bergfeld and colleagues[46] and a study by Cox[98] suggest that Type I and II injuries may cause more problems than previously recognized.

There are marked differences of opinion as to which type of conservative measures is indicated. Some authors routinely use the sling for 10 to 14 days to rest the injured shoulder, and this is followed by a gradual rehabilitation program. From this point on, things get pretty complicated, with various types of bandages and slings, adhesive tape strappings, braces, harnesses, traction techniques, and many, many types of plaster

casts. Allmann[13] recommended the use of the sling harness immobilizing device—the Kenny Howard sling—for three weeks (Fig. 12–31). Some authors recommended a plaster cast device as described by Urist,[411] with a strap over the top of the clavicle in an effort to depress the clavicle down to the acromion. However, the problem is a depressed upper extremity and not an elevated clavicle.

Whether adhesive tape, elastic strapping, cast, or harness is used, it must have uninterrupted continuous pressure over the top of the shoulder and around the elbow to compress the coracoclavicular space to allow for ligament healing. Some authors recommend three weeks and some recommend six weeks to prevent another injury from converting the weakened Type II subluxation into a Type III total dislocation. Heavy lifting or contact sports should be avoided for 8 to 12 weeks until the ligament has healed completely.

In nonlaborers and in patients who do not place any stress on their shoulders during daily activities, most authors manage a Type II sprain with only a sling for a few days and then encourage active use of the arm.

Operative Treatment

In some instances following the Type II sprain, pain persists in the acromioclavicular joint, and the injury could rightly be called internal derangement of the acromioclavicular joint. Since fibers of the joint were

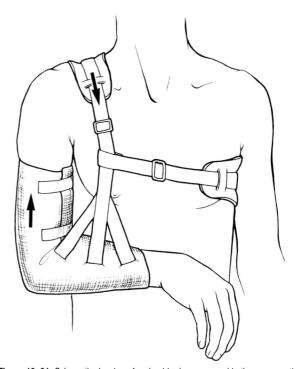

Figure 12–31. Schematic drawing of a shoulder harness used in the nonoperative treatment of injuries to the acromioclavicular joint (a modified Kenny Howard shoulder harness). The strap that runs over the top of the shoulder and under the elbow is tightened sufficiently to reduce the clavicle to the acromion. A halter strap around the trunk keeps the harness from slipping off the top of the shoulder.

initially disrupted, it is possible that shreds of the ligament or flakes of the articular cartilage are loose in the joint, causing symptoms. The meniscus may have been detached, and with motion it will pop and displace in and out of the joint like a torn meniscus in the knee. This internal derangement has been described by Bateman.[36] Brosgol[73] has described the technique of performing an arthrogram of the acromioclavicular joint, which may help to determine the integrity of the joint.

Ultimately, it may be necessary to do an arthroplasty of the acromioclavicular joint, a do-what-is-needed-when-you-get-there type of operation—that is, debridement and meniscectomy and, perhaps, if the degenerative arthritis is marked, excision of the outer 2.0 cm of the clavicle. The clavicle does not displace upward, because the coracoclavicular ligaments are still intact. This procedure has been described by Mumford.[275]

TREATMENT OF TYPE III INJURY

Historical Review

The controversy over conservative versus operative treatment of complete dislocation of the acromioclavicular joint seems to have had cyclic turns in the literature. Obviously, the earliest writings on the subject dealt with the closed reduction followed by strappings and bindings. The concepts developed by the fathers of medicine, Hippocrates, Galen, and Paul of Aegina, are still being used today. Hippocrates[2] recommended that the projecting part of the shoulder (the clavicle) be pushed down with compresses while the arm is kept elevated with sling and bandages. He went on to say that the end result would be good but that there would always be a deformity to the joint.

Following the discovery of anesthesia by Long and co-workers[450] in 1844, and following the development of antiseptic principles of surgery by Lister[450] in 1867, a great many operative procedures were described. Cadenat,[81] in a classic article in 1917, stated that the first operation on the acromioclavicular joint was performed by Samuel Cooper of San Francisco in 1861. Cooper used a loop of silver wire to repair the acromioclavicular joint. In 1886, Baum[81] used sutures in the acromioclavicular ligaments through the skin without an incision (a technique he learned from Volkmann). Paci,[81] in 1889, performed an arthrodesis of the acromioclavicular joint. In 1891, Poirier and Rieffel[319] used sutures in the joint and acromioclavicular ligament; Budinger[81] used a screw across the joint; Tuffier[81] used silk sutures in the acromioclavicular joint; Delbet[81] and Lambotte used acromioclavicular nailing; Morestin[81] resected the outer 2.5 cm of the clavicle. Cadenat[81] gives Baum credit for the first repair of the coracoclavicular ligaments in 1886 but states that Baum did it as a secondary step, because he felt repair of the acromioclavicular ligament was of primary importance.

Delbet,[81] in 1917, is credited with the first coracoclavicular reconstruction when, in three cases, he passed a loop of suture from under the coracoid through an anteroposterior drill hole in the clavicle. In the first case, he used a single strand of silver wire, but he had to explore it in 45 days when the deformity reappeared. He found that the wire had broken. He replaced the wire with two silk sutures and concluded that wire should not be used because it breaks. In two subsequent cases he used two strands of silk sutures tied over the top of the clavicle. Cadenat[81] used a strip of the short head of the biceps tendon to reconstruct the coracoclavicular ligament in cadavers but did not perform the operation on any patients because the coracoid was too far anterior from the clavicle. He found that when he vertically reduced the displaced clavicle with the biceps tendon, it displaced the clavicle anteriorly away from the acromion. However, in 1917, Cadenat did use the coracoacromial ligament to reconstruct the coracoclavicular ligament. He noted that the posterior attachment of this ligament was on the base of the coracoid, adjacent to the coracoclavicular ligament. After removing the acromial attachment, he also determined that if he detached the most anterior portion of the coracoacromial ligament from the coracoid, he would have enough length to suture the coracoacromial ligament into the clavicle, thus reestablishing a new coracoclavicular ligament.

In 1924, Henry[179] reported using an autogenous fascia lata graft to replace the coracoclavicular ligaments and repair and stabilize the acromioclavicular joints with two Kirschner wires. Bunnell,[77] in 1928, used fascia lata to reconstruct the acromioclavicular joint. Murray,[277] in 1940, recommended the use of one or two Kirschner wires across the acromioclavicular joint, and Phemister,[313] in 1942, recommended the use of heavier threaded pins across the joint. Bloom,[57] in 1945, recommended two 1/32-inch Steinmann pins. Caldwell,[83] in 1943, reported good results from an arthrodesis of the acromioclavicular joint in two patients.

In the 1930s and 1940s, the trend began to swing away from the surgical repairs and back to conservative forms of treatment. Conservative treatment using a plaster cast became particularly popular, and a sentence regarding the treatment of complete acromioclavicular joint injuries from Urist's[413] article of 1959 is worth quoting: "They range from the neatest and smallest to the largest and most grotesque seen in the whole field of traumatic and orthopaedic surgery." In the 1940s, new splints and harnesses were developed by Gibbens,[148] Morrison,[269] Batchelor,[35] Brandt,[70] and Varney and associates.[419]

Some authors still favored operative treatment. In 1941, Bosworth[62] described a technique, done under local anesthesia, of the blind insertion of a regular bone screw directed from the clavicle down into the coracoid process. Stewart[391] described a screw across the acromioclavicular joint, and Simmons and Martin[378] have described a special threaded screw pin across the joint.

In the 1950s, 1960s, and 1970s, there appeared to be more agreement by authors that the complete dislocation should be managed by operative means. Powers and Bach,[322] in a 1974 review, reported that the operative treatment of the complete acromioclavicular joint was most popular. They sent a questionnaire to all chairmen of approved residency programs in the United States and drew the following conclusions from their analysis of the responses:

1. The majority of program chairmen treated Type III injury by open reduction.

2. Surgical treatment varied, but 60 per cent used temporary acromioclavicular fixation, and 35 per cent used coracoclavicular fixation.

3. Nonoperative treatment was rarely advocated, as it was often inadequate.

Nonoperative Treatment

The two most commonly used forms of nonoperative treatment (Table 12–1) are (1) a sling and harness immobilization device and (2) "skillful neglect." Plaster casts have lost their popularity. Many authors recommend the nonoperative treatment of Type I, II, and III injuries. However, Type IV, V, and VI problems, because of the gross anatomical reasons, will be difficult, if not impossible, to treat without surgical reduction. Should the attempted closed reduction of Type IV and VI injuries be unsuccessful in removing the clavicle from the trapezius muscle or from under the coracoid, then an operative approach should be used.

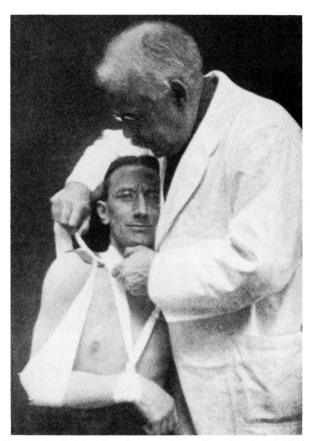

Figure 12–32. Sir Robert Jones is seen applying a sling and bandage that holds the arm elevated while depressing the lateral end of the clavicle (Reproduced from Jones R: Injuries of Joints. London: Oxford University Press, 1917.)

Table 12–1. NONOPERATIVE FORMS OF TREATMENT FOR ACROMIOCLAVICULAR DISLOCATION REPORTED IN THE LITERATURE

Form of Treatment	Authors
Adhesive strapping	Rawlings[333]
	Thorndike and Quigley[401]
	Benson[44]
	Bakalin and Wilppula[26]
Sling or bandage	Jones[203]
	Watson-Jones[430]
	Hawkins[177]
Brace and harness	Giannestras[147]
	Warner[426]
	Currie[101]
	Anderson and Burgess[17]
Crotch loops, stocking, garter, and strap	Darrow, Smith, and Lockwood[107]
	Spigelman[388]
	Varney[419]
Figure eight bandage	Usadel[414]
Sling and pressure dressing	Goldberg[154]
Abduction traction and suspension in bed	Caldwell[84]
Casts	Urist[411]
	Howard[191]
	Shaar[371]
	Hart[174]
	Trynin[405]
	Stubbins and McGaw[394]
	Dillehunt[117]
	Key and Cornwell[213]
	Gibbens[148]

Sling and Harness Device

The sling supports the forearm and arm. A strap or harness over the top of the shoulder and down and around the elbow is tightened so that it depresses the clavicle downward (Fig. 12–32). A separate halter strap around the trunk keeps the harness from slipping off the top of the shoulder. However, the sling and harness device must be continuously worn for six weeks, tightly enough to maintain the reduction. If the reduction cannot be accomplished, or if reduction cannot be maintained in the device, or if the patient will not wear and keep the device in position constantly, operative repairs should be considered. Allman reported that one of five patients, for reasons described above, cannot be treated with the sling and harness. In addition to shoulder harnesses, new devices using crotch loops, stocking, garter straps, and pads have been described.[107, 388, 419]

Skillful Neglect

Sometimes, this method of treatment is brought about by the patient's insistence, sometimes by circumstances, and sometimes by the physician who is dissatisfied with the results that were achieved by an operation or by the use of a sling and harness device. The

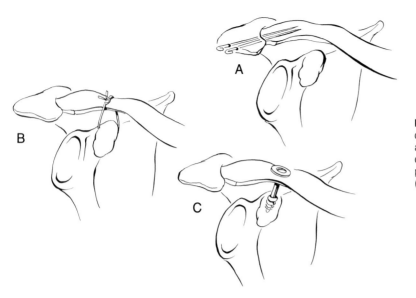

Figure 12–33. Operative procedures for the treatment of injuries of the acromioclavicular joint. *A*, Pins or screws across the acromioclavicular joint. *B*, Sutures between the clavicle and the coracoid. *C*, A coracoclavicular lag screw. (Reproduced with permission from Rockwood CA, and Green DP (eds): Fractures (3 vols), 2nd ed. Philadelphia: JB Lippincott, 1984.)

treatment consists of nothing more than a standard sling. Physicians who manage athletic injuries, especially those seen in soccer, rugby, and hockey, recommend a nonoperative treatment because they know that the players, within a few days or weeks or months, will be back in action and subjected to the same type of violent contact injury to their shoulders. Nicol,[288] in a philosophical editorial, states that conservative treatments cannot achieve the unattainable, and that operative procedures are unwarranted. He recommended a sling for only one to two weeks, followed by exercises. Glick[151] favors a skillful neglect form of treatment, especially for athletes, since it allows them to return to their event more rapidly and "just as safely." In 1977, Glick and associates[152] reported on 35 cases of unreduced Type III acromioclavicular dislocations in athletes. They concluded that a complete reduction is not necessary and that none of their athletes were disabled at follow-up. They recommended nonoperative treatment and stressed the need for a vigorous rehabilitation program to strengthen the shoulder.

Bjerneld and colleagues,[54] Dias and associates,[116] Sleeswijk and colleagues,[380] and Schwarz and Leixnering[365] have also reported series of patients with Type III injuries treated nonoperatively, with 90 to 100 per cent satisfactory results, with follow-up averaging five to seven years. Dias and colleagues[116] also reported good results in 52 of 53 patients treated conservatively for acromioclavicular dislocations (44) and subluxations (9).

Operative Treatment

During the 1800s and early 1900s, practically every conceivable operation was done to the acromioclavicular joint, to the coracoclavicular ligaments, and to both areas at the same time. Today, most surgeons use various combinations of the older procedures (Fig. 12–33). Four basic operations currently are being done.

Table 12–2. OPERATIVE TECHNIQUES FOR TYPE III INJURIES

Repair	Authors
Primary Acromioclavicular Joint Fixation With pins, screws, suture wires, plates, etc., or reconstruction, i.e., with or without coracoclavicular ligament and/or acromioclavicular ligament repair or reconstruction	Bateman,[36] Bundens and Cook,[76] Southmayd et al[236] Dannohl,[106] Ahstrom,[5] DePalma,[111] Dittel et al,[118] Aderhold,[4] McLaughlin,[248] O'Donoghue,[297] Stephens,[390] Sage and Salvatore,[353] Inman et al,[195] Zaricznyj,[447] Rowe,[348] Nevaiser,[284] Kaiser et al,[204] Bakalim and Wilppula,[26] Schindler et al,[361] Moshein and Elconin,[274] Augereau et al,[22] O'Carroll and Sheehan,[296] Barnhart,[31] Smith and Stewart,[383] Bargren et al,[29] Simmons and Martin,[378] Simeone,[377] Krawzak et al,[218] Holz and Weller,[187] Allman,[13] Schneppendahl and Ludolph,[363] Mikusev et al,[260] Muller and Schilling,[241] Bednarek et al,[42] Paavolainen et al[303]
Primary Coracoclavicular Ligament Fixation With screw, wire, fascia, conjoined tendon, or synthetic sutures With or without acromioclavicular ligament repair or reconstruction	Bosworth,[62] Weitzman,[434] Larsen and Peterson,[227] Kennedy and Cameron,[209] Orofinio and Stein,[302] Liang,[221] Baker and Stryker,[27] Bateman,[36] Jay and Monnet,[201] Alldredge,[11] Bearden et al,[39] Mumford,[275] Vargas,[418] Browne et al,[74] Rockwood,[340-342] Goldberg et al,[155] Grønmark,[159] Dahl,[104] Lowe and Fogarty,[238] Heitemeyer et al,[178] Linke and Moschinski,[236] Graves and Foster,[162] Bargren et al,[29] Vandekerckhove et al,[417] Burri and Neugebauer,[79] Burton,[80] Augereau et al,[22] Vargas,[418] Rauschning et al,[332] Sonnabend and Faithfull,[384] Ganz et al,[141] Shoji et al,[374] Kawabe et al,[208] Moravec et al,[266] Karlsson et al[206]
Excision of the Distal Clavicle With or without coracoclavicular ligament repair with fascia, suture, or coracoacromial ligament transfer	Gurd,[166] Mumford,[275] Urist,[412] Bateman,[36] Weaver and Dunn,[433] Rockwood,[342] Moseley[272]
Dynamic Muscle Transfers With or without excision of the distal clavicle	Dewar and Barrington,[114] Bailey and O'Connor,[24, 25] Berson et al,[48] Glorian and Delplace[153]

Each of the four procedures has been modified in many ways, and some authors have even combined modifications. However, other techniques such as synthetic materials used to reconstruct the acromioclavicular joint, metallic plates, or osteotomy of the clavicle are also being used (Table 12–2).

Intra-articular Acromioclavicular Repairs

Acromioclavicular repairs and stabilization remain popular procedures. Most authors do not use Kirschner wires, because there are only four sizes—0.028, 0.035, 0.045, and 0.062 inch—and all of them are small and liable to break and migrate. Most authors use the smaller, smooth or threaded Steinmann pins. These pins can be inserted from the lateral edge of the acromion through the joint and on into the clavicle, or they can be drilled retrograde from the joint out through the acromion and then back across the joint and into the clavicle. The portion of the pin that protrudes through the lateral acromion process should always be bent to prevent medial migration of the pin (Fig. 12–34).

Note: We must point out that despite the fact that the pin is bent, it can break, migrate, and create serious consequences (Fig. 12–35). See the section on Complications to read about pin migration to the spinal cord, lung, subclavian artery, pulmonary artery, mediastinum, heart, etc.

Blind pinning of the acromioclavicular joint has been mentioned occasionally in the literature, but it is difficult to perform. It is hard enough to drill a pin across the acromioclavicular joint under direct vision (Fig. 12–36).

Sage and Salvatore[353] recommended repair of the acromioclavicular ligament whenever possible. They used temporary pins across the joint and used the fibrocartilaginous meniscus to reinforce the superior acromioclavicular ligament. Stevens[353] stabilized the acromioclavicular joint with a Stuck nail. Smith and Stewart[383] reported less degenerative changes in the acromioclavicular joint following surgical repair when they repaired the acromioclavicular and coracoclavicular ligaments; they used an excision of the distal 1.0 cm of the clavicle and used two ³⁄₃₂-inch pins for 8 to 10 weeks across the joint as temporary internal fixation. Bundens and Cook,[76] after stabilizing the acromiocla-

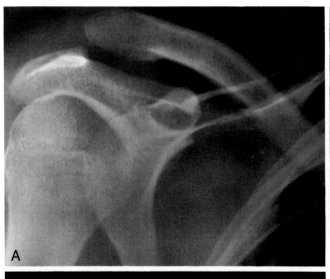

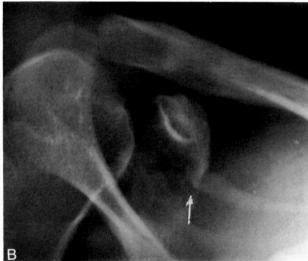

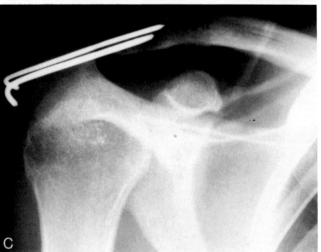

Figure 12–34. Dislocation of the right acromioclavicular joint associated with an avulsion fracture of the base of the coracoid process. *A,* The distal end of the clavicle is completely dislocated away from the acromion, but the coracoclavicular distance as compared with the normal shoulder is about the same. *B,* A cephalic tilt view of the shoulder reveals a fracture at the base of the coracoid. A Stryker notch view probably would have better defined the fracture of the base of the coracoid. *C,* Open reduction of the acromioclavicular joint and stabilization of that joint with two pins effectively reduced the fractured coracoid. Note that the distal ends of the pins have been bent to prevent medial migration. (Reproduced with permission from Rockwood CA, and Green DP (eds): Fractures (3 vols), 2nd ed. Philadelphia: JB Lippincott, 1984.)

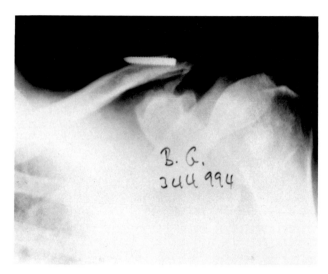

Figure 12–35. Type III dislocation was previously fixed with a threaded Steinmann pin. The reduction held satisfactorily but the pin broke, leaving the tip embedded in the distal end of the clavicle.

vicular joint with two pins, stressed the importance of reefing the attachment of the trapezius and deltoid muscles over each other on the top of the clavicle. Augereau and colleagues[22] used two pins to hold the acromioclavicular joint reduced and transfer the coracoacromial ligament up through and fastened to a clavicular tunnel. Ahstrom[5] transfixes the acromioclavicular joint with one ⁹⁄₆₄-inch threaded pin and then turns up a segment of the short head of the biceps to reinforce the coracoclavicular ligament. Simmons and Martin[378] use a special screw-pin that is inserted through a small stab wound on the posterolateral aspect of the acromion. With the distal clavicle reduced to the acromion, the pin is first drilled and then screwed across the joint. The threads on the pin near the screw head gain purchase in the acromion, which prevents medial migration of the pin. Mikusev and colleagues[260] advocate percutaneous pinning of the acromioclavicular joint and application of a plaster bandage for six weeks. Vainionpaa and colleagues[415] stabilized the acromioclavicular joint with an AO cortical screw. Bateman[36] creates a new suspensory ligament using fascia lata that passes from the coracoid around the clavicle and back to the spine of the acromion. If degenerative arthritis is present, he advises excision of the distal end of the clavicle. O'Donoghue[297] and Inman and associates[195] recommend acromioclavicular stabilization with pins and repair of the coracoclavicular ligaments. Linke and Moschinksi[236] recommend Kirschner wire with cerclage wire for acromioclavicular fixation and reconstruction of the coracoclavicular ligaments with a vicryl band. Paavolainen and colleagues[303] used a malleolar screw for acromioclavicular stabilization. Nevaiser[282–285] stabilized the acromioclavicular joint with one pin and then reconstructed a new superior acromioclavicular ligament by detaching the coracoacromial ligament from the coracoid process and swinging it up on top of the distal clavicle. He did

not recommend repair of the coracoclavicular ligaments. Moshein and Elconin[274] stabilize the acromioclavicular joint temporarily with small pins and repair the coracoclavicular ligament with the coracoacromial ligament.

Dittel and colleagues[118] Albrecht,[6] Kaiser and coworkers,[204] Schindler and colleagues,[361] and Dittmer and colleagues[119] have all reported good results with use of the Balser hook plate. Dannohl[106] supplements acromioclavicular wire fixation with an angulation osteotomy of the midclavicle, which is stabilized with a bent AO plate.

Postoperative Care. Patients are encouraged to move the hand and elbow but are discouraged from abducting the shoulder. Motion must be limited to prevent breakage or migration of the pins across the acromioclavicular joint. Rowe[348] recommends that abduction motion be limited to 40 degrees, and DePalma[111] recommends no abduction until the pins are removed. Most authors recommend that the pins be removed after six to eight weeks. After pins are removed, patients are instructed in range-of-motion and strengthening exercises.

Extra-articular Coracoclavicular Repairs

The technique of placing a screw between the clavicle and the coracoid was described by Bosworth[62] in 1941. The operation was performed under local anesthesia. With the patient in a seated position, a stab wound was made on the superior shoulder, 3.8 cm medial to the distal end of the clavicle. Under fluoroscopy and after a drill hole was made in the clavicle, an assistant depressed and reduced the clavicle with a special clavicle depressor instrument and elevated the arm to reduce the acromioclavicular joint. Under fluoroscopy, an awl was used to develop a hole in the superior cortex of the base of the coracoid, and then a regular bone screw was inserted. The screw was left indefi-

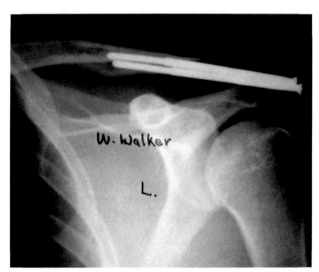

Figure 12–36. Type III dislocation has been managed by blind pinning of the acromioclavicular joint using two Deyerle hip screws.

nitely, unless specific indications for removal developed. In the original article,[62] Bosworth also described a newly developed lag screw with a broad head, which he preferred to the original regular bone screw. He referred to the procedure as a screw suspension operation, not a fixation (i.e., the screw suspends the scapula from the clavicle).

Bosworth, in all of his publications,[62–65] did not recommend repair of the coracoacromial ligaments, nor did he recommend exploration of the acromioclavicular joint. Kennedy and Cameron[209] in 1954 and Kennedy[210] in 1968 reported on a modified Bosworth technique. Under general anesthesia they recommended a thorough debridement of the acromioclavicular joint; preserved but did not repair the coracoclavicular ligament; overcorrected the acromioclavicular dislocation by compressing the clavicle down onto the top of the coracoid process with the Bosworth lag screw; and finally repaired the trapezius and deltoid muscles back to the clavicle. In acute cases, they placed the bone dust, created by drilling the hole in the clavicle, into the coracoclavicular joint area in an effort to gain a permanent bone fixation between the clavicle and the coracoid. Kennedy and Cameron[209] stated that the screw fixation of the clavicle to the coracoid process with ossification creates an extra-articular arthrodesis of the acromioclavicular joint, which did not interfere with the functional or normal clavicular rotation and produced an essentially normal range of motion in the shoulder.

Weitzman[434] reported the use of a Bosworth screw, which he inserted under general anesthesia. He did not expose or repair the coracoclavicular ligament but did expose and debride the acromioclavicular joint and imbricated the deltoid and trapezius muscle attachments. Jay and Monnet,[201] following the teaching of Amspacher, reviewed an excellent series of 31 cases from the University of Oklahoma Medical Center. In their technique, they debrided the acromioclavicular joint, repaired the coracoclavicular ligaments, used the

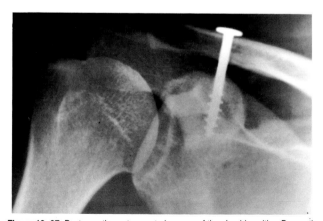

Figure 12–37. Postoperative anteroposterior x-ray of the shoulder with a Bosworth screw in place. Note that the acromioclavicular joint has been satisfactorily reduced and the coarse lag threads of the screw are well seated in the coracoid process. (Reproduced with permission from Rockwood CA, and Green DP (eds): Fractures (3 vols), 2nd ed. Philadelphia: JB Lippincott, 1984.)

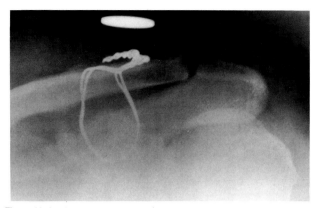

Figure 12–38. A postoperative x-ray of the acromioclavicular joint shows that two loops of wire have been used to reduce the joint. The loops of wire passed under the coracoid process can be passed over the clavicle, but preferably pass through a hole in the clavicle. A coin has been taped to the skin on the superior aspect of the shoulder to aid in the exact location of the loop of wire or the screw, which will be removed under local anesthesia.

Bosworth screw temporarily to hold the acromioclavicular joint reduced, and repaired the trapezius and deltoid muscle back to the clavicle (Fig. 12–37). They recommended that an x-ray be taken on the operating table to ensure that the screw is in the vertical position and that it is engaging both cortices of the coracoid process. Lowe and Fogarty[238] reported on 21 patients treated with the Bosworth technique, noting full recovery in all but one patient. They reported that ossification between the clavicle and the coracoid was not a problem. As in the report of Kennedy,[210] patients had a near full range of motion even though there was a bony bridge in the coracoclavicular space.

Bearden and co-workers[39] recommend two coracoclavicular loops of wire, repair of the coracoclavicular ligament, debridement of the acromioclavicular joint, and repair of the trapezius and deltoid muscles (Fig. 12–38). Alldredge[11] recommended ligament repair and used two loops of stainless steel wire around the coracoid and the clavicle. Tagliabue and Riva,[398] Park and colleagues,[304] Nelson,[281] Kappakas and Mc-Master,[205] Fleming and associates,[134] and Goldberg and colleagues[155] have all reported on the use of synthetic Dacron arterial graft or velour Dacron graft to repair dislocations of the acromioclavicular joint. However, they reported erosion of the material through the distal clavicle in some cases. Dahl[103, 104] has reported on the use of a synthetic velour or Dacron coracoclavicular loop for fixation and described marked clavicular erosion by the loop; in one case, the prosthesis had eroded through the entire clavicle, and in all seven of his cases, there was significant evidence of clavicular erosion (Fig. 12–39). Moneim and Balduini[264] reported a case of a coracoid fracture following reconstruction of the coracoclavicular ligaments through two drill holes in the clavicle. Park and associates[304] found superior results and no resorption in patients treated with double velour Dacron grafts compared with the older knitted Dacron vascular grafts.

Burton[80] favors the excision of the coracoclavicular

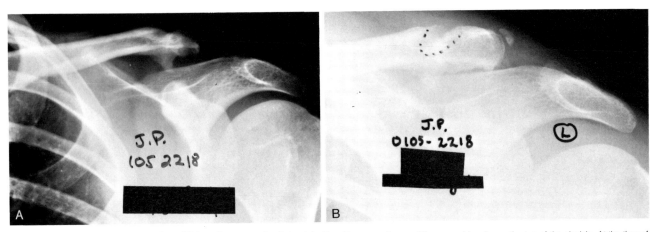

Figure 12–39. X-rays of patient with a Type III injury who was previously treated with a Dacron graft around the coracoid and over the top of the clavicle. At the time of secondary reconstruction, the Dacron graft was noted to be partially eroded down through the clavicle.

ligament and uses a transfer of the coracoacromial ligament to the clavicle, along with a meticulous repair of the trapezius and deltoid muscle back to the clavicle.

A combination of techniques is recommended by Copeland and Kessel,[95] who transfer the acromial attachment of the coracoacromial ligament, along with a piece of bone, to the superior surface of the clavicle and hold it in place with a Bosworth screw.

Vargas,[418] in 1942, reported on using a part of the conjoined tendon as a substitute for the coracoclavicular ligaments. Laing[221] reported on 30 cases in which he reconstructed a new coracoclavicular ligament by transferring the long head of the biceps up through a drill hole in the coracoid process into a drill hole in the clavicle. He states that this new ligament, with its own nerve and blood supplies, is sensitive to stress and is able to protect itself against stretching.

Postoperative Care. Bosworth[62] recommended a sling until the soft tissues are healed. However, he encouraged the patient to remove the sling daily to perform pendulum and crawling-up-the-wall exercises. He allowed the patient to bathe, dress, and feed himself, and, in general, care for himself from the day of surgery. The patient was restricted from heavy work for eight weeks. Kennedy[210] uses no form of external splintage and encourages a gradual range of motion. He looks for full abduction 7 to 10 days after the operation and returns the patient to vigorous athletic activities at six to eight weeks. Neither Bosworth nor Kennedy recommended removal of the screw.

Weitzman[434] recommended using a sling and swathe immediately after surgery, but on the first day after the operation, he applies a plaster shoulder Velpeau cast. This cast is worn for four weeks and is then removed to allow active exercises. He recommended removal of the screw under local anesthesia after three months. Bearden and colleagues[39] support the arm in a sling for 10 to 14 days after surgery. The patient is instructed to avoid strenuous activity such as lifting weights. After the skin sutures are removed, the patient is encouraged to regain range of motion. The

wire loops are removed at six to eight weeks. They are removed in the hospital under local anesthesia, if possible, or general anesthesia, if necessary. They recommend removing all the fragments if the wires are broken. Alldredge[10] recommends no postoperative immobilization beyond the second day and limiting the patient's activities for five to six weeks. If the wires are broken and there is full range of motion, the wires are not removed; otherwise, loops are removed after six to eight weeks. Jay and Monnet[201] recommend a sling for four weeks after operation, at which time active exercises are started. They remove the screw under local anesthesia at eight weeks.

Comparison of Acromioclavicular and Coracoclavicular Operative Repairs

Lancaster and associates[223] compared his results with acromioclavicular versus coracoclavicular fixation and found a higher minor complication rate with acromioclavicular fixation but a higher failure rate with coracoclavicular fixation. However, Bargren[29] had superior results with coracoclavicular fixation versus acromioclavicular fixation. Bargren and colleagues[29] compared the use of pins across the acromioclavicular joint with the use of the Dacron coracoclavicular loop and favored the latter. Taft and colleagues[395] reviewed 127 patients treated operatively and nonoperatively with an average follow-up of 9.5 to 10.8 years. They found that patients treated operatively with acromioclavicular fixation had a higher incidence of post-traumatic arthritis than those managed with a coracoclavicular screw. They further found a much greater incidence of post-traumatic arthritis in those patients who failed to maintain an anatomical acromioclavicular joint.

Kiefer and colleagues studied the biomechanics of some of the various surgical procedures that are used to stabilize the acromioclavicular joint, including (1) acromioclavicular joint tension band techniques, (2) the Streli plate, (3) Bosworth screw, (4) Wolter plate, (5) Rahmanzadeh plate, and (6) Balser plate and carbon fiber ligament. They found the Bosworth screw provided the most rigid fixation but noted that it has failed in fatigue clinically. They suggested either acromioclavicular fixation with Kirschner wires and a cerclage wire or a Wolter plate.

Excision of the Distal Clavicle

Exactly who performed the first excision of the outer end of the clavicle is not known. McLaughlin[248] states that it was first recommended by Facassini in 1902 but gives no reference, and Cadenat[81] states that it was first performed by Morestin but gives no reference or date. In 1941, Gurd[166] of Montreal and Mumford[275] of Indiana independently described their results of excision of the distal end of the clavicle. Mumford[275] recommended his operation for the symptomatic, incompletely dislocated, or Type II, acromioclavicular dislocation with arthritis of the joint (Fig. 12–40). Gurd[166] recommended his procedure for a symptomatic Type III completely dislocated acromioclavicular joint.

Currently, excision of the distal end of the clavicle is referred to as the Mumford[275] or the Gurd[166] operation, or by both eponyms combined. Strictly speaking, the simple excision of the distal clavicle should only be used for an old, symptomatic Type II injury, and the name that is associated with this procedure is Mumford. Furthermore, as pointed out by Mumford, if the problem is a symptomatic Type III injury in which the supporting coracoclavicular ligaments have been disrupted, then in addition to the excision of the distal clavicle, there must be a reconstruction of the coracoclavicular ligaments. This will be further discussed in the section on operative procedures for chronic, symptomatic complete acromioclavicular dislocation.

Weaver and Dunn,[433] in 1972, reported on 12 acute and 3 chronic Grade III acromioclavicular joint dislocations. Their procedure was to excise the distal 2.0 cm of the clavicle, and then, rather than use internal fixation, they recommended the transfer of the coracoacromial ligament from its acromial attachment to the intramedullary canal of the clavicle, as recommended by Cadenat in 1917.[81]

Rauschning and coworkers[332] performed the Weaver-Dunn procedure in 18 cases and reported stable and painless shoulders. Kawabe and associates[208] used the coracoacromial ligament with its bone insertion inserted with a screw into the distal clavicle without distal clavicle excision. Some cases were also supplemented with Kirschner wire acromioclavicular fixation. Shoji and associates[374] also transferred the coracoacromial ligament with a bone block in 12 acute and 3 chronic cases.

Browne and coworkers[74] reviewed a series of 25 patients, in which 12 had coracoclavicular fixation alone and 13 had coracoclavicular fixation, along with the resection of the distal 1 inch of the clavicle. They concluded that the distal clavicle resection did not offer any significant improvement over coracoclavicular fixation alone.

Smith[382, 383] compared acromioclavicular fixation and coracoclavicular ligament repair with and without distal clavicle excision. He found no difference in symptomatology, range of motion, or strength, although there was a higher incidence of degenerative changes in the patients without distal clavicle excision. Cook and Tibone[92] found that athletes treated with distal clavicle excision for chronic pain following Type II acromioclavicular separations had excellent subjective results. Sixteen of 17 patients returned to their preinjury performance level. The most common complaint was a decrease in maximum bench press strength. CYBEX testing demonstrated some weakness at slow speeds, but little or no weakness at faster speeds.

Postoperative Care. Weaver and Dunn[433] recommend a Velpeau dressing or a sling and beginning circumduction exercises on the first day after operation. At the end of four weeks, the patient is allowed full active use of the shoulder.

Dynamic Muscle Transfer

In 1964, Bailey,[25] at the annual meeting of the American Academy of Orthopaedic Surgeons, presented his results on the transfer of the coracoid process with the coracobrachialis and the short head of the biceps to the clavicle in nine patients with acute, complete acromioclavicular dislocation. He reported that the operation acted as a dynamic depressor of the clavicle. He did not state whether he excised the lateral end of the clavicle. He stated that in lower vertebrate forms, the coracobrachialis and short head of the biceps muscles have their origin from the clavicle, and that in a sense, the operation is a step backward in comparative vertebrate anatomy. In 1965, Dewar and Barrington[114] published a similar type procedure for chronic cases of acromioclavicular joint injuries. In 1972, Bailey and associates[25] reported on 38 cases. Berson and coworkers[48] reported satisfactory results in 23 acute and 6 chronic acromioclavicular dislocations. Glorian and Delplace[153] have reported satisfactory re-

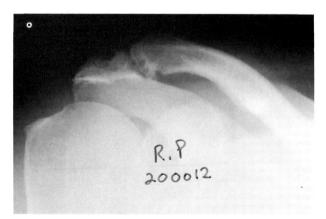

Figure 12–40. Degenerative arthritis in the right acromioclavicular joint. (Reproduced with permission from Rockwood CA, and Green DP (eds): Fractures (3 vols), 2nd ed. Philadelphia: JB Lippincott, 1984.)

sults in 36 cases and modified the procedure by temporarily using two pins across the acromioclavicular joint.

Treatment of Acromioclavicular Dislocation with a Fracture of the Coracoid Process

Acromioclavicular dislocation with a fracture of the coracoid process is not a common injury in adults. The mechanism of injury is essentially the same as for a Type II or III acromioclavicular dislocation, except that the coracoclavicular ligaments do not disrupt and a fracture occurs through the base of the coracoid, allowing a vertical displacement between the clavicle and the acromion. It is very difficult to internally stabilize the fracture of the base of the coracoid (Fig. 12–41). If surgery is indicated, pins across the acro-

mioclavicular joint are indicated (Fig. 12–42). Bernard and associates[47] reported on 4 new cases, only 3 of which were adults (ages 13, 15, 17, 28) and reviewed 13 cases from the literature. They concluded that, although surgery can produce good results, equally satisfactory function and minimal residual deformity could be achieved by immobilization of the shoulder in a sling for six weeks. Smith[382, 383] reported a good result in a single case treated operatively. Lasda and Murray[228] reported a good result in a conservatively treated case in which the coracoid fracture did not heal. Ishizuki and colleagues[198] treated three late cases of a fracture of the superior border of the scapula, fracture of the coracoid, and acromioclavicular dislocation with a Dewar and Barrington procedure with good results. The results of a fourth patient with similar injuries treated acutely with acromioclavicular stabilization were not reported.

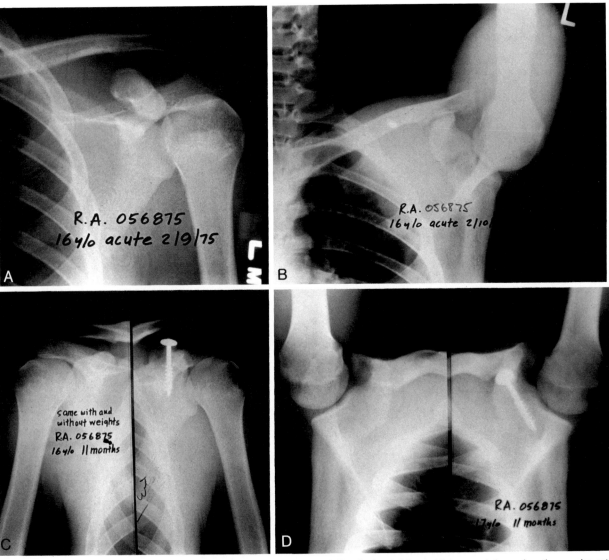

Figure 12–41. Fracture of the base of the coracoid with acromioclavicular joint dislocation. *A,* The distal end of the clavicle is separated away from the acromion, yet the coracoclavicular distance is essentially the same as the normal right shoulder. The appearance of the base of the coracoid is suspicious. *B,* The Stryker notch view reveals the fracture through the base of the coracoid. *C,* Open reduction and fixation of the fractured coracoid was accomplished using a special lag screw. *D,* A Stryker notch view reveals that the fracture of the base of the coracoid has healed.

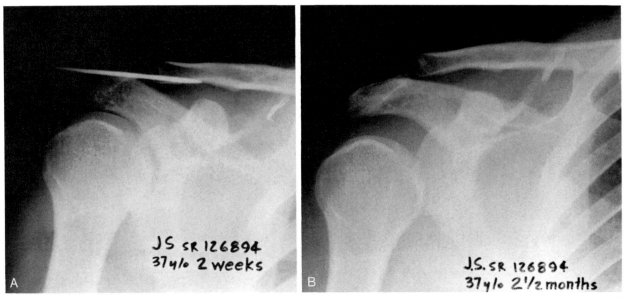

Figure 12–42. Fracture of the base of the coracoid with dislocation of the acromioclavicular joint. *A*, Satisfactory reduction of the acromioclavicular joint and hence the coracoid has been nicely obtained with pins across the acromioclavicular joint. *B*, Two and a half months following surgical repair, the coracoid fracture has healed and there is satisfactory alignment of the acromioclavicular joint.

Comparison Studies of Operative Versus Nonoperative Treatment of Injuries to the Acromioclavicular Joint

Indrekvam and colleagues[194] found an equal incidence of good results in a comparison study but felt operatively treated patients had less pain and could work longer. Park and colleagues[304] found a higher rating in shoulders treated operatively than nonoperatively. Larsen and colleagues[226] prospectively studied 84 patients randomized into operative and nonoperative treatment. They found a much higher complication rate with surgical management and recommended that surgery be considered in the patients with a prominent distal clavicle and in those who do heavy work or frequent overhead work.

Taft and colleagues[395] retrospectively compared 127 patients managed operatively and nonoperatively. They reported only slightly less good results with nonoperative management at an average followup of 9.5 years. The complication rate was significantly higher with operative management. Bakalim and Wilppula[26] concluded that surgical reconstruction of Type III injuries was superior to nonoperative management.

Hawkins[177] and Imatani and coworkers[193] have done comparison studies of operative versus nonoperative treatment and concluded that the nonoperative treatment gives an equal, if not better, end result.

TREATMENT OF TYPE IV AND V INJURIES

Because of the severe posterior displacement of the distal clavicle in a Type IV problem and the gross displacement in the Type V injury, most authors have recommended a surgical repair.[176, 290, 244, 352] Method of treatment of pure posterior dislocations of the clavicle is variable. Hastings and Horne[176] treated three patients. A 16-year-old hockey player with a posterior dislocation of the distal clavicle was treated with a figure-of-eight splint with a good result. A 16-year-old girl with an acute injury was treated with a Simmons screw across the acromioclavicular joint. A 30-year-old man with a chronic 10-year-old injury, weakness, and pain received nonoperative care. Nieminen and Aho[290] treated a 9-week-old posterior dislocation of the clavicle with reconstruction of the coracoclavicular ligaments and the dorsal acromioclavicular ligament, using the palmaris longus augmented with temporary acromioclavicular K-wire fixation. This patient was doing well one year postoperatively.

Malcapi and colleagues[244] and Sondegard-Petersen and Mikkelsen[352] reported an irreducible case which required excision of the distal clavicle but no further surgery, because the coracoclavicular ligaments were intact—stretched, but still intact. In a Type IV problem, the patient is quite symptomatic when the distal end of the clavicle penetrates the trapezius muscle (Fig. 12–43). If it were in an inactive patient and if the clavicle could be manipulated out of the trapezius muscle, a nonoperative approach could be used. However, if the clavicle cannot be manipulated out of the trapezius muscle, then one of the previously described surgical procedures could be performed. In a Type V problem, the deformity is so gross that a surgical repair is usually indicated (see Figs. 12–17, 12–29, and 12–54).

TREATMENT OF TYPE VI INJURY

Of the Type VI injuries described in the literature,[145, 254, 306, 354] all were treated with surgery. Initial attempts

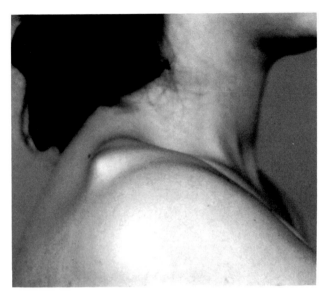

Figure 12–43. Patient with Type IV acromioclavicular joint injury. Note that the distal end of the clavicle is displaced posteriorly back into and through the trapezius muscle. (Courtesy of Louis Bigliani, M.D.)

at closed reduction failed. In one instance following open reduction by lateral retraction of the scapula, the clavicle was stabilized by suturing the deltoid and trapezius muscle avulsion and by repairing the acromioclavicular joint capsule. In one of the patients whose shoulder was operated on at 2.5 months, a Steinmann pin was used to stabilize the acromioclavicular joint. Following immobilization for three to six weeks, the patients had almost full range of motion and good power (Fig. 12–44). One patient with a recurrent subacromial dislocation was treated by an excision of the distal 1.0 cm of the clavicle, and at a five-year follow-up, the patient had no complaints or weakness. Gerber and Rockwood[145] reported using the extra-articular technique with a special coracoclavicular lag screw,* repair of the ligaments, and imbrication of the deltotrapezius fascia over the top of the clavicle.

TREATMENT FOR CHRONIC SYMPTOMATIC ACROMIOCLAVICULAR INJURY

Chronic, symptomatic acromioclavicular dislocation has not been very well discussed in the orthopedic literature, perhaps only in passing in some articles and textbooks. The usual recommended treatment for a chronic unreduced acromioclavicular dislocation is to excise the distal end of the clavicle, which, in the case of a Type III or greater injury, will give the patient more trouble and more symptoms than he or she had before the surgery. The excision of the distal clavicle as reported by Mumford[275] is indicated for a symptomatic Type I or II problem. Saranglia and associates[359]

*Howmedica Manufacturing Company—Special Products Division.

reported good or excellent results in all 19 cases they treated for late acromioclavicular injuries with a modified Cadenat procedure.

Excision of Distal Clavicle

As previously mentioned, the excision of the distal clavicle has been described by Mumford[275] and by Gurd.[166] The simple excision of the distal 1.5 to 2.0 cm of the clavicle is quite successful for chronic Type I and Type II injuries, but as the sole operative treatment, it should not be performed for Type III, IV, V, and VI injuries.

Dynamic Muscle Transfer

In 1965, Dewar and Barrington[114] published their results of a new procedure for chronic complete acromioclavicular dislocations, in which the tip of the coracoid process, along with the muscle attachments of the biceps, coracobrachialis, and a segment of the pectoralis minor tendon is detached and transferred up and fixed with a screw to the undersurface of the clavicle in the vicinity of the old coracoclavicular ligament attachments. This serves as a dynamic muscle transfer to hold the clavicle down. In two of five chronic acromioclavicular dislocations, they accompanied the coracoid transfer with lateral clavicular excision, and in three, they did not mention whether clavicular excision was performed. They recommend a Velpeau dressing after the operation and mobilization of the shoulder starting at four weeks. Bailey[25] reported on a similar procedure in patients with an acute injury to the acromioclavicular joint. Berson and co-workers[48] reported satisfactory results with this type of procedure in acute and chronic injuries to the acromioclavicular joint.

Excision of the Distal Clavicle and Transfer of the Coracoacromial Ligament

Weaver and Dunn[433] managed both acute and chronic injuries with distal clavicle excision and transfer of the coracoacromial ligament to the medullary canal of the clavicle. Boussaton and colleagues[66] performed this procedure on 15 patients with chronic Type II and III injuries with 80 per cent good or excellent and 20 per cent poor results. Burton[80] and Copeland and Kessel[95] have described a similar technique. Shoji and associates[374] modified the technique by harvesting the coracoacromial ligament with a bone block from the acromion transferred into the medullary canal of the clavicle and were pleased with their results in three patients. However, Larsen and Petersen[227] were unhappy with transfers of the coracoclavicular ligament with a bone block to the superior surface of the clavicle, because 50 per cent of their patients had complaints where the flake of bone was attached onto the clavicle. Rockwood, Guy, and Griffin[342] reported on 25 patients with chronic, symptomatic acromioclavicular Type III

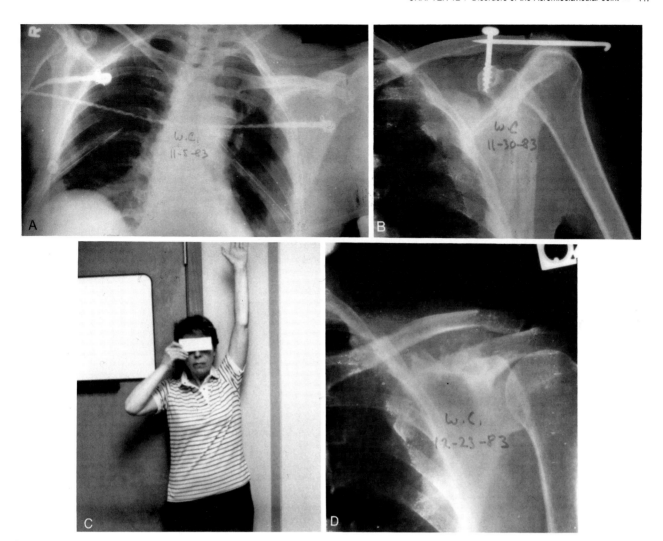

Figure 12–44. Type VI acromioclavicular dislocation. *A,* The distal end of the left clavicle is in the subcoracoid position. *B,* The injury was managed by open reduction and internal fixation with a coracoclavicular lag screw and pins across the acromioclavicular joint. *C,* Following the surgery, the patient had essentially a full range of motion of the left shoulder. *D,* X-ray 20 months after injury demonstrates an almost complete bar of bone between the coracoid and the clavicle. (Courtesy of Robert C. Erickson II, M.D.)

dislocations. They transferred the coracoacromial ligament using Cadenat's procedure and stabilized the clavicle to the coracoid with a lag screw for 12 weeks while the transferred ligament healed (Fig. 12–45).

Reconstruction of the Acromioclavicular or the Coracoclavicular Ligaments

Some authors have recommended reconstructions of the acromioclavicular joint which do not involve the excision of the distal clavicle. Zaricznyj[446] reconstructed the coracoclavicular and the superior acromioclavicular ligaments with tendon grafts. He used either the extensor tendon of the fifth toe or the palmaris longus. He supplemented his repair with temporary Kirschner wire acromioclavicular fixation and found that 15 of 16 patients were pain free an average of 5.1 years postoperatively. Bednarek and colleagues[42] treated 35 patients with injuries older than 2 weeks with reconstruction of both the coracoclavicular and acromioclavicular ligaments, using an intricate loop of thick fishing line in a Bunnell[77] fashion. All of his

patients were satisfied with their results. Fleming and colleagues[134] used a woven Dacron arterial loop in five patients with 80 per cent good results, although one patient with a good result required distal clavicle excision.

Miscellaneous Reconstructions

Dannohl[106] advised midclavicular osteotomy with plate fixation for the osteotomy and acromioclavicular fixation with Kirschner wires and a tension band wire.

Authors' Preferred Method of Treatment of Injuries

TYPE I INJURY

We recommend the use of an ice bag for the first 12 hours whenever it is convenient and give the patient a

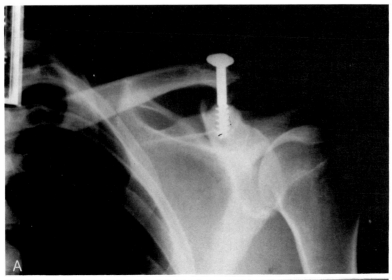

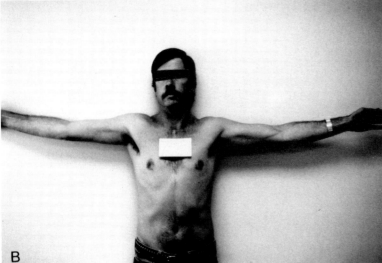

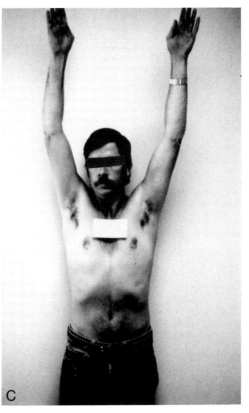

Figure 12–45. Reconstruction of chronic Type III injury of the left acromioclavicular joint. *A,* The coracoacromial ligament has been transferred into the medullary canal of the distal clavicle. A special coracoclavicular lag screw was inserted to temporarily suspend the upper extremity from the clavicle while the transferred ligament was healing. *B, C,* The patient had essentially a full range of motion with the screw in place. The screw was removed at 12 weeks.

sling to support the arm and to remind him and others that something is wrong with the shoulder. We encourage the patient to rest the shoulder but to gently maintain a normal range of motion. Usually, by seven days, the symptoms have subsided. Heavy stresses, lifting, and contact sports should be delayed until there is a full range of motion and no pain to joint palpation. This usually takes two weeks.

TYPE II INJURY

As in a Type I injury, rest is an important factor. Ice bags are used during the first 12 hours, followed by moist heat for 12 hours. The patient is given a sling to rest and support the arm. The sling is worn for one to two weeks, depending on the age of the patient, the symptoms, and the circumstances. We encourage the patient to begin gentle range-of-motion exercises of the shoulder and allow him to use the arm for dressing, eating, and necessary everyday living activities when

symptoms permit, which is usually about the seventh day. The average patient is instructed not to use the shoulder for any heavy lifting, pushing, pulling, or contact sports for at least six weeks. We do not want the patient to have another injury or stress the acromioclavicular joint and convert a Type II problem into a Type III problem.

For the average patient who only occasionally puts stress on the acromioclavicular joint, development of chronic problems are rare and usually can be resolved with anti-inflammatory drugs, moist heat, and maybe one or two injections of steroids into the joint. However, if the patient stresses the shoulder all day with heavy labor (i.e., pushes a wheelbarrow, swings a sledge hammer, does a lot of digging), chronic pain can develop in the acromioclavicular joint secondary to traumatic arthritis. If conservative measures fail, an arthroplasty may be required. Excision of the distal clavicle should not be skimpy, for the senior author has seen patients who, after excision of 1.0 cm of the distal clavicle, have continued to have pain in the joint

(Fig. 12–46). Films taken with the arm at the side revealed a clear acromioclavicular joint, but with an x-ray taken at 90 degrees of abduction, there was impingement of the clavicle into the acromion process. As a general rule, the senior author recommends the excision of a minimum of 2.0 to 2.5 cm of the distal clavicle. The excision of this much clavicle removes most of the trapezoid part of the coracoclavicular ligament, but as long as the conoid ligament remains, the distal clavicle will have a secure anchor to the coracoid process.

After the operation, the arm is carried in a sling until the sutures are removed; then the patient is instructed in pendulum exercises, followed by range-of-motion exercises, and finally, strengthening exercises. Laborers and athletes in contact sports usually can return to their activities after 8 to 10 weeks.

TYPE III ACUTE INJURY

Philosophy of Treatment

Our aim is either to restore the anatomy through an operative procedure or to put the arm into a sling for a few days and gradually allow the patient to begin functional use of the shoulder. We do not use casts, braces, or harnesses, nor do we use adhesive taping or strapping, which has the general tendency to irritate or ulcerate the tender skin on the top of the shoulder (Fig. 12–47). Some authors refer to these methods of care as conservative treatment, while others, including the authors, would call them radical forms of treatment. It seems unreasonable and impractical to immobilize the shoulder and upper extremity in a young, active person for the required six to eight weeks.

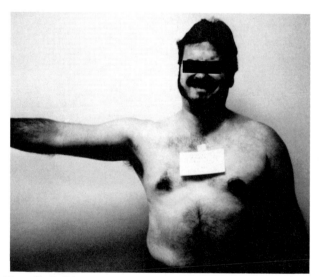

Figure 12–46. This patient with degenerative arthritis in the right shoulder had the distal 1.0 cm of the clavicle resected. Four months postoperatively he noted increasing pain with abduction. X-rays confirmed that during the abduction, the distal end of the clavicle again jammed into the acromion process, causing significant pain.

However, we do admire the physicians and patients who have the tenacity to achieve a good result with the various shoulder harness devices. The decision-making comes in when we have to determine whether we will use an operative repair or a nonoperative approach. We basically believe that, in a person who does heavy labor and in certain young people under the ages of 20 to 25 who have not made up their minds for their future plans for work or sports, a surgical repair should be performed. We also apply this philosophy to active older patients. We recall a cowboy from one of the large, south Texas ranches who was age 65 but who looked about 45. He worked 12 to 14 hours a day, rode horses, dug post holes, repaired fences, worked cattle, roped and threw calves, and truly demanded a strong, dominant functional shoulder all day long. He had a successful operative repair and returned to his usual job on the ranch. An exception to the rule for surgical repair in a young athlete would be in the case of a person who regularly subjects his shoulder to violent, repeated, and unprotected trauma (e.g., soccer and rugby players). There would be no sense to repair the injury only to have it recur a few months later when the patient again falls on the point of the shoulder. We prefer to repair the acutely injured Type III injury in many athletes, because we believe it will give a stronger shoulder that will stand up under repetitive stresses and heavy loads.

Nonoperative Treatment

We recommend a skillful neglect form of treatment for Type I, II, and III injuries for inactive, nonlaboring patients such as those who have only a mild interest in recreational activities, especially when the injury occurs in the nondominant shoulder (Fig. 12–48). If Type IV and VI injuries are seen early, we would recommend an attempted closed reduction to dislodge the clavicle from the trapezius muscle or from under the coracoid process. If this were successful, we would then apply the same indication as above for a Type III problem. If the reduction failed, an operative reduction and repair would be performed. Type IV, V, and VI injuries most likely will be treated with an operative repair.

If nonoperative treatment is to be used, we first explain the injury in detail to the patient by describing the ruptured ligaments and why there is the "bump" on the shoulder. We explain that, although surgery can correct the problem, he or she can, without the risks of surgery and anesthesia, end up with a very good functional shoulder. The shoulder is placed into a sling, and then during the first 12 hours or so, an ice bag is applied to decrease the discomfort. We may give the patient some mild analgesics and tell him or her that for the first three to four days the arm can be used for everyday living activities. Usually within seven days, a functional range of motion is achieved, and by two to three weeks, the patient has a full range of motion and little, if any, discomfort (see Fig. 12–48).

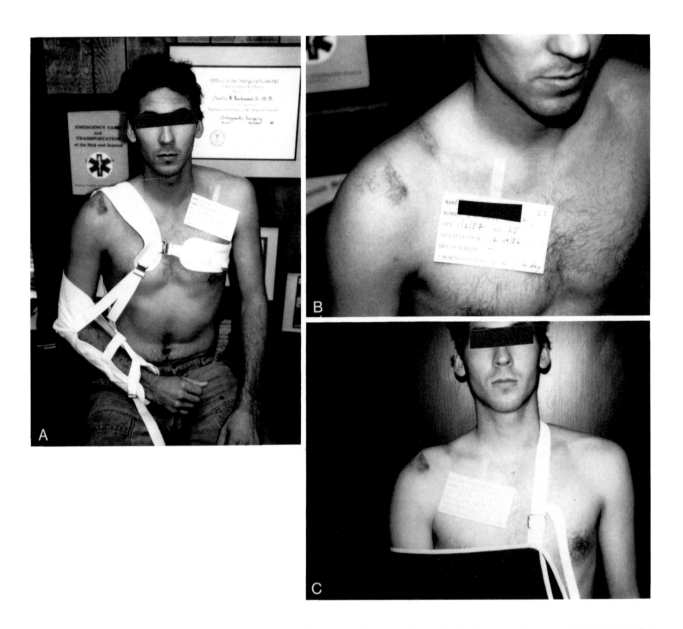

Figure 12–47. The continuous pressure of the strap over the top of the shoulder, which is attempting to depress the clavicle, in many instances will cause skin breakdown. *A,* This patient had been in a shoulder strap harness for a Type III acromioclavicular dislocation for four days, and said that the burning pain in the top of his shoulder was excessive. *B,* With the device removed, the skin breakdown on the top of his shoulder was obvious. *C,* The patient was not involved in any type of heavy-duty labor activities; he was simply placed into a sling and told he could remove the sling and begin to use the arm for everyday living activities whenever the shoulder felt comfortable.

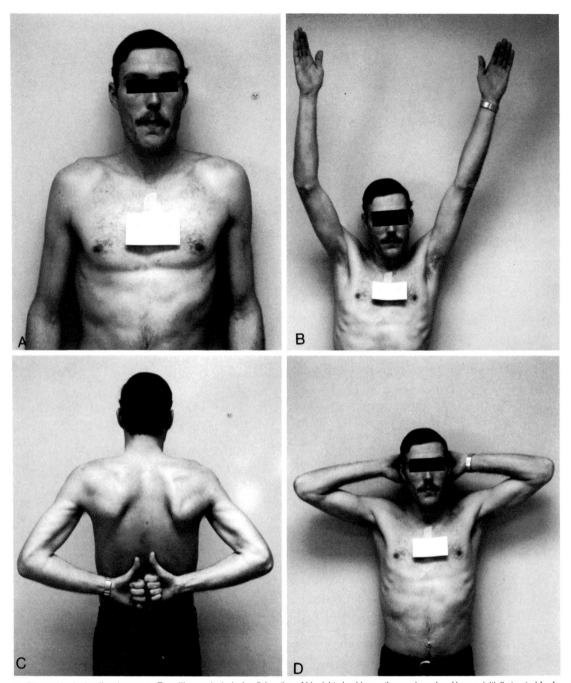

Figure 12–48. This patient had suffered an acute Type III acromioclavicular dislocation of his right shoulder on the previous day. He was initially treated for four days in a sling and then allowed to use the arm for everyday living activities. He still has a bump over the top of the right shoulder; however, he has a full range of motion and essentially no pain. He is not involved in heavy physical labor. (Reproduced with permission from Rockwood CA, and Green DP (eds): Fractures (3 vols) 2nd ed. Philadelphia: JB Lippincott, 1984.)

It really is amazing to see how fast the symptoms disappear and how fast the range of motion returns following an untreated Type III acromioclavicular joint dislocation. These patients are quite pleased with their end results and usually do not complain about the subsequent bump on the shoulder. However, if the patient changes jobs and has to put heavy stress on the acromioclavicular joint, he will begin to complain of a fatiguing, dull ache in the shoulder after four to six hours of heavy work. This may require that a reconstructive procedure be done.

Operative Treatment

As described above, the operative procedure is used primarily in people who perform heavy labor and who daily place stress on their shoulders, in athletes, and in certain young patients under the ages of 20 to 25 who have not made up their minds as to their future careers. The operative technique that the senior author has used for the past 27 years was learned from Dr. James Amspacher during the author's residency at the University of Oklahoma Medical Center. The operation currently encompasses the best ideas and qualities of several operative procedures. The acromioclavicular joint is explored and debrided, the coracoclavicular ligaments are reapproximated, and the vertical and horizontal stability of the acromioclavicular joint is restored through the use of temporary extra-articular screw fixation between the clavicle and the coracoid. The deltoid and trapezius muscles are imbricated and repaired back to the clavicle.

Preoperative Preparation

A small pad and a 10-inch × 12-inch x-ray cassette are placed under the patient's shoulder. The patient is put in the beach chair position on the operating room table. A special headrest is used so that the top of the patient's shoulder is completely free at the top of the corner of the table. The head should be slightly deviated toward the normal shoulder and stabilized to the headrest so that there is complete access to the superior aspect of the shoulder. The anesthesiologist and his or her equipment should be moved over toward the opposite shoulder so that the surgeon or an assistant can stand at the top of the table. Care must be taken during draping to allow access from the top of the shoulder over to the base of the neck.

Skin Incision

The strap-like incision is made in Langer's lines and is approximately 3 inches in length. It begins 1 inch posterior to the clavicle and then crosses the clavicle 1 inch medial to the acromioclavicular joint. It then extends downward to a point medial to the tip of the coracoid process (Fig. 12–49A). The incision is then undermined so that the acromioclavicular joint, the distal 2 inches of the clavicle, and the anterior deltoid can be visualized. This usually requires a coronal split or at least the completion of the coronal split in the deltotrapezius fascia and periosteum on the superior distal 2 inches of the clavicle.

The Anterior Deltoid

In some instances, the deltoid and trapezius muscle fasciae have been, as a result of the injury, stripped off the distal 2 or 3 inches of the clavicle. If not, this interval must be divided so that the clavicle can be grasped with a clamp and lifted upward, while the deltoid muscle is retracted anteriorly and distally to visualize the torn ends of the coracoclavicular ligament and the base of the coracoid process. If the deltoid has been stripped off the clavicle with an intact periosteal tube, it will be necessary to split the deltoid down 2 inches in line with its fibers and sometimes to detach the distal 2 inches from its insertion into the clavicle. This then will allow exposure of the coracoclavicular ligaments and the base of the coracoid process (Fig. 12–49B).

The Acromioclavicular Joint

The distal end of the clavicle is grasped with a towel clip, Lewin clamp, or a bone hook and lifted upward so that the acromioclavicular joint can be thoroughly debrided of the intra-articular disc and any loose frays and tags of the acromioclavicular ligament (Fig. 12–49B).

Reapproximation of the Coracoclavicular Ligaments

The torn ends of the ligament are freed up and tagged with two or three No. 1 cottony Dacron sutures. The sutures are not tied at this time (see Fig. 12–49B). This step is important to allow a reapproximation of the ligament ends after the screw is in its position of reducing the coracoclavicular space. This reapproximation is not like a nice 90 to 90 degree stitch that one uses in the repair of a lacerated tendon in the hand, but the stitches are secure enough so that when they are tied, they do reapproximate the torn ends of the ligament. Some authors do not believe that this step is important, because with the internal fixation, the whole area fills in with a "dense scar" that secures the distal clavicle down to the coracoid. However, we do not believe that this scar will give a consistent, good result. Although most coracoclavicular ligaments disrupt in the waist or in the middle of the ligament, we have noted at surgery that, on many occasions, the coracoclavicular ligament has been stripped off the coracoid and found lying parallel to and plastered underneath the clavicle, or it has pulled loose from the clavicle and then curled up in a ball down on the base of the coracoid. The coracoclavicular ligament is a dense, heavy, strong ligament almost the size of the small finger. It has a very definite purpose in the shoulder—to support the scapula and the upper extremity from the clavicle. If one is going to take the time and effort to operate on this joint, one might as well spend a few more minutes to expose the ends of the ligaments and reapproximate them with a few sutures, as opposed to depending on unreliable scar tissue to do the work.

Temporary Internal Fixation

With the superior surface of the clavicle exposed and the base of the coracoid visualized and palpated, the screw should ideally be placed vertically through the clavicle and then should penetrate both cortices of the *base of the coracoid*. The location of the drill hole in the clavicle is usually more medial to the acromioclavicular joint than one thinks, because the *base of the coracoid* is more medial than one thinks. Usually, the drill hole in the clavicle should be placed at least

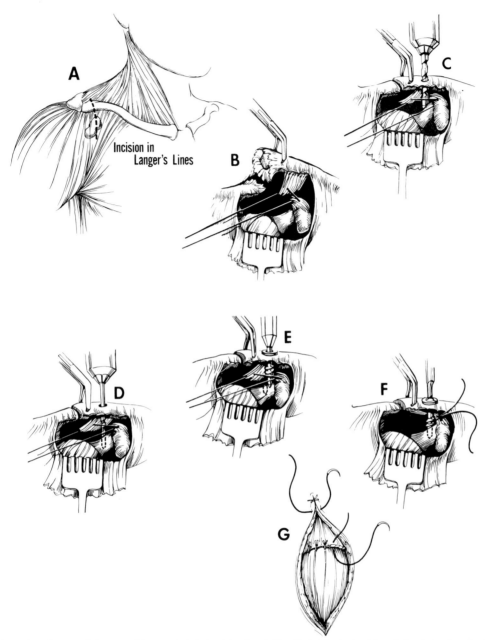

Figure 12–49. The senior author's repair for a complete acromioclavicular dislocation. *A,* The skin incision is about three inches in length and extends from the posterior edge of the clavicle, one inch medial to the acromioclavicular joint and then down in Langer's lines to a point just medial to the tip of the coracoid process. *B,* The deltoid secondary to the injury is usually subperiosteally stripped away from the distal clavicle. It may have to be surgically detached to aid in identification and reapproximation to the coracoclavicular ligaments and the base of the coracoid process. The distal end of the clavicle can be lifted up with a towel clip or a bone hook to aid in the placement of the sutures in the coracoclavicular ligament. The acromioclavicular joint is thoroughly debrided of the meniscus. If the acromioclavicular ligaments are amenable to repair, they are preserved and later repaired. *C,* The distal end of the clavicle is held reduced adjacent to the acromion with a towel clip. A ³⁄₁₆-inch drill bit is used to make a hole in the clavicle directly above the base of the coracoid. *D,* Through the ³⁄₁₆-inch hole in the clavicle, a ⁹⁄₆₄-inch drill bit is used to create a hole through both cortices of the base of the coracoid. *E,* The specially designed lag screw of appropriate length is then placed through the clavicle until the smooth shank of the screw is in the clavicle. The nonthreaded nipple end of the screw is then passed into the hole of the coracoid, and the screw is tightened home to depress the clavicle down to the level of the acromion. The stay sutures in the coracoclavicular ligaments are then tied and the screw tightened another half-turn to take any tension off the reapproximated ligaments. *G,* The muscle attachments of the deltoid and trapezius are carefully repaired and, if possible, are imbricated over the top of the clavicle and the acromioclavicular joint.

1½ inches medial to the distal end of the clavicle (Fig. 12–49C). While the clavicle is held reduced to the acromion, a ³⁄₁₆-inch hole is made through the distal clavicle, directly above the base of the coracoid. Next, a ⁹⁄₆₄-inch drill bit is then placed through the drill hole in the clavicle, and under direct vision by retracting the deltoid out of the way or by palpation, the hole is placed into and through both cortices of the *base of the coracoid* (Fig. 12–49D). Then, with the acromioclavicular joint still held reduced, the specially developed lag screw is inserted through the clavicle down into the coracoid. The screw that we are currently using for adult repairs is a modified Bosworth screw* (Fig. 12–50).

The screw developed by Bosworth is a 6.5 mm long-thread cancellous lag screw that comes in various lengths. It has a rather large head that keeps it from pulling through the clavicle but also prevents it from being used with a self-retaining screwdriver. It has a smooth shank and large built-up grooved threads. The tip end of the screw is quite rounded, and unless the screw hole in the coracoid is exactly perfect, the tip of the screw tends to skid medially or laterally off the coracoid. Without the screw attached to a self-retaining screwdriver, one does not have much control on the tip of the screw. For that reason, the senior author has modified the Bosworth screw by developing a screw with a regular size head that can be used with a standard self-retaining screwdriver. A washer is used to take the place of the large head of the original Bosworth screw. To avoid the problem of the rounded

tip end of the Bosworth screw sliding off the coracoid, the tip of the screw has been modified by creating a nonthreaded, nipple-like prominence on the distal end of the screw that is used like a probe to find the hole in the coracoid (see Fig. 12–49E). Even with these modifications, there still can be some aggravation if the screw holes in the clavicle and coracoid are not lined up in proper position.

A depth gauge determines the length of the screw to be used. Care must be taken to ensure that the screw engages both cortices of the coracoid. The screw is introduced through the clavicle; once the smooth part of the shank of the screw is in the clavicle, one then has some leeway to guide the smooth distal tip of the screw into the hole into the coracoid (see Fig. 12–49F). Before the final steps of repair are taken, an x-ray is taken using the preoperatively positioned cassette under the shoulder to be sure that the screw is properly in the coracoid (Fig. 12–51). When the screw is placed into the hole in the coracoid under direct vision, it is unlikely that the x-ray will reveal a misdirected screw. However, when the screw is inserted by palpation or blind technique, it is possible for the screw to skid off medially or laterally and be surprisingly stable because of the purchase of the heavy threads along the side of the coracoid.

As the screw is tightened, the clavicle is gradually reduced down to the level of the upper border of the acromion. At this point, the tagged sutures in the coracoclavicular ligaments are tied, and then another half turn is applied to the screw, which takes any tension off the sutures (Fig. 12–49F). The primary purpose of the screw is to temporarily hold the clavicle reduced vertically and horizontally to the scapula and to take tension off the coracoclavicular ligament reap-

---

*The screw is produced by the Special Products Division of Howmedica Manufacturing Company.

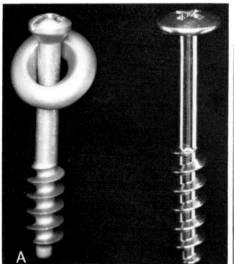
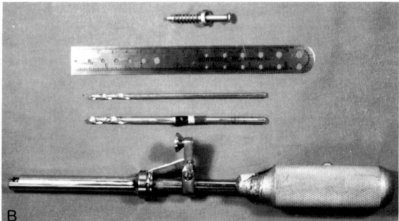

Figure 12–50. *A,* Comparison of the modified coracoclavicular lag screw with the original Bosworth screw. The large head of the original screw made it impossible to use the self-retaining screwdriver. Furthermore, the threads extended all the way down to the tip of the screw, making it difficult for the surgeon to place the screw into the hole in the base of the coracoid. The modified screw, which has a washer in place of the large head, can be used with a self-retaining screwdriver. The distal ¼ inch of the screw, which has no threads and is smooth-tipped, is used to seek out the hole in the base of the coracoid. *B,* Photograph of the type of self-retaining screwdriver that the senior author uses along with ³⁄₁₆- and ⁹⁄₁₆-inch drill bits. (Reproduced with permission from Rockwood CA, and Green DP (eds): Fractures (3 vols), 2nd ed. Philadelphia: JB Lippincott, 1984.)

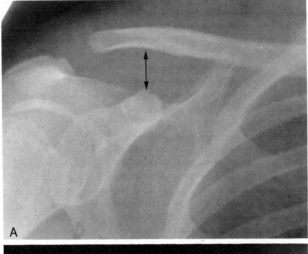
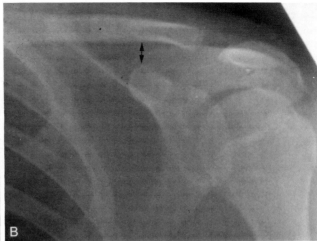
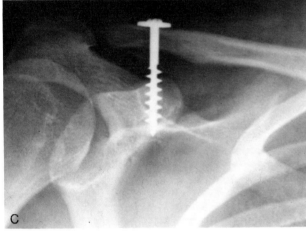

Figure 12–51. Use of the modified coracoclavicular lag screw. *A*, Anteroposterior stress x-ray of the right shoulder in a patient with a Type III acromioclavicular dislocation. *B*, A stress film of the normal left shoulder, revealing it to be normal. *C*, Postoperative x-ray showing the acromioclavicular joint reduced and held temporarily in place with a special modified coracoclavicular lag screw. (Reproduced with permission from Rockwood CA, and Green DP (eds): Fractures (3 vols), 2nd ed. Philadelphia: JB Lippincott, 1984.)

proximation until the coracoclavicular ligaments have healed.

Repair and Imbrication of the Deltotrapezius Muscle Fascia

The deltotrapezius muscle fascia interval must be repaired back to the clavicle. Not only should this be repaired, but also, if possible, the deltotrapezius fascia should be double-breasted or imbricated over the top of the clavicle to help support the shoulder and the repair (Fig. 12–49*G*).

Postoperative Care

Postoperatively, the arm is supported in a sling for one to two weeks, but the patient is allowed to use the arm for some gentle daily living activities, such as brushing teeth, eating, and bathroom care. After one to two weeks, the sling is discontinued, and the patient can use the arm for most everyday living activities but is cautioned to avoid any lifting, pushing, and pulling for the next six weeks. Ordinarily, by three weeks and certainly by six weeks from surgery, the patient has a very functional range of motion, i.e., up to 150 to 160 degrees of flexion and abduction without significant

discomfort (Fig. 12–52). The screw is routinely removed at six to eight weeks after surgery under local anesthesia. To aid in the screw removal, a small scratch is made with a 26-gauge hypodermic needle on the skin over the top of the shoulder where you think the screw head is located. This is usually 2 inches medial to the skin incision. Next, a small coin is then taped directly over the scratch mark, and an anteroposterior x-ray is made of the shoulder (Fig. 12–53). The location of the coin on the x-ray, as compared with the scratch mark on the skin, will reveal whether the stab wound was placed in the correct location or whether it needs to be moved medially or laterally to the scratch mark. Following screw removal, the patient is instructed not to perform any heavy lifting, pushing, pulling, or contact sports for 10 to 12 weeks from the initial operative repair. Athletes are not permitted to return to contact sports or undue stress until 12 weeks postoperatively, and only after they have recovered full strength of the shoulder and a full range of motion.

TYPE IV, V, AND VI INJURIES

In these three types of injuries, surgery is advised because the distal clavicle is so far displaced. However,

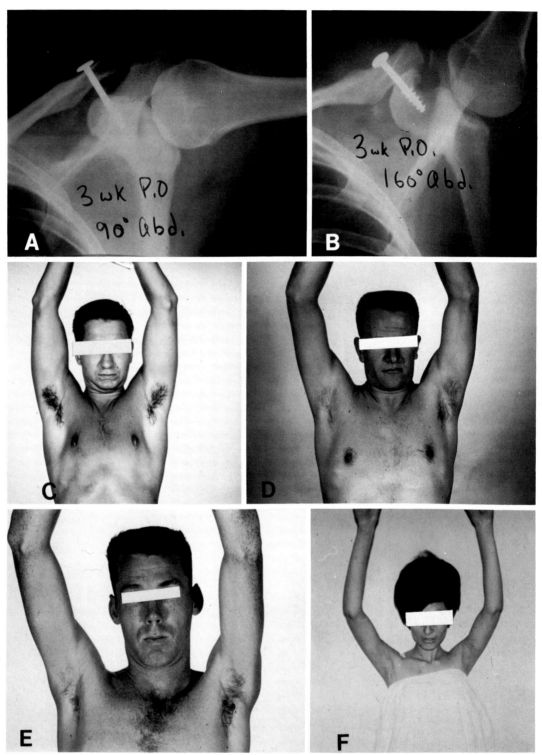

Figure 12–52. A functional range of motion can be attained with the coracoclavicular screw in place. *A* and *B*, Note that the x-ray demonstrates 160 degrees of elevation three weeks after surgery. A very functional range of motion is seen in patients with the screw in place *(C–F)*. (Reproduced with permission from Rockwood CA, and Green DP (eds): Fractures (3 vols), 2nd ed. Philadelphia: JB Lippincott, 1984.)

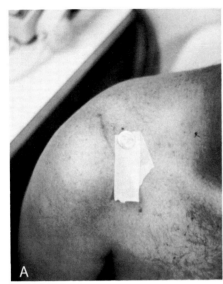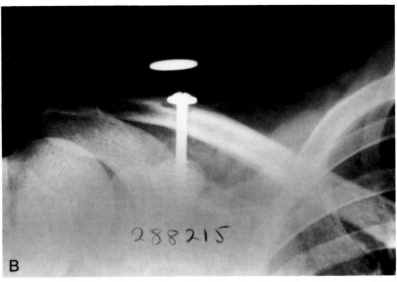

Figure 12–53. The screw is usually removed at six weeks after surgery using local anesthesia. A small scratch mark is made on the skin over the top of the shoulder at the approximate location of the head of the screw. A coin is taped over the top of the scratch. An x-ray is then taken to determine the relationship of the scratch mark to the head of the screw. (Reproduced with permission from Rockwood CA, and Green DP (eds): Fractures (3 vols), 2nd ed. Philadelphia: JB Lippincott, 1984.)

if, in a Type IV or VI injury under general anesthesia, the distal clavicle could be disengaged from the trapezius muscle or reduced from under the coracoid process, and if it was in an inactive, nonlaboring person, we would then treat the problem with the nonoperative skillful neglect method. If the patient were young or a laborer, we would surgically repair the problem as described for a Type III injury (see Fig. 12–51). Most of the patients with a Type V injury whom we have treated have had so much pain and cosmetic deformity that surgery was almost mandatory (Fig. 12–54). Patients with a Type VI injury have been treated with surgical correction (Fig. 12–55).[145]

AUTHORS' COMMENTS ON OTHER OPERATIVE PROCEDURES

Intra-articular Acromioclavicular Joint Fixation

We do not use intra-articular fixation unless there is a complete, symptomatic acromioclavicular dislocation that is associated with a fracture of the base of the coracoid. We prefer not to place two or more pins or a single large pin across this small joint, because the pins can produce traumatic degenerative changes in the joint. The pins also have a great tendency to migrate to another place. Another reason acromioclavicular pins are not used is that to be able to remove them at a later date, they must protrude from the lateral edge of the acromion. This irritates the deltoid muscle during movements of the shoulder.

Extra-articular Fixation

The use of fascia, suture, tape, vascular synthetic grafts, and other materials that pass under the coracoid and over or through the clavicle may be easier to apply

than the coracoclavicular lag screw. However, because the waist of the coracoid process is anterior to the base of the coracoid, the tightened loop of suture tends to displace the clavicle anteriorly away from the acromion. In other words, the loop of material reduces the vertical separation of the clavicle to the level of the acromion, but it does not restore the horizontal displacement of the acromioclavicular joint. Furthermore, if the loop of material is passed over the top of the clavicle, it may erode through the clavicle and produce a fracture (see Fig. 12–39). The coracoclavicular lag screw reduces the acromioclavicular joint in the vertical and horizontal planes, does not significantly interfere with clavicular rotation, and does allow the early restoration of shoulder motion.

Dynamic Muscle Transfers

The use of this technique for an acute injury seems to be bypassing the primary site of injury. Its purpose is to dynamically pull the clavicle *down*, through the pull of the coracobrachialis and the biceps muscles. However, the problem is *not* a high-riding clavicle, but a low hanging upper extremity. It is a major procedure and appears to have more risks than are necessary, i.e., injury to the musculocutaneous nerve, failure of the coracoid to heal to the clavicle, or loss of screw fixation or screw breakage.

Primary Excision of the Distal Clavicle

Of all the various operative procedures described for an acute injury to the acromioclavicular joint, primary excision of the distal clavicle seems to be the most unreasonable. If the distal clavicle is found to be fractured or the acromioclavicular joint is arthritic, a primary excision seems indicated. However, the clavi-

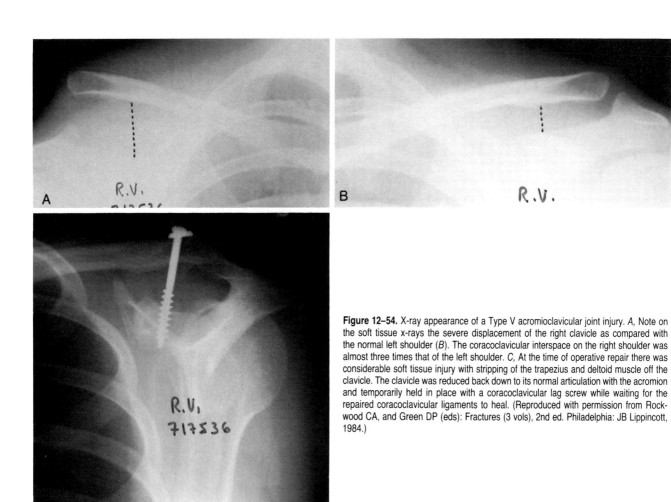

Figure 12–54. X-ray appearance of a Type V acromioclavicular joint injury. *A,* Note on the soft tissue x-rays the severe displacement of the right clavicle as compared with the normal left shoulder (*B*). The coracoclavicular interspace on the right shoulder was almost three times that of the left shoulder. *C,* At the time of operative repair there was considerable soft tissue injury with stripping of the trapezius and deltoid muscle off the clavicle. The clavicle was reduced back down to its normal articulation with the acromion and temporarily held in place with a coracoclavicular lag screw while waiting for the repaired coracoclavicular ligaments to heal. (Reproduced with permission from Rockwood CA, and Green DP (eds): Fractures (3 vols), 2nd ed. Philadelphia: JB Lippincott, 1984.)

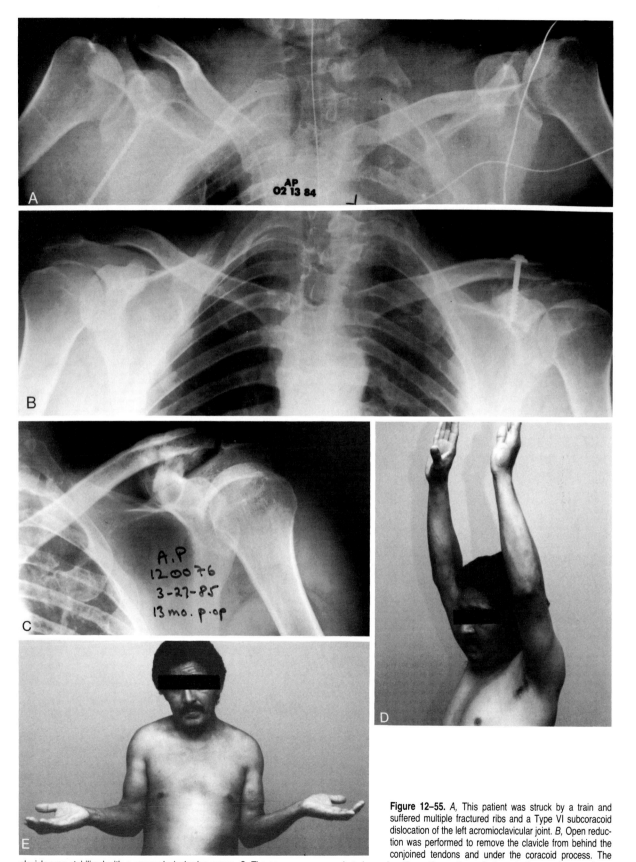

Figure 12–55. *A,* This patient was struck by a train and suffered multiple fractured ribs and a Type VI subcoracoid dislocation of the left acromioclavicular joint. *B,* Open reduction was performed to remove the clavicle from behind the conjoined tendons and under the coracoid process. The clavicle was stabilized with a coracoclavicular lag screw. *C,* The screw was removed at six weeks; 13 months postoperatively, note the massive new bone formation in the coracoclavicular ligaments. *D* and *E,* Despite the ossification between the clavicle and the coracoid, the patient demonstrated essentially a full range of motion compared with the normal right shoulder. He returned to his job as a laborer.

cle, through its articulation at the acromioclavicular joint, is important and should not be indiscriminately discarded.

AUTHORS' TREATMENT OF CHRONIC PROBLEMS OF THE ACROMIOCLAVICULAR JOINT

We are in agreement with other authors that the excision of the distal clavicle for a degenerated joint in a patient with an old, chronic Type II injury is appropriate. We recommend the excision of a minimum of 2.0 cm of the distal clavicle. Authors have recommended an excision of one-eighth, one-fourth, or one-half of the distal clavicle, and we do not think that is sufficient. With the excision of only one-quarter inch of the distal clavicle and with time, the distal clavicle may develop a spur; and with abduction, that spur again butts against the acromion, producing symp-

toms and pain just as before the operation (see Fig. 12–46). In many instances, the senior author has re-excised the distal clavicle because of the recurrence of symptoms. Excision of the distal 2.0 cm of the distal clavicle essentially removes that part of the clavicle that is attached to the coracoid by the trapezoid ligament. The remaining conoid ligament is sufficient to anchor the distal clavicle down to the coracoid process.

It is inappropriate to excise only the distal clavicle, even if it is 2.0 cm, in a chronic, symptomatic Type III, IV, V, or VI problem and expect to relieve the patient's symptoms. All that really does is take a displaced *long* clavicle and convert it into a displaced *short* clavicle, which will actually increase the patient's symptoms (Fig. 12–56). The remaining stump of the distal clavicle, without any attachment to the coracoid, is hypermobile, and thus tends to irritate the soft tissues about the shoulder and the base of the neck. Therefore,

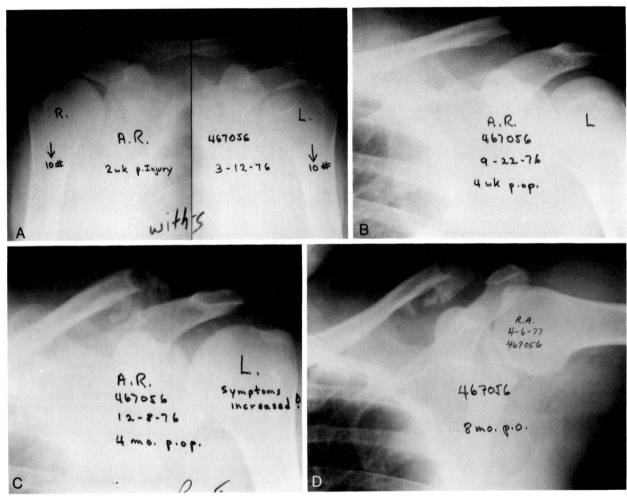

Figure 12–56. Complications of excising the distal end of the clavicle in a patient with an old, chronic Type III acromioclavicular dislocation. *A,* X-rays comparing the right shoulder with the injured left shoulder. *B,* Six months later, because of continued discomfort, the distal 2.5 cm of the clavicle was resected. The surgeon did not recognize that this was a Type III injury with loss of the coracoclavicular ligaments. Four weeks following surgery, the patient was noting increasing pain. Calcification is beginning to develop around the distal clavicle. *C,* Four months following the resection of the distal clavicle, the patient was more symptomatic and had more soft tissue calcification; there was greater disparity between the clavicle and the coracoid process. *D,* Eight months following surgery, the patient continued to have pain. (Reproduced with permission from Rockwood CA, and Green DP (eds): Fractures (3 vols), 2nd ed. Philadelphia: JB Lippincott, 1984.)

we strongly urge you to determine the status of the coracoclavicular ligaments before a simple excising of the distal clavicle.

If it is determined that the clavicle has lost its attachment to the coracoid (i.e., a chronic Type III, IV, V, or VI injury), a new coracoclavicular ligament must be constructed. Although fascia, suture, vascular grafts, and other materials can be used, we prefer to use the coracoacromial ligament, which already has an attachment on the base of the coracoid process, to replace the coracoclavicular ligament *and* to temporarily support the reconstruction with the senior author's special coracoclavicular lag screw. In a patient with a chronic dislocation, the use of the coracoacromial ligament alone is insufficient to maintain the reduction. In coracoclavicular reconstruction in a large, strong patient, the senior author has seen so much tension on the reconstruction that it caused the screw to bend (Fig. 12–57). The screw temporarily takes the tension off the deforming forces while the new ligament is healing in the clavicle. As mentioned, we prefer to use a structure that is already attached to the coracoid and, at the same time, get rid of a structure that could, in the future, produce an impingement syndrome in the shoulder. The coracoacromial ligament is attached to the base of the coracoid, adjacent to the site of the old coracoclavicular ligament, and is an ideal ligament

for the reconstruction and certainly could be involved in an impingement syndrome.

If, at the time of reconstruction, the coracoacromial ligament is absent or unsuitable, we then use the screw and either 1.0 mm or 3.0 mm cottony Dacron suture or a strip of conjoined tendons between the coracoid and the clavicle.

AUTHORS' METHOD FOR RECONSTRUCTING A CHRONIC COMPLETE ACROMIOCLAVICULAR DISLOCATION

The skin incision and much of the surgical approach is the same as described for an acute repair of a Type III injury (Fig. 12–58A). The distal 2.0 cm of the distal clavicle is excised. If a previous surgical procedure has removed part of the distal clavicle, enough more of the clavicle is removed so that the stump of the clavicle is located just above and at the lateral edge of the base of the coracoid (Fig. 12–58B). The medullary canal of the distal clavicle is then drilled and curetted to be able to receive the transferred coracoacromial ligament (Fig. 12–58C).

A No. 15 knife blade is used to carefully remove all of the acromial attachment of the coracoacromial ligament from the acromion (Fig. 12–58D,E). A small

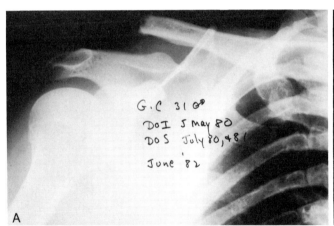

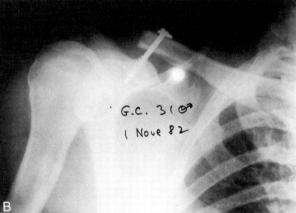

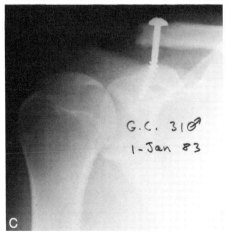

Figure 12–57. Complications of resecting the distal clavicle without reconstruction of the coracoclavicular ligament. *A,* Two years following injury and after two resections of the distal clavicle, the patient had continued pain and discomfort in the right shoulder. *B,* The superiorly and posteriorly displaced clavicle was reduced back to its normal position above the base of the coracoid with great effort. The clavicle was held reduced with a coracoclavicular lag screw, and the coracoacromial ligament was transferred into the medullary canal as described by Cadenat. At two months from surgery, the screw was removed under local anesthesia. The screw was bent because of the tremendous strain across the coracoclavicular interspace.

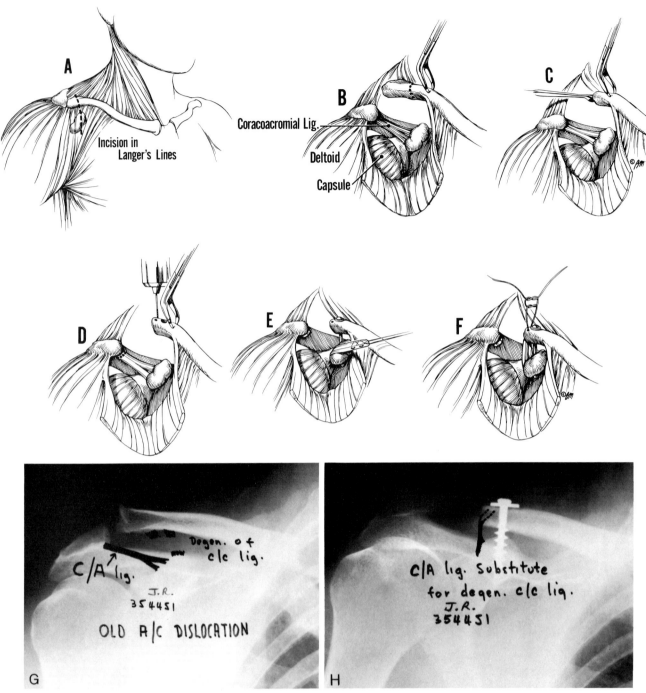

Figure 12–58. The senior author's method to reconstruct a chronic Type III, IV, V, or VI acromioclavicular dislocation. *A,* The incision is made in Langer's lines. *B,* The distal end of the clavicle is excised. *C,* The medullary canal is drilled out and curetted to receive the transferred coracoacromial ligament. *D,* Two small drill holes are made through the superior cortex of the distal clavicle. The coracoacromial ligament is carefully detached from the acromion process. *E* through *H,* With the coracoacromial ligament detached from the acromion, a heavy nonabsorbable suture is woven through the ligament. The ends of the suture are passed out through the two small drill holes in the distal end of the clavicle. The coracoclavicular lag screw is inserted, and when the clavicle is reduced down to its normal position, the sutures used to pull the ligament snugly up into the canal are tied. (*G* and *H* reproduced with permission from Rockwood CA, and Green DP (eds): Fractures (3 vols), 2nd ed. Philadelphia: JB Lippincott, 1984.)

fragment of the acromion may be removed with the ligament. If the patient happens to have any symptoms of an impingement syndrome, an anterior acromioplasty is done at this time. With the clavicle held reduced to just above the base of the coracoid, one must determine if there is sufficient length of the coracoacromial ligament to reach into the intramedullary canal of the clavicle. As has been pointed out by Cadenat,[81] further length to this ligament can be obtained by detaching the anterior fasciculus of the coracoacromial ligament from the waist of the coracoid process. A nonabsorbable No. 1 cottony Dacron suture is woven back and forth through the ligament so that both ends of the suture exit through the acromial end of the coracoacromial ligament (see Fig. 12–58E). Two small drill holes are then placed in the superior cortex of the distal stump of the clavicle, which connects into the medullary canal (see Fig. 12–58D). A 3/16-inch hole is drilled through the distal clavicle, which should be directly above the base of the coracoid. With the clavicle held to its correct position above the base of the coracoid, a 9/64-inch drill bit is inserted through the hole in the clavicle and drilled through both cortices of the coracoid process. Before the lag screw is inserted into the coracoid, the two ends of the suture through the coracoacromial ligament are passed into the medullary canal and out the two small drill holes in the superior cortex of the clavicle (Fig. 12–58F). The special lag screw is then inserted through the clavicle and into the coracoid and tightened to vertically reduce the clavicle down to just above the coracoid process (see Fig. 12–58E,F). The two ends of the suture through the coracoacromial ligament are tightened, and the coracoacromial ligament is fed into the curetted medullary canal of the distal clavicle. The suture is tied, thus securing the ligament into the clavicle (see Fig. 12–58F).

Postoperatively, the patient's arm is supported with a sling for four weeks. At 7 to 10 days, the patient can use the arm for everyday living activities but is instructed to avoid any heavy lifting, pushing, or pulling. After 10 to 12 weeks, the screw should be removed under local anesthesia.

Prognosis

TYPE I INJURY

In general, the prognosis for a Type I injury is excellent. Most patients recover full range of motion and have no pain by the end of the two-week period. However, Bergfeld and associates[46] and Cox[98] reported that significant symptoms may persist for six months to five years after Type I injury. Bergfeld and associates[46] reported nuisance symptoms in 30 per cent and significant symptoms in 9 per cent of midshipmen with Type I injuries. Cox[98] found nuisance symptoms in 28 per cent and significant symptoms in 8 per cent.

TYPE II INJURY

Again, most patients with Type II injury recover fully, leaving only a very small percentage who require debridement or excision of the outer end of the clavicle because of arthritis in the joint. Bergfeld and associates[46] and Cox[98] reported from the U.S. Naval Academy that 23 to 35 per cent of patients with a Type II injury had nuisance symptoms, and 13 to 42 per cent had significant symptoms six months to five years

following injury. Walsh and colleagues[425] also found residual pain and stiffness in some patients with Type II injuries. CYBEX-II evaluation of 9 patients with Type II injuries demonstrated a 24 per cent decrease in horizontal abduction strength at fast speeds. All other motions and speeds were not significantly different from the noninjured arm. Bjerneld and associates[54] found 100 per cent good or excellent results in 37 patients with Type II injuries, with an average follow-up of 6 years. Park and coworkers[304] found good results in 25 patients with Type II sprains treated nonoperatively.

TYPE III, IV, V, AND VI INJURIES

A review of the literature would suggest that excellent results can be obtained in patients with Type III injuries with operative and with nonoperative treatment. However, we believe that as physicians, we should use discrimination as to which patients we operate on and which ones we manage by nonoperative technique. We are quite confident that the nonoperative treatment in a nonlaboring white collar office worker will be successful, i.e., will result in essentially a full range of motion and minimal pain, and the patient can carry on with his usual activities. However, the senior author is quite certain that a patient whose work involves heavy labor and who is treated by a nonoperative technique will develop a dull, aching, dragging pain in the shoulder and will state that this causes difficulty in performing his usual job.[342] In general, given the proper treatment for a given patient, the end results tend to be completely acceptable in over 90 per cent of patients. In patients with Type III injuries, Walsh and coworkers[425] found decreased vertical abduction strength in operatively treated patients when compared with nonoperatively managed patients. All other strength parameters were not significantly different. However, endurance tests were not performed. Patients with Type IV, V, and VI injuries usually will require an open reduction and fixation. In our experience, the end results have been about the same as those in patients with a Type III injury (see Figs. 12–52 and 12–55).

Complications of Injuries to the Acromioclavicular Joint

COMPLICATIONS OF THE ACUTE INJURY

Associated Fractures and Injuries

Fractures associated with dislocation may include fractures of the midclavicle, the distal clavicle into the acromioclavicular joint, the acromion process, and the coracoid process. Barber[28] reported a patient with a Type IV acromioclavicular injury associated with a contralateral pneumothorax and an ipsilateral pulmonary contusion.

Coracoclavicular Ossification

Coracoclavicular ossification has been referred to as ossification and calcification. Urist[411] has demonstrated that bone does indeed form in the coracoclavicular interval. Although some authors have felt that the ossification was the result of operative treatment, most have shown that the ossification occurs regardless of whether the lesion is treated by conservative or operative means. Arner and associates[20] report that calcification or ossification of the acromioclavicular or coracoclavicular ligament is the rule rather than the exception. They report the incidence of calcification in their series and others as 14 of 17 cases, 62 of 109 cases, and 15 of 22 cases, respectively. Millbourn[261] states that calcium appears in the mild or severe sprain, regardless of whether the treatment is conservative or operative, and that it can be observed as early as the third or fourth week. It may be an isolated bone structure, or it may form a bridge of bone between the coracoid to the clavicle. In our experience, the ossification does not seem to affect the late functional results (see Fig. 12–4). In Weitzman's series,[434] 16 of 19 patients had calcification, and he could not correlate the end results with the presence of calcification. Alldredge[10] reported calcium in half of his operative cases, and there was no correlation with the end results.

Osteolysis of the Distal Clavicle

The condition may follow an acute injury, or it may occur in men who have repeated stress on the shoulder. Madsen,[243] in 1963, reported seven patients with the complication known as post-traumatic osteolysis of the distal clavicle. He stated there were eight cases in the literature at that time, and the first case was reported by Werder[436] in 1950. Ehricht[124] reported a case in a pneumatic toolworker. Cahill[82] reported 46 patients who were athletes, none of whom had an acute injury, but 45 lifted weights as part of their training. He used technetium bone scans and a 35-degree cephalic tilt x-ray to help make the diagnosis. Murphy and associates,[276] Orava and colleagues,[301] and Cooper and Cutter[94a] have reported this condition in women.

The x-ray changes consist of any or all of the following changes: osteoporosis, osteolysis, tapering, or osteophyte formation of the distal clavicle. Usually, bony changes do not occur in the acromion. Changes usually occur only in one shoulder (Fig. 12–59). If changes are noted in both shoulders, other conditions should be considered, such as rheumatoid arthritis, hyperparathyroidism, and scleroderma. The differential diagnosis of such a lesion in one shoulder should include Gorham's massive osteolysis, gout,[317] and a neoplasm such as multiple myeloma.

Most authors believe that the symptoms of dull ache, weakness, and pain with flexion and abduction are self-limited and resolve within a year or so. They recommend stopping the activities that strain the shoulder and rest. Should the symptoms not be relieved, then an excision of the distal clavicle is recommended. Levine and associates[233] reported that with rest, the distal clavicle may even reconstitute itself. Microscopic studies of the distal clavicle have been reported by Lamont,[222] Murphy and coworkers,[276] Madsen,[243] and Zsernaviczky.[452] They have described demineralization, subchondral cysts, and erosion of the distal clavicle. Griffiths and Glucksman[164] performed a biopsy eight months after injury, which showed patches of necrotic and reactive woven bone.

Nonunion Fracture of the Coracoid Process

This is a rare problem and can be quite disabling. The patient has discomfort when lifting or stressing the arm, and the shoulder is weak. Bone graft and stabilization of the nonunion is required (Fig. 12–60).

COMPLICATIONS FOLLOWING OPERATIVE TREATMENT

The following complications may result from operative treatment:
1. Wound infection.
2. Osteomyelitis.
3. Acromioclavicular arthritis.
4. Soft tissue calcification.
5. Erosion of the clavicle or coracoid by metal or sutures.
6. Late fracture through the implant holes in the bone.
7. Necessity of a second operative procedure to remove the fixation device.
8. Migration of pins or wires.
9. Metal failure.
10. Unsightly scar.
11. Inadequate purchase of the fixation.
12. Recurrent deformity.

Besides the obvious wound infection and osteomyelitis that might develop from the operative procedure, several other complications can occur: occurrence of a fracture through a drill hole, loss of purchase of the internal fixation, metal failure, and migration of the fixation device to all parts of the body (Fig. 12–61).

Migration of Pins

Mazet[246] reported migration of a 6.0 cm Kirschner wire into the lung 76 days after its insertion into the right acromioclavicular joint. Norrell and Llewellyn[293] reported migration of a Steinmann pin from the right acromioclavicular joint into the spinal cord. The pin was found in the subarachnoid space anterior to the spinal cord. It extended transversely through the spinal cord at the level of the first thoracic vertebra. It was easily removed in the direction from which it came.

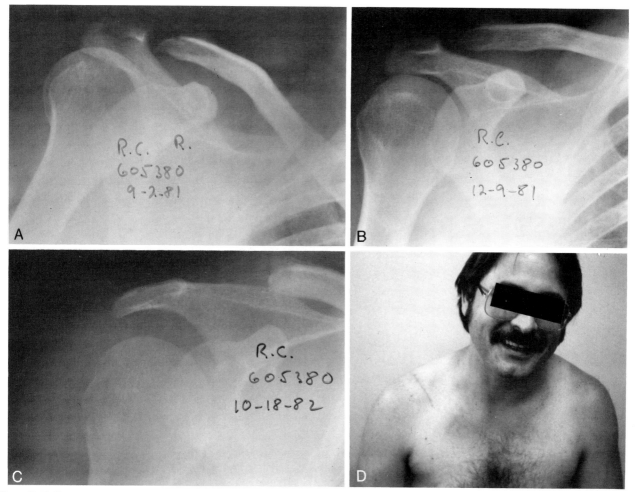

Figure 12–59. Traumatic osteolysis of the distal clavicle. *A,* An x-ray taken three months after a fall onto the right shoulder reveals resorption of the right distal clavicle and new bone formation on the dorsal aspect of the clavicle. *B,* An x-ray at six months reveals an increase in the resorption and new bone formation; the patient was experiencing pain. *C,* This x-ray was taken 14 months following the injury and two months after resection of the distal 2.5 cm of the clavicle. The remaining clavicle was held securely to the coracoid process through the conoid ligament. *D,* This skin incision was used for the arthroplasty. (Reproduced with permission from Rockwood CA, and Green DP (eds): Fractures (3 vols), 2nd ed. Philadelphia: JB Lippincott, 1984.)

Lindsey and Gutowski[235] reported migration of a Kirschner wire into the neck posterior to the carotid sheath. The pin was removed uneventfully. They concluded, as did Eaton and Serletti,[123] that CT scan was useful in planning removal of migratory pins. Eaton and Serletti[123] removed a migrated pin which had crossed the midline and was indenting the pleura posteriorly at the T2 level. Urban and Jaskiewicz[410] report a case of pin migration into the ipsilateral pleural cavity three months after surgery. Sethi and Scott[369] reported on the migration of a Hagie pin from the acromioclavicular joint, causing a laceration of the subclavian artery. Grauthoff and Klammer[161] reported five cases of migration of pins into the aorta, subclavian artery, or lung. Retief and Meintjes[334] reported a case in which a 12.0-cm Kirschner wire that had been placed into the acromioclavicular joint had migrated through the thoracic cavity and was lodged behind the liver. In the six-week period between the Kirschner wire insertion and its removal, the patient had suffered a pneumothorax secondary to the wire's penetration of the

lung. In most instances, migration of the pin can be prevented by bending a hook on the portion of the pin that protrudes from the acromion process. However, the pins can break, and then part of the pin is free to migrate. Patients must be prepared for and forewarned of the necessity of pin removal and the complications of pins that are not removed.

There are no reports of migration of loops or broken wire, and there are no reports of migrating Bosworth-type lag screws.

COMPLICATIONS OF NONOPERATIVE TREATMENT

The following complications may arise as a result of nonoperative treatment:

1. Tissues interposed in the acromioclavicular joint.
2. Joint stiffness as a result of immobilization.
3. The immobilization device may be restrictive and uncomfortable.

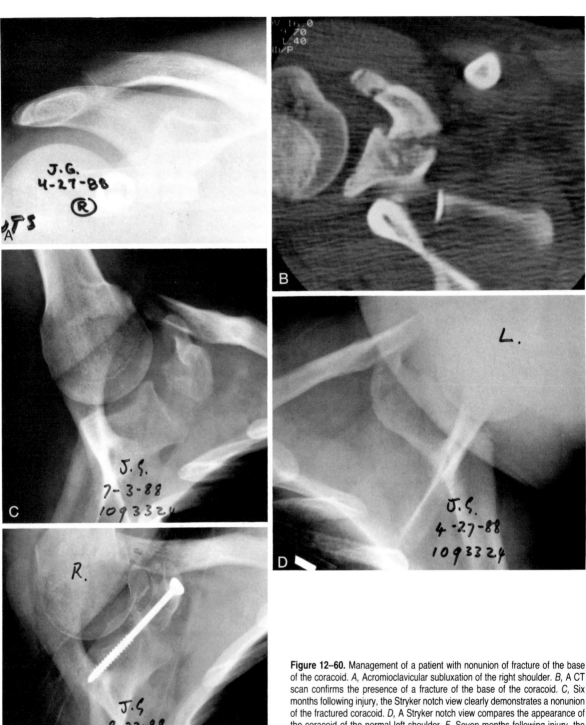

Figure 12–60. Management of a patient with nonunion of fracture of the base of the coracoid. *A,* Acromioclavicular subluxation of the right shoulder. *B,* A CT scan confirms the presence of a fracture of the base of the coracoid. *C,* Six months following injury, the Stryker notch view clearly demonstrates a nonunion of the fractured coracoid. *D,* A Stryker notch view compares the appearance of the coracoid of the normal left shoulder. *E,* Seven months following injury, the coracoid process was exposed, bone was grafted, and the process was held reduced with a lag screw. The patient had an uneventful recovery.

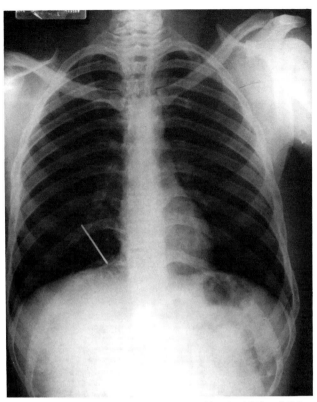

Figure 12–61. A broken Steinmann pin has migrated into the right lung field from its previous location in the right acromioclavicular joint. (Reproduced with permission from Rockwood CA, and Green DP (eds): Fractures (3 vols), 2nd ed. Philadelphia: JB Lippincott, 1984.)

4. Skin irritation, maceration, or ulcers over the shoulder secondary to the immobilization device.
5. Pressure sores on other parts of the body that are in contact with the immobilization device.
6. Possibility that patient can independently remove the immobilization device and lose the reduction.
7. Inability of patient to completely or properly bathe.
8. Everyday activities restricted.
9. Residual deformity.
10. Soft tissue calcification.
11. Acromioclavicular arthritis.

As described, patients with a Type I or II injury may develop degenerative changes in the joint which may be severe enough to require an excision of the distal clavicle. Following a Type III, IV, or V injury, the patient, if he is involved with heavy labor, may well develop chronic strain and ache in the shoulder and posterior neck muscles. This will require, in addition to an excision of the distal clavicle, a reconstruction of the coracoclavicular ligaments. Following a Type IV injury, chronic pain would be the most likely complication.

Degenerative Arthritis of the Acromioclavicular Joint

DePalma[110] pointed out that the deterioration of the fibrocartilaginous disc, which separates the two articular surfaces of the acromioclavicular joint, begins in the second decade of life. The disc may deteriorate entirely, and this is a natural process of aging. Petersson and Redlund-Johnell[308] found that the acromioclavicular joint space narrows with aging, and that a joint space of 0.5 mm in a 60-year-old patient is not necessarily abnormal. Petersson[310] performed dissections of the acromioclavicular joint in patients of all ages. He found increased severity of degenerative changes with age and suggested that this is a consequence of regression of the acromioclavicular disc. Horvath and Kéry[190] found x-ray changes of degeneration in 54 to 57 per cent of elderly patients and tenderness in the acromioclavicular joint in 42 to 45 per cent.

Waxman[432] evaluated the acromioclavicular joint in 100 patients presenting with osteoarthritis of other joints. He found that 70 per cent of patients had tenderness of one or both acromioclavicular joints and used intra-articular steroid injections with good results in 30 consecutive patients.

Grimes and Garner[165] managed six patients with refractory acromioclavicular arthritis with excision of three-quarters of an inch of the distal clavicle with good results. Taylor and Tooke[399] treated 20 patients with debridement of the meniscus and curettage of the cartilaginous endplates down to raw, bleeding bone, with good results in 18 patients.

Numerous authors have reported on the results of excision of the distal clavicle. Worchester and Green[444] followed 56 patients for an average of 4.5 years, with generally satisfactory results. Petersson[311] found good results in 10 patients and fair results in 4 out of 16 patients with nontraumatic acromioclavicular arthritis. Petersson[309] also reported on the possibility of distally pointing osteophytes off the acromioclavicular joint, causing rupture of the supraspinatus tendon. Wagner[422] reported good results in 20 of 22 patients. Sage and Salvatore[353] found that 91 per cent of patients with distal clavicle excisions had good or excellent results.

Rheumatoid Arthritis of the Acromioclavicular Joint

Petersson[312] studied 49 patients with rheumatoid arthritis and painful shoulders and found that the acromioclavicular joint is affected by rheumatoid arthritis in a fashion similar to that of other joints. He found acromioclavicular tenderness in 63 per cent and acromioclavicular x-ray changes in 85 per cent of symptomatic patients. He further reported that the incidence of acromioclavicular pathology increases with the severity of the underlying condition. He found resection of the acromioclavicular joint and subacromial bursectomy to be an effective procedure in selected patients at 18 to 62 months follow-up.

Septic Arthritis of the Acromioclavicular Joint

Septic arthritis of the acromioclavicular joint is rare. Two cases of pyogenic septic arthritis in otherwise healthy adults have been reported. Griffith and Boyadjis[163] managed a patient with *Staphylococcus aureus* acromioclavicular joint septic arthritis with arthrotomy and antibiotics with a good result, while Blankstein and colleagues[55] had a similar good result with joint excision and penicillin for a *Streptococcus viridans* infection. Adams and McDonald[3] reported a case of cryptococcal arthritis in a patient previously treated with prednisone for sarcoidosis. The patient did well on an antifungal medical regimen. Tuberculosis of the acromioclavicular joint has been reported by Richter and associates.[337]

Cysts of the Acromioclavicular Joint

Cystic changes may occur in the acromioclavicular joint. Involvement of the acromioclavicular joint in patients with rotator cuff disease is not uncommon. As the disease of the cuff progresses and the humeral head migrates superiorly, the head will erode the inferior aspect of the acromioclavicular joint. The resultant progressive cuff degeneration and accumulation of synovial fluid will push up through the acromioclavicular joint to produce the cyst superior to the joint. Craig[99] reported two cases of large cystic masses occurring in patients with rotator cuff tears. One patient's medical condition precluded surgery, and a second underwent acromioclavicular joint arthroplasty, acromioplasty, and cuff repair. Burns and Zvirbulis[78] excised a ganglion cyst over the acromioclavicular joint, which did not communicate with the glenohumeral joint, in a patient with no known cuff disease, and the cyst had not recurred at one year.

References

1. Abbott LC, Saunders JB, Hagey H, and Jones EW: Surgical approaches to the shoulder joint. J Bone Joint Surg 31A(2):235–255, 1949.
2. Adams FL: The Genuine Works of Hippocrates, Vols. 1 and 2. New York: William Wood, 1886.
3. Adams R, and McDonald M: Cryptococcal arthritis of the acromioclavicular joint. NC Med J 45(1):23–24, 1984.
4. Aderhold K: [A New Method of Therapy in Complete Separation of the Acromioclavicular Joint.] Unfallheilkunde 86:416–422, 1983.
5. Ahstrom JP, Jr: Surgical repair of complete acromioclavicular separation. JAMA 217(6):785–789, 1971.
6. Albrecht F: The Balser plate for acromioclavicular fixation. Chirurg 53(11):732–734, 1982.
7. Alexander OM: Dislocation of the acromio-clavicular joint. Radiography 15:260, 1949.
8. Alexander OM: Radiography of the acromio-clavicular joint. Radiography 14:139, 1948.
9. Alexander OM: Radiography of the acromio-clavicular articulation. Med Radiogr Photogr 30(2):34–39, 1954.
10. Alldredge RH: Surgical treatment of acromioclavicular dislocations (abstr). J Bone Joint Surg 47A:1278, 1965.
11. Alldredge RH: Surgical treatment of acromioclavicular dislocation. Clin Orthop 63:262–263, 1969.
12. Allen WC: Post-traumatic osteolysis of the distal clavicle. Postgrad Med 41:A73, 1967.
13. Allman FL, Jr: Fractures and ligamentous injuries of the clavicle and its articulation. J Bone Joint Surg 49A:774–784, 1967.
13a. Allmann F: Personal communication, 1984.
14. Alnor P: Die Posttraumatische Osteolyse des Lateralen Claviculaendes. Fortschr Rontgenstr 75:364, 1951.
15. Alpert M, and Myers MM: Osteolysis of the acromial end of the clavicles in rheumatoid arthritis. AJR 86:251, 1961.
16. Anderson ME: Treatment of dislocations of the acromioclavicular and sternoclavicular joints (abstr). J Bone Joint Surg 45A(3):657–658, 1963.
17. Anderson R, and Burgess E: Acromioclavicular dislocation: a conservative method of treatment. Northwest Med 38(2):40, 1939.
18. Anzel SH, and Streitz, WL: Acute acromioclavicular injuries: a report of nineteen cases treated non-operatively employing dynamic splint immobilization. Clin Orthop 103:143–149, 1974.
19. Appell HA: Acromioclavicular dislocation. Can Med Assoc J 43:23–25, 1940.
20. Arner O, Sandahl U, and Ohrling H: Dislocation of the acromioclavicular joint: review of the literature and a report of 56 cases. Acta Chir Scand 113:140–152, 1957.
21. Aufranc OE, Jones SN, and Harris WH: Complete acromioclavicular dislocation. JAMA 180(8):681–682, 1962.
22. Augereau B, Robert H, and Apoil A: Treatment of severe acromioclavicular dislocation: a coracoclavicular ligamentoplasty technique derived from Cadenat's procedure. Ann Chir 35(9):720–722, 1981.
23. Badgley CE: Sports injuries of the shoulder girdle. JAMA 172:444–448, 1960.
24. Bailey RW, O'Connor GA, Tilus PD, and Baril JD: A dynamic repair for acute and chronic injuries of the acromioclavicular area (abstr). J Bone Joint Surg 54A:1802, 1972.
25. Bailey RW: A dynamic repair for complete acromioclavicular joint dislocation (abstr). J Bone Joint Surg 47A:858, 1965.
26. Bakalim G, and Wilppula E: Surgical or conservative treatment of total dislocation of the acromioclavicular joint. Acta Chir Scand 141:43–47, 1975.
27. Baker DM, and Stryker WF: Acute complete acromioclavicular separations. JAMA 192(8):689–692, 1965.
28. Barber FA: Complete posterior acromioclavicular dislocation: a case report. Orthopedics 10(3):493–496, 1987.
29. Bargren JH, Erlanger S, and Dick HM: Biomechanics and comparison of two operative methods of treatment of complete acromioclavicular separation. Clin Orthop 130:267–272, 1978.
30. Barnhart JM, Fain RH, Dewar FP, and Stein AH: Acromioclavicular joint injuries. Clin Orthop 81:199, 1970.
31. Barnhart JM: Repair of acute acromioclavicular joint separation. Am J Orthop Surg 10:122–123, 1968.
32. Barr JS: Dislocations of the clavicle. In Wilson PD (ed): Experience in the Management of Fractures and Dislocations. Philadelphia: JB Lippincott Company, 1938.
33. Barrett J: The clavicular joints. Physiotherapy 57:268–269, 1971.
34. Basmajian JV: Acromioclavicular joint. In Grant's Method of Anatomy, 8th ed. Baltimore: Williams & Wilkins, 1971, pp 160–161.

35. Batchelor JS: Splint for fractured clavicle and acromioclavicular dislocation. Lancet 2:690, 1947.
36. Bateman JE: Athletic injuries about the shoulder in throwing and body-contact sports. Clin Orthop 23:75–83, 1962.
37. Bateman JE: The Shoulder and Neck. Philadelphia: WB Saunders Company, 1972.
38. Bayley I, and Kessel L: Shoulder Surgery. New York: Springer-Verlag, 1982.
39. Bearden JM, Hughston JC, and Whatley GS: Acromioclavicular dislocation: method of treatment. J Sports Med 1(4):5–17, 1973.
40. Bearn JG: Direct observations on the function of the capsule of the sternoclavicular joint in clavicle support. J Anat 101:159–170, 1967.
41. Beckman T: A case of simultaneous luxation of both ends of the clavicle. Acta Chir Scand 56:156–163, 1923.
42. Bednarek J, Kaczan Z, and Krochmalski M: [Results of treatment in acromio-clavicular dislocations] Chir Narzadow Ruchu Ortop Pol 46:13–16, 1981.
43. Behling F: Treatment of acromioclavicular separations. Orthop Clin North Am 4(3):747–757, 1973.
44. Benson RA: Acromioclavicular dislocation. US Naval Med Bull 34:341–342, 1936.
45. Benton J, and Nelson C: Avulsion of the coracoid process in an athlete. J Bone Joint Surg 53A(2):356–358, 1971.
46. Bergfeld JA, Andrish JT, and Clancy WG: Evaluation of the acromioclavicular joint following first- and second-degree sprains. Am J Sports Med 6(4):153–159, 1978.
47. Bernard TN Jr., Brunet ME, and Haddad RJ: Fractured coracoid process in acromioclavicular dislocations. Clin Orthop 175:227–232, 1983.
48. Berson BL, Gilbert MS, and Green S: Acromioclavicular dislocations: treatment by transfer of the conjoined tendon and distal end of the coracoid process to the clavicle. Clin Orthop 135:157–164, 1978.
49. Bertwistle AP: Acromio-clavicular dislocation and sprain. Clin J 66:76–77, 1937.
50. Besselaar PP, and Raaymakers ELFB: Operative treatment of acromioclavicular dislocation (abstr). Acta Orthop Scand 55(4):483–484, 1984.
51. Binet EF, and Markarian B: Asymptomatic clavicular lesion. NY State J Med 75(10):1710–1712, 1975.
52. Birkett AN: The result of operative repair of severe acromioclavicular dislocation. Br J Surg 32:103–105, 1944–1945.
53. Björkenheim JM, Paavolainen P, and Slätis P: Surgical treatment of acromioclavicular dislocation (abstr). Acta Orthop Scand 54(3):533, 1983.
54. Bjerneld H, Hovelius L, and Thorling J: Acromio-clavicular separations treated conservatively: a 5-year follow-up study. Acta Orthop Scand 54:743–745, 1983.
55. Blankstein A, Amsallem JL, Rubinstein E, Horoszowski H, et al.: Septic arthritis of the acromioclavicular joint (current problem case). Arch Orthop Trauma Surg 103:417–418, 1985.
56. Blazina ME: Letter to the editor re: Bearden's article: Acromioclavicular dislocation: method of treatment. J Sports Med 2:58–59, 1974.
57. Bloom FA: Wire fixation in acromioclavicular dislocation. J Bone Joint Surg 27(2):273–276, 1945.
58. Bohler L: Treatment of fractures, 4th ed. Baltimore: William Wood, 1935.
59. Bonnell F., and Mirfakhrai, AM: [Treatment of complete acromioclavicular luxation by coracoclavicular screw.] Acta Chir Acad Sci Hungaricae 22(1–2):69–74, 1981.
60. Bonnin JG: Complete Outline of Fractures. London: William Heinemann, 1941.
61. Bossart PJ, Joyce SM, Manaster BJ, and Packer SM: Lack of efficacy of 'weighted' radiographs in diagnosing acute acromioclavicular separation. Ann Emerg Med 17(1):47–51, 1988.
62. Bosworth BM: Acromioclavicular separation: new method of repair. Surg Gynecol Obstet 73:866–871, 1941.
63. Bosworth BM: Acromioclavicular dislocation: end-results of screw suspension treatment. Ann Surg 127:98–111, 1948.
64. Bosworth BM: Calcium deposits in the shoulder and subacro-
mial bursitis: a survey of 12,122 shoulders. JAMA 116(22):2477–2482, 1941.
65. Bosworth BM: Complete acromioclavicular dislocation. N Engl J Med 241:221–225, 1949.
66. Boussaton M, Julia F, Horvath E, Boudet J, et al.: [Transposition of the coracoacromial ligament according to the technique of Weaver and Dunn in the treatment of old acromioclavicular luxations: a report of 15 cases.] Acta Orthop Belg 51(1):80–90, 1985.
67. Bowers KD: Treatment of acromioclavicular sprains in athletes. Physician Sports Med 11(1):79–89, 1983.
68. Bowers RF: Complete acromioclavicular separation: diagnosis and operative treatment. J Bone Joint Surg 17(4):1005–1010, 1935.
69. Boyer DW: Trapshooter's shoulder: stress fracture of the coracoid process. J Bone Joint Surg 57A:862, 1975.
70. Brandt G: Die Behandlung der Verrenkung im Acromiolen Schlüsselbeingelenk. Klin Med 51(13):526–528, 1956.
71. Breitner S, and Wirth CJ: [Resection of the acromial and sternal ends of the clavicula.] Z Orthop 125(4):363–368, 1987.
72. Briggs JR: Acromio-clavicular dislocation (Proceedings). J Bone Joint Surg 44B(1):227, 1962.
73. Brosgol M: Traumatic acromioclavicular sprains and subluxations. Clin Orthop 20:98–107, 1961.
74. Browne JE, Stanley RF Jr, and Tullos HS: Acromioclavicular joint dislocations. Am J Sports Med 5(6):258–263, 1977.
75. Brunet ME, Reynolds MC, Cook SD, and Brown TW: Atraumatic osteolysis of the distal clavicle: histologic evidence of synovial pathogenesis: a case report. Orthopedics 9(4):557–559, 1986.
76. Bundens WD Jr, and Cook JI: Repair of acromioclavicular separations by deltoid-trapezius imbrication. Clin Orthop 20:109–114, 1961.
77. Bunnell S: Fascial graft for dislocation of the acromioclavicular joint. Surg Gynecol Obstet 46:563–564, 1928.
78. Burns SJ, and Zvirbulis RA: A ganglion arising over the acromioclavicular joint: a case report. Orthopedics 7(6):1002–1004, 1984.
79. Burri C, and Neugebauer R: Carbon fiber replacement of the ligaments of the shoulder girdle and the treatment of lateral instability of the ankle joint. Clin Orthop 196:112–117, 1985.
80. Burton ME: Operative treatment of acromioclavicular dislocations. Bull Hosp Jt Dis Orthop Inst 36(2):109–120, 1975.
81. Cadenat FM: The treatment of dislocations and fractures of the outer end of the clavicle. Int Clin 1:145–169, 1917.
82. Cahill BR: Osteolysis of the distal part of the clavicle in male athletes. J Bone Joint Surg 64A(7):1053–1058, 1982.
83. Caldwell GD: Treatment of complete permanent acromioclavicular dislocation by surgical arthrodesis. J Bone Joint Surg 25(2):368–374, 1943.
84. Caldwell GD: Treatment of Fractures. New York: Paul Hoeber, 1943.
85. Campbell WC: Operative Orthopaedics. St. Louis: CV Mosby Company, 1971.
86. Campos OP: Acromioclavicular dislocation. Am J Surg 43(2):287–291, 1939.
87. Carrell WB: Dislocation at the outer end of clavicle. J Bone Joint Surg 10:314–315, 1928.
88. Caspi I, Ezra E, Nerubay J, and Horoszovski H: Musculocutaneous nerve injury after coracoid process transfer for clavicle instability: report of three cases. Acta Orthop Scand 58(3):294–295, 1987.
89. Codman EA: Rupture of the supraspinatus tendon and other lesions in or about the subacromial bursa. In The Shoulder. Boston: Thomas Todd & Co., 1934.
90. Colson JHC, and Armour WJ: Sports Injuries and Their Treatment. Philadelphia: JB Lippincott Company, 1961.
91. Conway AM: Movements at the sternoclavicular and acromioclavicular joints. Phys Ther Rev 41(6):421–432, 1961.
92. Cook FF, and Tibone JE: The Mumford procedure in athletes: an objective analysis of function (abstr). Am Orthop Soc for Sports Med, San Francisco, CA, January 21, 1987.
93. Cooper A: A Treatise on Dislocations and Fractures of the

Joints, 2nd Am. ed. from 6th London ed. Boston: Lilly & Wait and Carter & Hendee, 1832.

94. Cooper ES: New method of treating long standing dislocations of the scapulo-clavicular articulation. Am J Med Sci 41:389–392, 1861.

94a. Cooper D, and Curtis R: Traumatic osteolysis in women: 1 case report. Personal communication, 1989.

95. Copeland S, and Kessel L: Disruption of the acromioclavicular joint: surgical anatomy and biological reconstruction. Injury 11:208–214, 1980.

96. Copher GH: A method of treatment of upward dislocation of the acromial end of the clavicle. Am J Surg 22:507–508, 1933.

97. Coues WP: Fracture of the coracoid process of the scapula. N Engl J Med 212:727, 1935.

98. Cox JS: The fate of the acromioclavicular joint in athletic injuries. Am J Sports Med 9(1):50–53, 1981.

99. Craig EV: The acromioclavicular joint cyst: an unusual presentation of a rotator cuff tear. Clin Orthop 202:189–192, 1986.

100. Crossan JF, and Macpherson IS: The role of the acromioclavicular joint in chronic shoulder impingement syndromes. J Bone Joint Surg 67B(1):161, 1985.

101. Currie DI: An apparatus for dislocation of the acromial end of the clavicle. Br Med J 1:570, 1924.

102. D'Ambrosia RD: Musculoskeletal Disorders. Philadelphia: JB Lippincott Company, 1977.

103. Dahl E: Follow-up after coracoclavicular ligament prosthesis for acromioclavicular joint dislocation (abstr). Acta Chir Scand [Suppl] 506:96, 1981.

104. Dahl E: Velour prosthesis in fractures and dislocations in the clavicular region. Chirurg 53:120–122, 1982.

105. Daniels S, Ellis E III, and Carlson DS: Histologic analysis of costochondral and sternoclavicular grafts in the TMJ of the juvenile monkey. J Oral Maxillofac Surg 45(8):675–682, 1987.

106. Dannöhl Ch: [Angulation osteotomy at the clavicle in old dislocations of the acromioclavicular joint.] Aktuel Traumatol 14(6):282–284, 1984.

107. Darrow JC, Smith JA, and Lockwood RC: A new conservative method for treatment of type III acromioclavicular separations. Orthop Clin North Am 11(4):727–733, 1980.

108. Dawe CJ: Acromioclavicular joint injuries. J Bone Joint Surg 62B:269, 1980.

109. de Sousa A, and Veiga A: Calcification of the coraco-clavicular ligaments after acromio-clavicular dislocation (proceedings). J Bone Joint Surg 33B(4):646, 1951.

110. DePalma AF, Callery G, and Bennett GA: Variational anatomy and degenerative lesions of the shoulder joint. AAOS Instructional Course Lectures 6:255–281, 1949.

111. DePalma AF: Surgery of the Shoulder, 2nd ed. Philadelphia: JB Lippincott Company, 1973.

112. DePalma AF: Surgical anatomy of the acromioclavicular and sternoclavicular joints. Surg Clin North Am 43:1540–1550, 1963.

113. DePalma AF: The role of the disks of the sternoclavicular and acromioclavicular joints. Clin Orthop 13:7–12, 1959.

114. Dewar FP, and Barrington TW: The treatment of chronic acromioclavicular dislocation. J Bone Joint Surg 47B(1):32–35, 1965.

115. Deyerle WM: Closed double rod fixation of complete acromioclavicular separation using image intensifier (abstr). Clin Orthop 133:266, 1978.

116. Dias JJ, Steingold RA, Richardson RA, Tesfayohannes B, et al.: The conservative treatment of acromioclavicular dislocation: review after five years. J Bone Joint Surg 69B(5):719–722, 1987.

117. Dillehunt RB: Luxation of the acromioclavicular joint. Surg Clin North Am 7(5):1307–1313, 1927.

118. Dittel KK, Pfaff G, and Metzger H: [Results after operative treatment of complete acromioclavicular separation (Tossy III injury).] Aktuel Traumatol 17(1):16–22, 1987.

119. Dittmer H, Jauch KW, and Wening V: [Treatment of acromioclavicular separations with Balser's hookplate.] Unfallheilkunde 87(5):216–222, 1984.

120. Dohn K: Luxatio acromio-clavicularis supraspinata. Acta Orthop Scand 25:183–189, 1956.

121. Dunlop J: Dislocations of the outer end of the clavicle. Calif West Med 26(1):38–40, 1927.

122. Dupus J, Badelon P, and Dayde G: Aspects radiologiques d'une osteolyse essentielle progressive de la main gauche. J Radiol 20:383–387, 1936.

123. Eaton R, and Serletti J: Computerized axial tomography—a method of localizing Steinmann pin migration: a case report. Orthopedics 4(12):1357–1360, 1981.

124. Ehricht HG: Die Osteolyse im Lateralen Claviculaende nach Pressluftschaden. Arch Orthop Unfallchirurg 50:576–589, 1959.

125. Eidman DK, Siff SJ, and Tullos HS: Acromioclavicular lesions in children. Am J Sports Med 9(3):150–154, 1981.

126. Eikenbary CF, and LeCocq JF: The operative treatment of acromioclavicular dislocations. Surg Clin North Am 13(6):1305–1314, 1933.

127. Ejeskär A: Coracoclavicular wiring for acromioclavicular joint dislocation: a ten year follow-up study. Acta Orthop Scand 45:652–661, 1974.

128. Elkin DC, and Cooper FW Jr: Resection of the clavicle in vascular surgery. J Bone Joint Surg 28(1):117–119, 1946.

129. Epps CH: Complications in Orthopaedic Surgery. Philadelphia: JB Lippincott Company, 1978.

130. Evans ET: Avascular necrosis—report of cases involving the distal end of the clavicle and the odontoid process. Minn Med 34:970, 1951.

131. Falstie-Jensen S, and Mikkelsen P: Pseudodislocation of the acromioclavicular joint. J Bone Joint Surg 64B(3):368–369, 1982.

132. Ferguson AB Jr, and Bender J: The ABC's of athletic injuries and conditioning. Baltimore: Williams & Wilkins, 1964.

133. Findlay RT: Fractures of the scapula and ribs. Am J Surg 38:489, 1937.

134. Fleming RE, Tomberg DN, and Kiernan HA: An operative repair of acromioclavicular separation. J Trauma 18(10):709–712, 1978.

135. Fukuda K, Craig EV, An K-N, Cofield RH, et al.: Biomechanical study of the ligamentous system of the acromioclavicular joint. J Bone Joint Surg 68A(3):434–439, 1986.

136. Fukuda K, Craig EV, An K-N, and Cofield RH: Anatomic and biomechanical studies of the ligamentous system of the acromioclavicular joint (abstr). Presented at AAOS Shoulder Meeting, Las Vegas, Nevada, January 1985.

137. Fulton WA: A treatment for greenstick fractures and for dislocations of the clavicle. Lancet 43:383–385, 1923.

138. Gaber O, Klima G, Lugger LJ, and Kostler G: Die Anatomische Struktur des Ligamentum Coracoacromiale als Voraussetzung für die Gestielte Bandplastik bei Luxationen de Articulatio Acromioclaviculars (abstr). Acta Anat 120:26, 1984.

139. Gallie WE: Dislocations. N Engl J Med 213(3):91–98, 1935.

140. Galpin RD, Hawkins RJ, and Grainger RW: A comparative analysis of operative versus nonoperative treatment of grade III acromioclavicular separations. Clin Orthop 193:150–155, 1985.

141. Ganz M, Gattlen W, Laffer U, and Regazzoni P: [Repair of acromioclavicular separation following Bosworth's technique: a follow-up study.] Z Unfallchir Versicherungsmed Berufskr 79(3):195–197, 1986.

142. Gardner E, and Gray DJ: Prenatal development of the human shoulder and acromioclavicular joints. Am J Anat 92:219–276, 1953.

143. Gartner W, and Schuier V: Die Posttraumatische Osteolyse des Schlusselbeines. Zentralbl Chir 80:953, 1955.

144. Gatewood LC: Dislocation of the outer end of the clavicle. Surg Clin North Am 3(5):1193–1197, 1919.

145. Gerber C, and Rockwood CA Jr.: Subcoracoid dislocation of the lateral end of the clavicle: a report of three cases. J Bone Joint Surg 69A(6):924–927, 1987.

146. Giancola R, Torretta F, and Burla S: [Reviewing of 41 cases of third type acromioclavicular luxation, surgically treated.] Chir Ital 37(3):345–352, 1985.

147. Giannestras NJ: A method of immobilization of acute acromioclavicular separation. J Bone Joint Surg 26(3):597–599, 1944.
148. Gibbens ME: An appliance for the conservative treatment of acromioclavicular dislocation. J Bone Joint Surg 28(1):164–165, 1946.
149. Gillespie HS: Excision of the outer end of the clavicle for dislocation of the acromioclavicular joint. Can J Surg 7:18, 1964.
150. Girard PM: Acute acromioclavicular dislocation. Bull U.S. Army Med Dept 82:5, 1944.
151. Glick J: Acromioclavicular dislocation in athletes: auto arthroplasty of the joint. Orthop Rev 1(4):31–34, 1972.
152. Glick JM, Milburn LJ, Haggerty JF, and Nishimoto D: Dislocated acromioclavicular joint: follow-up study of 35 unreduced acromioclavicular dislocations. Am J Sports Med 5(6):264–270, 1977.
153. Glorian B, and Delplace J: [Dislocations of the Acromioclavicular Joint Treated by Transplant of the Coracoid Process.] Rev Chir Orthop 59:667–679, 1973.
154. Goldberg D: Acromioclavicular joint injuries: a modified conservative form of treatment. Am J Surg 71(4):529–531, 1946.
155. Goldberg JA, Viglione W, Cumming WJ, Waddell FS, et al: Review of coracoclavicular ligament reconstruction using Dacron graft material. Aust NZ J Surg 57(7):441–445, 1987.
156. Goodley PH: The acromioclavicular joint and shoulder disability: arthrographic and anatomic studies (abstr). Arch Phys Med Rehabil 56:539, 1975.
157. Gorham LW, and Stout AD: Massive osteolysis (acute spontaneous absorption of bone): its relation to hemangiomatosis. J Bone Joint Surg 37A:985, 1955.
158. Gorham LW, Wright AW, Schultz HH, and Mascon FC: Disappearing bones: a rare form of massive osteolysis. Am J Med 17:674, 1954.
159. Grønmark T: Surgical treatment of acromioclavicular dislocation. Acta Orthop Scand 47:308–310, 1976.
160. Gradoyevitch B: Coracoclavicular joint. J Bone Joint Surg 21:918–920, 1939.
161. Grauthoff VH, and Klammer HL: [Complications due to migration of a Kirschner wire from the clavicle.] Fortschr Röntgenstr 128(5):591–594, 1978.
162. Graves SE, and Foster BK: Absorbable suture lasso in the treatment of complete disruption of the acromioclavicular joint (abstr). J Bone Joint Surg 66B(5):789–790, 1984.
163. Griffith PH III, and Boyadjis TA: Acute pyarthrosis of the acromioclavicular joint: a case report. Orthopedics 7(11):1727–1728, 1984.
164. Griffiths CJ, and Glucksman E: Posttraumatic osteolysis of the clavicle: a case report. Arch Emerg Med 3:129–132, 1986.
165. Grimes DW, and Garner RW: The degeneration of the acromioclavicular joint. Orthop Rev 9(1):41–44, 1980.
166. Gurd FB: The treatment of complete dislocation of the outer end of the clavicle: a hitherto undescribed operation. Ann Surg 113(6):1094–1098, 1941.
167. Gyr UF, Leutenegger A, and Rüedi Th: [Results of Bosworth procedures for Tossy III acromioclavicular luxations.] Z Unfallchir Versicherungsmed Berufskr 79(3):171–174, 1986.
168. Haggart GE: The treatment of acromioclavicular joint dislocation. Surg Clin North Am 13(3):683–688, 1933.
169. Halaby FA, and DiSalvo EL: Osteolysis: a complication of trauma: report of 2 cases. AJR 94:591–594, 1965.
170. Hall RH, Isaac F, and Booth CR: Dislocation of the shoulder with special reference to accompanying small fractures. J Bone Joint Surg 41A:489–494, 1959.
171. Hamill RC: Acromio-clavicular dislocation. Int Clin 3(30):130–132, 1920.
172. Hammond G: Complete acromionectomy in the treatment of chronic tendinitis of the shoulder. J Bone Joint Surg 44A(3):494–503, 1962.
173. Harrison RB, Riddervold HO, Willett ED, and Stamp WG: Acromio-clavicular separation masked by muscle spasm. Va Med 107:377–379, 1980.
174. Hart VL: Treatment of acute acromioclavicular dislocation. J Bone Joint Surg 23(1):175–176, 1941.
175. Hasselmann W: Die Sogen. Posttraumatische Osteolyse des lat. Claviculaendes. Monatsschr Kinderheilkd 58:242, 1955.
176. Hastings DE, and Horne JG: Anterior dislocation of the acromioclavicular joint. Injury 10:285–288, 1979.
177. Hawkins RJ: The acromioclavicular joint. Paper prepared for AAOS Summer Institute, Chicago, July 10–11, 1980.
178. Heitmeyer U, Hierholzer G, Schneppendahl G, and Haines J: The operative treatment of fresh ruptures of the acromioclavicular joint (Tossy III). Arch Orthop Trauma Surg 104:371–373, 1986.
179. Henry MD: Acromioclavicular dislocations. Minn Med 12:431–433, 1929.
180. Heppenstall RB: Fractures and dislocation of the distal clavicle. Orthop Clin North Am 6:477, 1975.
181. Heppenstall RB: Fracture Treatment and Healing. Philadelphia: WB Saunders Company, 1980.
182. Hierholzer G, and Caspers HD: [Chronic dislocation of the acromioclavicular joint: technique and results of treatment.] Unfallheilkunde 170:66–73, 1984.
183. Hill JA: Acromioclavicular separations need conservative treatment: same results achieved with surgical care. Orthopedics Today, p. 25, Sept. 1986.
184. Hill JA: Acromioclavicular dislocations: conservative treatment vindicated (editorial). Lancet 2(8515):1079, 1986.
185. Hohmann HG, and Parhofer R: Zur Differentialdiagnose der Erkrankungen des Schlussebeins. Munch Med Wochenschr 102:471, 1960.
186. Holstein A, Lewis GB, and Sturtz H: Experience in the treatment of acromioclavicular dislocation. J Bone Joint Surg 48A:1224, 1966.
187. Holz U, and Weller S: Luxationen im acromioclavicularen Gelenk. Hefte Unfallheilkd 160:222–229, 1982.
188. Holz U: Personal communication on acromioclavicular dislocations, 1984.
189. Horn JS: The traumatic anatomy and treatment of acute acromioclavicular dislocation. J Bone Joint Surg 36B(2):194–201, 1954.
190. Horvath F, and Kéry L: Degenerative deformations of the acromioclavicular joint in the elderly. Arch Gerontol Geriatr 3:259–265, 1984.
191. Howard NJ: Acromioclavicular and sternoclavicular joint injuries. Am J Surg 46(2):284–291, 1939.
192. Hoyt WA Jr.: Etiology of shoulder injuries in athletes. J Bone Joint Surg 49A(4):755–766, 1967.
193. Imatani RJ, Hanlon JJ, and Cady GW: Acute complete acromioclavicular separation. J Bone Joint Surg 57A(3):328–332, 1975.
194. Indrekvam K, Størkson R, Langeland N, and Hordvick M: [Acromioclavicular joint dislocation: surgical or conservative treatment?] Tidsskr Nor Laegeforen 106(15):1303–1305, 1986.
195. Inman VT, McLaughlin HD, Nevaiser J, and Rowe C: Treatment of complete acromioclavicular dislocation. J Bone Joint Surg 44A:1008–1011, 1944.
196. Inman VT, Saunders JB, and Abbott LC: Observations on the function of the shoulder joint. J Bone Joint Surg 26:1–30, 1944.
197. Inman VT, and Saunders JB: Observations on the function of the clavicle. California Med 65(4):158–166, 1946.
198. Ishizuki M, Yamaura I, and Isobe Y: Avulsion fracture of the superior border of the scapula. J Bone Joint Surg 63A9(5):820–822, 1981.
199. Jacobs B, and Wade PA: Acromioclavicular joint injury: an end-result study. J Bone Joint Surg 48A(3):475–486, 1966.
200. Jacobs P: Post-traumatic osteolysis of the outer end of the clavicle. J Bone Joint Surg 46B:705–707, 1964.
201. Jay GR, and Monnet JC: The Bosworth screw in acute dislocations of the acromioclavicular joint. Presented at Clinical Conference, University of Oklahoma Medical Center, April 1969.
202. Johnston TB, Davies DV, and Davies F (eds.): Gray's Anatomy, 32nd ed. London: Longmans, Green, and Co., 1958.
203. Jones R: Injuries of Joints. London: Henry Frowde, Hodder & Stoughton, 1917, pp. 56–58.
204. Kaiser W, Ziemer G, and Heymann H: [Treatment of acro-

mioclavicular luxations with the Balser hookplate and ligament suture.] Chururg 55(11):721–724, 1984.

205. Kappakas GS, and McMaster JH: Repair of acromioclavicular separation using a Dacron prosthesis graft. Clin Orthop 131:247–251, 1978.

206. Karlsson J, Arnarson H, and Sigurjonsson K: Acromioclavicular dislocations treated by coracoacromial ligament transfer. Arch Orthop Trauma Surg 106(1):8–11, 1986.

207. Katznelson A, Nerubay J, and Oliver S: Dynamic fixation of the avulsed clavicle. J Trauma 16(10):841–844, 1976.

208. Kawabe N, Watanabe R, and Sato M: Treatment of complete acromioclavicular separation by coracoacromial ligament transfer. Clin Orthop 185:222–227, 1984.

209. Kennedy JC, and Cameron H: Complete dislocation of the acromioclavicular joint. J Bone Joint Surg 36B(2):202–208, 1954.

210. Kennedy JC: Complete dislocation of the acromioclavicular joint: 14 years later. J Trauma 8(3):311–318, 1968.

211. Kery L, and Wouters HW: Massive osteolysis. J Bone Joint Surg 52B:452, 1970.

212. Kessel L: Clinical Disorders of the Shoulder. London: Churchill Livingstone, 1982.

213. Key JA, and Conwell HE: The Management of Fractures, Dislocations, and Sprains, 3rd ed. St. Louis: CV Mosby Company, 1942.

214. Kiefer H, Claes L, Burri C, and Holzworth J: The stabilizing effect of various implants on the torn acromioclavicular joint: a biomechanical study. Arch Orthop Trauma Surg 106(1):42–46, 1986.

215. Kleinfeld F, and Pemsel W: [Primary ligament replacement with autologous corium in the surgical treatment of acromioclavicular joint injuries.] Aktuel Traumatol 10(1):15–21, 1980.

216. Kolesnikon IuP, and Dubrovich GM: [Treatment of dislocation of the acromial end of the clavicle.] Orthop Travmatol Protez 12:41–42, 1986.

217. Krawczyk E: [Reposition-reconstruction in dislocations of acromioclavicular joints.] Chir Narzadow Ruchu Ortop Pol 49(4):335–338, 1984.

218. Krawzak HW, Lindecken KD, Gütgemann U, and Schlenkhoff D: [Surgical treatment of acromioclavicular separation, using Balser's hookplate.] Zentralbl Chir 111(24):1509–1514, 1986.

219. Kurock W, and Sennerich Th: Injuries of the acromioclavicular joint in sport (abstr). Int J Sports Med 8:127, 1987.

220. Lagier R: [Anatomico-radiological study of an ununited intracapsular fracture of the femoral neck dating back 47 years: data relevant to osteoarthritis, bone infarct, and Paget's disease of the bone. Arch Orthop Trauma Surg 104:155–160, 1985.

221. Laing PG: Transplantation of the long head of the biceps in complete acromioclavicular separations (Proceedings). J Bone Joint Surg 51A(8):1677–1678, 1969.

222. Lamont MK: Letter to the editor re "Osteolysis of the outer end of the clavicle." NZ Med J 95:241–242, 1982.

223. Lancaster S, Horowitz M, and Alonso J: Complete acromioclavicular separations: a comparison of operative methods. Clin Orthop 216:80–88, 1987.

224. Lancourt JE: Acromioclavicular dislocation with adjacent clavicular fracture (report of a case with a method of repair). Personal communication, 1985.

225. Landoff GA: Une Bisher Nicht Beschriebene Schadigung am Processus Coracoideus. Acta Chir Scand 89:401, 1943–44.

226. Larsen E, Bjerg-Nielsen A, and Christensen P: Conservative or surgical treatment of acromioclavicular dislocation: a prospective, controlled, randomized study. J Bone Joint Surg 68A(4):552–555, 1986.

227. Larsen E, and Petersen V: Operative treatment of chronic acromioclavicular dislocation. Injury 18(1):55–56, 1987.

228. Lasda NA, and Murray DG: Fracture separation of the coracoid process associated with acromioclavicular dislocation: conservative treatment—a case report and review of the literature. Clin Orthop 134:222–224, 1978.

229. Lasher WW: Cartilage injuries: a clinical study. Am J Surg 6:493–500, 1929.

230. Lazcano MA, Anzel SH, and Kelly PJ: Complete dislocation and subluxation of the acromioclavicular joint: end result in seventy-three cases. J Bone Joint Surg 43A(3):379–391, 1961.

231. Lei MX, Liu H, and Yang KH: [Coracoclavicular ligamentplasty in the treatment of acromioclavicular dislocation.] Chung Hua Wai Ko Tsa Chih 25(2):70–71, 124, 1987.

232. LeNoir JL: Treatment of acromioclavicular separation. Iowa Orthop J 4:69–71, 1984.

233. Levine AH, Pais MJ, and Schwartz EE: Posttraumatic osteolysis of the distal clavicle with emphasis on early radiologic changes. AJR 127:781–784, 1976.

234. Liberson F: The role of the coracoclavicular ligaments in affections of the shoulder girdle. Am J Surg 44(1):145–157, 1939.

235. Lindsey RW, and Gutowski WT: The migration of a broken pin following fixation of the acromioclavicular joint: a case report and review of the literature. Orthopedics 9(3):413–416, 1986.

236. Linke R, and Moschinski D: [Combined method of operative treatment of ruptures of the acromioclavicular joint.] Unfallheilkunde 87:223–225, 1984.

237. Litton LO, and Peltier LR: Athletic Injuries. Boston: Little, Brown, 1963.

238. Lowe GP, and Fogarty MJP: Acute acromioclavicular joint dislocation: results of operative treatment with the Bosworth screw. Aust NZ J Surg 47(5):664–667, 1977.

239. Lucas DB: Biomechanics of the shoulder joint. Arch Surg 107:425–432, 1973.

240. Lugger LJ, Gaber O, and Klima G: Structure and suitability of the coracoacromial ligament for the band transfer treating delayed acromioclavicular luxation (abstr). Langenbecks Arch Chir 366:718, 1985.

241. Müller HW, and Schilling H: [Importance of traction-wiring osteosynthesis as dynamic stabilization after acromioclavicular joint dislocation: a critical view.] Aktuel Traumatol 16(3):94–96, 1986.

242. Macey HB: Separation of acromioclavicular joint: report of a case. Proc Staff Meet Mayo Clin 11:683–684, 1936.

243. Madsen B: Osteolysis of the acromial end of the clavicle following trauma. Br J Radiol 36(431):822, 1963.

244. Malcapi C, Grassi G, and Oretti D: Posterior dislocation of the acromioclavicular joint: a rare or an easily overlooked lesion? Ital J Orthop Traumatol 4:79–83, 1978.

245. Marcove RC, Wolfe SW, Healey JH, Huvos AG, et al.: Massive solitary tophus containing calcium pyrophosphate dihydrate crystals at the acromioclavicular joint. Clin Orthop 227:305–309, 1988.

246. Mazet RJ: Migration of a Kirschner wire from the shoulder region into the lung: report of two cases. J Bone Joint Surg 25A(2):477–483, 1943.

247. McCurrich HJ: Calcification of the bursa of the coracoclavicular ligament. Br J Surg 26:329–332, 1938.

248. McLaughlin HL: Trauma. Philadelphia: WB Saunders Company, 1959.

249. McLaughlin HL, and Cavallaro WU: Primary anterior dislocation of the shoulder. Am J Surg 80:615–621, 1950.

250. McLaughlin HL: On the frozen shoulder. Bull Hosp Jt Dis Orthop Inst 12:383–393, 1951.

251. McLaughlin HL: Rupture of the rotator cuff. J Bone Joint Surg 44A(5):979–983, 1962.

252. McMurray TP: A Practice of Orthopaedic Surgery. Baltimore: William Wood, 1937.

253. McNealy RW: Dislocations and fracture-dislocations occurring at the acromioclavicular articulation. Illinois Med J 41:202–205, 1922.

254. McPhee IB: Inferior dislocation of the outer end of the clavicle. J Trauma 20(8):709–710, 1980.

255. McPherson J, Black J, and Reed MH: Traumatic 'pseudodislocation' of the acromioclavicular joint in children. J Bone Joint Surg 69B(3):507, 1987.

256. Meixner J: [Dislocations and juxtaarticular fractures of the acromioclavicular joint in childhood.] Zentralbl Chir 108:793–797, 1983.

257. Meyerding HW: The treatment of acromioclavicular dislocations. Surg Clin North Am *17*:1199–1205, 1937.
258. Michele AA: New treatment of acromioclavicular dislocation. Clin Orthop *63*:245, 1969.
259. Mikhelson ER, and Chaika IA: [Surgical treatment of dislocations of the acromial end of the clavicle.] Ortop Travmatol Protez *6*:42–43, 1987.
260. Mikusev IE, Zainulli RV, and Skvortso AP: [Treatment of dislocations of the acromial end of the clavicle.] Vestn Khir *139*(8):69–71, 1987.
261. Millbourn E: On injuries to the acromioclavicular joint: treatment and results. Acta Orthop Scand *19*:349–382, 1950.
262. Mitchell AB: Dislocation of outer end of clavicle. Br Med J *2*:1097, 1926.
263. Moffat BM: Separation of the acromioclavicular joint. Surg Gynecol Obstet *41*:73–74, 1925.
264. Moneim MS, and Balduini FC: Coracoid fractures as a complication of surgical treatment by coracoclavicular tape fixation. Clin Orthop *168*:133–135, 1982.
265. Montgomery SP, and Loyd RD: Avulsion fracture of the coracoid epiphysis with acromioclavicular separation. J Bone Joint Surg *59A*(7):963–965, 1977.
266. Moravec O, Lexa C, Sykora F, and Sedivy J: [Dynamic stabilization of acromioclavicular luxation.] Acta Chir Orthop Traumatol Cech *53*(3):225–227, 1986.
267. Mordeja J: Die Posttraumatische Osteolyse des Lat. Schlusselbeinendes. Arch Orthop Unfallchirurg *49*:289, 1957.
268. Morisi M, and Ferrabosch P: Treatment of acromioclavicular dislocation with percutaneous synthesis of the axis. Arch Orthop *68*:1148–1156, 1955.
269. Morrison GM: Cast of acromioclavicular dislocation. J Bone Joint Surg *39A*:238–239, 1948.
270. Moschinski D, Linke R, and Drüke V: [Surgery of acute dislocation of the acromioclavicular joint using a resorbable implant.] Aktuel Chir *22*(5):183–186, 1987.
271. Moseley HF, and Templeton J: Dislocation of acromioclavicular joint (Proceedings). J Bone Joint Surg *51B*:196, 1969.
272. Moseley HF: Athletic injuries to the shoulder region. Am J Surg *98*:401–422, 1959.
273. Moseley HF: Shoulder Lesions, 2nd ed. New York: Paul Hoeber, 1953.
274. Moshein J, and Elconin KB: Repair of acute acromioclavicular dislocation, utilizing the coracoacromial ligament (Proceedings). J Bone Joint Surg *51A*:812, 1969.
275. Mumford EB: Acromioclavicular dislocation. J Bone Joint Surg *23*:799–802, 1941.
276. Murphy OB, Bellamy R, Wheeler W, and Brower TD: Posttraumatic osteolysis of the distal clavicle. Clin Orthop *109*:108–114, 1975.
277. Murray G: Fixation of dislocations of the acromioclavicular joint and rupture of the coracoclavicular ligament. Can Med Assoc J *43*:270–273, 1940.
278. Murray G: The use of longitudinal wires in the treatment of fractures and dislocations. Am J Surg *67*:156–167, 1945.
279. Naumann Th: [The rare case of habitual lateral dislocation of the clavicle in dorsal subacromial direction: a case report.] Z Orthop *124*:34–35, 1986.
280. Nell W: Die Posttraumatische Osteolyse des Schlusselbeins und ihr Verlauf. Monatsschr Kinderheilkd *44*:151, 1953.
281. Nelson CL: Repair of acromio-clavicular separations with knitted Dacron graft. Clin Orthop *143*:289, 1979.
282. Neviaser JS: Acromioclavicular dislocation treated by transference of the coracoacromial ligament. Bull Hosp Jt Dis Orthop Int *12*(1):46–54, 1951.
283. Neviaser JS: Acromioclavicular dislocation treated by transference of the coracoacromial ligament. Arch Surg *64*:292–297, 1952.
284. Neviaser JS: Acromioclavicular dislocation treated by transference of the coraco-acromial ligament: a long-term follow-up in a series of 112 cases. Clin Orthop *58*:57–68, 1968.
285. Neviaser JS: Complicated fractures and dislocations about the shoulder joint. J Bone Joint Surg *44A*(5):984–998, 1962.
286. Neviaser JS: Injuries of the clavicle and its articulations. Orthop Clin North Am *11*(2):233–237, 1980.
287. Nickel VL: Orthopedic Rehabilitation. London: Churchill Livingstone, 1982.
288. Nicoll EE: Annotation: miners and mannequins (editorial). J Bone Joint Surg *36B*(2):171–172, 1954.
289. Nielsen WB: Injury to the acromioclavicular joint (Proceedings). J Bone Joint Surg *45B*:207, 1963.
290. Nieminen S, and Aho AJ: Anterior dislocation of the acromioclavicular joint. Ann Chir Gynaecol *73*(1):21–24, 1984.
291. Norfray JF, Tremaine MJ, Groves HC, and Bachman DC: The clavicle in hockey. Am J Sports Med *5*:275–280, 1977.
292. Norfray JF: Bone resorption of the distal clavicle. JAMA *241*(18):1922–1934, 1979.
293. Norrell H, and Llewellyn RC: Migration of a threaded Steinmann pin from an acromioclavicular joint into the spinal canal: a case report. J Bone Joint Surg *47A*:1024–1026, 1965.
294. Nutter PD: Coracoclavicular articulations. J Bone Joint Surg *23*(1):177–179, 1941.
295. Nygaard ØP, and Reikeras O: [Acromionectomy in chronic shoulder pain.] Tidsskr Nor Laegeforen *107*(6):560–561, 1987.
296. O'Carroll PF, and Sheehan JM: Open reduction and percutaneous Kirschner wire fixation in complete disruption of the acromioclavicular joint. Injury *13*:299–301, 1982.
297. O'Donoghue DH: Treatment of Injuries to Athletes. Philadelphia: WB Saunders Company, 1970.
298. Odelberg A: Operative method for dislocation of the acromioclavicular joint. Acta Chir Scand *98*:507–510, 1949.
299. Oh WH: Anterior subluxation of the distal clavicle. Orthop Clin North Am *11*(4):813–818, 1980.
300. Olsson D: Degenerative changes of the shoulder joint and their connection with shoulder pain. Acta Chir Scand [Suppl] *181*:1–130, 1953.
301. Orava S, Virtanen K, and Holopainen YVO: Posttraumatic osteolysis of the distal ends of the clavicle. Ann Chir Gynaecol *73*:83–86, 1984.
302. Orofinio CS, and Stein AH Jr: Operative treatment for recent and complete tears of the acromioclavicular ligaments. Am J Surg *85*:760–763, 1953.
303. Paavolainen P, Björkenheim JM, Paukku P, and Slätis P: Surgical treatment of acromioclavicular dislocation: a review of 39 patients. Injury *14*:415–420, 1983.
304. Park JP, Arnold JA, Coker TP, Harris WD, et al.: Treatment of acromioclavicular separations: a retrospective study. Am J Sports Med *8*(4):251–256, 1980.
305. Paton DF: Complete acromioclavicular dislocation treated by transfer of the origin of coracobrachialis and short head of biceps to the clavicle. J Bone Joint Surg *62B*:117, 1980.
306. Patterson WR: Inferior dislocation of the distal end of the clavicle. J Bone Joint Surg *49A*:1184–1186, 1967.
307. Pearson GR: Radiographic technic for acromioclavicular dislocation. Radiology *27*:239, 1936.
308. Petersson CJ, and Redlund-Johnell I: Radiographic joint space in normal acromioclavicular joints. Acta Orthop Scand *54*:431–433, 1983.
309. Petersson CJ, and Gentz CF: The significance of distally pointing acromioclavicular osteophytes in ruptures of the supraspinatus tendon. Acta Orthop Scand *54*(3):490–491, 1983.
310. Petersson CJ: Degeneration of the acromioclavicular joint: a morphological study. Acta Orthop Scand *54*:434–438, 1983.
311. Petersson CJ: Resection of the lateral end of the clavicle: a 3 to 30-year follow-up. Acta Orthop Scand *54*:904–907, 1983.
312. Petersson CJ: The acromioclavicular joint in rheumatoid arthritis. Clin Orthop *223*:86–93, 1987.
313. Phemister DB: The treatment of dislocation of the acromioclavicular joint by open reduction and threaded-wire fixation. J Bone Joint Surg *24*(1):166–168, 1942.
314. Pilcher M: Dislocation of the acromial end of the clavicle (Proceedings). NY State J Med *43*:419–420, 1886.
315. Pillay VK: Significance of the coracoclavicular joint (Proceedings). J Bone Joint Surg *49B*:390, 1967.
316. Piterman L: Sports medicine quiz: "the dropped shoulder." Aust Fam Physician *11*(6):469, 1982.

317. Podgorski MR, Ibels LS, and Webb J: Case report 445: diagnosis—bilateral acromioclavicular gouty arthritis with pseudo-tumor of the outer end of the right clavicle: saturnine gout. Skeletal Radiol *16*:589–591, 1987.

318. Poigenfürst J: The infraclavicular soft tissue ossification following the tearing of the shoulder joint. Personal communication re article in Acta Med Austriaca *11(1)*:A16, 1984.

319. Poirier P, and Rieffel H: Mechanisme des luxations sur acromiales de la clavicule. Arch Gen Med *1*:396–422, 1891.

320. Post M: Current concepts in the diagnosis and management of acromioclavicular dislocations. Clin Orthop *200*:234–247, 1985.

321. Post M: The Shoulder. Philadelphia: Lea & Febiger, 1978.

322. Powers JA, and Bach PJ: Acromioclavicular separations—closed or open treatment. Clin Orthop *104*:213–223, 1974.

323. Pridie K: Dislocation of acromio-clavicular and sterno-clavicular joints (Proceedings). J Bone Joint Surg *41B(2)*:429, 1959.

324. Pritchett JW: Ossification of the coracoclavicular ligaments in ankylosing spondylitis: a case report. J Bone Joint Surg *65A(7)*:1017–1018, 1983.

325. Protass JJ, Stampfli FV, and Osmer JC: Coracoid process fracture diagnosis in acromioclavicular separation. Radiology *116*:61, 1975.

326. Pulles HJW: Operative treatment of acromio-clavicular dislocation (abstr). Acta Orthop Scand *55(4)*:483, 1984.

327. Quesada F: Technique for the roentgen diagnosis of fractures of the clavicle. Surg Gynecol Obstet *42*:424–428, 1926.

328. Quigley TB, and Banks H: Progress in the Treatment of Fractures and Dislocations. Philadelphia: WB Saunders Company, 1960.

329. Quigley TB: Correspondence. N Engl J Med *241*:431, 1949.

330. Quigley TB: Injuries to the acromioclavicular and sternoclavicular joints sustained in athletics. Surg Clin North Am *43*:1551–1554, 1963.

331. Rüegger R, Bleuler P, and Fehr JL: [Primary surgical treatment of fresh acromioclavicular dislocation (Tossy III): results of treatment in 50 patients.] Helv Chir Acta *54(4)*:425–429, 1987.

332. Rauschning W, Nordesjö LO, Nordgren B, Sahlstedt B, et al.: Resection arthroplasty for repair of complete acromioclavicular separations. Arch Orthop Traumatol Surg *97*:161–164, 1980.

333. Rawlings G: Acromioclavicular dislocations and fractures of the clavicle. A simple method of support. Lancet *2*:789, 1939.

334. Retief PJ, and Meintjes FA: Migration of a Kirschner wire in the body—a case report. S Afr Med J *53*:557–558, 1978.

335. Richards RR, Herzenberg JE, and Goldner JL: Bilateral nontraumatic anterior acromioclavicular joint dislocation: a case report. Clin Orthop *209*:255–258, 1986.

336. Richardson WF: "Acromion" in ancient Greek medical writers. Med History *20(1)*:52–58, 1976.

337. Richter R, Hahn H, Naaubling W, and Kohler G: [Tuberculosis of the shoulder girdle.] Z Rheumatol *44*:87–92, 1985.

338. Riddel J: Dislocation of the acromioclavicular joint. Br Med J *1*:697, 1926.

339. Roberts SM: Acromioclavicular dislocation: anatomical exposure of the outer end of the clavicle and the coracoid process. Am J Surg *23(2)*:322–324, 1934.

340. Rockwood CA Jr: Acromioclavicular dislocation. *In* Fractures, Vol. 1, 1st ed. Philadelphia: JB Lippincott Company, 1975, pp 721–756.

341. Rockwood CA Jr: Injuries to the acromioclavicular joint. In Fractures in Adults, Vol. 1, 2nd ed. Philadelphia: JB Lippincott Company, 1984, pp 860–910.

342. Rockwood CA Jr, Guy DK, and Griffin JL: Treatment of chronic, complete acromioclavicular dislocation. Orthop Trans *12(3)*:735, 1988.

343. Rodnan GP (ed.): Primer on the rheumatic diseases. JAMA *224(5)*:662–749, 1973.

344. Roper BA, and Levack B: The surgical treatment of acromioclavicular dislocations. J Bone Joint Surg *64B(5)*:597–599, 1982.

345. Rosenørn M, and Pedersen EB: A comparison between conservative and operative treatment of acute acromioclavicular dislocation. Acta Orthop Scand *45*:50–59, 1974.

346. Rosenørn M, and Pedersen EB: The significance of the coracoclavicular ligament in experimental dislocation of the acromioclavicular joint. Acta Orthop Scand *45*:346–358, 1974.

347. Rounds RC: Isolated fracture of the coracoid process. J Bone Joint Surg *31A*:662, 1949.

348. Rowe CR: Symposium on surgical lesions of the shoulder: acute and recurrent dislocation of the shoulder. J Bone Joint Surg *44A*:977–1012, 1962.

349. Rowe MJ: Nylon bone suture. Surgery *18*:764–768, 1945.

350. Roy SP: The nature and frequency of rugby injuries: a pilot study of 300 injuries at Stellenbosch. S Afr Med J *48*:2341, 1974.

351. Ryan AJ: Medical Care of the Athlete. New York: McGraw-Hill, 1962.

352. Søndergard-Petersen P, and Mikkelsen P: Posterior acromioclavicular dislocation. J Bone Joint Surg *64B(1)*:52–53, 1982.

353. Sage FP, and Salvatore JE: Injuries of acromioclavicular joint: study of results in 96 patients. South Med J *56*:486–495, 1963.

354. Sage J: Recurrent inferior dislocation of the clavicle at the acromioclavicular joint. Am J Sports Med *10(3)*:145–146, 1982.

355. Sage MR, and Allen PW: Massive osteolysis. J Bone Joint Surg *56B*:130, 1974.

356. Salter EG, Nasca RJ, and Shelley BS: Anatomical observations on the acromioclavicular joint and supporting ligaments. Am J Sports Med *15(3)*:199–206, 1987.

357. Salter EG, Shelley BS, and Nasca R: A morphological study of the acromioclavicular joint in humans (abstr). Anat Rec *211(3)*:353, 1985.

358. Sandrock AR: Another sports fatigue fracture: stress fracture of the coracoid process of the scapula. Radiology *117*:274, 1975.

359. Saranglia D, Julliard R, Marcone L, and Butel J: [The results of the modified Cadenat procedure in old acromioclavicular dislocations: 26 cases.] Rev Chir Orthop *73*:187–190, 1987.

360. Schildhaus AIE, and Meyers WJ: Stabilization of the clavicle in acromioclavicular separation. Orthop Rev *16(3)*:85–87, 1987.

361. Schindler A, Schmid JP, and Heyse C: [Hookplate fixation for repair of acute complete acromioclavicular separation: review of 41 patients.] Unfallchirurg *88(12)*:533–540, 1985.

362. Schneider CC: Acromioclavicular dislocation: autoplastic reconstruction. J Bone Joint Surg *15*:957–962, 1933.

363. Schneppendahl G, and Ludolph E: [Posttraumatic chronic instability of the shoulder joint.] Unfallchirurgie *13(1)*:19–21, 1987.

364. Schwarz B, and Heisel J: [Causes, treatment and results of surgery of fresh and old breaks of the acromioclavicular joint. Aktuel Traumatol *16*:97–109, 1986.

365. Schwarz N, and Leixnering M: [Results of nonreduced acromioclavicular Tossy III separations.] Unfallchirurg *89*:248–252, 1986.

366. Schwarz von B, and Heisel J: [Late results of inveterate cleavages of the acromioclavicular joint.] Orthop Praxis *3*:159–168, 1986.

367. Scott JC, and Orr MM: Injuries to the acromioclavicular joint. Injury *5*:13–18, 1973.

368. Seddon HJ: Nerve lesions complicating certain closed bone injuries. JAMA *135*:691–694, 1947.

369. Sethi GK, and Scott SM: Subclavian artery laceration due to migration of a Hagie pin. Surgery *80(5)*:644–646, 1976.

370. Seymour EQ: Osteolysis of the clavicular top associated with repeated minor trauma to the shoulder. Radiology *123(1)*:56, 1977.

371. Shaar CM: Upward dislocation of acromial end of clavicle: treatment by elastic traction splint. JAMA *92(23)*:2083–2085, 1929.

372. Shands AR Jr: An analysis of the more important orthopaedic information. Surgery *16*:569–616, 1944.

373. Shands AR Jr: Handbook of Orthopaedic Surgery, 2nd ed. St. Louis: CV Mosby Company, 1940.

374. Shoji H, Roth C, and Chuinard R: Bone block transfer of coracoacromial ligament in acromioclavicular injury. Clin Orthop *208*:272–277, 1986.

375. Siegling CW, and Jahn K: [Dislocation of the acromio-clavicular joint. Results of surgical treatment.] Zentralbl Chir *107(14)*:858–862, 1982.

376. Silloway KA, McLaughlin RE, Edlich RC, and Edlich RF: Clavicular fractures and acromioclavicular joint dislocations in lacrosse: preventable injuries. J Emerg Med 3:117–121, 1985.

377. Simeone L: Le lussazioni acromio-claveari: il cerchiaggio dinamico. Minerva Ortopedica 36(11):805–812, 1985.

378. Simmons EH, and Martin RF: Acute dislocation of the acromioclavicular joint. Can J Surg 11:479, 1968.

379. Simmons EH, and Roscoe MWA: The treatment of complete acromioclavicular dislocation (abstr). J Trauma 23(7):664, 1983.

380. Sleeswijk Visser SV, Haarsma SM, and Speeckaert MTC: Conservative treatment of acromioclavicular dislocation: Jones strap versus mitella (abstr). Acta Orthop Scand 55(4):483, 1984.

381. Smart MJ: Traumatic osteolysis of the distal ends of the clavicles. J Can Assoc Radiol 23:264–266, 1972.

382. Smith DW: Coracoid fracture associated with acromioclavicular dislocation. Clin Orthop 108:165, 1975.

383. Smith MJ, and Stewart MJ: Acute acromioclavicular separations. Am J Sports Med 7(1):62–71, 1979.

384. Sonnabend DH, and Faithfull DK: Operative repair of acromioclavicular dislocation (abstr). J Bone Joint Surg 66B(5):789, 1984.

385. Soule AB Jr: Ossification of the coracoclavicular ligament following dislocation of the acromioclavicular articulation. AJR 56(5):607–615, 1946.

386. Southmayd WW, Scheller AD, and Tesner RJ: Surgical treatment of grade III acromioclavicular separations. Sports Med Clin 2(3):1–3, 7, 1985.

387. Speed K: A Textbook of Fractures and Dislocations, 4th ed. Philadelphia: Lea & Febiger, 1942.

388. Spigelman L: A harness for acromioclavicular separation. J Bone Joint Surg 51A(3):585–586, 1969.

389. Stahl F: Considerations on post-traumatic absorption of the outer end of the clavicle. Acta Orthop Scand 23:9, 1954.

390. Stephens HEG: Stuck nail fixation for acute dislocation of the acromio-clavicular joint. J Bone Joint Surg 51B(1):197, 1969.

391. Stewart R: Acute acromioclavicular joint dislocation: internal fixation of the clavicle and coracoid process of the scapula with a vitallium screw. Minn Med 29:357–360, 1946.

392. Stimson LA: Fracture and Dislocations. Philadelphia: Lea & Febiger, 1941.

393. Strauch W: Posttraumatische Osteolysen des Lateralen Klavikulaendes. Radiol Diagn 11:221–229, 1970.

394. Stubbins SG, and McGaw WH: Suspension cast for acromio-clavicular separations and clavicle fractures. JAMA 169(7):672–675, 1959.

395. Taft TN, Wilson FC, and Oglesby JW: Dislocation of the acromioclavicular joint: an end-result study. J Bone Joint Surg 69A(7):1045–1051, 1987.

396. Taga I, Yondea M, and Ono K: Epiphyseal separation of the coracoid process associated with acromioclavicular sprain: a case report and review of the literature. Clin Orthop 207:138–141, 1986.

397. Tagliabue D, and Riva A: La cleidopessi coraco-claveare nella lussazione acromion-claveare. Minerva Ortop 36(11):817–23, 1985.

398. Tagliabue D, and Riva A: [Current approaches to the treatment of acromioclavicular joint separation in athletes.] Ital J Sports Traumatol 3(1):15–24, 1981.

399. Taylor GM, and Tooke M: Degeneration of the acromioclavicular joint as a cause of shoulder pain. J Bone Joint Surg 59B:507, 1977.

400. Thiemeyer JS Jr: Method of repair of symptomatic chronic acromioclavicular dislocation. Ann Surg 140(1):75–85, 1954.

401. Thorndike A Jr, and Quigley TB: Injuries to the acromioclavicular joint: a plea for conservative treatment. Am J Surg 55:250–261, 1942.

402. Thorndike A: Athletic Injuries. Philadelphia: Lea & Febiger, 1956.

403. Tossy JD, Mead NC, and Sigmond HM: Acromioclavicular separations: useful and practical classification for treatment. Clin Orthop 28:111–119, 1963.

404. Toumey JW: Surgery of the acromioclavicular joint. Surg Clin North Am 29:905–912, 1949.

405. Trynin AH: Conservative treatment for complete dislocation of the acromioclavicular joint. J Bone Joint Surg 16(1):713–715, 1934.

406. Tucker WE, and Armstrong JR: Injury in Sport. Springfield IL: Charles C Thomas, 1964.

407. Twigg HL, and Rosenbaum RC: Duplication on the clavicle. Skeletal Radiol 6(4):281, 1981.

408. Tyler GT: Acromioclavicular dislocation fixed by a vitallium screw through the joint. Am J Surg 58:245–247, 1942.

409. Tyurina TV: [Age-related characteristics of the human acromioclavicular joint.] Arkh Anat Gistol Embriol 89(11):75–81, 1985.

410. Urban J, and Jaskiewicz A: [Idiopathic displacement of Kirschner wire to the thoracic cavity after the osteosynthesis of acromioclavicular joint.] Chir Narzadow Ruchu Ortop Pol 49(4):399–402, 1984.

411. Urist MR: Complete dislocation of the acromioclavicular joint: the nature of the traumatic lesion and effective methods of treatment with an analysis of 41 cases. J Bone Joint Surg 28:813–837, 1946.

412. Urist MR: Complete dislocation of the acromioclavicular joint (follow-up notes). J Bone Joint Surg 45A:1750–1753, 1963.

413. Urist MR: The treatment of dislocation of the acromioclavicular joint. Am J Surg 98:423–431, 1959.

414. Usadel G: Zur Behandlung der Luxatio claviculae supraacromialis. Arch Klin Chir 200:621–626, 1940.

415. Vainionpää S, Kirves P, and Laike E: Acromioclavicular joint dislocation—surgical results in 36 patients. Ann Chir Gynaecol 70:120–123, 1981.

416. van der Werf GGIM, and Tonino AJ: Dacron as ligament graft in the treatment of acromioclavicular dislocation (abstr). Acta Orthop Scand 55(4):484, 1984.

417. Vandekerckhove B, Van Meirhaeghe J, Van Steenkiste M, De Groote, W, et al.: Surgical treatment of acromioclavicular dislocations: long-term follow-up study. Acta Orthop Belg 51(1):66–79, 1985.

418. Vargas L: Repair of complete acromioclavicular dislocation, utilizing the short head of the biceps. J Bone Joint Surg 24(4):772–773, 1942.

419. Varney JH, Coker JK, and Cawley JJ: Treatment of acromioclavicular dislocation by means of a harness. J Bone Joint Surg 34A(1):232–233, 1952.

420. Viehweger G: Die Posttraumatische Claviculaosteolyse. Chirurg 30:313, 1959.

421. Vogel H, Thomä J, and Jungbluth KH: [Plain film diagnosis of the acromioclavicular dislocation.] Röntgen 33:564–570, 1980.

422. Wagner C: Partial claviculectomy. Am J Surg 85:259–265, 1953.

423. Wakeley CPG: Stabilization of the acromioclavicular joint. Lancet 2:708–710, 1935.

424. Waldrop JI, Norwood LA, and Alvarez RG: Lateral roentgenographic projections of the acromioclavicular joint. Am J Sports Med 9(5):337–341, 1981.

425. Walsh WM, Peterson DA, Shelton G, and Newmann RD: Shoulder strength following acromioclavicular injury. Am J Sports Med 13(3):153–158, 1985.

426. Warner AH: A harness for use in the treatment of acromioclavicular separation. J Bone Joint Surg 19(4):1132–1133, 1937.

427. Warren-Smith CD, and Ward MW: Operation for acromioclavicular dislocation: a review of 29 cases treated by one method. J Bone Joint Surg 69B(5):715–718, 1987.

428. Wasylenko MJ, and Busse EF: Posterior dislocation of the clavicle causing fatal tracheoesophageal fistula. Can Med J 24(6):626–627, 1981.

429. Watkins JT: An operation for the relief of acromio-clavicular luxations. J Bone Joint Surg 7:790–792, 1925.

430. Watson-Jones R: Fractures and Joint Injuries, Vol. II, 4th ed. Baltimore: Williams & Wilkins, 1956.

431. Watson-Jones R: Fractures and Joint Injuries. London: Churchill Livingstone, 1982.

432. Waxman J: Acromioclavicular disease in rheumatologic practice—the forgotten joint. J La State Med Soc *129*(1):1–3, 1977.
433. Weaver JK, and Dunn HK: Treatment of acromioclavicular injuries, especially complete acromioclavicular separation. J Bone Joint Surg *54A*(6):1187–1197, 1972.
434. Weitzman G: Treatment of acute acromioclavicular joint dislocation by a modified Bosworth method: report on twenty-four cases. J Bone Joint Surg *49A*(6):1167–1178, 1967.
435. Wenner SM: Dislocation of the acromioclavicular joint: a review of the literature and a pathologic series of thirteen joint dissections. Orthop Rev *3*(7):35–42, 1974.
436. Werder H: Posttraumatische Osteolyse des Schlusselbeinendes. Schweiz Med Wochenschr *80*:912, 1950.
437. Wertheimer LG: Coracoclavicular joint: surgical treatment of a painful syndrome caused by an anomalous joint. J Bone Joint Surg *30A*(3):570–578, 1948.
438. Weston WJ: Arthrography of the acromio-clavicular joint. Aust Radiol *18*(2):213–214, 1974.
439. Weston WJ: Erosions of the acromion process of the scapula in rheumatoid arthritis. Aust Radiol *17*(2):219–220, 1973.
440. Wilber MC, and Evans EB: Fractures of the scapula. J Bone Joint Surg *59A*:358, 1977.
441. Wilson PD, and Cochrane WA: Immediate management, after care, and convalescent treatment, with special reference to the conservation and restoration of function. *In* Fractures and Dislocations. Philadelphia: JB Lippincott Company, 1925.
442. Wolff EF: Transposition of the biceps brachii tendon to repair luxation of the canine shoulder joint (review of a procedure). Vet Med/Small Anim Clin *69*:51–53, 1974.
443. Wolin I: Acute acromioclavicular dislocation: a simple effective method of conservative treatment. J Bone Joint Surg *26*(3):589–592, 1944.
444. Worchester JN, and Green DP: Osteoarthritis of the acromioclavicular joint. Clin Orthop *58*:69–73, 1968.
445. Zanca P: Shoulder pain: involvement of the acromioclavicular joint: analysis of 1,000 cases. AJR *112*(3):493–506, 1971.
446. Zaricznyj B: Injuries and treatment of the acromioclavicular joint. Orthop Rev *10*(4):41–51, 1981.
447. Zaricznyj B: Late reconstruction of the ligaments following acromioclavicular separation. J Bone Joint Surg *58A*(6):792–795, 1976.
448. Zaricznyj B: Reconstruction for chronic scapuloclavicular instability. Am J Sports Med *11*(1):17–25, 1983.
449. Zettas JP, and Muchnic PD: Fractures of the coracoid process base in acute acromioclavicular separation. Orthop Rev *5*:77, 1976.
450. Zimmerman LM, and Veith I: Great Ideas in the History of Surgery. Baltimore: Williams & Wilkins, 1961.
451. Zlotsky NA: Treatment of acromioclavicular separations in athletics. Conn Med *40*(1):15–17, 1976.
452. Zsernaviczky J, and Horst M: Kasuistischer Beitrag zur Osteolyse am Distalen Klavikulaende. Arch Orthop Unfallchirurg *89*:163–167, 1977.

Disorders of the Sternoclavicular Joint

Charles A. Rockwood, Jr., M.D.

Historical Review

A review of the early literature on this subject indicates that in the 19th century, dislocations of the sternoclavicular joint were managed essentially the same way as fractures of the medial clavicle.[57, 127] Sir Astley Cooper,[57] in his 1824 text, recommended that the injury be treated not only with a clavicle bandage but also with a sling "which through the medium of the os humeri and scapula supports it and prevents the clavicle from being drawn down by the weight of the arm."

Cooper reported that he had never seen an isolated traumatic posterior dislocation of the sternoclavicular joint but suggested that it might happen from excessive force.[57] However, he did describe a posterior dislocation of the sternoclavicular joint in a patient who had such a severe scoliosis that, as the scapula advanced laterally around the chest wall, it pushed the medial end of the clavicle behind the sternum. The patient finally developed so much pressure on the esophagus and had such difficulty swallowing that Davie, a surgeon in Suffolk, resected the medial end of the clavicle. He must have been an excellent surgeon, for in 1824 he resected one inch of the medial clavicle using a saw! He protected the vital structures in the area from the saw by introducing "a piece of well beaten sole leather under the bone whilst he divided it." The patient recovered and had no more problems with swallowing. This case probably represents the first resection of the medial end of the clavicle, either for trauma or for arthritis.

Rodrigues,[220] in 1843, may have published the first case of traumatic posterior dislocation of the sternoclavicular joint in the literature, "a case of dislocation inward of the internal extremity of the clavicle." The patient's left shoulder was against a wall when the right side of the chest and thorax were compressed and rolled forward almost to the midline by a cart. Immediately, the patient experienced shortness of breath, which persisted for three weeks. When first seen by the physician, he appeared to be suffocating and his face was blue. The left shoulder was swollen and painful, and there was "a depression on the left side of the superior extremity of the sternum." Pressure on the depression greatly increased the sensation of suffocation. Rodrigues observed that when the outer end of the shoulder was displaced backward, the inner end of the clavicle was displaced forward, which relieved the asphyxia. Therefore, treatment consisted of binding the left shoulder backward with a cushion between the two scapulae, but only after the patient had been bled twice within the first 24 hours. Rodrigues may have seen other cases of posterior dislocation, since he stated that the patient "retained a slight depression of the internal extremity of the clavicle; such, however, is the ordinary fate of the patients who present this form of dislocation."

In the late 19th century, a number of articles appeared from England, Germany, and France, and it was not until the 1930s that articles by Duggan,[69] Shafer,[119] and Lowman[156] appeared in the American literature.

Surgical Anatomy

The sternoclavicular joint is a diarthrodial type of joint and is the only true articulation between the clavicle of the upper extremity and the axial skeleton (Fig. 13–1). The articular surface of the clavicle is much larger than that of the sternum, and both are covered with fibrocartilage. The enlarged bulbous medial end of the clavicle is concave front to back and

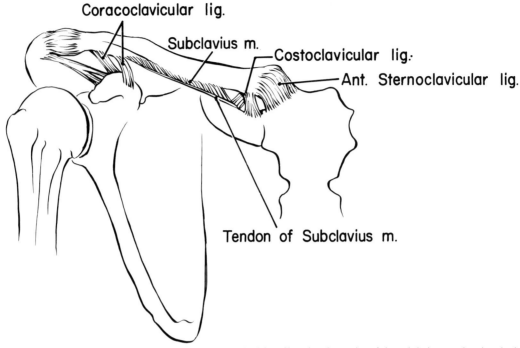

Figure 13–1. Normal anatomy around the sternoclavicular and acromioclavicular joints. Note that the tendon of the subclavius muscle arises in the vicinity of the costoclavicular ligament from the first rib and has a long tendon structure. (Reproduced with permission from Rockwood CA, and Green DP (eds): Fractures (3 vols), 2nd ed. Philadelphia: JB Lippincott, 1984.)

convex vertically and, therefore, creates a saddle-type joint with the clavicular notch of the sternum.[97, 98] The clavicular notch of the sternum is curved, and the joint surfaces are not congruent. Cave[47] has demonstrated that in 2.5 per cent of patients, on the inferior aspect of the medial clavicle there is a small facet which articulates with the superior aspect of the first rib at its synchondral junction with the sternum.

Because less than half of the medial clavicle articulates with the upper angle of the sternum, the sternoclavicular joint has the distinction of having the least amount of bony stability of the major joints of the body. Grant[97] remarks, "The two (make) an ill fit." If a finger is placed in the superior sternal notch, one can feel that, with motion of the upper extremity, a large part of the medial clavicle is completely above the articulation with the sternum.

LIGAMENTS OF THE STERNOCLAVICULAR JOINT

There is so much joint incongruity that the integrity has to come from its surrounding ligaments, i.e., the intra-articular disc ligament, the extra-articular costoclavicular ligament (rhomboid ligament), the capsular ligament, and the interclavicular ligament.

Intra-articular Disc Ligament

The intra-articular disc ligament is a very dense, fibrous structure that arises from the synchondral junction of the first rib to the sternum and passes through

the sternoclavicular joint, which divides the joint into two separate joint spaces (Fig. 13–2).[97, 98] The upper attachment is on the superior and posterior aspects of the medial clavicle. DePalma[66] has shown that the disc is perforated only rarely; the perforation allows a free

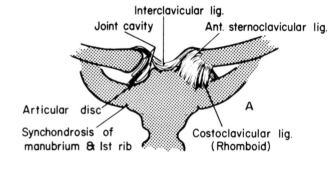

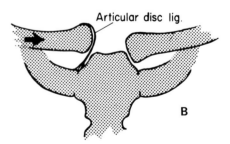

Figure 13–2. A, Normal anatomy around the sternoclavicular joint. Note that the articular disc ligament divides the sternoclavicular joint cavity into two separate spaces and inserts onto the superior and posterior aspects of the medial clavicle. B, The articular disc ligament acts as a checkrein for a medial displacement of the proximal clavicle.

communication between the two joint compartments. Anteriorly and posteriorly, the disc blends into the fibers of the capsular ligament. The disc acts as a checkrein against medial displacement of the inner clavicle (Fig. 13–2).

Costoclavicular Ligament

The costoclavicular ligament, also called the rhomboid ligament, is short and strong and consists of an anterior and a posterior fasciculus (see Fig. 13–1).[23, 47, 98] Cave[47] reports that the average length is 1.3 cm, with 1.9 cm maximum width, and it is 1.3 cm thick. Bearn[23] has shown that there is always a bursa between the two components of the ligament. Because of the two different parts of the ligament, it has a twisted appearance.[98] The costoclavicular ligament attaches below to the upper surface of the first rib and at the adjacent part of the synchondral junction with the sternum, and above to the margins of the impression on the inferior surface of the medial end of the clavicle, sometimes known as the rhomboid fossa.[97, 98] Cave[47] has shown, from a study of 153 clavicles, that the attachment of the costoclavicular ligament to the clavicle can be any of three types: (1) a depression, the rhomboid fossa (30 per cent); (2) flat (60 per cent); and (3) an elevation (10 per cent).

The fibers of the anterior fasciculus arise from the anterior medial surface of the first rib and are directed upward and laterally. The fibers of the posterior fasciculus are shorter and arise lateral to the anterior fibers on the rib and are directed upward and medially. The fibers of the anterior and posterior components cross and allow for stability of the joint during rotation and elevation of the clavicle. The two-part costoclavicular ligament is in many ways similar to the two-part configuration of the coracoclavicular ligament on the outer end of the clavicle.

Bearn[23] has shown experimentally that the anterior fibers resist excessive upward rotation of the clavicle and that the posterior fibers resist excessive downward rotation. Specifically, the anterior fibers also resist lateral displacement, and the posterior fibers resist medial displacement.

Interclavicular Ligament

The interclavicular ligament connects the superomedial aspects of each clavicle with the capsular ligaments and the upper sternum (see Fig. 13–2). According to Grant,[97] this band may be homologous with the wishbone of birds. This ligament assists the capsular ligaments to produce "shoulder poise," that is, to hold up the shoulder. This can be tested by putting a finger in the superior sternal notch; with elevation of the arm, the ligament is quite lax, but as soon as both arms hang at the sides, the ligament becomes tight.

Capsular Ligament

The capsular ligament covers the anterosuperior and posterior aspects of the joint and represents thickenings of the joint capsule (see Figs. 13–1 and 13–2). The anterior portion of the capsular ligament is heavier and stronger than the posterior portion.

According to the original work of Bearn,[23] this may be the strongest ligament of the sternoclavicular joint, and it is the first line of defense against the upward displacement of the inner clavicle caused by a downward force on the distal end of the shoulder. The clavicle attachment of the ligament is primarily onto the epiphysis of the medial clavicle, with some secondary blending of the fibers into the metaphysis. I have demonstrated this, as have Poland,[203] Denham and Dingley,[64] and Brooks and Henning.[36] Although some authors report that the intra-articular disc ligament greatly assists the costoclavicular ligament in preventing upward displacement of the medial clavicle, Bearn[23] has shown that the capsular ligament is the most important structure in preventing upward displacement of the medial clavicle. In experimental postmortem studies, he evaluated the strength and the role of each of the ligaments at the sternoclavicular joint to see which one would prevent a downward displacement of the outer clavicle. He attributed the lateral "poise of the shoulder" (i.e., the force that holds the shoulder up) to a locking mechanism of the ligaments of the sternoclavicular joint (Fig. 13–3). To accomplish his experiments, Bearn[23] dissected all the muscles attaching onto the clavicle, the sternum, and the first rib and left all the ligaments attached. He secured the sternum to a block in a vise. He then loaded the outer end of the clavicle with 10 to 20 pounds of weight and cut the ligaments of the sternoclavicular joint, one at a time and in various combinations, to determine each ligament's effect on maintaining the clavicle poise, that is, which ligament was most important in holding up the lateral end of the shoulder, or, thinking of it in another way, which ligament would rupture first when a force was applied to the outer end of the clavicle.

He determined, after cutting the costoclavicular, intra-articular disc, and interclavicular ligaments, that they had no effect on clavicle poise. However, the division of the capsular ligament alone resulted in a downward depression on the distal end of the clavicle. He also noted that the intra-articular disk ligament tore under 5 pounds of weight, once the capsular ligament had been cut. Bearn's article has many clinical implications for the mechanisms of injury of the sternoclavicular joint.

RANGE OF MOTION OF THE STERNOCLAVICULAR JOINT

The sternoclavicular joint is freely movable and functions almost like a ball-and-socket joint in that the joint has motion in almost all planes, including rotation.[123, 157] The clavicle, and therefore the sternoclavicular joint, in normal shoulder motion is capable of 30 to 35 degrees of upward elevation, 35 degrees of combined forward and backward movement, and 45 to 50 degrees of rotation around its long axis (Fig. 13–4).

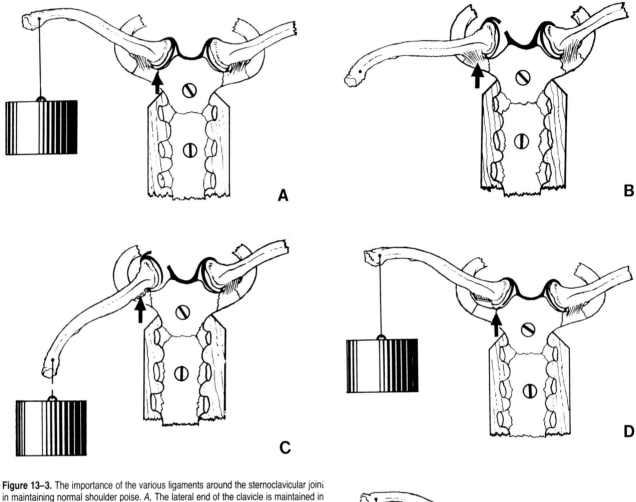

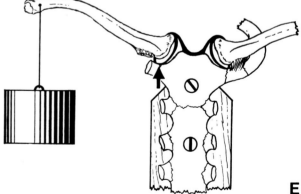

Figure 13–3. The importance of the various ligaments around the sternoclavicular joint in maintaining normal shoulder poise. *A,* The lateral end of the clavicle is maintained in an elevated position through the sternoclavicular ligaments. The *arrow* indicates the fulcrum. *B,* When the capsule is divided completely, the lateral end of the clavicle descends under its own weight without any loading. The clavicle will seem to be supported by the intra-articular disc ligament. *C,* After division of the capsular ligament, it was determined that a weight of less than 5 pounds was enough to tear the intra-articular disc ligament from its attachment on the costal cartilage junction of the first rib. The fulcrum was transferred laterally so that the medial end of the clavicle hinged over the first rib in the vicinity of the costoclavicular ligament. *D,* After division of the costoclavicular ligament and the intra-articular disc ligament, the lateral end of the clavicle could not be depressed, as long as the capsular ligament was intact. *E,* After resection of the medial first costal cartilage along with the costoclavicular ligament, there was no effect on the poise of the lateral end of the clavicle, as long as the capsular ligament was intact. (Reproduced with permission from Bearn JG: Direct observation on the function of the capsule of the sternoclavicular joint in clavicular support. J Anat *101:*159–170, 1967.)

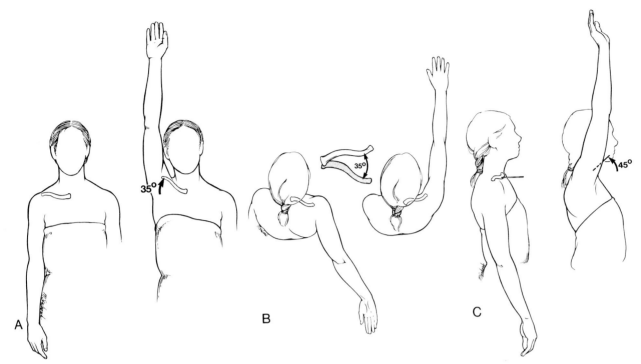

Figure 13–4. Motions of the clavicle and the sternoclavicular joint. *A,* With full overhead elevation the clavicle elevates 35 degrees. *B,* With adduction and extension the clavicle displaces anteriorly and posteriorly 35 degrees. *C,* The clavicle rotates on its long axis 45 degrees as the arm is elevated to the full overhead position.

Figure 13–5. Tomogram demonstrating the thin, waferlike disc of the epiphysis of the medial clavicle. (Reproduced with permission from Rockwood CA, and Green DP (eds): Fractures (3 vols), 2nd ed. Philadelphia: JB Lippincott, 1984.)

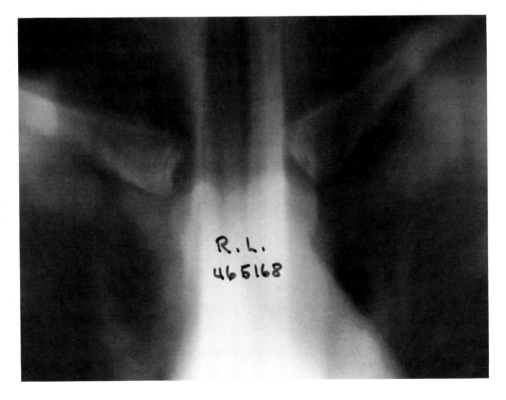

It is most likely the most frequently moved joint of the long bones in the body, because almost any motion of the upper extremity is transferred proximally to the sternoclavicular joint.

EPIPHYSIS OF THE MEDIAL CLAVICLE

Although the clavicle is the first long bone of the body to ossify (fifth intrauterine week), the epiphysis at the medial end of the clavicle is the last of the long bones in the body to appear and the last epiphysis to close (Fig. 13–5).[97, 98, 203] The medial clavicular epiphysis does not ossify until the 18th to 20th year, and it fuses with the shaft of the clavicle around the 23rd to 25th year.[97, 98, 203] Webb and Suchey,[259] in an extensive study of the physis of the medial clavicle in 605 males and 254 females at autopsy, reported that complete unions may not be present until 31 years of age. This knowledge of the epiphysis is important, because I believe that many of the so-called sternoclavicular dislocations are fractures through the physeal plate.

Posterior Dislocation of the Clavicle

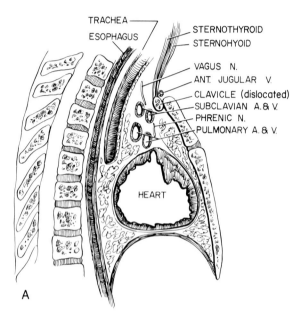

A

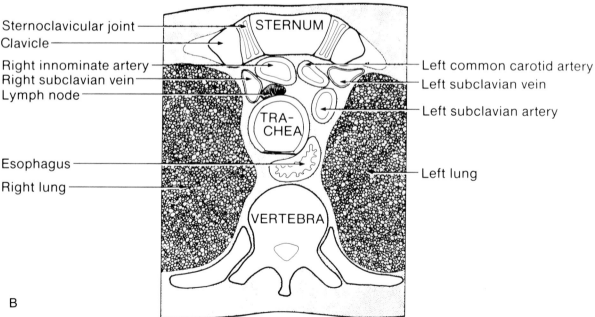

B

Figure 13–6. Applied anatomy of the vital structures posterior to the sternoclavicular joint. *A, B,* Sagittal views in cross-section demonstrating the structures posterior to the sternoclavicular joint.

APPLIED SURGICAL ANATOMY

The surgeon who is planning an operative procedure on or near the sternoclavicular joint should be completely knowledgeable about the vast array of anatomical structures immediately posterior to the sternoclavicular joint. There is a "curtain" of muscles, the sternohyoid, sternothyroid, and scaleni, which is posterior to the sternoclavicular joint and the inner third of the clavicle, and this curtain blocks the view of the vital structures. Some of these vital structures include the innominate artery, innominate vein, vagus nerve, phrenic nerve, internal jugular vein, trachea, and esophagus (Fig. 13–6). If one is considering the possibility of stabilizing the sternoclavicular joint by running a pin down from the clavicle and into the sternum, it is important to remember that the arch of the aorta, the superior vena cava, and the right pulmonary artery are also very close at hand.

Another structure to be aware of is the anterior jugular vein, which is between the clavicle and the curtain of muscles. The anatomy books state that it can be quite variable in size; I have seen it as large as 1.5 cm in diameter. This vein has no valves, and when it is nicked, it looks like someone has opened up the flood gates.

Mechanism of Injury

Because the sternoclavicular joint is subject to practically every motion of the upper extremity, and because the joint is so small and incongruous, one would think that it would be the most commonly dislocated joint in the body. However, the ligamentous supporting structure is so strong and so designed that it is one of the least commonly dislocated joints in the body. The

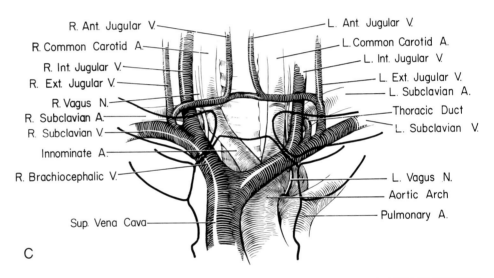

R. Ant. Jugular V.
R. Common Carotid A.
R. Int. Jugular V.
R. Ext. Jugular V.
R. Vagus N.
R. Subclavian A.
R. Subclavian V.
Innominate A.
R. Brachiocephalic V.
Sup. Vena Cava

L. Ant. Jugular V.
L. Common Carotid A.
L. Int. Jugular V.
L. Ext. Jugular V.
L. Subclavian A.
Thoracic Duct
L. Subclavian V.
L. Vagus N.
Aortic Arch
Pulmonary A.

C

Figure 13–6 *Continued. C,* A diagram demonstrates the close proximity of the major vessels that are posterior to the sternoclavicular joint. *D,* An aortogram showing the relationship of the medial end of the clavicle to the major vessels in the mediastinum. (*A* and *C* reproduced with permission from Rockwood CA, and Green DP (eds): Fractures (3 vols), 2nd ed. Philadelphia: JB Lippincott, 1984.)

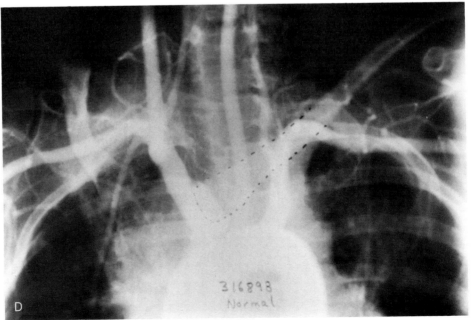

D

traumatic dislocation of the sternoclavicular joint usually occurs only after tremendous forces, either direct or indirect, have been applied to the shoulder.

DIRECT FORCE

When a force is applied directly to the anteromedial aspect of the clavicle, the clavicle is pushed posteriorly behind the sternum and into the mediastinum (Fig. 13–7). This may occur in a variety of ways: an athlete lying on his back on the ground is jumped on and the knee of the jumper lands directly on the medial end of the clavicle; a kick is delivered to the front of the medial clavicle; a person is run over by a vehicle; or a person is pinned between a vehicle and a wall. Because of our anatomy, it would be most unusual for a direct force to produce an anterior sternoclavicular dislocation.

INDIRECT FORCE

A force can be applied indirectly to the sternoclavicular joint from the anterolateral or posterolateral aspects of the shoulder. This is the most common mechanism of injury to the sternoclavicular joint. Mehta and coworkers[169] reported that three of four posterior sternoclavicular dislocations were produced by indirect force, and Heinig[110] reported that indirect force was responsible for eight of nine cases of posterior sternoclavicular dislocations. It was the most common mechanism of injury in our series of 168 patients. If the shoulder is compressed and rolled forward, an ipsilateral posterior dislocation results; if the shoulder is compressed and rolled backward, an ipsilateral anterior dislocation results (Fig. 13–8). One of the most common causes that I have seen is a pile-on in a football game. In this instance, a player falls on the ground, landing on the lateral shoulder; before he can get out of the way, several players pile on top of his opposite shoulder, which applies significant compressive force on the clavicle down toward the sternum. If, during the compression, the shoulder is rolled forward, the force directed down the clavicle produces a posterior dislocation of the sternoclavicular joint. If the shoulder is compressed and rolled backward, the force directed down the clavicle produces an anterior dislocation of the sternoclavicular joint. Other types of indirect forces that can produce sternoclavicular dislocation are a cave-in on a ditch digger, with lateral compression of the shoulders by the falling dirt; lateral compressive forces on the shoulder when a person is pinned between a vehicle and a wall; and a person's falling on the outstretched abducted arm, which drives the shoulder medially in the same manner as a lateral compression on the shoulder.

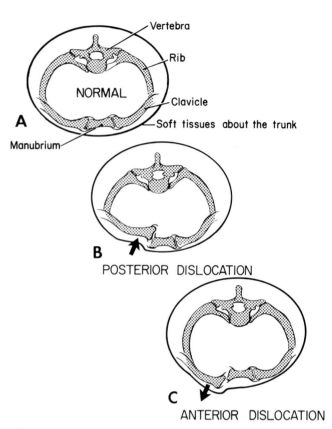

Figure 13–7. A cross-section through the thorax at the level of the sternoclavicular joint. A, Normal anatomical relations. B, Posterior dislocation of the sternoclavicular joint. C, Anterior dislocation of the sternoclavicular joint. (Reproduced with permission from Rockwood CA, and Green DP (eds): Fractures (3 vols), 2nd ed. Philadelphia: JB Lippincott, 1984.)

MOST COMMON CAUSE OF INJURY TO THE STERNOCLAVICULAR JOINT

The most common cause of dislocation of the sternoclavicular joint is vehicular accidents; the second is an injury sustained during participation in sports.[178, 190, 255] Omer,[190] in his review of patients from 14 military hospitals, accumulated 82 cases of dislocation to the sternoclavicular joint. He reported that almost 80 per cent of these cases occurred as the result of vehicular accidents (47 per cent) and athletics (31 per cent).

Probably the youngest patient to have a traumatic sternoclavicular dislocation was reported by Wheeler and associates.[262] They reported an anterior dislocation in a seven-month-old infant girl. The injury occurred when she was lying on her left side and her older brother accidentally fell on her, compressing her shoulders together. The closed reduction was unstable, and the child was immobilized in a figure-of-eight bandage for five weeks. At 10 weeks the child had a full range of motion, and there was no evidence of instability. I have seen an anterior injury in a three-year-old patient that occurred as a result of an automobile accident (Fig. 13–9).

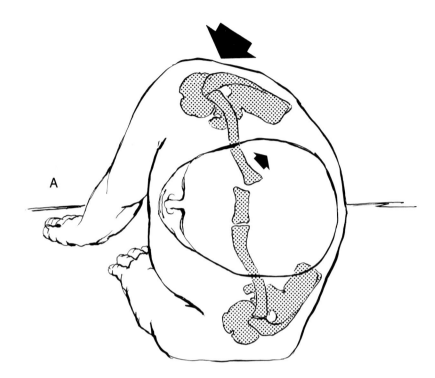

Figure 13–8. Mechanisms that produce anterior or posterior dislocations of the sternoclavicular joint. *A,* If the patient is lying on the ground and a compression force is applied to the posterior lateral aspect of the shoulder, the medial end of the clavicle will be displaced posteriorly. *B,* When the lateral compression force is directed from the anterior position, the medial end of the clavicle is dislocated posteriorly. (Reproduced with permission from Rockwood CA, and Green DP (eds): Fractures (3 vols), 2nd ed. Philadelphia: JB Lippincott, 1984.)

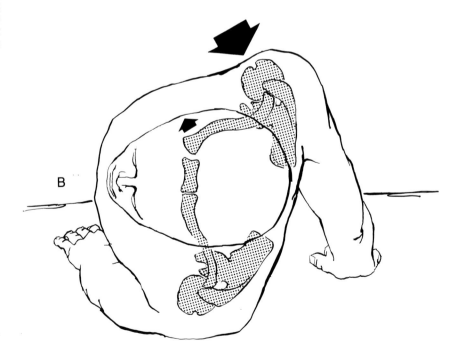

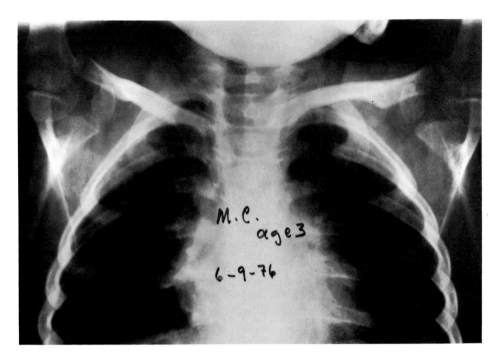

Figure 13–9. X-ray of a three-year-old child with traumatic anterior dislocation of the left sternoclavicular joint. The chest film demonstrates that the left clavicle is superior to the right, suggesting an anterior displacement of the left medial clavicle. (Reproduced with permission from Rockwood CA, and Green DP (eds): Fractures (3 vols), 2nd ed. Philadelphia: JB Lippincott, 1984.)

Classification of Problems of the Sternoclavicular Joint

There are two types of classifications. One is based on the etiology of the dislocation, and the other on the anatomical position that the dislocation assumes.

CLASSIFICATION BASED ON ANATOMY

Detailed classifications are confusing and difficult to remember, and the following classification is suggested.

Anterior Dislocation

The anterior dislocation is the most common type of sternoclavicular dislocation. The medial end of the clavicle is displaced anteriorly or anterosuperiorly to the anterior margin of the sternum (see Fig. 13–18).

Posterior Dislocation

Posterior sternoclavicular dislocation is uncommon. The medial end of the clavicle is displaced posteriorly or posterosuperiorly with respect to the posterior margin of the sternum (see Figs. 13–19 and 13–24).

CLASSIFICATION BASED ON ETIOLOGY

Traumatic Injury

Sprain or Subluxation

The acute sprains to the sternoclavicular joint can be classified as mild, moderate, or severe. In a *mild*

sprain, all the ligaments are intact and the joint is stable. In a *moderate* sprain, there is subluxation of the sternoclavicular joint. The capsular, intra-articular disc, and costoclavicular ligaments may be partially disrupted. The subluxation may be anterior or posterior. In a *severe* sprain, there is complete disruption of the sternoclavicular ligaments, and the dislocation may be anterior or posterior.

Acute Dislocation

In a dislocated sternoclavicular joint, the capsular and intra-articular ligaments are ruptured. Occasionally, the costoclavicular ligament is intact but stretched out enough to allow the dislocation.

Recurrent Dislocation

If the initial acute traumatic dislocation does not heal, mild to moderate forces may produce recurrent dislocations. This is a rare entity.

Unreduced Dislocation

The original dislocation may go unrecognized, it may be irreducible, or the physician may decide not to reduce certain dislocations.

Atraumatic Problems

For a variety of nontraumatic reasons, the sternoclavicular joint may sublux or enlarge.

Spontaneous Subluxation or Dislocation

One or both of the sternoclavicular joints may spontaneously sublux or dislocate anteriorly during over-

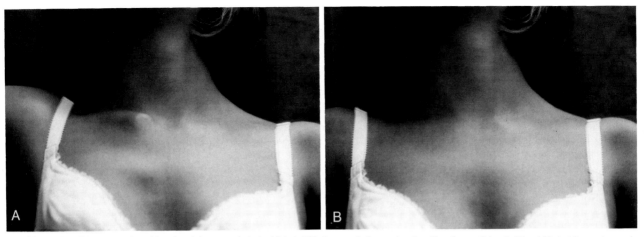

Figure 13–10. Spontaneous anterior subluxation of the sternoclavicular joint. *A,* With the arms in the overhead position, the medial end of the right clavicle spontaneously subluxes out anteriorly without any trauma. *B,* When the arm is brought back down to the side, the medial end of the clavicle spontaneously reduces. This is usually associated with no significant discomfort.

head motion. The problem is usually nonpainful (Fig. 13–10).

Congenital or Developmental Subluxation or Dislocation

Newlin[180] reported a case of a 25-year-old man who had bilateral congenital posterior dislocation of the medial ends of the clavicle that simulated an intrathoracic mass. Guerin[100] first reported congenital luxations of the sternoclavicular joint in 1841. Congenital defects with loss of bone substance on either side of the joint can predispose to subluxation or dislocation. Cooper[57] described a patient with scoliosis so severe that the shoulder was displaced forward enough to posteriorly dislocate the clavicle behind the sternum.

Arthritis

Arthritis involving the sternoclavicular joint can come in many forms:

- Osteoarthritis
- Arthropathies
- Condensing osteitis of the medial clavicle
- Sternocostoclavicular hyperostosis
- Postmenopausal arthritis

Osteoarthritis. Osteoarthritis[107, 137, 139] is characterized by narrowing of the joint space, osteophytes, subchondral sclerosis, and cysts on both sides of the joint (Fig. 13–11). Because most of the wear occurs in the inferior part of the head of the medial clavicle, most of the degenerative changes occur in that region. The sometimes discrete degenerative changes are best seen on tomograms and CT scans.[13, 137] Kier, Wain, Apple, and Martinez[137] correlated the x-ray and the pathological specimens of patients with osteoarthritis of the sternoclavicular joint. Sternoclavicular joint arthritis and hypertrophy can develop following radical neck surgery, particularly when the spinal accessory nerve is sacrificed.[46, 95] The incidence is reported to be as high

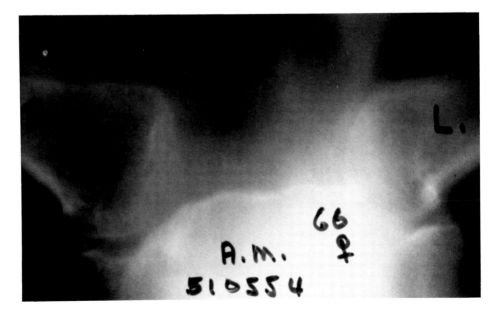

Figure 13–11. Tomogram of the sternoclavicular joints in a 66-year-old patient with degenerative arthritis of the sternoclavicular joint.

as 54 per cent.[46] The reason for the arthritis is the downward and forward droop of the shoulder, which puts an extra stress on the sternoclavicular joint. I followed one patient who had such stress on the sternoclavicular joint following a radical neck and spinal accessory nerve sacrifice that he developed a posterior dislocation of the sternoclavicular joint. The posterior displacement was so severe that the medial end of the clavicle compressed his trachea and esophagus. In order for him to swallow he had to hold the right shoulder back and up, which relieved the pressure on his esophagus. Baker, Martinez, Kier, and Wain[13] reported that the CT scan was very useful in evaluating the pathological changes in the degenerative disease of the sternoclavicular joint.

Arthropathies. Some of the disease processes that produce degenerative changes in the sternoclavicular joint are rheumatoid arthritis,[40, 74, 268] rheumatoid spondylitis,[210] scleroderma,[74] Reiter's syndrome,[137] psoriasis,[241] polymyalgia rheumatica,[192] secondary hyperparathyroidism,[210, 251] gout,[59, 163] leprosy,[183] syringomyelia,[62] metastatic carcinoma,[221] condensing osteitis,[37] Friedreich's disease[150] (aseptic necrosis of medial end of the clavicle), and sternoclavicular hyperostosis (Fig. 13–12).

Condensing Osteitis of the Medial Clavicle. This was first described in detail by Brower, Sweet, and Keats[37] and is a rather rare condition. It usually occurs in women over the age of 40 and may occur secondary to chronic stress on the joint. The joint is swollen and tender, and radionuclide studies reveal an increased uptake of the isotope. X-rays show sclerosis and slight expansion of the medial one-third of the clavicle. The inferior portion of the sternal end of the clavicle shows sclerotic changes. Some osteophytes may be present, but the joint space is preserved. The changes of the medial clavicle are best detected with a CT scan. The differential diagnosis includes Paget's disease, sternoclavicular hyperostosis, Friedreich's avascular necrosis of the medial clavicle epiphysis, infection, Tietze's syndrome, and osteoarthritis. The condition has been

described by many authors.[55, 82, 128, 140] Most patients do well with conservative treatment, i.e., anti-inflammatory medications. However, Kruger, Rock, and Munro[140] recommend incisional or excisional biopsy in refractory cases.

Sternocostoclavicular Hyperostosis. According to most authors,* the condition was first described by Sonozaki in 1974.[238–240] The majority of cases reported are from Japan.

This condition, usually bilateral, involves adults of both sexes between 30 and 50 years. The process begins at the junction of the medial clavicle, the first rib, and the sternum as an ossification in the ligaments and later involves the bones. Lagier, Arroyo, and Fallet[142] reported a very excellent review of the x-ray and pathology from an autopsy specimen. In some cases, the hyperostosis is extensive and forms a solid block of bone of the sternum, ribs, and clavicle. Patients may have peripheral arthritis. Subperiosteal bone changes have been noted in the x-rays of other bones of the skeleton, i.e., humerus, pelvis, tibia, ribs, and vertebral bodies.[91] The condition has been graded into Stage I, II, and III by Sonozaki.[238, 239, 240] Stage I is mild ossification in the costoclavicular ligaments. Stage II is characterized by an ossific mass between the clavicle and the first rib. In Stage III, a bone mass exists between the clavicle, sternum, and first rib. As might be expected with the fusion of the sternoclavicular joint, shoulder motion is severely restricted. Dohler[61] reported that as a result of the fusion of the sternoclavicular joint, his patient developed compensatory dislocation of the acromioclavicular joint.

Pustular cutaneous lesions of the palmar and plantar surfaces of skin may be seen. There is no specific laboratory test, except for an occasional elevation of the serum alkaline phosphatase.[91]

Postmenopausal Arthritis. This type of arthritis is primarily seen in postmenopausal women. Bremner[35]

---

*See references 4, 53, 91, 94, 129, 142, 225.

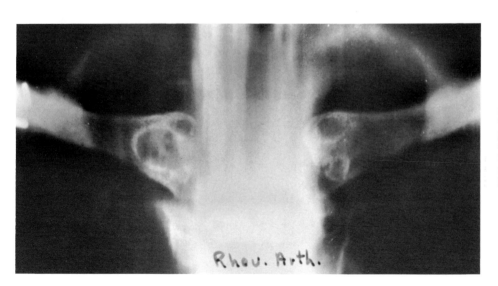

Figure 13–12. Tomogram of a patient with rheumatoid arthritis with bilateral degenerative changes in the medial clavicles. (Reproduced with permission from Rockwood CA, and Green DP (eds): Fractures (3 vols), 2nd ed. Philadelphia: JB Lippincott, 1984.)

and Bonnin[30] both have reported on this condition. Sadr and Swann[223] reported on 22 patients with this problem who were seen in a five-year study. Twenty of the cases were in women, and the majority involved the sternoclavicular joint of the dominant arm. Nonoperative treatment was recommended. The condition is the result of normal degeneration of a frequently moved joint. It is almost without symptoms; a lump develops at the sternoclavicular joint and, occasionally, a vague ache (Fig. 13–13). There is no previous history of injury or disease. X-rays reveal sclerosis and enlargement of the medial end of the clavicle, reactive sclerosis of the sternum, and subluxation of the joint. The pathological changes are those of degenerative arthritis.

Infection

Wohlgethan and Newberg[264] reviewed 39 cases of infection of the sternoclavicular joint. Fifteen were in drug addicts, and 24 were in nonaddicts. Common causes of the infection in nonaddicts are bacteremia, invasion from surrounding bone, rheumatoid arthritis, alcoholism, and chronic debilitating diseases. Lindsey and Leach[152] reported on sternoclavicular osteomyelitis as a complication of subclavian vein catheterization and in patients undergoing dialysis. There are many case reports of isolated infections of the sternoclavicular joint that have been caused by a variety of microorganisms, i.e., *Staphylococcus aureus*,[60, 113, 153, 165] *Escherichia coli*,[63, 153] *Citrobacter diversus*,[84] coliform bacilli,[63] *Pasteurella multocida*,[182] *Streptococcus sanguis*,[182] *Streptococcus anginosus-constellatus*,[122] *Streptococcus pyogenes*,[176] *Pseudomonas aeruginosa*,[83, 247] *Brucella*,[268, 15] and *Neisseria gonorrhoeae* (Fig. 13–14). Blankstein and associates[28] reported a septic sternoclavicular joint that cultured *Staphylococcus aureus* secondary to bacteremia infection from a paronychia of the finger. Farrer[77] reported a case involving a 66-year-old man who had a septic sternoclavicular joint that cultured *Staphylococcus aureus*. Tabatabai and colleagues[249] reported infection of the sternoclavicular joint caused by Group B *Streptococcus*. The CT scan is very helpful in making an early diagnosis of a septic sternoclavicular joint.[152, 176, 264]

Richter, Hahn, Nubling, and Kohler[212] reported on nine patients with infection of the sternoclavicular joint secondary to tuberculosis. The average time from onset of the disease until diagnosis was 1.4 years.

For some reason, drug addicts who use the intravenous route seem to have a high incidence of acute gram-negative infection of the sternoclavicular joint.[83, 93] Friedman and colleagues[83] reported four cases of sternoclavicular infection in intravenous drug abusers. In three cases, *Staphylococcus aureus* was recovered, and in the fourth case, *Streptococcus pneumoniae* was isolated.

Higoumenakis[114] has reported that unilateral enlargement of the sternoclavicular joint is a diagnostic sign of congenital syphilis. The enlargement of the sternoclavicular joint can be mistaken for an anterior dislocation. He reported the sign to be positive in 170 of 197 cases of congenital syphilis. Glickman and Minsky[92] have reported on the same condition. The enlargement is a hyperostosis of the medial clavicle occurring in the sternoclavicular joint of the dominant extremity, which reaches its permanent stage and size at puberty. The theory of why it affects the sternoclavicular joint relates it to spirochete invasion of the sternal end of the clavicle at the time of its early ossification.

Incidence of Injury to the Sternoclavicular Joint

Sternoclavicular injuries are rare, and many of the authors apologize for reporting only three or four cases. Attesting to this rarity is the fact that some orthopedists have never treated or seen a dislocation of the sternoclavicular joint.[117, 224]

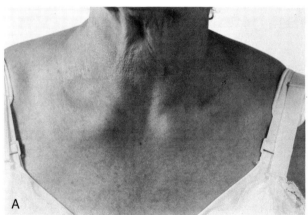
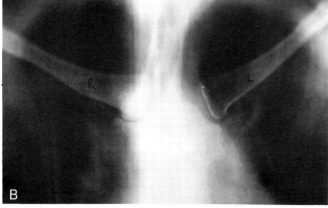

Figure 13–13. *A,* Bilateral anterior swelling of the sternoclavicular joints in a 67-year-old postmenopausal female. The right medial clavicle was more prominent because she was right handed. *B,* The tomogram demonstrates sclerosis and degenerative changes in the right sternoclavicular joint consistent with ordinary degenerative arthritis. (Reproduced with permission from Rockwood CA, and Green DP (eds): Fractures (3 vols), 2nd ed. Philadelphia: JB Lippincott, 1984.)

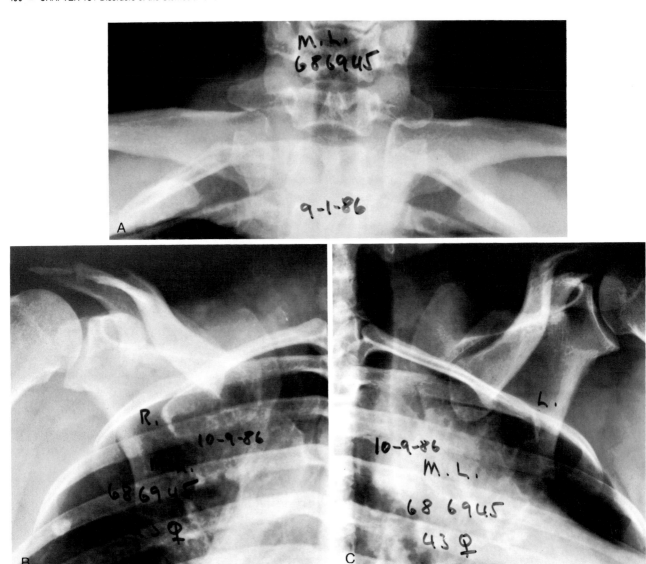

Figure 13–14. Infection in the right sternoclavicular joint. *A,* On the initial x-ray there is little difference between the right and left medial clavicles, as seen on the 30 degree cephalic tilt view. *B, C,* Thirty-eight days later, the medial end of the right clavicle is seen to be dissolving away compared with the medial end of the left clavicle. The patient had a *Staphylococcus aureus* infection in the right sternoclavicular joint, which was managed by open debridement.

The incidence of sternoclavicular dislocation, based on the series of 1603 injuries of the shoulder girdle reported by Cave,[48] is 3 per cent. (The total incidence in the study was glenohumeral dislocations, 85 per cent; acromioclavicular, 12 per cent; and sternoclavicular, 3 per cent.) In the series by Cave and in my own experience, dislocation of the sternoclavicular joint is not as rare as posterior dislocation of the glenohumeral joint.

RATIO OF ANTERIOR TO POSTERIOR INJURIES

Undoubtedly, anterior dislocations of the sternoclavicular joint are much more common than the posterior type. However, the ratio of anterior to posterior dislocations is only rarely reported. Theoretically, one could survey the literature and develop the ratio of anterior dislocations to posterior dislocations, but most of the published material on sternoclavicular dislocations is on the rare posterior dislocation. Of the references listed at the end of this chapter that deal with injuries of the sternoclavicular joint, more than 60 per cent discuss only the rare posterior dislocation of the sternoclavicular joint and the various complications associated with it. The largest series from a single institution is reported by Nettles and Linscheid,[178] who studied 60 patients with sternoclavicular dislocations (57 anterior and 3 posterior). This gives a ratio of anterior dislocations to posterior dislocations of the sternoclavicular joint of approximately 20 to 1. Waskowitz[255] reviewed 18 cases of sternoclavicular dislocations, none of which was posterior. However, in my series of 273 traumatic injuries, there have been 121 patients with anterior dislocation and 41 patients with posterior dislocation.

In 1896, Hotchkiss[118] reported a bilateral traumatic dislocation of the sternoclavicular joint. A 28-year-old man was run over by a cart and received an anterior dislocation of the right shoulder and a posterior dislocation of the left one. I have had experience in treating four cases of bilateral sternoclavicular dislocation.

Signs and Symptoms of Injuries to the Sternoclavicular Joint

MILD SPRAIN

In a mild sprain, the ligaments of the joint are intact. The patient complains of a mild to moderate amount of pain, particularly with movement of the upper extremity. The joint may be slightly swollen and tender to palpation, but instability is not noted.

MODERATE SPRAIN (SUBLUXATION)

A moderate sprain results in a subluxation of the sternoclavicular joint. The ligaments are either partially disrupted or severely stretched. Swelling is noted and pain is marked, particularly with any movement of the arm. Anterior or posterior subluxation may be obvious to the examiner when the injured joint is compared with the normal sternoclavicular joint.

SEVERE SPRAIN (DISLOCATION)

A severe sprain is analogous to a joint dislocation. The dislocation may be anterior or posterior. The capsular ligament and the intra-articular disc ligament are ruptured. Regardless of whether the dislocation is anterior or posterior, there are characteristic clinical findings of sternoclavicular joint dislocation.

Signs Common to Both Anterior and Posterior Injuries

The patient has severe pain that is increased with any movement of the arm, particularly when the shoulders are pressed together by a lateral force. The patient usually supports the injured arm across the trunk with the normal arm. The affected shoulder appears to be shortened and thrust forward when compared with the normal shoulder. The head may be tilted toward the side of the dislocated joint. The patient's discomfort increases when he or she is placed into the supine position, at which time it will be noted that the involved shoulder will not lie back flat on the table.

Signs and Symptoms of Anterior Injury

The medial end of the clavicle is visibly prominent anterior to the sternum (see Fig. 13–18) and can be palpated anterior to the sternum. It may be fixed anteriorly or be quite mobile.

Signs and Symptoms of Posterior Injury

The patient with a posterior dislocation has more pain than a patient with anterior sternoclavicular dislocations. Stankler[243] reported on two patients with unrecognized posterior dislocations which developed venous engorgement of the ipsilateral arm. The anterosuperior fullness of the chest produced by the clavicle is less prominent and visible when compared with the normal side. The usually palpable medial end of the clavicle is displaced posteriorly. The corner of the sternum is easily palpated as compared with the normal sternoclavicular joint. Venous congestion may be present in the neck or in the upper extremity. Breathing difficulties, shortness of breath, or a choking sensation may be noted. Circulation to the ipsilateral arm may be decreased. The patient may complain of difficulty in swallowing or a tight feeling in the throat or may be in a state of complete shock or possibly have a pneumothorax.

I have seen six patients who clinically had an anterior dislocation of the sternoclavicular joint but, by x-ray, were shown to have complete posterior dislocation. The point is that one cannot always rely on the clinical findings of observing and palpating the joint to make a distinction between the anterior and posterior dislocations.

X-ray Findings of Injury to the Sternoclavicular Joint

ANTEROPOSTERIOR VIEWS

The older literature reflects that routine x-rays of the sternoclavicular joint, regardless of the special views, are difficult to interpret. Special oblique views of the chest have been recommended, but because of the distortion of one of the clavicles over the other, interpretation is difficult (Fig. 13–15). The older literature on dislocation of the sternoclavicular joint indicates that the diagnosis is best made from a clinical examination of the patient and not from the x-rays. However, it goes on to say that tomography offers more detailed information, often showing small fractures in the vicinity of the sternoclavicular joint. Occasionally, the routine anteroposterior or posteroanterior x-ray of the chest or sternoclavicular joint suggests that something is wrong with one of the clavicles, because it appears to be displaced as compared with the normal side. It would be ideal to take a view at right angles to the anteroposterior plane, but because of our anatomy, it is impossible to take a true 90-degree cephalic-to-caudal lateral view. Lateral x-rays of the chest are at right angles to the anteroposterior plane, but they cannot be interpreted because

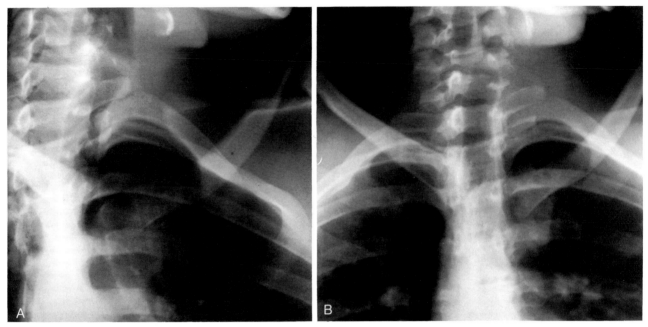

Figure 13-15. Routine x-rays of the sternoclavicular joint are difficult to interpret, even though this patient has a classical posterior dislocation of the left sternoclavicular joint. See Fig. 13–33 for further information on and treatment of this patient. (Reproduced with permission from Rockwood CA, and Green DP (eds): Fractures (3 vols), 2nd ed. Philadelphia: JB Lippincott, 1984.)

of the density of the chest and the overlap of the medial clavicles with the first rib and the sternum.

Note: Regardless of the clinical impression that suggests an anterior dislocation, x-rays must be obtained to confirm one's suspicions. I have seen six patients with anterior swelling and pain following an injury, which suggested anterior dislocation, but on x-ray, it proved to be a posterior dislocation.

SPECIAL PROJECTED VIEWS

Kattan[133] has recommended a special projection, as have Ritvo and Ritvo,[213] Schmitt,[230] Fedoseev,[78] and Fery and Leonard.[76] Kurzbauer[141] has recommended special lateral projections. Hobbs,[115] in 1968, recommended a view that comes close to being a 90-degree cephalocaudal lateral view of the sternoclavicular joints. In the Hobbs' view, the patient is seated at the x-ray table, high enough to lean forward over the table. The cassette is on the table, and the lower anterior rib cage is against the cassettes (Fig. 13–16). The patient leans forward so that the nape of his flexed neck is almost parallel to the table. The flexed elbows straddle the cassette and support the head and neck. The x-ray source is above the nape of the neck, and the beam passes through the cervical spine to project the sternoclavicular joints onto the cassette on the table.

Serendipity View

This view is rightfully called the serendipity technique because that is the way it was developed. I

found, accidentally, that the next best thing to having a true cephalocaudal lateral view of the sternoclavicular joint is a 40-degree cephalic tilt view. The patient is positioned on his back squarely and in the center of the x-ray table. The tube is tilted at a 40-degree angle off the vertical and is centered directly on the sternum (Fig. 13–17). A nongrid 11 × 14 inch cassette is placed squarely on the table and under the patient's upper

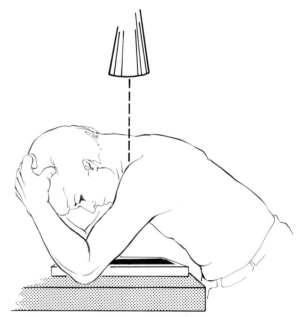

Figure 13-16. Positioning of the patient for x-ray evaluation of the sternoclavicular joint, as recommended by Hobbs. (Modified from Hobbs DW: The sternoclavicular joint: a new axial radiographic view. Radiology 90:801, 1968.)

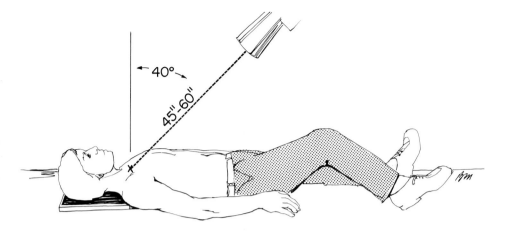

Figure 13–17. Positioning of the patient to take the "serendipity" view of the sternoclavicular joints. The x-ray tube is tilted 40 degrees from the vertical position and is aimed directly at the manubrium. The nongrid cassette should be large enough to receive the projected images of the medial halves of both clavicles. In children the tube distance from the patient should be 45 inches; in thicker-chested adults the distance should be 60 inches. (Reproduced with permission from Rockwood CA, and Green DP (eds): Fractures (3 vols), 2nd ed. Philadelphia: JB Lippincott, 1984.)

shoulders and neck so that the beam aimed at the sternum will project both clavicles onto the film. The tube is adjusted so that the medial one-half of both clavicles is projected onto the film. It is important to note that the cassette should be placed squarely on the x-ray table (i.e., not angulated or rotated) and that the patient should be positioned squarely on top of the cassette.

For children, the distance from the tube to the cassette is 45 inches; for adults, whose anteroposterior chest diameter is greater, the distance should be 60 inches. The technical setting of the machine is essentially the same as for a posteroanterior view of the chest.

For example, imagine that your eyes are down at the level of the patient's knees and you are looking up toward his clavicles at a 40-degree angle. If the right sternoclavicular joint were dislocated anteriorly, the right clavicle would appear to be displaced more anteriorly or riding higher on an imaginary horizontal line when compared with the normal left clavicle (Fig. 13–18). The reverse is true if the left sternoclavicular joint is dislocated posteriorly (i.e., the left clavicle would be displaced inferiorly or riding lower on an

imaginary horizontal plane than the normal right clavicle) (Fig. 13–19). The idea, then, is to take a 40-degree cephalic tilt x-ray of both medial clavicles and compare the relationship of the injured clavicle to the normal clavicle (Fig. 13–20).

SPECIAL TECHNIQUES

Tomograms

Tomograms can be very helpful in distinguishing between a sternoclavicular dislocation and a fracture of the medial clavicle. They are also helpful in questionable anterior and posterior dislocation of the sternoclavicular joint to distinguish fractures from dislocations and to evaluate arthritis changes (Fig. 13–21).

In 1959, Baker[12] recommended the use of tomography, which was developed in the late 1920s, and said it was far more valuable than routine films and the fingertips of the examining physician. Morag and Shahin,[173] in 1975, reported on the value of tomography, which they used in a series of 20 patients, and recommended that it be used routinely to evaluate

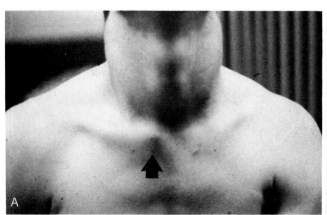
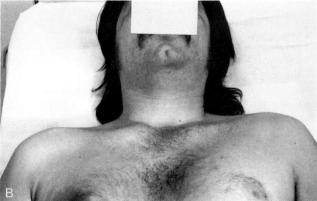

Figure 13–18. *A*, Clinically there is an evident anterior dislocation of the right sternoclavicular joint (*arrow*). *B*, When the clavicles are viewed from down around the level of the patient's knees, it is apparent that the right clavicle is dislocated anteriorly. (Reproduced with permission from Rockwood CA, and Green DP (eds): Fractures (3 vols), 2nd ed. Philadelphia: JB Lippincott, 1984.)

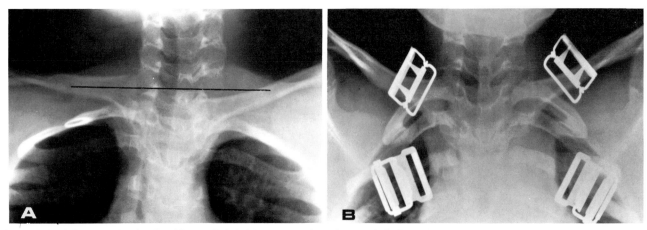

Figure 13–19. *A,* Posterior dislocation of the left sternoclavicular joint as seen on the 40-degree cephalic tilt x-ray in a 12-year-old boy. The left clavicle is displaced inferiorly to a line drawn through the normal right clavicle. Following the closed reduction, the medial ends of both clavicles are in the same horizontal position. The buckles are a part of the figure-of-eight clavicular harness that is used to hold the shoulders back after reduction. (Reproduced with permission from Rockwood CA, and Green DP (eds): Fractures (3 vols), 2nd ed. Philadelphia: JB Lippincott, 1984.)

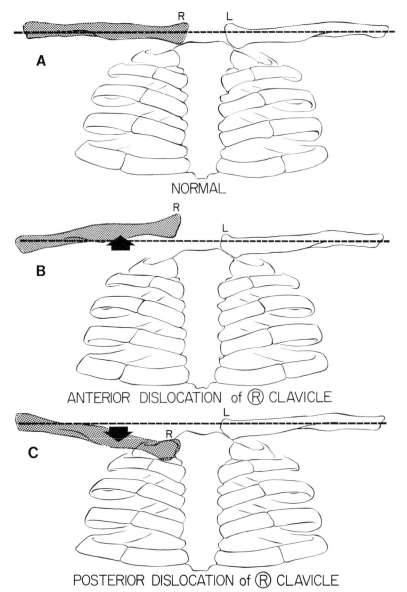

Figure 13–20. Interpretation of the cephalic tilt x-rays of the sternoclavicular joints. *A,* In the normal person, both clavicles appear on the same imaginary line drawn horizontally across the film. *B,* In a patient with anterior dislocation of the right sternoclavicular joint, the medial half of the right clavicle is projected above the level of the normal left clavicle. *C,* If the patient has a posterior dislocation of the right sternoclavicular joint, the medial half of the right clavicle is displaced below the imaginary line drawn through the normal left clavicle. (Reproduced with permission from Rockwood CA, and Green DP (eds): Fractures (3 vols), 2nd ed. Philadelphia: JB Lippincott, 1984.)

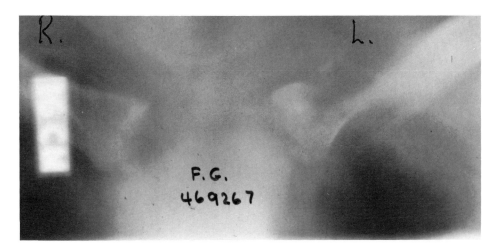

Figure 13–21. Tomogram demonstrating a fracture of the left medial clavicle. The clinical pre–x-ray diagnosis was an anterior dislocation of the left sternoclavicular joint. (Reproduced with permission from Rockwood CA, and Green DP (eds): Fractures (3 vols), 2nd ed. Philadelphia: JB Lippincott, 1984.)

problems of the sternoclavicular joint. From a study of normal sternoclavicular joints, they pointed out the variation in the x-ray appearance in different age groups.

CT Scans

Without question, the CT scan is the best technique to study any or all problems of the sternoclavicular joint (Fig. 13–22). It clearly distinguishes injuries of the joint from fractures of the medial clavicle and defines minor subluxations of the joint. The orthopedist must remember to ask for CTs of both sternoclavicular joints and the medial one-half of both clavicles so that the injured side can be compared with the normal side. The patient should lie flat in the supine position. If one requests a study of the right sternoclavicular joint, the x-ray technician may rotate the patient to the affected side and provide views of only the one joint.

Hartman and Dunnagan[108] reported on the use of CT arthrography to demonstrate capsular disruption in a patient following a traumatic injury to the joint.

Treatment

TRAUMATIC INJURIES

Mild Sprain

The joint is stable but painful. Application of ice for the first 12 to 24 hours followed by heat is helpful. The upper extremity should be immobilized in a sling for three to four days, and then, gradually, the patient can regain use of the arm in everyday activities. I recently had a fascinating case of a young mother who had a semi-acute or semi-chronic strain to both sternoclavicular joints. Her bra size, over a period of four weeks, had jumped from a 36B to a 38EE. The increase in weight depressed both shoulders and produced pain while upright in both sternoclavicular joints. I could

completely relieve the discomfort by pushing both elbows up, thus elevating the distal clavicles, which in turn took the strain off her sternoclavicular joints. I suggested she consult her gynecologist and surgeon to determine the quickest way to reduce the size of her breasts.

Moderate Sprain (Subluxation)

For subluxation of the sternoclavicular joint, application of ice is recommended for the first 12 hours, followed by heat for the next 24 to 48 hours. The joint may be subluxed anteriorly or posteriorly, which may be reduced by drawing the shoulders backward as if reducing and holding a fracture of the clavicle. A clavicle strap can be used to hold the reduction. A sling and swath should also be used to hold up the shoulder and to prevent motion of the arm. The patient should be protected from further possible injury for four to six weeks. DePalma[65] suggests a plaster figure-of-eight dressing, and McLaughlin[168] recommended the same type of treatment that would be used for fracture of the clavicle, with the addition of a sling to support the arm. Allman[7] prefers the use of a soft figure-of-eight bandage with a sling and occasionally uses adhesive strapping over the medial end of the clavicle. When in certain circumstances the subluxation cannot be reduced, some authors[20, 65] have recommended repair of the ligaments and temporary internal fixation of the sternoclavicular joint with pins drilled from the clavicle into the sternum. Postoperatively, DePalma[67] applies a plaster figure-of-eight cast and, in addition, supports it with a sling and swath; the pins and the cast are removed after six weeks.

As will be pointed out later in the section on author's preferred method of treatment, the use of pins across the sternoclavicular joint has too many serious complications.

Occasionally, following conservative treatment of a Type II injury, the pain lingers on and the symptoms of popping and grating persist. This may require joint exploration. Bateman[20] has commented on the possi-

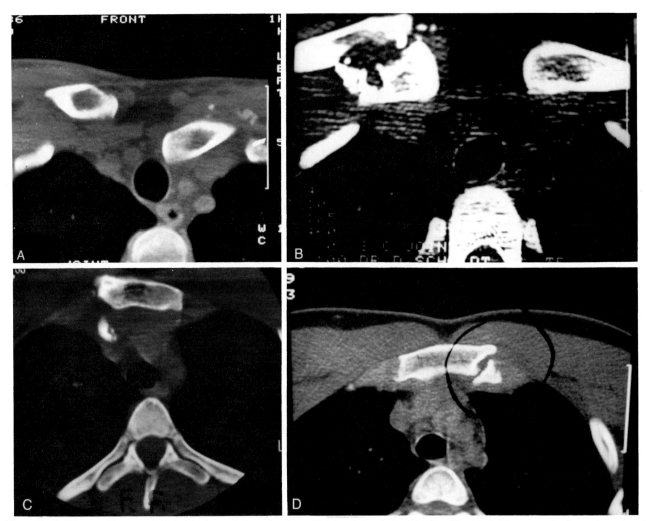

Figure 13–22. CT scans of the sternoclavicular joint demonstrating various types of injuries. *A,* A posterior dislocation of the left clavicle compressing the great vessels and producing swelling of the left arm. *B,* A fracture of the medial clavicle that does not involve the articular surface. *C,* A fragment of bone displaced posteriorly into the great vessel. *D,* A fracture of the medial clavicle into the sternoclavicular joint.

bility of finding a tear of the intra-articular disc, which should be excised. Duggan[69] reported a case in which, several weeks after an injury to the sternoclavicular joint, the patient still had popping in the joint.

Through a small incision, Duggan exposed the capsule and out through the capsule popped the intra-articular disc, which looked like "an avulsed fingernail." Following repair of the capsule, the patient had no more symptoms. If degenerative changes become severe in the sternoclavicular joint, an excision of the medial end of the clavicle may be required.

Severe Sprain (Dislocation)

The dislocation of the sternoclavicular joint may be anterior or posterior.

Nonoperative Treatment

Anterior Dislocation

There still is some controversy regarding the treatment of acute or chronic anterior dislocation of the sternoclavicular joint. Most acute anterior dislocations are unstable following reduction, and many operative procedures have been described to repair or reconstruct the joint.

Technique of Closed Reduction. Closed reduction of the sternoclavicular joint may be accomplished with local or general anesthesia or, in stoic patients, without anesthesia. Most authors recommend the use of narcotics or muscle relaxants. The patient is placed supine on the table, lying on a three- to four-inch-thick pad between the shoulders. In this position, the clavicle may reduce with direct gentle pressure over the anteriorly displaced clavicle. However, when the pressure is released, the clavicle usually dislocates again.

Occasionally, the clavicle will remain reduced. Sometimes, the physician will need to push both shoulders back to the table while an assistant applies pressure to the anteriorly displaced clavicle. Laidlaw[143] treated an interesting case of a patient who had a dislocated clavicle. The sternoclavicular joint was dislocated anteriorly and was mildly symptomatic. The acromioclavicular joint was most symptomatic and was treated by excision of the distal clavicle. Surprisingly, the anteriorly dislocated sternoclavicular joint reduced and became pain free.

Postreduction Care. If, with the shoulders held back, the sternoclavicular joint remains reduced, the shoulders can be stabilized with a soft figure-of-eight dressing, a commercial clavicle strap harness, or a plaster figure-of-eight cast. Some authors recommend a bulky pressure pad over the anterior medial clavicle that is held in place with elastic tape. A sling might be used because it holds up the shoulder and prevents motion of the arm. Immobilization should be maintained at least six weeks, and then the arm should be protected for another two weeks before strenuous activities are undertaken. If the sternoclavicular joint again dislocates when the reduction pressure is released, as it usually does, a figure-of-eight dressing or a sling can be used until the patient's symptoms subside. Most anterior closed reductions of the sternoclavicular joint are unstable, and even with the shoulders held back, the joint is unstable. Although some authors have recommended operative repair of anterior dislocations of the sternoclavicular joint, I believe that the operative complications are too great and the end results are too unsatisfactory to consider an open reduction. Certainly in children, in whom many if not most of the injuries are physeal fractures, a nonoperative approach should be strongly considered.

Posterior Dislocation

A careful examination of the patient is extremely important. Complications are common with posterior dislocation of the sternoclavicular joint, and the patient should receive prompt attention.

A very careful history and physical examination should be done to rule out damage to the pulmonary and vascular systems. The sternoclavicular joint must be carefully evaluated by all available x-ray techniques including, when indicated, combined aortogram-CT scan for potential vascular injuries. If specific complications are noted, appropriate consultants should be called in before reduction is performed. Worman and Leagus[266] reported a posterior dislocation of the sternoclavicular joint in which it was noted at surgery that the displaced clavicle had put a hole into the right pulmonary artery. The clavicle had prevented exsanguination, because the vessel was still impaled by the clavicle. Had a closed reduction been performed in the emergency department, the result could have been disastrous.

General anesthesia is usually required for reduction of a posterior dislocation of the sternoclavicular joint because the patient has so much pain and muscle spasm. However, for the stoic patient, some authors have performed the reduction under intravenous narcotics and muscle relaxants. Heinig[110] has successfully used local anesthesia in a posterior dislocation reduction.

From a review of the earlier literature, it would appear that the treatment of choice for posterior sternoclavicular dislocation was by operative procedures. However, since the 1950s, the treatment of choice of posterior sternoclavicular dislocation is closed reduction.* Some authors[196, 245] who had previously done open reductions reported that they were amazed at how easily the dislocation reduced under direct vision, and thereafter, they used closed reductions with complete success.

Techniques of Closed Reduction. Many different techniques have been described for closed reduction of a posterior dislocation of the sternoclavicular joint.

Abduction Traction Technique. For the abduction traction technique,[66, 79, 167, 171, 215, 224] the patient is placed on his back with the dislocated shoulder near the edge of the table. A three- to four-inch-thick sandbag is placed between the shoulders (Fig. 13–23). Lateral traction is applied to the abducted arm, which is then gradually brought back into extension. This may be all that is necessary to accomplish the reduction. The clavicle usually reduces with an audible snap or pop, and it is almost always stable. Too much extension can bind the anterior surface of the dislocated medial clavicle on the back of the manubrium. Occasionally, it may be necessary to grasp the medial clavicle with one's fingers to dislodge it from behind the sternum. If this fails, the skin is prepared, and a sterile towel clip is used to grasp the medial clavicle to apply lateral and anterior traction (Fig. 13–24).

Adduction Traction Technique. In this technique,[41] the patient is supine on the table with a three- to four-inch bolster between the shoulders. Traction is then applied to the arm in adduction, while a downward pressure is exerted on the shoulders. The clavicle is levered over the first rib into its normal position. Buckerfield and Castle[41] reported that this technique has succeeded when the abduction traction technique has failed. Butterworth and Kirk[44] used a similar adducted position, except they applied lateral traction on the upper humerus. Heinig[110] and Elting[72] have reported that they have accomplished reduction by placing the patient supine on the table with three or four folded towels between the two shoulders. Forward pressure is then applied on both shoulders, which accomplished the reduction. Other authors have put their knee between the shoulders of the seated patient and, by pulling back on both shoulders, have accomplished a reduction. Stein[245] used skin traction on the abducted and extended arm to accomplish the reduction gently and gradually. Many authors have reported that closed reduction usually cannot be accomplished after 48 hours. However, others[41, 146] have reported closed reduction as late as four and five days after the injury.

Postreduction Care. After reduction, to allow ligament healing, the shoulders should be held back for four to six weeks with a figure-of-eight dressing or one

*See references 44, 54, 79, 102, 110, 167, 168, 171, 196, 224, 245.

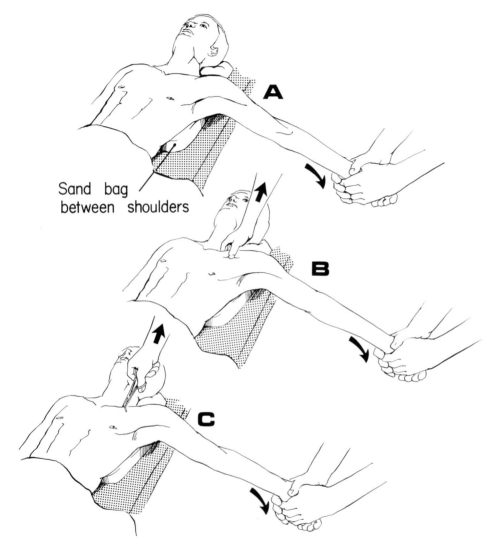

Sand bag
between shoulders

Figure 13–23. Technique of closed reduction of the sternoclavicular joint. *A,* The patient is positioned supine with a sandbag placed between the two shoulders. Traction is then applied to the arm against countertraction in an abducted and slightly extended position. In anterior dislocations, direct pressure over the medial end of the clavicle may reduce the joint. *B,* In posterior dislocations, in addition to the traction it may be necessary to manipulate the medial end of the clavicle with the fingers to dislodge the clavicle from behind the manubrium. *C,* In stubborn cases of posterior dislocations, it may be necessary to sterilely prepare the medial end of the clavicle and use a towel clip to grasp *around* the medial clavicle to lift it back into position. (Reproduced with permission from Rockwood CA, and Green DP (eds): Fractures (3 vols), 2nd ed. Philadelphia: JB Lippincott, 1984.)

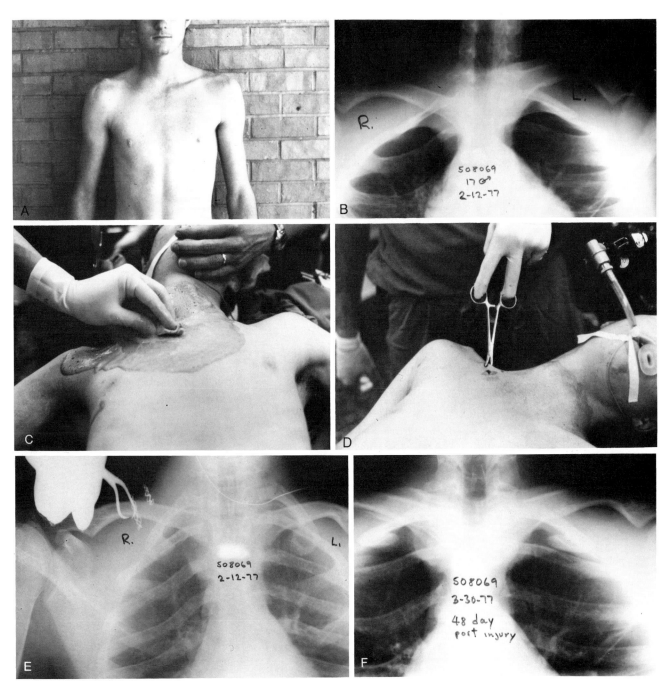

Figure 13–24. Posterior dislocation of the right sternoclavicular joint. *A,* A 16-year-old boy has a 48-hour-old posterior displacement of the right medial clavicle that occurred from direct trauma to the anterior right clavicle. He noted immediate onset of difficulty in swallowing and some hoarseness in his voice. *B,* The 40-degree cephalic tilt x-ray confirmed the presence of the posterior displacement of the right medial clavicle as compared with the left clavicle. Because of the patient's age, this was considered most likely to be a physeal injury of the right medial clavicle. *C,* Because the injury was 48 hours old, we were unable to reduce the dislocation with simple traction on the arm. The right shoulder was surgically cleansed so that a sterile towel clip could be used. *D,* With the towel clip securely around the clavicle and with continued lateral traction, a visible and audible reduction occurred. *E,* Postreduction x-rays showed that the medial clavicle had been restored to its normal position. The reduction was quite stable, and the patient's shoulders were held back with a figure-of-eight strap. *F,* The right clavicle has remained reduced. Particularly note the periosteal new bone formation along the superior and inferior borders of the right clavicle. This is the result of a physeal injury whereby the epiphysis remains adjacent to the manubrium while the clavicle is displaced out of a split in the periosteal tube. (Reproduced with permission from Rockwood CA, and Green DP (eds): Fractures (3 vols), 2nd ed. Philadelphia: JB Lippincott, 1984.)

of the commercially available figure-of-eight straps used to treat fractures of the clavicle.

Should closed maneuvers fail in the adult, an operative procedure should be performed since most adult patients cannot tolerate the posterior displacement of the clavicle in the mediastinum. Gangahar and Flogaites[86] reported a case of late thoracic outlet syndrome following an unreduced posterior dislocation, and Borrero[33] reported late and significant vascular problems. I recently was asked to evaluate a patient who, following a significant injury, complained of swelling and bluish coloration of his left arm after any

type of physical activity. He really did not have many local sternoclavicular joint symptoms, but by physical examination, the left clavicle was displaced posteriorly. The CT scan demonstrated a major posterior displacement of the left clavicle (Fig. 13–25). Because of the marked displacement and the vascular compromise, arteriography combined with the CT scan was performed, which did not reveal any vascular leak. With the help of the chest surgeon, the clavicle was removed from the mediastinum, the medial 1½ inches were removed, and the shaft was stabilized to the first rib. The greatest displacement that I have seen was in

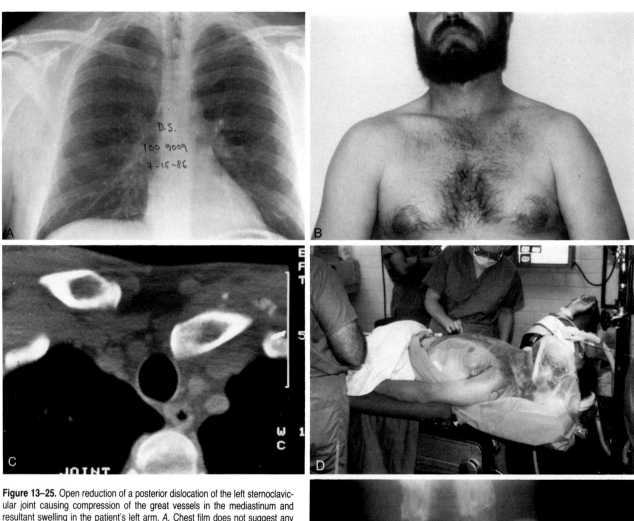

Figure 13–25. Open reduction of a posterior dislocation of the left sternoclavicular joint causing compression of the great vessels in the mediastinum and resultant swelling in the patient's left arm. *A,* Chest film does not suggest any serious problem with the left medial clavicle. *B,* Clinically the patient had a depressed medial end of the left clavicle compared with the right. *C,* The CT scan reveals posterior displacement of the medial clavicle back into the mediastinum, compressing the great vessels and slightly displacing the trachea. *D,* The patient was carefully prepared for a surgical repair in cooperation with a cardiovascular surgeon. The patient was prepared from the base of his neck down to the umbilicus so that we could manage any type of vascular problem or complication. Open reduction was accomplished without any vascular incident. The medial end of the clavicle was totally unstable, so the medial 2.0 cm was resected and the remaining clavicle stabilized to the first rib. *E,* Four months following surgery, the patient's slight anterior displacement of the clavicle was essentially asymptomatic and the remaining clavicle was stable.

a patient with a posteroinferior dislocation of the medial clavicle down into an intrathoracic position (Fig. 13–26).

However, Louw and Louw[155] reported a case in which a 30-year-old patient with a T3-T4 paraplegia and posterior dislocation of the left sternoclavicular joint had essentially no problems. He underwent an extensive rehabilitation program and could lower himself from his wheelchair to the floor and back again without assistance, and he could transfer from his wheelchair to the bed, bath, and car without difficulty.

If children and young adults under the age of 23 to 25 have symptoms from the pressure of the posteriorly displaced clavicle into the mediastinum, an operative procedure should likewise be performed. However, children may have no symptoms, and the physician can wait and watch to see if the physeal plate remodeling process removes the posteriorly displaced bone.

Technique of Operative Treatment

The operative procedure should be performed in a manner that disturbs as few of the anterior ligament structures as possible. If the procedure can be performed with the anterior ligaments intact, then, with the shoulders held back in a figure-of-eight dressing, the reduction may be stable. If all the ligaments are disrupted, a significant decision has to be made to try to stabilize the sternoclavicular joint or to resect the medial 1 to 1½ inches of the medial clavicle and stabilize the remaining clavicle to the first rib.

Some of the older literature in the 1960s and 1970s recommended stabilization of the sternoclavicular joint with pins. Elting[72] used Kirschner wires to stabilize the joint and supplemented ligament repairs with a short toe extensor tendon. Denham and Dingley[64] and Brooks and Henning[36] used Kirschner wires. DePalma[65] and Brown[38] recommended repair of the ligaments and stabilized the sternoclavicular joint with one or two Steinmann pins.

Habernek and Hertz,[105] Nutz,[186] Pfister and Weller,[201] Kennedy,[134] Tagliabue and Riva,[250] Hartman and Dunnagan,[108] Bankart,[14] Ecke,[71] and Stein[245] avoided the use of pins across the sternoclavicular joint and used loops of various types of suture wires across the joint. Burri and Neugebauer[42] recommended the use of a figure-of-eight loop of carbon fiber. Maguire,[160] Booth and Roper,[31] Barth and Hagen,[18] and Lunseth, Chapman, and Frankel[159] reconstructed the sternoclavicular joint using local tendons of the sternocleidomastoid, subclavius, or pectoralis major tendons for repair. Haug[109] reported on the use of a special plate to stabilize the joint. The complications of fixation of the sternoclavicular joint with Kirschner wires or Steinmann pins are horrendous and are discussed in the section on complications.

Recurrent or Unreduced Dislocation

Nonoperative Approach. It has been stressed by many authors that most patients who have recurrent long-standing sternoclavicular joint dislocation are asymptomatic and require no treatment. Holmdahl,[117] Louw and Louw,[155] and Borrero[33] have reported complications following unreduced posterior dislocations.

Surgical Reconstructions. There are several basic procedures to maintain the medial end of the clavicle in its normal articulation with the sternum. Fascia lata,

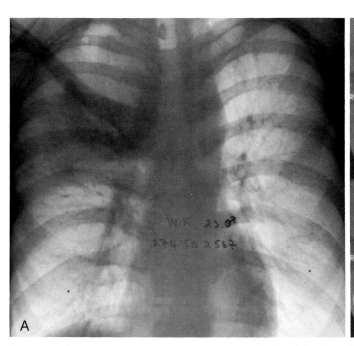 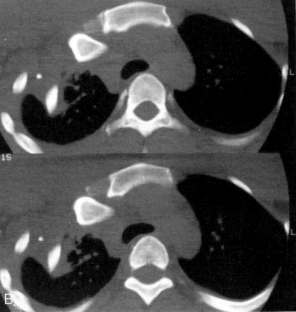

Figure 13–26. A most unusual posterior, inferior, intrathoracic dislocation of the right medial clavicle. *A,* On the chest film the clavicle is displaced behind the manubrium down into the parenchyma of the lung. *B,* The CT scan shows the clavicle down into the lung field with partial collapse of the lung.

suture, internal fixation across the joint, subclavius tendons, osteotomy of the medial clavicle, and resection of the medial end of the clavicle have been advocated.

Fascia Lata. Bankart[14] and Milch[170] used fascia lata between the clavicle and the sternum. Lowman[156] used a loop of fascia in and through the sternoclavicular joint so that it acts like the ligamentum teres in the hip. Speed[242] and Key and Conwell[136] reported on the use of a fascial loop between the clavicle and the first rib. Allen[6] uses fascia lata to reconstruct a new sternoclavicular ligament.

Subclavius Tendon. Burrows[43] recommended that the subclavius tendon be used to reconstruct a new costoclavicular ligament. The origin of the subclavius muscle is from the first rib just 6 mm lateral and 1.3 mm anterior to the attachment of the costoclavicular ligament.[97, 98] The insertion of the tendon is to the inferior surface of the junction of the middle third with the outer third of the clavicle, and the muscle fibers arising from the tendon insert into the inferior surface of the mid-third of the clavicle (Fig. 13–27). The muscle fibers coming off the tendon look like feathers on a bird's wing. Burrows detaches the muscle fiber from the tendon, does not disturb the origin of the tendon, and then passes the tendon through drill holes in the anterior proximal clavicle.

In comparing his operation with the use of free strips of fascia, Burrows said that it is "safer and easier to

pick up a mooring than to drop anchor; the obvious mooring is the tendon of the subclavius separated from its muscle fiber and suitably realigned." Lunseth and associates[159] have reported a modified Burrows procedure with the additional use of a threaded Steinmann pin across the joint.

Osteotomy of the Medial Clavicle. As previously described, Omer,[190] following repair or reconstruction of the ligaments, creates a step-cut osteotomy lateral to the joint and detaches the clavicular head of the sternocleidomastoid muscle from the proximal fragment.

Resection of the Medial End of the Clavicle. McLaughlin,[168] Breitner and Wirth,[34] Pridie,[205] Bateman,[20] and Milch[170] all have recommended excision of the medial clavicle when degenerative changes are noted in the joint. If the medial end of the clavicle is to be removed because of degenerative changes, the surgeon should be careful not to damage the costoclavicular ligament.

Arthrodesis. Arthrodesis was once reported[211] in the treatment of a habitual dislocation of the sternoclavicular joint. However, this procedure should *not* be done because it prevents the previously described normal elevation, depression, and rotation of the clavicle. The end result would be a severe restriction of shoulder movement (Fig. 13–28).

PHYSEAL INJURIES

As has been described earlier in the chapter, the epiphysis on the medial end of the clavicle is the last epiphysis in the body to appear on x-ray and the last one to close. The epiphysis on the medial end of the clavicle does not appear on x-rays until about the 18th year and does not unite with the clavicle until the 23rd to 25th year (Fig. 13–29; see also Fig. 13–5).[97, 98, 259]

This is important information to remember because many of the "dislocations of the sternoclavicular joint" are not dislocations but physeal injuries. Most of these injuries will heal with time, without surgical intervention. In time, the remodeling process eliminates any bone deformity or displacement. Anterior physeal injuries can certainly be left alone without problem. Posterior physeal injuries should be reduced. If the posterior dislocation cannot be reduced and the patient is having no significant symptoms, the displacement can be observed while remodeling occurs. If the posterior displacement is symptomatic and cannot be reduced closed, the displacement must be reduced during surgery.

In 1967, Denham and Dingley[64] reported three cases of medial clavicle physeal injury in patients aged 14 to 16. They demonstrated at surgery that the pathology was indeed a physeal fracture of the medial clavicle. In 1972, Brooks and Henning[36] presented a paper in which they concluded from a review of nine cases that many "sternoclavicular dislocations" and "fractures of the medial clavicle" were indeed medial clavicle

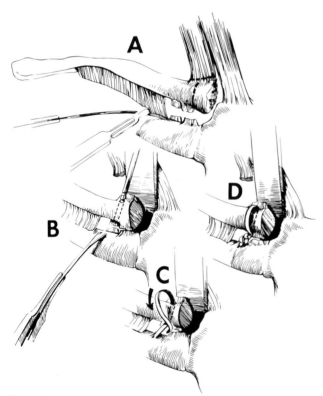

Figure 13–27. The technique of Jackson Burrows using the subclavius tendon to reconstruct the coracoclavicular ligament. (Modified from Burrows HJ: Tenodesis of the subclavius in the treatment of recurrent dislocation of the sternoclavicular joint. J Bone Joint Surg *33B*:240–243, 1951.)

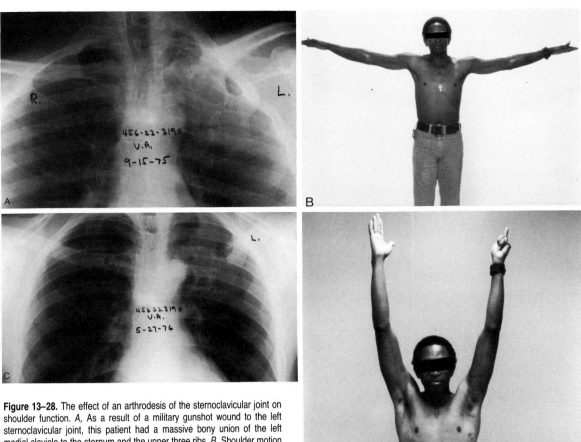

Figure 13–28. The effect of an arthrodesis of the sternoclavicular joint on shoulder function. *A,* As a result of a military gunshot wound to the left sternoclavicular joint, this patient had a massive bony union of the left medial clavicle to the sternum and the upper three ribs. *B,* Shoulder motion was limited to 90 degrees of flexion and abduction. *C,* An x-ray following resection of the bony mass, freeing up the medial clavicle. *D,* Function of the left shoulder was essentially normal following the elimination of the sternoclavicular arthrodesis. (Reproduced with permission from Rockwood CA, and Green DP (eds): Fractures (3 vols), 2nd ed. Philadelphia: JB Lippincott, 1984.)

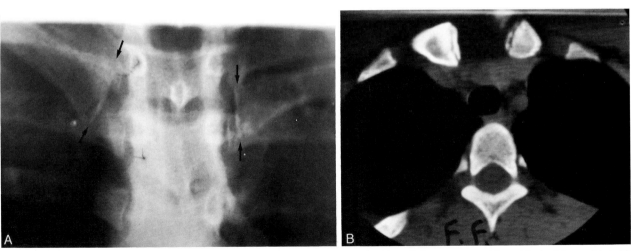

Figure 13–29. *A,* An anteroposterior view of the medial ends of both clavicles demonstrates the thin, waferlike appearance of the epiphysis of the medial clavicle. (Reproduced with permission from Rockwood CA, and Green DP (eds): Fractures (3 vols), 2nd ed. Philadelphia: JB Lippincott, 1984.) *B,* A CT scan of the sternoclavicular joints demonstrates the epiphysis of both medial clavicles.

physeal injuries. In 1984, Lemire and Rosman[147] reported a case of "double fracture" of the medial clavicle in a 15-year-old patient. One fracture was through the physis and the other through the medial third of the clavicle. They surgically restored the clavicle into the periosteal tube, and the patient returned to normal activity without any further problems.

Anterior Displacement of the Medial Clavicle

If the physeal injury is recognized, or if the patient is under the age of 25, closed reduction, as has been described for anterior dislocation of the sternoclavicular joint, should be performed. The shoulders should be held back in a clavicular strap of figure-of-eight dressing for three to four weeks, even if the reduction is unstable. Healing is prompt, and remodeling will occur at the site of the deformity.

Posterior Displacement of the Medial Clavicle

Closed reduction of this injury should be performed in the manner described for posterior dislocation of the sternoclavicular joint. The reduction is usually stable with shoulders held back in a figure-of-eight dressing or strap. Immobilization should continue for three to four weeks. If the posterior physeal injury cannot be reduced, and if the patient is not having symptoms, and if the patient is a child or an adult under the age of 23, one could wait and watch to see if remodeling eliminates the posteriorly displaced clavicle.

ATRAUMATIC INJURIES

Spontaneous Subluxation or Dislocation

This usually occurs in young people under the age of 20, and most often occurs in females. Without significant trauma, one or both of the medial clavicles spontaneously displace anteriorly during abduction or flexion to the overhead position (see Fig. 13–10). The clavicle reduces when the arm is returned to the side. It usually is associated with laxity in other joints of the extremities. I have reviewed 37 cases from my own practice and have found it to be a self-limiting condition.[219] The conditions should not be treated with *attempted* surgical reconstruction, because the joint will continue to sublux or dislocate and may indeed cause more pain, discomfort, and an unsightly scar (Fig. 13–30). The condition should be carefully explained to the patient and the family, and they should be told that it will ultimately not be a problem and the symptoms may disappear.

Congenital or Developmental

Congenital or developmental problems (e.g., absence or partial absence of bone or muscles) can produce subluxation or dislocation of the sternoclavicular joint. Specific rehabilitation or surgical procedures are usually unnecessary.[100, 180]

Arthritis

The management of patients with osteoarthritis and of patients with postmenopausal osteoarthritis can usually be done with conservative nonoperative treatment, i.e., heat, anti-inflammatory agents, and rest.[30, 35] However, the patient must be thoroughly evaluated to rule out other conditions that mimic the changes in the sternoclavicular joint, i.e., tumor, metabolic, infectious, or collagen disorders, and so forth. Patients with post-traumatic arthritic changes in the sternoclavicular joint, which follow fractures of the sternoclavicular joint and previous attempts at reconstruction, may require a formal arthroplasty of the joint and careful stabilization of the remaining clavicle to the first rib.

Patients with collagen disorders, such as rheumatoid arthritis, and some patients with condensing osteitis of the medial clavicle may require an arthroplasty. In operating on the sternoclavicular joint, care must be taken to evaluate the residual stability of the medial clavicle. It is the same analogy as used when resecting the distal clavicle for a complete old acromioclavicular joint problem. If the coracoclavicular ligaments are intact, an excision of the distal clavicle is indicated. If the coracoclavicular ligaments are gone, then, in addition to the excision of the distal clavicle, you must reconstruct the coracoclavicular ligaments. If the costoclavicular ligaments are intact, the clavicle medial to the ligaments should be resected and beveled smooth (Fig. 13–31). If the ligaments are gone, the clavicle must be stabilized to the first rib. If too much clavicle is resected, or if the clavicle is not stabilized to the first rib, an increase in symptoms can occur (Fig. 13–32).

Patients with sterno-costal-clavicular hyperostosis have a very difficult problem to manage.* The condition cannot be arrested with drugs. Treatment is largely dependent on analgesic and anti-inflammatory medications and physical therapy. Occasionally, surgical excision of the bony mass to allow an increase in function of the upper extremity is indicated.

Infection

Infections of the sternoclavicular joint should be managed as they are in other joints, except that during aspiration and surgical drainage, great care and respect must be directed to the vital structures that lie posterior to the joint. If aspiration or a high index of suspicion demonstrates purulent material in the joint, a formal arthrotomy should be carried out. The anterior sternoclavicular ligament will need to be removed, but the posterior and interclavicular ligaments should be spared. Occasionally, the infection will arise in the medial end of the clavicle or the manubrium, which

---

*See references 4, 53, 91, 94, 129, 142, 225, 238–240.

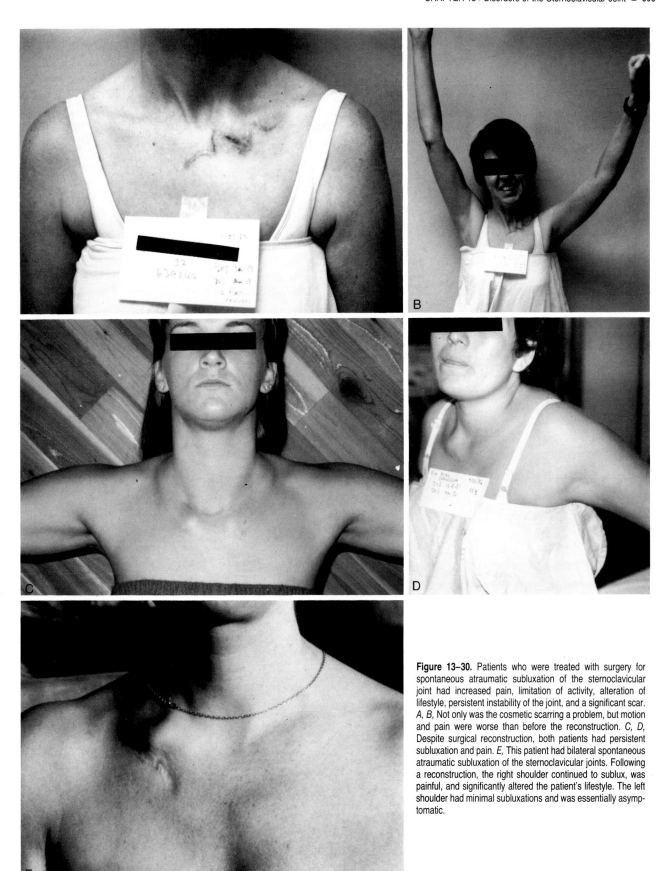

Figure 13–30. Patients who were treated with surgery for spontaneous atraumatic subluxation of the sternoclavicular joint had increased pain, limitation of activity, alteration of lifestyle, persistent instability of the joint, and a significant scar. *A, B,* Not only was the cosmetic scarring a problem, but motion and pain were worse than before the reconstruction. *C, D,* Despite surgical reconstruction, both patients had persistent subluxation and pain. *E,* This patient had bilateral spontaneous atraumatic subluxation of the sternoclavicular joints. Following a reconstruction, the right shoulder continued to sublux, was painful, and significantly altered the patient's lifestyle. The left shoulder had minimal subluxations and was essentially asymptomatic.

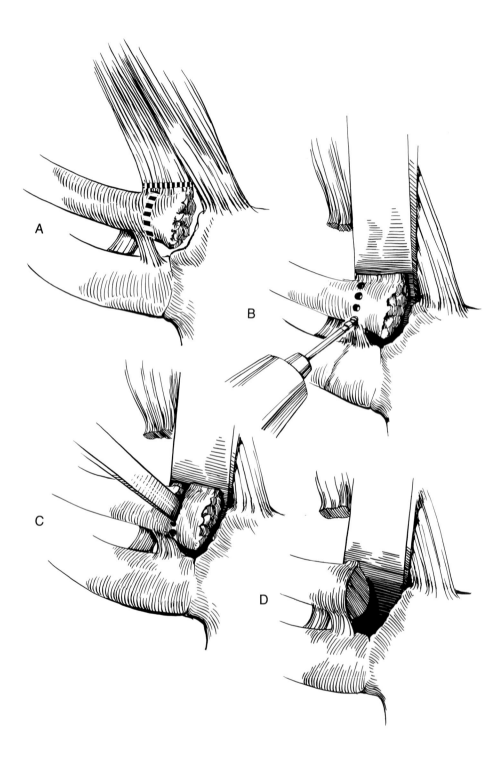

Figure 13–31. Technique of resecting the medial clavicle for degenerative arthritis. *A,* Care must be taken to remove only that part of the clavicle that is medial to the costoclavicular (rhomboid) ligaments. There must be adequate protection for the vital structures that lie posterior to the medial end of the clavicle. *B, C,* An air drill with a side cutting bur can be used to perform the osteotomy. *D,* When the fragment of bone has been removed, the dorsal and anterior borders of the clavicle should be smoothed down to give a better cosmetic appearance. (Reproduced with permission from Rockwood CA, and Green DP (eds): Fractures (3 vols), 2nd ed. Philadelphia: JB Lippincott, 1984.)

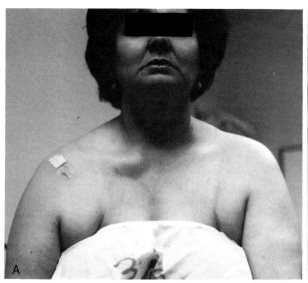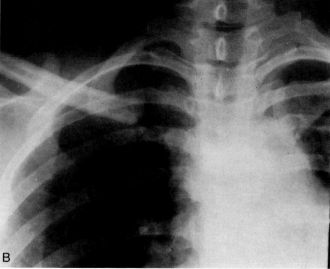

Figure 13–32. *A,* This postmenopausal right hand–dominant woman had a resection of the right medial clavicle because of preoperative diagnosis of "possible tumor." The postoperative microscopic diagnosis was degenerative arthritis of the right medial clavicle. Following surgery, the patient complained of pain and discomfort, marked prominence, and gross instability of the right medial clavicle. *B,* An x-ray confirms that the excision of the medial clavicle extended lateral to the costoclavicular ligaments, hence the patient had an unstable medial clavicle. (Reproduced with permission from Rockwood CA, and Green DP (eds): Fractures (3 vols), 2nd ed. Philadelphia: JB Lippincott, 1984.)

will necessitate the resection of some of the dead bone. Depending on the status of the wound following the debridement, one can either close the wound loosely over a drain or pack the wound open and close it at a later time.

Author's Preferred Method of Treatment

TRAUMATIC PROBLEMS

Type I Injury (Mild Sprain)

I recommend the use of cold packs for the first 12 to 24 hours and a sling to rest the joint. Ordinarily, after five to seven days, the patient can use the arm for everyday living activities.

Type II Injury (Subluxation)

In addition to the cold pack, I may use a soft, padded figure-of-eight clavicle strap to gently hold the shoulders back to allow the sternoclavicular joint to rest. The figure-of-eight harness can be removed after a week or so, and then either put the patient into a sling for a week or so, or allow the patient to gradually return to everyday living activities.

Type III Injury (Dislocation)

In general, I manage almost all dislocations of the sternoclavicular joint in children and in adults by either a closed reduction or by a nonoperative skillful neglect form of treatment. The acute traumatic posterior dislocations are reduced closed and become stable when

the shoulders are held back in a figure-of-eight dressing. Most of the anterior dislocations are unstable, but I accept the deformity since I believe it is less of a problem than the potential problems of operative repair and internal fixation.

Anterior Dislocation

Method of Reduction. In most instances, knowing that the anterior dislocation will be unstable, I will still try to reduce the anterior displacement. Muscle relaxants and narcotics are administered intravenously, and the patient is placed supine on the table with a stack of three or four towels between the shoulder blades. While an assistant gently applies downward pressure on the anterior aspect of both shoulders, I will push the medial end of the clavicle backward where it belongs. On some occasions, rare as they may be, the anterior displacement may stay adjacent to the sternum. However, in most cases, either with the shoulders still held back or when they are relaxed, an anterior displacement promptly occurs. I explain to the patient that the joint is unstable and that the hazards of internal fixation are too great, and I prescribe a sling for a couple of weeks and allow the patient to begin using the arm as soon as the discomfort is gone.

Most of the anterior injuries that I have treated in children and in adults under the age of 25 are not dislocations of the sternoclavicular joint but Type I or II physeal injuries, which heal and remodel without operative treatment. Patients over the ages 23 to 25 with anterior dislocations of the sternoclavicular joint do have persistent prominence of the anterior clavicle. However, this does not seem to interfere with usual activities and, in some cases, has not even interfered with heavy manual labor.

I wish to re-emphasize that I do not recommend open reduction of the joint, and I would never recommend transfixing pins across the sternoclavicular joint.

Postreduction Care. If the reduction happens to be stable, I place the patient in either a figure-of-eight dressing or in whatever device or position the clavicle is most stable. If the reduction is unstable, the arm is placed into a sling for a week or so, and then the patient can begin to use the arm for gentle everyday activities.

Posterior Dislocation

It is very important to take a very careful history and to perform a very careful physical examination. The physician should obtain x-rays, tomograms or CT scans, or angio-CT scans to document whether there is any compression of the great vessels in the neck or arm or any difficulty in swallowing or breathing. It is also important to determine if the patient has any feeling of choking or hoarseness. If any of these symptoms are present, indicating pressure on the mediastinum, the appropriate specialist should be consulted.

I do not believe that operative techniques are usually required to reduce the acute posterior sternoclavicular joint dislocation. Furthermore, once the joint has been reduced closed, it is usually stable (Fig. 13–33).

Although I used to think that I could always make the diagnosis of anterior or posterior injury of the sternoclavicular joint on physical examination, I know now that one cannot rely on the anterior swelling and firmness as being diagnostic of an anterior injury. I have been fooled on six occasions when, from physical examination, the patient appeared to have an anterior dislocation, but x-rays have documented a posterior problem. Therefore, I recommend that the clinical impression *always* be documented with appropriate x-rays before any decision to treat or not to treat is made.

Method of Closed Reduction. The patient is placed in the supine position with a three- to four-inch thick sandbag or three to four folded towels between the scapulae to extend the shoulders. The dislocated shoulder should be over toward the edge of the table so that the arm and shoulder can be abducted and extended. If the patient is having extreme pain and muscle spasm and is quite anxious, I use general anesthesia; otherwise, narcotics, muscle relaxants, or tranquilizers are given through an established intravenous route in the normal arm. First, gentle traction is applied on the abducted arm in line with the clavicle while countertraction is applied by an assistant who steadies the patient on the table. The traction on the abducted arm is gradually increased while the arm is brought into extension.

Reduction of an acute injury usually occurs with an audible pop or snap and the relocation can be noted visibly. If the traction in abduction and extension is not successful, an assistant grasps or pushes down on the clavicle in an effort to dislodge it from behind the sternum. Occasionally, in a stubborn case, especially in a thick-chested person or a patient with extensive swelling, it is impossible to obtain a secure grasp on the clavicle with the assistant's fingers. The skin should then be surgically prepared and a sterile towel clip used to gain purchase on the medial clavicle percutaneously (see Fig. 13–24). The towel clip is used to grasp completely around the shaft of the clavicle. The dense cortical bone prevents the purchase of the towel clip into the clavicle. Then the combined traction through the arm plus the anterior lifting force on the towel clip will reduce the dislocation. Following the reduction, the sternoclavicular joint is stable, even with the patient's arms at the side. However, I always hold the shoulders back in a well-padded figure-of-eight clavicle strap for three to four weeks to allow for soft tissue and ligamentous healing.

I have not used the technique described by Butterworth and Kirk[44] of traction on the arm in adduction, but I believe this technique is valid and will use it should the traction abduction technique fail.

Technique of Open Reduction. The complications of an unreduced posterior dislocation are numerous, e.g., thoracic outlet syndrome[86] and vascular compromise[33] and erosion of the medial clavicle into any one of the many vital structures that lie posterior to the sternoclavicular joint. Therefore, in adults, if closed reduction fails, an open reduction should be performed.

The patient is supine on the table and the three to four towels or the sandbag should be left between the scapulae. The upper extremity should be draped out free so that lateral traction can be applied during the open reduction. In addition, a folded sheet around the patient's thorax should be left in place so that it could be used for countertraction during the traction on the involved extremity. An anterior incision is used that parallels the superior border of the medial three to four inches of the clavicle, and then extends downward over the sternum just medial to the involved sternoclavicular joint. As previously described, this should usually be done with a thoracic surgeon. The trick is to remove sufficient soft tissues to expose the joint but to leave the anterior capsular ligament intact. The reduction can usually be accomplished with traction and countertraction while lifting up anteriorly with a clamp around the medial clavicle. Along with the traction and countertraction, it may be necessary to use an elevator to pry the clavicle back to its articulation with the sternum. When the reduction has been obtained, and with the shoulders held back, the reduction will be stable because the anterior capsule has been left intact. If the anterior capsule is damaged or is insufficient to prevent anterior displacement of the medial end of the clavicle, I recommend an excision of the medial 1 to 1½ inches of the clavicle and securing the residual clavicle to the first rib with 1.0 mm Dacron tape. Postoperatively, the patient should be held with

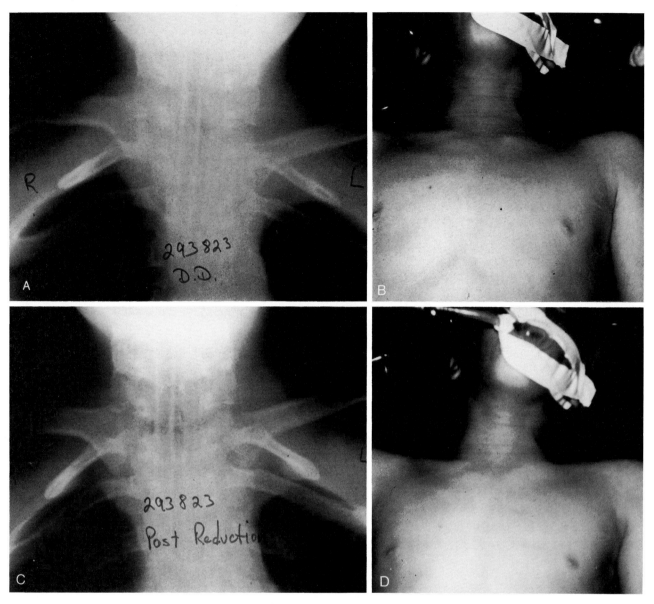

Figure 13–33. Posterior dislocation or Type I epiphyseal separation of the left sternoclavicular joint in a 12-year-old boy. *A,* The 40-degree cephalic tilt "serendipity" x-ray reveals that the left clavicle is significantly lower on the horizontal plane than the normal right clavicle. *B,* Prior to reduction, the medial end of the left clavicle was displaced posteriorly compared with the normal right clavicle. The only remaining prominence of the left sternoclavicular joint was the prominence of the superomedial corner of the manubrium. *C,* Under general anesthesia, a closed reduction was performed by traction on the arm out into abduction and extension. The clavicle reduced with an audible pop back into position. It was restored to the same horizontal level as the normal right clavicle. *D,* Clinically both clavicles were palpable at the same level following reduction.

his shoulders back in a figure-of-eight dressing for four to six weeks to allow for healing of the soft tissues.

Note: I do not recommend the use of Kirschner wires or Steinmann pins or any other type of metallic pins to stabilize the sternoclavicular joint. The complications are horrendous; see section on complications for details.

Physeal Injuries of the Medial Clavicle

I believe that many of the anterior and posterior injuries of the sternoclavicular joint in patients under the age of 25, which are thought to be "dislocations" of the sternoclavicular joint, are injuries to the medial physis of the clavicle. Many authors have observed at the time of surgery that the intra-articular disc ligament stays with the sternum, and I agree with them. In addition, I submit that the unossified or ossified epiphyseal disk, depending on the age of the patient, also stays with the sternum. Anatomically, the epiphysis is lateral to the articular disc ligament, and it is held in place by the capsular ligament and can be mistaken for the intra-articular disc ligament.

As previously described, the medial epiphysis does not ossify and thus does not appear on the x-ray until the age of 18. Therefore, the diagnosis cannot be "documented" until after ossification occurs. However,

I would still perform the closed reduction maneuvers as described above for a suspected anterior or posterior injury. Open reduction of the physeal injury is seldom indicated except for the possibility of an irreducible posterior displacement in a patient who was having significant symptoms of compression of the vital structures in the mediastinum. After reduction, the shoulders are held back with a figure-of-eight strap or dressing for three to four weeks.

In 1966, I first treated a 16-year-old boy with a fracture of the medial one-third of the clavicle and a "dislocation" of the sternoclavicular joint which turned out to be a Type I epiphyseal injury (Fig. 13–34). I thought then that it might be an original observation. Since I could not find any references on the problem, I was ready to publish my observation when my good friend Lee Rogers, M.D. (now Professor and Chairman of the Department of Radiology at Northwestern Medical School) recommended that I review the text by John Poland that had been written in 1898. As happens with most "new ideas" in orthopedics, my observation was not new. Poland,[203] in his text entitled *Traumatic Separation of Epiphyses of the Upper Extremity,* described the entity in detail. He reviewed several French articles that evaluated more than 60 cases of fracture of the medial epiphysis of the clavicle that clinically appeared as sternoclavicular dislocations. He discussed the anatomy of the joint and the classifications of the injury and described methods of treatment. He described in detail an article by Verchere, written in 1886, which probably represents the first published report of a death caused by posterior dislocation of the sternoclavicular joint:

A 20-year-old man, following a severe crushing injury, died on the seventh day, of subcutaneous emphysema. Autopsy revealed that the inner third of the right clavicle was detached of its periosteum, and its smooth rounded end was displaced posteriorly and had produced a perforation of the pleural sac about the size of a 2-franc piece. The hole was in the left lung, whereas the ipsilateral lung escaped injury. The report very clearly described that the sternoclavicular joint was not injured and that the 5-mm-wide epiphyseal plate was held firmly in place by the ligaments about the joint. The specimen of the separated epiphysis was placed in the Dupuytren Museum.

Poland went on to describe that the capsular ligament is primarily attached to the epiphysis of the medial clavicle and stated that with injury the epiphysis is held by the capsular ligament and stays with its articulation with the sternum.

In treating the 16-year-old boy with the fracture of the medial clavicle and the "dislocation" of the sternoclavicular joint, I figured that I needed to, at least, line up the clavicle and put the sternoclavicular joint in better approximation (see Fig. 13–37). The fragment was 3.7 cm long and had rotated 90 degrees from the long axis of the clavicle. In my eagerness to explore the anatomy, the fragment of clavicle, which had been completely stripped of its periosteum, fell onto the floor. However, the sternal end of the fragment did not have a smooth cartilaginous articular surface. It was rough and had the appearance of the end of a chicken leg when your last bite took off the epiphysis. The costoclavicular ligaments were intact to the periosteum inferiorly, and in the most medial corner of the periosteal tube was a dense structure that could be

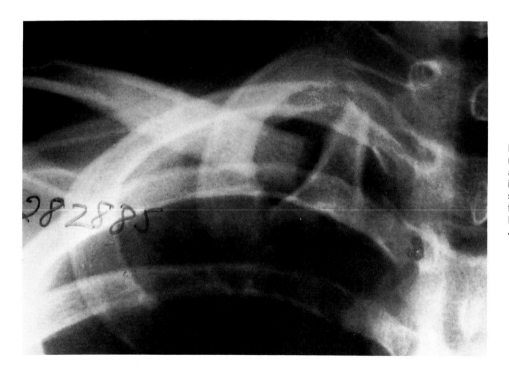

Figure 13–34. Type I epiphyseal separation of the right medial clavicle associated with fracture of the shaft of the clavicle with 90-degree rotation of the segment. (Reproduced with permission from Rockwood CA, and Green DP (eds): Fractures (3 vols), 2nd ed. Philadelphia: JB Lippincott, 1984.)

taken for the intra-articular disc ligament—or it could have been the unossified epiphysis.

Treatment consisted of closing the periosteal tube and hoping that the epiphysis was still present adjacent to the sternum (Fig. 13–35). Later, microscopic studies of the most medial end of the fragment revealed the provisional zone of calcification of the metaphysis, indicating that indeed there had been a separation through the physeal plate and that it had occurred through the zone of hypertrophy (Fig. 13–36). Serial x-rays revealed a gradual replacement of the medial clavicle, and after 18 months, the entire defect had been replaced with bone (Fig. 13–37A). The patient returned to his former job as a manual laborer (Fig. 13–37B).

Since 1966, in other cases of "dislocation of the sternoclavicular joint," I have been able to document with the 40-degree cephalic tilt x-ray and CT scans that the injury really was a physeal fracture, because the thin wafer-like disc has remained in its normal articulation with the sternum, while the metaphysis and shaft were displaced. Some of the physeal fractures have been Type II injuries, with a small fragment of the

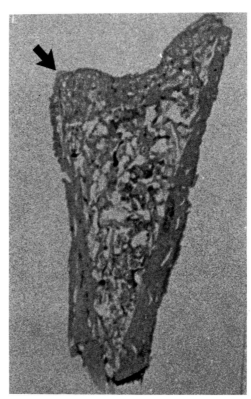

Figure 13–36. Microscopic examination of the fragment of clavicle that was removed from the patient in Figure 13–34. The medial end of the fragment revealed the provisional zone of calcification of the metaphysis. This indicates that the epiphysis of the medial clavicle was still in its normal position adjacent to the manubrium. The physeal injury occurred through the zone of hypertrophy. (Reproduced with permission from Rockwood CA, and Green DP (eds): Fractures (3 vols), 2nd ed. Philadelphia: JB Lippincott, 1984.)

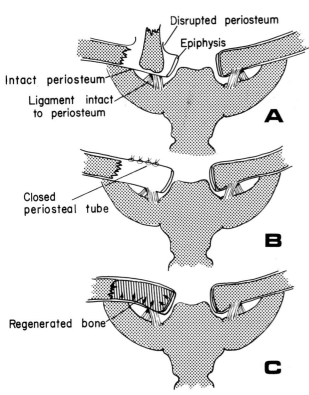

Figure 13–35. Schematic drawing of the injury and healing of the patient in Figure 13–34. A, The fragment, with its metaphysis, has been separated from the epiphyseal plate and partially displaced out of the periosteal tube. B, The fragment was removed, and the defect in the periosteal tube was closed. The coracoclavicular ligaments were intact and were attached inferiorly to the periosteal tube. The epiphysis remained in its normal anatomical position by the sternoclavicular capsular ligaments. C, At 18 months, the medial end of the clavicle was replaced by new bone formation from the epiphysis and the periosteum. (Reproduced with permission from Rockwood CA, and Green DP (eds): Fractures (3 vols), 2nd ed. Philadelphia: JB Lippincott, 1984.)

metaphysis remaining with the epiphysis. Obviously, before the epiphysis ossifies at the age of 18, one cannot be sure whether a displacement about the sternoclavicular joint is a dislocation of the sternoclavicular joint or a fracture through the physeal plate.

Despite the fact that there is significant displacement of the shaft with either a Type I or Type II physeal fracture, the periosteal tube remains in its anatomical position and the attaching ligaments are intact to the periosteum, i.e., the costoclavicular ligaments inferiorly and the capsular and inter-articular disc ligaments medially (Fig. 13–38).

Recurrent Traumatic Dislocation of the Sternoclavicular Joint

Recurrent anterior or posterior dislocation of the sternoclavicular joint following an acute injury is extremely rare. I have not seen or read of a patient with recurrent anterior or posterior subluxation or dislocation following a traumatic injury. Usually the joint is stable following reduction, or it remains permanently anteriorly or posteriorly displaced. This entity should not be confused with the problem of spontaneous subluxation or dislocation.

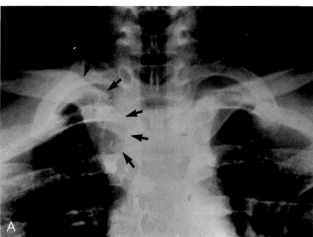
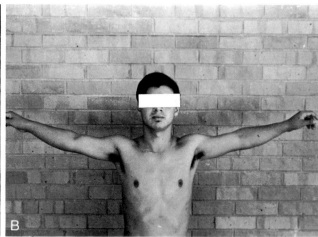
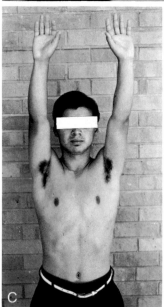

Figure 13–37. *A,* The x-ray of the sternoclavicular joint taken 18 months after the removal of the medial clavicle (Fig. 13–34). There has been total regeneration of the medial clavicle by the periosteal tube and the retained epiphysis. *B, C,* Eighteen months after the injury and a regrowth of the medial clavicle, the patient had a full range of motion, was asymptomatic, and was performing manual labor. (Reproduced with permission from Rockwood CA, and Green DP (eds): Fractures (3 vols), 2nd ed. Philadelphia: JB Lippincott, 1984.)

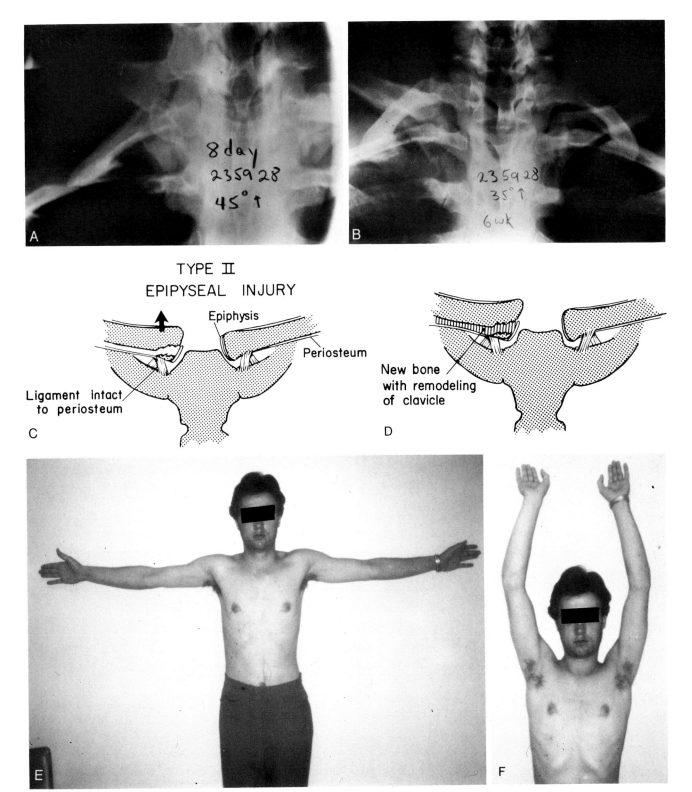

Figure 13–38. A Type II physeal injury of the right medial clavicle. *A,* The x-ray at eight days reveals that the right medial clavicle is displaced superiorly from the left clavicle. The inferior medial corner of the clavicle is still located in its normal position adjacent to the epiphysis. *B,* The x-ray at six weeks reveals new bone formation along the inferior periosteal tube. Note the thin epiphyseal plate of the normal left medial clavicle. *C,* A schematic of the healing process with a Type II physeal injury to the medial clavicle. The medial clavicle splits out of the periosteal tube, leaving a small fragment (Thurston-Holland sign) behind. The costoclavicular ligaments are intact to the inferior periosteal tube. *D,* Through remodeling from the retained epiphysis and the periosteal tube, the fracture heals itself. *E, F,* Clinically, at eight weeks the physeal injury was healed and the patient had a full range of motion.

Unreduced Traumatic Dislocation of the Sternoclavicular Joint

Anterior Dislocation

As previously described, most patients with an un-reduced and permanent anterior dislocation of the sternoclavicular joint are not very symptomatic, have almost a complete range of motion, and can work and even perform manual labor without many problems (Fig. 13–39). Because the joint is so small and incon-gruous and because the results I have seen in patients who have had attempted reconstructions are so miser-able, I usually recommend a nonoperative skillful neglect type of treatment. In patients who have had a previous failed sternoclavicular operative procedure, I will perform a repeat arthroplasty with a resection of the medial clavicle in an attempt to reduce and stabilize the joint with suture, fascia, tendons, and so on.

If the patient has persistent symptoms of traumatic arthritis for 6 to 12 months following a dislocation, and if the symptoms can be completely relieved by injection of local anesthesia into the sternoclavicular joint re-gion, I would perform an arthroplasty of the sternocla-vicular joint. This would include a resection of the medial one inch of the clavicle with a beveling of the superoanterior corner for cosmetic purposes, a de-bridement of the intra-articular disc ligament, and stabilization of the remaining clavicle to the first rib with either 1.0 mm or 3.0 mm cotton Dacron tape. If the costoclavicular ligaments do not stabilize the medial clavicle, it is essential to reconstruct a ligament-like structure between the clavicle and the first rib. I also detach the clavicular head of the sternocleidomastoid to temporarily resist the upward pull of the clavicle by this muscle.

Unreduced Posterior Dislocation

In the adult, because of the potential problems that can be associated with the clavicle's remaining dis-placed posteriorly into the mediastinum, an open re-duction is usually indicated. This requires the excision of the medial one inch of the clavicle and stabilization to the first rib as described above.

ATRAUMATIC PROBLEMS

Spontaneous Subluxation or Dislocation of the Sternoclavicular Joint

I have seen 37 patients with this problem, and about the only symptom they have is that the medial end of the clavicle subluxes or dislocates anteriorly when they raise their arms over their heads.[219] This occurs spon-taneously and without any significant trauma. It might be considered a voluntary or an involuntary problem, because it occurs whenever the patient raises the arms to the overhead position. Some patients seen for an-other shoulder problem are completely unaware that with the overhead motion the medial end of the clavicle subluxes or dislocates. I have never seen a posterior spontaneous subluxation of the sternoclavicular joint. Only occasionally does the patient with atraumatic anterior displacement complain of pain during the displacement. Because I do not believe that I can stabilize the joint and prevent the subluxation or dislocation and end up with a pain-free range of motion, I manage the problem with nonoperative skill-ful neglect. I very carefully explain the anatomy of the problem to the patient and the family. I explain further that surgery is of little benefit, that they should discon-

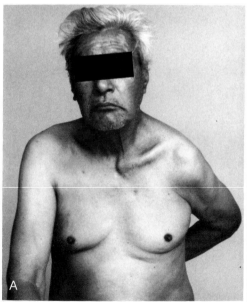
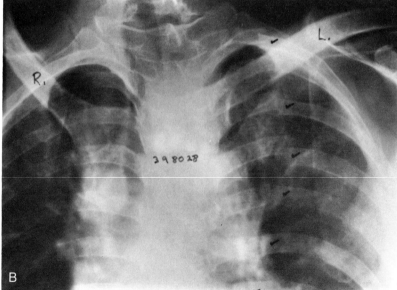

Figure 13–39. Unreduced anterior traumatic dislocations of the sternoclavicular joint. *A,* This patient has an anterior unreduced dislocation of the left sternoclavicular joint. He works as a laborer and has few if any complaints. *B,* The injury occurred five years prior to the photograph when he had a dislocation and multiple fractures of his ribs.

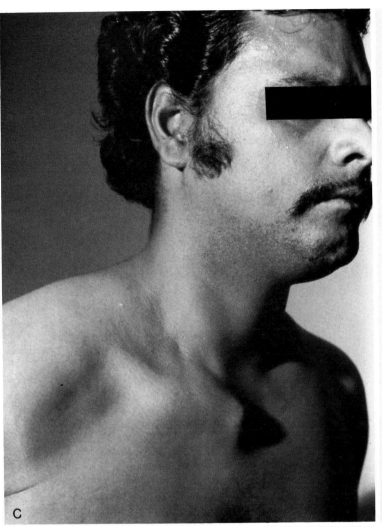

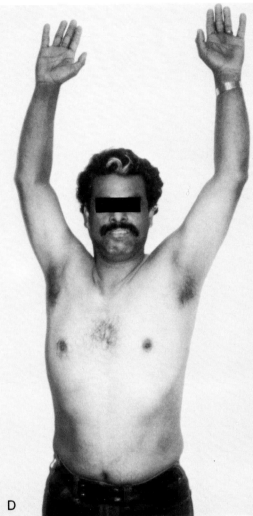

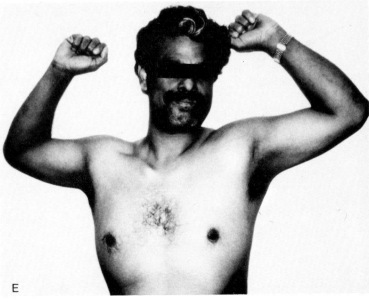

Figure 13–39 *Continued. C,* This patient suffered an unre-duced traumatic anterior dislocation in his right shoulder following an automobile accident. At the time of the injury the medial clavicle could be manually reduced, but it would not stay in position. *D, E,* Fifteen years later the patient continues to have prominence of his right medial clavicle, but he works as a day laborer unloading and loading 50-pound sacks of cement. (*A* and *C* reproduced with permission from Rockwood CA, and Green DP (eds): Fractures (3 vols), 2nd ed. Philadelphia: JB Lippincott, 1984.)

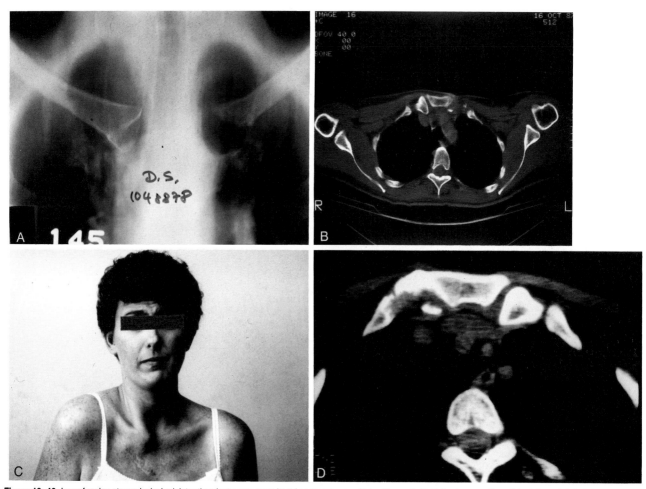

Figure 13–40. In performing sternoclavicular joint arthroplasty, care must be taken to remove sufficient bone. *A, B,* Following resection of the left medial clavicle, this patient continued to have pain with shoulder motion. The CT scan confirms fragments of bone in the site of the arthroplasty. *C,* Following arthroplasty of the right sternoclavicular joint, the medial clavicle was still quite prominent and painful. *D,* A CT scan confirms the medial right clavicle butting into the manubrium and a loose fragment of bone in the joint.

tinue the voluntary aspect of the dislocation, and that in time the symptoms will either disappear or they will completely forget that the dislocation is a problem.

In the review by Rockwood and Odor of 37 patients with spontaneous atraumatic subluxation, 29 were managed without surgery and 8 were treated with a surgical reconstruction elsewhere.[219] With an average follow-up of more than 8 years, all of the 29 nonoperated patients were doing just fine without limitations of activity or lifestyle. The 8 patients who were treated with surgery had increased pain, limitation of activity, alteration of lifestyle, persistent instability, and a significant scar.

In many instances, the patient, before a previous reconstruction or resection, had minimal discomfort, an excellent range of motion, and only complained of the "bump" that slipped in and out of place with certain motions. Postoperatively, the patient still had the bump, along with a scar and a painful range of motion (see Fig. 13–30).

Arthritis

Most patients with simple degenerative arthritis or postmenopausal osteoarthritis can be managed with rest, moist heat, and anti-inflammatory medications (see Figs. 13–12 and 13–13). As previously described, it is very important to do a good work-up of the patient with arthritis of the sternoclavicular joint to rule out tumor, arthropathies, condensing osteitis of the medial clavicle, and sternocostoclavicular hyperostosis. Patients with post-traumatic osteoarthritis or sternocostoclavicular hyperostosis may require resection of the medial clavicle. Care must be taken to remove sufficient, but not too much, bone of the medial clavicle (Fig. 13–40).

Infection

I believe that pus in this joint should be managed by arthrotomy and exploration of the joint. If the procedure is done soon after the onset of the infection, the arthrotomy and joint clean-out is usually sufficient. If the infection is long-standing and there is destruction of the cartilage and bone, a resection of the medial clavicle or the involved manubrium should be performed. Care should be taken to preserve the posterior, interclavicular, and costoclavicular ligaments (see Fig. 13–14).

Complications of Injuries to the Sternoclavicular Joint

The serious complications that occur at the time of dislocation of the sternoclavicular joint are primarily limited to the posterior injuries. About the only complication that occurs with the anterior dislocation of the sternoclavicular joint is a "cosmetic bump" or late degenerative changes.

Many complications have been reported secondary to the retrosternal dislocation: pneumothorax and laceration of the superior vena cava,[194] venous congestion in the neck, rupture of the esophagus with abscess and osteomyelitis of the clavicle,[32] pressure on the subclavian artery in an untreated patient,[119, 243] occlusion of the subclavian artery late in a patient who was not treated,[243] compression of the right common carotid artery by a fracture-dislocation of the sternoclavicular joint,[119] brachial plexus compression,[167] and hoarseness of the voice, onset of snoring, and voice changes from normal to falsetto with movement of the arm (Figs. 13–25, 13–41).[32, 134, 171, 224, 253] Wasylenko and Busse[256] reported a posterior dislocation of the medial clavicle that caused a fatal tracheoesophageal fistula. Gangahar and Flogaites[86] reported a case of posterior dislocation of the clavicle that produced a severe thoracic outlet syndrome with swelling and cyanosis of the upper extremity. Gardner and Bidstrup[87] reported on three patients who had severe great vessel injuries following

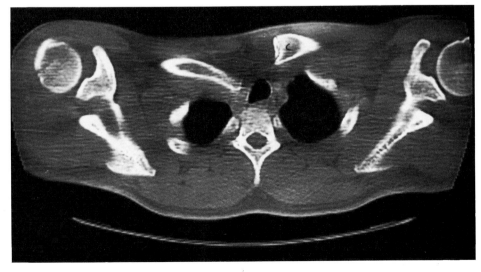

Figure 13–41. A CT scan demonstrates posterior dislocation of the clavicle back into the mediastinum, displacing the trachea.

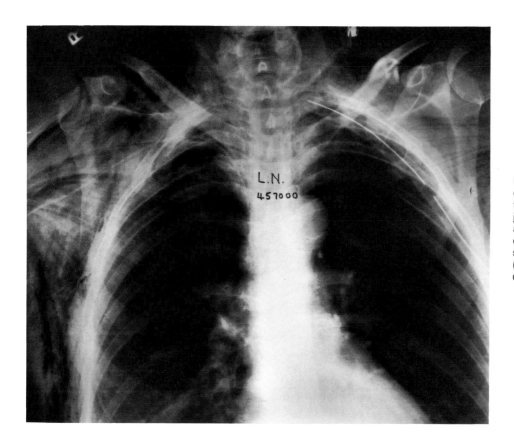

Figure 13–42. Complications of sterno-clavicular dislocation. As a result of posterior dislocation of the sternoclavicular joint, the patient had a lacerated trachea and developed massive subcutaneous emphysema. (Reproduced with permission from Rockwood CA, and Green DP (eds): Fractures (3 vols), 2nd ed. Philadelphia: JB Lippincott, 1984.)

Figure 13–43. Complications of sterno-clavicular joint dislocation. This patient had an anterior dislocation on the right and a posterior dislocation on the left. As a result of the posterior dislocation, he had sufficient pressure on the mediastinal structures to cause significant hypotension. When the posterior dislocation was reduced, the blood pressure on the continuous monitor promptly returned to normal. (Reproduced with permission from Rockwood CA, and Green DP (eds): Fractures (3 vols). Philadelphia: JB Lippincott, 1984.)

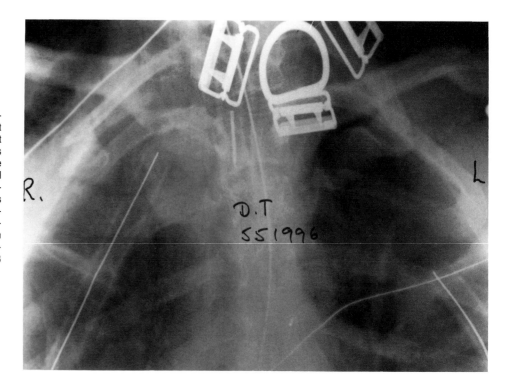

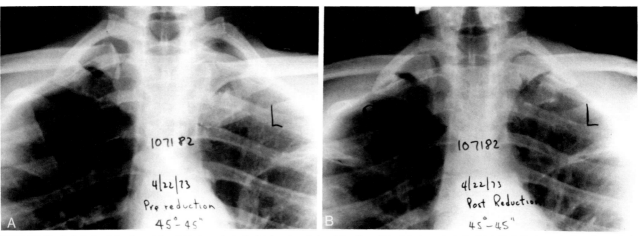

Figure 13–44. *A,* Anterior dislocation of the right sternoclavicular joint and posterior dislocation of the left sternoclavicular joint. *B,* Following reduction, the posterior dislocation was stable and the right remained slightly anteriorly displaced.

blunt chest trauma and posterior dislocation of the sternoclavicular joint. Two cases involved the innominate artery, and one case involved the carotid and subclavian arteries.

Several of my patients have had unusual complications that have resulted from traumatic injuries to the sternoclavicular joint. One patient, as the result of a posterior dislocation and rupture of the trachea, developed massive subcutaneous emphysema (Fig. 13–42). Another patient had an anterior dislocation on the right and a posterior dislocation on the left. When first seen, his blood pressure was very low. Following reduction of the posterior dislocation, his blood pressure, as recorded on his monitor, instantly returned to normal (Fig. 13–43). It was theorized that the posteriorly displaced clavicle was irritating some of the vital structures of the mediastinum. Another patient, who had vascular compromise, was discussed in the section on Treatment of Posterior Dislocations (see Fig. 13–25). Another patient had a traumatic injury to both sternoclavicular joints—the left was posterior and the right was anterior. Following reduction of the left posterior dislocation, the right side remained unstable. However, he developed a painless full range of motion (Fig. 13–44).

Worman and Leagus,[266] in an excellent review of the complications associated with posterior dislocations of the sternoclavicular joint, reported that 16 of 60 patients reviewed from the literature had suffered complications of the trachea, esophagus, or great vessels. I should point out that even though the incidence of complications was 25 per cent, only four deaths have been reported as a result of the injury.[99, 134, 203]

Complications of Operative Procedures

Until 1984, four deaths[51, 148, 178, 224] and three near deaths[38, 193, 266] from complications of transfixing the

sternoclavicular joint with Kirschner wires or Steinmann pins had been reported. The pins, either intact or broken, migrated into the heart, pulmonary artery, innominate artery, or into the aorta. Tremendous leverage force is applied to pins that cross the sternoclavicular joint, and fatigue breakage of the pins is common. All but one of the seven deaths or near deaths were reported in the 1960s.[38, 148, 178, 193, 224, 266] One was reported in 1974.[51] To my knowledge, there were no deaths reported that occurred as a result of migrating pins from the sternoclavicular joint, until the report in 1984 by Gerlach, Wemhoner, and Ogbuihi[90] from West Germany. They reported on two deaths that resulted from migrating nails that caused cardiac tamponade. The physicians were charged with manslaughter by negligence. *I do not recommend any type of transfixing pins—large or small—across the sternoclavicular joint.*

Brown[38] has reported an incidence of 3 complications in 10 operative cases: 2 from broken pins which had to be removed from a window in the sternum, and 1, a near death, in which the pin penetrated the back of the sternum and entered into the right pulmonary artery. Nordback and Markkula[185] removed a pin that migrated completely inside the aorta. Jelesijevic and associates,[126] Pate and Wilhite,[193] Rubenstein and colleagues,[222] and Schechter and Gilbert[229] reported cases where the pin migrated into the heart. Leonard and Gifford[148] reported on migration to the pulmonary artery. Sethi and Scott[232] reported on migration of the pin to lacerate the subclavian artery. Clark and associates;[51] S. Gaston, in the report by Nettles and Linscheid;[178] and Salvatore[224] reported migration of pins into the aorta and resultant death. Grabski[96] reported on the migration of the pin to the opposite breast in a 37-year-old female. In addition, I personally have treated patients in whom the pin has migrated into the chest and up into the base of the neck.

Omer,[190] in a review of 14 military hospitals, reported on 15 patients who had elective surgery for

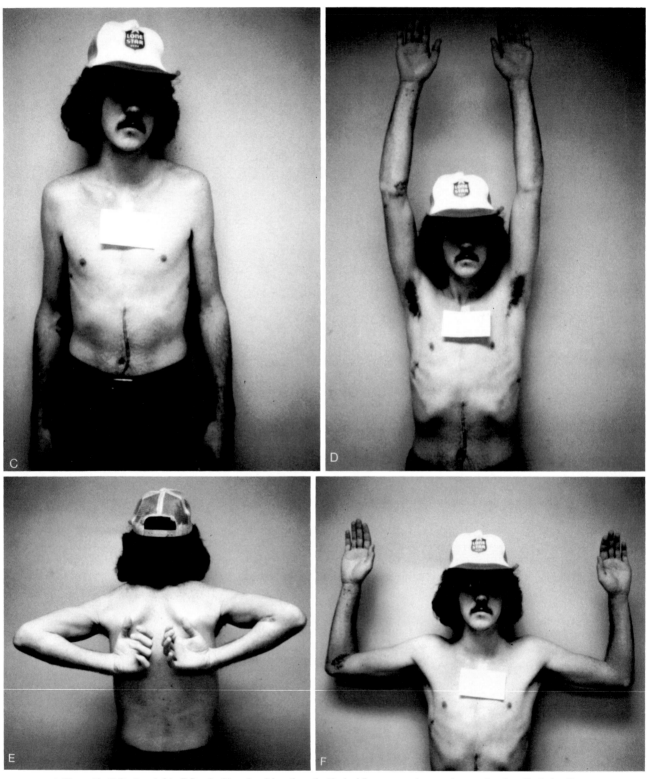

Figure 13–44 *Continued. C* to *F*, Despite this serious injury, the patient had a full recovery and a normal range of motion of both shoulders.

reduction and reconstruction of the sternoclavicular joint. Eight patients were followed by the same house staff for more than six months with the following complications: of the five patients who had internal fixation with metal, two developed osteomyelitis, two had fracture of the pin with recurrent dislocation, and one had migration of the pin into the mediastinum with recurrent dislocation. Of the three patients who had soft tissue reconstructions, one developed recurrent dislocation with drainage, one developed recurrent dislocation, and the third developed arthritis and extremity weakness and was discharged from military service. Omer commented on this series of complications: "It would seem that complications are common in this rare surgical problem." To Omer's comment I can only add, amen.

References

1. Abbott LC, and Lucas DB: The function of the clavicle: its surgical significance. Ann Surg 140:583–599, 1954.
2. Abbott LC, Saunders JB, Hagey H, and Jones EW: Surgical approaches to the shoulder joint. J Bone Joint Surg 31A(2):235–255, 1949.
3. Abel MS: Symmetrical anteroposterior projections of the sternoclavicular joints with motion studies. Radiology 132:757–759, 1979.
4. Aberle DR, Milos MJ, Aberle AM, and Bassett LW: Case report 407. Diagnosis: sternocostoclavicular hyperostosis affecting the sternum, medial ends of the clavicles and upper segments of the anterior ribs. Skeletal Radiol 16:70–73, 1987.
5. Adunsky A, Yaretzky A, and Klajman A: Letter to the editor re malignant lymphoma presenting as sternoclavicular joint arthritis. Arthritis Rheum 2:1330–1331, 1980.
6. Allen AW: Living suture grafts in the repair of fractures and dislocations. Arch Surg 16:1007–1020, 1928.
7. Allman FL: Fracture and ligamentous injuries of clavicle and its articulations. J Bone Joint Surg 49A(4):774–784, 1967.
8. Anderson ME: Treatment of dislocations of the acromioclavicular and sternoclavicular joints (Proceedings). J Bone Joint Surg 45A(3):657–658, 1963.
9. Böhler L: Dislocations of the clavicle at the sternal end. In The Treatment of Fractures, Vol. 1. New York: Grune & Stratton, 1956, pp 540–545.
10. Bachmann M: Swelling of the sternoclavicular joint. Isr J Med Sci 17:65–72, 1958.
11. Badgley CE: Sports injuries of the shoulder girdle. JAMA 172:444–448, 1960.
12. Baker EC: Tomography of the sternoclavicular joint. Ohio State Med J 55:60, 1959.
13. Baker ME, Martinez S, Kier R, and Wain S: Computed tomography of the cadaveric sternoclavicular joint: technique, findings, and significance in degenerative disease. Presented at the 33rd Annual Meeting of the AUR, Nashville, Tennessee, 1985.
14. Bankart ASB: An operation for recurrent dislocation (subluxation) of the sternoclavicular joint. Br J Surg 26:320–323, 1938.
15. Baranda MM, Pascual JB, Gomez-Escolar IA, et al.: Letter to the editor re sternoclavicular septic arthritis as first manifestation of brucellosis. Br J Rheumatol 25(3):322, 1986.
16. Barrett J: The clavicular joints. Physiotherapy 57:268–269, 1971.
17. Barth E, and Hagen R: Surgical treatment of recurrent dislocation of the sternoclavicular joint. Acta Orthop Scand 53(4):709, 1982.
18. Barth E, and Hagen R: Surgical treatment of dislocations of the sternoclavicular joint. Acta Orthop Scand 54:746–747, 1983.
19. Basmajian JV: Joints of the upper limb. In Grant's Method of Anatomy, 8th ed. Baltimore: Williams & Wilkins, 1971, pp 158–159.
20. Bateman JE: The Shoulder and Neck. Philadelphia: WB Saunders Company, 1972.
21. Bateman JE: The Shoulder and Neck, 2nd ed. Philadelphia: WB Saunders Company, 1978.
22. Bayley I, and Kessel L: Shoulder Surgery. New York: Springer-Verlag, 1982.
23. Bearn JG: Direct observations on the function of the capsule of the sternoclavicular joint in clavicular support. J Anat 101(1):159–170, 1967.
24. Beckman T: A case of simultaneous luxation of both ends of the clavicle. Acta Chir Scand 56:156–163, 1923.
25. Beller RD, Grana WA, and O'Donoghue DH: Recurrent posterior dislocation of the shoulder: a method of reconstruction. Orthopedics 1:384–388, 1978.
26. Berkhina FO: [Traumatic dislocations of clavicle.] Orthop Traumatol 9:11–26, 1935.
27. Bernard TN Jr, and Haddad RJ Jr: Enchondroma of the proximal clavicle: an unusual cause of pathologic fracture-dislocation of the sternoclavicular joint. Clin Orthop 167:239–247, 1982.
28. Blankstein A, Nerubay J, Lin E, et al: Septic arthritis of the sternoclavicular joint. Orthop Rev 15(7):41–43, 1986.
29. Bloom FA: Wire fixation in acromioclavicular dislocation. J Bone Joint Surg 27:273–276, 1945.
30. Bonnin JG: Spontaneous subluxation of the sternoclavicular joint. Br Med J 2:274–275, 1960.
31. Booth CM, and Roper BA: Chronic dislocation of the sternoclavicular joint: an operative repair. Clin Orthop 140:17–20, 1979.
32. Borowiecki B, Charow A, Cook W, et al: An unusual football injury (posterior dislocation of the sternoclavicular joint). Arch Otolaryngol 95:185–187, 1972.
33. Borrero E: Traumatic posterior displacement of the left clavicular head causing chronic extrinsic compression of the subclavian artery. Physician Sports Med 15(7):87–89, 1987.
34. Breitner S, and Wirth CJ: [Resection of the acromial and sternal ends of the clavicula.] Z Orthop 125:363–368, 1987.
35. Bremner RA: Nonarticular, non-infective subacute arthritis of the sterno-clavicular joint. J Bone Joint Surg 41B(4):749–753, 1959.
36. Brooks AL, and Henning GD: Injury to the proximal clavicular epiphysis (Proceedings). J Bone Joint Surg 54A(6):1347–1348, 1972.
37. Brower AC, Sweet DE, and Keats TE: Condensing osteitis of the clavicle: a new entity. AJR 121:17–21, 1974.
38. Brown JE: Anterior sternoclavicular dislocation—a method of repair. Am J Orthop 31:184–189, 1961.
39. Brown R: Backward and inward dislocation of sternal end of clavicle. Surg Clin North Am 7(5):1263, 1927.
40. Buchmann M: Swelling of the sternoclavicular joint. Acta Med Orient 17(3–4):65–72, 1958.
41. Buckerfield CT, and Castle ME: Acute traumatic retrosternal dislocation of the clavicle. J Bone Joint Surg 66-A(3):379–384, 1984.
42. Burri C, and Neugebauer R: Carbon fiber replacement of the ligaments of the shoulder girdle and the treatments of lateral instability of the ankle joint. Clin Orthop 196:112–117, 1985.
43. Burrows HJ: Tenodesis of subclavius in the treatment of recurrent dislocation of the sterno-clavicular joint. J Bone Joint Surg 33B(2):240–243, 1951.
44. Butterworth RD, and Kirk AA: Fracture dislocation sternoclavicular joint—case report. Va Med 79:98–100, 1952.
45. Camus JP, Prier A, and Cassou B: [Sternocostoclavicular hyperostosis.] Rev Rhum Mal Osteoartic 47(5):361–363, 1980.
46. Cantlon GE, and Gluckman JL: Sternoclavicular joint hypertrophy following radical neck dissection. Head Neck Surg 5:218–221, 1983.
47. Cave AJE: The nature and morphology of the costoclavicular ligament. J Anat 95:170–179, 1961.
48. Cave EF: Fractures and Other Injuries. Chicago: Year Book Medical Publishers, Inc., 1958.

49. Cave ER, Burke JF, and Boyd RJ: Trauma Management. Chicago: Year Book Medical Publishers, Inc., 1974, pp 409–411.
50. Christensen EE, and Dietz GW: The supraclavicular fossa. Radiology 118(1):37–39, 1976.
51. Clark RL, Milgram JW, and Yawn DH: Fatal aortic perforation and cardiac tamponade due to a Kirschner wire migrating from the right sternoclavicular joint. South Med J 67(3):316–318, 1974.
52. Codman EA: Rupture of the supraspinatus tendon and other lesions in or about the subacromial bursa. In The Shoulder. Boston: Thomas Todd, 1934.
53. Colhoun EN, Hayward C, and Evans KT: Inter-sterno-costo-clavicular ossification. Clin Radiol 38:33–38, 1987.
54. Collins JJ: Retrosternal dislocation of the clavicle (Proceedings). J Bone Joint Surg 54B(1):203, 1972.
55. Cone RO, Resnick D, Goergen TG, et al.: Condensing osteitis of the clavicle. AJR 141:387–388, 1983.
56. Conway AM: Movements at the sternoclavicular and acromioclavicular joints. Phys Ther Rev 41(6):421–432, 1961.
57. Cooper A: A Treatise on Dislocations and Fractures of the Joints, 2nd Am. ed. from the 6th London ed. Boston: Lilly & Wait and Carter & Hendee, 1832.
58. Cooper A: Dislocation of the clavicle. In A Treatise on Dislocations and Fractures of the Joints, 2nd Am. ed. from the 6th London ed. Boston: Lilly & Wait and Carter & Hendee, 1832, pp 367–373.
59. Currey H: Letter to the editor re primary gout affecting the sternoclavicular joint. Br Med J 1(6009):583–584, 1976.
60. D'Ambrosia RD: Musculoskeletal Disorders. Philadelphia: JB Lippincott Company, 1977.
61. Döhler JR: [Ankylosing hyperostosis of the sternoclavicular joint.] Dtsch Med Wochenschr 112(8):304–305, 1987.
62. Daffner RH, and Gehweiler JA Jr: Case report 236. Diagnosis: neuropathic arthropathy of the sternoclavicular joint, secondary to syringomyelia. Skeletal Radiol 10:113–116, 1983.
63. Delevette AF, and Monahan DT: Acute arthritis of the sternoclavicular joint due to coliform bacillus. Conn Med 34(9):629–630, 1970.
64. Denham RH Jr, and Dingley AF Jr: Epiphyseal separation of the medial end of the clavicle. J Bone Joint Surg 49A(6):1179–1183, 1967.
65. DePalma AF: Surgery of the Shoulder, 2nd ed. Philadelphia: JB Lippincott Company, 1973, pp 328–240.
66. DePalma AF: Surgical anatomy of acromioclavicular and sternoclavicular joints. Surg Clin North Am 43:1541–1550, 1963.
67. DePalma AF: The role of the disks of the sternoclavicular and the acromioclavicular joints. Clin Orthop 13:222–233, 1959.
68. Destouet JM, Gilula LA, Murphy WA, and Sagel SS: Computed tomography of the sternoclavicular joint and sternum. Radiology 138(1):123–128, 1981.
69. Duggan N: Recurrent dislocation of sternoclavicular cartilage. J Bone Joint Surg 13:365, 1931.
70. Duthie RB, and Ferguson AB Jr: Dislocations of the medial end of the clavicle. In Mercer's Orthopaedic Surgery, 7th ed. Baltimore: Williams & Wilkins, 1973, pp 958–959.
71. Ecke H: Sternoclavicular dislocations. Personal communication, 1984.
72. Elting JJ: Retrosternal dislocation of the clavicle. Arch Surg 104:35–37, 1972.
73. Epps CH: Complications in Orthopaedic Surgery. Philadelphia: JB Lippincott Company, 1978.
74. Epstein BS: Sternoclavicular arthritis in patients with scleroderma and rheumatoid arthritis. AJR 89:1236–1240, 1963.
75. Eskola A: Sternoclavicular dislocation: a plea for open treatment. Acta Orthop Scand 57:227–228, 1986.
76. Féry A, and Léonard A: [Transsternal sternoclavicular projection. Diagnostic value in sternoclavicular dislocations.] J Radiol 62(3):167–170, 1981.
77. Farrer WE: Case report: sternoclavicular pyarthrosis. J Med Soc NJ 82(9):735–737, 1985.
78. Fedoseev VA: [Method of radiographic study of the sternoclavicular joint.] Vestn Rentgenol Radiol 3:88–91, 1977.
79. Ferry AM, Rook FW, and Masterson JH: Retrosternal dislocation of the clavicle. J Bone Joint Surg 39A(4):905–910, 1957.
80. Fisk GH: Some observations of motion at the shoulder joint. Can Med Assoc J 50:213–216, 1944.
81. Fitchet SM: Cleidocranial dysostosis: hereditary and familial. J Bone Joint Surg 11:838–866, 1929.
82. Franquet T, Lecumberri F, Rivas A, et al: Condensing osteitis of the clavicle: report of two new cases. Skeletal Radiol 14:184–187, 1985.
83. Friedman RS, Perez HD, and Goldstein IM: Septic arthritis of the sternoclavicular joint due to gram-positive microorganisms. Am J Med Sci 282:91–93, 1981.
84. Fuxench-Chiesa X, Mejias E, and Ramirez-Ronda CH: Letter to the editor re septic arthritis of the sternoclavicular joint due to Citrobacter diversus. J Rheumatol 10(1):162–164, 1983.
85. Gallie WE: Dislocations. N Engl J Med 213:91–98, 1935.
86. Gangahar DM, and Flogaites T: Retrosternal dislocation of the clavicle producing thoracic outlet syndrome. J Trauma 18(5):369–372, 1978.
87. Gardner NA, and Bidstrup BP: Intrathoracic great vessel injury resulting from blunt chest trauma associated with posterior dislocation of the sternoclavicular joint. Aust NZ J Surg 53:427–430, 1983.
88. Gartland JJ: Disorders of the sternoclavicular joint. In Fundamentals of Orthopaedics, 3rd ed. Philadelphia: WB Saunders Company, 1979, pp. 249–250.
89. Gazak S, and Davidson SJ: Posterior sternoclavicular dislocations: two case reports. J Trauma 24(1):80–82, 1984.
90. Gerlach D, Wemhöner SR, and Ogbuihi S: [On two cases of fatal heart tamponade due to migration of fracture nails from the sternoclavicular joint.] Z Rechtsmed 93(1):53–60, 1984.
91. Gerster JC, Lagier R, and Nicod L: Case report 311: open-quiz solution. Skeletal Radiol 14:53–60, 1985.
92. Glickman LG, and Minsky AA: Case reports—enlargement of one sternoclavicular articulation: a sign of congenital syphilis. Radiology 28:85–86, 1937.
93. Goldin RH, Chow AW, Edwards JE Jr, et al: Sternoarticular septic arthritis in heroin users. N Engl J Med 289(12):616–618, 1973.
94. Goossens M, Vanderstraeten CV, and Claessens H: Sternoclavicular hyperostosis: a case report and review of the literature. Clin Orthop 194:164–168, 1985.
95. Gorman JB, Stone RT, and Keats TE: Changes in the sternoclavicular joint following radical neck dissection. AJR 111:584–587, 1971.
96. Grabski RS: [Unusual dislocation of a fragment of Kirschner wire after fixation of the sternoclavicular joint.] Wiad Lek 40(9):630–632, 1987.
97. Grant JCB: Method of Anatomy, 7th ed. Baltimore: Williams & Wilkins, 1965.
98. Gray H: Anatomy of the Human Body, 28th ed (CM Goss, ed). Philadelphia: Lea & Febiger, 1966, pp 324–326.
99. Greenlee DP: Posterior dislocation of the sternal end of the clavicle. JAMA 125:426–428, 1944.
100. Guerin M: Recherches sur les luxations congenitales. Gaz Med Paris 9:97, 1841.
101. Gunson EF: Radiography of sternoclavicular articulation. Radiog Clin Photog 19(1):20–24, 1943.
102. Gunther WA: Posterior dislocation of the sternoclavicular joint. J Bone Joint Surg 31A(4):878–879, 1949.
103. Gurd FB: Surplus parts of skeleton: recommendation for excision of certain portions as means of shortening period of disability following trauma. Am J Surg 74:705–720, 1947.
104. Haas SL: The experimental transplantation of the epiphysis. JAMA 65:1965–1971, 1915.
105. Habernek H, and Hertz H: [Origin, diagnosis and treatment of traumatic dislocation of sternoclavicular joint.] Aktuel Traumatol 17(1):23–28, 1987.
106. Haenel LC, Bradway WR, and Costantini PJ: Thrombophlebitis complicating sternoclavicular hyperostosis (case report). Postgrad Med J 68(5):113–118, 1980.
107. Hamilton-Wood C, Hollingworth P, Dieppe P, et al: The painful swollen sterno-clavicular joint. Br J Radiol 58:941–945, 1985.

108. Hartman TJ, and Dunnagan WA: Cinearthrography of the sternoclavicular joint (abstr). Personal communication, 1979.
109. Haug W: Retention Einer Seltenen Sterno-clavicular-Luxationsfraktur Mittels Modifizierter Y-Platte der AO. Aktuel Traumatol 16:39–40, 1986.
110. Heinig CF: Retrosternal dislocation of the clavicle: early recognition, x-ray diagnosis, and management. J Bone Joint Surg 50A(4):830, 1968.
111. Heppenstall RB: Sternoclavicular dislocations. In Fracture Treatment and Healing. Philadelphia: WB Saunders Company, 1980, pp 417–419.
112. Hermann G, Rothenberg RR, and Spiera H: The value of tomography in diagnosing infection of the sternoclavicular joint. Mt Sinai J Med 50(1):52–55, 1983.
113. Hernandez LA, Watson JD, and Sturrock RD: Septic arthritis of the sternoclavicular joint complicated by fistula formation. Rheumatol Rehabil 15:292–294, 1976.
114. Higoumenakis GK: Neues Stigma der kongenitalen Lues. Die Vergrösserung des sternalen Endes des rechten Schlüsselbeins, seine Beschreibung, Deutung und Ätiologie. Deutsche Ztschr Nervenh 114:288–299, 1930.
115. Hobbs DW: Sternoclavicular joint: a new axial radiographic view. Radiology 90:801–802, 1968.
116. Hollinshead WH: Sternoclavicular joint. Pectoral region, axilla, and shoulder. Back and limbs. Anatomy for Surgeons 3:265–268, 1958.
117. Holmdahl HC: A case of posterior sternoclavicular dislocation. Acta Orthop Scand 23:218–222, 1953–1954.
118. Hotchkiss LW: Double dislocation of the sternal end of the clavicle. Ann Surg 23:600, 1896.
119. Howard FM, and Shafer SJ: Injuries to the clavicle with neurovascular complications: a study of fourteen cases. J Bone Joint Surg 47A:1335–1346, 1965.
120. Howard NJ: Acromioclavicular and sternoclavicular joint injuries. Am J Surg 46:284–291, 1939.
121. Hoyt WA: Etiology of shoulder injuries in athletes. J Bone Joint Surg 49A(4):755–766, 1967.
122. Hynd RF, Klofkorn RW, and Wong JK: Case report: Streptococcus anginosus-constellatus infection of the sternoclavicular joint. J Rheumatol 11(5):713–715, 1984.
123. Inman VT, Saunders JB, and Abbott LC: Observations on the function of the shoulder joint. J Bone Joint Surg 26:1–30, 1944.
124. Inman VT: Observations on the function of the clavicle. California Med 65(4):158–166, 1946.
125. Jönsson G: A method of obtaining structural pictures of the sternum. Acta Radiol 18:336–340, 1937.
126. Jelesijevic V, Knoll D, Klinke F, et al: Penetrating injuries of the heart and intrapericardial blood vessels caused by migration of a Kirschner pin after osteosynthesis. Acta Chir Iugosl 29:274, 1982.
127. Jones R: Injuries of Joints, 2nd ed. London: Oxford University Press, 1917, pp 53–55.
128. Jurik AG, De Carvalho A, and Graudal H: Sclerotic changes of the sternal end of the clavicle. Clin Radiol 36:23–25, 1985.
129. Jurik AG, and De Carvalho A: Sterno-clavicular hyperostosis in a case with psoriasis and HLA-B27 associated arthropathy. Fortschr Rontgenstr 142(3):345–347, 1985.
130. Köhler H, Uehlinger E, Kutzner J, and West TB: Sternoclavicular hyperostosis: painful swelling of the sternum, clavicles, and upper ribs—report of two new cases. Ann Intern Med 87:192–194, 1977.
131. Kalliomäki JL, Viitanen SM, and Virtama P: Radiological findings of sternoclavicular joints in rheumatoid arthritis. Acta Rheum Scand 14:233–240, 1969.
132. Kanoksikarin S, and Wearne WM: Fracture and retrosternal dislocation of the clavicle. Aust NZ J Surg 48(1):95–96, 1978.
133. Kattan KR: Modified view for use in roentgen examination of the sternoclavicular joints. Radiology 108(3):8, 1973.
134. Kennedy JC: Retrosternal dislocation of the clavicle. J Bone Joint Surg 31B(1):74–75, 1949.
135. Kessel L: Clinical Disorders of the Shoulder. London: Churchill Livingstone, 1982.
136. Key JA, and Conwell HE: The Management of Fractures, Dislocations, and Sprains, 5th ed. St. Louis: CV Mosby Company, 1951, pp 458–461.
137. Kier R, Wain S, Apple J, and Martinez S: Osteoarthritis of the sternoclavicular joint: radiographic features and pathologic correlation. Invest Radiol 21:227–33, 1986.
138. King JM Jr, and Holmes GW: A review of four hundred and fifty roentgen ray examinations of the shoulder. AJR 17:214–218, 1927.
139. Kofoed H, Thomsen P, and Lindenberg S: Serous synovitis of the sternoclavicular joint: differential diagnostic aspects. Scand J Rheumatol 14:61–64, 1985.
140. Kruger GD, Rock MG, and Munro TG: Condensing osteitis of the clavicle: a review of the literature and report of three cases. J Bone Joint Surg 69A(4):550–557, 1987.
141. Kurzbauer R: The lateral projection in roentgenography of the sternoclavicular articulation. AJR 56(1):104–105, 1946.
142. Lagier R, Arroyo J, and Fallet GH: Sternocostoclavicular hyperostosis: radiological and pathological study of a specimen with ununited clavicular fracture. Pathol Res Pract 181:596–603, 1986.
143. Laidlaw JT: Personal communication on treatment of dislocated clavicle, 1985.
144. Lasher WW: Cartilage injuries: a clinical study. Am J Surg 6:493–500, 1929.
145. Lee HM: Sternoclavicular dislocations. Minn Med 20:480–482, 1937.
146. Leighton RK, Buhr AJ, and Sinclair AM: Posterior sternoclavicular dislocations. Can J Surg 29(2):104–106, 1986.
147. Lemire L, and Rosman M: Sternoclavicular epiphyseal separation with adjacent clavicular fracture: a case report. J Pediatr Orthop 4:118–120, 1984.
148. Leonard JW, and Gifford RW: Migration of a Kirschner wire from the clavicle into pulmonary artery. Am J Cardiol 16:598–600, 1965.
149. Levinsohn EM, Bunnell WP, and Yuan HA: Computed tomography in the diagnosis of dislocations of the sternoclavicular joint. Clin Orthop 140:12–16, 1979.
150. Levy M, Goldberg I, and Fischel RE, et al: Friedrich's disease: aseptic necrosis of the sternal end of the clavicle. J Bone Joint Surg 63B(4):539–541, 1981.
151. Lewin KW: Letter to the editor re rhomboid fossa or inflammation? Arch Intern Med 138:658–659, 1978.
152. Lindsey RW, and Leach JA: Sternoclavicular osteomyelitis and pyoarthrosis as a complication of subclavian vein catheterization: a case report and review of the literature. Orthopedics 7(6):1017–1021, 1984.
153. Linscheid RL, Kelly PJ, Martin WJ, and Fontana RS: Monarticular bacterial arthritis of the sternoclavicular joint. JAMA 178(4):421–422, 1961.
154. Lourie JA: Tomography in the diagnosis of posterior dislocations of the sterno-clavicular joint. Acta Orthop Scand 51:579–580, 1980.
155. Louw JA, and Louw JA: Posterior dislocation of the sternoclavicular joint associated with major spinal injury. S Afr Med J 71(12):791–792, 1987.
156. Lowman CL: Operative correction of old sternoclavicular dislocation. J Bone Joint Surg 10(3):740–741, 1928.
157. Lucas DB: Biomechanics of the shoulder joint. Arch Surg 107:425–432, 1973.
158. Lucas GL: Retrosternal dislocation of the clavicle. JAMA 193(10):850–853, 1965.
159. Lunseth PA, Chapman KW, and Frankel VH: Surgical treatment of chronic dislocation of the sterno-clavicular joint. J Bone Joint Surg 57B(2):193–196, 1975.
160. Maguire WB: Safe and simple method of repair of recurrent dislocation of the sternoclavicular joint (abstr). J Bone Joint Surg 68B(2):332, 1986.
161. Marsh HO, Shellito JG, and Callahan WP: Synovial sarcoma of the sternoclavicular region. J Bone Joint Surg 45A(1):151–155, 1963.
162. Martinez S, Khoury MB, and Harrelson J: Imaging of condensing osteitis of the clavicle: new observations (abstr). The Proceedings of the 33rd Annual Meeting of the AUR, 1986.

163. Mathews JG: Primary gout affecting the sternoclavicular joint. Br Med J *1*(6004):262, 1976.

164. Mazet R: Migration of a Kirschner wire from the shoulder region into the lung: report of two cases. J Bone Joint Surg *25A*(2):477–483, 1943.

165. McCarroll JR: Isolated staphylococcal infection of the sternoclavicular joint. Clin Orthop *156*:149–150, 1981.

166. McCaughan JS, and Miller PR: Letter to the editor re migration of Steinmann pin from shoulder to lung. JAMA *207*(10):1917, 1969.

167. McKenzie JMM: Retrosternal dislocation of the clavicle: a report of two cases. J Bone Joint Surg *45B*(1):138–141, 1963.

168. McLaughlin H: Trauma. Philadelphia: WB Saunders Company, 1959.

169. Mehta JC, Sachdev A, and Collins JJ: Retrosternal dislocation of the clavicle. Injury *5*(1):79–83, 1973.

170. Milch H: The rhomboid ligament in surgery of the sternoclavicular joint. J Int Coll Surg *17*(1):41–51, 1952.

171. Mitchell WJ, and Cobey MC: Retrosternal dislocation of clavicle. Med Ann DC *29*(10):546–549, 1960.

172. Moncada R, Matuga T, Unger E, et al: Migratory traumatic cardiovascular foreign bodies. Circulation *57*:186–189, 1978.

173. Morag B, and Shahin N: The value of tomography of the sternoclavicular region. Clin Radiol *26*:57–62, 1975.

174. Moseley HF: Athletic injuries to the shoulder region. Am J Surg *98*:401–422, 1959.

175. Mouchet A: Luxation sterno-claviculaire en avant: reduction sanglante. Rev Orthop *28*(1–2):99–100, 1942.

176. Muir SK, Kinsella PL, Trevilcock RG, and Blackstone IW: Infectious arthritis of the sternoclavicular joint. Can Med Assoc J *132*(11):1289–1290, 1985.

177. Nair V: Case report: sternoclavicular arthritis: an unusual complication of drug abuse. J Med Soc NJ *72*(6):519–520, 1975.

178. Nettles JL, and Linscheid R: Sternoclavicular dislocations. J Trauma *8*(2):158–164, 1968.

179. Neviaser JS: Injuries of the clavicle and its articulations. Orthop Clin North Am *11*(2):233–237, 1980.

180. Newlin NS: Congenital retrosternal subluxation of the clavicle simulating an intrathoracic mass. AJR *130*:1184–1185, 1978.

181. Nickel VL: Orthopedic rehabilitation. London: Churchill Livingstone, 1982.

182. Nitsche JF, Vaughan JH, Williams G, and Curd JG: Septic sternoclavicular arthritis with *Pasteurella multocida* and *Streptococcus sanguis*. Arthritis Rheum *25*(4):467–469, 1982.

183. Nittis S: Prominence of the right sterno-clavicular junction in lepers. Urol Cutan Rev *41*:625–630, 1937.

184. Noonan TR: Personal communication on sternoclavicular dislocation, July 30, 1984.

185. Nordback I, and Markkula H: Migration of Kirschner pin from clavicle into ascending aorta. Acta Chir Scand *151*:177–179, 1985.

186. Nutz V: [Fracture dislocation of the sternoclavicular joint.] Unfallchirurg *89*(3):145–148, 1986.

187. O'Donoghue DH: Treatment of Injuries to Athletes, 2nd ed. Philadelphia: WB Saunders Company, 1970.

188. O'Donoghue DH: Treatment of Injuries to Athletes, 3rd ed. Philadelphia: WB Saunders Company, 1976, pp 144–151.

189. Ogden JA, Conlogue GJ, and Bronson ML: Radiology of postnatal skeletal development: the clavicle. Skeletal Radiol *4*:196–203, 1979.

190. Omer GE: Osteotomy of the clavicle in surgical reduction of anterior sternoclavicular dislocation. J Trauma *7*(4):584–590, 1967.

191. Orsini G, Guercio N, and Paschero B: Retrosternal dislocation of the clavicle. Observations on three cases. Ital J Orthop Traumatol *10*(4):533–539, 1984.

192. Paice EW, Wright FW, and Hill AGS: Sternoclavicular erosions in polymyalgia rheumatica. Ann Rheum Dis *42*:379–383, 1983.

193. Pate JW, and Wilhite J: Migration of a foreign body from the sternoclavicular joint to the heart: a case report. Am Surg *35*(6):448–449, 1969.

194. Paterson DC: Retrosternal dislocation of the clavicle. J Bone Joint Surg *43B*(1):90–92, 1961.

195. Pauleau JL, and Baux S: Les disjonctions sternoclaviculaires: presentation d'un cas de disjonction sternoclaviculaire posterieure. Revue de la litterature. J Chir *117*(8–9):453–456, 1980.

196. Peacock HK, Brandon JR, and Jones OL: Retrosternal dislocation of the clavicle. South Med J *63*(11):1324–1328, 1970.

197. Peltier LF: The classic: separations of the epiphyses: Jean Timothee Emile Foucher. Clin Orthop *188*:3–9, 1984.

198. Pendergrass EP, and Hodes PJ: The rhomboid fossa of the clavicle. AJR *38*:152–155, 1937.

199. Percy EC: Sternoclavicular dislocation. Can Med Assoc J *104*:1016–1017, 1971.

200. Persoons D, Copin G, and Dosch J: [Retrosternal dislocation of the clavicle: contribution of computertomography in diagnosis and treatment—a case report. Acta Orthop Belg *51*(1):103–109, 1985.

201. Pfister U, and Weller S: [Luxation of the sternoclavicular joint.] Unfallchirurgie *8*(2):81–87, 1982.

202. Pierce RO Jr: Internal derangement of the sternoclavicular joint. Clin Orthop *141*:247–250, 1979.

203. Poland J: Separation of the epiphyses of the clavicle. *In* Traumatic Separation of Epiphyses of the Upper Extremity. London: Smith, Elder, and Co., 1898.

204. Post M: The Shoulder. Philadelphia: Lea & Febiger, 1978.

205. Pridie K: Dislocation of acromio-clavicular and sterno-clavicular joints (Proceedings). J Bone Joint Surg *41B*(2):429, 1959.

206. Quigley TB: Injuries to the acromioclavicular and sternoclavicular joints sustained in athletics. Surg Clin North Am *43*:1551–1554, 1963.

207. Raney RB, Brashear HR, and Shands AR Jr: Old sternoclavicular dislocation. *In* Shands' Handbook of Orthopaedic Surgery. St. Louis: The C. V. Mosby Company, 1971, p 421.

208. Reeves BD: Postpartum sternoclavicular joint pain. J Am Med Assoc *248*(22):3030–3031, 1982.

209. Resnick D: Sternocostoclavicular hyperostosis. AJR *135*(6):1278–1280, 1980.

210. Reuler JB, Girard DE, and Nardone DA: Sternoclavicular joint involvement in ankylosing spondylitis. South Med J *71*(12):1480–1481, 1978.

211. Rice EE: Habitual dislocation of the sternoclavicular articulation—a case report. J Okla State Med Assoc *25*:34–35, 1932.

212. Richter R, Hahn H, Nübling W, and Kohler G: [Tuberculosis of the Shoulder Girdle.] Z Rheumatol *44*:87–92, 1985.

213. Ritvo M, and Ritvo M: Roentgen study of the sternoclavicular region. AJR *53*(5):644–650, 1947.

214. Rockwood CA Jr: Dislocations of the sternoclavicular joint. AAOS Instructional Course Lectures *24*:144–159, 1975.

215. Rockwood CA Jr: Dislocation of the sternoclavicular joint. *In* Fractures, Vol. 1. Philadelphia: JB Lippincott Company, 1975, pp 756–787.

216. Rockwood CA Jr: Fracture of the clavicle and injuries of the sternoclavicular joint. Orthop Trans *6*(3):422, 1982.

217. Rockwood CA Jr: Injuries to the sternoclavicular joint. Orthop Trans *1*:96, 1977.

218. Rockwood CA Jr: Injuries to the sternoclavicular joint. *In* Fractures in Adults, Vol. 1, 2nd ed. Philadelphia: JB Lippincott Company, 1984, pp 910–948.

219. Rockwood CA Jr, and Odor JM: Spontaneous atraumatic anterior subluxations of the sternoclavicular joint in young adults. Report of 37 cases. Orthop Trans *12*(3):557, 1988.

220. Rodrigues H: Case of dislocation inwards of the internal extremity of the clavicle. Lancet *1*:309–310, 1843.

221. Rozboril MB, Good AE, Zarbo RJ, and Schultz DA: Sternoclavicular joint arthritis: an unusual presentation of metastatic carcinoma. J Rheumatol *10*(3):499–502, 1983.

222. Rubenstein ZR, Moray B, and Itzchak Y: Percutaneous removal of intravascular foreign bodies. Cardiovasc Intervent Radiol *5*:64–68, 1982.

223. Sadr B, and Swann M: Spontaneous dislocation of the sternoclavicular joint. Acta Orthop Scand *50*:269–274, 1979.

224. Salvatore JE: Sternoclavicular joint dislocation. Clin Orthop 58:51–54, 1968.
225. Sanmarti Sala R, and Munoz Gomez R: [Sterno-costo-clavicular hyperostosis: presentation of one case and review of the literature. Medicina Clinica 84(12):483–486, 1985.
226. Sante LR: Manual of Roentgenological Technique, 9th ed. Ann Arbor, MI: Edwards Brothers, Inc., 1942, pp 160–161.
227. Sartoris DJ, Schreiman JS, Kerr R, et al: Sternocostoclavicular hyperostosis: a review and report of 11 cases. Radiology 158:125–128, 1986.
228. Savastano AA, and Stutz SJ: Traumatic sternoclavicular dislocation. Int Surg 63(1):10–13, 1978.
229. Schechter DC, and Gilbert L: Injuries of the heart and great vessels due to pins and needles. Thorax 24:246–253, 1969.
230. Schmitt WGH: Articulatis sternoclavicularis: Darstellung in Einer Zweiter Ebene. Röntgenpraxis 34:262–267, 1981.
231. Selesnick FH, Jablon M, Frank C, and Post M: Retrosternal dislocation of the clavicle: report of four cases. J Bone Joint Surg 66A(2):287–291, 1984.
232. Sethi GK, and Scott SM: Subclavian artery laceration due to migration of a Hagie pin. Surgery 80(5):644–646, 1976.
233. Silberberg M, Frank EL, Jarrett SR, and Silberberg R: Aging and osteoarthritis of the human sternoclavicular joint. Am J Pathol 35(4):851–865, 1959.
234. Silverman M: Sternocostoclavicular hyperostosis. Ann Intern Med 87:797, 1977.
235. Simurda MA: Retrosternal dislocation of the clavicle: a report of 4 cases and a method of repair. Can J Surg 11:487–490, 1968.
236. Snyder CC, Levine GA, and Dingman DL: Trial of a sternoclavicular whole joint graft as a substitute for the temporomandibular joint. Plast Reconstr Surg 48(5):447–452, 1971.
237. Sokoloff L, and Gleason IO: The sternoclavicular articulation in rheumatic diseases. Am J Clin Pathol 24(1):406–414, 1954.
238. Sonozaki H, Azuma A, Okai K, et al: Inter-sterno-costo-clavicular ossification with a special reference to cases of unilateral type. Kanto J Orthop Traumatol 9:196–200, 1978.
239. Sonozaki H, Azuma A, Okai K, et al: Clinical features of 22 cases with inter-sterno-costo-clavicular ossification. Arch Orthop Trauma Surg 95:13–22, 1979.
240. Sonozaki H, Furusawa S, Seki H, et al: Four cases with symmetrical ossifications between the clavicles and the first ribs of both sides. Kanto J Orthop Traumatol 5:244–247, 1974.
241. Spar I: Psoriatic arthritis of the sternoclavicular joint. Conn Med 42(4):225–226, 1978.
242. Speed K: A Textbook of Fractures and Dislocations, 4th ed. Philadelphia: Lea & Febiger, 1942, pp 282–290.
243. Stankler L: Posterior dislocation of clavicle: a report of 2 cases. Br J Surg 50:164–168, 1962.
244. Stapelmohr SV: Ueber Die Habituelle Luxatio Sternoclavicularis und Eine Neue Operative Behandlungsmethode Dersleben. Acta Orthop Scand 3:1–42, 1932.
245. Stein AH: Retrosternal dislocation of the clavicle. J Bone Joint Surg 39A(3):656–660, 1957.
246. Stimson LA: Dislocations of the clavicle. In Fractures and Dislocations. Philadelphia: Lea & Febiger, 1912, pp 588–589.
247. Streifler J, Gartz M, Rosenfeld JB, et al.: Sternoclavicular arthritis and osteomyelitis due to Pseudomonas aeruginosa, not related to drug abuse. Israel J Med Sci 21:458–459, 1985.
248. Szilvaasy J: Age determination of the sternal articular faces of the clavicula. J Human Evol 9(8):609–610, 1980.
249. Tabatabai MF, Sapico FL, Canawati HN, and Harley HAJ: Letter to the editor re sternoclavicular joint infection with Group B Streptococcus. J Rheumatol 13(2):466, 1986.
250. Tagliabue D, and Riva A: Le lussazioni sterno-claveari. Minerva Ortopedica 36(11):876–871, 1985.
251. Teplick JG, Eftekhari F, and Haskin ME: Erosion of the sternal ends of the clavicles: a new sign of primary and secondary hyperparathyroidism. Radiology 113(2):323–326, 1974.
252. Turek SL: Orthopaedics: Principles and Their Application, 2nd ed. Philadelphia: JB Lippincott Company, 1967, pp 568–570.
253. Tyler HDD, Sturrock WDS, and Callow FM: Retrosternal dislocation of the clavicle. J Bone Joint Surg 45B(1):132–137, 1963.
254. Von Stapelmohr S: Ueber die Habituelle Luxatio Sterno clavicularis und eine Neue Operative Behandlungsmethode Derselben. Acta Orthop Scand 3:1–42, 1932.
255. Waskowitz WJ: Disruption of the sternoclavicular joint: an analysis and review. Am J Orthop 3:176–179, 1961.
256. Wasylenko MJ, and Busse EF: Posterior dislocation of the clavicle causing fatal tracheoesophageal fistula. Can J Surg 24(6):626–627, 1981.
257. Watson-Jones R: Fractures and Joint Injuries, Vol. 2, 4th ed. Baltimore: Williams & Wilkins, 1956.
258. Watson-Jones R: Fractures and Joint Injuries. London: Churchill Livingstone, 1982, pp 462–463.
259. Webb PAO, and Suchey JMM: Epiphyseal union of the anterior iliac crest and medial clavicle in a modern multiracial sample of American males and females. Am J Phys Anthropol 68:457–466, 1985.
260. Weiner SN, Levy M, Bernstein R, and Morehouse H: Condensing osteitis of the clavicle: a case report. J Bone Joint Surg 66A(9):1484–1486, 1984.
261. Weingarten M, Tash R, Klein RM, and Kearns RJ: Posterior dislocation of the sternoclavicular joint. NY State J Med 85(5):226–229, 1985.
262. Wheeler ME, Laaveg SJ, and Sprague BL: S-C joint disruptions in an infant. Clin Orthop 139:68–69, 1979.
263. Williams HH: Oblique views of the clavicle. Radiog Clin Photog 5:191–194, 1929.
264. Wohlgethan JR, and Newberg AH: Clinical analysis of infection of the sternoclavicular joint (abstr). Clin Res 32(2):666A, 1984.
265. Wolford LM, and Smith BR: Sternoclavicular grafts for temporomandibular joint reconstruction (abstr). J Oral Maxillofac Surg 45(11):M3, 1987.
266. Worman LW, and Leagus C: Intrathoracic injury following retrosternal dislocation of the clavicle. J Trauma 7(3):416–423, 1967.
267. Worrell J, and Fernandez GN: Retrosternal dislocation of the clavicle: an important injury easily missed. Arch Emerg Med 3:133–135, 1986.
268. Yood RA, and Goldenberg DL: Sternoclavicular joint arthritis. Arthritis Rheum 23(2):232–239, 1980.
269. Zucman J, Robinet L, and Aubart J: [Treatment of sternal dislocations of the clavicle.] Rev Chir Orthop 64:35–44, 1978.

Anterior Glenohumeral Instability

Frederick A. Matsen III, M.D.
Steven C. Thomas, M.D.
Charles A. Rockwood, Jr., M.D.

Historical Review

EARLY DESCRIPTIONS

The first report of a shoulder dislocation is found in humankind's oldest book, the Edwin Smith Papyrus (3000–2500 B.C.).[574] Hussein[238] reported that in 1200 B.C. in the tomb of Upuy, an artist and sculptor to Ramses II, there was a drawing of a scene that was strikingly similar to Kocher's method of reduction (Fig. 14–1).

The most detailed early description of anterior dislocations came from the father of medicine, Hippocrates, who was born in 460 B.C. on the island of Cos.[2] Hippocrates described the anatomy of the shoulder, the types of dislocations, and the first surgical procedure. In one of his classic procedures for reduction, he stressed the need for suitably sized leather-covered balls to be placed into the axilla, for without them the heel could not reach the head of the humerus in his reduction maneuver. Other hippocratic techniques are described by Brockbank and Griffiths (Fig. 14–2).[67]

Hippocrates wrote,

It deserves to be known how a shoulder which is subject to frequent dislocations should be treated. For many persons owing to this accident have been obliged to abandon gymnastic exercises, though otherwise well qualified for them; and from the same misfortune have become inept in warlike practices, and have thus perished. And this subject deserves to be noticed, because I have never known any physician [to] treat the case properly; some abandon the attempt altogether, and others hold opinions and practice the very reverse of what is proper.

Hippocrates criticized his contemporaries for improper burning of the shoulder, a treatment popular at the time. In this first description of a surgical procedure for recurrent dislocation of the shoulder, he described how physicians had burned the top, anterior, and posterior aspects of the shoulder, which only caused scarring in those areas and promoted the downward dislocation. He advocated the use of cautery in which an oblong, red-hot iron was inserted through the axilla to make eschars, but only in the lower part of the joint. Hippocrates displayed considerable knowledge of the anatomy of the shoulder, and he warned the surgeon not to let the iron come in contact with the major vessels and nerves since this would cause great harm. Following the burnings, he bound the arm to the side, day and night for a long time, "for thus more especially will cicatrization take place, and the wide space into which the humerus used to escape will become contracted."

In the centuries that followed, more refined descriptions of shoulder conditions and their management were published. The text by H. F. Moseley[359] has a particularly good section on the historical aspects of management of shoulder instability.

HUMERAL HEAD DEFECT

The defect created by the anterior margin of the glenoid in the posterolateral aspect of the humeral head has long been recognized. In 1861, Flower[163] described the anatomical and pathological changes found in 41 traumatically dislocated shoulders from specimens in London museums. He wrote that "where

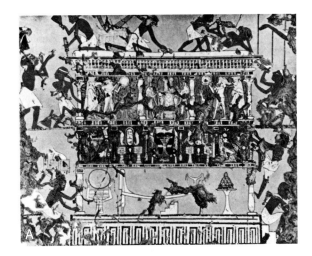

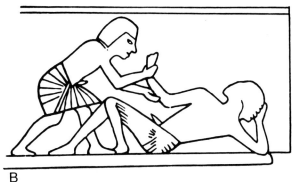

Figure 14–1. The Kocher technique is 3000 years old. *A*, Drawing from the tomb of Upuy in the year 1200 B.C. (From The Metropolitan Museum of Art.) *B*, Schematic drawing of the picture in the upper right corner of the tomb painting depicting a patient on the ground while a man—possibly a physician—is manipulating a dislocated shoulder in the technique of Kocher. (Reproduced with permission from Hussein MK: Kocher's method is 3,000 years old. *J Bone Joint Surg 50B*:669–671, 1968.)

the head of the humerus rests upon the edge of the glenoid fossa absorption occurs, and a groove is evacuated, usually between the articular head and the greater tuberosity." In 1880, Eve[148] reported an autopsy on a patient who died 12 hours after an acute anterior dislocation in which he found the deep groove in the posterolateral aspect of the head. Joessel[247] also observed the defect. According to Hill and Sachs,[221] beginning in 1882 publications appeared by Kuster,[277] Cramer,[106] Löbker,[307] Schüller,[492] Staffel,[512] and Francke[165] that described the finding of a posterolateral defect in humeral heads resected for relief of chronic or recurrent dislocation.

In 1887, Caird[71] of Edinburgh concluded that in the true subcoracoid dislocation there must be an indentation fracture of the humeral head that is produced by the dense, hard anterior lip of the glenoid fossa. In cadaver experiments, he was able to produce the head defect. He said that the hard, dense glenoid lip would cut into the soft cancellous bone like a knife.

Hermodsson's text[217] on radiographic studies of anterior dislocations of the shoulder offers the best review of the changes that were detectable by radiography.

Largely through the efforts of Moseley of Montreal, the text was translated from German to English in 1963. Hermodsson's work has shown that the posterolateral humeral head defect is the result of a compression fracture caused by the anterior glenoid rim following the exit of the humeral head from the glenoid fossa. He also made several observations about fresh, acute traumatic anterior dislocations: (1) the defect is seen in the majority of cases, (2) the longer the head is dislocated, the larger the defect will be, (3) the defects generally are larger with anteroinferior dislocations than with anterior dislocations, and (4) the defect generally is larger in recurrent anterior dislocations of the shoulder.

Hermodsson reported that in 1898 Franke made the first mention of radiographic changes in the humeral head associated with recurrent dislocation of the shoulder. In 1925, Pilz[432] reported the first detailed radiographic examination of recurrent dislocation of the shoulder and stated that routine radiographs were of little help. He stressed the need for an angled-beam projection to observe the defect. Currently, all of the special views that demonstrate the posterolateral humeral head defect involve an angled projection of the x-ray beam.

In 1940 Hill and Sachs[221] published a very clear and concise review of the available information on the humeral head compression fracture defect that now carries their names.

ANTERIOR CAPSULE DEFECTS

According to the Hunterian Lecture given by Reeves in 1967, Roger of Palermo in the 13th century taught that the lesion in an acute dislocation was a capsular rupture. This concept was later challenged by Hunter, Flower,[163] Caird,[71] Broca and Hartmann,[66] Perthes,[430] and Bankart,[27, 28] who noted that the lesion in traumatic anterior instability was caused by the shearing off of the anterior soft tissue structures from the glenoid resulting from forward translation of the humeral head.

ROTATOR CUFF INJURIES

In 1880, Joessel[247] reported on his careful postmortem studies of four cases of known recurrent dislocations of the shoulder. In all cases he found a rupture of the posterolateral portion of the rotator cuff from the greater tuberosity and a greatly increased shoulder joint capsule volume. He also noted fractures of the humeral head and the anterior glenoid rim. He concluded that cuff disruptions that did not heal predisposed to recurrence of the problem; that recurrences were facilitated by the enlarged capsule; and that fractures of the glenoid or head of the humerus resulted in a smaller articular surface, which may tend to produce recurrent dislocation. However, his four patients were elderly and may have had the degenerative cuff changes so common in older people.

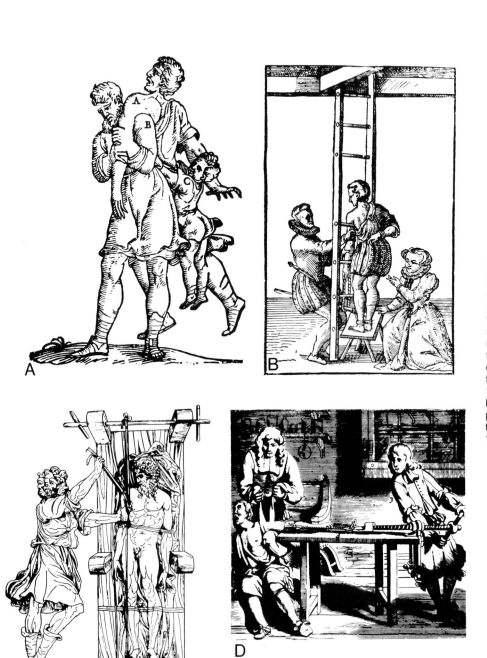

Figure 14–2. Modified techniques of Hippocrates to reduce dislocations of the shoulder. *A,* Reduction over the operator's shoulder (from the Venice edition of Galen in 1625). *B,* Reduction over the rung of the ladder. When the step stool on which the patient is standing is withdrawn, the weight of the patient's body produces a reduction of the dislocation (from deCruce in 1607). *C,* The use of the rack to reduce the shoulder dislocation (Vidius). *D,* Reduction of the dislocation by a medieval type of screw traction (from Scultetus in 1693). (Reproduced with permission from Brockbank W, and Griffiths DL: Orthopaedic surgery in the 16th and 17th centuries. J Bone Joint Surg *30B*:365–375, 1948.)

THE "ESSENTIAL LESION" OF RECURRING DISLOCATIONS: BONE DEFECTS VERSUS SOFT TISSUE DEFECTS AND OTHERS ·

Roentgen's discovery of x-ray in 1895 ushered in new evaluations and studies on the anatomy of the anterior glenoid and on humeral head defects. These studies gave further impetus to the theory that the posterolateral defect of the humeral head was the essential lesion that produced recurrent anterior dislocations. Bankart,[27] following the concepts of Broca and Hartmann[66] and Perthes,[430] continued to claim that the essential lesion was the detached labrum and capsule from the anterior glenoid (referred to by subsequent authors as the Bankart lesion) (Fig. 14–3). Later experimental and clinical work by Reeves[447] and Townley[536] has suggested that other lesions can be responsible for recurrent dislocation, such as lack of bleeding at the time of the initial traumatic dislocation, detachment of the subscapularis tendon, and variance in the attachment of the inferior glenohumeral ligament.

Moseley and Overgaard[362] found laxity in 25 consecutive cases, and DePalma and associates[129] reported subscapularis laxity, ruptures, and decreased muscle tone in 38 consecutive cases. Several of their cases, as did those of Hauser,[204] revealed a definite defect along the anterior or inferior aspect of the subscapularis tendon, as if it had been partially torn from its bone attachment, along with separation of those muscle fibers that insert into the humerus directly below the lesser tuberosity. McLaughlin,[332] DePalma and associates,[129] Jens,[244] and Reeves,[446] have noted, at the time of surgery but before arthrotomy, that with abduction and external rotation the humeral head would dislocate under the lower edge of the subscapularis tendon. Symeonides[523] biopsied the subscapularis muscle tendon unit at the time of surgery and found microscopic evidence of "healed post-traumatic lesions." He stated that the lengthening of the subscapularis muscle, which leads to a decrease in power, is the prime factor producing instability of the shoulder.

TREATMENT OF ACUTE TRAUMATIC DISLOCATIONS

Hippocrates[224] discussed in detail at least six different techniques to reduce the dislocated shoulder. From century to century the literature has included woodcuts, drawings, and redrawings, illustrating modifications of Hippocrates' teachings by such investigators as Paré, de Cruce, Vidius, and Scultetus. Some of Hippocrates' techniques are still in use today.

In 1870 Theodore Kocher,[269] a Nobel Prize winner

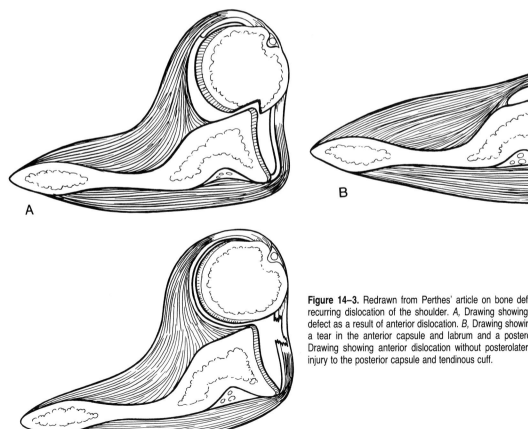

Figure 14–3. Redrawn from Perthes' article on bone defects versus soft tissue effects in recurring dislocation of the shoulder. *A*, Drawing showing the posterolateral humeral head defect as a result of anterior dislocation. *B*, Drawing showing the humeral head reduced with a tear in the anterior capsule and labrum and a posterolateral humeral head defect. *C*, Drawing showing anterior dislocation without posterolateral humeral head defect but with injury to the posterior capsule and tendinous cuff.

for medicine in 1909, gave a somewhat confusing report of his technique for levering in the anteriorly dislocated shoulder. Had Kocher not been so famous as a thyroid surgeon, his article might have received only scant attention.

OPERATIVE RECONSTRUCTIONS FOR ANTERIOR INSTABILITY

Most of the published literature on shoulder dislocations is concerned with the problem of recurrent anterior dislocations. As mentioned previously, Hippocrates[224] described the use of a white-hot poker to scar the anteroinferior capsule. Since then more than 100 different operative procedures have been developed to manage the recurrent anterior dislocation. The reader who has a yearning for the detailed history should read the classic texts by Moseley[359] and Hermodsson.[217]

Various operative techniques have been based on the posterolateral defect and the soft tissue disruptions on the front of the shoulder. Bardenheuer[30] in 1886 and Thomas[527, 528] from 1909 to 1921 discussed capsular plication or shrinking; in 1888, Albert[9] performed arthrodesis; and in 1901, Hildebrand[220] deepened the glenoid socket.

In 1906, Perthes[430] wrote a classic paper on the operative treatment of recurrent dislocations. He stated that the operation should be directed to a repair of the underlying lesion (i.e., repair of the capsule, the glenoid labrum detachment from the anterior bony rim, and the rotator cuff tear). He repaired the capsule with suture to the anterior glenoid rim through drill holes and in several cases used staples to repair the anterior capsular structures. This report gave the first description of repair of the anterior labrum and capsule to the anterior glenoid rim. Two patients were followed for 17 years, one for 12 years, two for 3 years, and one for 1 year and 9 months. All had excellent function with no recurrences.

The muscle-sling myoplasty operation was used in 1913 by Clairmont and Ehrlich.[85] The posterior third of the deltoid, with its innervation left intact, was removed from its insertion on the humerus, passed through the quadrilateral space, and sutured to the coracoid process. When the arm was abducted the deltoid contracted, which held up the humeral head. Finsterer,[158] in a similar but reversed procedure, used the coracobrachialis and the short head of the biceps from the coracoid and transferred them posteriorly. Both operations failed because of high recurrence rates.

In 1923 Bankart[27] first published his operative technique, noting that only two classes of operations were used at that time for recurrent dislocations of the shoulder: (1) those designed to diminish the size of the capsule by plication or pleating,[527, 528] and (2) those designed to give inferior support to the capsule.[85, 86] Bankart condemned both in preference to his proce-

dure. He stated that the essential lesion was the detachment or rupture of the capsule from the glenoid ligament. He recommended repair using interrupted sutures of silkworm gut passed between the free edge of the capsule and the glenoid ligament. At that time he did not repair the lateral capsule to the bone of the anterior glenoid rim. In his 1939 article, Bankart[28] described the essential lesion as a "detachment of the glenoid ligament from the anterior margin of the glenoid cavity" and stated that "the only rational treatment is to reattach the glenoid ligament (or the capsule) to the bone from which it has been torn." He further wrote that "the glenoid ligament may be found lying loose either on the head of the humerus or the margin of the glenoid cavity" and that "in every case the anterior margin of the glenoid cavity will be ound to be smooth, rounded, and free of any attachments, and a blunt instrument can be passed freely inwards over the bone on the front of the neck of the scapula." He recommended the repair of the lateral capsule down to the raw bone of the anterior glenoid and held it in place with suture through drill holes made in the anterior glenoid rim with sharp, pointed forceps. Although no references were listed in either article, Bankart must have been greatly influenced by the previously published work of Broca and Hartmann[66] and particularly of Perthes,[430] which described virtually identical pathology and repair.

Beginning in 1929, Nicola[380–384] published a series of articles on management of recurrent dislocations of the shoulder. He used the long head of the biceps tendon and the coracohumeral ligament as a suspension checkrein to the front of the shoulder. Because of technical difficulties and the high rate of recurrences, this procedure has been abandoned. Henderson[213, 214] described another checkrein operation that looped half of the peroneus longus tendon through drill holes in the acromion and the greater tuberosity. The Henderson tenosuspension operation also has been abandoned. Gallie and LeMesurier[175] described the use of autogenous fascia lata suture in the treatment of recurrent dislocations of the shoulder in 1927. This procedure has been modified and has been recently used by Bateman.[35]

POSTERIOR GLENOHUMERAL INSTABILITY

In 1839, in a Guy's Hospital report,[102] Sir Astley Cooper described in detail a dislocation of the os humeri upon the dorsum scapulae. This report is a classic, for Cooper presented most of the characteristics associated with posterior dislocations: the dislocation occurred during an epileptic seizure; pain was greater than with the usual anterior dislocation; external rotation of the arm was entirely impeded, and the patient could not elevate his arm from his side; the shoulder had an anterior void or flatness and a posterior fullness; and the patient was "unable to use or move his arm to any extent." In this report of a case in which Cooper had acted as a consultant, a reduction could not be accomplished and the patient never recovered the use of his shoulder. A postmortem examination of the shoulder, performed seven years later, revealed that the subscapularis tendon was detached and the infraspinatus muscles were stretched posteriorly about the head of the humerus. The report suggested that the detached subscapularis was "the cause of the symptoms." Cooper further described a resorption of the anterior aspect of the humeral head where it was in contact with the posterior glenoid—probably the first description of the so-called reversed Hill-Sachs lesion.

Another classic article on the subject was published in 1855 by Malgaigne,[321] who reported on 37 cases of posterior dislocations of the shoulder. Three cases were his own and 34 were reviewed from literature. This series of cases was collected 40 years before the discovery of x-rays, and it points out that with adequate physical examination of the patient the correct diagnosis can be made.

Anatomy of the Glenohumeral Joint

SURGICAL ANATOMY

The Skin

Shoulder stabilization surgery usually can be accomplished through cosmetically acceptable incisions in the lines of the skin. Anteriorly the surgeon can identify the prominent anterior axillary crease by adducting the shoulder. An incision placed in the lower part of this crease provides excellent access to the shoulder for anterior repair and yet heals nicely with a subcuticular closure (Figs. 14–4 to 14–6). When cosmesis is a concern, the incision can be made more into the axilla as described by Leslie and Ryan.[298]

Posteriorly, an analogous vertical incision in line with the extended posterior axillary crease (best visualized by extending the shoulder backwards) also heals

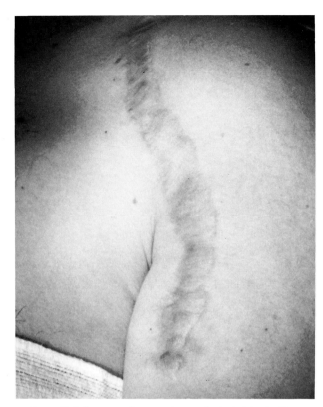

Figure 14–5. A noncosmetic approach across the front of the shoulder.

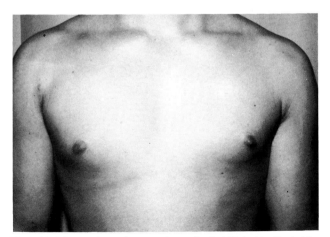

Figure 14–4. A cosmetic anterior approach on patient's right shoulder. The incision is made in the skin crease.

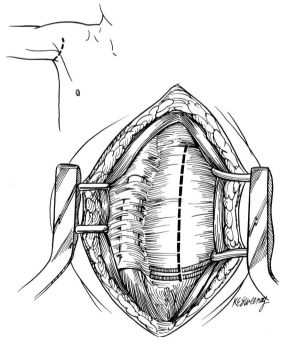

Figure 14–6. Anterior approach to the shoulder. Note the skin incision in the axillary line (*inset*). Also note the position of the subscapularis incision 1 cm medial to its insertion. (Reproduced with permission from Matsen FA, and Thomas SC: Glenohumeral instability. *In* Evarts CM (ed): Surgery of the Musculoskeletal System, 2nd ed. New York: Churchill Livingstone, 1989.)

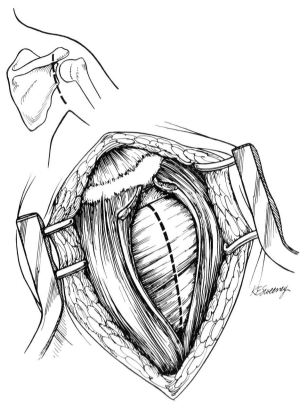

Figure 14–7. Posterior approach for treatment of posterior glenohumeral instability. The skin incision is centered over the posterior glenoid rim (*inset*). Note the deltoid-splitting approach to minimize the amount of deltoid origin that must be released. Also note the incision in the infraspinatus and teres minor tendons. (Reproduced with permission from Matsen FA, and Thomas SC: Glenohumeral instability. *In* Evarts CM (ed): Surgery of the Musculoskeletal System, 2nd ed. New York: Churchill Livingstone, 1989.)

well (Fig. 14–7). Fortuitously, these creases lie directly over the joint to which the surgeon needs access.

The First Muscle Layer

The shoulder is covered by the deltoid muscle arising from the clavicle, acromion, and scapular spine. The anterior deltoid extends to a line running approximately from the midclavicle to the midlateral humerus. This line passes over the cephalic vein, the anterior venous drainage of the deltoid, and over the coracoid process. The deltoid is innervated by the axillary nerve, whose branches swoop upward as they extend anteriorly. The commonly described "safe zone" 5 cm distal to the acromion does not take into account these anterior branches, which may come as close as 2 cm to the acromion. The deltoid abuts against the pectoralis major muscle, the clavicular head of which assists the anterior deltoid in forward flexion. Its medial and lateral pectoral nerves are not in the surgical field of shoulder stabilization. Splitting the deltopectoral interval just medial to the cephalic vein preserves the deltoid's venous drainage and takes the surgeon to the next layer. It is important to note that extension of the shoulder tightens the pectoralis major and the anterior

deltoid as well as the coracoid muscles, compromising the exposure. Thus assistants must be reminded to hold the shoulder in slight flexion to relax these muscles and facilitate exposure.

Posteriorly, the medial edge of the deltoid is too medial to provide useful access to the glenohumeral joint. Access must be achieved by splitting the deltoid, which is most conveniently done at the junction of its middle and posterior thirds. This junction is marked by the posterior corner of the acromion. The site is favorable for a split because it overlies the joint and also because the axillary nerve exiting the quadrangular space divides into two trunks (its anterior and posterior branches) in an inferior location.

The Coracoacromial Arch and the Clavipectoral Fascia

The coracoid process is the "lighthouse" of the anterior shoulder, providing a palpable guide to the deltopectoral groove, a locator for the coracoacromial arch, and an anchor for the coracoid muscles (the coracobrachialis and short head of the biceps) that separate the lateral "safe side" from the medial "suicide" where the brachial plexus and major vessels lie. The surgeon fully appreciates the value of such a lighthouse when it is lacking—for example, when re-exploring a shoulder for complications of a coracoid transfer procedure. The clavipectoral fascia covers the floor of the deltopectoral groove and can be easily identified by rotating the humerus. This permits the surgeon to observe the moving subscapularis beneath the fascial layer. Incising the fascia up to but not through the coracoacromial ligament preserves the stabilizing function of the coracoacromial arch. The bursa separates the structures that do not move on humeral rotation (the deltoid, coracoid muscles, acromion, and coracoacromial ligament) from those that do (the rotator cuff, long head of the biceps tendon, and humeral tuberosities). Posteriorly a similar plane exists between the nonrotating and the rotating structures. Anteriorly or posteriorly, this plane provides a convenient place for medial and lateral retractors.

The Zone of the Nerves

The axillary nerve runs between the deltoid and the coracoid muscles on one hand and the rotator cuff on the other. Sweeping a finger from superior to inferior along the anterior aspect of the subscapularis muscle catches the axillary nerve, hanging like a chain passing beneath the shoulder joint. Tracing this nerve proximal and medial leads the finger to the bulk of the brachial plexus. Tracing it laterally and posteriorly leads the finger beneath the shoulder capsule toward the quadrangular space. From a posterior vantage the axillary nerve is felt exiting the quadrangular space beneath the teres minor and extending laterally, where it is applied to the deep surface of the deltoid muscle. By virtue of its prominent location in close proximity to

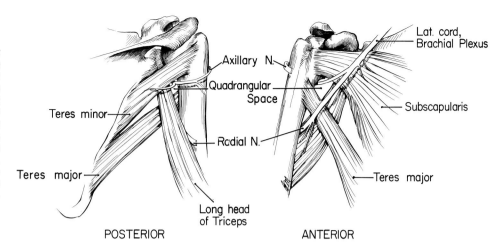

Figure 14–8. Relations of the axillary nerve to the subscapularis muscle, the quadrangular space, and the neck of the humerus. With anterior dislocations the subscapularis is displaced forward, which creates a traction injury to the axillary nerve. The nerve cannot move out of the way because it is held above by the brachial plexus and below where it wraps around behind the neck of the humerus. (Reproduced with permission from Rockwood CA, and Green DP (eds): Fractures (3 vols), 2nd ed. Philadelpha: JB Lippincott, 1984.)

the shoulder joint anteriorly, inferiorly, and posteriorly, the axillary nerve is the most frequently injured structure in shoulder surgery (Fig. 14–8). The musculocutaneous nerve lies on the deep surface of these coracoid muscles and penetrates the coracobrachialis with one or more branches lying a variable distance distal to the coracoid. (Again, the often-described 5-cm "safe zone" for the nerve beneath the process refers only to the average position of the main trunk and not to an area that can be entered recklessly.) The musculocutaneous nerve is vulnerable to injury from retractors placed under the coracoid muscles and to traction injury in coracoid transfer. Knowledge of the position of these nerves can make the shoulder surgeon both more comfortable and more effective.

The Rotator Cuff

The next layer of the shoulder is the rotator cuff. The tendons of these muscles blend in with the capsule as they insert to the humeral tuberosities. Thus, in reconstructions that require splitting of these muscles from the capsule, this splitting is more easily accomplished medially, before the blending becomes complete. The nerves to these muscles run on their deep surfaces: the upper and lower subscapular to the subscapularis and the suprascapular to the supraspinatus and infraspinatus. Medial dissection on the deep surface of these muscles may jeopardize their nerve supply.

The cuff is relatively thin between the supraspinatus and the subscapularis (the "rotator interval"). This allows the cuff to pass around the coracoid process as the arm is elevated and lowered. Splitting this interval toward the glenoid may be helpful when mobilization of the subscapularis is needed.

The tendon of the long head of the biceps originates from the supraglenoid tubercle. It runs beneath the cuff in the area of the rotator interval and exits the shoulder beneath the transverse humeral ligament and between the greater and lesser tuberosities. In the bicipital groove of the humerus this tendon is endan-

gered by procedures that involve lateral transfer of the subscapularis tendon across the groove.

The Scapulohumeral Ligaments

These capsular reinforcements are usually five in number: the coracohumeral and the superior, middle, anteroinferior, and posteroinferior glenohumeral ligaments. As will be discussed in greater detail, these ligaments are important static stabilizers of the shoulder when they are under tension. Considerable variation has been noted in the size of these ligaments and in their attachment to the scapula. These variations may explain why certain shoulders appear more prone to instability. The anteromedial and anteroinferior glenohumeral ligaments are often avulsed from the glenoid or glenoid labrum in traumatic anterior insta-

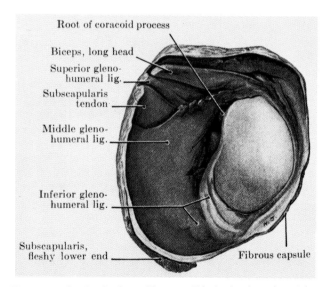

Figure 14–9. Anterior glenohumeral ligaments. This drawing shows the anterior-superior, anterior middle, and anterior-inferior glenohumeral ligaments. The middle and inferior anterior glenohumeral ligaments are often avulsed from the glenoid or glenoid labrum in traumatic anterior instability. (Reproduced with permission from Grant's Atlas of Anatomy, 4th ed. Baltimore: Williams & Wilkins, 1956.)

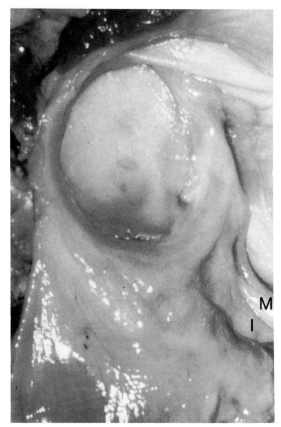

Figure 14–10. Cadaver dissection of the glenoid and associated glenohumeral ligaments. This dissection demonstrates the anterior glenohumeral ligaments. Note the relationship of the anterior inferior (I) and the anterior middle (M) glenohumeral ligaments to the anterior rim of the glenoid.

bility. Secure repair of these avulsions is an important aspect of management of recurrent traumatic glenohumeral instability (Figs. 14–9 and 14–10).

FACTORS IN GLENOHUMERAL STABILITY

The glenohumeral joint is suited for mobility. The large spherical head of the humerus articulates with the small, shallow glenoid fossa of the scapula. The glenoid provides little coverage of the head, particularly when the shoulder is (1) adducted, flexed and internally rotated, (2) abducted and elevated, or (3) adducted at the side with the scapula rotated downward.[116, 320, 483, 541] In spite of this lack of coverage, the normal shoulder precisely constrains the humeral head to within 1 mm of the center of the glenoid cavity throughout most of the arc of movement.[235, 434, 435] It is amazing that this seemingly unstable joint is able to provide this precise centering, resist the gravitational pull on the arm hanging at the side for long periods, allow for the lifting of large loads, permit throwing a baseball at speeds approaching 100 miles an hour, and hold together during the application of an almost infinite variety of forces of differing magnitude, direction, duration, and abruptness. Rather than asking

why the shoulder dislocates in some subjects, perhaps we should ask how it can be so stable in most individuals. We suggest that glenohumeral stability results from a hierarchy of mechanisms, including those that do not require the expenditure of energy by muscles ("passive" mechanisms) and those that do ("active" mechanisms). In this way Nature conserves energy while reserving the ability to call up muscular reinforcement as needed.

Passive Mechanisms

It is apparent that muscle activity is not required to hold the shoulder together. The intact shoulder of a fresh anatomical specimen is quite stable. The anesthetized and paralyzed shoulder does not fall apart in the operating room. Basmajian and Bazant[34] used electromyography of the deltoid, supraspinatus, infraspinatus, biceps, and triceps in a series of young men to show that *none* of these muscles is active when the arm hangs quietly at the side. In cadaver studies Kumar and Balasubramaniam[275] found that the position of the humeral head was maintained without muscle activity (with the entire arm hanging down) in 18 of 24 cadaver shoulders. Thus it is appropriate to discuss "passive" stabilizing mechanisms of the glenohumeral joint, which include joint conformity, finite joint volume, adhesion/cohesion, ligamentous and capsular restraints, and the glenoid labrum.

Joint Conformity

Saha[483] has demonstrated that there is considerable variation in the radii of the curvature of the glenoid fossa. The contour may be almost flat or slightly curved or may have a definite socket-like appearance. The stability of the glenohumeral joint is affected by the size, shape, and tilt of the glenoid fossa.

Cyprien and coworkers[112] studied the humeral retrotorsion and glenohumeral relationship in a group of normal patients and in patients with recurrent anterior dislocation and found essentially no difference. However, when they studied the affected and unaffected shoulders in the group of patients with recurrent dislocation, they found that the diameter of the glenoid and the contact index were smaller in the dislocated shoulder than in the normal shoulder. Whether these changes were the cause or the effect of the instability is unclear. Brewer and associates[65] measured the "retroversion" of the glenoid in 10 adolescents with 17 posteriorly unstable shoulders. The authors concluded that "excessive retroversion is a developmental deformity and is considered the primary etiology of posterior instability of the shoulder." However, their data are also consistent with the hypothesis that the deformity is a result (rather than a cause) of the instability: a major right-left difference in glenoid tilt (>10 degrees) was found only when one shoulder had experienced numerous dislocations and the other none. Perhaps even more important is the fact that the apparent tilt

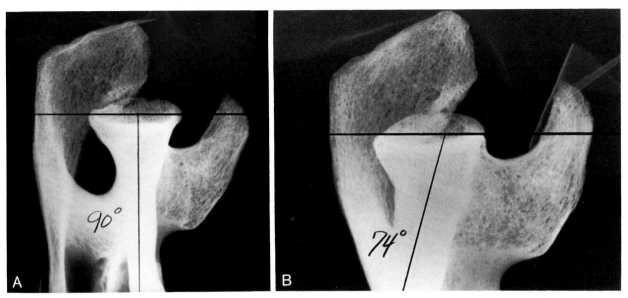

Figure 14–11. Two radiographs of the same cadaver scapula showing the variation in apparent glenoid retroversion depending on the radiographic projection.

of the glenoid surface on the axillary view varies with the angle at which the radiograph is obtained (Fig. 14–11).

Randelli and Gambrioli[442] used computed tomography (CT) to perform glenohumeral osteometry. They found no significant developmental differences in glenohumeral index, glenoid anteroposterior orientation, and humeral retrotorsion between 50 normal subjects and 40 patients with recurrent anterior dislocations. They concluded that erosions and fractures may affect the apparent orientation and anteroposterior diameter of the glenoid.

The depth of the bony glenoid is enhanced by the contributions of the articular cartilage and the glenoid labrum, which, by virtue of their relative compliance, provide an element of plasticity that can enhance the quality of the glenohumeral fit (not dissimilar from the "feathered" edge of a contact lens) (Fig. 14–12). The

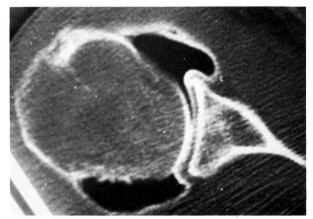

Figure 14–12. CT arthrogram of glenohumeral joint. The depth of the bony glenoid is enhanced by contributions of the articular cartilage and the glenoid labrum. This further increases the stability of the glenohumeral joint.

concavity and the fit of the glenoid to the humeral head provide stability to the joint, which is enhanced by forces pressing the ball into the socket (see Active Mechanisms).

Finite Joint Volume

When one pulls on the plunger of a plugged syringe, a relative vacuum is created that resists displacement of the plunger. Anatomical studies, surgical findings, attempts at aspiration, and magnetic resonance images all confirm that there is minimal (less than 1 cc) free fluid in the normal shoulder joint. The normal shoulder is sealed by the capsule so that outside fluid cannot enter it. Thus, like the syringe, the shoulder joint is stabilized by its limited joint volume. As long as the joint is a closed space containing minimal free fluid, the joint surfaces cannot be easily distracted or subluxated. Small translations of the humerus on the glenoid can be balanced by fluid flow in the opposite direction, allowing a nonuniform gap to open in the joint space. This gap can increase until all available fluid has been mobilized, at which point further motion of the joint is resisted by negative fluid pressure in the joint. This negative pressure pulls the capsule inward toward the joint space, putting its fibers "on the stretch." Individuals with more stretchy capsules (see the discussion of the AMBRI syndrome) will allow greater translation than those with stiff joint capsules.

This mechanism is aided by the fact that intra-articular pressure is normally slightly negative.[300, 364, 504] This negative intra-articular pressure is likely to be the result of the high osmotic pressure in interstitial tissues, which draws water from the joint. For example, if the colloid osmotic pressure of normal synovial fluid is 10 mm Hg and the colloid osmotic pressure of the synovial interstitium is 14 mm Hg, the equilibrium pressure in the joint fluid will be -4 mm Hg.[504] This negative intra-articular pressure adds a small amount of resistance to distraction (about one ounce per square inch) to the limited joint volume effect. The greater importance of these osmotic effects lies in the fact that they provide a mechanism by which free fluid is scavenged from the joint space.

Adhesion/Cohesion

The stabilization mechanism changes when the gap between the articular surfaces becomes very small. Viscous and intermolecular forces begin to dominate, preventing ready fluid motion and providing a cohesive bond between the glenoid and humerus. We term this the *adhesion/cohesion mechanism*. A familiar example is provided by two wet microscope slides pressed together. Water is held to their surfaces by *adhesion*. They can readily slide on each other but cannot be pulled apart easily by forces applied at right angles to their flat surfaces—the water holds them together by *cohesion*. Joint surfaces are wet with joint fluid that holds them together by adhesion/cohesion as well. This joint fluid interface has the highly desirable properties of (1) having high tensile strength (difficult to pull apart), and (2) having little shear strength (allows sliding of the two joint surfaces on each other with low resistance).[504] An important distinction is that the adhesion/cohesion mechanism does not put the capsular fibers on the stretch, as viscous forces suffice to prevent fluid from entering the joint space. Thus stability is provided entirely by forces exerted by and on the articular surfaces. It is also noteworthy that adhesion/cohesion forces do not stabilize a prosthetic shoulder replacement, because metal and polyethylene are insufficiently compliant to provide the necessary near-perfect congruence and because water does not adhere to their surfaces.

Both the limited joint volume effect and the effect of adhesion/cohesion would be reduced or eliminated by the addition of excess fluid (gas or liquid) to the joint. This phenomenon was well described by Humphry in 1858:[237]

In many joints—the ball and socket joints for instance—though the ligaments assist, as just mentioned, in preventing dislocation, it is quite clear that the articular surfaces cannot, under ordinary circumstances, be directly held in apposition by them, inasmuch as they must be loose in the whole circumference to permit the movements of the joint in every direction. If the ligament were sufficiently tight at any one part to hold the bones together, it must of necessity prevent the movement in one direction, which we know is not the case. The experiments of Weber upon the hip-joint were, I believe, the first to prove the fact that atmospheric pressure is the real power by which the head of the femur is held in the acetabulum when the muscles are at rest. One convincing experiment is easily repeated; hold up a side of the pelvis, with its appended lower extremity, the joint not having been opened, and then bore a hole through the acetabulum, so as to admit air into the hip-joint. The weight of the limb causes it to drop from half an inch to an inch, the head of the thigh-bone is pulled out of the acetabulum, as soon as the air is permitted to pass between the articular surfaces. In the unopened state of the joint, therefore, the weight of the limb is entirely borne by atmospheric pressure, so that both ligaments and muscles, the latter especially, are relieved in a corresponding manner. The same fact may be shown with regard to the shoulder and other joints, in a greater or less degree, though obviously the illustration is easiest in the hip and shoulder. The advantages of this construction, and the facilities it affords for easy movement by leaving all the muscles free to act upon the joint, need no demonstration. We have only to remember that this power is in continual operation to appreciate the amount of animal force that is economized by it.

The contribution of atmospheric pressure to shoulder stability is also described in *Gray's Anatomy* (second edition, 1963): "The looseness of the capsule is so great that the arm will fall about an inch from the scapula when the muscles are dissected and a hole made in it to remove the atmospheric pressure." Kumar and Balasubramaniam again demonstrated this effect in cadaver shoulders.[275] They fixed the scapula to a frame in the vertical position while the arm hung free. Radiographs were taken to determine the presence of glenohumeral subluxation. The results of these studies are so striking that they are quoted here:

In none of the shoulders was any subluxation of the joint demonstrable radiographically after dividing the muscles; but, when the capsule was then punctured [with an 18 gauge needle], marked inferior subluxation of the humeral head was seen. This occurred regardless of where the capsule was punctured. Provided atmospheric air was able to gain access into the glenohumeral joint, subluxation was always noted. As soon as the capsule was punctured percutaneously a hissing sound was heard as air rushed into the joint and it subluxated: the subluxation was confirmed radiographically. The point of puncture of the capsule did not affect these findings. No further subluxation beyond the position reached after percutaneous puncture of the capsule occurred when the overlying muscles were subsequently divided.

They found that once air had been admitted, the intact shoulder could be subluxated manually into any position with minimal force. Before air had been admitted, "a fair amount of force" was necessary to produce subluxation. It seems likely that the air admitted to the joint eliminated the stabilizing effect of the limited joint volume and also interrupted the continuity of the fluid cohesion holding the wet joint surfaces together. The change in shoulder stability with admission of air has been quantitated by Sidles and coworkers.[503a] The addition of blood to the joint in an intracapsular fracture may produce inferior subluxation by similar mechanisms.* It is of note that finite volume and adhesion/cohesion also operate in the subacromial bursa, providing additional resistance to inferior displacement of the humerus.

These stabilizing mechanisms may be overwhelmed by the application of traction, as in the cracking of the

---

*See references 103, 153, 371, 404, 405, 529, 530.

metacarpophalangeal joint. A "crack" is produced as the joint cavitates: subatmospheric pressure within the joint releases gas (>80 per cent carbon dioxide) from solution in the joint fluid. This is accompanied by a sudden jump in the joint separation. Once a joint has cracked it cannot be cracked again until about 20 minutes later when all the gas has been reabsorbed.[460, 543] (We are indebted to Peter Simkin of the University of Washington, Division of Rheumatology, who pointed us to the important literature on joint volume and adhesion/cohesion effects in joint stability.)

Ligamentous and Capsular Restraints

Ligamentous and capsular restraints are a fourth passive mechanism of joint stability. The joint capsule is large, loose, and redundant. The capacity of the glenohumeral joint capsule is larger than that of the humeral head to allow for the full and free range of motion of the shoulder. By virtue of their mandatory redundancy, the capsule and its ligaments cannot prevent glenohumeral translation when the joint is in most of its range. This is because the capsular ligaments must be under tension to exert an effect, and this occurs only when the joint approaches the end of its range of motion. Kaltsas[258] has studied some of the material properties of the shoulder capsule and found it to be more elastic and stronger than the capsule of the elbow.

The three anterior glenohumeral ligaments were first described by Schlemm.[490] Whereas Codman[90] believed that the ligaments are only a variable thickening of the capsule, Fick,[157] Weitbrecht,[561] Delorme,[121] Moseley and Overgaard,[362] Reeves,[448] Turkel and associates,[541] DePalma,[126] and McLaughlin[332] agreed that the superior, middle, and inferior glenohumeral ligaments are distinguishable and important for joint stability (see Fig. 14–9).

The constant yet diminutive *superior glenohumeral ligament* extends from the anterosuperior edge of the glenoid (near the origin of the tendon of the long head of the biceps) to the top of the lesser tuberosity of the humerus (with a portion of the coracohumeral ligament).

The dense but variable *middle glenohumeral ligament* originates from the supraglenoid tubercle, the superior labrum, or the scapular neck. It attaches to the base of the lesser tuberosity of the humerus with the posterior aspect of the subscapularis muscle. Its distal half is fused with the tendon of the subscapularis. It is usually 1 to 2 cm wide and 4 mm thick. It is poorly defined or absent in 30 per cent of shoulders.[128] In four cases of recurrent dislocation, Moseley and Overgaard found the middle glenohumeral ligament either was not discernible or was attached to the neck of the scapula rather than the labrum.[362]

The *inferior glenohumeral ligament* extends from the anteroinferior labrum and glenoid lip to the lesser tuberosity of the humerus just inferior to the middle glenohumeral ligament. The inferior glenohumeral ligament reinforces the capsular area between the subscapularis and the origin of the long head of the triceps. The experimental work on primates that was reported by Reeves[446, 447] demonstrated the importance of the inferior glenohumeral ligament in preventing anterior dislocation of the shoulder. He further pointed out that in most instances the anteroinferior glenohumeral ligament inserted primarily into the inferior labrum and only partially into bone. Turkel and associates[541] pointed out three parts of this ligament: the superior band, the anterior axillary pouch, and the posterior axillary pouch. They proposed that the superior band of the inferior glenohumeral ligament was a major stabilizer of the joint.

Delorme,[121] DePalma,[127] and Moseley and Overgaard[362] documented variability in the glenohumeral ligaments, which sometimes were very poorly defined (see Fig. 14–9). They also demonstrated a great variation in the size and number of synovial recesses that form in the anterior capsule above, below, and between the glenohumeral ligaments. They have shown from dissections that if the capsule arises at the labrum, there are few if any synovial recesses (in this situation there is a generalized blending of all three ligaments, which leaves no room for synovial recesses or weaknesses, and hence the anterior glenohumeral capsule is stronger). However, the more medially the capsule arises from the glenoid (i.e., from the anterior scapular neck), the larger and more numerous are the synovial recesses. The end result can be a thin, weak anterior capsule. Uhthoff and Piscopo[544] demonstrated in an embryological study that in 52 specimens the anterior capsule inserted into the glenoid labrum in 77 per cent and into the medial neck of the scapula in 23 per cent. These congenital variations may play a major role in the relative frequency of bilateral glenohumeral instability (see Bilateral Shoulder Instability, p. 540).

Ovesen and coworkers,[404–410] Turkel and colleagues,[541] and Warren and associates[555] have demonstrated the role of the anterior and posterior capsule and capsular ligaments in limiting the translation and rotation of the humerus. We emphasize that glenohumeral ligaments can exert an effect only if they are under tension. Thus these ligaments provide a check-rein function that is the last guardian of shoulder stability after all other passive and dynamic mechanisms have been overwhelmed. Examples of restraint provided by capsular ligaments have been demonstrated in cadaver studies as follows:

1. The anteroinferior capsule restrains anterior subluxation of the abducted arm.[405]

2. The middle glenohumeral ligament limits external rotation at 45 degrees of abduction.[541]

3. The inferior glenohumeral ligament limits external rotation at 45 to 90 degrees of abduction.[541]

4. The posterior capsule and the teres minor restrain internal rotation.[406, 409]

5. The lower two-thirds of the anterior capsule and the lower subscapularis restrain abduction and external rotation.[406, 408]

Schwartz and coworkers[494] performed selective arthroscopic cutting experiments on cadaver shoulders to quantitate the contribution of the capsular structures to glenohumeral stability. They pointed out that clinically, instability usually was accompanied by both anterior and posterior lesions. They concluded:

1. The inferior glenohumeral ligament in concert with the posteroinferior capsule provided the primary restraint to anterior translation.

2. The middle glenohumeral ligament (when present) provided a secondary restraint to anterior dislocation.

3. The posteroinferior capsule provided the primary posterior restraint to posterior dislocation.

4. The posterosuperior capsule and superior glenohumeral ligament provided secondary restraint to posterior dislocation.

Howell and associates[235] used axillary roentgenograms to document the anteroposterior position of the humeral head on the glenoid. They found that *posterior* translation of the humeral head occurs in normal subjects with the arm in extension and external rotation. This posterior translation is absent in shoulders with anterior instability. These authors suggest that this posterior translation is the result of the tension in the intact anterior capsule and ligaments.

The *coracohumeral ligament* extends from the lateral border of the horizontal arm of the coracoid process, below the coracoacromial ligament, to the transverse humeral ligament bridging the greater and lesser tuberosities between the supraspinatus and subscapularis tendon insertions.[195] Basmajian and Bazant[34] have carried out cadaver dissections demonstrating that the coracohumeral ligament and the superior capsule became quite taut when the arm was in adduction, and suggested that this tension helped to stabilize the humeral head in the glenoid. In contrast, when the shoulder was abducted to the mid range, the superior capsule became more lax and the humeral head became more unstable. They proposed that this ligament held the humeral head on the slope of the glenoid, providing substantial stability that was further enhanced by upward rotation (abduction) of the scapula and by supraspinatus contraction. Ovesen and Nielsen[404] demonstrated that cutting the coracohumeral ligament gave rise to distal subluxation of the humerus in the vertically mounted shoulder. The authors concluded that the superior capsuloligamentous structures are the most important structures preventing distal subluxation of the humeral head. However, they did not consider that cutting the superior capsuloligamentous structures must have admitted air to the joint—an action that in itself can produce downward subluxation (see sections on Finite Joint Volume and Adhesion/Cohesion). Thus, although the coracohumeral ligament provides stability to the adducted shoulder, it is probably insufficient by itself, as was demonstrated in the 24 shoulders studied by Kumar and Balasubramaniam that became downwardly unstable with only the admission of air into the joint.

Glenoid Labrum

The glenoid labrum is a fibrous rim that serves to deepen the glenoid fossa and allow attachment of the glenohumeral ligaments and the biceps tendon to the glenoid. It is the interconnection of the periosteum of the glenoid, the glenoid bone, the glenoid articular cartilage, the synovium, and the capsule. At the posterosuperior section the labrum is continuous with the long head tendon of the biceps. Anteriorly it is continuous with the inferior glenohumeral ligament (see Figs. 14–9 and 14–10).[195, 357, 361, 538] Bankart deemed its detachment from the glenoid the essential lesion responsible for the high incidence of recurrent anterior dislocations. The labrum is detached in most cases of traumatic anterior instability (Fig. 14–13).

DePalma[127] and Olsson[399] have shown that the incidence of severe recurrent dislocations is low in elderly patients in whom the labral degeneration is more common. Townley[536] and Reeves[446, 447] removed the anterior glenoid labrum through a posterior approach and found that as long as the anterior capsular mechanism remained a strong structural unit, anterior displacement of the humeral head was prevented. Thus the integrity of the labrum itself may not be as important as the security of the attachment of glenohumeral ligaments to the glenoid.

Microscopic studies by Moseley and Overgaard,[362] Townley,[536] and Gardner[182] have shown that a small amount of fibrocartilage exists at the junction of the hyaline cartilage of the glenoid and fibrous capsule. The vast majority of the labrum consists of dense fibrous tissue with a few elastic fibers. A defect in the glenoid labrum lessens the effective depth of the fossa and thus can be expected to diminish the constraint of the head and facilitate the translation of the head in the direction of the defect. In fresh cadavers, Sidles and coworkers[503a] showed that excision of the labrum reduced by just over 50 per cent the stabilization provided by glenoid geometry against distal subluxation.

Bony Restraints

The glenoid prevents the humerus from moving medially. It faces anteriorly at an angle of about 45 degrees with the coronal plane, which places it behind the humeral head for most forward uses of the arm. The acromion, coracoid, and coracoacromial ligament limit the extent of posterosuperior, superior, and anterosuperior motion of the humeral head, "backstopping" the other stabilizing mechanisms.

Active Mechanisms

The role of dynamic stability can easily be demonstrated in the normal subject. When the subject is completely relaxed, the humerus can be pushed forward and backward with respect to the scapula. If the subject contracts the muscles (for example, by slightly

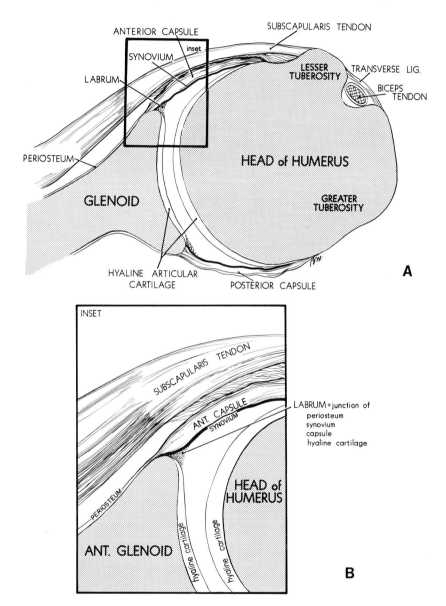

Figure 14–13. Normal shoulder anatomy. *A,* A horizontal section through the middle of the glenohumeral joint demonstrating normal anatomical relationships. Note the close relation of the subscapularis tendon to the anterior capsule. *B,* A close-up view in the area of the labrum. The labrum is essentially devoid of fibrocartilage and is composed of tissues from the nearby hyaline cartilage, capsule, synovium, and periosteum. (Reproduced with permission from Rockwood CA, and Green DP (eds): Fractures (3 vols), 2nd ed. Philadelphia: JB Lippincott, 1984.)

abducting the shoulder), the anteroposterior excursion is virtually eliminated.

Dynamic glenohumeral stability is provided by the long head of the biceps and the muscles of the rotator cuff: the subscapularis, the supraspinatus, the infraspinatus, and the teres minor. The cuff muscles serve several stabilizing functions. First, by virtue of the blending of their tendons with the glenohumeral capsule and ligaments, selective contraction of the cuff muscles can adjust the tension in these structures, producing "dynamic" ligaments, as proposed by Cleland in 1866.[88] Second, by contracting together, they press the humeral head into the glenoid fossa, locking it into position and thus providing a secure scapulohumeral link for upper extremity function.[434] Sidles and associates[503a] have demonstrated that the resistance of the shoulder to distal subluxation is proportionally increased by 67 per cent of the applied compressive load. Thus a 3-kg increase in the forces pushing the head into the glenoid increases the resistance to distal subluxation by 2 kg. Third, by contracting selectively, the rotator cuff muscles can resist displacing forces resulting from contraction of the principal shoulder motors.[362, 523] For example, when the pectoralis major and anterior deltoid muscles elevate and flex the shoulder, they tend to push the humeral head out the back of the glenoid fossa; this displacement is resisted by contraction of the subscapularis, infraspinatus, and teres minor muscles. Similarly, when the lateral deltoid initiates shoulder abduction, the supraspinatus and the long head of the biceps actively resist upward displacement of the humeral head relative to the glenoid fossa. Patients who can consciously relax these stabilizing muscles can achieve voluntary glenohumeral subluxation and dislocation. Conversely, patients with capsular instability can increase the security of their glenohumeral joints by strengthening the rotator muscles. Dynamic stability is most effective if the contractions of all shoulder muscles are coordinated with one another; strength alone is insufficient. Thus, repetitive coordination exercises such as swimming are an important tool for enhancing dynamic stability.[245]

Conclusion

We conclude that the shoulder has a hierarchy of supporting mechanisms. Minimal loads, such as the gravitational pull on the arm, are resisted by passive mechanisms such as the concavity of the joint surface provided by the glenoid and its labrum, the finite joint volume, and the adhesion/cohesion of joint fluid. Larger loads, such as those encountered in serving a tennis ball, washing a car, or picking up a child, are resisted by the action of cuff muscles whose contraction is coordinated with that of the prime movers to balance displacing forces. These mechanisms cost the body some energy but do not threaten its integrity. Finally, the ability of the shoulder to resist massive loads depends on the ligaments, the capsule, and the bony support of the joint. For example, the severe abduc-

tion–external rotation forces of a fall in skiing or a "clothesline" tackle in football challenge the anteroinferior glenohumeral ligaments. If these ligaments do not hold, a subluxation or dislocation occurs.

The function, movements, and biomechanics of the shoulder joint are further detailed in articles by Inman and colleagues,[241] Lucas,[310] Saha,[479, 483] Bechtol,[40] Colachis and Strohm,[93] Dvir and Berme,[141] Engin,[146] Poppen and Walker,[435] Turkel and coworkers,[541] Jobe and associates,[246] and Gainor and colleagues.[170]

BILATERAL SHOULDER INSTABILITY

Some of the factors contributing to joint stability are congenitally determined, such as the particular collagen makeup of the patient's ligaments, the arrangement of the glenohumeral ligaments and their method of attachment to the glenoid, the tilt of the glenoid face, the size and depth of the glenoid, the thickness of the glenoid labrum, the torsion of the humerus, and the variations in cuff muscle anatomy. These factors are likely to affect both shoulders similarly. Thus variations in these factors among individuals could have a major effect on the propensity of *both* of their shoulders to be unstable. Other factors affecting both of the patient's shoulders include the patient's age, predilection for trauma, and presence of seizures. In light of these considerations, it is not surprising that the incidence of bilateral glenohumeral instability is higher than would be expected if instability were distributed randomly among shoulders. Hovelius and coworkers[229] found that 17 per cent of their patients aged 23 to 29 with shoulder instability had this problem in both shoulders. In further support of a genetic predisposition, they found that incidence of dislocation in other family members was 5 per cent as compared with the population-wide incidence of 1.7 per cent. O'Driscoll and Evans[397] reviewed a series of 257 patients having DuToit capsulorrhaphy for recurrent instability; 13 per cent developed contralateral instability within 15 years (Fig. 14–14).

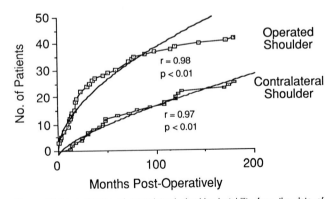

Figure 14–14. Incidence of contralateral shoulder instability from the data of O'Driscoll and Evans.[397] Thirteen per cent of the patients with normal contralateral shoulders at the time of surgery developed contralateral instability within the next 15 years.

Classification of Glenohumeral Instability

Glenohumeral instability may be classified according to the degree of instability, the chronology of instability, whether substantial force initiated the process (i.e., traumatic or atraumatic), whether the patient intentionally contributes to the shoulder's instability (i.e., voluntary or involuntary), and the direction in which the humeral head translates in relation to the glenoid fossa.

DEGREE OF INSTABILITY

Dislocation of the glenohumeral joint is the complete separation of the articular surfaces; immediate, spontaneous relocation does not occur. Glenohumeral *subluxation* is defined as symptomatic translation of the humeral head on the glenoid without complete separation of the articular surfaces. This is in contrast to the small amount of glenohumeral translation that occurs in normal shoulder function.[235, 434] Subluxation of the glenohumeral joint is transient and often momentary: the humeral head quickly and spontaneously returns to its normal position in the glenoid fossa. In a series of patients with anterior shoulder subluxation reported by Rowe and Zarins,[470] 87 per cent were traumatic and over 50 per cent were not aware that their shoulders were unstable. Like dislocations, subluxations may be traumatic or atraumatic, anterior, posterior, or inferior, acute or recurrent, or they may occur after previous surgical repairs that did not achieve complete shoulder stability. Recurrent subluxations may coexist with or be initiated by glenohumeral dislocation. Rowe and Zarins[461, 471] reported seeing a Hill-Sachs compression fracture in 40 per cent of the patients in their series on subluxation of the shoulder, an observation indicating that at some time these shoulders had been completely dislocated. *Apprehension* refers to the fear that the shoulder will subluxate or dislocate. This fear may be more functionally limiting than the instability itself.

CHRONOLOGY OF INSTABILITY

Congenital instability may result from absence or abnormalities of the proximal humerus or glenoid, such as excessive retroversion of the head of the humerus or malformation of the glenoid. A glenohumeral dislocation is *acute* if seen within the first day or so after its occurrence; otherwise, it is *chronic*. A dislocation is *locked* (or fixed) if the humeral head has been impaled on an edge of the glenoid, making reduction of the dislocation difficult. If a glenohumeral joint has been unstable on multiple occasions, the instability is *recurrent*. Recurrent instability may consist of repeated glenohumeral dislocations, subluxations, or both.

CONTRIBUTING FACTORS

Rowe[461] carefully analyzed 500 dislocations of the glenohumeral joint and determined that 96 per cent were *traumatic* (caused by a major injury) and the remaining 4 per cent were *atraumatic*. DePalma,[128] Rockwood,[456] and Collins and Wilde[94] also recognized the importance of distinguishing between traumatic and atraumatic instability of the shoulder. This distinction is critical in the selection of treatment. Patients with the *traumatic* shoulder instability problem usually have a *unilateral* problem, usually have a *Bankart* lesion, and *surgery* is usually required to manage the problem—acronym of TUBS. Patients with the *atraumatic* shoulder problem usually have an *atraumatic* initial injury, may have *multidirectional* instability, usually have *bilateral* shoulder instability, and usually respond to a *rehabilitation* program. However, should surgery be performed, the surgeon must pay particular attention to performing an *inferior* capsular shift—acronym of AMBRI. If a patient intentionally subluxates or dislocates his or her shoulder, instability is described as *voluntary*. If the instability occurs unintentionally, it is *involuntary*. Voluntary and involuntary instability may coexist. Voluntary anterior dislocation may occur with the arm at the side or in abduction/external rotation. Voluntary posterior dislocation may occur with the arm in flexion, adduction and internal rotation, or with the arm at the side. The relatively frequent association of voluntary dislocations of the shoulder with emotional instability and psychiatric problems has been noted by several authors.[74, 467] The desire to voluntarily dislocate the shoulder cannot be treated surgically.

Neuromuscular causes of shoulder instability have been reported as well. Percy[428] described a woman who, following an episode of encephalitis, developed a posterior dislocation. Kretzler and Blue[272] have discussed the management of posterior dislocations of the shoulder in children with cerebral palsy. Sever,[500] Fairbank,[152] L'Episcopo,[296] Zachary,[572] and Wickstrom[565] have reported techniques for the management of neurological dislocation of the shoulder caused by upper brachial plexus birth injuries.

DIRECTIONS OF INSTABILITY

Anterior Dislocations

Subcoracoid dislocation is the most common type of anterior dislocation. The usual mechanism that causes subcoracoid dislocations is a combination of shoulder abduction, extension, and external rotation producing forces that challenge the anterior capsule and ligaments, the glenoid rim, and the rotator cuff mechanism. The head of the humerus is displaced anteriorly with respect to the glenoid and is inferior to the coracoid process (Fig. 14–15). Other types of anterior dislocation include *subglenoid* (the head of the humerus lies anterior and below the glenoid fossa),

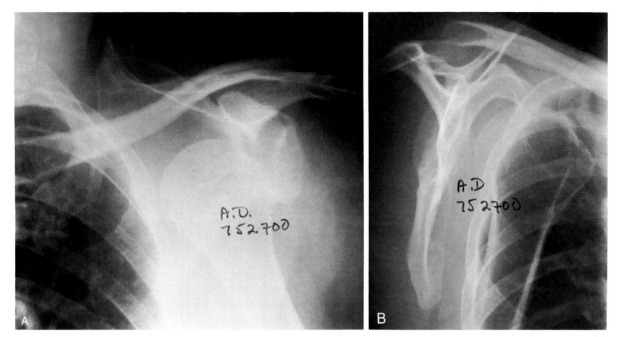

Figure 14–15. Subcoracoid dislocation. *A,* Anteroposterior view reveals that the head is medially displaced away from the glenoid fossa. On this view it is impossible to tell whether the head is anteriorly or posteriorly dislocated. *B,* On the true scapular lateral view the humeral head is completely anterior to the glenoid fossa. (Reproduced with permission from Rockwood CA, and Green DP (eds): Fractures (3 vols), 2nd ed. Philadelphia: JB Lippincott, 1984.)

subclavicular (the head of the humerus lies medial to the coracoid process, just inferior to the lower border of the clavicle), and *intrathoracic* (the head of the humerus lies between the ribs and the thoracic cavity).[190, 360, 423, 489, 563] These rarer types of dislocation are usually associated with severe trauma. There is a high incidence of fracture of the greater tuberosity of the humerus and rotator cuff avulsion. Neurological, pulmonary, and vascular complications can occur, as can subcutaneous emphysema. West[563] reported a case of intrathoracic dislocation in which with reduction the

humerus was felt to slip out of the chest cavity with a sensation similar to that of slipping a large cork from a bottle. His patient, who had an avulsion fracture of the greater tuberosity and no neurological deficit, regained a functional range of motion and returned to his job as a carpenter.

Posterior Dislocations

Posterior dislocations may leave the humeral head in a subclavicular (head behind the glenoid and beneath

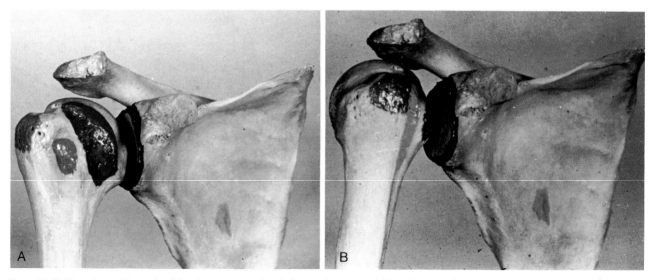

Figure 14–16. The subacromial posterior dislocation can appear deceptively normal on x-rays. *A,* Normal position of the humeral head in the glenoid fossa. *B,* In the subacromial type of posterior shoulder dislocation, the arm is in full internal rotation, and the articular surface of the head is completely posterior, leaving only the lesser tuberosity in the glenoid fossa. This positioning explains why abduction—and particularly external rotation—is blocked in posterior dislocations of the shoulder. (Reproduced with permission from Rockwood CA, and Green DP (eds): Fractures (3 vols), 2nd ed. Philadelphia: JB Lippincott, 1984.)

the acromion), subglenoid (head behind and beneath the glenoid), or subspinous (head medial to acromion and beneath the spine of the scapula) location. The subacromial dislocation is the most common by far (Fig. 14–16). Posterior dislocations are frequently locked. Hawkins and coworkers[208] reviewed 41 such cases related to motor vehicle accidents, surgeries, and electroshock therapy.

Inferior Dislocations

Inferior dislocation of the glenohumeral joint was first described by Middeldorpf and Scharm[343] in 1859. Lynn[312] in 1921 carefully reviewed 34 cases, and Roca and Ramos-Vertiz[454] in 1962 reviewed 50 cases from the world literature. Laskin and Sedlin[285] reported a case in an infant. Three bilateral cases have been reported by Murrard,[366] Langfritz,[284] and Peiro and coworkers.[427]

Severe soft tissue injury or fractures about the proximal humerus occur with this dislocation (Fig. 14–17). At the time of surgery or autopsy, various authors have found avulsion of the supraspinatus, pectoralis major, or teres minor muscles and fractures of the greater tuberosity.[273, 285, 312, 343, 366, 454]

Superior Dislocations

Speed[511] reports that Langier, in 1834, was the first to record a case of superior dislocation of the glenohumeral joint, and Stimson[518] has reviewed 14 cases that had been reported in the literature prior to 1912. In current literature little is mentioned about this type of dislocation, but undoubtedly occasional cases occur. The usual cause is an extreme forward and upward force on the adducted arm. With displacement of the

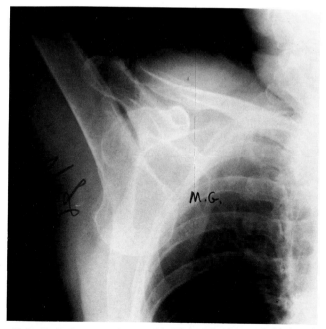

Figure 14–17. Anteroposterior x-ray of the inferior dislocation reveals that the entire humeral head and surgical neck of the humerus are inferior to the glenoid fossa.

humerus upward, fractures may occur in the acromion, acromioclavicular joint, clavicle, coracoid process, or humeral tuberosities. Extreme soft tissue damage occurs to the capsule rotator cuff, biceps tendon, and surrounding muscles. Clinically, the head rides above the level of the acromion. The arm is short and adducted to the side. Shoulder movement is restricted and quite painful. Neurovascular complications are usually present. Treatment consists of closed reduction and restoration of the damaged tissues.

Incidence and Mechanism of Injury

INCIDENCE OF SHOULDER INSTABILITY

The shoulder is the most commonly dislocated major joint in the body, accounting for 45 per cent of 8056 dislocations at the Central Outpatient Department of the Injured of Budapest.[261] Cave[80] demonstrated that, in a series of 1600 shoulder injuries, 394 were dislocations; of these 84 per cent were anterior glenohumeral dislocations, 12 per cent were acromioclavicular, 2.5 per cent were sternoclavicular, and only 6 of the 394, or 1.5 per cent, were posterior dislocations.

The incidence of posterior dislocations is estimated at 2 per cent but is difficult to ascertain because of the frequency with which this diagnosis is missed. Thomas[526] reported seeing only 4 cases of posterior shoulder dislocation in 6000 x-ray examinations. The literature reflects that the diagnosis of posterior dislocation of the shoulder is missed in over 60 per cent of cases.[145, 211, 425, 550] A 1982 article by Rowe and Zarins[471] indicates that the diagnosis was missed in 79 per cent of cases! McLaughlin[330] stated that posterior shoulder dislocations are sufficiently uncommon that their occurrence creates a "diagnostic trap."

The largest reported and complete series of posterior dislocations of the shoulder (37 cases) was recorded by Malgaigne[321] in 1855, 40 years before the discovery of x-rays. He and his colleagues made the diagnosis by performing a *proper physical examination!* Cooper[102] stated that the physical findings are so classic that he called it "an accident which cannot be mistaken."

MECHANISMS OF SHOULDER INSTABILITY

Atraumatic Instability

In patients with constitutionally lax shoulders, instability can develop with no or minimal injury.[184, 438, 470] If the shoulder muscles become deconditioned, the dynamic stability may be lost, so that the joint is launched on a self-perpetuating cycle of more instability → less use → more shoulder dysfunction → more instability. This situation is reminiscent of the interrelationship of patellar instability and quadriceps weakness.

Traumatic Instability

The previously normal shoulder can become unstable as a result of trauma. Although the shoulder can be dislocated by *direct* trauma such as a blow directed at the proximal humerus, *indirect* force is the most common cause of shoulder sprain, subluxation, or dislocation. The combination of abduction, extension, and external rotation forces applied to the arm may result in an anterior dislocation. Axial loading of the adducted, internally rotated arm may produce a posterior dislocation.[353]

Dislocations may result from violent muscle contraction, by electrical shock or convulsive seizures.* Although the resulting dislocation may be anterior, it is usually posterior. The combined strength of the internal rotators (latissimus dorsi, pectoralis major, and subscapularis muscles) simply overwhelms the external rotators (infraspinatus and teres minor muscles) (Fig. 14–18).

Inferior dislocation may be produced by a hyperabduction force that causes impingement of the neck of the humerus against the acromion process, which levers the head out inferiorly. The humerus is then locked with the head below the glenoid fossa and the humeral shaft pointing overhead. The force may be so great as to force the head out through the soft tissues and the skin. Lucas and Peterson[311] have reported a case of a 16-year-old boy who caught his arm in the power take-off of a tractor and suffered an open luxatio erecta injury.

Clinical Presentation

DISLOCATIONS

History

Glenohumeral instability may present in a wide variety, ranging from a vague sense of shoulder dysfunction to an obvious fixed dislocation.[438, 470, 471] The history should attempt to define the *mechanism of injury* including the position of the arm, the amount of applied force, and the point of force application. Injury with the arm in extension, abduction, and external rotation favors anterior dislocation. Electroshock, seizures, or a fall on the flexed and adducted arm is more consistent with posterior dislocation. It is important to determine the *amount of trauma* that initiated the instability as well as the force required to produce subsequent episodes. A violent injury from a fall while skiing is associated with a quite different pathological process and requires different management than a shoulder that becomes unstable without any particular precipitating episode, i.e., swinging a badminton racket or throwing a ball. When there is a *prior history of instability* we inquire how long the

---

*See references 6, 74, 159, 209, 304, 324, 347, 400, 438, 497.

shoulder was "out," whether radiographs were taken, and what was done to reduce the shoulder. Previous radiographs and medical records are frequently most helpful in supporting the diagnosis. The history should also solicit evidence of *neurological or rotator cuff* problems after previous episodes of shoulder instability. Finally the *previous treatment* and its effectiveness needs to be investigated, including rehabilitation and surgery.

Physical Examination of the Dislocated Shoulder

Anterior Dislocation

The physical examination of the anteriorly dislocated shoulder should be diagnostic. The acutely dislocated shoulder is very painful. Muscles are in spasm in an attempt to stabilize the joint. The humeral head may be palpable anteriorly. The posterior shoulder shows a hollow beneath the acromion. The arm is held in slight abduction and external rotation. Anterior dislocation usually produces a shoulder incapable of complete internal rotation and abduction. Because of the frequent association of nerve injury, particularly the axillary nerve, and, to a lesser extent, vascular injuries,[49] an essential part of the physical examination of the anteriorly dislocated shoulder is the assessment of the neurovascular status of the upper extremity and the charting of the findings prior to reduction.

Posterior Dislocation

Recognition of a posterior dislocation may be impaired by the lack of a striking deformity of the shoulder and by the fact that the shoulder is held in the traditional sling position of adduction and internal rotation. However, a directed physical examination will reveal the diagnosis. The classical features of a posterior dislocation include:

1. Limited external rotation of the shoulder (often to less than zero degrees).
2. Limited elevation of the arm (often to less than 90 degrees).
3. Posterior prominence and rounding of the shoulder compared with normal.
4. Flattening of the anterior aspect of the shoulder.
5. Prominence of the coracoid process on the dislocated side.

Asymmetry of the shoulder contours can often be best visualized by viewing the shoulders from above while standing behind the patient (Fig. 14–19).

The motion is limited because the head of the humerus is fixed on the posterior glenoid rim by muscle forces, or the head may actually be impaled on the glenoid rim. With the passage of time, the posterior rim of the glenoid may further impact the fracture of the humeral head and produce a deep hatchet-like defect or V-shaped compression fracture, which engages the head even more securely. Patients with old, unreduced posterior dislocations of the shoulder may have 30 to 40 degrees of glenohumeral abduction and

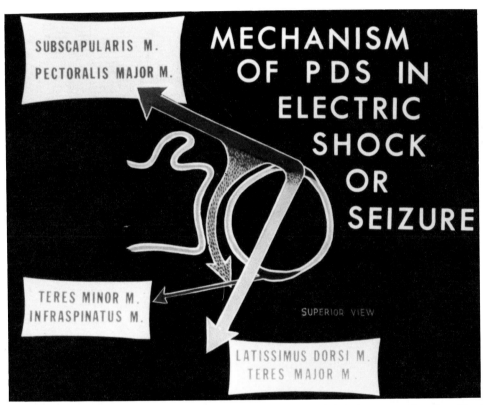

Figure 14–18. Mechanism of posterior dislocation of the shoulder that is caused by an accidental electrical shock or a convulsive seizure. The strong internal rotators simply overpower the weak external rotators.

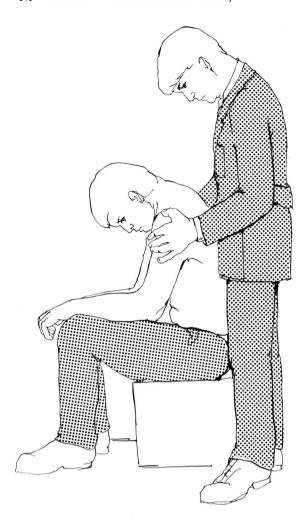

Figure 14–19. Visualization of the anterior and posterior aspects of the shoulders can best be accomplished by having the patient sit on a low stool, with the examiner standing behind him. Then the injured shoulder can easily be compared with the uninjured one. (Reproduced with permission from Rockwood CA, and Green DP (eds): Fractures (3 vols), 2nd ed. Philadelphia: JB Lippincott, 1984.)

some humeral rotation owing to enlargement of the groove. With long-standing disuse of the muscles about the shoulder, atrophy will be present, which accentuates the flattening of the anterior shoulder, the prominence of the coracoid, and the fullness of the posterior shoulder.

Proper physical examination is essential. Rowe and Zarins[471] reported 23 cases of unreduced dislocation of the shoulder, of which 14 were posterior. Hill and McLaughlin[223] reported that in their series the average time from injury to diagnosis was eight months. In the interval before the diagnosis of posterior dislocation of the shoulder is made, the injury may be misdiagnosed as "frozen shoulder"[223, 334, 335] for which vigorous therapy may be mistakenly instituted in an attempt to restore the range of motion.

Inferior Dislocation

In a subglenoid dislocation the arm is abducted about 30 degrees, internally rotated, and shortened. Nobel[387] reported a case of this rare type of dislocation in which the acromion–olecranon distance was shortened by 1.5 inches.

A patient with luxatio erecta usually has the humerus locked in a position somewhere between 110 and 160 degrees of abduction (see Fig. 14–17). The head of the humerus may be palpated on the lateral chest wall. Pain is quite severe. The condition is more common among the elderly.

Bilateral Dislocations

Mynter[367] first described the condition in 1902; according to Honner,[225] only 20 cases were reported prior to 1969. Bilateral dislocations have been reported by McFie,[324] Yadav,[570] Onabowale and Jaja,[400] Segal and colleagues,[497] and Carew-McColl.[74] Most of these cases were the result of convulsions or violent trauma. Peiro and coworkers[427] reported bilateral erect dislocation of the shoulders in a man caught in a cement mixer. Bilateral dislocation of the shoulder secondary to accidental electrical shock has been reported by Carew-McColl[74] and Fipp.[159] Nicola and coworkers[379] have reported cases of bilateral posterior fracture-dislocation following a convulsive seizure. Ahlgren and associates[6] reported three cases of bilateral posterior fracture-dislocation associated with a convulsion. Lind-holm and Elmstedt[304] reported a case of bilateral posterior fracture-dislocation following an epileptic seizure, which was treated by open reduction and internal fixation with screws. Parrish and Skiendzielewski[418] reported a patient with bilateral posterior fracture-dislocations after status epilepticus. The diagnosis was missed for over 12 hours. Pagden and associates[413] reported two cases of posterior shoulder dislocation following seizures related to regional anesthesia.

RECURRENT INSTABILITY

History

The challenge of diagnosis is greater in the shoulder with recurrent instability. Particularly in the shoulder with recurrent subluxation, the condition is much less obvious to the patient and the physician. Yet the same diagnostic steps—the history, the physical examination, and the roentgenograms—usually will point to the diagnosis. With traumatic instability the patient usually can describe the initial injury in great detail, i.e., a sharp stabbing pain, a closed reduction done by a physician usually with sedation, and a residual aching shoulder for several weeks. In most cases of recurrent traumatic anterior instability, the injury results from a forced abduction and external rotation of the shoulder. A classic example is the defender who tries to make an arm tackle on the ball carrier and ends up having his arm pulled back into extension, abduction, and external rotation. Similarly a skier may fall on the abducted arm or a kayaker may have the arm pulled back over the head while bracing in white water. This movement is associated with a sharp, stabbing pain in the shoulder. Spontaneous reduction may occur immediately or the patient may require a manipulative reduction. Records and roentgenograms from this initial episode are most valuable. Subsequently the shoulder may demonstrate recurrent subluxation,[456] "dead arm syndrome,"[471] or frank dislocation when it resumes the extended, abducted, and externally rotated position. Recurrent traumatic posterior instability may begin with a fall on the outstretched arm or a blow on the front of the shoulder.

Recurrent instability may also have an *atraumatic* onset. Without a major injury the humeral head starts to slide out of its normal position. This instability may be anterior, posterior, inferior, or multidirectional. Patients with atraumatic instability may describe aggravation of their problem by trauma. Careful questioning usually reveals that the original injury was minor in nature and occurred with such things as taking an overhead swing at a tennis ball, lifting up a garage door, a minor fall on the shoulder, or swinging a baseball bat. Several important clues that suggest the diagnosis of atraumatic subluxation or dislocation can be obtained from the patient: the original injury was a minor one and was usually not associated with signifi-

cant pain; the subluxation or dislocation reduced spontaneously; the patient returned to his or her activities without much pain or problem; and the patient has generalized ligament laxity, i.e., the opposite shoulder, the metacarpophalangeal joints, elbows, knees, and so forth. The symptoms include feelings of recurrent instability, apprehension, or dislocation. A good history of the onset, positions of instability, and past treatment is very helpful in diagnosis.

We routinely ask whether the patient can dislocate the shoulder voluntarily. If the answer is "yes," the surgeon must determine whether *voluntary* instability is the preponderant problem (in which case surgical stabilization is unlikely to succeed) or just a minor facet of a shoulder that usually goes out involuntarily. The patient with voluntary instability usually has no history of injury but can remember since childhood the ability to slip one or both shoulders out of place with minimal discomfort. In the late teens or twenties the patient may note that the shoulder begins to slip out of place when a stress is placed on it (Fig. 14–20).

Physical Examination

Like the history, physical examination of the shoulder with suspected recurrent instability is challenging. We usually start by seeking evidence of generalized ligamentous laxity, such as contralateral shoulder instability, hyperextension of the knees, elbows, and the metacarpophalangeal joints, thumb flexibility, and flat feet. The strength of the anterior, middle, and posterior deltoid and the external rotators is next checked; a screening neurological examination is also performed. Weakness of external rotation suggests the possibility of a rotator cuff tear or a suprascapular nerve injury. Perhaps the most important part of the examination is the performance of stress tests to challenge the stability of the joint in various directions, observing both the resulting translation and the degree of apprehension demonstrated by the patient with each test. It is particularly helpful if a particular test reproduces the sensation that is problematic for the patient ("That's the thing that happens!"). In the performance of these tests, it is important that the patient be as relaxed as possible so that the examiner is testing static (capsular) and not dynamic (muscular) stability. In interpreting the significance of the degree of translation on a given test, it is helpful to use the contralateral shoulder and previous examinations of other shoulders as a standard of what is normal.

Drawer Test (Fig. 14–21). The patient is seated with the forearm resting on the lap and the shoulder relaxed. The examiner stands behind the patient. One of the examiner's hands stabilizes the shoulder girdle (scapula and clavicle) while the other grasps the proximal humerus. The humeral head is pressed gently toward the scapula to center it in the glenoid, assuring a neutral starting position. Starting from this neutral position, the humerus is first pushed forward to determine the

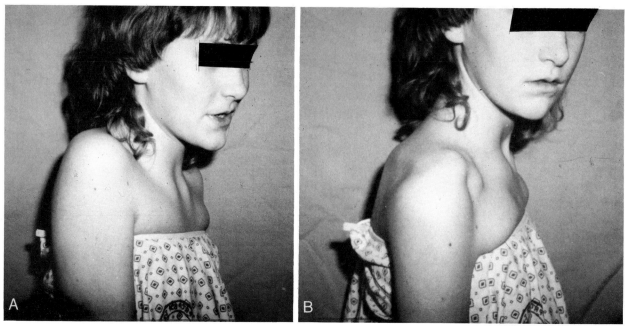

Figure 14–20. Voluntary instability. This patient had no significant history of injury but could voluntarily dislocate her shoulder with minimal discomfort. Patient with the right shoulder reduced (A) can posteriorly dislocate voluntarily (B).

amount of anterior displacement relative to the scapula. The normal shoulder reaches a firm end-point with only slight anterior translation, no clunking, and no pain or apprehension. A clunk or snap on anterior subluxation or reduction may suggest a labral tear or Bankart lesion. The humerus is returned to the neutral position and then pulled backward to determine the amount of posterior translation relative to the scapula. The normal shoulder allows posterior translation up to

about one-half of the humeral head diameter. Increased anterior and posterior translation suggests multidirectional instability. This test has the advantage of eliciting evidence of capsular laxity without threatening the patient with dislocation—a threat that may lead to a false negative test from protective muscle contraction.

Sulcus Test (Figs. 14–22 and 14–23). The patient sits with the arm relaxed at the side. The examiner pulls

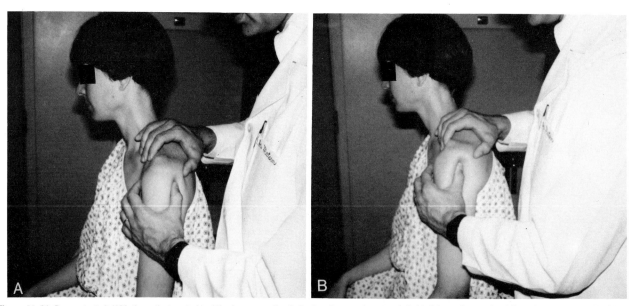

Figure 14–21. Drawer test. A, With the patient seated and the forearm resting in the lap, the examiner stands behind the patient and stabilizes the shoulder girdle with one hand while grasping the proximal humerus with the other, pressing the humeral head gently toward the scapula to center it in the glenoid. B, The head is then pushed forward to determine the amount of anterior displacement relative to the scapula. It can then be returned to the neutral position and a posterior force applied to determine the amount of posterior translation relative to the scapula.

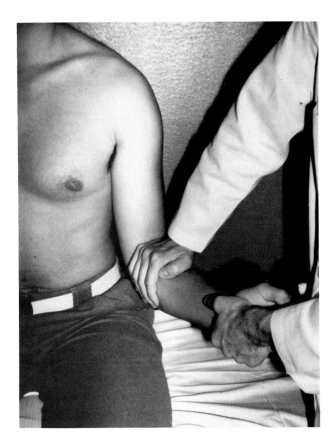

Figure 14–22. Sulcus test. The patient is seated with his arm relaxed and at the side. The examiner pulls downward on the arm. Inferior instability is demonstrated if a sulcus (or hollow) appears inferior to the acromion. This patient has a negative sulcus test.

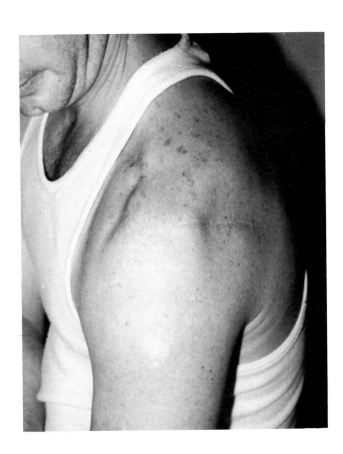

Figure 14–23. Positive sulcus sign. This patient had a posterior repair for glenohumeral instability. However, he continues to have inferior instability and demonstrates the sulcus (or hollow) just inferior to the anterior acromion during this sulcus test. A capsular shift is indicated.

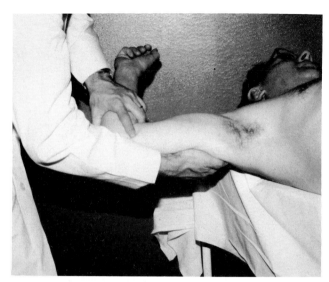

Figure 14–24. Fulcrum test. With the patient supine and the shoulder at the edge of the examination table, the arm is abducted to 90 degrees. The examiner's right hand is used as a fulcrum while the arm is gently and progressively extended and externally rotated. In the presence of anterior instability, the patient becomes apprehensive or the shoulder translates with this maneuver.

the arm downward. Inferior instability is demonstrated if a sulcus or hollow appears inferior to the acromion. This test is often positive in multidirectional instability.

Fulcrum Test (Fig. 14–24). The patient lies supine at the edge of the examination table with the arm abducted to 90 degrees. The examiner places one hand on the table under the glenohumeral joint to act as a fulcrum. The arm is gently and progressively extended and externally rotated over this fulcrum. Maintaining gentle passive external rotation for a minute fatigues the subscapularis, challenging the capsular contribution to the anterior stability of the shoulder. The patient with anterior instability will usually become apprehensive as this maneuver is carried out (watch the eyebrows for a clue that the shoulder is getting ready to dislocate).

Crank or Apprehension Test (Fig. 14–25). The patient sits with the back toward the examiner. The arm is held in 90 degrees of abduction and external rotation. The examiner pulls back on the patient's wrist with one hand while stabilizing the back of the shoulder with the other. The patient with anterior instability usually will become apprehensive with this maneuver. Again, we refer to apprehension as a feeling that the shoulder is getting ready to dislocate, rather than just pain (which could come from other conditions such as impingement).

Jerk Test (Posterior Instability) (Figs. 14–26 and 14–27). The patient sits with the arm internally rotated and flexed forward to 90 degrees. The examiner grasps the elbow and axially loads the humerus in a proximal direction. While axial loading of the humerus is maintained, the arm is moved horizontally across the body. In many patients with recurrent posterior instability this test will produce a sudden jerk when the humeral head slides off the back of the glenoid. When the arm

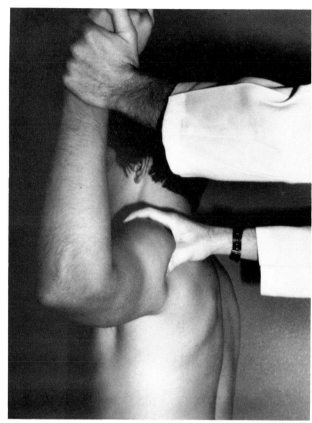

Figure 14–25. Crank test. The arm is held in 90-degree abduction and external rotation. The examiner's left hand is pulling back on the patient's wrist while his right hand stabilizes the back of the shoulder. The patient with anterior instability becomes apprehensive with this maneuver.

is returned to the original position of 90-degree abduction, a second jerk may be observed, that of the humeral head returning to the glenoid.

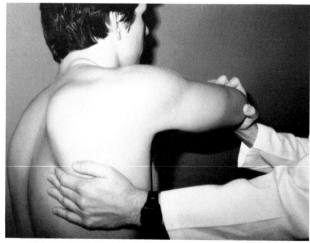

Figure 14–26. Jerk test. The patient's arm is abducted to 90 degrees and internally rotated. The examiner axially loads the humerus while the arm is moved horizontally across the body. The left hand stabilizes the scapula. Patients with recurrent posterior instability may demonstrate a sudden jerk as the humeral head slides off the back of the glenoid or when it is reduced by moving the arm back to the starting position.

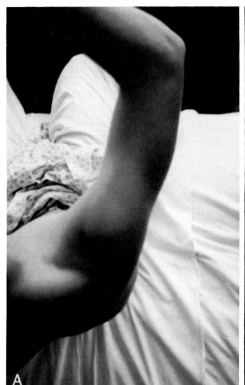
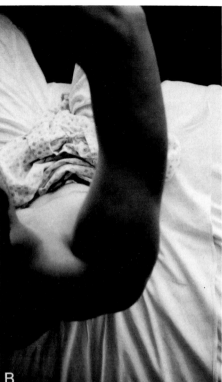

Figure 14–27. Positive jerk test. *A,* Normal appearance of the shoulder before the patient performs a jerk test. *B,* With axial loading and movement of the arm horizontally across the body, the humeral head slides off the back of the glenoid, as is demonstrated by the prominence in the posterior aspect of the patient's shoulder. This maneuver resulted in a sudden jerk and some discomfort.

Push-Pull Test (Posterior Instability (Fig. 14–28). The patient lies supine with the shoulder off the edge of the table. The arm is in 90 degrees of abduction and 30 degrees of flexion. Standing next to the patient's hip, the examiner pulls up on the wrist with one hand while pushing down on the proximal humerus with the other. The shoulders of normal, relaxed patients often will allow 50 per cent posterior translation on this test.

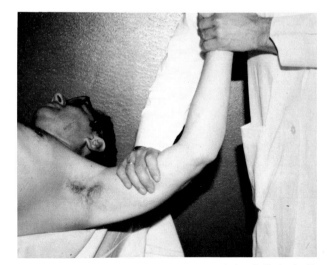

Figure 14–28. Push-pull test. The patient lies supine and relaxed with the shoulder at the edge of the examination table. The examiner pulls up on the wrist with one hand while pushing down on the proximal humerus with the other. Approximately 50 per cent posterior translation of the humerus on the glenoid is normal in relaxed patients.

Greater degrees of translation, apprehension, or reproduction of the patient's symptoms suggest pathological posterior instability. This test should be performed on both sides to compare the degrees of translation and the patient's response.

If apprehension on these tests cannot be easily differentiated from painful subacromial impingement, a subacromial injection of lidocaine can help eliminate the symptoms of impingement.[375] The reader should refer to Chapter 26, The Shoulder in Sports, for description of other tests to differentiate shoulder instability from the impingement problem.

Instability in more than one direction (multidirectional instability) is not uncommon. Thus, all directions of glenohumeral instability are routinely examined, even in the patient with documented recurrent anterior shoulder dislocations.

Radiographic and Laboratory Evaluation

Note: The reader should refer to Chapter 5, X-Ray Evaluation of Shoulder Problems, for the details of obtaining radiographs for shoulder instability.

PLAIN RADIOGRAPHY

In the situation of the dislocated shoulder, the physician needs to know the following: (1) the direction of the dislocation, (2) the existence of associated fractures (displaced or not), and (3) possible barriers to relocation. If a dislocation is confirmed, reduction and postreduction films can be accomplished on the x-ray table. (The patient certainly appreciates not being moved for each of these steps!)

Radiographs in the Plane of the Body

Radiographs of the shoulder are most conveniently identified by the plane of the projection. For many years the standard shoulder films have been taken with the film in the plane of the body.

Anteroposterior View

The anteroposterior view has been obtained with the patient's back flat on the cassette and the x-ray beam at right angles to this plane and centered on the shoulder. This may be called the "AP in the plane of the body." This is not a true anteroposterior view of the glenohumeral joint, because the scapula lies on the posterolateral chest wall at an angle of 30 to 45 degrees from the frontal plane. Hence the glenoid is open or faces anteriorly 45 degrees, and the view projects a significant overlap of the humeral head on three-fourths to seven-eighths of the glenoid (Fig. 14–29).

Although the anteroposterior view in the plane of the body may provide sufficient information to diagnose the various types of anterior dislocations and the subspinous and subglenoid types of posterior dislocations, it is insufficient to diagnose the most common type of posterior dislocation, the subacromial. Frequently, this dislocation is missed on this view because the displacement is essentially at right angles to the plane of the film. Even posterior dislocations associated with a fracture can appear deceptively normal.

We do not recommend the use of radiographic views in the plane of the body to routinely evaluate the glenohumeral joint. McLaughlin has said that the reliance on anteroposterior radiographs will lead the unwary orthopedist into a "diagnostic trap."[330] However, a number of radiographic signs that suggest dislocation have been described on the anteroposterior view in the plane of the body. These signs include the following:

1. Absence of the normal elliptical overlap shadow. Normally on the routine anteroposterior view an overlap shadow is created by the head of the humerus superimposed on the glenoid fossa of the scapula. The shadow is a smooth-bordered ellipse. In posterior dislocations, the articular surface of the humeral head is posterior to the glenoid and the elliptical overlap shadow is distorted.

2. Vacant glenoid sign. Normally on the routine anteroposterior view the head fills the majority of the glenoid cavity. However, in posterior dislocations with the head resting behind the glenoid, the glenoid fossa appears to be partially vacant. Arndt and Sears[15] refer to this as a positive rim sign and state that if the space between the anterior rim and the humeral head is greater than 6 mm, it is highly suggestive of a posterior dislocation.

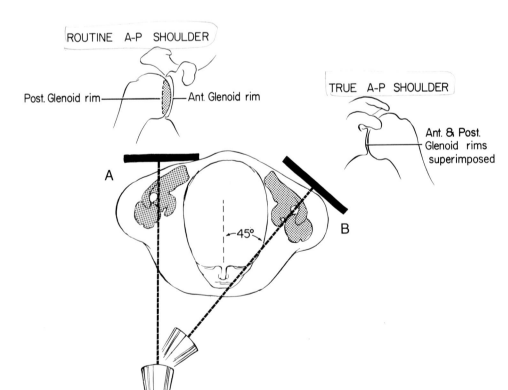

Figure 14–29. Positioning of the patient for a routine anteroposterior x-ray and for the true anteroposterior view of the shoulder. *A*, In the routine view of the shoulder, the glenoid fossa faces anteriorly, because the scapula is sitting on the posterolateral aspect of the thoracic cavity. Both the anterior and posterior rims of the glenoid fossa, as well as the head of the humerus, are visualized on the x-ray. *B*, In a true anteroposterior view of the shoulder, the anterior and posterior glenoid rims are superimposed on each other into a single articular surface.

3. The "trough line." Cisternino and colleagues[84] and Demos[122] have reported on the high incidence of a "trough line" on the anteroposterior x-ray. This is a result of the impaction fracture of the humeral head caused by the posterior rim of the glenoid and is analogous to the Hill-Sachs impaction fracture line that is seen with anterior dislocation of the shoulder. These authors reported that the trough line on the anteroposterior x-rays was present in 75 per cent of their 20 cases of posterior dislocation.

4. Loss of profile of the neck of the humerus. In posterior dislocations of the shoulder, the arm is in full internal rotation; thus, a profile of the neck of the humerus is not seen. However, the same is true for the normal shoulder when the radiograph is taken with the arm in internal rotation. If anteroposterior films of an injured shoulder in internal or external rotation do not show the profile of the neck of the humerus on either view, then posterior dislocation of the shoulder is suggested.

5. Void in the inferior or superior glenoid fossa. With posterior dislocation the humeral head is occasionally displaced upward or downward, leaving a void in the inferior or superior third of the glenoid fossa. This is not seen in the normal shoulder.

Transthoracic Lateral View

As with the anteroposterior view in the plane of the scapula, we discuss this view for the reader's interest but do not recommend it for the analysis of glenohumeral pathology. In this view, the lateral aspect of the involved arm and shoulder is placed against the cassette and the normal arm over the head of the patient. The x-ray beam is directed through the chest.

Dorgan[138] reported that, in addition to obesity, technical factors may prevent accurate identification of the glenohumeral joint in the transthoracic lateral view. He credits Dr. Albert Moloney of Boston with interpreting a "break in the normal scapulohumeral arch" (Moloney's line). Normally in this projection a smooth or rounded dome type of arch is created by the shaft of the humerus, the head of the humerus, and the lateral or axillary border of the scapula. In posterior dislocations of the shoulder, the head and neck of the humerus are behind and superimposed on the glenoid fossa; hence, the smooth dome shape is obliterated. Consequently, the top of the arch comes to a narrow apex created by the shaft of the humerus, which meets the axillary border of the scapula. In anterior dislocations the opposite is true; that is, the dome of the arch becomes quite wide. This widening occurs (1) because the head is displaced anteriorly and (2) because the arm is in external rotation and places more of the neck on profile, which widens the arch.

Radiographs in the Plane of the Scapula

Rather than views referred to the plane of the body, we suggest a standard series of radiographs referred to

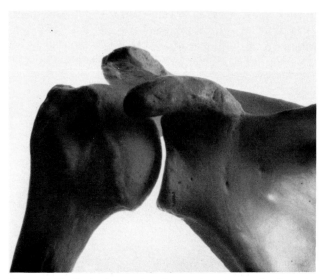

Figure 14–30. Simulated x-ray view of a scapular anteroposterior view using backlighted skeletal models. This view reveals the radiographic glenohumeral joint space and provides a good opportunity to detect fractures of the humerus or glenoid lip.

the plane of the scapula for all injured shoulders: an anteroposterior view in the plane of the scapula, a scapular lateral, and an axillary view.

Anteroposterior View

In 1923 Grashey[196] recognized that in order to take a true anteroposterior radiograph of the shoulder joint, the direction of the x-ray beam must be perpendicular to the plane of the scapula. This view is most easily accomplished by placing the scapula flat on the cassette (a position the patient can help achieve) and passing the x-ray beam at right angles to this plane, centering it on the coracoid process. We refer to this view as an "AP in the plane of the scapula" (Fig. 14–30). In the

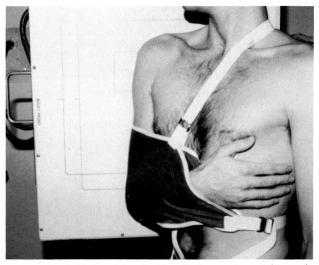

Figure 14–31. Positioning of the patient in a sling for an anteroposterior x-ray in the plane of the scapula. The scapula is placed flat on the cassette. The x-ray beam is positioned at right angles to the cassette and centered on the coracoid process.

normal shoulder the articular surface of the humeral head is separated clearly from the glenoid fossa by a radiographic joint space. This view can be taken with the arm in a sling and only requires positioning of the entire body rather than the arm (Figs. 14–31 and 14–32).

Lateral View

The view at right angles to the anteroposterior in the plane of the scapula is the "scapular lateral" (Figs. 14–33 and 14–34).[330, 334, 335, 370, 455] Like the anteroposterior view, it can be obtained by positioning the body and not the arm. Here the cassette is placed anterolateral to the deltoid and the scapula is positioned perpendicular to it (Fig. 14–34). Since the posterior aspect of the body of the scapula is easy to palpate, this position can be reliably achieved. The beam is placed parallel to the spine of the scapula and perpendicular to the cassette. To aid the radiological technician the physician can draw a line along the spine of the scapula with a marking pen. The x-ray cassette is placed

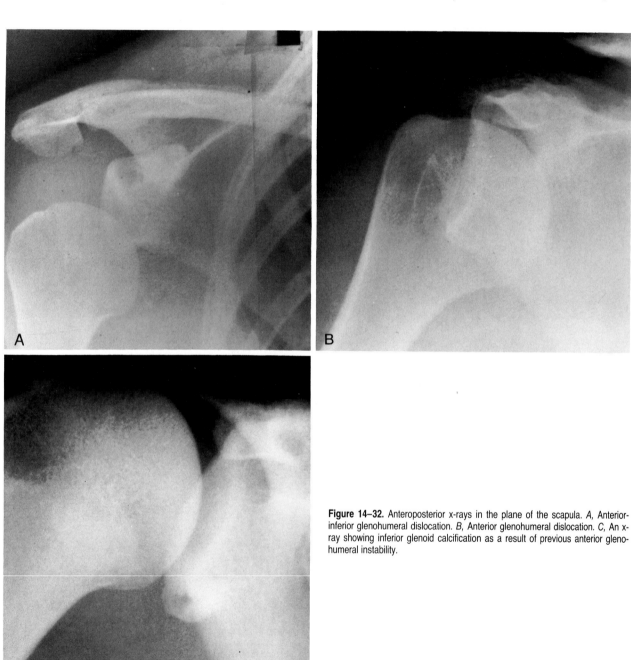

Figure 14–32. Anteroposterior x-rays in the plane of the scapula. *A,* Anterior-inferior glenohumeral dislocation. *B,* Anterior glenohumeral dislocation. *C,* An x-ray showing inferior glenoid calcification as a result of previous anterior glenohumeral instability.

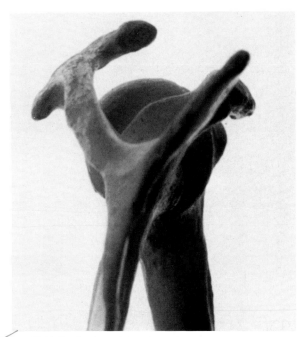

Figure 14-33. Simulated scapulolateral x-ray view with backlighted skeletal model. The x-ray beam is passed parallel to the plane of the scapula and is centered on the scapular spine. The view reveals the anteroposterior relationship of the head of the humerus in the glenoid fossa. The glenoid fossa is identified as the intersection of the spine of the scapula, the coracoid process, and the body of the scapula.

anterolateral to the shoulder, which will be perpendicular to the line on the scapula. The x-ray beam is directed down the line on the spine onto the cassette.[455] In this view, the contour of the scapula projects as the letter Y.[475] The downward stem of the Y is projected by the body of the scapula; the upper forks are projected by the coracoid process anteriorly and by the spine and acromion posteriorly (Figs. 14–35 and 14–36). The glenoid is located at the junction of the stem and the two arms of the Y and appears as a dense circle of bone. In obese people the circular density of

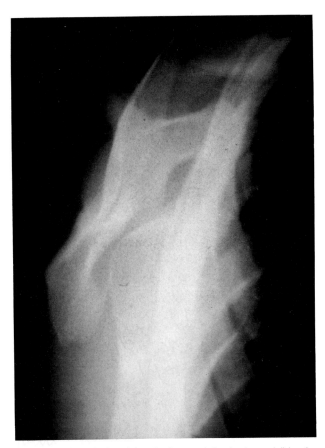

Figure 14-35. Scapular lateral view showing an anterior glenohumeral dislocation. Note that the humerus is no longer centered at the base of the Y.

the glenoid may not be seen, but it is always located at this intersection. In the normal shoulder the humeral head is at the center of the arms of the Y, that is, about the glenoid fossa. In posterior dislocations the head is seen posterior to the glenoid; in anterior dislocations it is anterior to the glenoid.

Axillary View

In this view, first described by Lawrence in 1915,[290, 342] the cassette is placed on the superior aspect of the shoulder. The arm is abducted enough to allow the radiographic beam to pass between the chest and the arm in a direction perpendicular to the cassette (Fig. 14–37A). In the presence of shoulder trauma, this view is usually obtained with the patient supine and the beam horizontal, but it may also be obtained with the patient prone or standing. In some situations when the patient cannot abduct the arm more than 30 to 40 degrees, a curved cassette or a rolled cardboard cassette can be placed in the axillae; then the radiographic beam would come from a superior position (Fig. 14–37B). An effort should always be made to take the axillary radiograph since it not only is diagnostic of shoulder dislocation but also offers a special premium in that it will often demonstrate the presence and size of the head compression fractures, as well as

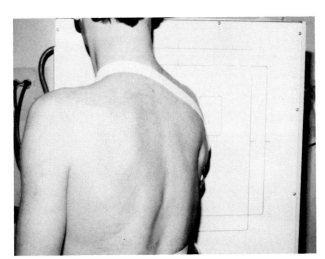

Figure 14-34. Position of the patient in the sling for a scapular lateral x-ray. The scapula is positioned perpendicular to the cassette. The beam should be placed parallel to the spine of the scapula and perpendicular to the cassette.

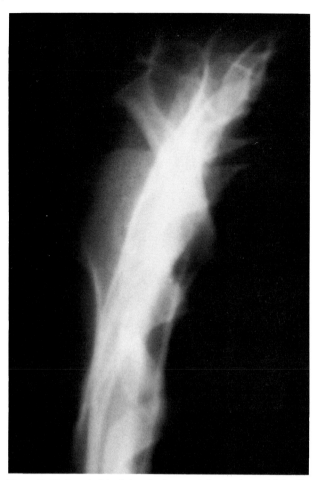

Figure 14–36. Scapular lateral view showing a posterior glenohumeral dislocation. The head of the humerus is dislocated posterior to the glenoid fossa and in this view appears to be sitting directly below the spine of the scapula.

fractures of the glenoid or of the lesser tuberosity of the humerus (Figs. 14–38 to 14–42).

Some modifications of the axillary view have been described. In his text on radiographic positioning, Jordan demonstrated the various techniques for obtaining axillary lateral views.[257] Cleaves[87, 342] and Teitge and Ciullo[436] have described variations on this view. Bloom and Obata[50] have modified the axillary technique so that the arm does not have to be abducted. They call this the Velpeau axillary lateral view. While wearing a sling or Velpeau dressing, the patient leans backward 30 degrees over the cassette on the table (Fig. 14–43). The x-ray tube is placed above the shoulder and the beam projected vertically down through the shoulder onto the cassette.

In summary, in the evaluation of a possibly dislocated shoulder or a fracture-dislocated shoulder we recommend the three orthogonal projections of the shoulder (anteroposterior and lateral in the plane of the scapula and axillary views), which provide a sensitive assessment of shoulder dislocation. The use of fewer views or other less interpretable projections may obscure significant pathological processes. If the three views cannot be taken, or if there is a question regard-

ing the diagnosis, then a CT scan will be of great assistance.

RADIOGRAPHIC EVALUATION OF RECURRENT GLENOHUMERAL INSTABILITY

The radiographic evaluation of recurrent glenohumeral instability is more subtle. The approaches may be grouped into stress views and views seeking fixed abnormalities. *Stress views* may serve to document the amount of glenohumeral translation with loading in various directions. Inferior translation may be documented by taking an anteroposterior view in the plane of the scapula while a "sulcus test" is performed.

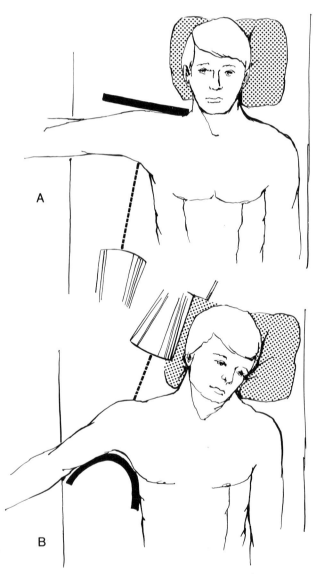

Figure 14–37. *A,* Positioning of the patient for taking an axillary x-ray of the glenohumeral joint. If the patient can abduct the arm 90 degrees, the cassette is placed above the shoulder. *B,* If the injured shoulder cannot be abducted 90 degrees, a curved cassette can be placed below the tube above the shoulder. (Reproduced with permission from Rockwood CA, and Green DP (eds): Fractures (3 vols), 2nd ed. Philadelphia: JB Lippincott, 1984.)

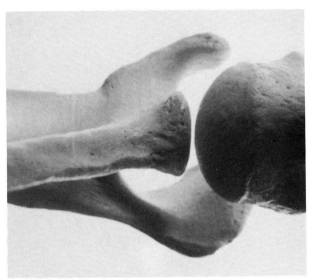

Figure 14–38. Simulated axillary view using backlighted skeletal model. An x-ray beam is passed up the axilla, projecting the glenoid fossa between the coracoid process anteriorly and the scapular spine posteriorly. This projection reveals the radiographic glenohumeral joint space, the anteroposterior position of the head of the humerus relative to the glenoid, and a view of fractures of the glenoid lip and humerus.

Anterior translation is best demonstrated on an axillary view taken while the "fulcrum test" is performed. Posterior translation is most easily documented on an axillary view taken while the "push-pull test" is performed. Although these tests may demonstrate translation, they do not confirm that the translation is causing the patient's problem (for example, asymptomatic shoulders may demonstrate substantial posterior translation). Furthermore, the inability to achieve a positive stress view does not necessarily exclude the diagnosis of instability (muscle action or incorrect technique may produce a falsely negative test).

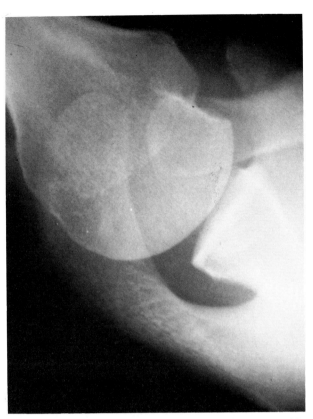

Figure 14–40. Axillary view. This patient has an anterior humeral head defect, which occurred as a result of a posterior glenohumeral dislocation.

Fixed abnormalities may provide valuable clues to the direction of instability and the contributing factors to this instability. The anteroposterior view in the plane of the scapula and the axillary view may reveal anterior or posterior glenoid lip fractures, new bone formation, or rounding of the glenoid lip in the presence of recurrent instability. Modifications of the axillary view may help the identification of glenoid rim changes. Rokous[458] and colleagues described what has become known as the "West Point" axillary view.[455] In this technique the patient is placed prone on the x-ray table with the involved shoulder on a pad raised 7.5 cm from the top of the table. The head and neck are turned away from the involved side. With the cassette held against the superior aspect of the shoulder, the x-ray beam is centered at the axilla, 25 degrees downward from the horizontal and 25 degrees medial. The resulting x-ray is a tangential view of the anteroinferior rim of the glenoid (Fig. 14–44). Using this view, Rokous and associates demonstrated bony abnormalities of the anterior glenoid rim in 53 of 63 patients whose histories indicated traumatic subluxation of the shoulder. Cyprien and coworkers[112] demonstrated lessening of the glenoid diameter and shortening of the anterior glenoid rim in shoulders with recurrent anterior dislocation. Blazina and Satzman[48] also reported anteroinferior glenoid rim fractures seen on the axillary view in nine of their cases.

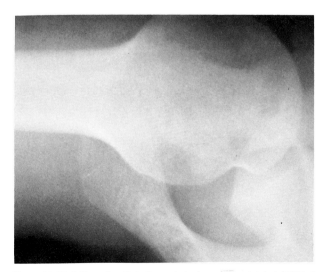

Figure 14–39. Axillary view. Note the posterior humeral head defect (Hill-Sachs lesion), secondary to an anterior glenohumeral dislocation.

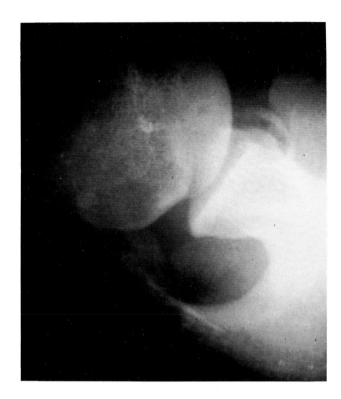

Figure 14–41. Axillary view showing an anterior glenoid defect and calcification as a result of an anterior glenohumeral dislocation.

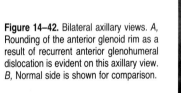

Figure 14–42. Bilateral axillary views. *A,* Rounding of the anterior glenoid rim as a result of recurrent anterior glenohumeral dislocation is evident on this axillary view. *B,* Normal side is shown for comparison.

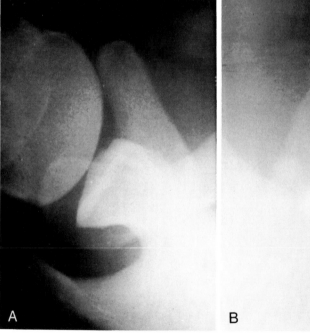

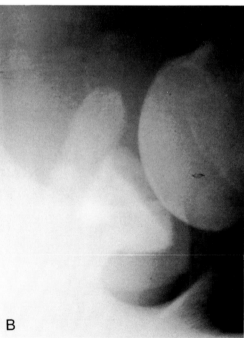

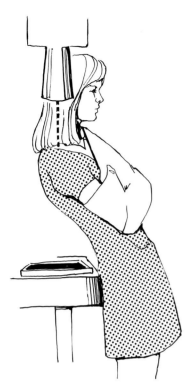

Figure 14–43. Positioning of the patient for the Velpeau axillary lateral view as described by Bloom and Obata. (Reproduced with permission from Rockwood CA, and Green DP (eds): Fractures (3 vols), 2nd ed. Philadelphia: JB Lippincott, 1984.)

Humeral Head Defects

Humeral head defects may also be seen, confirming previous anterior dislocations in the case of posterolateral defects and posterior dislocations in the case of anteromedial defects. A number of special views have been described for identifying humeral head defects.

1. Hermodsson's internal rotation technique (anteroposterior radiograph in internal rotation). Hermodsson recommended that the patient be supine and that a sandbag be placed under the elbow to put the humerus horizontal to the top of the table. The arm is adducted to the side of the patient, the humerus is internally rotated 45 degrees and the forearm lies across the anterior trunk. The x-ray beam is tilted 15 degrees toward the feet and centered over the humeral head.[217]

2. Adams' modification of the internal rotation view. Adams' modification[4] is essentially the same view recommended by Hermodsson but with internal rotation increased from 70 to 100 degrees.

3. Hermodsson's tangential view technique. To obtain marked internal rotation of the humerus, the elbow is flexed 90 degrees and the dorsum of the hand placed behind the trunk, over the upper lumbar spine. The thumb points upward. The film cassette is held superior to the adducted arm, and the x-ray tube is placed posterior, lateral, and inferior to the elbow joint, making a 30-degree angle with the humeral axis.[359]

4. Hill-Sachs view. An anteroposterior radiograph is made of the shoulder with the arm in marked internal rotation.

5. Stryker notch view. The patient is supine on the table with the cassette placed under the shoulder.[202] The palm of the hand of the affected shoulder is placed on top of the head, with the fingers directed toward the back of the head. The elbow of the affected shoulder should point straight upward. The x-ray beam tilts 10 degrees toward the head, centered over the coracoid process (Fig. 14–45). This technique was developed by William S. Stryker and reported by Hall and coworkers.[202] They stated that they could demon-

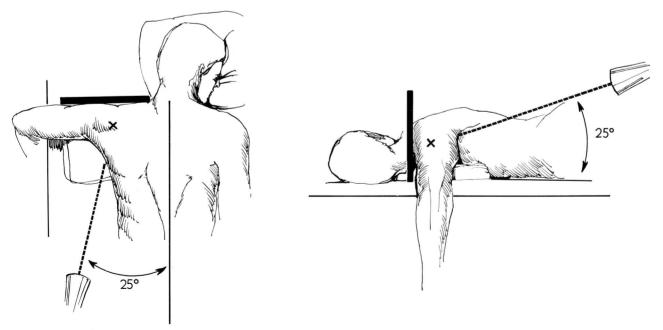

Figure 14–44. Positioning of the patient for taking the West Point view (a modified axillary view) to visualize the anteroinferior glenoid rim in subluxations of the shoulder. (Reproduced with permission from Rockwood CA, and Green DP (eds): Fractures (3 vols), 2nd ed. Philadelphia: JB Lippincott, 1984.)

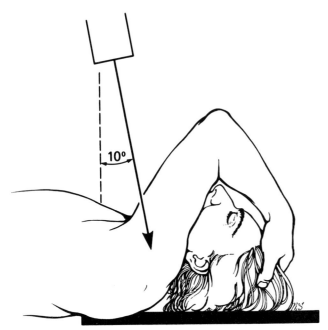

Figure 14–45. Technique of making the Stryker notch view. Position of the patient and the x-ray tube for making the notch view of the humerus.

strate the humeral head defect in 90 per cent of 20 patients with a history of recurring anterior dislocation of the shoulder.

6. Didiee view. The patient is prone on the table with the cassette under the shoulder.[134, 359, 425] The forearm is behind the trunk, as for the tangential view of Hermodsson. The arm is parallel to the top of the table with a 3-inch pad placed under the elbow. The dorsum of the hand is on the iliac crest with the thumb directed upward. The x-ray tube is directly lateral to the shoulder joint, and the beam is angled 45 degrees.

7. Cephaloscapular projection. Oppenheim and coworkers[401] have described a view in which the x-ray beam is passed from superior to inferior across the glenoid face to a cassette behind the patient, who is leaning forward.

8. Garth and coworkers[184, 185] described the apical oblique projection of the shoulder. In this technique the patient sits with the scapula flat against the cassette (as for the anteroposterior view in the plane of the scapula). The arm may be in a sling. The x-ray beam is directed perpendicular to the cassette (45 degrees to the coronal plane) and 45 degrees caudally and is centered on the coracoid. The beam then passes tangential to the articular surface of the glenohumeral joint and the posterolateral aspect of the humeral head. This view will also reveal both anterior glenoid lip defects and posterior lateral impression fractures of the humeral head.

In their classic article, Hill and Sachs[221] evaluated the relationship of humeral head defects to shoulder instability. They concluded that more than two-thirds of anterior shoulder dislocations are complicated by a bony injury of the humerus or scapula. We quote:

Compression fractures as a result of impingement of the weakest portion of the humeral head, that is, the posterior lateral aspect of the articular surface against the anterior rim of the glenoid fossa are found so frequently in cases of habitual dislocation that they have been described as a typical defect . . . These defects are sustained at the time of the original dislocation . . . A special sign is the sharp, vertical, dense medial border of the groove known as the line of condensation, the length of which is correlated with the size of the defect.

They reported the defect in only 27 per cent of 119 acute anterior dislocations and in 74 per cent of 15 recurrent anterior dislocations. However, they stated that the incidence of the groove defect was low, undoubtedly because it was only in the last 6 months of their 10-year study (1930 to 1940) that they used the special radiographic views. The size of the defect varied in length (cephalocaudal) from 5 mm to 3 cm, in width from 3 mm to 2 cm, and in depth from 10 mm to 22 mm.[221]

Using the Adams technique, Symeonides[523] reported the humeral head defect in 23 of 45 patients who had recurrent anterior dislocations of the shoulder—an incidence of 50 per cent. However, at the time of surgery he could confirm only 18 of 45, bringing the incidence of the defect down to 40 per cent. In the remaining five cases he was only able to palpate the groove, which is normally located between the greater tuberosity and the humeral head.

Eyre-Brook[151] reported an incidence of the defect of 64 per cent in 17 recurrent anterior dislocations, and Brav[63] recorded a rate of 67 per cent in 69 recurrent dislocations. Rowe[465] noted the defect in 38 per cent of 125 acute dislocations and in 57 per cent of 63 recurrent dislocations. Adams[3] noted that the defect was found at the time of surgery in 82 per cent of 68 patients. Palmar and Widen[414] found the defect at surgery in all of 60 patients.

Danzig, Greenway, and Resnick[114] reported that in cadaveric and clinical studies no single view will always reveal the humeral head compression fracture. Pavlov and coworkers[425] found that the Stryker notch view taken in internal rotation best revealed the posterolateral humeral head defect, while the anterior glenoid lip was best evaluated by the Didiee and West Point views. Rozing and associates[473] found that the humeral head defect was most often seen by the Stryker notch view and that glenoid rim defects were most easily seen on a coronal projection with the beam angled 45 degrees craniocaudal.

The demonstration of a humeral head defect confirms that the shoulder has been dislocated and reveals in which direction. Furthermore, the presence of such a defect usually suggests a traumatic cause of the instability. When these factors are already known—for example, in a 17-year-old whose recurrent anterior dislocations began with a well-documented abduction-external rotation injury in football—we tend not to spend a great deal of effort demonstrating the humeral head defect because (1) it is very likely to be present even if not seen on the radiographs, and (2) the existence of such a lesion does not in itself alter our management of the patient.

SPECIAL RADIOGRAPHIC INVESTIGATIONS

Arthrography

Single- and double-contrast arthrograms can be used to evaluate previously dislocated shoulders for rotator cuff tears. This is especially important if a patient fails to regain strength of flexion and rotation after a shoulder dislocation. (See Chapter 16 for a complete discussion of cuff tears and arthrography.)

Computed Tomography

Through the use of computed tomographic (CT) scans, we can study the cross-sectional anatomy of the shoulder in great detail. They are helpful in revealing the extent of fractures of the glenoid or humeral head compression fractures. Gould and colleagues[194] used CT to demonstrate a loose body blocking reduction of the shoulder. CT offers a method for determining the size and locations of glenoid rim defects.[498] When previous glenoid bone blocks have been carried out or hardware inserted, CT is useful for examining the possibility of their encroachment on the humeral head.[106, 107, 115] Injecting small amounts of air- and radio-

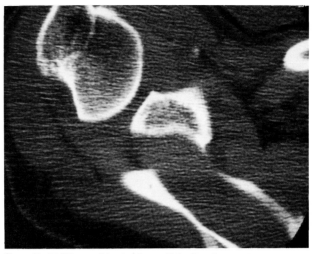

Figure 14-47. CT scan of the glenohumeral joint. Note the posterior humeral head defect and the anterior glenoid defect, well demonstrated on this scan.

opaque contrast into the joint prior to CT scanning often highlights the glenoid labrum. This imaging technique may permit the preoperative identification of attenuation, tears, and displacement of the labrum as well as stripping and stretching of the anterior shoulder joint capsule (Figs. 14-46 to 14-48).*

OTHER DIAGNOSTIC TESTS

Fluoroscopy

Norris[389] has described a technique for the fluoroscopic evaluation of the shoulder under anesthesia. This examination is performed in the axillary projection while the shoulder is stressed anteriorly or posteriorly. Norris found that any anterior subluxation was

---

*See references 61, 107, 144, 262, 267, 325, 338, 440, 441, 502.

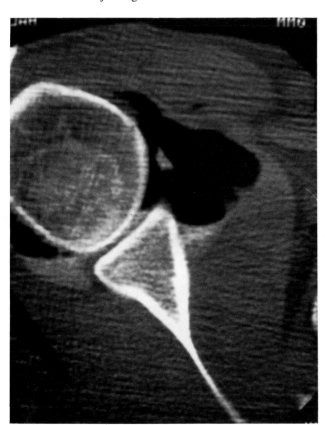

Figure 14-46. CT scan of the glenohumeral joint with air contrast. This study demonstrates a bony avulsion from the anterior glenoid rim.

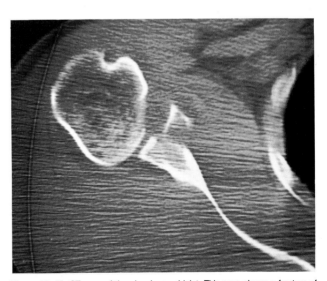

Figure 14-48. CT scan of the glenohumeral joint. This scan shows a fracture of the anterior glenoid rim secondary to anterior glenohumeral dislocation.

likely to be abnormal but that posterior displacement of up to 50 per cent of the humeral head may be normal. If surgeons recognize this normal posterior laxity, unnecessary posterior tightening can be avoided. Other tests may be indicated in the evaluation of the patient with glenohumeral instability, such as electromyography if there is a concern about brachial plexus injury.

Arthroscopy

Shoulder arthroscopy is being used by some to evaluate glenohumeral instability. This technique allows inspection of the humeral head and anteromedial or posterolateral defects. It also allows observation of the anterior glenoid for the scuffing that often accompanies recurrent anterior instability and for labral or ligamentous anomalies and injuries.* We currently reserve this technique for the rare instances in which substantial question concerning the diagnosis remains even after a thorough history, physical examination, and radiographic studies.

---

*See references 12, 76, 168, 184, 201, 251, 303, 338, 351, 398, 416, 566, 567, 575.

Complications of Injury

COMPLICATIONS OF TRAUMATIC ANTERIOR DISLOCATIONS OF THE SHOULDER

Ligaments and Capsular Changes

Because the ligament and capsule are stretched or stripped off the rim and neck of the scapula, the most common complication following a traumatic anterior dislocation of the shoulder is a recurrence of the shoulder instability.

Fractures and Bony Changes

Bony injuries have been discussed briefly in earlier parts of this chapter. Essentially they consist of compression fractures of the humeral head (the Hill-Sachs lesion), fractures of the anterior glenoid lip, fractures of the greater tuberosity, and fractures of the acromion or coracoid process associated with the superior dislocation of the shoulder (Figs. 14–49 to 14–53). Benchetrit and Friedman[42] and Wong-Pack and associates[569] have reported on fractures of the coracoid process that may not be recognized on a routine anteroposterior

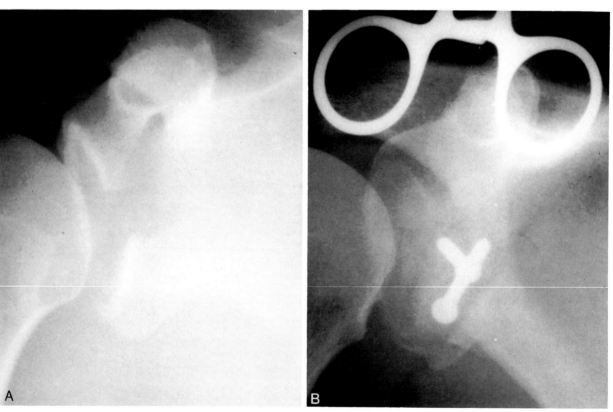

Figure 14–49. Anterior glenoid rim fracture. *A*, An anteroposterior x-ray demonstrates an anterior glenoid rim fracture secondary to traumatic anterior dislocation. *B*, An intraoperative anteroposterior x-ray shows reduction and screw fixation of an anterior glenoid rim fracture.

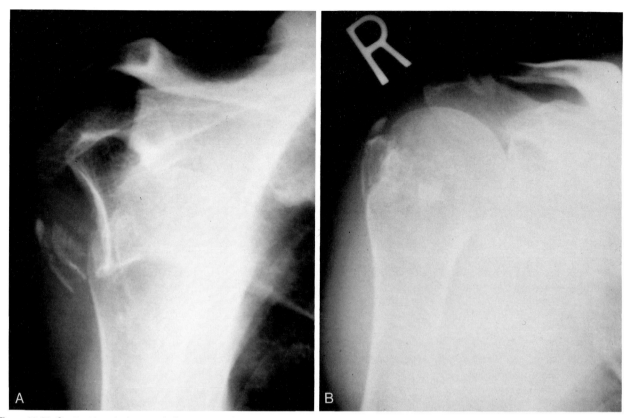

Figure 14–50. Greater tuberosity fracture. *A,* An anteroposterior x-ray prior to reduction showing a fracture of the greater tuberosity. *B,* A postreduction anteroposterior x-ray of a greater tuberosity fracture.

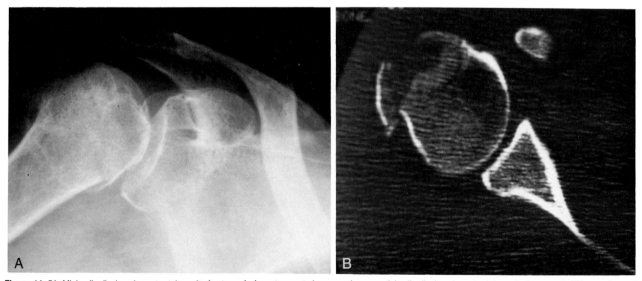

Figure 14–51. Minimally displaced greater tuberosity fracture. *A,* An anteroposterior x-ray shows a minimally displaced greater tuberosity fracture. *B,* CT scan shows the position of the greater tuberosity.

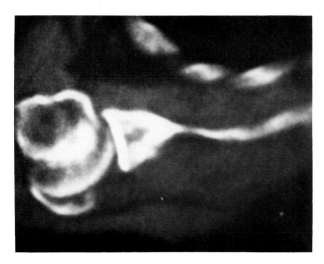

Figure 14–52. CT scan of significantly displaced greater tuberosity fracture.

x-ray. Verrina[550] reported a patient who developed voluminous ossification of the joint following an easily reduced anterior dislocation of the shoulder.

Ferkel and coworkers[156] have pointed out the risk of creating displaced fractures at the time of reduction of an anterior shoulder dislocation. Both their patients were in their 50s and had subcoracoid dislocations with greater tuberosity fractures. Each attempted reduction using simple traction created a displaced fracture of the anatomical neck (Fig. 14–54).

Cuff Tears

Rotator cuff tears may accompany anterior and inferior glenohumeral dislocations.[421, 431, 446, 523] Pettersson reported 27 ruptures of the rotator cuff in 47 patients with anterior dislocation.[431] Tijmes and coworkers[533] reported cuff rupture in 28 per cent of anterior dislocations.

The frequency of this complication increases with age: in patients over 40 years of age, the incidence exceeds 30 per cent; over age 60, it exceeds 80 per cent. Rotator cuff tears may present as pain or weakness on external rotation and abduction.[207, 431, 447, 564] Johnson and Bayley,[249] in a series of 12 complications following acute anterior dislocation, stressed that rotator cuff injury can be obscured by an axillary nerve injury. Shoulder ultrasonography[314] or arthrography is considered in patients over age 40, in those with substantial initial displacement of the humeral head (such as in a subglenoid dislocation), and in those demonstrating a slow return of active function after a glenohumeral dislocation. Prompt operative repair of this tendon rupture is usually indicated.

McLaughlin and MacLellan[337] point out that the incidence of recurrence is low when shoulder dislocation occurs by disruption of the posterior structures—the greater tuberosity and cuff. Their series of 90 shoulder dislocations associated with tuberosity fractures showed only 1 recurrence. In Rowe's series[461, 467] there were only 3 recurrences among 75 such cases.

Vascular Injuries

Vascular damage most frequently occurs in elderly patients with stiffer, more fragile vessels. The injury may be to the axillary artery or vein or to the branches of the axillary artery—the thoracoacromial, subscapular, circumflex, and rarely the long thoracic. Approximately 200 cases have been reported in the literature. Injury may occur at the time of either dislocation or reduction.[14, 111, 197, 243]

Anatomy

The axillary artery is divided into three parts that lie medial to, behind, and lateral to the pectoralis minor

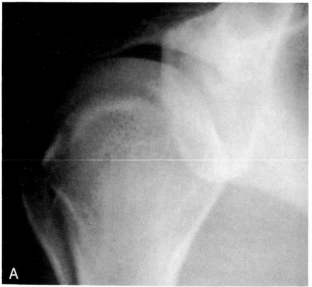
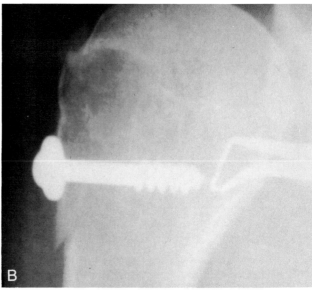

Figure 14–53. *A,* An x-ray showing a displaced greater tuberosity fracture. *B,* An intraoperative x-ray showing screw fixation of a greater tuberosity fracture.

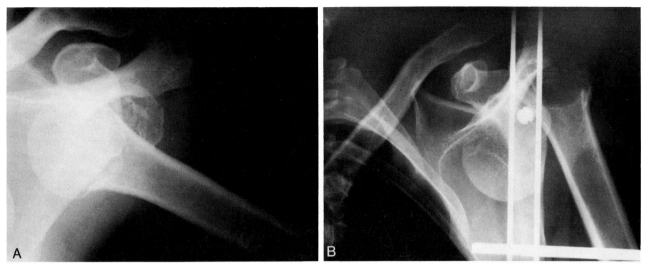

Figure 14–54. *A,* An anteroposterior view showing an anteroinferior dislocation with an associated greater tuberosity fracture. *B,* An anteroposterior view after reduction attempt showing displacement of a humeral neck fracture.

muscle (Fig. 14–55). The sites most commonly injured are in the second part, when the thoracoacromial trunk is avulsed, and in the third part, when subscapular and circumflex branches are avulsed or the axillary artery is totally ruptured.

Mechanism of Injury

Damage to the axillary artery can take the form of a complete transection, a linear tear of the artery caused by avulsion of one of its branches, or an intravascular thrombus, perhaps related to an intimal tear. Brown and Navigato[69] observed that the artery is relatively fixed at the lateral margin of the pectoralis minor muscle. With abduction and external rotation, the artery is taut; when the head dislocates, it dislocates the axillary artery forward, and the pectoralis minor

acts as a fulcrum over which the artery is deformed and ruptured. Milton[349] proposed that the axillary artery is fixed in its third part by the circumflex and subscapular branches and that these branches hold the axillary artery in place and prevent it from escaping injury when the humeral head displaces forward. Jardon and coworkers[243] reported two cases in which the axillary artery was fixed by scar to the pericapsular tissues and transected during displacement of the capsule. Watson-Jones[558] reported the case of a man who had multiple anterior dislocations that he reduced himself. Finally, when the man was older, the axillary artery ruptured during one of the dislocations and he died.

Injury at the Time of Dislocation

Vascular injuries are commonly associated with inferior dislocation.[181, 299, 312, 341] Gardham and Scott[181] reported an axillary artery occlusion with an erect dislocation of the shoulder in a 40-year-old patient who had fallen headfirst down an escalator. Although we often consider vascular complications as a phenomenon of older patients, they can occur at any age. Banatta and coworkers[29] reported the case of a 13-year-old boy who ruptured his axillary artery with a subcoracoid dislocation sustained while wrestling. Vascular injuries also have been reported by Drury and Scullion,[139] Fitzgerald and Keates[160] and coworkers,[488] Bertrand and colleagues,[44] and Lescher and Andersen.[297, 513]

Injury at the Time of Reduction

Vascular damage at the time of reduction occurs primarily in the elderly, particularly when an old anterior dislocation is mistaken for an acute injury and

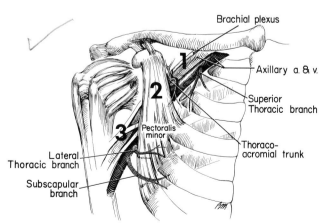

Figure 14–55. The axillary artery is divided into three parts by the pectoralis minor muscle; the second part is behind it and the third part is lateral to it. (Reproduced with permission from Rockwood CA, and Green DP (eds): Fractures (3 vols), 2nd ed. Philadelphia: JB Lippincott, 1984.)

a closed reduction is performed. The axillary artery is bound down by the pectoralis minor muscle and frequently by anterior pericapsular scarring; it is brittle and cannot withstand the traction required to reduce an old dislocation. The injury can also occur during any forceful manipulation in younger patients who, because of locked acute dislocation, have excessive forces applied during reduction.

The largest series of vascular complications associated with closed reduction of the shoulder has been reported by Calvet and coworkers,[72] who in 1941 collected 90 cases. This paper, revealing the tragic end results, must have accomplished its purpose because there have been very few reports in the literature since then dealing with the complications that occur during reduction. In their series, in which 64 of 91 reductions were performed many weeks after the initial dislocation, the mortality rate was 50 per cent. The other patients either lost the arm or the function of the arm. Besides the long delay from dislocation to reduction, Guibe[198] stated that excessive forces were commonly used to reduce difficult dislocations of the shoulder. He quotes Delpeche, who observed a case in which the force of 10 men was used to accomplish the shoulder reduction, damaging the axillary vessel. Kirker[265] described a case of rupture of the axillary artery and axillary vein and brachial plexus palsy, but he was uncertain as to when the complication occurred (at the time of dislocation or reduction). Stener[515] also has reported a case of axillary artery damage in which he could not determine when the injury occurred.

Signs and Symptoms

Vascular damage may be obvious or subtle. Findings may include pain, expanding hematoma, pulse deficit, peripheral cyanosis, peripheral coolness and pallor, neurological dysfunction, and shock. An arteriogram should confirm the diagnosis and locate the site of injury.

Treatment and Prognosis

Patients suspected of having major arterial injury need a large-bore intravenous line and blood must be sent for type and cross-match. Jardon and coworkers[243] reported that the bleeding can be controlled before operation by digital pressure on the axillary artery over the first rib. The patient in severe shock or ischemia should be taken promptly to the operating room, where emergent treatment can be rendered. Jardon and coworkers[243] have recommended that the axillary artery be explored through the subclavicular operative approach, as described by Steenburg and Tavitch.[514] The results of simple ligation of the vessels in the elderly patient have been disappointing, probably because of poor collateral circulation and the presence of arteriosclerotic vascular disease.[253, 265, 546] Even when ligation has been performed in younger patients with good collateral circulation, approximately two-thirds of these

patients have lost some of the function of the upper extremity—some by developing upper extremity claudication. The treatment of choice is to restore normal circulation to the arm; this can be done by repair of the lesion or by using a graft or prosthesis. The authors agree that it is most important to resect the damaged artery back to normal intima before the vessel is repaired in order to prevent a late thrombus from occurring. Lev-el and associates[299] reported a patient who had an injury to the axillary artery and who subsequently developed a thrombus that required resection and vein graft. Gardham and Scott[181] reported a case in 1980 in which the axillary artery was damaged in its third part and was managed by a bypass graft using the saphenous vein. Excellent results have been reported by Henson,[216] Cranley and Krause,[109] Stevens,[516] McKenzie and Sinclair,[327] Brown and Navigato,[69] Gibson,[189] Rob and Standeven,[452] and Jardon and coworkers.[243]

Neural Injuries

The brachial plexus and the axillary artery lie immediately anterior, inferior, and medial to the glenohumeral joint.[195] It is not surprising, therefore, that neurovascular injuries frequently accompany traumatic anterior glenohumeral dislocations.

Anatomy

The axillary nerve originates off the posterior cord of the brachial plexus. It crosses the anterior surface of the subscapularis muscle and angulates sharply posteriorly to travel along the inferior shoulder joint capsule. It then leaves the axilla to exit through the quadrangular space below the lower border of the teres minor muscle, where it hooks around the posterior and lateral humerus on the deep surface of the deltoid muscle.

Mechanism of Injury

According to Milton,[348, 349] McGregor has postulated that the nerve is crushed between the head of the humerus and the axillary border of the scapula (Fig. 14–56). Stevens[516] pointed out that in normal anatomy the path of the axillary nerve is directly across the anterior surface of the subscapularis muscle. In an anterior dislocation the head displaces the subscapularis tendon and muscle forward, creating traction and direct pressure on the nerve. Nerve injuries are divided into three groups:

1. *Neurapraxia*—transient denervation produced by a mild injury to the nerve. Recovery is usually complete in one to two months.

2. *Axonotmesis*—complete denervation produced by a moderate to severe injury of the nerve, in which the nerve cells die but regeneration can be accomplished through the intact nerve sheaths. The recovery rate is approximately 2.5 cm per month.

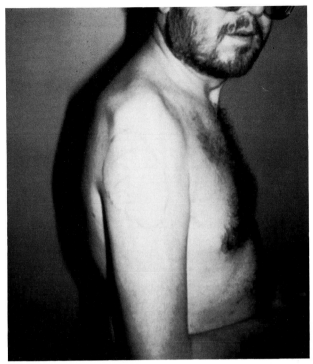

Figure 14–56. This patient sustained an axillary nerve palsy secondary to glenohumeral dislocation. Note the area of decreased sensation diagrammed on the lateral aspect of the proximal humerus. Also note the presence of significant wasting.

3. *Neuronotmesis*—complete denervation that occurs when the axons and the sheaths are transected. Recovery is poor without careful nerve repair. This rarely occurs as a result of anterior dislocation of the shoulder.

Incidence

McLaughlin reported nerve injuries in 2 per cent of recurrent dislocations and in 10 per cent of acute dislocations. Watson-Jones[556] reported 14 per cent and Rowe[461] 5.4 per cent. DePalma[127] reported 5 per cent; Mumenthaler and Schliack[365] 15 per cent, and Brown[68] 25 per cent of 76 cases. Gariepy[183] stated that the nerve injury is more common than is realized. Tuszynski[542] has written on two patients with temporary injury to the brachial plexus following anterior dislocation of the shoulder. Pasila and coworkers,[422] in a review of 226 patients with acute dislocation of the shoulder, found an incidence of complications of 25 per cent. There were 25 brachial plexus injuries and 19 axillary nerve injuries. Parsons and Rowley[419] demonstrated that delayed reduction of a shoulder dislocation could cause deterioration of neurological function.

The axillary is the most commonly involved nerve: between 1 out of 20 and 1 out of 3 first-time anterior glenohumeral dislocations is accompanied by a significant axillary nerve injury.[49, 197, 293, 422, 462] The likelihood of an axillary nerve injury increases with the age of the patient, the duration of the dislocation, and the amount of trauma that initiated the dislocation.[49, 421]

Other nerves injured are the radial, musculocutaneous, median, ulnar, and the entire brachial plexus.

Livson[306] presented an extensive electromyographic analysis of 11 cases of shoulder dislocation with nerve injury. The axillary nerve was most commonly injured, but more proximal involvement of the posterior and median cords of the brachial plexus was also observed.

Blom and Dahlback,[49] in a very careful electromyographic study of 73 patients with anterior dislocation or fracture of the humeral neck, showed that the incidence of nerve injury was 35 per cent. Of the 73 patients studied, 26 had nerve damage (17 partial injuries and 9 complete denervations). Of the 26 nerve injuries, 22 were confined to the axillary nerve. In the remaining 4 the breakdown was as follows: axillary and musculocutaneous nerves, 1; axillary and radial nerves, 1; radial nerve, 1; and musculocutaneous and median nerves, 1. In their series over half of the patients over the age of 50 had damage to the axillary nerve. They observed that the transient, partial denervations of the axillary nerve were responsible for the poor recovery following an anterior dislocation. They noted that if a patient's recovery is delayed beyond one to three months it may well be the result of an unrecognized partial axillary nerve injury.

Diagnosis

The diagnosis of nerve injury is considered in any patient having neurological symptoms or signs such as weakness or numbness. Nerve injury may also present as delayed recovery of active shoulder motion after glenohumeral dislocation. Blom and Dahlback[49] demonstrated that the usual sensory testing of the axillary nerve (i.e., checking the skin sensation just above the deltoid insertion on the lateral shoulder) is unreliable. An electromyogram provides objective evaluation of neurological function, provided that three or four weeks have intervened between the injury and the evaluation.[49]

Treatment and Prognosis

It is generally agreed that most axillary nerve injuries resulting from anterior dislocation are traction neurapraxias and will recover completely. Blom and Dahlback[49] have shown full functional and electromyographic recovery at three to five months in 26 cases of partial and complete axillary nerve denervation. Brown[68] has shown almost complete recovery in 76 cases. His treatment consisted of "watchful expectancy," without galvanic stimulation or exploration of the nerve. Assmus and Meinel[20] reported that patients with partial axillary nerve palsy frequently recovered in two to six weeks and that complete reinnervation could be expected by one year. However, a poor prognosis resulted if the axillary nerve did not recover after 10 weeks.

In summary, damage to the axillary nerve is a common complication of anterior dislocations of the shoulder; regardless of whether the damage is partial or complete, the result is usually a normal, functioning shoulder. The incidence of axillary nerve denervation is higher in elderly patients, and the overall incidence is probably in the range of 30 per cent. The classic technique of checking the lateral shoulder for abnormal skin sensation is an unreliable indicator of axillary nerve damage.

Recurrence

Recurrent dislocation is the most common complication following an acute traumatic anterior dislocation of the shoulder. The *age* of the patient at the time of the initial dislocation has a major effect on the incidence of redislocation.[461, 468] McLaughlin and Mac-Lellan[337] observed that 95 per cent of 181 primary traumatic dislocations in teenagers recurred. Henry and Genung[215] found an 85 to 90 per cent redislocation rate for acute traumatic anterior dislocations in young patients (average age of 19). Under the age of 20, the incidence is reported by Rowe,[461] McLaughlin and Cavallaro,[336] and others[359] to be between 80 and 92 per cent. Over the age of 40 the incidence drops sharply to 10 to 15 per cent. The majority of all recurrences occur within the first two years after the first traumatic dislocation.*

Simonet and Cofield[505] found an overall incidence of recurrence in 116 patients followed for over 4 years to be 33 per cent; 66 per cent in patients under 20 years of age, 17 per cent in patients 20 to 40, and zero in patients over 40 years old. However, they did point out that the recurrence rate in athletes under the age of 20 was 80 per cent but only 30 per cent in nonathletes of a similar age group. Hovelius[229] followed 257 primary shoulder dislocations in 254 patients between the ages of 12 and 40 years. They found two or more recurrences in 55 per cent of patients 22 years old or younger, 37 per cent in patients 23 to 29 years old, and 12 per cent in patients 30 to 40 years old.

Kiviluoto and coworkers[266] again emphasized that patients under 30 are more prone to recurrent dislocations, while patients over 30 are more likely to develop shoulder stiffness. Rowe and Sakellarides[468] reported on 66 patients with an average age of 60 in which the recurrence rate was 4.5 per cent. McLaughlin and MacLellan reported a recurrence rate of 1.1 per cent in a similar population.[337]

Recurrences are more common in men than in women. Moseley[359] quotes several series in which the ratios range from four to one to six to one. Rowe[460] reports that recurrent dislocations are neither more nor less common in the dominant shoulder, nor does the weaker shoulder tend to suffer primary or recurrent dislocations more frequently than does the stronger, dominant one. Rowe[461, 468] also has pointed out that the recurrence rate varies inversely with the severity of the original trauma; in other words, the more easily

the dislocation occurred initially, the more easily it recurs.

In many clinical series, the incidence of recurrence seems to be affected very little by the type and length of *immobilization* of the shoulder following initial dislocation. In the series of 573 dislocations of the shoulder reported by McLaughlin and Cavallaro,[336] they concluded that the length of time that the shoulder was immobilized after initial anterior dislocation was of little importance. Hovelius and associates[230] compared 112 patients whose shoulders were immobilized for three to four weeks with 104 patients who used the shoulder as early and as freely as possible and found an equal recurrence rate after two years of follow-up. Ehgartner[143] found the same recurrence rate in patients who were immobilized in plaster of paris Velpeau and in patients who used a sling. Rowe and Sakellarides[468] were unable to document that prolonged immobilization lessened the incidence of redislocation.

By contrast, Stromsoe and coworkers[520] reported in a follow-up of 99 patients a 6.4 per cent recurrence rate if patients were immobilized for three weeks and 12 per cent recurrence if immobilized for less than three weeks. Kazar and Relovszky[261] reported a 10 to 15 per cent incidence of recurrence. They found that the rate of recurrence was less for those immobilized longer than one week.

Aronen and Regan[17] reported on 20 naval midshipmen with first-time shoulder dislocations who were treated with a specific, aggressive postdislocation program and followed for an average of 35.8 months (age averaged 19.2 years). The shoulders were immobilized in a sling for three weeks. Isometric deltoid and internal rotation exercises were started at two weeks. The patients were not allowed to return to activity until there was no evidence of weakness or atrophy and no apprehension on abduction and external rotation. Patients required an average of three months to reach these goals. These patients had no recurrent dislocations; two had recurrent subluxations. This is comparable to the result of Yoneda,[571] who found good results in 83 per cent of patients in a program emphasizing postimmobilization exercises.

Hovelius[229] reported on 256 shoulders with primary dislocations in patients 12 to 40 years of age. Although age exerted the primary effect as described earlier, the presence of *fractures* also seemed to have an effect. A moderate humeral head defect was correlated with an increased incidence of recurrence in patients over 22 years of age. Out of 32 shoulders with fractures of the greater tuberosity, dislocations recurred only in 1. These two factors may be related. These fractures were four times as common in patients over 30: 23 per cent compared with 8 per cent among patients under 30. Other series noted fracture of the greater tuberosity with anterior glenohumeral joint dislocations in approximately 15 to 35 per cent of their patients.[124, 337, 460] The redislocation rates of shoulders with greater tuberosity fractures were low in these series as well.

We conclude that the injuries sustained by young

---

*See references 3, 28, 127, 150, 336, 357, 360, 461, 462, 536.

patients in traumatic dislocations are relatively unlikely to heal in a manner yielding a stable shoulder. Probably the most important of these unhealing injuries is the avulsion of the glenohumeral ligament from the anterior glenoid lip and neck of the scapula. Older patients tend to stretch the capsule or avulse the greater tuberosity, either of which is likely to heal leaving a stable shoulder. In atraumatic instability, there is no lesion and thus a high chance of recurrence. The degree of trauma and the age of the patient seem to be more important than the specifics of past dislocation management in determining the recurrence rate.

COMPLICATIONS OF TRAUMATIC POSTERIOR DISLOCATIONS OF THE SHOULDER

Fractures

Fractures of the posterior glenoid rim and of the proximal humerus (upper shaft, tuberosities, and head) are quite common in traumatic posterior dislocations of the shoulder.[395, 396, 526, 568] Vichard and Arnould[552] reported 11 cases of posterior dislocation associated with fractures. The commonly associated compression fracture of the anteromedial portion of the humeral head is produced by the posterior cortical rim of the glenoid. It is best visualized on an axillary view or a CT scan. This lesion, sometimes called a "reversed Hill-Sachs lesion," often occurs at the time of the original posterior dislocation. It becomes larger with multiple posterior dislocations of the shoulder. Large humeral head defects are seen in the patient with an old, unreduced posterior dislocation.

The posterior rim of the glenoid may be fractured and displaced in posterior dislocations (Fig. 14–57). This occurs not only with direct forces from an anterior direction that push the humeral head out posteriorly,

but also with indirect types of dislocations such as occur during seizures or accidental electrical shock.

Fracture of the lesser tuberosity of the humerus may accompany posterior dislocations. The subscapularis muscle comes under considerable tension in this dislocation and may avulse the lesser tuberosity onto which it inserts. Although the fracture may be seen on the anteroposterior and lateral x-rays of the glenohumeral joint, it is best seen on the axillary view and on CT scan.

When the x-rays reveal a comminuted fracture of the proximal humerus, one should be aware that the head fragment may be displaced posteriorly. Because of the distortion of the fragments, it is impossible to determine the exact position of the head without axillary lateral x-rays or CT scan studies. In the series of 16 cases of posterior dislocation of the shoulder reported by O'Conner and Jacknow,[396] 12 had comminuted fractures of the proximal humerus. In 8 of the 12 cases of fracture, the diagnosis of posterior dislocation was initially missed. Kavanaugh[260] reported posterior dislocation of the shoulder associated with a fracture of the shaft of the humerus.

Other Complications

Neurovascular injuries and cuff tears are much less common after posterior dislocations than after anterior dislocations. Recurrence is very common with (1) atraumatic posterior dislocation and (2) large bony defects of the humerus and/or glenoid resulting from traumatic posterior dislocation.

Differential Diagnosis

The differential diagnosis of the acute dislocation includes contusion, fracture, and acute rotator cuff tear, all of which may coexist. Radiographs in three planes should resolve the diagnosis of dislocation. The differential diagnosis of recurrent instability is more difficult. It includes all causes of recurrent shoulder dysfunction, such as impingement, cuff tear, loose bodies, glenohumeral joint surface roughness, and snapping scapula. A careful history of the first episode and circumstances of recurrence, plus repeated physical examinations that include stress tests and radiographs to look for clues of instability, should lead to the correct diagnosis.

Treatment

ACUTE DISLOCATIONS

Anterior Dislocations

Acute Traumatic Anterior Dislocations

Acute dislocations of the glenohumeral joint should be reduced as quickly and gently as possible. Whenever

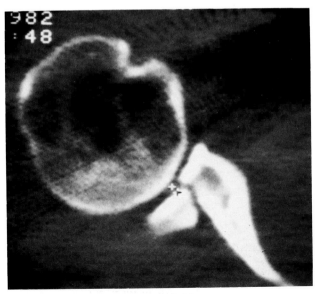

Figure 14–57. A CT scan of the glenohumeral joint demonstrates a fracture of the posterior glenoid rim as a result of posterior dislocation of the glenohumeral joint.

possible, a complete set of radiographs should be obtained prior to reduction to rule out associated bony injuries. Early relocation promptly eliminates the stretch and compression of neurovascular structures, minimizes the amount of muscle spasm that must be overcome to effect reduction, and prevents progressive enlargement of the humeral head defect in locked dislocations. The extent of anesthesia required to accomplish a gentle reduction depends on many factors, including the amount of trauma that produced the dislocation, the duration of the dislocation, the number of previous dislocations, whether the dislocation is locked, and to what extent the patient can voluntarily relax the shoulder musculature. When seen acutely, some dislocations can be reduced without the use of medication. At the other extreme, reduction of a long-standing, locked dislocation may require a brachial plexus block or general anesthetic with muscle relaxation. Many practitioners use narcotics and muscle relaxants to aid in the reduction of shoulder dislocations. A potential trap exists: the dosages required to produce muscle relaxation while the shoulder is dislocated may be sufficient to produce respiratory depression once the shoulder is reduced. Our recommendation is that if these medications are to be used, they should be administered through an established intravenous line. This produces a more rapid onset, a short duration of action, and the opportunity to adjust the required dose more appropriately. Furthermore, resuscitation (if necessary) is facilitated by the prospective presence of such a route of access. Airway management tools should be readily available.

Two different principles have been used in the reduction of shoulder dislocation—traction and leverage. Many of the older texts and some of the more current ones prefer the leverage techniques, but more recently concern has grown over the possibility of damaging the capsule, axillary vessels, and the brachial plexus when applying the great force used during leverage.

Hippocratic Technique. Hippocrates' original technique[2] is still effective when only one person is available to reduce the shoulder. The stockinged foot of the physician is used as countertraction. The heel should not go into the axilla (i.e., between the anterior and posterior axillary folds) but should extend across the folds and against the chest wall. Traction should be slow and gentle; as with all traction techniques, the arm may be gently rotated internally and externally to disengage the head.

Stimson's Technique. Although Lewis A. Stimson[517, 518] of New York City is given credit for this method of reduction, he attributed it to a Dr. Cole, a house-staff physician of the Chambers Street Hospital. It was a variation of Stimson's technique of obtaining muscle relaxation in the prone position to reduce a posterior dislocation of the hip. The patient is placed prone on the edge of the examining table while downward traction is gently applied.[517] McLaughlin felt that the weight of the arm may be sufficient to reduce the shoulder. The use of weights is a subsequent modification of the original technique. Appropriate weights are taped to the wrist of the dislocated shoulder, which hangs free off the edge of the table. Five pounds is usually sufficient, but more or less weight may be used depending on the size of the patient. When using this technique, one should be patient since it may take 15 to 20 minutes for the reduction to occur. It is important that patients not be left unattended in this position, particularly if narcotics and muscle relaxants have been administered.

Milch's Technique. In 1938 Milch[344] described a technique for reduction that employed abduction and external rotation. With the patient supine, the arm is abducted and externally rotated, and the thumb is used to gently push the head of the humerus back in place. Lacey[278] modified the technique by performing the maneuver with the patient prone on an examining table. Russell and associates[477] have reported on the ease and success of this technique.

Kocher's Leverage Technique. In this maneuver, the humeral head is levered on the anterior glenoid and the shaft is levered against the anterior thoracic wall until the reduction is completed. We do not recommend it for routine use because of the complications that can occur during the leverage and manipulation.[453] DePalma[127] warned that undue forces used in rotation leverage can damage the soft tissues of the shoulder joint, the vessels, and the brachial plexus. Beattie and coworkers[39] reported a fracture of the humeral neck during a Kocher procedure. Other authors have reported spiral fractures of the upper shaft of the humerus and further damage to the anterior capsular mechanism when the Kocher leverage technique of reduction was used. McMurray[339] reported that of 64 dislocations reduced by the Kocher method, 40 per cent became recurrent, whereas of 112 dislocations reduced by gently lifting the head in place, only 12 per cent became recurrent.

Since 1975 numerous articles have appeared in the literature describing simple techniques to reduce the dislocated shoulder: the forward elevation maneuver,[242, 553] the external rotation method,[294, 350] the scapular manipulation,[10] the modified gravity method,[305] the crutch and chair technique,[417] the chair and pillow technique.[564] and others.[89, 322]

Chronic Anterior Traumatic Dislocations

A glenohumeral joint that has been dislocated for several days is a chronic dislocation. As the chronicity of the dislocation increases, so do the difficulties and complications of reduction. The old, persistent, unreduced chronic dislocation is usually a very difficult problem to handle. When one encounters an elderly patient with pain in the shoulder whose x-rays reveal an anterior dislocation, a very careful history is needed to determine whether the initial injury occurred acutely or a week to several months earlier.

The condition is noted most commonly in elderly

people and in those whose general mental status may prevent them from seeking help at the time of the injury. Ten of the 14 patients presented by Bennett[43] were over the age of 50. The dislocation may be produced by a trivial injury, since with increasing age there is weakness and degeneration of the soft tissues.[350] In younger patients, the late diagnosis of an old unreduced anterior dislocation of the shoulder is unusual but may occur when the patient is unconscious for a period with severe multiple injuries.

McLaughlin[328] describes this type of dislocation of the shoulder as the most difficult of all. It is difficult to establish criteria for when to attempt a closed reduction, when to operate and reduce the shoulder, and when to simply leave it alone. There are no established rules because conditions (the age of patient, length of time from dislocation, degree of symptoms, range of motion, radiographic findings, and general stability of the patient) can vary so much. If a closed reduction is to be performed, it should be done with minimal traction, without leverage, and with total muscle relaxation under controlled general anesthesia. Usually by two to three weeks after the dislocation the humeral head is firmly impaled on the anterior glenoid, and there is so much soft tissue contraction and interposition that it is impossible to perform a gentle closed reduction. If a gentle closed reduction fails, an open procedure should be considered. This can be a very difficult procedure because of the distorted anatomy of the axillary artery and nerves and because the structures are tight and "scarred down." Some older patients' old dislocations produce minimal symptoms so that nontreatment is selected owing to the hazards of open treatment. Ganel and coworkers[179] reported on four elderly patients with long-standing persistent dislocations of the shoulder who had relatively good functional results.

In performing an open reduction, the subscapularis and anterior capsule are incised near their insertion. External rotation and lateral traction will usually disimpact the humerus from the glenoid. The humerus is then gently internally rotated while lateral traction is applied to reduce the head. Leverage is avoided because the head is usually very soft. If the posterolateral head defect is greater than 40 per cent or if the head collapses during reduction, a humeral head prosthesis is inserted. The subscapularis and capsule are then repaired. The shoulder is carefully inspected for cuff tears and vascular damage.

Schulz and associates[493] reported that of 61 chronic dislocations in 58 patients, 17 (24 per cent) were posterior and 44 (76 per cent) were anterior. These dislocations occurred primarily among elderly people; more than half of the dislocations were associated with fracture of the tuberosities, head or neck of the humerus, glenoid, or coracoid process, and more than one third involved neurological deficits. Closed reduction was attempted in 40 shoulders and was successful in 20. Of the 20 shoulders successfully reduced (3 posterior and 17 anterior), the duration of dislocation exceeded four weeks in only one instance. Open reduction was performed in 20 and humeral head excision in 6. Eight patients were not treated, and five shoulders were irreducible.

Perniceni and coworkers[429] described the reinforcement of the anterior shoulder complex in three patients with old unreduced anterior dislocations of the shoulder. They used the Gosset[193] technique, which places a rib graft between the coracoid and the glenoid rim. Rowe and Zarins[471] reported on 24 patients with unreduced dislocations of the shoulder and operated on 14 of them. They concluded that the operative treatment gave better results than previously reported.

Management After Reduction of an Anterior Dislocation

After reducing the glenohumeral joint, repeat anteroposterior and lateral x-ray views are obtained in the plane of the scapula to verify the adequacy of the reduction and to provide an additional opportunity to detect fractures of the glenoid and proximal humerus. The patient's neurological status is checked, including the sensory and motor functions of all five major nerves in the upper extremity. The strength of the pulse is verified and evidence of bruits or an expanding hematoma is sought.[197] The integrity of the rotator cuff is initially evaluated by observing the strength of isometric external rotation and abduction.

Trimmings[539] demonstrated that aspiration of the hemarthrosis from the shoulder can be an effective means of reducing discomfort after the shoulder is reduced.

Since recurrent glenohumeral instability is the most common complication of a glenohumeral dislocation, postreduction treatment focuses on optimizing shoulder stability. Thus, two potentially important elements in postreduction treatment are protection and muscle rehabilitation. Reeves demonstrated in primates that three months were required before normal capsular patterns of collagen bundles were observed, five months before subscapularis tendon was histologically normal, and four to five months before tensile strength was regained.[447] It is unknown whether labral tears or ligamentous avulsions from the glenoid heal or how long this might take. In any event, it is apparent that the shoulder should not be immobilized for the length of time required for complete healing. Traumatic anterior dislocations in young patients are usually managed by two to five weeks of postreduction immobilization; shorter periods are indicated for patients over 30 years of age owing to their lesser predilection for recurrence and greater tendency for shoulder stiffness.[266, 336, 337, 461, 571] (See the section Complications of Injury for further discussion of the relationship between the period of immobilization and the incidence of recurrence.)

Indications for Early Surgery in Shoulders Dislocated Anteriorly

In addition to the need for open reduction for the rare irreducible dislocation, a few other situations exist in which early surgery may be indicated in the early management of shoulder dislocations.

Soft Tissue Interposition. If the rotator cuff, capsule, or biceps tendon prevents reduction, operative reduction will be required. Tietjen[532] reported a case of avulsion of the supraspinatus, infraspinatus, and teres minor, which at the time of surgery were interposed between the humeral head and the glenoid.

Displaced Fracture of the Greater Tuberosity. Although fractures of the greater tuberosity are not uncommonly associated with anterior shoulder dislocation, the tuberosity usually reduces into an acceptable position when the shoulder is reduced. Occasionally the greater tuberosity fragment displaces up under the acromion process or is pulled posteriorly by the cuff muscles. If the greater tuberosity remains displaced following reduction of the shoulder joint, consideration should be given to anatomical reduction and internal fixation of the fragment and repair of the attendant split in the tendons of the rotator cuff. It is relatively easy to determine the amount of superior displacement of the tuberosity fragment on the anteroposterior roentgenogram in the plane of the scapula. The scapular lateral radiograph is helpful to determine the amount of posterior displacement. If the tuberosity is allowed to heal with posterior displacement, it may produce not only the functional equivalent of a rotator cuff tear but also a bony block to external rotation. Norris and coworkers[392] found that CT scans were necessary to define the anteroposterior position of displaced tuberosity fragments in 10 out of 18 cases.

Glenoid Rim Fracture. Aston and Gregory[21] reported three cases in which a large anterior fracture of the glenoid occurred as a result of a fall on the lateral aspect of the abducted shoulder. A fracture of the anterior glenoid lip may be associated with an anterior dislocation, recurring subluxation, or recurrent anterior dislocation. Open reduction and internal fixation of displaced lip fractures offers the opportunity to anatomically restore the capsule and ligamentous attachments to the glenoid.

Special Problems

Occasionally it may be necessary to perform an early surgical reconstruction in a patient who requires absolute and complete shoulder stability before being able to return to his or her occupation (i.e., a person who is involved in the construction of a high-rise building who has to walk and balance on steel beams, or an outstanding young athlete whose income depends on his having a full, complete stable range of motion). A surgical repair done two weeks after the initial traumatic injury will more reliably allow the patient to have full function and stability than the usual treatment of three to four weeks in a shoulder immobilizer.

Matsen's Preferred Method of Anterior Reduction

I find that reduction of either anterior or posterior glenohumeral dislocations usually can be effected by traction on the abducted and flexed arm. The elbow is also flexed to relax the neurovascular structures of the arm. This maneuver may be carried out with the patient in either a prone or supine position, as long as the body is fixed to resist the traction force. The only drawback with the prone position (Stimson's maneuver) is the discomfort the patient experiences in assuming it. I commonly place the patient supine with a sheet around the thorax, with the loose ends on the side opposite the shoulder dislocation where they are held by an assistant (Fig. 14–58). The surgeon stands on the side of the dislocated shoulder near the waist of the patient. The elbow of the dislocated shoulder is flexed to 90 degrees. A second sheet tied loosely around the waist of the surgeon is looped over the patient's forearm so that it lies just distal to the flexed elbow. While the assistant provides countertraction by pulling on the sheet around the patient's thorax, the surgeon applies traction to the shoulder by leaning back against the sheet around his waist and grasping the forearm. Steady traction along the axis of the arm will usually effect reduction. Anesthesia, muscle relaxants, and analgesics are often unnecessary with this gentle method. To this basic maneuver, one may add gentle rocking of the humerus from internal to external rotation or outward pressure on the proximal humerus

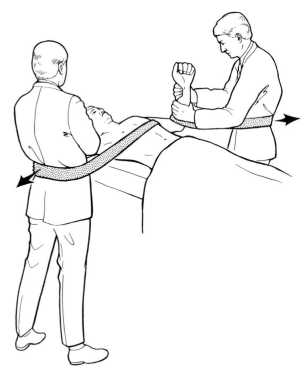

Figure 14–58. Reduction technique for anterior glenohumeral dislocation. The patient lies supine with a sheet placed around the thorax, then around the assistant's waist; this provides countertraction. The surgeon stands on the side of the dislocated shoulder near the patient's waist with the elbow of the dislocated shoulder flexed to 90 degrees. A second sheet is tied loosely around the waist of the surgeon and looped over the patient's forearm, thereby providing traction while the surgeon leans back against the sheet, grasping the forearm. Steady traction along the axis of the arm will usually cause reduction. The surgeon's hands are free to gently rock the humerus from internal to external rotation or to provide gentle outward pressure on the proximal humerus from the axilla.

from the axilla. These additions are particularly useful if prereduction axillary roentgenograms show the humeral head to be impaled on the glenoid rim. Postreduction roentgenograms are used to confirm reduction and to detect fractures. A postreduction neurovascular check is routine.

Rockwood's Preferred Method of Anterior Reduction

I prefer the use of the traction and countertraction method (Fig. 14–59). I use a combination of narcotics, with muscle relaxants or tranquilizers, and perform the reduction in the emergency department. An intravenous line is routinely established in the normal arm. Half of the narcotics are given intramuscularly, and half are given intravenously into the intravenous tubing, followed by administration of a tranquilizer or a muscle relaxant. A sheet folded to form a 5-inch swathe is used as the countertraction to stabilize the chest. After 5 to 6 minutes have passed, very gentle traction is applied to the involved arm in line with the deformity and the traction is increased very gradually against the countertraction. Occasionally gentle internal and external rotation is used to disengage the head from the glenoid rim. With very gentle and gradual traction, the reduction can be accomplished without pain and sometimes even without any palpable sensation of reduction. In some larger patients, the reduction may be so atraumatic that neither the physician nor the patient feels or sees the reduction. It is only after traction has been discontinued that the patient moves his arm about, stating that everything is all right. If this technique is unsuccessful and there are no other contraindications, I prefer to use general anesthesia, again with traction–countertraction maneuvers, instead of the leverage type of reduction.

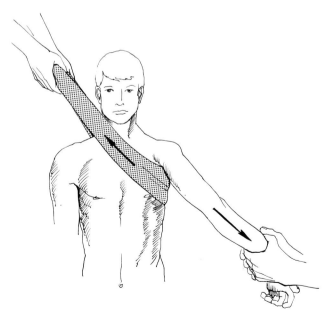

Figure 14–59. Closed reduction of the left shoulder with traction against countertraction. (Reproduced with permission from Rockwood CA, and Green DP (eds): Fractures (3 vols), 2nd ed. Philadelphia: JB Lippincott, 1984.)

Postreduction Management

The position of immobilization after the reduction of an anterior dislocation of the joint should be one of comfortable adduction and internal rotation. This position relaxes the injured anterior structures. Tight bandaging is not required and the immobilization need not be absolute. The elbow should be fully extended at least several times a day. Allowing the arm to externally rotate to zero degrees twice a day is helpful in preventing "sling soreness." It is again emphasized that persons over 30 tend to develop stiffness of the shoulder, elbow, and hand with immobilization. Thus in the older population mobilization may be instituted within a week after anterior dislocation. In this approach external rotation is allowed to 30 degrees and flexion to 90 degrees for the first three weeks and to 40 degrees and 140 degrees, respectively, for the second three weeks.

During the period of protection, the patient is instructed in progressive isometric exercises, particularly of the internal and external shoulder rotator muscles. The patient will not be well served by the atrophy of disuse. After the period of immobilization, more vigorous rotator-strengthening exercises using rubber tubing or weights are prescribed. Strong subscapularis and infraspinatus muscles are ideally situated to increase glenohumeral stability.[483] Range-of-motion exercises are rarely needed after a routine glenohumeral dislocation in a young patient. Swimming is recommended at six weeks to enhance endurance and coordination. By three months after the dislocation, most patients should have almost full flexion and rotation of the shoulder. The patient is not allowed to use the injured arm in sports or for over-the-head labor until normal rotator strength and nearly full forward elevation are achieved. Any deviation from the expected course of recovery requires careful re-evaluation for occult fractures, loose bodies, rotator cuff tears, peripheral nerve injuries, and glenohumeral arthritis. Matsen's management of first dislocations in a 17-year-old and a 38-year-old are contrasted in Table 14–1.

In the very rare situation in which a locked anterior dislocation cannot be managed as described here, open reduction may be accomplished after the subscapularis and anterior capsule are incised from the lesser tuberosity. After open reduction, the subscapularis and capsule are repaired.

Posterior Dislocations

Reduction

Patients with acute, traumatic posterior dislocation of the shoulder usually have much more pain than do those with acute, traumatic anterior dislocation. The use of intravenous narcotics combined with muscle relaxants or tranquilizers to reduce the dislocation may be unsuccessful; general anesthesia with muscle relaxation may be required. Closed reduction can usually

Table 14–1. COMPARISON OF MANAGEMENT OF FIRST ANTERIOR DISLOCATION IN PATIENTS OF TWO AGES

	17-Year-Old Patient	38-Year-Old Patient
Pathology anticipated	Inferior glenohumeral ligament avulsion from glenoid	Capsule and/or cuff tear
Neurovascular check	x	x
Three radiographic views relative to plane of scapula	x	x
Radiographic findings	Posterior lateral head defect Possible anteroinferior glenoid chip	Possible greater tuberosity fracture —
Reduction by two-sheet method	x	x
Postreduction neurovascular examination	x	x
Postreduction radiographs	x	x
Possible cuff tear	—	x
Possible axillary palsy	x	x
Sling	x	x
Elbow straightening twice daily	x	x
Immediate isometrics for rotator muscles	x	x
Concern about stiffness	—	x
Avoid external rotation beyond 0° and flexion beyond 90° for	6 weeks	2 weeks
Start vigorous range-of-motion exercises	3 months	6 weeks
Start vigorous internal and external strengthening	6 weeks	2 weeks
Start swimming	6 weeks	Earlier if possible
Concern about redislocation	High	Low

be accomplished once the muscle spasm has been eliminated. With the patient in the supine position, traction should be applied to the adducted arm in the line of the deformity along with a gentle lifting of the head back into the glenoid fossa. Care should be taken not to force the arm into external rotation; if the head is locked posteriorly on the glenoid rim, the forced rotation could produce a fracture of the head or shaft of the humerus. If the maneuver is done gently after good muscle relaxation has been achieved, the reduction is atraumatic. If the prereduction radiographs show that the head is locked on the posterior glenoid, distal traction on the arm should be combined with lateral traction on the upper arm. A folded towel or soft roller bandage can be used by an assistant to apply the lateral traction. In locked posterior dislocations, reduction may be facilitated by gently internally rotating the humerus to stretch out the posterior capsule and cuff musculature before reduction is attempted.

If gentle closed reduction of a locked posterior glenohumeral dislocation is not possible, open reduction may be accomplished through an anterior deltopectoral approach.* Because local anatomy is significantly distorted, the tendon of the long head of the biceps is used as a guide to the lesser tuberosity. The subscapularis is released either by lesser tuberosity osteotomy or by direct incision. With the glenoid thus exposed, open reduction is carried out. After reduction, the humeral head defect may be rendered extra-articular by filling it with the subscapularis tendon[329, 331, 335] or the lesser tuberosity.[455] If the humeral head defect involves over 30 per cent of the articular surface, prosthetic replacement may be indicated.

Moeller[353] reported on a patient who had an open acute posterior dislocation of the left shoulder. The shoulder was totally unstable following reduction with tears of the rotator cuff, biceps tendon, and subscapularis tendons. The patient had associated injury to the axillary and suprascapular nerves.

Hawkins and coworkers[208] reviewed 41 cases of locked posterior shoulder dislocations. The average interval between injury and diagnosis was one year! In seven shoulders the deformity was accepted. Closed reduction was successful in only 6 of the 12 cases in which it was attempted.

Postreduction Care

If the shoulder is stable after closed reduction, McLaughlin recommended that the shoulder be immobilized in a sling-and-swathe position. However, if the shoulder tends to sublux or redislocate in the sling-and-swathe position, a shoulder spica or some type of modification should be used. The amount of external rotation is determined by applying the cast with the arm in its most stable position. Cautilli and colleagues[78, 79] do not recommend the sling and swathe (internal rotation), since it places the injured posterior structures under tension. Their immobilization technique consists of a padded plaster cast around the waist and a padded circle of plaster around the wrist. These two casts are then connected by a wooden bar and held in place with plaster. The shoulder is usually immobilized in neutral to slight external rotation. A sling of stockinette may be used to support the arm.

Wilson and McKeever[568] stated that many of the acute traumatic posterior dislocations are unstable and recommended the use of Steinmann pins to maintain their reduction. In their technique, after the shoulder has been reduced, two pins are drilled in cruciate fashion down from the acromion process into the reduced humeral head. The pins are removed after three weeks and rehabilitation is instituted. There is a

---

*See references 110, 136, 208, 248, 274, 279, 335, 589.

danger of pin breakage when the pins are placed from the acromion into the head or from the head into the glenoid.

A large anteromedial humeral head defect, as is occasionally seen on axillary lateral x-rays, may predispose to recurrent dislocations. Therefore the shoulder can best be immobilized with the arm in external rotation to allow posterior capsular healing. Scougall[496] has shown experimentally in monkeys that a surgically detached posterior glenoid labrum and capsule heal soundly without repair. He concluded that the best position of immobilization, to allow healing for all of the posterior structures, was in abduction, external rotation, and extension and that the position should be maintained for four weeks.

Early Surgery in Acute Traumatic Posterior Dislocation

Indications for surgery include a major displacement of an associated lesser tuberosity fragment, a major fragment off the posterior glenoid, an irreducible dislocation, open dislocation, or an unstable reduction.

The specific indication for the McLaughlin operation is the presence of a large anteromedial humeral head defect so that a stable reduction cannot be achieved. Through an anterior approach, the subscapularis is detached from the lesser tuberosity; the shoulder is reduced and the subscapular tendon is transferred into the head defect.[299, 330] Neer[455] has modified this operation by transferring the lesser tuberosity with the tendon into the defect. The added fragment of the lesser tuberosity helps fill the space in the defect, and it is simpler to perform because the lesser tuberosity can be secured into the defect with a bone screw. Nicola and coworkers[384] reported a successful result in a patient who had bilateral posterior fracture-dislocation following a seizure and who was treated with Neer's modification of the McLaughlin procedure.

In their series of locked posterior dislocations, Hawkins and associates[208] used subscapularis transfer into the defect, lesser tuberosity transfer, hemiarthroplasty, and total shoulder arthroplasty according to the specific problem.

McLaughlin recommended a sling-and-swathe position following the transfer of the subscapularis muscle for two weeks. Rockwood[455] recommends the immobilization of the arm in a position of neutral rotation in a modified shoulder spica cast for six weeks. The rehabilitation program following removal of the cast consists of three to four weeks' gentle use of the shoulder for everyday living activities, followed by gentle stretching exercises and finally resistive exercises to gain strength in the internal and external rotators and the deltoid muscles. The patient should not return to any heavy lifting or heavy work before three to six months and not until full range of motion and strength have been regained.

Rowe and Zarins[471] did not use a postoperative cast or brace following reconstruction of unreduced posterior dislocation. Instead, they positioned the arm at the side of the body, posterior to the coronal plane, and held it with a strip of Elastoplast tape or a canvas restraint.

Chronic Posterior Dislocation

If a patient, especially an older patient, has had a chronic posterior dislocation for months or years and if there is minimal pain and a functional range of motion, then surgery may not be indicated. However, if disability exists and there is good bone stock to the glenohumeral joint, then a reconstruction should be considered. Rowe and Zarins,[471] in a review of 23 patients with chronic dislocations that had been unreduced over three weeks, found that 14 were posterior and 8 were anterior. Fourteen of these shoulders were operated upon. Seven patients had open reduction with preservation of the humeral head; one had a total shoulder replacement, a humeral head prosthesis was used in two, and four were treated with humeral head resection.

Authors' Preferred Method of Treatment

Our management of acute traumatic posterior dislocations begins with a definition of the extent and chronicity of the injury. A complete radiographic evaluation is necessary, including anteroposterior and lateral views in the plane of the scapula and an axillary view. Careful note is made of associated fractures, including the extent of the impression fracture of the anteromedial humeral head. A gentle closed reduction is attempted using axial traction on the arm. If the head is locked on the glenoid rim, gentle internal rotation may stretch out the posterior capsule to facilitate reduction. Lateral traction on the proximal humerus may unlock the humeral head. Once it is unlocked, the humerus is gently externally rotated. After reduction is achieved and confirmed by postreduction radiographs, the reduction is maintained for three weeks by a cummerbund "handshake" cast in neutral rotation and slight extension (Fig. 14-60). This position relaxes the injured structures. External rotation and deltoid isometrics are carried out during this period of immobilization. After removal of the cast, a vigorous internal and external rotator–strengthening program is initiated. Range of motion is allowed to return with active use. Vigorous physical activities are not resumed until the shoulder is strong and three months have elapsed since reduction. Swimming is encouraged to develop endurance and muscle coordination.

RECURRENT INSTABILITY

Recurrent Anterior Instability

In the management of recurrent glenohumeral instability, perhaps the greatest challenge is to be sure of what condition is being treated. At the risk of oversim-

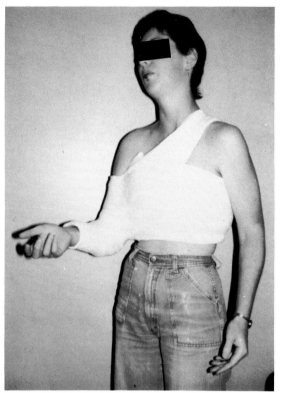

Figure 14–60. Handshake cast. After closed reduction of an acute traumatic posterior dislocation is confirmed by x-rays, a cast is applied in neutral rotation and slight extension for three weeks.

plifying, we have found it useful to recognize that most patients with recurrent instability fall into one of two large groups. The first is characterized by a history of definite *trauma* initiating a problem of *unidirectional* shoulder instability. These shoulders usually have definite structural damage. When the direction of traumatic instability is anterior, the shoulders commonly have ruptures of the glenohumeral ligaments at their glenoid attachments, referred to as *Bankart* (Perthes) lesions. Finally, these shoulders frequently require *surgery* to achieve stability. To help remember this grouping, we use the acronym TUBS (Table 14–2). A typical patient is a 17-year-old skier whose recurrent anterior instability began with a fall on an abducted, externally rotated arm.

The second group of patients have no history of significant trauma; thus instability is *atraumatic*. These patients are much more prone to have *multidirectional*

Table 14–2. TWO TYPES OF RECURRENT INSTABILITY

Traumatic
Unidirectional
Bankart lesion (avulsion of glenohumeral ligaments from glenoid)
Surgery is often necessary

Atraumatic
Multidirectional
Bilateral
Rehabilitation enhances stability
Inferior capsular shift should be a part of repair if surgery is necessary

instability that is *bilateral. Rehabilitation,* especially rotator cuff strengthening and coordination exercises, is the first line of treatment. If surgery is performed, laxity of the *inferior* capsule must be managed with an inferior capsular shift. The acronym for this group is AMBRI (Table 14–2). A typical patient is a 15-year-old swimmer whose shoulders are becoming painful and on examination are found to be loose in all directions.

Although many variants of these basic themes exist, it is essential to differentiate the shoulder that goes out because it has suffered a major injury from one that goes out because it is constitutionally loose. This fundamental distinction can become obscured in some of the very involved classifications that have been proposed.

Nonoperative Management

Coordinated, strong contraction of the muscles of the rotator cuff is one of the important mechanisms of shoulder stability. Sidles and coworkers[503a] have shown that a compressive load applied to the glenohumeral joint is able to resist a translational force two-thirds as large as the compressive force. Shoulders with looser capsules, such as those of pitchers, swimmers, and gymnasts, have a greater relative dependence on this dynamic stabilizing mechanism. Saha and associates[479–483, 486] point to deficiencies of the posterior shoulder depressor or steering muscles as a major factor in recurrent instability. Many if not most of these deficiencies in muscle strength should respond to vigorous internal and external rotator–strengthening exercises. Both internal and external rotator strength contribute to anterior and posterior stability. Coordinated contractions of the cuff muscles help hold the humerus in the glenoid and resist potentially displacing forces. Rotator-strengthening exercises are most effectively performed by keeping the humerus close to the body and rotating the arm against the resistance of rubber tubing, spring exercises, or weights in the sidelying position. A useful goal is to strive for sufficient strength in both directions to rotate 20 times against a resistance of 20 per cent of the body weight of the patient (the 20-20 goal). Rockwood and colleagues[457] found that 12 per cent of patients with traumatic subluxation, 80 per cent of those with anterior atraumatic subluxation, and 90 per cent of those with posterior instability responded to a special rehabilitation program (see Fig. 14–94).

Although any form of glenohumeral instability may benefit from this rehabilitation, it is particularly indicated in patients with atraumatic, multidirectional, bilateral instability (the AMBRI syndrome). Nonoperative management is desirable for patients with voluntary instability, for those with posterior glenohumeral instability, and for those requiring a supranormal range of motion (such as baseball pitchers and gymnasts) in whom surgical management often does not permit return to a competitive level of function.[207, 467, 483]

Because the coordination of muscle contraction is a key element of dynamic stability, smooth repetitive activities such as swimming play an essential role in this treatment program. In addition to rotator strengthening and coordination exercises, those patients with voluntary shoulder instability require a careful explanation of the importance of avoiding intentional glenohumeral subluxation or dislocation: "Each time you let your shoulder go out of joint it makes it looser and more prone to unpredictable instability."

Operative Management

In contemplating a surgical approach to anterior glenohumeral instability, it is essential to identify preoperatively any factors that may compromise the surgical results, such as generalized ligamentous laxity, multidirectional instability, or significant bony defects of the humeral head or glenoid. When these conditions exist, it is necessary to tailor the surgical procedure to the specific pathology.

Surgical stabilization of the glenohumeral joint is considered if instability or apprehension repeatedly compromises shoulder comfort or function in spite of a reasonable trial of internal and external rotator strengthening and coordination exercises. A vigorous effort to stabilize the shoulder with exercises is particularly indicated in patients with multidirectional or posterior instability and in athletes requiring a completely normal or supranormal range of motion. Surgical stabilization is not indicated in patients with a refractory desire to voluntarily subluxate or dislocate the glenohumeral joint. Surgery is especially not indicated in patients with atraumatic instability who are emotionally unstable.

Many surgical procedures have been described for the treatment of recurrent anterior glenohumeral instability. Tightening and to some degree realigning the subscapularis tendon and partially eliminating external rotation are the goals of the Magnuson-Stack and the Putti-Platt procedures. The Putti-Platt operation also tightens and reinforces the anterior capsule. Reattachment of the capsule and glenoid labrum to the glenoid lip is the goal of the Bankart repair, the DuToit staple capsulorrhaphy, and the Eyre-Brook capsulorrhaphy.[149, 150] Augmentation of the bony anterior glenoid lip is the objective of anterior bone block procedures. The Bristow procedure transfers the tip of the coracoid process with its muscle attachments and also creates a musculotendinous sling across the anteroinferior tendon at the front of the glenohumeral joint. An anterior glenoid bone buttress procedure is the objective of the Oudard and Trillat procedure. A large posterolateral humeral head defect may be approached by limiting external rotation, by filling the defect with the infraspinatus tendon, or by performing a rotational osteotomy of the humerus.[78, 79, 521, 559]

Capsular Repairs
Bankart Procedure. This repair was apparently first

done by Perthes[430] in 1906, who recommended the repair of the anterior capsule to the anterior glenoid rim. He was not in doubt about the pathology of traumatic instability: "In every case the anterior margin of the glenoid cavity will be found to be smooth, rounded, and free of any attachments, and a blunt instrument can be passed freely inwards over the bare bone on the front of the neck of the scapula." He reattached the capsule to the glenoid rim by placing drill holes through the bone. Credit for this type of repair should go to Perthes, but the popularity of the technique is due to the work of Bankart,[27, 28] who first performed the operation in 1923 on one of his former house surgeons. The procedure commonly used today is based on Bankart's 1939 article in which he discusses the repair of the capsule to the bone of the anterior glenoid through the use of drill holes and suture. The subscapularis muscle, which is carefully divided to expose the capsule, is reapproximated without any overlap or shortening. Bankart reported 27 consecutive cases with "full movements of the joint and in no case has there been any recurrence of the dislocation."[48, 458, 462, 470]

Hovelius and coworkers[233] found a 2 per cent redislocation rate after the Bankart procedure compared with a 19 per cent redislocation after the Putti-Platt. Over one-third of patients under 25 years of age were dissatisfied with the results of the Putti-Platt. Rowe and Zarins[470] reported a series of 50 subluxating shoulders with good or excellent results in 94 per cent after a Bankart repair. A Bankart lesion was found in 32 of these shoulders.

Rowe and coworkers[465] reported on 51 shoulders with a fracture of the anterior rim of the glenoid. Eighteen shoulders had a fracture involving one-sixth or less of the glenoid, 26 involved one-fourth of the glenoid, and 7 had one-third of the anterior glenoid fractured off. In this group of patients who were treated with a Bankart repair without particular attention being given to the fracture, the overall incidence of failure was 2 per cent.

Many shoulder surgeons consider this the procedure of choice for management of traumatic unidirectional instability, which is almost always associated with an avulsion of the glenohumeral ligaments from the glenoid.

Staple Capsulorrhaphy. In the DuToit staple capsulorrhaphy, the detached capsule is secured back to the glenoid using staples.[140, 510] Actually, the staple repair had been described 50 years earlier by Perthes. Rao and associates[445] reported follow-up on 65 patients having a DuToit staple repair of the avulsion of the capsule from the glenoid rim. Of these, 94 per cent had separation of the labrum from the rim. Good to excellent results were obtained in 98 per cent; 58 per cent were able to return to athletics. Two patients showed radiographic evidence of loose staples.

O'Driscoll and Evans[397] reviewed 269 consecutive DuToit capsulorrhaphies in 257 patients for a median follow-up of 8.8 years. Eighty-eight per cent of the procedures were performed for dislocations and 12 per

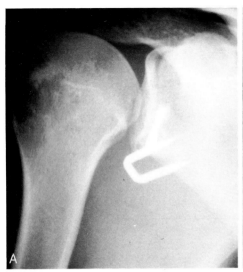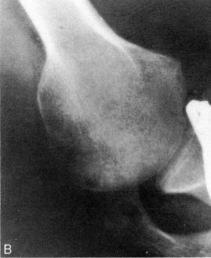

Figure 14–61. Complications of staple capsulorrhaphy. *A,* An anteroposterior x-ray showing a prominent staple on the inferior glenoid rim. *B,* An axillary view showing staple impingement on the head of the humerus.

cent for subluxations. Fifty-three per cent of the patients had postoperative pain. Internal and external rotation were limited. Recurrence was reported in 28 per cent if stapling alone was done and in 8 per cent if a Putti-Platt procedure was added; 11 per cent had staple loosening, migration, or penetration of cartilage. Staple complications contributed to pain, physical restrictions, and osteoarthritis.

The use of staples for surgical repairs may be associated with major complications (Figs. 14–61 and 14–62).[576]

Subscapularis Muscle Procedures

Putti-Platt Procedure. In 1948 Osmond-Clark[402] described this procedure, which was used by Sir Harry Platt of England and Vittorio Putti of Italy. Platt first used this technique in November 1925. Some years later Osmond-Clarke saw Putti perform essentially the same operation that had been his standard practice since 1923. Scaglietta, one of Putti's pupils, revealed that the operation may well have been performed first by Codivilla, Putti's teacher and predecessor. Neither Putti nor Platt ever described the technique in the literature.

In the Putti-Platt procedure, the subscapularis tendon is divided 2.5 cm from its insertion. The anterior shoulder joint capsule, which adheres to the posterior surface of the subscapularis tendon, may be opened in the same plane as the tendon is divided so that the joint can be inspected. The lateral stump of the tendon is attached to the "most convenient soft-tissue structure along the anterior rim of the glenoid cavity." If the capsule and labrum have been stripped from the anterior glenoid and the neck of the scapula, the tendon is sutured to the deep surface of the capsule, and "it is advisable to raw the anterior surface of the neck of the scapula, so that the sutured tendo-capsule will adhere to it." After the lateral tendon stump is secured, the medial muscle stump is lapped over the lateral stump, producing a substantial shortening of the capsule and subscapularis muscle.

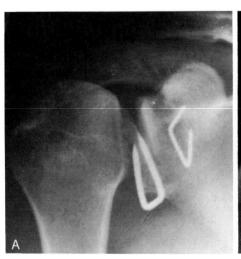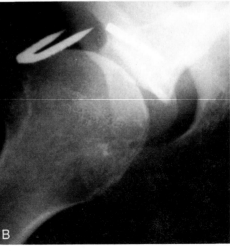

Figure 14–62. Loose staple after staple capsulorrhaphy. *A,* An anteroposterior x-ray showing a loose staple in the glenohumeral joint. *B,* Axillary view.

In those instances when the medial capsule can be separated from the medial muscle tendon unit, the capsule is sutured on top of the secured lateral tendon and the medial muscle tendon unit is then secured over the capsule laterally in the area of the greater tuberosity of the humerus. The exact placement of the lateral stump into the anterior soft tissues and of the medial stump into the greater tuberosity is determined so that, after conclusion of the procedure, the arm should externally rotate to the neutral position.

Blazina and Satzman[48] described the use of the Putti-Platt procedure to manage anterior shoulder subluxation. Watson-Jones[557] and other authors have recommended that the Bankart and the Putti-Platt procedures be combined (i.e., following the meticulous repair of the capsule to the glenoid, they "double-breast" the subscapularis rather than merely reapproximating it). Muller[559] reattaches the capsule with screws and then shortens the subscapularis.

Symeonides[523] reported 33 cases in which the subscapularis and anterior capsule were overlapped without attempting to suture the lateral flap to the glenoid.

Quigley and Freedman[439] reported the results of 92 Putti-Platt operations; of these patients, 11 had more than a 30 per cent loss of motion. Seven had recurrent instability after their surgery.

Leach and coworkers[291] in 1981 reported a series of 78 patients who had been treated with a modified Putti-Platt procedure. The only failure was in a diabetic who had a recurrence during a seizure following an insulin reaction. Loss of external rotation averaged between 12 and 19 degrees.

Collins and associates[95] reviewed a series of 58 Putti-Platt procedures and 48 Putti-Platt–Bankart procedures. The redislocation rate was 11 per cent (some because of significant trauma), 20 per cent had residual pain, and the average restriction of external rotation was 20 degrees.

Hovelius and colleagues,[233] in a follow-up of 114 patients who underwent either a Bankart or Putti-Platt reconstruction, found a recurrence rate of 2 per cent in 46 patients treated with the Bankart procedure and of 19 per cent in 68 patients treated with a Putti-Platt procedure. The follow-up was between 1.5 and 10 years.

Since the description of the Putti-Platt technique by Osmond-Clarke in 1948, authors have described the technique as securing the lateral tendon into the "*rawed*" *anterior glenoid rim of the scapula.* In effect, this would create a tenodesis of the subscapularis tendon. With only a 2.5-cm lateral stump of the tendon to work with, there is no way that one can attach the lateral stump of the subscapularis tendon to the anterior glenoid of the neck of the scapula and have the patient be able to externally rotate the arm beyond the neutral position or flex, extend, abduct, or elevate the upper extremity. Since the radius of the humerus is approximately 2.5 cm, a 2.5-cm stump of subscapularis fused to the anterior glenoid would limit the total humeral rotation to one radian, or 57 degrees. If the

lateral stump of the subscapularis tendon is attached to the raw bone of the anterior glenoid and if the patient develops a functional range of motion, this suggests that the tendon was disrupted from the glenoid. This was confirmed by Symeonides, who performed an autopsy on a patient who had had a Putti-Platt procedure 22 months before his unexpected death.

Angelo and Hawkins[13] presented a series of eight patients who developed osteoarthritis an average of 15 years after a Putti-Platt repair. A common feature of these shoulders is that they had never gained more than zero degrees of external rotation after their shoulder repair. The authors hypothesized that the excessive tightness of the anterior repair changed the joint mechanics so that increased wear was the result.

The Putti-Platt procedure is contraindicated in multidirectional instability (AMBRI); tightening the front of the shoulder will only increase the likelihood of posterior instability. In traumatic instability (TUBS) the data suggest that such a procedure, which limits external rotation, is not necessary if the Bankart lesion is solidly repaired.

Magnuson-Stack Procedure. Transfer of the subscapularis tendon from the lesser tuberosity across the bicipital groove to the greater tuberosity was originally described by Paul Magnuson and James Stack in 1940.[259, 317–319, 346, 445] In 1955, Magnuson[445] recommended that in some cases the tendon should be transferred not only across the bicipital groove but also distally into an area between the greater tuberosity and the upper shaft. In this manner, when the arm is abducted the subscapularis muscle tendon unit would act more effectively as a sling to support the head of the humerus. DePalma[127] also recommended that the tendon be transferred to the upper shaft below the greater tuberosity. He interpreted this procedure as being designed to strengthen the anterior muscle barrier to the front of the shoulder and to produce a dynamic force that, on elevation of the arm, forces and holds the head of the humerus in the glenoid fossa. The tendon has been attached to the shaft into a bone trough with sutures, a staple, or a boat nail. Karadimas,[259] in the largest single series of Magnuson-Stack procedures (154 patients), reported a 2 per cent recurrence rate.

Badgley and O'Connor[24] and Bailey[25] have reported on a combination of the Putti-Platt and the Magnuson-Stack operations; they used the upper half of the subscapularis muscle to perform the Putti-Platt procedure and the lower half of the muscle to perform the Magnuson-Stack procedure.

Although the Magnuson-Stack procedure has been successfully applied, it is losing favor to more specific anatomical surgical repairs. If isolated laxity of the subscapularis were the problem in recurrent instability, it should be manageable by internal rotation–strengthening exercises. The capsular avulsion common to most cases of traumatic instability can be specifically repaired without loss of rotation. The complications

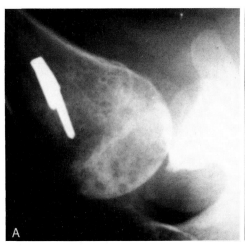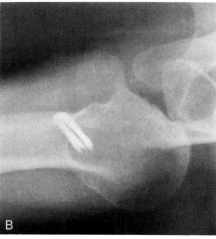

Figure 14–63. Magnuson-Stack procedure. *A,* This axillary view shows posterior subluxation of the humeral head on the glenoid as a result of excessive anterior tightening with the Magnuson-Stack procedure. *B,* Another patient's axillary view shows excessive anterior tightening from the Magnuson-Stack procedure, resulting in posterior glenohumeral displacement of the humeral head.

observed after this procedure include excessive anterior tightening with posterior subluxation or dislocation (Fig. 14–63), damage to the biceps (Fig. 14–64), and recurrent instability.

Bone Block

Eden-Hybbinette Procedure. The Eden-Hybbinette procedure was performed independently by Eden[142] in 1918 and by Hybbinette[239] in 1932. Eden first used tibial grafts, but both authors finally recommended the use of iliac grafts. This procedure is supposed to extend the anterior glenoid. It has been used by Palmar and Widen,[414] Lavik,[289] and Hovelius[230] in treating shoulder subluxation and dislocation. Lavik modified the procedure by inserting the graft into the substance of the anterior glenoid rim. Lange[283] inserted the bone graft into an osteotomy on the anterior glenoid. Hehne and Hubner[211] reported a comparison of the Eden-Hybbinette–Lange and the Putti-Platt procedures in 170 patients; their results seemed to favor the latter. Paa-

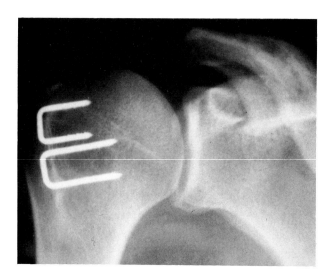

Figure 14–64. Staple impingement on the long head of the biceps tendon. This anteroposterior x-ray shows the position of the staple resulting in tendon impingement. Anterior shoulder pain resolved on staple removal.

volainen and coworkers[412] reported on 41 cases of Eden-Hybbinette procedures; 3 had recurrent instability, and external rotation was diminished an average of 10 per cent. They found the results similar to their series of Putti-Platt operations. Ten per cent in each group developed degenerative joint disease!

Oudard Procedure. In 1924 Oudard[403] described a method in which the coracoid process was prolonged with a bone graft from the tibia. The graft (4 × 3 × 1 cm) was inserted between the sawed-off tip and the remainder of the coracoid and was directed laterally and inferiorly. The graft acted as an anterior buttress that served to prevent recurrent dislocations. Oudard also shortened the subscapular tendon. Later he published another method of obtaining the elongation of the coracoid by performing an oblique osteotomy of the coracoid and displacing the posterolateral portion to serve as a bone block.

Bone blocks rarely seem to be the procedure of choice for increasing shoulder stability. One must be concerned about procedures that may bring the humeral head into contact with bone that is not covered by articular cartilage because of the high risk of degenerative joint disease. Soft tissue repairs and reconstructions would appear to be safer and more effective for dealing with all but the most unusual situation.

Coracoid Transfer

Trillat Procedure. Trillat and Leclerc-Chalvet[51, 388, 537, 538] performed an osteotomy at the base of the coracoid process and then displaced the coracoid downward and laterally. The displaced coracoid is held in position by a special nail-pin or screw. The pin is passed into the scapula above the inferiorly displaced subscapularis muscle, which effectively shortens the muscle.

Bristow-Helfet Procedure. This procedure was developed, used, and reported by Arthur Helfet[212] in 1958 and was named the Bristow operation after his former chief at St. Thomas Hospital, W. Rowley Bristow of South Africa. Helfet originally described detaching the tip of the coracoid process from the scapula just distal to the insertion of the pectoralis minor muscle, leaving the conjoined tendons (i.e., the short head of the biceps and the coracobrachialis) attached. Through a vertical slit in the subscapularis tendon, the joint is exposed and the anterior surface of the neck of the scapula is "rawed up." The coracoid process with its attached tendons is then passed through the slit in the subscapularis and kept in contact with the raw area on the scapula by suturing the conjoined tendon to the cut edges of the scapularis tendon.

In 1958, T. B. McMurray (son of T. P. McMurray of hip osteotomy fame) visited Dr. Newton Mead[340] of Chicago and described modifications of the Bristow operation that were being used in Capetown, Johannesburg, and Pretoria. Mead and Sweeney[340] reported the modifications in over 100 cases. The modifications consist of splitting the subscapularis muscle and tendon unit in line with its fibers to open the joint and firmly securing the coracoid process to the anterior glenoid rim with a screw. May[323] has modified the Bristow procedure further by vertically dividing the entire subscapularis tendon from the lesser tuberosity; after exploring the joint, he attaches the tip of the coracoid process with the conjoined tendon to the anterior glenoid with a screw. The subscapularis tendon is then split horizontally and reattached—half of the tendon above and half below the transferred conjoined tendon—to the site of its original insertion.

Helfet[212] reported that the procedure not only "reinforced" the defective part of the joint but also had a "bone block" effect. Mead,[340] however, does not regard the bone block as being a very important part of the procedure and believes that the transfer adds a muscle reinforcement at the lower anterior aspect of the shoulder joint that prevents the lower portion of the subscapularis muscle from displacing upward as the humerus is abducted. Bonnin[53, 54] has modified the Bristow procedure in the following way: he does not shorten or split the subscapularis muscle tendon unit but for exposure he divides the subscapularis muscle at its muscle-tendon junction and, following the attachment of the coracoid process to the glenoid with a screw, he reattaches the subscapularis on top of the conjoined tendon. Results with this modification in 81 patients have been reported by Hummel and associates.[236]

Torg and coworkers[535] reported their experience with 212 cases of the Bristow procedure. In their modification the coracoid was passed over the superior border rather than through the subscapularis. Their postoperative instability rate was 8.5 per cent (3.8 per cent redislocation and 4.7 per cent subluxation). Ten patients required reoperation for screw-related problems; 34 per cent had residual shoulder pain and 8 per cent were unable to do overhead work. Only 16 per cent of athletes were able to return to their preinjury level of throwing. Carol and associates[75] reported on the results of the Bristow procedure performed for 32 recurrent dislocating shoulders and 15 "spontaneous" shoulder instabilities. At an average follow-up of 3.7 years, only

one patient had recurrent instability and the average limitation of external rotation was 12 degrees. Hovelius and coworkers[230] reported follow-up on 111 shoulders treated with the Bristow procedure. At 2.5 years their postoperative instability rate was 13 per cent (6 per cent dislocation and 7 per cent subluxation). External rotation was limited an average of 20 degrees, and 6 per cent required reoperation because of screw-related complications. Muscle strength was 10 per cent less in the operated shoulder. Chen and colleagues[83] found that after the Bristow procedure, the reduced strength of the short head of the biceps was compensated for by increased activity in the long head.

Lamm and coworkers[280] and Lemmens and de Waal Malefijt[295] have described four special x-ray projections to evaluate the position of the transplanted coracoid process: anteroposterior, lateral, oblique lateral, and modified axial. Lower and coworkers[309] used CT to demonstrate the impingement of a Bristow screw on the head of the humerus. Collins and Wilde[94] and Nielsen and associates[385] reported that while they had minimal problems with recurrence of dislocation, they did encounter problems with screw breakage, migration, and nonunion of coracoid to scapula. Hovelius and colleagues[227, 228] reported only a 50 per cent union of the coracoid to the scapula.

Norris and associates[392] evaluated 24 patients with failed Bristow repairs; only two had union of the transferred coracoid. Causes of failure included (1) residual subluxation and (2) osteoarthritis from screw or bone impingement or overtight repair. They pointed to the difficulty of reconstructing a shoulder after a failed Bristow procedure.

There also appears to be a significant problem with recurrent subluxation after the Bristow procedure.[228, 316, 324] Hill and coworkers[222] and MacKenzie[315] noted failures to manage subluxation with this procedure.

Latarjet Procedure. The Latarjet procedure,[286–288, 420] described in 1954, involves the transfer of a larger portion of the corocoid process than used with the Bristow procedure with the biceps and coracobrachialis tendons to the anteroinferior aspect of the neck of the scapula. Instead of the raw cut surface of the tip of the coracoid process being attached to the scapula as is done in the Bristow-Helfet procedure, the coracoid is laid flat on the neck of the scapula and held in place with one or two screws. Tagliabue and Esposito[524] have reported on the Latarjet procedure in 94 athletes. Vittori has modified the procedure by turning downward the subscapularis tendon and holding it displaced downward with the transferred coracoid. Pascoet and associates reported on the Vittori modification in 36 patients with one recurrence.

Although many surgeons use coracoid transfer procedures, the redislocation rates after these operations appear to be no lower than those of other operations for shoulder instability. Yet complications are frequent and can have major consequences (see Complications of Injury) (Figs. 14–65 to 14–70). Coracoid transfer

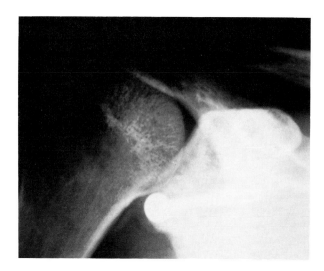

Figure 14–65. This anteroposterior x-ray shows screw impingement on the humeral head after the Bristow procedure.

Figure 14–66. Nonunion of coracoid process after the Bristow procedure. *A,* An anteroposterior x-ray shows nonunion of the coracoid process. *B,* An axillary view of a different patient shows nonunion of the coracoid process after the Bristow procedure.

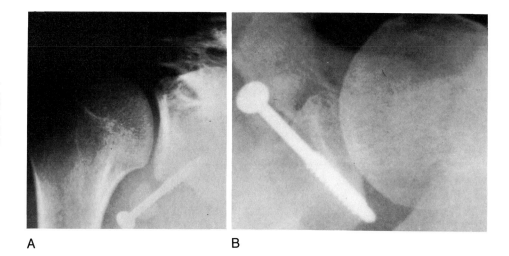

A   B

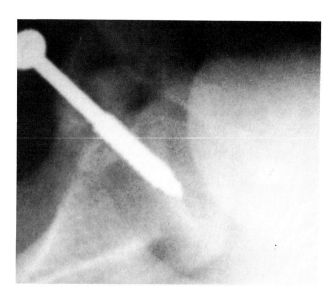

Figure 14–67. Axillary view shows the screw backing out of the glenoid after the Bristow procedure.

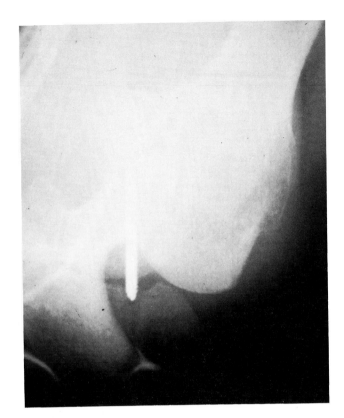

Figure 14–68. Axillary view shows an excessively long screw used during the Bristow procedure. The patient had an infraspinatus palsy as a result of injury to the nerve to this muscle.

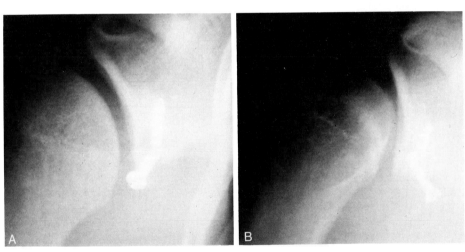

Figure 14–69. Anteroposterior x-rays showing broken screws with the humerus in external rotation (*A*) and internal rotation (*B*).

Figure 14–70. Late screw loosening after the Bristow procedure. *A*, An anteroposterior x-ray shows the position of the screw in the transferred coracoid process. *B*, An anteroposterior x-ray taken five years later shows the screw backed out and significant glenohumeral arthropathy.

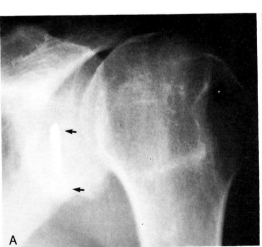
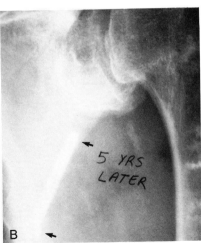

does not address the primary pathology of either traumatic or atraumatic glenohumeral instability and presents the risks of hardware and bone blocks. Finally, coracoid transfer procedures are extremely difficult and hazardous to revise. The subscapularis and axillary neurovascular structures are scarred in abnormal positions. It is also difficult to regain normal suppleness of the subscapularis muscle. In addition, the axillary and musculocutaneous nerves are at risk in the revision of failed transfers.

Other Open Repairs

Gallie Procedure. Gallie and LeMesurier[175, 176] originally described the use of autogenous fascia lata to create new ligaments between the anteroinferior aspect of the capsule and the anterior neck of the humerus in 1927. Bateman[35] of Toronto has also used this procedure.

Nicola Procedure. Toufick Nicola's name is usually associated with this operation, but the procedure was first described by Rupp[476] in 1926 and Heymanowitsch[219] in 1927. In 1929, Nicola[379] published his first article in which he described the use of the long head of the biceps tendon as a checkrein ligament. The procedure has been modified several times.[379, 381-383] Recurrence rates have been reported to be between 30 and 50 per cent.[73, 255, 559]

Saha Procedure. A. K. Saha[479-481, 483, 484, 486] has reported on the transfer of the latissimus dorsi posteriorly into the site of the infraspinatus insertion on the greater tuberosity. He reports that, during abduction, the transferred latissimus reinforces the subscapularis muscle and the short posterior steering and depressor muscles by pulling the humeral head backward. He has used the procedure for traumatic and atraumatic dislocations, and in 1969 he reported 45 cases with no recurrence.

Boytchev Procedure. Boytchev first reported this procedure in 1951 in the Italian literature,[58, 59] and later modifications were developed by Conforty.[96] The muscles that attach to the coracoid process along with the tip of the coracoid are rerouted deep to the subscapularis muscle between it and the capsule. The tip of the coracoid with its muscles is then reattached to its base in the anatomical position. Conforty[96] reported on 17 patients, none of whom had a recurrence of dislocation. Ha'eri and associates[200] reported 26 cases with a minimum of two years' follow-up.

Osteotomy of the Proximal Humerus. Debevoise and associates[119] have shown that humeral torsion is abnormal in the repeatedly dislocating shoulder. B. G. Weber[260, 346, 445, 559, 560] of Switzerland reported a rotational osteotomy whereby he increased the retroversion of the humeral head. He also shortened the subscapularis muscle. The indications were a moderate to severe posterior lateral humeral head defect, which he found in 65 per cent of his patients with recurrent anterior instability. By increasing the retroversion, the posterolateral defect is delivered more posteriorly and the anterior undisturbed portion of the articular surface of the humeral head then articulates against the gle-

noid. Following this procedure, even with external rotation of the arm, the posterolateral defect no longer engages the glenoid cavity. Weber and colleagues[560] reported a redislocation rate of 5.7 per cent with good to excellent results in 90 per cent. Most patients required reoperation for plate removal.

This procedure also includes an anterior capsular reefing, making it difficult to determine the effect of the osteotomy itself. Although posterior lateral humeral head defects are common in recurrent traumatic instability, we do not usually find this head defect to be a significant factor if the capsular pathology is managed appropriately.

Osteotomy of the Neck of the Glenoid. In 1933, Meyer-Burgdorff reported on decreasing the anterior tilt of the glenoid by a posterior wedge closing osteotomy.[479] Saha has written[479] about an anterior opening wedge osteotomy with bone graft into the neck of the glenoid to decrease the tilt.

Caution must be observed in determining the glenoid version from plane roentgenograms. Change in angulation of the beam can change the apparent version substantially (see Fig. 14–11). There is little evidence that glenoid version is the primary problem in recurrent glenohumeral instability. Glenoid osteotomy is too hazardous a procedure for use in ordinary situations.

Arthroscopic Repair

The reader is referred to Chapter 8, Shoulder Arthroscopy, for greater details.

Arthroscopic repair of the Bankart lesion using a staple was performed by Johnson as early as 1982.[250] In this procedure a metal staple is used to reattach the torn labrum or capsule to the roughened edge of the glenoid. Johnson recommends at least three weeks of immobilization. Concern about the safety of using staples and the high redislocation rate has given rise to other arthroscopic techniques (Fig. 14–71). Morgan and Bodenstab[354] reported 25 arthroscopic shoulder stabilizations using a transglenoid absorbable suture.

Our experience with open repairs leads us to predict that arthroscopic repair of atraumatic multidirectional instability (the AMBRI condition) is too extensive a procedure to be performed under arthroscopic control. However, the traumatic tearing of the glenohumeral ligaments from the glenoid (TUBS condition) is suited to arthroscopic repair, once a safe technique is developed that yields results comparable with those obtained with an open Bankart repair.

Postoperative Treatment

Postoperatively the arm is immobilized in adduction and internal rotation. This can be accomplished by supporting the arm in a standard sling and then securing the arm to the trunk with a soft roller bandage, or by using one of the standard shoulder immobilizers that are commercially available. Some authors recommend postoperative immobilization for four to six weeks, after which a rehabilitation program is begun. This may be too long in that limitation of external

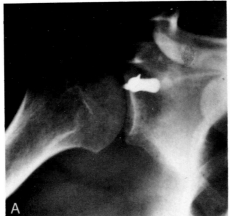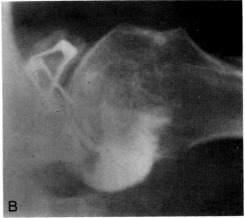

Figure 14–71. *A,* An anteroposterior x-ray shows the position of an arthroscopically placed staple. Impingement on humeral head is suggested by this view. *B,* An axillary x-ray with contrast material demonstrates impingement of the staple on the humeral head.

rotation is a problem after shoulder repair, particularly in the older patient or in the throwing athlete. Rowe and associates[466] recommend immobilization for just two to three days, after which the arm is completely free. Their patients are instructed to gradually increase the motion and function of the extremity.

Results

Most of the reported series on the various types of reconstructions have yielded "excellent" results. However, it is very difficult to determine how each author graded his results. For example, if the patient has no recurrences after repair but has loss of 45 degrees of external rotation and cannot throw, is that a fair, good, or excellent result? The simple fact that the shoulder no longer dislocates cannot be equated with an excellent result. Although the older literature suggested that the goal of surgery for anterior dislocations of the shoulder was to limit external rotation, more modern literature suggests that a reconstruction can both prevent recurrent dislocation and allow a nearly normal range of motion and comfortable function.

Complications of Surgical Procedures

Complications of surgical repairs for anterior glenohumeral instability may be grouped into several categories. The first includes complications that may follow any surgical procedure. Of primary importance in this category is postoperative *infection*. Thorough skin preparation, adhesive plastic drapes, and prophylactic antibiotics are useful in reducing contamination by axillary bacterial flora. It also is important to prevent the accumulation of a significant hematoma by achieving good hemostasis, obliterating any dead space, and using a suction drain if significant bleeding persists. Finally, it is important to keep the axilla clean and dry postoperatively by using a gauze sponge as long as the arm is held at the side.

The second category of complications consists of postoperative *recurrent instability*. The published incidence of recurrent dislocation after the standard an-

terior repairs ranges from zero to 11 per cent. A 1975 review of 1634 reconstructions compiled from the literature revealed that the incidence of recurrence averaged 3 per cent.[455] In a 1983 review of 3076 procedures this incidence was unchanged.[454] This review included 432 Putti-Platt operations, 571 Magnuson-Stack operations or modifications, 513 Bankart operations or modifications, 45 Saha operations, 203 Bankart–Putti-Platt combinations, 639 Bristow operations, 115 Badgley combined procedures, 254 Eden-Hybbinette operations, 277 Gallie operations or modifications, and 27 Weber operations. However, for the most part the results were based on whether or not the patient's shoulder redislocated after the operative procedure.

Morrey and Jones,[355] in a long-term follow-up study of 176 patients that averaged 10.2 years, found a recurrence rate of 11 per cent. The operative reconstructions were of the Bankart and Putti-Platt types. Among the 20 patients with recurrences, half of the failures were related to athletic activities, inadequate immobilization, a history of contralateral dislocation, and a family history of shoulder dislocation. In 7 of the 20 patients, recurrence of dislocation occurred two years or more after surgery. The need for long-term follow-up was further emphasized in a recent study by O'Driscoll and Evans,[397] who followed 269 consecutive staple capsulorrhaphies for a minimum of 8.8 years. Twenty-one per cent experienced recurrent instability; this incidence increased progressively with the length of follow-up.

Rowe and colleagues[472] reported on the management of 39 patients with recurrence of instability after various surgical repairs. Of 32 who were reoperated upon, 84 per cent had unrepaired avulsions of the capsule and labrum from the anterior glenoid rim. Excessive laxity was thought to be the primary cause of instability in four shoulders. Twenty-two of the 24 shoulders reoperated on with a Bankart repair and followed for at least two years had a good or excellent result. Our experience is similar: recurrence rarely follows anterior repairs unless the initial procedure fails to treat significant pathology, such as capsular avulsions from the glenoid, huge bony defects from the glenoid and humeral head, or generalized laxity.

The third major category of complications arises from *failure of diagnosis*. It is essential to differentiate traumatic unidirectional instability (TUBS syndrome) from atraumatic multidirectional instability (AMBRI syndrome) before carrying out any surgical repair. The consequences of mistaking multidirectional instability for pure anterior instability are substantial. In this situation, if only the anterior structures are tightened, limited external rotation and posterior subluxation may lead to the rapid loss of glenohumeral articular cartilage and postsurgical degenerative joint disease. This complication can be prevented only by accurate preoperative diagnosis. It also points out the necessity for preserving external rotation during the postoperative period and reassessing with axillary roentgenograms any shoulder that appears to vary from the expected course.

The fourth category of operative complications consists of *neurovascular injuries*. The musculocutaneous nerve runs as a single or multipartite structure obliquely through the coracobrachialis, a variable distance distal to the coracoid process. In this location it may be injured by (1) dissection to free up the coracoid process, (2) retraction, or (3) inclusion in suture.[502] Helfet[212] described one case in which the nerve had a high penetration into the coracobrachialis and became impinged where the conjoined tendon entered the slit made in the subscapularis tendon. The axillary nerve may be injured in dissection and suture of the inferior capsule and subcapularis. Rockwood specifically recommends that the axillary nerve be routinely palpated and protected with a retractor during anterior reconstructions, especially during a capsular shift reconstruction.[455] Richards and associates[451] presented nine patients sustaining brachial plexus injuries during anterior shoulder repair (three Bristows and six Putti-Platts). Seven involved the musculocutaneous nerve and two the axillary nerve. Two of the nerves were lacerated, five injured by suture, and two injured by traction. These nerve injuries are relatively more common during reoperation after a previous repair; in this situation the nerves are tethered by scar tissue and thus are more difficult to mobilize out of harm's way. Neurovascular complications can best be avoided by good knowledge of local anatomy (including the possible normal variations), good surgical technique, and a healthy respect for the change in position and mobility of the neurovascular structures after a previous surgical procedure in the area.

The fifth category of complications includes those related to *hardware* inserted about the glenohumeral joint.[81, 210] The screw used to fix the coracoid fragment in Bristow procedures has a particular potential for being problematic.[385, 439] This may be because the coracoid muscles tend to rotate the fragment as the arm is raised and lowered; this rotation may contribute to screw loosening. Artz and Huffer[19] have reported a devastating complication following use of a screw to

secure the coracoid process. The screw became loose and caused a false aneurysm of the axillary artery with a subsequent compression of the brachial plexus and paralysis of the upper extremity.

The axillary artery has been injured by screws placed for Bristow procedures; a false aneurysm of this vessel has been reported as late as three years after surgery.[155] In other instances the screw has damaged the articular surface of the glenoid and humeral head when placed too close to the glenoid lip, irritated the infraspinatus or its nerve when too long, or affected the brachial plexus when it became loose. Staples used to attach the capsule to the glenoid may miss their target, damaging the humeral or glenoid articular cartilage. Staples also may become loose from repeated pull of the muscles and capsule during shoulder usage, particularly if they were not well seated in the first place. O'Driscoll and Evans[397] reported an 11 per cent incidence of staple complications after the DuToit procedure. If screws and staples migrate into the intra-articular region, significant damage to the joint surfaces may result. Metal fixation may injure the biceps tendon in a Magnuson-Stack procedure.

Zuckerman and Matsen[576] reported a series of patients with problems related to the use of screws and staples about the glenohumeral joint; 21 had problems related to the Bristow procedure and 14 to the use of staples (either for capsulorrhaphy or subscapularis advancement). The time between placement and symptom onset ranged from 4 weeks to 10 years. Screws and staples had been incorrectly placed in 10 patients, had migrated or loosened in 24, and had fractured in 3. Almost all patients required reoperation, at which time 41 per cent had a significant injury to one or both of the joint surfaces.

One can only conclude that hardware-free methods of managing glenohumeral instability are safer. The recurrence rates of techniques using screws and staples are no better than with hardware-free repairs. Risks are incurred with hardware that simply do not exist with other repair techniques. The depth and variable orientation of the glenoid at surgery provides substantial opportunity for hardware misplacement (into the joint, under the articular cartilage, subperiosteally, out the back, too high, too low, too medial, too prominent anteriorly, and too insecurely). The large range of motion of the shoulder with frequent vigorous challenges to its stability creates an opportunity for hardware loosening and for irreversible surface and neurovascular damage.

The sixth category of complications is *limited motion*. Limited range of motion, especially external rotation, has been reported after the Magnuson-Stack and the Putti-Platt procedures. It has also been noted after the Bristow procedure, which was supposed to be free of this problem.[30, 60, 223] Hovelius and colleagues[233] reported an average loss of external rotation of 21 degrees with the arm in abduction. This loss of range compromises function. In their series of 46 patients with continuing problems after shoulder reconstruc-

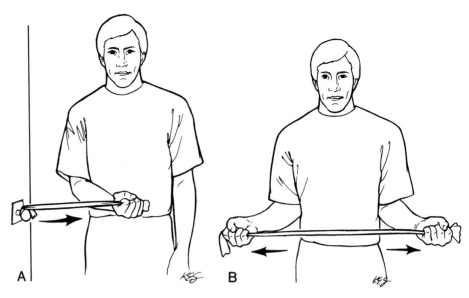

Figure 14–72. Internal and external rotator–strengthening exercises using rubber band. *A,* Internal rotator–strengthening exercise with rubber tube secured to the door. The elbow must be maintained close to the patient's side and flexed at 90 degrees. *B,* External rotator–strengthening exercise. Elbows are held close to the patient's side and in 90 degree flexion.

tion, Hawkins and Hawkins[209] found that 10 had stiffness related to limited external rotation. Excessive limitation of external rotation has a high association with the subsequent development of osteoarthritis. Angelo and Hawkins[13] reported eight patients with disabling degenerative arthritis presenting an average of 15.1 years after a Putti-Platt procedure. None of the patients had ever developed external rotation beyond zero degrees after their repair.

Matsen's Preferred Method of Surgical Treatment for Recurrent Traumatic Shoulder Instability

My approach to traumatic anterior instability (TUBS syndrome) is discussed here.[526a] The treatment of atraumatic instability (AMBRI syndrome) is presented in the earlier section on atraumatic instability. My nonoperative program for recurrent anterior instability includes vigorous rotator strengthening and coordina-

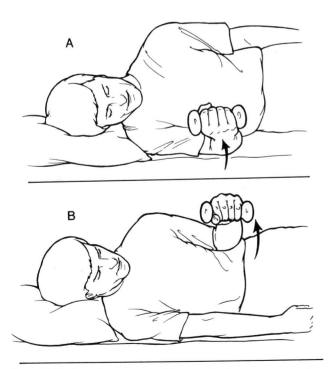

Figure 14–73. Internal and external rotator–strengthening exercises using free weights. *A,* Internal rotator strengthening. *B,* External rotator strengthening.

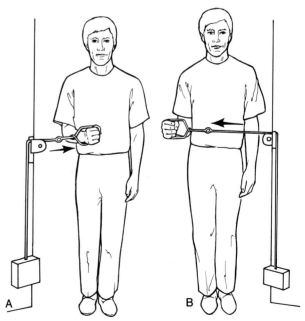

Figure 14–74. Internal and external rotator–strengthening exercises using wall weights. *A,* Internal rotator strengthening. The elbow is held close to the side in 90-degree flexion. *B,* External rotator strengthening. The elbow is held close to the patient's side and flexed 90 degrees.

Table 14–3. FOUR STAR EXERCISE PROGRAM
FOR OPTIMIZING SHOULDER STABILITY

★1. Develop shoulder rotator strength.
Perform internal and external rotator–strengthening exercises.
Rubber tubing (Fig. 14–72).
Decubitus curls (Fig. 14–73).
Wall weights (Fig. 14–74).
Perform exercises two to five times per day, selecting a resistance that
will allow 20 repetitions.
Advance until the patient can perform 20 repetitions against 20 per cent
of body weight.

★2. Develop shoulder coordination and endurance.
Swim three to five times per week.
Avoid breast stroke if it causes symptoms of posterior instability.
Avoid back stroke and butterfly if they cause symptoms of anterior
instability.
Work up to an average of ½ hour every other day.

★3. Avoid competitive basketball, volleyball, football, kayaking, and other
violent overhead sports until goals of Steps 1 and 2 are attained.

★4. Maintain general conditioning with aerobic workouts such as brisk walking,
jogging, swimming, biking, and rowing. Sustain these exercises for ½
hour at least four times per week.

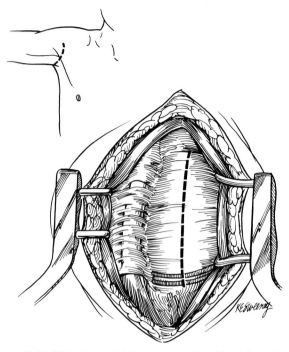

Figure 14–75. Skin incision and deltopectoral split. Dotted line indicates incision through subscapularis and capsule. (Reproduced with permission from Matsen FA, and Thomas SC: Glenohumeral instability. *In* Evarts CM (ed): Surgery of the Musculoskeletal System, 2nd ed. New York: Churchill Livingstone, 1989.)

tion exercises (for example, swimming). I present this to the patient as the Four Star program (Table 14–3). Although this program will not cure most cases of traumatic instability, it will frequently enhance function. At a minimum it introduces the patient to the rehabilitation program that would be used after a surgical repair.

The patient desiring surgical stabilization is presented with a frank discussion of the risks and alternatives. The relative importance to the patient of (1) a full range of motion and (2) stability is determined so that the procedure and postoperative care can be biased in the desired direction. Baseball pitchers have a requirement for more shoulder capsular laxity. Skiers or football linemen require more stability. A preoperative arthrogram is obtained in patients over 30 years of age if there is pain between episodes of dislocation or weakness of external rotation. Electromyograms are obtained if nerve injury is suspected.

After a thorough preoperative evaluation the patient is taken to the operating room, where either a brachial plexus block or a general anesthetic is administered. The glenohumeral joint is examined under anesthesia. Although this examination rarely changes the procedure performed, it provides helpful confirmation of the diagnosis. The direction of translation may be documented by axillary and/or anteroposterior roentgenograms taken while the surgeon stresses the glenohumeral joint. Most normal shoulders translate posteriorly for a distance of about 50 per cent of the humeral head diameter.

The patient is positioned in a slight head-up position (approximately 20 degrees) with the scapula off the edge of the operating table. This position provides a full range of humeral and scapular mobility, and, if necessary, access to the posterior aspect of the shoulder. The major axillary skin crease is marked with ink or dye. The neck, chest, axilla, and entire arm are

prepared with iodine solution. Draping includes application of adherent, transparent plastic to the exposed area to minimize contact with the axillary skin.

The 8-cm skin incision is centered on the inferior border of the pectoralis major tendon and located in the previously marked axillary skin crease.[24] This incision heals with a very pleasing cosmetic result if closed with subcuticular suture and sterile paper tape (Fig. 14–75). The skin and subcutaneous tissue are undermined up to the level of the coracoid process, which is then used as a guide to the cephalic vein and the deltopectoral groove (Fig. 14–76). The groove is

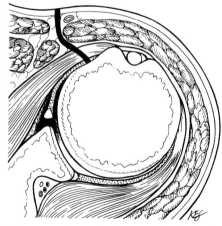

Figure 14–76. Transverse plane section from a superior view showing the incision and the plane for exposure. Note that the deltopectoral interval is utilized. The subscapularis tendon and the underlying joint capsule are incised as a unit 1 cm medial to the insertion. (Reproduced with permission from Matsen FA, and Thomas SC: Glenohumeral instability. *In* Evarts CM (ed): Surgery of the Musculoskeletal System, 2nd ed. New York: Churchill Livingstone, 1989.)

opened by spreading with the two index fingers medial to the cephalic vein. A consistent neurovascular bundle (a branch of the thoracoacromial artery and the lateral pectoral nerve) is identified in the upper third of the groove;[195] this bundle is cauterized and transected. The clavipectoral fascia is seen lateral to the coracoid muscles (the coracobrachialis and the short head of the biceps). This fascia is divided up to but not through the coracoacromial ligament, exposing the subjacent subscapularis tendon and lesser tuberosity.

The surgeon's index finger is then passed medially along the subscapularis to palpate the axillary nerve coursing inferolaterally. At this point it is useful to insert a self-retaining retractor, with one blade on the deltoid muscle and the other on the coracoid muscles (Fig. 14–77). Rotating the arm from internal to external rotation reveals, in succession, the greater tuberosity, the bicipital groove, the lesser tuberosity, and the subscapularis. The anterior circumflex humeral vessels marking the inferior border of the subscapularis may be cauterized, but we prefer to retract them inferiorly.

The interval between the supraspinatus and subscapularis tendons is identified by palpation, and a blunt elevator is inserted through this interval into the joint. This elevator brings the upper subscapularis into the incision. The subscapularis tendon is tagged with a suture 2 cm medial to the lesser tuberosity. The subscapularis tendon and subjacent capsule are then incised together approximately 1 cm medial to the lesser tuberosity, beginning at the superior rounded edge of the tendon and extending inferiorly to the anterior circumflex humeral vessels (see Fig. 14–75). If necessary for greater exposure, the joint capsule may be

further divided along the coracohumeral ligament, just medial to the intra-articular biceps tendon. Without separating them, the subscapularis tendon and anterior shoulder capsule are reflected medially, providing an excellent view of the joint. Visualization of the capsule and glenoid is facilitated by the careful insertion of a humeral head retractor, which leans on the posterior glenoid lip and pushes the humeral head posterolaterally. The capsule is pulled tight by applying traction to its cut edge while the junction of the capsular ligaments to the glenoid is palpated. This area is also exposed for inspection using a narrow right-angle retractor (Fig. 14–78). A small (less than 1 cm) defect is normally found in the capsule just below the coracoid process, the articular opening of the subcoracoid recess. This should not be confused with a Bankart lesion. In the TUBS syndrome, the vast majority of shoulders demonstrate detachment of the glenohumeral ligaments from the anterioinferior bony rim of the glenoid. The labrum usually remains attached to the capsular ligaments but may remain on the glenoid side of the rupture, may be a separate ("bucket handle") fragment, or may be absent.

The glenohumeral joint is inspected thoroughly for loose bodies, defects of the bony glenoid, tears of the glenoid labrum, and tears of the rotator cuff. In traumatic anterior instability, a posterolateral humeral head defect is usually palpable by passing an index finger over the top of the head while putting longitudinal traction on the arm. Approximately 50 per cent of my TUBS patients have moderate to large humeral head defects; this finding does not change my treatment. Massive humeral head defects in this location may require tightening of the anterior structures to

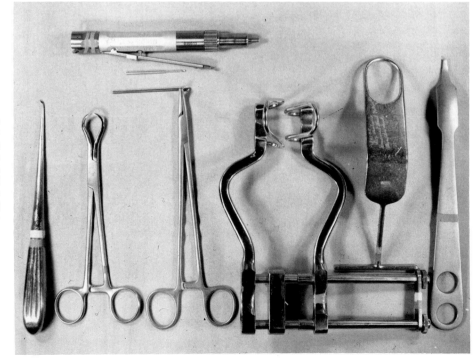

Figure 14–77. Instruments for surgical repairs of recurrent glenohumeral instability. *Top:* high-speed drill used for drilling holes in the glenoid rim. *Left* to *right:* small angled curette and reaming tenaculum used to connect the holes drilled in the glenoid rim; curved-nosed needle holder for passing a No. 5 Mayo needle through these holes; self-retaining retractor; humeral head retractor; and sharp-tipped levering retractor.

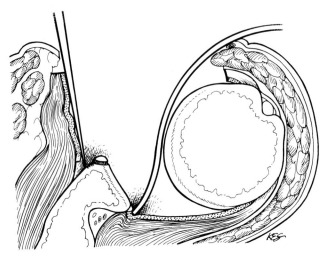

Figure 14–78. Transverse plane section showing placement of retractors and location of drill holes. Note the area roughened by curette along the anterior glenoid neck; also note the position of the drill hole relative to the anterior glenoid rim. (Reproduced with permission from Matsen FA, and Thomas SC: Glenohumeral instability. *In* Evarts CM (ed): Surgery of the Musculoskeletal System, 2nd ed. New York: Churchill Livingstone, 1989.)

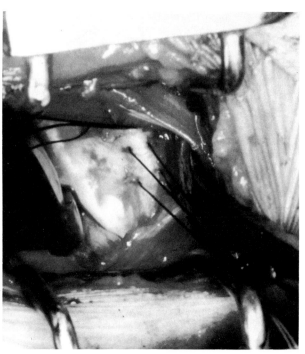

Figure 14–79. Intraoperative photograph of the Bankart procedure showing the placement of sutures through holes in the glenoid rim.

keep them from entering the joint on external rotation, but this is highly unusual. The supraspinatus and infraspinatus tendons are palpated to check their integrity, especially in patients over the age of 30. Finally, the biceps tendon is inspected and note taken of the integrity of the transverse humeral ligament. At this point the surgeon has a complete idea of the anatomical factors contributing to the glenohumeral instability.

In my experience, 97 per cent of patients with the TUBS syndrome have a rupture of the glenoid attachment of the middle and/or inferior glenohumeral ligaments. In my view, the repair of these ligamentous detachments is necessary and sufficient for the repair of the traumatic instability. This repair is carried out from inside the joint, without needing to separate the capsule from the subscapularis muscle and tendon.

The glenoid is well exposed by a humeral head retractor laterally and a sharp-tipped levering retractor inserted through the capsular defect onto the neck of the glenoid. Bucket handle or flap tears of the glenoid labrum are excised.[1, 32] The anterior, nonarticular surface of the glenoid is prepared by curettage down to bleeding bone. A 1.8-mm drill is used to make holes for the passage of suture. Holes are spaced 6 mm apart; the number of holes is determined by the size of the capsular defect (Fig. 14–79). On the articular side, the holes are placed 4 mm from the anterior edge of the glenoid. On the anterior aspect, corresponding holes are also made 4 mm from the anterior edge of the glenoid edge. These pairs of holes are then connected using a 000 angled curette (Fig. 14–80). No. 2 nonabsorbable suture is then passed through these holes using a No. 5 Mayo needle and a curved needle holder (Figs. 14–77 and 14–81). Traction is applied to each suture to ensure that it has a firm purchase on the bony glenoid.

When sufficient sutures have been placed to repair the capsular defect, the sharp-tipped levering retractor is removed and replaced by a right-angled retractor positioned to show the detached medial edge of the capsule, which is most easily identified by tracing the capsular edge from where it remains attached to the

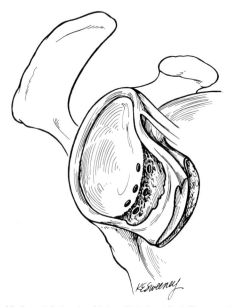

Figure 14–80. Anteroinferior glenoid rim with holes drilled. The nonarticular edge has been curetted, and the holes have been carefully placed 4 mm from the glenoid rim to afford strong fixation. Note the reflection of the capsule in the typical location of the Bankart lesion, 3 to 6 o'clock. (Reproduced with permission from Matsen FA, and Thomas SC: Glenohumeral instability. *In* Evarts CM (ed): Surgery of the Musculoskeletal System, 2nd ed. New York: Churchill Livingstone, 1989.)

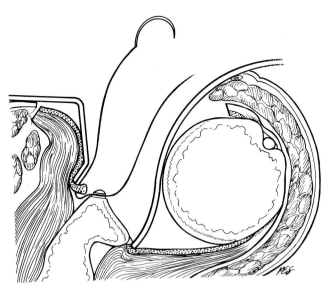

Figure 14–81. Transverse plane section showing passage of a No. 2 nonabsorbable suture through the drill hole and into the capsule. Note the use of a deep right-angle retractor on the subscapularis and superficial capsule to afford the necessary exposure for proper placement of the suture. (Reproduced with permission from Matsen FA, and Thomas SC: Glenohumeral instability. *In* Evarts CM (ed): Surgery of the Musculoskeletal System, 2nd ed. New York: Churchill Livingstone, 1989.)

glenoid. The limb of each suture exiting the holes in the anterior glenoid is then passed through the detached medial edge of the capsule, taking just enough tissue to ensure a secure bite. The capsular repair is completed by tying these sutures so that the knots lie against the articular surface of the capsule (Fig. 14–82). The capsular repair is checked by palpation and

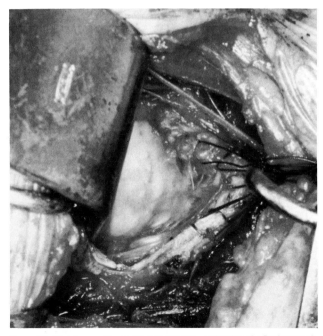

Figure 14–82. Intraoperative photograph during re-exploration of a Bankart repair. This patient ruptured his subscapularis tendon repair several months after a Bankart procedure. At the time of reoperation for repair of the subscapularis tendon, the anterior glenoid rim was explored and the Bankart repair was intact. The repair sutures were covered by synovium.

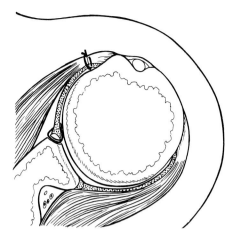

Figure 14–83. Transverse plane section showing the completed repair of a Bankart lesion and the anatomical repair of an incision through the subscapularis and the capsule. (Reproduced with permission from Matsen FA, and Thomas SC: Glenohumeral instability. *In* Evarts CM (ed): Surgery of the Musculoskeletal System, 2nd ed. New York: Churchill Livingstone, 1989.)

under direct vision to ensure that it is complete and strong.

Approximately 10 per cent of TUBS patients have fractures or deficiencies of the anterior bony lip of the glenoid. Anterior glenoid deficiencies of up to 33 per cent of the articular surface are managed in a similar way with direct repair of capsular ligaments to the edge of the articular surface. I am reluctant to use bone blocks because of the adverse effects of nonphysiological contact with the articular surface of the humeral head.

Once the capsular avulsion is repaired, the lateral capsule and subscapularis tendons are repaired back to the lesser tuberosity in their anatomical positions (Fig. 14–83). This repair minimizes any restriction of external rotation. Once this repair has been completed, the shoulder stability is examined. If anterior laxity remains (which is rarely the case), the lateral capsular and subscapularis reattachment may be advanced laterally or superolaterally as desired (Fig. 14–84).

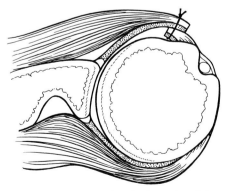

Figure 14–84. Transverse plane section showing reefing of the subscapularis tendon and capsule in a situation where no Bankart lesion is found with isolated anterior instability. Note the intact anterior glenoid rim and the strong repair of the subscapularis tendon. (Reproduced with permission from Matsen FA, and Thomas SC: Glenohumeral instability. *In* Evarts CM (ed): Surgery of the Musculoskeletal System, 2nd ed. New York: Churchill Livingstone, 1989.)

In the rather unusual situation (3 per cent of cases or less) in which a shoulder with the TUBS syndrome is found not to have capsular detachment, the anterior laxity is treated by reefing the anterior capsule and the subscapularis tendon. Shortening these structures by 1 cm limits external rotation of the humerus by approximately 20 degrees. Generally, restricting external rotation to 30 degrees at the operating table will permit a very functional shoulder after rehabilitation is complete. If the patient has marked anterior ligamentous laxity, proportionately greater anterior tightening may be necessary, although the surgeon must be certain that the patient does not have multidirectional laxity before a unidirectional tightening is carried out.

After the operation, the shoulder is held for two weeks in a conventional sling. The elbow is straightened twice daily to avoid sling soreness. This period of immobilization may be lengthened in young patients, particularly those with generalized ligamentous laxity, or if patients are unreliable. The period is shortened in patients over the age of 30, when chronic shoulder stiffness is more likely. During immobilization, the tone of the shoulder musculature is maintained by isometric abduction and external rotation exercises. These are started on the first day after surgery. The repaired subscapularis tendon is protected for six weeks by avoiding active internal rotation against resistance. The Four Star rehabilitation program is initiated six weeks after surgery. My goal is near-normal motion 12 weeks after surgery.

It is important to be observant for excessive anterior tightness. If anterior stiffness appears to be a potential problem (such as external rotation limited to zero degrees in a 35-year-old four weeks postoperatively), forward flexion and external rotation stretching exercises are started. An axillary roentgenogram should be taken to exclude the possibility of posterior displacement of the humeral head. Patients are allowed to return to sports and vigorous labor after three months and after they have regained full forward elevation and excellent rotator strength of the operated shoulder. Patients are advised that maintaining rotator strength will increase the dynamic stability of the glenohumeral joint and decrease the likelihood of further injury. Swimming is routinely recommended to develop and maintain coordination and endurance of the shoulder. This exercise is usually started six to eight weeks after operation.

In a 5.5-year follow-up of my first group of repairs of this type, I found 97 per cent good to excellent results based on Rowe's[462] grading system. One of 39 shoulders had a single redislocation four years after repair while the patient was practicing karate. He has been rendered asymptomatic by a strengthening program and is back to full activities including karate. The average range of motion at follow-up was 171 degrees of elevation, 68 degrees of external rotation with the arm at the side, and 85 degrees of external rotation at 90 degrees of abduction. Ninety-five per cent of my patients reported that their shoulder felt stable with all activities; 80 per cent had no shoulder pain while 20 per cent had occasional pain with activity. None had complications of posterior subluxation due to excessive anterior tightness. None had complications related to hardware!

Rockwood's Preferred Method of Surgical Treatment of Traumatic Shoulder Instability

Prior to surgery, all of my patients are instructed in a series of exercises designed to strengthen the rotator cuff, deltoid, and the scapular stabilizers (see Fig. 14–94). Currently and for the past ten years, my preferred method of surgical repair has been an anatomical reconstruction, i.e., repair of the Perthes/Bankart lesion and/or a double-breasting of the capsule. I rarely have to overlap and thus shorten the subscapularis tendon.

The standard anterior axillary incision begins in the anterior axillary crease, extending up toward and usually stopping at the coracoid process (Fig. 14–85A). In large muscular men, the incision may extend proximally as far as the clavicle. In women, I use the modified axillary incision as described by Leslie and Ryan.[298] The skin is undermined subcutaneously in the proximal medial corner and the distal lateral corner so as to expose the deltopectoral interval (Fig. 14–85B). Usually this interval is identified by the presence of the cephalic vein (Fig. 14–85C), which may be either absent or lying deep in the interval out of sight. When the vein is not present I can define the deltopectoral interval proximally, because in this area it is easier to see the difference in angles of the muscle fibers between the pectoralis major and the deltoid. The interval should be very carefully opened, taking the vein *laterally* with the deltoid muscle. To routinely ligate the vein produces venous congestion in the area and in the upper extremity and increases the postoperative discomfort. Preservation of the vein contributes to an easier postoperative course (i.e., less pain and less swelling). I use 8-0 nylon suture to repair an inadvertent nick in the vein. The deltopectoral interval is developed all the way up to the clavicle, and there is no need to detach any of the deltoid from the clavicle. I usually detach the upper 2 cm of the pectoralis major tendon. This allows for better visualization of the inferior capsule and makes it easier to locate and protect the axillary nerve, which passes *just inferior* to the capsule. I do not find it necessary to detach the coracoid process or the conjoined tendons (Fig. 14–85D). With the deltopectoral muscles retracted out of the way, the clavipectoral fascia is seen covering the conjoined tendons. This fascia is divided vertically along the lateral border of the conjoined tendons. Proximally, the clavipectoral fascia blends into the coracoacromial ligament; I always divide this ligament at the time of a surgical procedure about the shoulder as it may prevent future symptoms of the impingement syndrome.

Before a Richardson retractor is placed in the medial

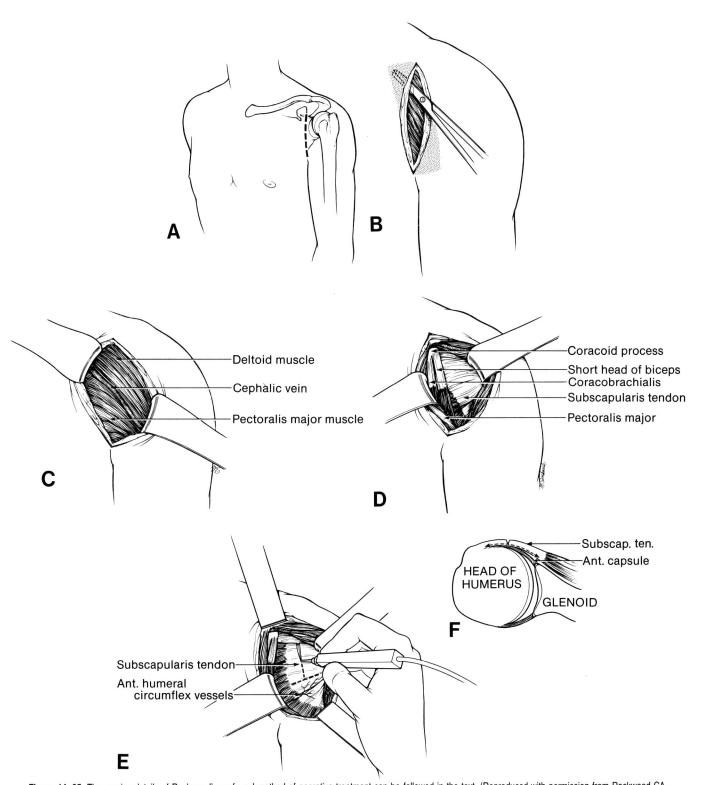

A

B

C

- Deltoid muscle
- Cephalic vein
- Pectoralis major muscle

D

- Coracoid process
- Short head of biceps
- Coracobrachialis
- Subscapularis tendon
- Pectoralis major

E

- Subscapularis tendon
- Ant. humeral circumflex vessels

F

- Subscap. ten.
- Ant. capsule

HEAD OF HUMERUS

GLENOID

Figure 14–85. The precise details of Rockwood's preferred method of operative treatment can be followed in the text. (Reproduced with permission from Rockwood CA, and Green DP (eds): Fractures (3 vols), 2nd ed. Philadelphia: JB Lippincott, 1984.)

Illustration continued on following page

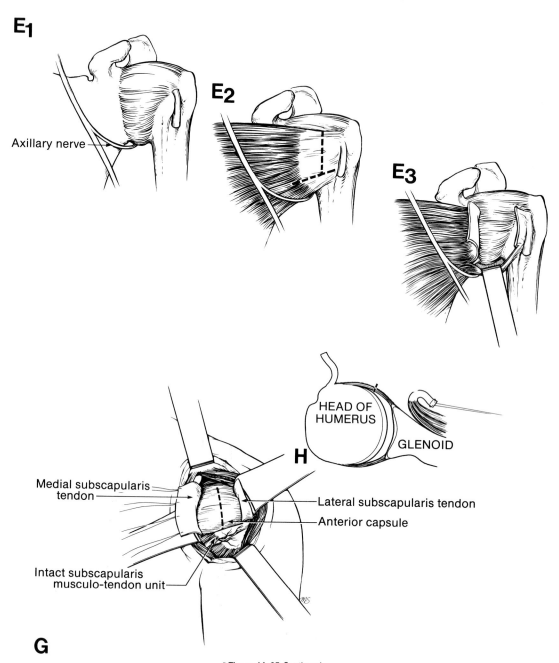

E₁

Axillary nerve

E₂

E₃

H

HEAD OF
HUMERUS

GLENOID

Medial subscapularis
tendon

Lateral subscapularis tendon

Anterior capsule

Intact subscapularis
musculo-tendon unit

G

`Figure 14–85 Continued

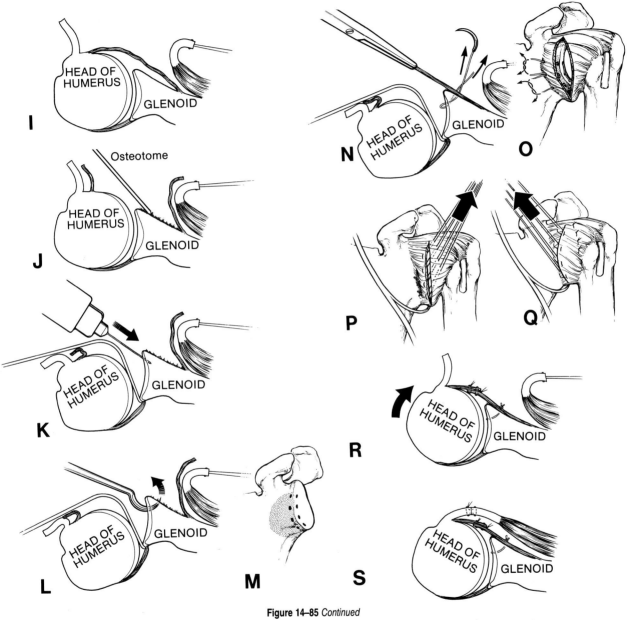

Figure 14–85 *Continued*

side of the incision to retract the conjoined muscles and pectoralis major muscle, I palpate for the location of the musculocutaneous nerve as it enters the conjoined tendon. Ordinarily the nerve enters the coracobrachialis and biceps muscles from the medial aspect approximately 5 cm distal to the tip of the coracoid process. However, it must be remembered that it might penetrate immediately below the tip of the coracoid. I have even seen the nerve visible on the lateral aspect of the conjoined tendon! Usually, by palpating just medial to the conjoined tendon and muscles, one can feel the entrance of the musculocutaneous nerve.

Next, I locate the axillary nerve—an especially important step when performing the capsular shift procedure. This is done by passing the finger down and along the lower and intact subscapularis muscle tendon unit (Fig. 14–85E_1–E_3). The right index finger should be used to locate the nerve in the left shoulder and the left index finger should be used to locate the nerve in the right shoulder. When the finger is as deep as it will go, the volar surface of the finger should be on the anterior surface of the muscle. Then the distal phalanx is flexed and rotated anteriorly, which will hook under the axillary nerve before it dives back posteriorly under the inferior capsule. With the arm in external rotation the nerve is displaced medially, making it difficult to locate. This large nerve can be easily located with the arm in adduction and in neutral rotation. With the upper 2 cm of the pectoralis major tendon taken down, not only can the nerve be palpated, it also can be visualized. The nerve is at least 5/32 inch in size.

With the arm in external rotation, the upper and lower borders of the subscapularis tendon can be visualized and palpated. The "soft spot" at the superior border of the subscapularis tendon is the interval between the subscapularis and supraspinatus tendons. The lower border of the tendon is identified by the presence of the anterior humeral circumflex artery and veins. The upper three-fourths of the subscapularis tendon will be vertically transected usually ¾ to 1 inch medial to its insertion into the lesser tuberosity. I cut only the upper three-fourths of the subscapularis tendon and prefer to do this with the electric cautery (Fig. 14–85E, F). I am very careful to divide only the tendon. I usually try to leave a little of the subscapularis tendon on the capsule to add to its strength. I avoid transecting the lower fourth of the subscapularis tendon, leaving it in place to prevent injury to the anterior humeral circumflex artery and veins and protect the axillary nerve. The anterior humeral circumflex artery is the primary blood supply to the head of the humerus, and I believe that it should be preserved. Once the vertical cut in the tendon has been completed, I very carefully reflect the medial part of the tendon off the capsule, using curved Mayo scissors, until there are no further connections between the tendon and the capsule. When applying lateral traction on the tendon, it should have a rubbery bounce to it. Three or four stay sutures of No. 2 cottony Dacron are placed in the

medial edge of the tendon; these are used initially for retraction and later at the time of tendon repair. The lateral stump of the subscapularis tendon is reflected off the capsule with a small sharp knife. This is rather easy with the capsule intact when the arm is in external rotation and difficult when the capsule has been divided. Failure to perform this step will make the two-layer closure of the capsule and the subscapularis tendon more difficult.

With the divided portions of the subscapularis tendon reflected medially *and* laterally and with the arm in mild external rotation, I use an elevator to gently strip the intact lower fourth of the subscapularis muscle tendon unit off the anteroinferior capsule (Fig. 14–85E_3). A narrow deep retractor (i.e., Scofield) should be used to retract the lower part of the subscapularis muscle anteriorly and distally, which allows for easy visualization of the inferior capsule. The retractor holds not only the lower part of the subscapularis muscle but also the axillary nerve anteriorly and distally out of the way, preventing injury when the inferior capsule is opened and divided and repaired.

Next, the capsule is divided vertically *midway* between its usual attachment on the glenoid rim and the humeral head (Fig. 14–85G, H). I have found that is it easier to divide the capsule midway between the humeral head and glenoid attachments. This allows for repair of the capsule if there is a Perthes-Bankart lesion. Furthermore, after the medial capsule is reattached to the glenoid rim I have plenty of room to add strength to the anterior and inferior capsule by double-breasting it with the planned capsular reconstruction. This vertical incision begins at the superior glenohumeral ligament and extends all the way down to the most inferior aspect of the capsule. I prefer to insert the horizontal mattress sutures in the medial capsule *just* as I complete the division of the most interior portion of the capsule. I explore the joint carefully, removing loose bodies and glenoid labrum tears. Close attention should be paid for stripping of the labrum, capsule, and periosteum off their normal attachments on the glenoid rim and neck of the scapula, i.e., the Perthes-Bankart lesion (Fig. 14–85I).

If the capsule has a secure fixation on the glenoid rim, the capsular reconstruction can then be performed (Fig. 14–85P–Q). However, if stripping of the capsule and periosteum off the glenoid rim and neck of the scapula has occurred, this must first be reattached before proceeding to the capsular reconstruction (Fig. 14–85I–O). Formerly I believed that if there was a stripping of the capsule off the neck of the scapula, all that was needed was to roughen this up with a curette or osteotome to create bleeding and then the capsule would spontaneously reattach or heal itself back to the glenoid rim. However, because of failures I had to reoperate, and I found that this area had not healed and the capsule was still stripped off the glenoid neck. I am sure that synovial fluid inhibits the usual healing process and prevents a *consistent* firm reattachment of the capsule and periosteum to the bony glenoid rim.

In some situations it may be necessary to horizontally split the medial part of the capsule in its midportion to be able to better visualize and decorticate the anterior rim and neck of the scapula with an osteotome or an air bur. There is a special retractor, developed by Dr. Carter Rowe, that I call the "dinner fork" because of its shape and its three sharp teeth. It is used to retract the capsule and muscles out of the way while the anterior glenoid rim and neck of the scapula are decorticated and while the drill holes are being placed in the glenoid rim. I have tried a number of devices, including angle-dental drills and Hall drills, curved cutting gouges, clamps, and the Ellison glenoid rim punch; no matter what instrument is used, it always seems to be difficult to place these holes in the dense glenoid rim. With the Bowen, Rowe, or Fukuda retractor holding the humeral head out of the way and the "dinner fork" holding the medial capsule and muscles out of the way, I prefer to first use an osteotome to decorticate the anterior surface of the neck of the scapula down to raw cancellous bone. Usually three holes are then made between 3 and 6 o'clock on the anterior *articular* surface of the glenoid. These holes are made with a small drill bit approximately ⅛ inch in, from the rim of the glenoid on the articular surface (Fig. 14–85K). Next, a curved Carter Rowe awl and tenaculum are used to connect the drill holes with the decorticated neck of the anterior glenoid (Fig. 14–85L, M). I pass the No. 2 nonabsorbable cottony Dacron sutures through these holes so that there are two loops of intra-articular sutures through the three holes (the center hole has two sutures through it) (Fig. 14–85N, O).

The medial capsule is then pulled laterally and the needles on the intra-articular loops of sutures are passed up and through the medial capsule so that when they are tied, the capsule is reapproximated to the raw bone of the glenoid rim (Fig. 14–85N, O). I believe this step is absolutely critical to eliminate the abnormal pouch in the capsule.

With the medial capsule secured back to the glenoid rim, I proceed with the capsular reconstruction. Prior to closure of the capsule, the joint is thoroughly irrigated with saline. The medial capsule will be double-breasted laterally and superiorly under the lateral capsule (Fig. 14–85P). All of the sutures should be placed and tied, being sure that during this step the arm is held in neutral to 15 to 20 degrees of external rotation. In order to carry out this step, the lateral stump of the subscapularis tendon must have been separated from the lateral portion of the capsule. It is critical that the capsular reconstruction sutures be placed under the proper tension so that the arm may easily rotate to the desired position. Next, the lateral capsule is double-breasted by taking it medially and superiorly and suturing it down to the anterior surface of the medial capsule (Fig. 14–85Q, R). These sutures are also placed with the arm in the desired rotation. This type of capsular reconstruction not only eliminates all of the laxity in the anterior and inferior capsular

ligaments, but because of the double-breasting of the capsule it is much stronger. The wound is again carefully irrigated with several liters of saline.

With the arm held in 15 to 20 degrees of external rotation or in the neutral rotation position, the medial subscapularis tendon is then brought into view by pulling on the previously placed sutures. The two borders of the tendon are easily approximated with gentle traction, and tendon is repaired without any overlapping (Fig. 14–85S). If the tendon is noted to be loose with the arm in neutral rotation, then a double-breasting or overlapping of the tendon can be performed by using a two-layer closure with No. 2 Dacron horizontal mattress sutures.

Prior to closure of the wound I carefully irrigate with antibiotic solution and then infiltrate the joint, muscles, and subcutaneous tissue with about 25 to 30 ml of 0.5 per cent bupivacaine (Marcaine). This aids in decreasing the amount of immediate postoperative pain. I am impressed that the use of bupivacaine prior to wound closure gives the patient an easier postoperative recovery period. The effect of the bupivacaine will last from six to eight hours, which allows the patient, as he or she is waking up, to have relatively little pain; later in the day, as the anesthesia begins to wear off, he or she can request pain medications. Care should be taken not to overuse the bupivacaine or to inject it directly into vessels. It is usually unnecessary to put any sutures in the deltopectoral interval. The deep subcutaneous layer is closed with 2-0 nonabsorbable sutures, which helps to prevent widening of the scar. The subcutaneous fat is closed with absorbable sutures, and a running subcuticular nylon suture is used in the skin.

Postoperatively the patient's arm is stabilized in a shoulder immobilizer. As soon as the patient is awake, I assess and chart the neurovascular status of the extremity. Depending on the anesthesia, this can often be done on the operating room table before the patient is taken to the recovery room. The status of the pulses and the *axillary*, musculocutaneous, median, ulnar, and radial nerves can be determined and recorded within a few seconds.

Postoperatively I prefer to use a commercial shoulder immobilizer because it is comfortable, quick, and simple to apply and prevents abduction, flexion, and external rotation. Regardless of the type of immobilization, it is very important to temporarily remove the device when the patient is seen on the afternoon or evening of the day of surgery. For some reason, a patient who awakens from surgery with the arm in the "device" does not want to wiggle any part of the arm—almost as if it were frozen in the sling-and-swathe position. The commercial immobilizer can be easily removed; this allows the patient to move the hand and wrist and then gradually extend the elbow down to the side and lay it on the bed. This almost always relieves the aching pain in the arm and the muscle tension pain. I then tell the patient to flex and extend the elbow several times, which also relieves the generalized arm and shoulder discomfort. In many instances, a patient has related that the vague ache in the shoulder and elbow is more of a problem than pain at the operative site and that this simple release of the immobilizer, allowing movement of the elbow and wrist, eliminates the discomfort. I allow the patient to remove the immobilizer three to four times a day to exercise the elbow, but otherwise I instruct him or her to always keep the immobilizer in place. Specific instructions are given to the patient to avoid abduction, flexion, and external rotation when the device is removed.

Patients are usually dismissed on the second or third postoperative day, and I allow them to remove the immobilizer two or three times a day while at home when sitting, reading, or watching television. The patient can return to school or work any time after discharge from the hospital. At five days following surgery the patient can remove the small dressing, take a shower, and reapply the new bandage. I usually delay removing the running subcuticular nylon stitch for two weeks since this seems to help prevent a wide scar.

As a general rule, the older the patient, the shorter the postoperative immobilization; the younger the patient, the longer the immobilization. In young patients under the age of 20 or in the competitive, aggressive athlete, I immobilize the shoulder for three to four weeks; in young, semiathletic people under 30, shoulders are immobilized for three weeks; shoulders of patients under 50 are immobilized for two weeks; shoulders of patients over 50 are immobilized for one to two weeks. Following removal of the shoulder immobilizer, I allow the patient to gently use the arm for everyday living activities but do not allow any rough use (*e.g.,* lifting, moving furniture, pushing, pulling). At the end of the immobilization period, I start the patient on a stretching exercise program using an overhead pulley and rope set. Following the return of motion I institute a resisted weight exercise and shoulder-strengthening program to strengthen the deltoid, internal rotators, external rotators and the scapular stabilizers (see Fig. 14–94). Athletes are not permitted to return to competitive sports until they have reached a full and functional range of motion and have regained normal muscle strength; this usually requires four to six months.

Recurrent Posterior Instability

Nonoperative Management

As with anterior glenohumeral instability, strong subscapularis and infraspinatus muscles can significantly augment glenohumeral stability even in the presence of capsular laxity.[371] Voluntary instability is relatively common among patients with recurrent posterior glenohumeral instability;[371] in this population, nonoperative treatment is indicated. These patients may be helped by informing them of the nature of the problem, counseling them to avoid dislocation, and giving them exercises for strengthening the rotator muscles.

Operative Management

Surgical stabilization of posterior glenohumeral instability may be considered when recurrent involuntary posterior subluxations or dislocations occur in spite of a reasonable effort at the rehabilitation program. Prior to surgery it is essential to identify all directions of instability and any anatomical factors that may predispose the joint to recurrent instability, such as humeral head or glenoid defects, abnormal glenoid version, rotator cuff tears, neurological injuries, or generalized ligamentous laxity. It is important to consider the high recurrence and complication rates associated with attempted surgical correction of posterior instability. Hawkins and associates[209, 270] reported a 50 per cent failure rate following surgical procedures on recurrent posterior dislocation of the shoulder. Since functional limitations and pain can be minimal, they suggested that some of these patients may do better without reconstructive procedures. Tibone and coworkers[531] stated that recurrent posterior dislocation of the shoulder is not a definite indication for surgery and stressed the need for careful patient selection prior to surgical reconstruction. They reported a failure rate of 30 per cent following posterior staple capsulorrhaphy. Bayley and Kessel[38] stated that the failure to distinguish between traumatic and habitual (atraumatic) types of instability led to inappropriate surgery and was a major cause of recurrence following the operative repairs.

Several surgical approaches have been described for treatment of recurrent posterior glenohumeral instability. These approaches include scapular osteotomy,* posterior bone block,[369] and posterior soft tissue procedures.[191, 234, 301, 374, 472, 545]

Reverse Putti-Platt Procedure. The infraspinatus muscle and tendon is used in this muscle-shortening or muscle-plication procedure. In some cases the infraspinatus and teres minor tendon may be used together in the plication. Care must be taken not to injure the axillary nerve when the teres minor muscle tendon unit is used.

Boyd-Sisk[57] Procedure. The long head biceps tendon is transplanted posteriorly around the humerus to the posterior glenoid rim.

Glenoid Osteotomy and Bone Blocks. Kretzler and coworkers,[271, 272] Scott,[495] English and Macnab,[147] Bestard,[45] Vegter,[549] and Ahlgren and associates[7] have all reported using an opening, posterior wedge, glenoid osteotomy in recurrent posterior dislocations of the shoulder. In 1966 Kretzler and Blue[272] reported on the use of a posterior opening glenoid osteotomy in six patients with cerebral palsy. They used the acromion as the source of the graft to hold the wedge open. Kretzler[271] reported on 31 cases of the posterior glenoid osteotomy in voluntary (15 cases) and involuntary (16 cases) posterior dislocations with recurrences in 4 patients, 2 from each category. Extreme care must be taken during this procedure to prevent the osteotome

---

*See references 152, 188, 191, 199, 271, 272, 369, 495.

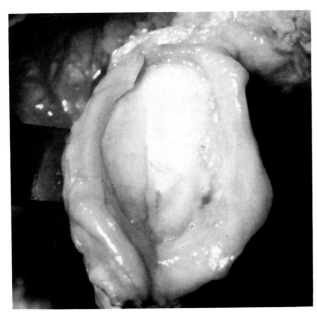

Figure 14–86. Cadaver dissection showing a fracture of the glenoid created during a posterior opening wedge osteotomy of the glenoid.

from entering into or causing a fracture of the posterior half of the glenoid (Fig. 14–86). The suprascapular nerve above and the axillary nerve below are also at risk. English and Macnab[147] have pointed out that there is a tendency for the humeral head to subluxate anteriorly after the osteotomy of the glenoid. Gerber and associates[186] demonstrated that posterior glenoid osteotomy thrusts the humeral head forward and potentially causes impingement of the humeral head on the coracoid, producing pain and dysfunction. Their cadaver studies demonstrated that glenoplasty "consistently produced impingement of the subscapularis between the coracoid tip and the humeral head."

The posterior bone block or the glenoid osteotomy has been combined with the various soft tissue reconstructions.[133] Mowery and associates[363] reported a series of five patients having a bone block for recurrent posterior dislocation. One patient had a subsequent anterior dislocation.

Hawkins and coworkers[207] presented 50 shoulders in 35 patients treated for recurrent posterior instability. Only 11 of the 50 followed a traumatic event; 41 demonstrated voluntary and involuntary instability. Of those operated upon, 17 patients had glenoid osteotomy, 6 had a reverse Putti-Platt procedure, and 3 had biceps tendon transfers. The dislocation rate after surgery was 50 per cent; complications occurred in 20 per cent of the operated cases. Two patients developed substantial degenerative osteoarthritis after glenoid osteotomy.

Matsen's Preferred Method of Treatment for Recurrent Posterior Glenohumeral Instability

Care is taken to identify the circumstances and directions of instability, the presence of generalized ligamentous laxity, and any anatomical factors that might potentially compromise the surgical result. I evaluate the possibilities of atraumatic and voluntary instability in each patient with posterior instability. All patients with posterior instability are placed on the Four Star rehabilitation program. A substantial number of patients with recurrent posterior instability respond to this program. Only straightforward patients who continue to have major symptomatic posterior instability after a reasonable rehabilitation effort are considered for surgery. These patients are told that the risks of surgery include excessive laxity (recurrent instability) and excessive tightness with limited flexion and internal rotation. A stress examination under anesthesia is routinely performed to confirm the diagnosis; stress x-rays are frequently used for documentation. The patient is placed almost prone with the shoulder off the operating table to allow a full range of humeral and scapular motion. After routine preparation of the arm, shoulder, neck, and back, a 10-cm incision is made in the extended line of the posterior axillary crease (Fig. 14–87A). The deltoid muscle is split for a distance of 4 cm between its middle and posterior thirds. If necessary, additional exposure may be obtained by carefully dissecting the muscle for a short distance from the scapular spine and posterior acromion. Retraction of the deltoid muscle inferiorly and laterally reveals the infraspinatus muscle, the teres minor muscle, and the axillary nerve emerging from the quadrangular space. The spinoglenoid notch is palpated to determine the location of the important nerve to the infraspinatus.

The infraspinatus, the teres minor, and the attached capsule are incised 1 cm from the greater tuberosity to expose the posterior glenohumeral joint (Fig. 14–87A–C). Excessive traction on the axillary nerve and the nerve to the infraspinatus is carefully avoided. The joint is inspected for humeral head defects, wear of the anterior or posterior glenoid, tears in the glenoid labrum, loose bodies, and tears of the rotator cuff. Posterior capsular avulsions are uncommon but, when present, are repaired by a technique similar to that described for anterior repair. In the usual case, the shoulder is stabilized by reefing the capsule along with the attached infraspinatus and teres minor tendons. This may be accomplished by overlapping the medial and lateral flaps by the desired amount or by advancing the capsule and tendon into a bony groove at the desired length (Fig. 14–87D). We usually try to limit internal rotation of the adducted humerus to 45 degrees. Internal rotation is limited by approximately 20 degrees for each centimeter of shortening of the posterior capsule and tendon (Fig. 14–87E). Greater tightening may be used in patients with generalized ligamentous instability.

If the patient demonstrates posteroinferior capsular laxity, the capsule is released from the inferior neck of the humerus under direct visualization as the humerus is progressively internally rotated. The capsule and muscle tendons are then advanced superiorly as well

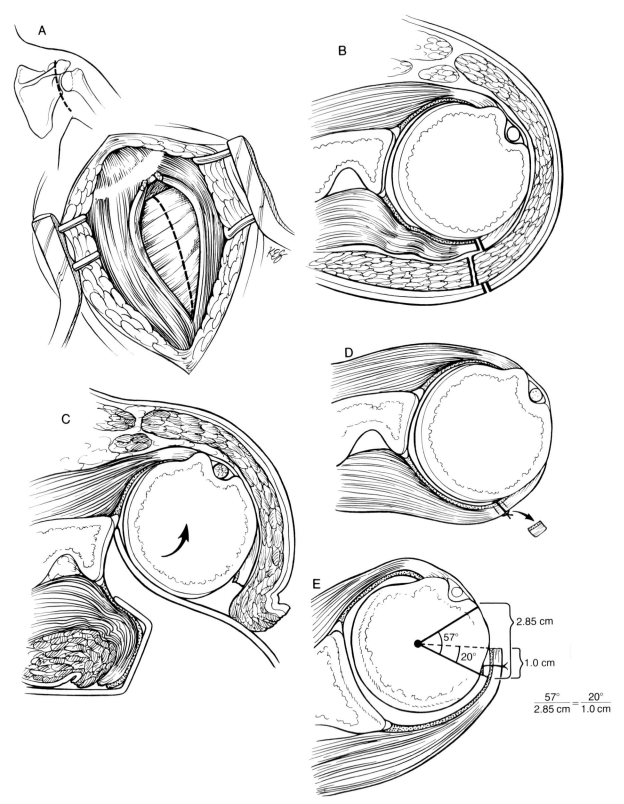

Figure 14–87. Operative repair for recurrent posterior glenohumeral instability. *A,* A 10-cm skin incision is made in the extended line of the posterior axillary crease (*inset*). The deltoid muscle is split between its middle and posterior thirds. *B,* A transverse plane section shows the interval through the deltoid muscle and the infraspinatus tendon. *C,* A transverse plane section shows placement of the retractors exposing the glenoid. *D,* A transverse plane section shows repair of the infraspinatus tendon after resecting the desired amount for capsular and tendon advancement. Shortening the posterior capsule and tendon by 1 cm will limit internal rotation by approximately 20 degrees. *E,* The effect of shortening capsular structures on limitation to rotation. The average radius of the humerus is 2.85 cm; this is the length of an arc equal to one radian, or approximately 57 degrees. Shortening the capsule by 2.85 cm would restrict rotation by 57 degrees. Proportionally, a 1-cm shortening of the capsule would restrict rotation by 20 degrees. Shown here is a posterior reefing of approximately 1 cm, decreasing internal rotation by approximately 20 degrees.

as laterally, tightening the axillary recess. If significant multidirectional instability is present, a formal inferior capsular shift may be performed.[371]

Anteromedial humeral head defects of moderate size are managed by tightening the posterior capsule so that internal rotation is limited to 30 degrees. A shoulder with an anterior humeral head defect constituting more than a third of the articular surface often cannot be stabilized by soft tissue surgery. In these instances insertion of a prosthetic head through the anterior approach will be required to restore stability and function to the glenohumeral joint. Because it changes the surgical approach a lesion of this size needs to be identified preoperatively.

When the indicated repair is complete, the deltoid is carefully repaired to the scapular spine and acromion. After surgery, the patient is immobilized in a "handshake" cummerbund cast with the shoulder in adduction, neutral rotation, and slight extension for three weeks, during which time internal rotation isometric exercises are instituted. After the cast is removed, the patient is allowed to perform more vigorous rotator-strengthening exercises and to use the shoulder below the horizontal. The patient is encouraged to regain forward flexion strength and range in concert with increases in external rotation strength, so that the repair has the backup of strong posterior cuff muscles. Patients are placed on the Four Star rehabilitation program (see Table 14–3) six to eight weeks after surgery. Vigorous shoulder activity is prohibited until normal rotator strength is achieved. The patient is advised to continue rotator strengthening–exercises on a daily basis to optimize dynamic shoulder stability.

Rockwood's Technique of Posterior Reconstruction

The patient is placed in the lateral decubitus position with the operative shoulder upward. The best way to support the patient in this position is to use the kidney supports and the "bean bag."

The incision begins 1 inch medial to the posterolateral corner of the acromion and extends downward 3 inches toward the posterior axillary creases[70a] (Fig. 14–88A). If a bone graft is to be taken from the acromion, the incision extends a little farther superiorly so that the acromion can be exposed (Fig. 14–88L). Next, the subcutaneous tissues are dissected medially and laterally so that the skin can be retracted to visualize the fibers of the deltoid (Fig. 14–88B).

A point 1 inch medial to the posterior corner of the acromion is selected, and the deltoid is then split distally 4 inches in the line of its fibers (Fig. 14–88C). The deltoid can be easily retracted medially and laterally to expose the underlying infraspinatus and teres minor muscles. This deltoid split can be made down to the midportion of the teres minor muscle. Remember that the axillary nerve exits the quadrangular space at the lower border of the teres minor muscle.

In performing a posterior reconstruction, the teres minor tendon should be reflected inferiorly down to the level of the inferior joint capsule. If the infraspinatus tendon is divided and reflected medially and laterally, care should be taken not to injure the suprascapular nerve. When the infraspinatus tendon is very lax, it can be reflected off the capsule and retracted superiorly without having to divide the tendon (Fig. 14–88D).

With the infraspinatus and teres minor muscles retracted out of the way, a vertical incision can be made in the posterior capsule to expose and explore the joint. I prefer to make the incision midway between the humeral and glenoid attachment so that at closure I can double-breast it and make it stronger (Fig. 14–88E, F). In doing the posterior capsular shift procedure, it is essential to have the teres minor muscle reflected sufficiently inferior so that the vertical cut in the capsule will go all the way down to the most inferior recess of the capsule. If the capsule is thin and friable, and it appears that a capsular shift alone will be insufficient, then the infraspinatus tendon can be divided so that it can be double-breasted to shorten it.

With the capsule divided all the way down inferiorly, horizontal mattress sutures of No. 2 cottony Dacron are inserted in the edge of the medial capsule. The arm should be held in neutral rotation and the medial capsule is sutured laterally and superiorly under the lateral capsule (Fig. 14–88N). Next, the lateral capsule is reflected and sutured medially and superiorly over the medial capsule and again held in place with horizontal mattress sutures (Fig. 14–87O). This capsular shift procedure has effectively eliminated any of the posterior and inferior capsular redundancy.

The infraspinatus tendon is next repaired; this should also be done with the arm in neutral rotation. If laxity exists, the tendon can be double-breasted (Fig. 14–88P). The wound is thoroughly irrigated, and the muscle and subcutaneous tissues are infiltrated with 25 to 30 ml of 0.5 per cent bupivacaine (Marcaine). Care must be taken not to overuse the bupivacaine or inject it directly into vascular channels.

When the retractors are withdrawn, the deltoid falls nicely together and a subcutaneous closure is performed. Care must be taken throughout the closure of the capsule, infraspinatus tendon, and skin to maintain the arm in neutral rotation. The patient is then gently rolled into the supine position, making sure that the arm is in neutral rotation. When the anesthetic is completed, the patient is transferred to his or her bed, where the arm is maintained in the neutral position and supported by skin traction. Usually within 24 hours following surgery the patient can stand, and a modified shoulder immobilizer cast is applied.

Posterior Glenoid Osteotomy. I do not use this as a routine part of my posterior reconstruction. Occasionally when there is a posterior glenoid deficiency, or in cases where there is a congenital retrotilt of the glenoid (i.e., greater than 30 degrees), then a posterior osteotomy should be considered. Care must be taken not to overcorrect the retroversion, as it may force the head out anteriorly. However, if a posterior osteotomy

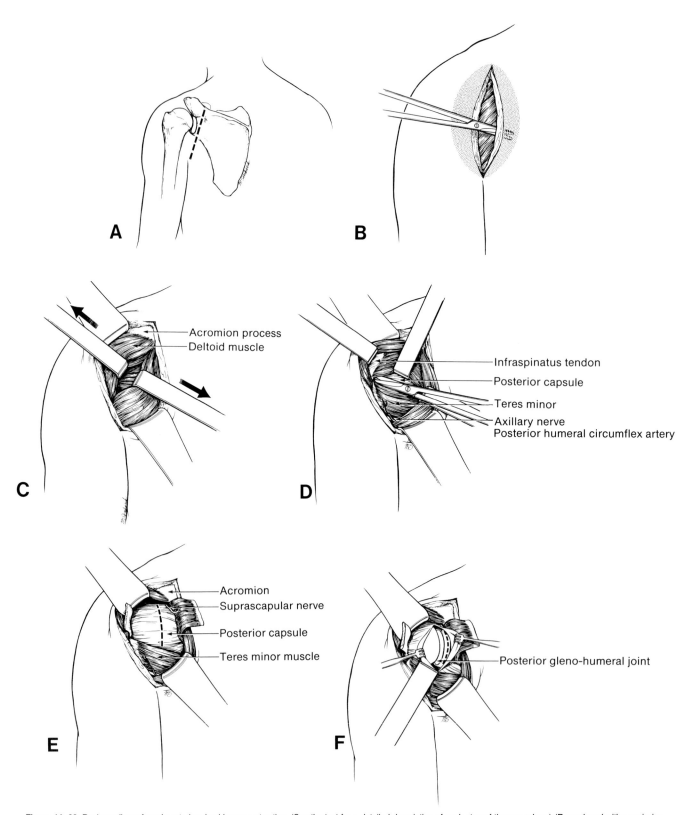

Figure 14–88. Rockwood's preferred posterior shoulder reconstruction. (See the text for a detailed description of each step of the procedure.) (Reproduced with permission from Rockwood CA, and Green DP (eds): Fractures (3 vols), 2nd ed. Philadelphia: JB Lippincott, 1984.)

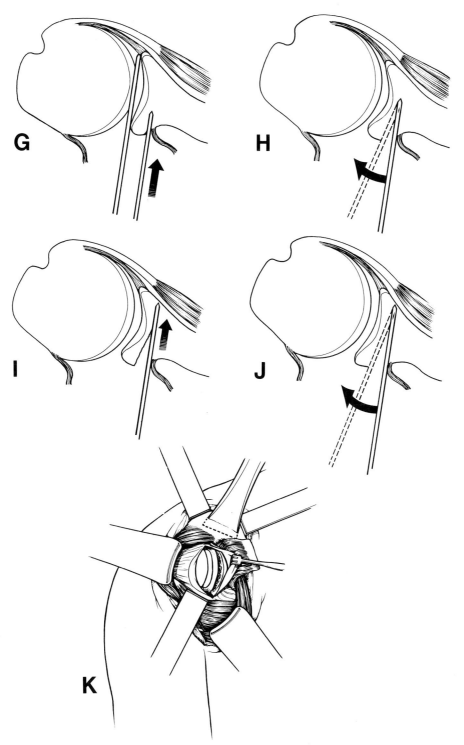

Figure 14–88 *Continued*

Illustration continued on following page

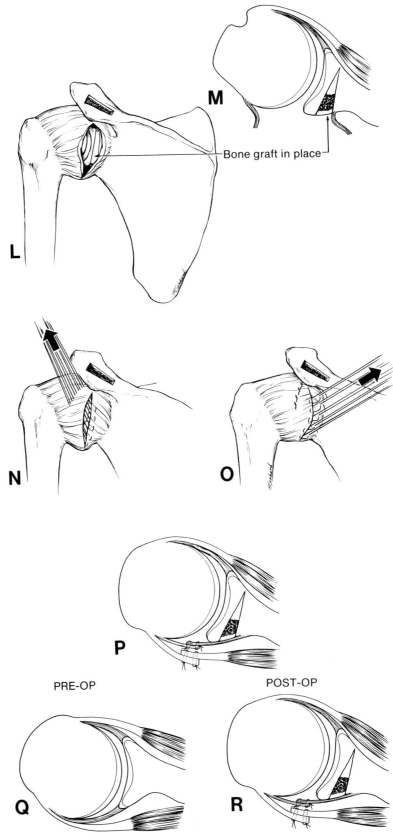

Bone graft in place

Figure 14–88 *Continued*

PRE-OP

POST-OP

is to be performed, it is absolutely essential to know the anatomy and angle of the slope of the glenoid. This can best be determined by placing a straight, blunt instrument into the joint so that it lies on the anterior and posterior glenoid rim (Fig. 14–88G). Next, the osteotome is placed intracapsularly and directed parallel to the blunt instrument. If one is unsure of the angle and does not have a guide instrument in place, there is the possibility of the osteotomy entering the joint (see Fig. 14–86). The osteotomy site is not more than ¼ inch medial to the articular surface of the glenoid. If the osteotomy is more medial than this, the possibility exists of injuring the suprascapular nerve as it passes around the base of the spine of the scapula to supply the infraspinatus muscle. Each time the osteotome is advanced, the osteotomy site is pried open (Fig. 14–88H, I); this helps to create a lateral plastic deformation of the posterior glenoid. The osteotomy should *not* exit anteriorly but should stop just at the anterior cortex of the scapula (Fig. 14–88J). The intact anterior cortex periosteum and soft tissue will act as a hinge, which allows the graft to be secure in the osteotomy without the need for internal fixation. I usually use an osteotome that is 1 inch wide to make the original cut and then use smaller ½-inch osteotomes superiorly and inferiorly to complete the posterior division of bone. Osteotomes are used to open up the osteotomy site, and the bone graft is placed into position (Fig. 14–88K and M). If the anterior cortex is partially intact, there is no need for any internal fixation of the graft because it is held securely in place by the osteotomy. The technique of the osteotomy has been described by Kretzler and associates,[271, 272] Scott,[495] and English and Macnab.[147] I prefer to take the bone graft from the acromion (Fig. 14–88K, L). Either a small piece (8 × 30 mm) for the osteotomy or a large piece (15 × 30 mm) for a posteroinferior bone block can be taken from the top or the posterior edge of the acromion. If a larger piece of graft is required, it should be taken from the ilium. Following completion of the osteotomy, the capsular shift, as described above, is performed.

As mentioned, following surgery the patient is supine with the forearm supported by the overhead bed frame, holding the arm in neutral rotation. I usually let the patient sit up on the bed the evening of surgery while maintaining the arm in neutral rotation. I let him or her sit up in a chair the next day, again holding the arm in neutral rotation. Either 24 or 48 hours after surgery, when the patient can stand comfortably, I apply a lightweight long arm cast. Next, a well-padded iliac crest band that sits around the abdomen and iliac crest is applied. The arm is then connected to the iliac crest band with a broom handle support to maintain the arm in 10 to 15 degrees of abduction and in neutral rotation. The cast is left in place for six to eight weeks. Following removal of the plaster, the patient is allowed to use the arm for four to six weeks for everyday living activities. A rehabilitation program is begun that includes pendulum exercises, isometric exercises, and stretching of the shoulder with the use of an overhead pulley, after which resistive exercises are gradually increased.

Complications

The principal cause of failure after a posterior repair is recurrent instability.[207, 374] As the patient begins to use the shoulder and to regain the normal flexion range, the posterior capsule must stretch out. Unless good dynamic stability is regained, dependence on the repaired capsule will continue and stretch it out. This loosening is hastened if the posterior soft tissues are of poor quality, if the patient voluntarily or habitually tries to translate the shoulder posteriorly, or if large bony defects excessively load the soft tissues.

Occasionally the opposite outcome can occur—posterior repair may produce a shoulder that is too tight, which may push the shoulder out anteriorly. Insufficient posterior laxity can limit flexion, cross-body adduction, and internal rotation.

Technical problems may occur in the surgical treatment of posterior glenohumeral instability. Posterior opening wedge osteotomy of the glenoid is difficult to perform without cracking through the subchondral bone. Posterior glenoid osteotomy may result in avascular necrosis or may push the humeral head too far anteriorly and give rise to postsurgical degenerative joint disease. Posterior bone blocks placed in an excessively prominent position may cause severe degenerative joint disease. The axillary nerve may be injured as it exits the quadrangular space, or the nerve to the infraspinatus may be injured in the spinoglenoid notch.[241, 374]

Recurrent Multidirectional Inferior and Voluntary Instability

Matsen's Approach to Treatment of Recurrent Inferior and Multidirectional Glenohumeral Instability

Inferior displacement of the head of the adducted humerus may indicate a torn or lax superior rotator cuff, suprascapular nerve palsy,[120] deltoid atony, or deltoid palsy. These specific lesions must be sought for since their presence may substantially affect treatment.

Inferior glenohumeral instability is a common component of multidirectional instability (AMBRI syndrome). Inferior instability produces symptoms primarily when loads are carried at the side. This condition may be documented on an anteroposterior x-ray of each shoulder taken with the shoulders relaxed and a weight of 10 pounds held in each hand (Fig. 14–89). The effects of generalized capsular instability can often be ameliorated by vigorous rotator strengthening. I again use the Four Star rehabilitation program (see Table 14–3). The results are often most satisfying in this group of patients, particularly if they are well informed about the need for dynamic stability in the presence of lax soft tissues about the joint.

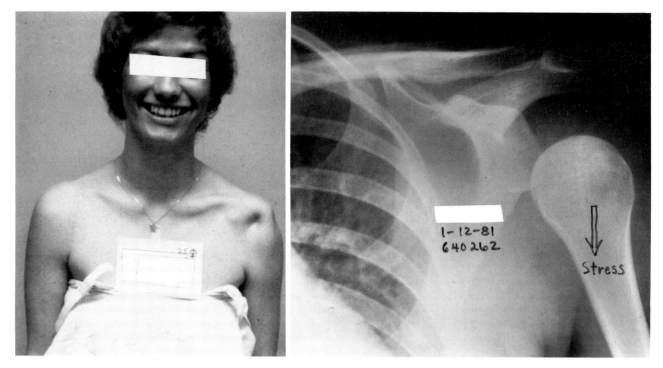

Figure 14–89. *A,* Patient with voluntary anteroinferior subluxation of the left shoulder. She can perform this maneuver without any discomfort. The left shoulder has become so unstable that she is unable to carry out her daily activities. The scar on the right shoulder is a result of a successful capsular shift reconstruction. *B,* Anteroposterior x-ray taken at the time of her voluntary anteroinferior subluxation. (Reproduced with permission from Rockwood CA, and Green DP (eds): Fractures (3 vols), 2nd ed. Philadelphia: JB Lippincott, 1984.)

When the history and physical examination indicate that the shoulder is loose in all directions and when the patient has failed to respond to vigorous internal and external rotator–strengthening, endurance, and coordination exercises, an inferior capsular shift procedure may be considered.[371] The principle of the procedure is to symmetrically tighten the anterior, inferior, and posterior aspects of the capsule by advancing its humeral attachment. We prefer to carry out this procedure from the anterior approach, advancing the capsular anteriorly on the humerus. In this way, shoulder flexion produces additional posterior

capsular tightening (Fig. 14–90). In contrast, when the procedure is performed from a posterior approach the capsule is advanced posteriorly on the humerus. In this situation the tightened capsule loosens as the shoulder is flexed (Fig. 14–91).

The approach is identical with that used for an anterior repair. The skin incision is made in the anterior axillary crease (Fig. 14–92). The deltopectoral interval is developed, exposing the clavipectoral fascia. This is divided and the muscles attached to the coracoid process are retracted medially. The axillary nerve is identified and protected during this procedure. The

CAPSULAR SHIFT TO FRONT

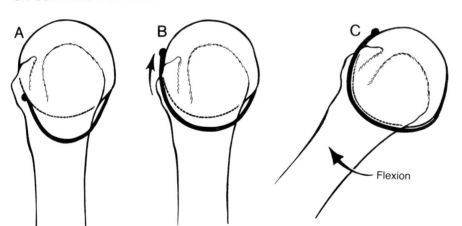

Figure 14–90. Inferior capsular shift, when performed from the anterior approach, advances the capsule anteriorly on the humerus. This produces additional posterior capsular tightening with shoulder flexion. *A,* Lax inferior capsule. *B,* Inferior capsule brought anteriorly on the humerus on an anterior approach. *C,* With humeral flexion, the posterior and inferior capsule are further tightened.

CAPSULAR SHIFT TO BACK

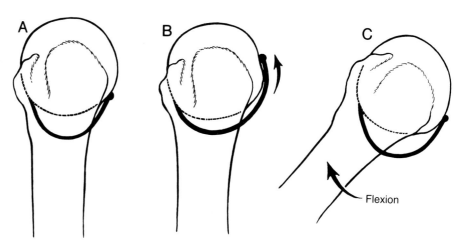

Figure 14–91. When the inferior capsular shift is performed from the posterior approach and the capsule is advanced posteriorly on the humerus, the tightened capsule loosens with shoulder flexion. *A,* Lax inferior capsule. *B,* From the posterior approach the lax inferior capsule is advanced posteriorly on the humerus. *C,* Humeral flexion loosens the posterior and inferior capsule.

arm is held in external rotation and the subscapularis tendon is divided near its insertion to the lesser tuberosity, leaving 1 cm of tendon laterally for reattachment. The subscapularis is split from the capsule in the coronal plane, leaving some tendon on the anterior capsule to reinforce it.

While the arm is progressively externally rotated, the anterior, inferior, and posterior aspects of the capsule are incised from the neck of the humerus up to the midposterior part of the humeral head. The joint is inspected. Capsular detachments from the glenoid and labral tears are uncommon in the AMBRI syndrome. The detached lateral margin of the capsule is then rotated from posterior to anterior, reducing the

volume of the joint symmetrically (Fig. 14–93). Tension of the capsular flap must reduce the inferior axillary pouch and posterior capsule redundancy until *symmetrical* shoulder stability is restored. The advanced capsule is sutured into a bony groove created at the humeral neck. Redundant superior capsule is used to reinforce the anterior repair. The anterior repair must not be excessively tight; a 30-degree range of external rotation is desired to prevent excessive anterior tightness. The subscapularis tendon is then brought over the capsular repair and reattached at its normal location.

Postoperatively the arm is held at the side in a sling. If posterior instability was a major problem preopera-

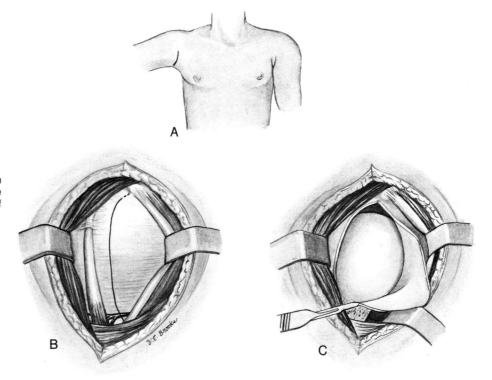

Figure 14–92. *A,* Axillary incision. *B,* Incision through the subscapularis. *C,* Release of the anterior and inferior capsule from the neck of the humerus.

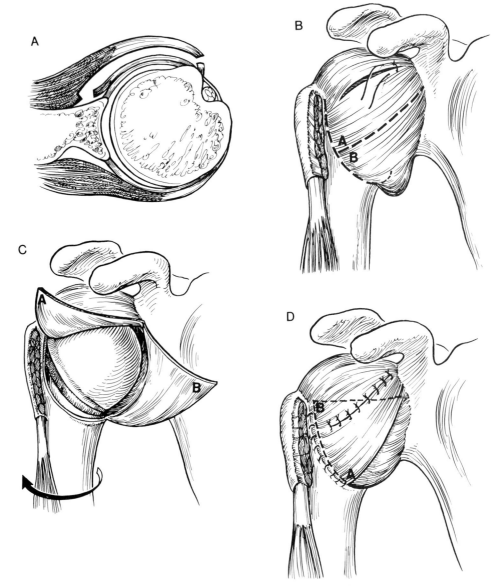

Figure 14–93. *A,* The subscapularis split, leaving part of the tendon to reinforce the anterior capsule. *B,* The split in the rotator internal is closed. *C,* Capsular flaps A and B are created. *D,* Flap B is brought superiorly and flap A inferiorly, eliminating capsular redundancy. (Reproduced with permission from Matsen FA, and Thomas SC: Glenohumeral instability. *In* Evarts CM (ed): Surgery of the Musculoskeletal System, 2nd ed. New York: Churchill Livingstone, 1989.)

tively, the shoulder is held in neutral flexion-extension and in neutral rotation, using a "handshake" cast. Immobilization is usually continued for three weeks, during which isometric exercises are carried out to prevent atrophy. After immobilization is discontinued, the Four Star rehabilitation program (see Table 14–3) is instituted. Motion is allowed to progress under active control of strong, coordinated muscles.

Rockwood's Approach to Treatment of Atraumatic and Multidirectional Glenohumeral Instability

In 1956 Rowe[461] carefully analyzed 500 dislocations of the glenohumeral joint and determined that 96 per cent were caused by trauma and only 4 per cent were atraumatic. However, recent evidence indicates that atraumatic lesions are more commonly recognized currently than were reported in the older literature. The patient with the atraumatic instability may have instability anteriorly, posteriorly, inferiorly, or in all directions. Atraumatic instability can be voluntary, involuntary, or combined voluntary and involuntary.

In voluntary instability the patient places the shoulder into the "right" position so that with selective muscle contraction and relaxation he or she can subluxate or dislocate the shoulder anteriorly, posteriorly, or inferiorly (see Fig. 14–89). This can become habit forming. Voluntary subluxation and dislocation can be associated with emotional and psychiatric disorders. Patients with a voluntary problem usually do not have a history of a significant injury and usually can remember that since early childhood they have been able to slip one or both shoulders out of position. The patient can subluxate or dislocate the shoulder without significant pain.

The involuntary type of subluxation is not quite so obvious and only occurs when the patient puts stress on the shoulder, such as while carrying a suitcase. This type of instability may be associated with congenital abnormalities or developmental problems such as the Ehlers-Danlos syndrome, aplasia of the shoulder joint, following a nerve injury to the shoulder, or following a stroke with flail shoulder. The patient notes that when stress is applied the shoulder will slip out of place, and when the stress is removed the shoulder relocates. There is no history of significant injury and the patient describes the shoulder slipping in and out of place without significant discomfort.

On physical examination, in the voluntary and the involuntary type, the involved shoulder will be quite lax to examination. The patient may demonstrate unilateral instability (i.e., the shoulder may be unstable anteriorly, posteriorly, or inferiorly, or may have multidirectional instability). Not only is the involved shoulder lax to examination, but laxity is also noted in the normal shoulder and in other major joints. The elbows and knees may be hyperextended and the patient may have extreme laxity of the metacarpophalangeal joints. Radiographic evaluation of the involved shoulder will be essentially normal; even the special x-rays fail to show any evidence of anterior glenoid rim fractures or compression fractures of the posterolateral humeral head. A stress view with the shoulder voluntarily subluxated or with weight attached to the wrist will show displacement of the glenohumeral joint.

The treatment of patients with atraumatic instability requires that the physician differentiate between the voluntary and the involuntary types. Certainly, the patient with voluntary instability who has psychiatric problems should never be treated with surgery. Rowe and Yee[469] reported on disasters in patients with psychiatric problems who had been treated with surgical reconstructions. Patients with emotional disturbances and psychiatric problems should be referred for psychiatric help. Rowe and Yee also pointed out that there are patients with voluntary instability who do not have psychiatric problems who can be significantly helped with a rehabilitation program. If the emotionally stable patient fails to respond to 6 to 12 months of rehabilitation, a specific capsular shift reconstruction should be performed. Neer and Foster[373] have reported on their specific capsular shift procedure.

I place all patients with atraumatic instability problems on a very specific rehabilitation program used to strengthen the three parts of the deltoid, the rotator cuff, and the scapular stabilizers. If the patient has an obvious psychiatric or emotional problem, I do my best to explain the problem to the patient and the family and help them seek psychiatric help. Under no circumstances do I ever tell the patient or family that surgery is a possibility for the emotionally disturbed

patient. When I have ruled out congenital or developmental causes for the instability problem, I personally teach the patient how to perform the shoulder-strengthening exercises and give him or her a copy of the exercise diagrams (Fig. 14–94). I give the patient a set of Therabands, which includes yellow, red, green, blue, and black bands, and the diagrams of the exercises to be performed. Each Theraband is a strip 3 inches wide and 5 feet long that is tied into a loop. The loop can be fastened over a doorknob or any fixed object to offer resistance to the pull. The patient does five basic exercises to strengthen the deltoid and the rotator cuff. The yellow Theraband is the weakest and offers 1 pound of resistance; the red, two pounds; the green, 3 pounds; the blue, 4 pounds; and, finally, the black offers 5 pounds of resistance to the pull. The patient is instructed to do the five exercises two to three times a day. Each exercise should be done five to ten times and each held for a count of five to ten. The patient is instructed to gradually increase the resistance (i.e., yellow to red and green, and so on) every two to four weeks. After the black Theraband becomes easy to use, the patient is given a pulley kit and is instructed to do the same five basic exercises, but now lifting weights, as shown in Figure 14–94. The pulley kit consists of a pulley, an open eye screw hook, a handle, and a piece of rope, all in a plastic bag. The patient begins by attaching 7 to 10 pounds of weight to the end of the rope and proceeds on to the five basic exercises. Gradually over several months, the patient increases the weights of resistance, up to 15 pounds for women and 20 to 25 pounds for men. When we start the basic strengthening of the rotator cuff and the deltoid, I also instruct the patient how to do the exercises to strengthen the scapular stabilizer muscles. The push-ups (i.e., wall push-ups, knee push-ups, and regular push-ups) are used to strengthen the serratus anterior, rhomboids, etc., and the shoulder-shrugging exercises are done to strengthen the trapezius muscles. We have learned that the rehabilitation program is 80 per cent successful in managing anterior instability problems and 90 per cent successful in managing the atraumatic posterior instability problems.[457] Regardless of any prior "rehabilitation program" that the patient has participated in, I always start the patient on our strengthening routine.

If the patient still has the signs and symptoms of instability after 6 months of doing the exercises, a very specific capsular shift procedure is performed. One must always remember that it is possible for a patient with laxity of the major joints to have a superimposed traumatic episode, which ordinarily does not respond to a rehabilitation program. A patient with atraumatic instability who has a history of significant trauma, pain, swelling, and so forth, probably will require a surgical reconstruction, but only after a trial with the rehabilitation program.

The details of the incision, surgical approach, protection of the axillary nerve, and preservation of the anterior humeral circumflex vessels are essentially the

Shoulder Strengthening Exercises

Shoulder Service - Department of Orthopaedics
University of Texas Health Science Center
at San Antonio

Do each exercise _____ times. Hold each
time for _____ counts. Do exercise program
_____ times per day.

Begin with _____ Theraband for _____ weeks.
Then use _____ Theraband for _____ weeks.
Then use _____ Theraband for _____ weeks.

EXERCISE 3

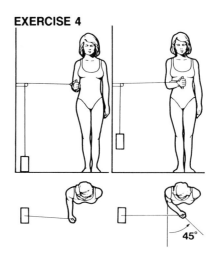

EXERCISE 1

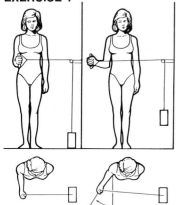

EXERCISE 4

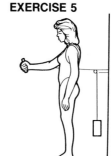

Figure 14–94. *A,* Shoulder strengthening exercises. Initially the patient is given rubber Therabands to strengthen the rotator cuff muscles and the three parts of the deltoid. When the patient is proficient with the rubber resistance with exercises 1 to 5, then the patient is given an exercise kit that consists of a pulley, hook, rope, and a handle. The pulley is attached to the hook, which is fixed to the wall, and the five exercises are performed. Initially the patient is instructed to use 5 or 10 pounds of weight; this is gradually increased over a period of several months to as much as 25 pounds. The purpose of the five exercises is to strengthen the three parts of the deltoid muscles, the internal rotators, and the external rotators.

EXERCISE 2

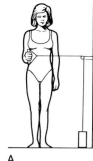

EXERCISE 5

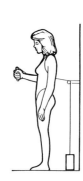

A

Shoulder Strengthening and Stretching Exercises

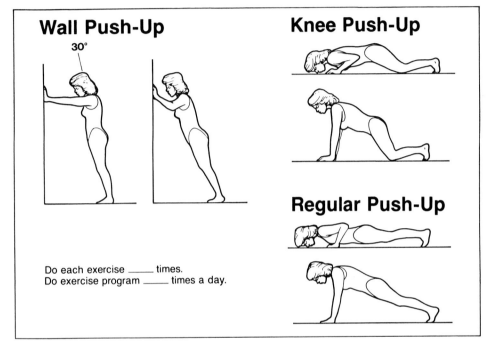

Wall Push-Up

30°

Do each exercise _____ times.
Do exercise program _____ times a day.

Knee Push-Up

Regular Push-Up

Figure 14–94 *Continued B,* In addition, the patient is instructed in exercises to strengthen the scapular stabilizer muscles. To strengthen the serratus anterior and rhomboids, the patient is instructed first to do wall push-ups and then is instructed gradually to do knee push-ups and then regular push-ups. The shoulder shrug exercise is used to strengthen the trapezius and the levator scapulae muscles.

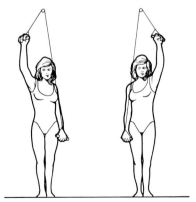

Do each exercise _____ times.
Hold each time for _____ counts.
Do exercise program _____ times a day.

Shoulder Shrug

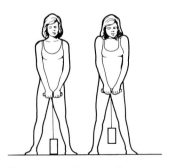

Do each exercise _____ times.
Hold each time for _____ counts.
Use _____ pounds of weight.
Do exercise program _____ times a day.

B

same as I use for the management of a recurrent traumatic anterior instability problem (see Fig. 14–85*A–S*). The main difference is noted after the capsule is opened and the surgeon notices that there is no Perthes-Bankart lesion (Fig. 14–95*A*). The deficiency is simply a very redundant capsule anteriorly, inferiorly, or posteroinferiorly. The principle of the capsular shift is to divide the capsule all the way down inferiorly, midway between its attachment on the humerus and

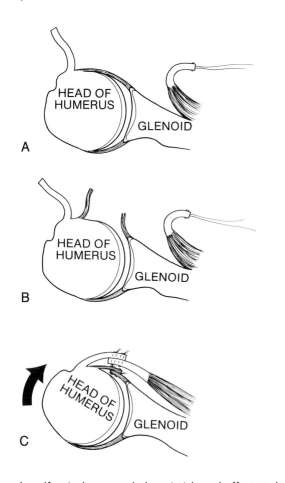

Procedure if anterior capsule is not stripped off scapula.

Capsular Repair

D Before   E After

Figure 14–95. Capsular shift reconstruction for atraumatic anterior subluxation or dislocation. The Bankort/Perthes lesion is not present, and the capsule is shifted to eliminate the anterior inferior laxity.

on the glenoid rim. The joint is carefully inspected and then the shift is performed. As is demonstrated in Figure 14–85*P* and *Q*, I prefer to take the medial capsule superiorly and laterally under the lateral capsule, and then take the lateral capsule superiorly and medially over the medial capsule. I am careful that the placement and tying of the sutures are done with the arm in approximately 15 to 20 degrees of external rotation for an anterior reconstruction and in neutral rotation for a posterior reconstruction. Ordinarily, the subscapularis is simply repaired to itself, but should there be laxity of the subscapularis with the arm in 15 to 20 degrees of external rotation, then the subscapularis can be double-breasted (Fig. 14–95*C*). Ordinarily, in doing the posterior capsular shift, the infraspinatus tendon can be reflected superiorly and the teres minor reflected inferiorly off the posterior capsule. As with the anterior shift, the posterior capsule is divided midway between its attachments (Fig. 14–95*B*), thus allowing a double-breasting or strengthening of the midportion of the capsule (Fig. 14–95*C*). The reader must remember, however, that posterior shifts are rarely required because most patients do so well with the rehabilitation program.

The surgical management of patients with atraumatic instability demands that the shoulder not be put up too tight, as can be done with the Magnuson-Stack, Putti-Platt, or Bristow procedure. If the surgeon fails to recognize that the patient has an atraumatic instability problem, and if a routine muscle-tightening procedure is performed, the result may be that the humeral head will be pushed out in the opposite direction. The surgeon must also be careful, even in patients with atraumatic instability, not to perform a capsular shift that is so tight as to force the head out in the opposite direction. As mentioned, I prefer to place and tie the sutures in the anterior capsular shift procedure with the arm in 15 to 20 degrees of external rotation and held in neutral rotation during the posterior capsular shift reconstruction. The reader must also be warned that it is essential to isolate and protect the axillary nerve when doing the anterior or posterior capsular shift (Fig. 14–95*D, E*).

References

1. Adams F: The Genuine Works of Hippocrates, Vol 2. New York: William Wood, 1891.
2. Adams FL: The Genuine Works of Hippocrates, Vols 1 and 2. New York: William Wood, 1886.
3. Adams JC: Recurrent dislocation of the shoulder. J Bone Joint Surg *30B*:26, 1948.
4. Adams JC: The humeral head defect in recurrent anterior dislocations of the shoulder. Br J Radiol *23*:151–156, 1950.
5. Adler H, and Lohmann B: The stability of the shoulder in stress radiography. Arch Orthop Trauma Surg *103*:83–84, 1984.
6. Ahlgren O, Lorentzon R, and Larsson SE: Posterior dislocation of the shoulder associated with general seizures. Acta Orthop Scand *52*:694–695, 1981.
7. Ahlgren SA, Hedlund T, and Nistor L: Idiopathic posterior instability of the shoulder joint. Acta Orthop Scand *49*:600–603, 1978.
8. Ahmadain AM: The Magnuson-Stack operation for recurrent

anterior dislocation of the shoulder. A review of 38 cases. J Bone Joint Surg (Br) *69*(1):111–114, 1987.

9. Albert E: Arthodese bei einer Habituellen Luxation der Schultergelenkes. Klin Rundschau *2*:281–283, 1898.

10. Anderson D, Zvirbulis R, and Ciullo J: Scapular manipulation for reduction of anterior shoulder dislocations. Clin Orthop *164*:181–183, 1982.

11. Andrews JR, and Carson WG: Shoulder joint arthroscopy. Orthopedics *6*:1157–1162, 1983.

12. Andrews J, Carson WCM, and Hughston JC: Operative shoulder arthroscopy. Paper presented at the annual meeting of the American Orthopaedic Association, Homestead, VA, June 1983.

13. Angelo RL, and Hawkins RJ: Osteoarthritis following an excessively tight Putti-Platt repair. American Shoulder and Elbow Surgeons 4th Open Meeting, Atlanta, 1988.

14. Antal CS, Conforty B, Engelberg M, et al: Injuries to the axillary due to anterior dislocation of the shoulder. J Trauma *13*:564, 1973.

15. Arndt JH, and Sears AD: Posterior dislocation of the shoulder. Am J Roentgenol *94*:639–645, 1965.

16. Aronen JG: Shoulder rehabilitation. Clin Sports Med *4*(3):477–493, 1985.

17. Aronen JG, and Regan K: Decreasing the incidence of recurrence of first time anterior shoulder dislocations with rehabilitation. Am J Sports Med *12*(4):283–291, 1984.

18. Aronen JG: Anterior shoulder dislocations in sports. Sports Med *3*(3):224–234, 1986.

19. Artz T, and Huffer JM: A major complication of the modified Bristow procedure for recurrent dislocation of the shoulder. A case report. J Bone Joint Surg *54A*:1293–1296, 1972.

20. Assmus H, and Meinel A: Schulterverletzung und Axillarparese. Hefte Unfallheilkd *79*:183–187, 1976.

21. Aston JW, and Gregory CF: Dislocation of the shoulder with significant fracture of the glenoid. J Bone Joint Surg *55A*:1531–1533, 1973.

22. Aufderheide TP, Frascone RJ, and Cicero JJ: Simultaneous bilateral anterior and posterior shoulder dislocations. Am J Emerg Med *3*(4):331–333, 1985.

23. Badgley CE: Sports injuries of the shoulder girdle. JAMA *172*:444–448, 1960.

24. Badgley CE, and O'Connor GA: Combined procedure for the repair of recurrent anterior dislocation of the shoulder. J Bone Joint Surg *47A*:1283, 1965.

25. Bailey RW: Acute and recurrent dislocation of the shoulder. Instr Course Lect *18*(J1):70–74, 1962–1969.

26. Baker LL, and Parker K: Neuromuscular electrical stimulation of the muscles surrounding the shoulder. Phys Ther *66*(12):1930–1937, 1986.

27. Bankart ASB: Recurrent or habitual dislocation of the shoulder joint. Br Med J *2*:1132–1133, 1923.

28. Bankart ASB: The pathology and treatment of recurrent dislocation of the shoulder joint. Br J Surg *26*:23–29, 1939.

29. Baratta JB, Lim V, Mastromonaco E, and Edillon E: Axillary artery disruption secondary to anterior dislocation of the shoulder. J Trauma *23*(11):1009–1011, 1983.

30. Bardenheuer BA: Die Verletzungen Der Oberen Extremitaten. Deutsche Chir *63*:268–418, 1886.

31. Barquet A, Schimchak M, Carreras O, et al: Dislocation of the shoulder with fracture of the ipsilateral shaft of the humerus. Injury *16*(5):300–302, 1985.

32. Barrett J: The clavicular joints. Physiotherapy *57*:268–269, 1971.

33. Barry TP, Lombardo SJ, Kerlan RK, et al: The coracoid transfer for recurrent anterior instability of the shoulder in adolescents. J Bone Joint Surg *67*(3):383–387, 1985.

34. Basmajian JV, and Bazant FJ: Factors preventing downward dislocation of the adducted shoulder joint. J Bone Joint Surg *41A*:1182–1186, 1959.

35. Bateman JE: Gallie technique for repair of recurrent dislocation of the shoulder. Surg Clin North Am *43*:1655–1662, 1963.

36. Bateman JE: The Shoulder and Neck. Philadelphia: WB Saunders, 1972.

37. Bateman JE: The Shoulder and Neck, 2nd ed. Philadelphia: WB Saunders, 1978.

38. Bayley JIL, and Kessel L: Posterior dislocation of the shoulder: the clinical spectrum. J Bone Joint Surg *60B*:440, 1978.

39. Beattie TF, Steedman DJ, McGowan A, and Robertson CE: A comparison of the Milch and Kochner techniques for acute anterior dislocation of the shoulder. Injury *17*(5):349–352, 1986.

40. Bechtol CO: Biomechanics of the shoulder. Clin Orthop *146*:37–41, 1980.

41. Beckers L: Sub-deltoid approach to the shoulder. Acta Orthop Belg *51*(5):847–851, 1985.

42. Benechetrit E, and Friedman B: Fracture of the coracoid process associated with subglenoid dislocation of the shoulder. J Bone Joint Surg *61A*:295–296, 1979.

43. Bennett GE: Old dislocations of the shoulder. J Bone Joint Surg *18*:594–606, 1936.

44. Bertrand JC, Maestro M, Pequignot JP, and Moviel J: Les complications vasculaires des luxations arterieures fermes de l'épaule. Ann Chir *36*:329–333, 1981.

45. Bestard EA: Glenoplasty: a simple reliable method of correcting recurrent posterior dislocation of the shoulder. Orthop Rev *5*:29–34, 1976.

46. Billington RW: A new (plaster yoke) dressing for fracture of the clavicle. South Med J *24*:667, 1931.

47. Bjelland JC, and Freundlich IM: Radiology case of the month. Case number five. Arizona Med *32*:961–962, 1975.

48. Blazina ME, and Satzman JS: Recurrent anterior subluxation of the shoulder in athletes—a distinct entity. J Bone Joint Surg *51A*:1037–1038, 1969.

49. Blom S, and Dahlback LO: Nerve injuries in dislocations of the shoulder joint and fractures of the neck of the humerus. Acta Chir Scand *136*:461–466, 1970.

50. Bloom MH, and Obata WG: Diagnosis of posterior dislocation of the shoulder with use of Velpeau axillary and angle-up roentgenographic views. J Bone Joint Surg *49A*:943–949, 1967.

51. Bodey WN, and Denham RA: A free bone block operation for recurrent anterior dislocation of the shoulder joint. Injury *15*:184, 1983.

52. Böhler L: Die Behandlung von Verrenkungsbrüchen der Schulter. Deutsche Zschr Chir *219*:238–245, 1929.

53. Bonnin JG: Transplantation of the tip of the coracoid process for recurrent anterior dislocation of the shoulder. J Bone Joint Surg *51B*:579, 1969. (Proceedings.)

54. Bonnin JG: Transplantation of the coracoid tip: a definitive operation for recurrent anterior dislocation of the shoulder. R Soc Med *66*:755–758, 1973.

55. Bost F, and Inman VT: The pathologic changes in recurrent dislocation of the shoulder. A report of Bankart's operative procedure. J Bone Joint Surg *24*:595–613, 1942.

56. Boyd HB, and Hunt H: Recurrent dislocation of the shoulder. J Bone Joint Surg *47A*:1514–1520, 1965.

57. Boyd HB, and Sisk TD: Recurrent posterior dislocation of the shoulder. J Bone Joint Surg *54A*:779, 1972.

58. Boytchev B: Treatment of recurrent shoulder instability. Minerva Orthopedica *2*:377–379, 1951.

59. Boytchev B, Conforty B, and Tchokanov K: Operatiunaya Ortopediya y Travatologiya, 2nd ed. Sofia: Meditsina y Fizkultura, 1962.

60. Braly WG, and Tullos HS: A modification of the Bristow procedure for recurrent anterior shoulder dislocation and subluxation. Am J Sports Med *13*:81, 1985.

61. Braunstein EM, and O'Conner G: Double-contrast arthrotomography and the shoulder. J Bone Joint Surg *64A*:192–195, 1982.

62. Brav EA: An evaluation of Putti-Platt reconstruction procedure for recurrent dislocation of the shoulder. J Bone Joint Surg *37A*:731–741, 1955.

63. Brav EA: Ten years' experience with Putti-Platt reconstruction procedure. Am J Surg *100*:423–430, 1960.

64. Brennike P, Bro-Rasmussen F, and Bro-Rasmussen P: Dislocation and/or congenital malformation of the shoulder joint. Observations on a medieval skeleton from Denmark. Anthropol Anz *45*(2):117–129, 1987.

65. Brewer BJ, Wubben RC, and Carrera GF: Excessive retroversion of the glenoid cavity. A cause of non-traumatic posterior instability of the shoulder. J Bone Joint Surg *68*(5):724–731,

1986 (published erratum appears in J Bone Joint Surg 68(7):1128, 1986).

66. Broca A, and Hartmann H: Contribution à l'étude des luxations de l'épaule. Bull Soc Anat Paris 4:312–336, 416–423, 1890.

67. Brockbank W, and Griffiths DL: Orthopaedic surgery in the 16th and 17th centuries. J Bone Joint Surg 30B:365–375, 1948.

68. Brown JT: Nerve injuries complicating dislocation of the shoulder. J Bone Joint Surg 34B:526, 1952.

69. Brown FW, and Navigato WJ: Rupture of the axillary artery and brachial plexus palsy associated with anterior dislocation of the shoulder—report of a case with successful vascular repair. Clin Orthop 60:195–199, 1968.

70. Burri C, and Neugebauer R: Carbon fiber replacement of the ligaments of the shoulder girdle and the treatment of lateral instability of the ankle joint. Clin Orthop (196):112–117, 1985.

70a. Butters KP, Curtis RJ, and Rockwood CA Jr: Posterior deltoid splitting shoulder approach. J Bone Joint Transactions 11:233, 1987.

71. Caird FM: The shoulder joint in relation to certain dislocations and fractures. Edinb Med J 32:708–714, 1887.

72. Calvet J, Leroy M, and Lacroix L: Luxations de l'épaule et lesions vasculaires. J Chir 58:337–346, 1942.

73. Carpenter GI, and Millard PH: Shoulder subluxation in elderly inpatients. J Am Geriatr Soc 30(7):441–446, 1982.

74. Carew-McColl M: Bilateral shoulder dislocations caused by electrical shock. Br J Clin Prac 34:251–254, 1980.

75. Carol EJ, Falke LM, Kortmann JH, et al: Bristow-Laterjet repair for recurrent anterior shoulder instability; an 8-year study. Neth J Surg 37(4):109–113, 1985.

76. Caspari RB: Shoulder arthroscopy: a review of the present state of the art. Contemp Orthop 4:523–531, 1982.

77. Caspri I, Ezra E, Oliver S, et al: Treatment of avulsed clavicle and recurrent subluxations of the ipsilateral shoulder by dynamic fixation. J Trauma 27(1):94–95, 1987.

78. Cautilli RA, Joyce MF, and Mackell JV Jr: Posterior dislocation of the glenohumeral joint. Jefferson Orthop J 7:15–20, 1978.

79. Cautilli RA, Joyce MF, and Mackell JV Jr: Posterior dislocations of the shoulder: a method of postreduction management. Am J Sports Med 6:397–399, 1978.

80. Cave EF, Burke JF, and Boyd RJ: Trauma Management. Chicago: Year Book Medical Publishers, 1974, p 437.

81. Cayford EH, and Tees FJ: Traumatic aneurysm of the subclavicular artery as a late complication of fractured clavicle. Can Med Assoc J 25:450–452, 1931.

82. Chaco J, and Wolf E: Subluxation of the glenohumeral joint in hemiplegia. Am J Phys Med 50:139–143, 1971.

83. Chen SK, Perry J, Jobe FW, et al: Elbow flexion analysis in Bristow patients. A preliminary report. Am J Sports Med 12(5):347–350, 1984.

84. Cisternino SJ, Rogers LF, Stufflebam BC, and Kruglik GD: The trough line: a radiographic sign of posterior shoulder dislocation. AJR 130:951–954, 1978.

85. Clairmont P, and Ehrlich H: Ein Neues Operations-Verfahren zur Behandlung der Habituellen Schulterluxation Mittels Muskelplastik. Verh Deutsch Ges Chir 38:79–103, 1909.

86. Clark KC: Positioning in Radiography, 2nd ed. London: William Heinemann, 1941.

87. Cleaves EN: A new film holder for roentgen examination of the shoulder. Am J Roentgenol Rad Ther Nucl Med 45:288–290, 1941.

88. Cleland J: On the actions of muscles passing over more than one joint. J Anat Physiol 1:85–93, 1866.

89. Clotteau JE, Premont M, and Mercier V: A simple procedure for reducing dislocations of the shoulder without anesthesia. Nouv Presse Med 11:127–128, 1982.

90. Codman EA: Rupture of the Supraspinatus Tendon and Other Lesions in or about the Subacromial Bursa. Boston: Thomas Todd & Co, 1934.

91. Cofield RH, Kavanagh BF, and Frassica FJ: Anterior shoulder instability. Instr Course Lect 34:210–227, 1985.

92. Cofield RH, and Simonet WT: The shoulder in sports. Mayo Clin Proc 59:157–164, 1984.

93. Colachis SC, and Strohm BR: Effects of suprascapular and axillary nerve blocks on muscle force in upper extremity. Arch Phys Med Rehabil 52:22–29, 1971.

94. Collins HR, and Wilde AH: Shoulder instability in athletes. Orthop Clin North Am 4:759–773, 1973.

95. Collins KA, Capito C, and Cross M: The use of the Putti-Platt procedure in the treatment of recurrent anterior dislocation, with special reference to the young athlete. Am J Sports Med 14(5):380–382, 1986.

96. Conforty B: The results of the Boytchev procedure for treatment of recurrent dislocation of the shoulder. Int Orthop 4:127–132, 1980.

97. Connolly JF: Humeral head defects associated with shoulder dislocation—their diagnostic and surgical significance. AAOS Instr Course Lect 21:42, 1972.

98. Connolly JF: Personal communication, 1972.

99. Conwell HE: Fractures of the clavicle. JAMA 90:838–839, 1928.

100. Conwell HE, and Reynolds FC: Key and Conwell's Management of Fractures, Fractures, Dislocations, and Sprains, 7th ed. St. Louis: CV Mosby, 1961.

101. Cooper A: A Treatise on Dislocations and Fractures of the Joints, 2nd American ed from the 6th London ed. Boston: Lilly, Wait, Carter, & Hendee, 1832, pp 375–377.

102. Cooper A: On the dislocation of the os humeri upon the dorsum scapula, and upon fractures near the shoulder joint. Guy's Hosp Rep 4:265–284, 1839.

103. Cotton FJ: Subluxation of the shoulder downward. Boston Med Surg J 185:405–407, 1921.

104. Cotton FJ, and Brickley WJ: Treatment of fracture of neck of scapula. Boston Med Surg J 185A:326–329, 1921.

105. Craig EV: The posterior mechanism of acute anterior shoulder dislocations. Clin Orthop (190):212–216, 1984.

106. Cramer F: Resection des Oberamkopfes wegen Habitueller Luxation (Nach einem im Arzlichen Verein zu Wiesbaden Gehaltenen Vortrage). Berliner Klin Wochenschr 19:21–25, 1882.

107. Cramer F, Von BM, Kramps HA, et al: [CT diagnosis of recurrent subluxation of the shoulder.] Fortschr Rontgenstr 136(4):440–443, 1982.

108. Cranley JJ, and Krause RF: Injury to the axillary artery following anterior dislocation of the shoulder. Am J Surg 95:524–526, 1958.

109. Cubbins W, Callahan H, and Scuderi C: The reduction of old or irreducible shoulder dislocation. Surg Gynecol Obstet 58:129–135, 1934.

110. Cunningham's Textbook of Anatomy, 11th ed (Romanes GJ, ed). London: Oxford University Press, 1972.

111. Curr JF: Rupture of the axillary artery complicating dislocation of the shoulder. Report of a case. J Bone Joint Surg 52B:313–317, 1970.

112. Cyprien JM, Vasey HM, Burdet A, et al: Humeral retrotorsion and glenohumeral relationship in the normal shoulder and in recurrent anterior dislocation. Clin Orthop 175:8–17, 1983.

113. Dannaeus C, and Liedberg G: Traumatic disruption of the axillary artery. Acta Chir Scand 148:549–550, 1982.

114. Danzig LA, Greenway G, and Resnick D: The Hill-Sachs lesion: an experimental study. Am J Sports Med 8:328–332, 1980.

115. Danzig LA, Resnick D, and Greenway G: Evaluation of unstable shoulders by computed tomography. Am J Sports Med 10:138–141, 1982.

116. Das SP, Roy GS, and Saha AK: Observations on the tilt of the glenoid cavity of scapula. J Anat Soc India 15:114, 1966.

117. Day AJ, MacDonell JA, and Pederson HE: Recurrent dislocation of the shoulder. Clin Orthop 45:123–126, 1966.

118. DeAnquin CE: Recurrent dislocation of the shoulder: roentgenographic study. J Bone Joint Surg 47A:1085, 1965.

119. Debevoise NT, Hyatt GW, and Townsend GB: Humeral torsion in recurrent shoulder dislocations. Clin Orthop 76:87–93, 1971.

120. Dehne E: Fractures of the upper end of the humerus: a classification based on the etiology of trauma. Surg Clin North Am 25:28–47, 1945.

121. Delorme D: Die Hemmungsbander des Schultergelenks und

ihre Bedeutung fur die Schulterluxationen. Arch Klin Chir *92*:79–101, 1910.

122. Demos TC: Radiologic case orthopedics study: Bilateral posterior shoulder dislocations. Orthopedics *3*:887–897, 1980.

123. Dempster WT: Mechanisms of shoulder movement. Arch Phys Med Rehabil *46*:49–70, 1965.

124. DePalma AF: Recurrent dislocation of the shoulder joint. Ann Surg *132*:1052–1065, 1950.

125. DePalma AF: Factors influencing the choice of a modified Magnuson procedure for recurrent anterior dislocation of the shoulder. With a note on technique. Surg Clin North Am *43*:1647–1649, 1963.

126. DePalma AF: The Management of Fractures and Dislocations. An Atlas, 2nd ed, Vol 1. Philadelphia: WB Saunders, 1970.

127. DePalma AF: Surgery of the Shoulder, 2nd ed. Philadelphia: JB Lippincott, 1973.

128. DePalma AF: Surgery of the Shoulder, 3rd ed. Philadelphia: JB Lippincott, 1983.

129. DePalma AF, Cooke AJ, and Prabhakar M: The role of the subscapularis in recurrent anterior dislocations of the shoulder. Clin Orthop *54*:35–49, 1967.

130. DePalma AF, and Silberstein CE: Results following a modified Magnuson procedure in recurrent dislocation of the shoulder. Surg Clin North Am *43*:1651–1653, 1963.

131. Deutsch AL, Resnick D, and Mink JH: Computed tomography of the glenohumeral and sternoclavicular joints. Orthop Clin North Am *16*:497–511, 1985.

132. De Waal Malefijt J, Doms AJ, and Van Rens TJ: A comparison of the results of the Bristow-Latarjet procedure and the Bankart/Putti-Platt operation for recurrent anterior dislocations of the shoulder. Acta Orthop Belg *51*(5):831–842, 1985.

133. Dick W, and Baumgartner R: Hypermobilitat und Wilkurliche Hintere Schulterluxation. Orthop Prax *16*:328–330, 1980.

134. Didiee J: Le radiodiagnostic dans la luxation recidivante de l'épaule. J Radiol Electrol *14*:209–218, 1930.

135. Dimon JH, III: Posterior dislocations and posterior fracture-dislocation of the shoulder: a report of 25 cases. South Med J *60*:661–666, 1967.

136. Doege KW: Irreducible shoulder joint dislocations. Lancet *49*:191–195, 1929.

137. Dolk T, and Gremark O: Arthroscopy and stability testing of the shoulder joint. Anthroscopy *2*(1):35–40, 1986.

138. Dorgan JA: Posterior dislocation of the shoulder. Am J Surg *89*:890–900, 1955.

139. Drury JK, and Scullion JE: Vascular complications of anterior dislocation of the shoulder. Br J Surg *67*:579–581, 1980.

140. DuToit GT, and Roux D: Recurrent dislocation of the shoulder. A 24-year study of the Johannesburg stapling operation. J Bone Joint Surg *38A*:1–12, 1956.

141. Dvir Z, and Berme N: The shoulder complex in elevation of the arm: a mechanism approach. J Biomech *11*:219–225, 1978.

141a. Edeland HG, and Stefansson T: Block of the suprascapular nerve in reduction of acute anterior shoulder dislocation. Case reports. Acta Anaesthesiol Scand *17*(1):46–49, 1973.

142. Eden R: Zur Operation der Habituellen Schulterluxation unter Mitteilung Eines Neuen Verfahrens bei Abriss am Inneren Pfannenrande. Dtsch Ztschr Chir *144*:269, 1918.

143. Ehgartner K: Has the duration of cast fixation after shoulder dislocations an influence on the frequency of recurrent dislocation? Arch Orthop Unfallchir *89*:187–190, 1977.

144. El-Khoury GY, Kathol MH, Chandler JB, and Albright JP: Shoulder instability: impact of glenohumeral arthrotomography on treatment. Radiology *160*(3):669–673, 1986.

145. Engelhardt MB: Posterior dislocation of the shoulder: report of six cases. South Med J *71*:425–427, 1978.

146. Engin AE: On the biomechanics of the shoulder complex. Biomechanics *13*:575–590, 1980.

147. English E, and Macnab I: Recurrent posterior dislocation of the shoulder. Can J Surg *17*:147–151, 1974.

148. Eve FS: A case of subcoracoid dislocation of the humerus with the formation of an indentation on the posterior surface of the head. Medico-Chirurg Trans Soc London *63*:317–321, 1880.

149. Eyre-Brook AL: Recurrent dislocation of the shoulder. Lesions discovered in seventeen cases. Surgery employed, and intermediate report on results. J Bone Joint Surg *30B*:39, 1948.

150. Eyre-Brook AL: The morbid anatomy of a case of recurrent dislocation of the shoulder. Br J Surg *29*:32–37, 1943.

151. Eyre-Brook AL: Recurrent dislocation of the shoulder. Physiotherapy *57*:7–13, 1971.

152. Fairbank HAT: Birth palsy: subluxation of the shoulder joint in infants and young children. Lancet *1*:1217–1223, 1913.

153. Fairbank TJ: Fracture-subluxations of the shoulder. J Bone Joint Surg *30B*:454–460, 1948.

154. Farrugia PD: Superior glenohumeral dislocation—a case report. Injury *16*(7):489–490, 1985.

155. Fee HJ, McAvoy JM, and Dainko EA: Pseudoaneurysm of the axillary artery following a modified Bristow operation: report of a case and review. J Cardiovasc Surg *19*:65, 1978.

156. Ferkel RD, Hedley AK, and Eckardt JJ: Anterior fracture-dislocations of the shoulder: pitfalls in treatment. J Trauma *24*(4):363–367, 1984.

157. Fick R: Handbuch der Anatomie und Mechanik der Gelenke unter Berücksichtigung der Bewegenden Muskeln. Jena: Fischer, 1904.

158. Finsterer H: Die Operative Behandlung der Habituellen Schulterluxation. Deutsch Ztschr Chir *141*:354–497, 1917.

159. Fipp GJ: Simultaneous posterior dislocation of both shoulders. Clin Orthop *44*:191–195, 1966.

160. Fitzgerald JF, and Keates J: False aneurysm as a late complication of anterior dislocation of the shoulder. Ann Surg *181*:785–786, 1975.

161. Fitzgerald-Finch OP, and Gibson IIJM: Subluxation of the shoulder in hemiplegia. Age Ageing *4*:16–18, 1975.

162. Flood V: Discovery of a new ligament of the shoulder joint. Lancet *1*:672–673, 1829.

163. Flower WH: On pathologic changes produced in the shoulder joint by traumatic dislocation. Trans Path Soc London *12*:179–200, 1861.

164. Foster WS, Ford TB, and Drez D Jr: Isolated posterior shoulder dislocation in a child. A case report. Am J Sports Med *13*(3):198–200, 1985.

165. Franke GH: Dislocations of shoulder. Dtsch Ztschr Chir *48*:399, 1898.

166. Frankel VH, and Nordin M: Basic Biomechanics of the Skeletal System. Philadelphia: Lea and Febiger, 1980.

167. Freeland AE, and Higgins RW: Anterior shoulder dislocation with posterior displacement of the long head of the biceps tendon. Arthrographic findings. A case report. Orthopaedics *8*(4):468–469, 1985.

168. Frizziero L, Zizzi F, Facchini A, et al: Arthroscopy of the shoulder joint: a review of 23 cases. Rheumatologie *11*:267–276, 1981.

169. Fronek J, Bowen M, Pavlov H, and Warren R: Posterior subluxation of the glenohumeral joint: non-surgical and surgical treatment. American Shoulder and Elbow Surgeons 2nd Open Meeting, New Orleans, 1986.

170. Gainor BJ, Piotrowski G, Puhl J, et al: The throw: biomechanics and acute injury. Am J Sports Med *8*:114–118, 1980.

171. Galenus: On the Usefulness of the Parts of the Body, Vol 2 (May MT, trans and ed). Ithaca, New York: Cornell University Press, 1968.

172. Galinat BJ, Howell SM, and Kraft TA: The glenoid-posterior acromion angle: an accurate method of evaluating glenoid version. American Shoulder and Elbow Surgeons 4th Open Meeting, Atlanta, 1988.

173. Galinat LBJ, Murphy JM, and MacEwen GD: Shoulder arthrodesis: a long term functional evaluation. American Shoulder and Elbow Surgeons 4th Open Meeting, Atlanta, 1988.

174. Gallen J, Wiss DA, Cantelmo N, and Menzoin JO: Traumatic pseudoaneurysm of the axillary artery: report of three cases and literature review. J Trauma *24*:350–354, 1984.

175. Gallie WE, and LeMesurier AB: An operation for the relief of recurring dislocations of the shoulder. Trans Am Surg Assoc *45*:392–398, 1927.

176. Gallie WE, and LeMesurier AB: Recurring dislocation of the shoulder. J Bone Joint Surg *30B*:9–18, 1948.

177. Gambrioli PL, Magg F, and Radelli M: Computerized tomography in the investigation of scapulohumeral instability. Ital J Orthop Traumatol *11*(2):223–232, 1985.

178. Gandin J, and Gandin R: Oudard's operation and its variants in recurrent dislocation of shoulder—statistical study of 139 late results. Chirurgie *99*:779–786, 1973.

179. Ganel A, Horoszowski H, Heim M, et al: Persistent dislocation of the shoulder in elderly patients. J Am Geriatr Soc *28*:282–284, 1980.

180. Garcia-Elias M, and Salo JM: Non-union of a fractured coracoid process after dislocation of the shoulder. A case report. J Bone Joint Surg *67*(5):722–723, 1985.

181. Gardham JRC, and Scott JE: Axillary artery occlusion with erect dislocation of the shoulder. Injury *11*(2):155–158, 1980.

182. Gardner E: The prenatal development of the human shoulder joint. Surg Clin North Am *43*:1465–1470, 1963.

183. Gariepy R, Derome A, and Laurin CA: Brachial plexus paralysis following shoulder dislocation. Can J Surg *5*:418–421, 1962.

184. Garth WP, Allman FL, and Armstrong WS: Occult anterior subluxations of the shoulder in noncontact sports. Am J Sports Med *15*(6):579–585, 1987.

185. Garth WP Jr, Slabbey CE, and Och CW: Roentgenographic demonstration of instability of the shoulder: the apical oblique projection. A technical note. J Bone Joint Surg *66*(9):1450–1453, 1984.

186. Gerber C, Ganz R, and Vinh TS: Glenoplasty for recurrent posterior shoulder instability. Clin Orthop Rel Res *216*:70–79, 1987.

187. Gerlev C, and Ganz R: Clinical assessment of instability of the shoulder. J Bone Joint Surg *66B*:551–556, 1984.

188. Ghormley RK, Black JR, and Cherry JH: Ununited fractures of the clavicle. Am J Surg *51*:343–349, 1941.

189. Gibson JMC: Rupture of the axillary artery following anterior dislocation of the shoulder. J Bone Joint Surg *44B*:114–115, 1962.

190. Glessner JR: Intrathoracic dislocation of the humeral head. J Bone Joint Surg *42A*:428–430, 1961.

191. Gold AM: Fractured neck of the humerus with separation and dislocation of the humeral head (fracture-dislocation of the shoulder, severe type). Bull Hosp Joint Dis *32*(1):87–99, 1971.

192. Goss TP: Factors to consider in chronic symptomatic shoulder instability. Orthopedic Rev *10*:27–32, 1985.

193. Gosset J: Une technique de greffe coraco-glenordienne dans le traitement des luxations recidivantes de l'époule. Mem Acad Chir *86*:445–447, 1960.

194. Gould R, Rosenfield AT, and Friedlaender GE: Loose body within the glenohumeral joint in recurrent anterior dislocation: CT demonstration. J Comput Assist Tomogr *9*(2):404–405, 1985.

195. Grant JCB: Grant's Atlas of Anatomy, 6th ed. Baltimore: Williams & Wilkins, 1972.

196. Grashey R: Atlas Typischer Rontgenfilder. 1923.

197. Gugenheim S, and Sanders RJ: Axillary artery rupture caused by shoulder dislocation. Surgery *95*:55, 1984.

198. Guibe M: Des lesions des vaisseaux de l'aiselle qui compliquent les luxations de l'épaule. Rev Chir *4*:580–583, 1911.

199. Guilfoil PH, and Christiansen T: An unusual vascular complication of fractured clavicle. JAMA *200*:72–73, 1967.

200. Ha'eri GB: Boytchev procedure for the treatment of anterior shoulder instability. Clin Orthop *May* (206):196–201, 1986.

201. Ha'eri GB, and Maitland A: Arthroscopy findings in the frozen shoulder. J Rheumatol *8*:149–152, 1981.

202. Hall RH, Isaac F, and Booth CR: Dislocations of the shoulder with special reference to accompanying small fractures. J Bone Joint Surg *41A*:489–494, 1959.

203. Hastings DE, and Coughlin LP: Recurrent subluxation of the glenohumeral joint. Am J Sports Med *9*:352–355, 1981.

204. Hauser EDW: Avulsion of the tendon of the subscapularis muscle. J Bone Joint Surg *36A*:139–141, 1954.

205. Hawkins RJ: Unrecognized dislocations of the shoulder. Instr Course Lect *34*:258–63, 1985.

206. Hawkins RJ, Bell RH, Hawkins RH, and Koppert GJ: Anterior dislocation of the shoulder in the older patient. Clin Orthop *206*:192, 1986.

207. Hawkins RJ, Koppert G, and Johnston G: Recurrent posterior instability (subluxation) of the shoulder. J Bone Joint Surg *66A*:169, 1984.

208. Hawkins RJ, Neer CS, Pianta RM, and Mendoza FX: Locked posterior dislocation of the shoulder. J Bone Joint Surg *69A*:9, 1987.

209. Hawkins RH, and Hawkins RJ: Failed anterior reconstruction for shoulder instability. J Bone Joint Surg *67*(5):709–714, 1985.

210. Hawkins RJ, Neer CS II, Pianta R, and Mendoza FX: Missed posterior dislocations of the shoulder. Paper presented at the American Academy of Orthopaedic Surgery Meeting, New Orleans, January 1982.

211. Hehne HJ, and Hubner H: Die Behandlung der Rezidivierenden Schulterluxation nach Putti-Platt-Bankart und Eden-Hybinette-Lange. Orthop Prax *16*:331–335, 1980.

212. Helfet AJ: Coracoid transplantation for recurring dislocation of the shoulder. J Bone Joint Surg *40B*:198–202, 1958.

213. Henderson MS: Habitual or recurrent dislocation of the shoulder. Surg Gynecol Obstet *33*:1–7, 1921.

214. Henderson MS: Tenosuspension operation for recurrent or habitual dislocation of the shoulder. Surg Clin North Am *5*:997–1007, 1949.

215. Henry JH, and Genung JA: Natural history of glenohumeral dislocation—revisited. Am J Sports Med *10*:135–137, 1982.

216. Henson GF: Vascular complications of shoulder injuries: a report of two cases. J Bone Joint Surg *38B*:528–531, 1956.

217. Hermodsson I: Rontgenologische Studein uber die Traumatischen und Habituellen Schultergelenk-Verrenkungen Nach Vorn und Nach Unten. Acta Radiol (Suppl) *20*:1–173, 1934.

218. Hernandez A, and Drez D: Operative treatment of posterior shoulder dislocations by posterior glenoidplasty, capsulorraphy, and infraspinatus advancement. Am J Sports Med *14*(3):187–191, 1986.

219. Heymanowitsch Z: Ein Beitrag zur Operativen Behandlung der Habituellen Schulterluxationen. Zbl Chir *54*:648–651, 1927.

220. Hildebrand: Zur Operativen Behandlung der Habituellen Schulterluxation. Arch Klin Chir *66*:360–364, 1902.

221. Hill HA, and Sachs MD: The grooved defect of the humeral head. A frequently unrecognized complication of dislocations of the shoulder joint. Radiology *35*:690–700, 1940.

222. Hill JA, Lombardo SJ, Kerlan RK, et al: The modified Bristow-Helfet procedure for recurrent anterior shoulder subluxations and dislocations. Am J Sports Med *9*:283–287, 1981.

223. Hill NA, and McLaughlin HL: Locked posterior dislocation simulating a "frozen shoulder." J Trauma *3*:225–234, 1963.

224. Hippocrates: Works of Hippocrates with an English Translation by WHS Jones and ET Withington. London: William Heinemann, 1927.

225. Honner R: Bilateral posterior dislocation of the shoulder. Aust NZ J Surg *38*:269–272, 1969.

226. Hoofwijk AG, and Hoogmartens M: The Putti-Platt operation for recurrent anterior dislocation of the shoulder. Acta Orthop Belg *50*(4):481–488, 1984.

227. Hovelius L: Incidence of shoulder dislocation in Sweden. Clin Orthop *166*:127–131, 1982.

228. Hovelius L: Recurrences after initial dislocation of the shoulder. J Bone Joint Surg *65A*:343–349, 1983.

229. Hovelius L: Anterior dislocation of the shoulder in teenagers and young adults. Five-year prognosis. J Bone Joint Surg *69A*:393, 1987.

230. Hovelius L, Akermark C, Albrektsson B, et al: Bristow-Latarjet procedure for recurrent anterior dislocation of the shoulder. Acta Orthop Scand *54*:284–290, 1983.

231. Hovelius L, Eriksson K, Fredin H, et al: Recurrences after initial dislocation of the shoulder: results of a prospective study of treatment. J Bone Joint Surg *65A*:343–349, 1983.

232. Hovelius L, Korner L, Lundberg B, et al: The coracoid transfer for recurrent dislocation of the shoulder. Technical aspects of the Bristow Latarjet procedure. J Bone Joint Surg *65A*:926–934, 1983.

233. Hovelius L, Thorling J, and Fredin H: Recurrent anterior

dislocation of the shoulder. Results after the Bankart and Putti-Platt operations. J Bone Joint Surg *61A*:566–569, 1979.

234. Howard FM, and Shafer SJ: Injuries to the clavicle with neurovascular complications. J Bone Joint Surg *47A*:1335–1346, 1965.

235. Howell SM, Galinat BJ, Renzi AJ, and Marone PJ: Normal and abnormal mechanics of the glenohumeral joint in the horizontal plane. J Bone Joint Surg *70A*(2):227–232, 1988.

236. Hummel A, Bethke RO, and Kempf L: Die Behandlung der Habituellen Schulterluxation Nach dem Bristow-Verfahren. Unfallheilkunde *85*:482–484, 1982.

237. Humphry GM: A Treatise on the Human Skeleton (Including the Joints). Cambridge: Macmillan and Co, 1858.

238. Hussein MK: Kocher's method is 3,000 years old. J Bone Joint Surg *50B*:669–671, 1968.

239. Hybbinette S: De la transplantation d'un fragment osseux pour remedier aux luxations recidivantes de l'épaule; constations et resultats operatoires. Acta Chir Scand *71*:411–445, 1932.

240. Iftikhar TB, Kaminski RS, and Silva I: Neurovascular complications of the modified Bristow procedure. J Bone Joint Surg *66A*:951, 1984.

241. Inman VT, Saunders JB, and Abbott LC: Observations on the function of the shoulder joint. J Bone Joint Surg *26*:1–30, 1944.

242. Janecki CJ, and Shahcheragh GH: The forward elevation maneuver for reduction of anterior dislocations of the shoulder. Clin Orthop *164*:177–180, 1982.

243. Jardon OM, Hood LT, and Lynch RD: Complete avulsion of the axillary artery as a complication of shoulder dislocation. J Bone Joint Surg *55*:189, 1973.

244. Jens J: The role of the subscapularis muscle in recurring dislocation of the shoulder (abstract). J Bone Joint Surg *34B*:780, 1964.

245. Jobe FW: Unstable shoulders in the athlete. Instr Course Lect *34*:228–231, 1985.

246. Jobe FW, Tibone JE, Perry J, and Moynes D: An EMG analysis of the shoulder in throwing and pitching. Am J Sports Med *11*:3–5, 1983.

247. Joessel D: Ueber die Recidine der Humerus-Luxationen. Deutsch Ztschr Chir *13*:167–184, 1880.

248. Johnson HF: Unreduced dislocation of the shoulder. Nebr State Med J *16*:220–224, 1931.

249. Johnson JR, and Bayley JIL: Loss of shoulder function following acute anterior dislocation. J Bone Joint Surg *63B*:633, 1981.

250. Johnson JR, and Bayley JIL: Early complications of acute anterior dislocation of the shoulder in the middle-aged and elderly patient. Injury *13*:431–434, 1982.

251. Johnson LL: Arthroscopy of the shoulder. Orthop Clin North Am *11*:197–204, 1980.

252. Johnston GH, Hawkins RJ, Haddad R, and Fowler PJ: A complication of posterior glenoid osteotomy for recurrent posterior shoulder instability. Clin Orthop *187*:147, 1984.

253. Johnston GW, and Lowry JH: Rupture of the axillary artery complicating anterior dislocation of the shoulder. J Bone Joint Surg *44B*:116–118, 1962.

254. Jones D: The Role of Shoulder Muscles in the Control of Humeral Position (An Electromyographic Study). Master's Thesis, Case Western Reserve University, 1970.

255. Jones FW: Attainment of upright position of man. Nature *146*:26–27, 1940.

256. Jones V: Recurrent posterior dislocation of the shoulder. Report of a case treated by posterior bone block. J Bone Joint Surg *40B*:203–207, 1958.

257. Jordan H: New technique for the roentgen examination of the shoulder joint. Radiology *25*:480–484, 1935.

258. Kaltsas DS: Comparative study of the properties of the shoulder joint capsule with those of other joint capsules. Clin Orthop *173*:20–26, 1983.

259. Karadimas J, Rentis G, and Varouchas G: Repair of recurrent anterior dislocation of the shoulder using transfer of the subscapularis tendon. J Bone Joint Surg *62A*:1147–1149, 1980.

260. Kavanaugh JH: Posterior shoulder dislocation with ipsilateral humeral shaft fracture. Clin Orthop *131*:168–172, 1978.

261. Kazar B, and Relovszky E: Prognosis of primary dislocation of the shoulder. Acta Orthop Scand *40*:216, 1969.

262. Kelley JP: Fractures complicating electroconvulsive therapy and chronic epilepsy. J Bone Joint Surg *36B*:70–79, 1954.

263. Kinnard P, Gordon D, Levesque RW, and Bergeron D: Computerized arthrotomography in recurring shoulder dislocations and subluxations. Can J Surg *27*(5):487–488, 1984.

264. Kinnard P, Tricoire JL, Levesque, and Bergeron D: Assessment of the unstable shoulder by computer arthrography. Am J Sports Med *11*:157–159, 1983.

265. Kirker JR: Dislocation of the shoulder complicated by rupture of the axillary vessels. J Bone Joint Surg *34B*:72–73, 1952.

266. Kiviluoto O, Pasila M, Jaroma H, and Sundholm A: Immobilization after primary dislocation of the shoulder. Acta Orthop Scand *51*:915–919, 1980.

267. Kleinman PD, Kanzaria PK, Goss TP, and Pappas AM: Axillary arthrotomography of the glenoid labrum. AJR *142*:993–999, 1984.

268. Kline DG, Kott J, Barnes G, and Bryant L: Exploration of selected brachial plexus lesions by the posterior subscapular approach. J Neurosurg *49*:872–880, 1978.

269. Kocher T: Eine Neue Reductionsmethode fur Schulterverrenkung. Berlin Klin *7*:101–105, 1870.

270. Koppert G, and Hawkins RJ: Recurrent posterior dislocating shoulder. J Bone Joint Surg *62B*:127–128, 1980.

271. Kretzler HH: Posterior glenoid osteotomy. Paper presented to the American Academy of Orthopaedic Surgeons Meeting, Dallas, TX, January 17–22, 1944.

272. Kretzler HH, and Blue AR: Recurrent posterior dislocation of the shoulder in cerebral palsy. J Bone Joint Surg *48A*:1221, 1966.

273. Kubin Z: Luxatio humeri erecta: kasuisticke sdeleni. Acta Chir Orthop Traumatol Cech *31*:565, 1964.

274. Kuhnen W, and Groves RJ: Irreducible acute anterior dislocation of the shoulder: case report. Clin Orthop *139*:167–168, 1979.

275. Kumar VP, and Balasubramaniam P: The role of atmospheric pressure in stabilising the shoulder. An experimental study. J Bone Joint Surg (Br) *67*(5):719–721, 1985.

276. Kummel BM: Fractures of the glenoid causing chronic dislocation of the shoulder. Clin Orthop *69*:189–191, 1970.

277. Kuster E: Ueber Habituelle Schulter Luxation. Verh Deutsch Ges Chir *11*:112–114, 1882.

278. Lacey T II: Reduction of anterior dislocation of the shoulder by means of the Milch abduction technique. J Bone Joint Surg *34A*:108–109, 1952.

279. Lam SJS: Irreducible anterior dislocation of the shoulder. J Bone Joint Surg *48B*:132, 1966.

280. Lamm CR, Zaehrisson BE, and Korner L: Radiography of the shoulder after Bristow repair. Acta Radiol Diagn *23*:523–528, 1982.

281. Lance S, and Putkonen M: Positioning of the painful patient for the axial view of the glenohumeral joint. Rontgenblatter *38*(12):380–382, 1985.

282. Landsmeer JMF, and Meyers KAW: The shoulder region exposed by anatomical dissection. Arch Chir Neerl *11*:274–296, 1959.

283. Lange M: Die Operative Behandlung der Gewohnheitsmabigen Verrenkung an Schulter, Knie und Fub. Z Orthop *75*:162, 1944.

284. Langfritz HV: Die Doppelseitige Traumatische Luxatio Humeri Erecta eine Seltene Verletzungsform. Monatschr Unfallheilkunde *59*:367, 1956.

285. Laskin RS, and Sedlin ED: Luxatio erecta in infancy. Clin Orthop *80*:126–129, 1971.

286. Latarjet M: Technique de la butee coracoidienne preplenoidienne dans le traitement des luxations recidivantes de l'épaule. Lyon Chir *54*:604–607, 1958.

287. Latarjet M: Techniques chirurgicales dans le traitement de la luxation anterointerne recidivante de l'épaule. Lyon Chir *61*:313–318, 1965.

288. Latarjet M, and Vittori P: Resultat du traitement des luxations recidivantes de l'épaule par le procede de Latarjet, a propos de 42 cas. Lyon Chir *64*:964–968, 1968.

289. Lavik K: Habitual shoulder luxation. Acta Orthop Scand *30*:251–264, 1961.

290. Lawrence WS: New position in radiographing the shoulder joint. Am J Roentgenol 2:728–730, 1915.
291. Leach RE, Corbett M, Schepsis A, and Stockel J: Results of a modified Putti-Platt operation for recurrent shoulder dislocations and subluxations. Clin Orthop 164:20–25, 1982.
292. LeClerk J: Chronic subluxation of the shoulder. J Bone Joint Surg 51B:778, 1969.
293. Leffert RD, and Seddon H: Infraclavicular brachial plexus injuries. J Bone Joint Surg 47B:9–22, 1965.
294. Leidelmeyer R: Letter to the editor: external rotation method of shoulder dislocation reduction. Ann Emerg Med 10:228, 1981.
295. Lemmens JA, and de Waal Malefijt J: Radiographic evaluation of the modified Bristow procedure for recurrent anterior dislocation of the shoulder. Diagn Imaging Clin Med 53(5):221–225, 1984.
296. L'Episcopo JB: Restoration of muscle balance in the treatment of obstetrical paralysis. NY J Med 39:357–363, 1939.
297. Lescher TJ, and Andersen OS: Occlusion of the axillary artery complicating shoulder dislocation: case report. Milit Med 144:621–622, 1979.
298. Leslie JT, and Ryan TJ: The anterior axillary incision to approach the shoulder joint. J Bone Joint Surg 44A:1193–1196, 1962.
299. Lev-el A, and Rubinstein Z: Axillary artery injury in erect dislocation of the shoulder. J Trauma 21:323–325, 1981.
300. Levick JR: Joint pressure-volume studies: their importance, design and interpretation. J Rheumatol 10:353–357, 1983.
301. Leyder P, Augereau B, and Apoil A: Traitement des luxations posterieures inveterees de l'epaule par double abord et butée osseuse retro-glenoidienne. Ann Chir 34:806–809, 1980.
302. Liberson F: Os acromiale—a contested anomaly. J Bone Joint Surg 19A:683–689, 1937.
303. Lilleby H: Arthroscopy of the shoulder joint. Acta Orthop Scand 53:708–709, 1982.
304. Lindholm TS, and Elmstedt E: Bilateral posterior dislocation of the shoulder combined with fracture of the proximal humerus. Acta Orthop Scand 51:485–488, 1980.
305. Lippert FG: A modification of the gravity method of reducing anterior shoulder dislocations. Clin Orthop 165:259–260, 1982.
306. Liveson JA: Nerve lesions associated with shoulder dislocation: an electrodiagnostic study in 11 cases. J Neurol Neurosurg Psychiatry 47:742–744, 1984.
307. Löbker K: Einige Präparate von habitueller Schulterluxation. Arch Klin Chir 34:658–667, 1887.
308. Lombardo SJ, Kerlan RK, Jobe FW, et al: The modified Bristow procedure for recurrent dislocation of the shoulder. J Bone Joint Surg 58A:256–261, 1976.
309. Lower RF, McNiesh LM, and Callaghan JJ: Computed tomographic documentation of intra-articular penetration of a screw after operations on the shoulder. A report of two cases. J Bone Joint Surg 67(7):1120–1122, 1985.
310. Lucas DB: Biomechanics of the shoulder joint. Arch Surg 107:425–432, 1973.
311. Lucas GL, and Peterson MD: Open anterior dislocation of the shoulder. J Trauma 17:883–884, 1977.
312. Lynn FS: Erect dislocation of the shoulder. Surg Gynecol Obstet 39:51–55, 1921.
313. MacArthur BJ: Arthroscopy of the shoulder. Orthop Nurs 5(4):26–28, 1986.
314. Mack LA, Matsen FA, Kilcoyne RF, et al: Ultrasound: US evaluation of the rotator cuff. Radiology 157:205, 1985.
315. Mackenzie DB: The Bristow-Helfet operation for recurrent anterior dislocation of the shoulder. J Bone Joint Surg 62B:273–274, 1980.
316. Mackenzie DB: The treatment of recurrent anterior shoulder dislocation by the modified Bristow-Helfet procedure. S Afr Med J 65:325, 1984.
317. Magnuson PB: Treatment of recurrent dislocation of the shoulder. Surg Clin North Am 25:14–20, 1945.
318. Magnuson PB, and Stack JK: Bilateral habitual dislocation of the shoulders in twins, a familial tendency. JAMA 144:2103, 1940.
319. Magnuson PB, and Stack JK: Recurrent dislocation of the shoulder. JAMA 123:889–892, 1943.
320. Maki S, and Gruen T: Anthropomorphic studies of the glenohumeral joint. Trans Orthop Res Soc 1:173, 1976.
321. Malgaigne JF: Traite des Fractures et des Luxations. Paris: JB Bailliere, 1855; Philadelphia: JB Lippincott, 1859.
322. Manes HR: A new method of shoulder reduction in the elderly. Clin Orthop 147:200–202, 1980.
323. May VR: A modified Bristow operation for anterior recurrent dislocation of the shoulder. J Bone Joint Surg 52A:1010–1016, 1970.
324. McFie J: Bilateral anterior dislocation of the shoulders: a case report. Injury 8:67–69, 1976.
325. McGlynn FJ, El-Khoury G, and Albright JP: Arthrotomography of the glenoid labrum in shoulder instability. J Bone Joint Surg 64A:506–518, 1982.
326. McGlynn FJ, and Caspari RB: Arthroscopic findings in the subluxating shoulder. Clin Orthop 183:173–178, 1984.
327. McKenzie AD, and Sinclair AM: Axillary artery occlusion complicating shoulder dislocation. Am Surg 148:139–141, 1958.
328. McLaughlin HL: Discussion of acute anterior dislocation of the shoulder by Toufick Nicola. J Bone Joint Surg 31A:172, 1949.
329. McLaughlin HL: On the "frozen" shoulder. Bull Hosp Joint Dis 12:383–393, 1951.
330. McLaughlin HL: Posterior dislocation of the shoulder. J Bone Joint Surg 34A:584, 1952.
331. McLaughlin HL: Trauma. Philadelphia: WB Saunders, 1959.
332. McLaughlin HL: Recurrent anterior dislocation of the shoulder. I. Morbid anatomy. Am J Surg 99:628–632, 1960.
333. McLaughlin HL: Follow-up notes on articles previously published in the journal. Posterior dislocation of the shoulder. J Bone Joint Surg 44A:1477, 1962.
334. McLaughlin HL: Dislocation of the shoulder with tuberosity fractures. Surg Clin North Am 43:1615–1620, 1963.
335. McLaughlin HL: Locked posterior subluxation of the shoulder—diagnosis and treatment. Surg Clin North Am 43:1621, 1963.
336. McLaughlin HL, and Cavallaro WU: Primary anterior dislocation of the shoulder. Am J Surg 80:615–621, 1950.
337. McLaughlin HL, and MacLellan DI: Recurrent anterior dislocation of the shoulder: II. A comparative study. J Trauma 7:191–201, 1967.
338. McMaster WC: Anterior glenoid labrum damage: a painful lesion in swimmers. Am J Sports Med 14(5):383–387, 1986.
339. McMurray TB: Recurrent dislocation of the shoulder (proceedings). J Bone Joint Surg 43B:402, 1961.
340. Mead NC, and Sweeney HJ: Bristow procedure. Spectator Letter, July 9, 1964.
341. Meadowcroft JA, and Kain TM: Luxatio erecta shoulder dislocation: report of two cases. Jefferson Orthop J 6:20–24, 1977.
342. Merrill V: Atlas of Roentgenographic Positions and Standard Radiologic Procedures, 4th ed, Vol 1. St. Louis: CV Mosby, 1975.
343. Middeldorpf M, and Scharm B: De Nova Humeri Luxationis Specie. Clinique Europenne, Vol. II. Dissert Inag. Breslau, 1859.
344. Milch H: Treatment of dislocation of the shoulder. Surgery 3:732–740, 1938.
345. Milgram JE: Shoulder anatomy (the Shoulder Symposium). American Academy of Orthopaedic Surgeons Instr Course Lect 3:55–68, 1946.
346. Miller LS, Donahue JR, Good RP, and Staerk AJ: The Magnuson-Stack procedure for treatment of recurrent glenohumeral dislocations. Am J Sports Med 12:133, 1984.
347. Mills KLG: Simultaneous bilateral posterior fracture dislocation of the shoulder. Injury 6:39–41, 1974–1975.
348. Milton GW: The circumflex nerve and dislocation of the shoulder. Br J Phys Med 17:136–138, 1954.
349. Milton GW: The mechanism of circumflex and other nerve injuries in dislocation of the shoulder and the possible mechanism of nerve injuries during reduction of dislocation. Aust NZ J Surg 23:24–30, 1953–1955.
350. Mirick MJ, Clinton JE, and Ruiz E: External rotation method

of shoulder dislocation reduction. J Am Coll Emerg Physicians 8:528–531, 1979.

351. Mital MA, and Karlin LI: Diagnostic arthroscopy in sports injuries. Orthop Clin North Am 11:771–785, 1980.

352. Mizuno K, and Hirahote K: Diagnosis of recurrent traumatic anterior subluxation of the shoulder. Clin Orthop 179:160–167, 1983.

353. Moeller JC: Compound posterior dislocation of the shoulder. J Bone Joint Surg 57A:1006–1007, 1975.

354. Morgan CD, and Bordenstab AB: Arthroscopic Bankart suture repair: technique and early results. Arthroscopy 3(2):111–122, 1987.

355. Morrey BF, and Jones JM: Recurrent anterior dislocation of the shoulder. Long-term follow-up of the Putti-Platt and Bankart procedures. J Bone Joint Surg 58A:252, 1976.

356. Morton KS: The unstable shoulder: recurrent subluxation. In Proceedings of the Canadian Orthopaedic Association. J Bone Joint Surg 59B:508, 1977.

357. Moseley HF: Shoulder Lesions. Springfield IL: Charles C Thomas, 1945.

358. Moseley HF: Recurrent Dislocation of the Shoulder. London: E. and S. Livingstone, 1961, p 112.

359. Moseley HF: Recurrent Dislocations of the Shoulder, Montreal: McGill University Press, 1961.

360. Moseley HF: The basic lesions of recurrent anterior dislocation. Surg Clin North Am 43:1631–1634, 1963.

361. Moseley JF: Shoulder Lesions. Edinburgh: Churchill Livingstone, 1972.

362. Moseley HF, and Overgaard B: The anterior capsular mechanism in recurrent anterior dislocation of the shoulder. J Bone Joint Surg 44B:913–927, 1962.

363. Mowery CA, Garfin SR, Booth RE, and Rothman RH: Recurrent posterior dislocation of the shoulder: treatment using a bone block. J Bone Joint Surg 67(5):777–781, 1985.

364. Müller W: Über den negativen Luftdruck im Gelenkraum. Dtsch A Chir 217:395–401, 1929.

365. Mumenthaler M, and Schliack H: Lasionen Peripherer Nerven. Stuttgart: Georg Thieme Verlag, 1965.

366. Murrard J: Un cas de luxatio erecta de l'épaule double et symetrique. Rev Orthop 7:423, 1920.

367. Mynter H: Subacromial dislocation from muscular spasm. Ann Surg 36:117–119, 1902.

368. Najenson T, and Pilielny SS: Malalignment of the glenohumeral joint following hemiplegia. A review of 500 cases. Ann Phys Med 8:96–99, 1965.

369. Neer CS II: Degenerative lesions of the proximal humeral articular surface. Clin Orthop 20:116–124, 1961.

370. Neer CS II: Fractures of the distal third of the clavicle. Clin Orthop 58:43–50, 1968.

371. Neer CS II: Displaced proximal humeral fractures. I. Classification and evaluation. J Bone Joint Surg 52A:1077–1089, 1970.

372. Neer CS II: Involuntary inferior and multidirectional instability of the shoulder: etiology, recognition, and treatment. Instr Course Lect 34:232–238, 1985.

373. Neer CS, and Foster CR: Inferior capsular shift for involuntary inferior and multidirectional instability of the shoulder. A preliminary report. J Bone Joint Surg 62A:897–907, 1980.

374. Neer CS II, and Horwitz BS: Fractures of the proximal humeral epiphyseal plate. Clin Orthop 41:24–31, 1965.

375. Neer CS II, and Welsh RP: The shoulder in sports. Symposium on injuries in sports: recent developments. Orthop Clin North Am 8B:583, 1977.

376. Neviaser JS: An operation for old dislocation of the shoulder. J Bone Joint Surg 30A:997–1000, 1948.

377. Neviaser JS: Complicated fractures and dislocations about the shoulder joint. American Academy of Orthopaedic Surgeons Instr Course Lect 44A:984–998, 1962.

378. Neviaser JS: The treatment of old unreduced dislocations of the shoulder. Surg Clin North Am 43:1671–1678, 1963.

379. Nicola FG, Ellman H, Eckardt J, and Finerman G: Bilateral posterior fracture-dislocation of the shoulder treated with a modification of the McLaughlin procedure, J Bone Joint Surg 63A:1175–1177, 1981.

380. Nicola T: Recurrent anterior dislocation of the shoulder. J Bone Joint Surg 11:128–132, 1929.

381. Nicola T: Recurrent dislocation of the shoulder—its treatment by transplantation of the long head of the biceps. Am J Surg 6:815, 1929.

382. Nicola T: Anterior dislocation of the shoulder: the role of the articular capsule. J Bone Joint Surg 24:614–616, 1942.

383. Nicola T: Acute anterior dislocation of the shoulder. J Bone Joint Surg 31A:153–159, 1949.

384. Nicola T: Recurrent dislocation of the shoulder. Am J Surg 86:85–91, 1953.

385. Nielsen AB, and Nielsen K: The modified Bristow procedure for recurrent anterior dislocation of the shoulder. Acta Orthop Scand 53:229–232, 1982.

386. Nixon JR, and Young WS: Arthrography of the shoulder in anterior dislocation: a study of African and Asian patients. Injury 9:287–293, 1977.

387. Nobel W: Posterior traumatic dislocation of the shoulder. J Bone Joint Surg 44A:523–538, 1962.

388. Noesberger B, and Mader G: Die Modifizierte Operation nach Trillat bei Habitueller Schulterluxation. Zschr Unf Med Berufskr 69:34–36, 1976.

389. Norris TR: C-arm fluoroscopic evaluation under anesthesia for glenohumeral subluxations. In Bateman JE, and Welsh RP (eds): Surgery of the Shoulder. Philadelphia: BC Decker, 1984, pp 22–25.

390. Norris TR: Diagnostic techniques for shoulder instability. Instr Course Lect 34:239–257, 1985.

391. Norris TR, and Bigliani LU: Analysis of failed repair for shoulder instability; a preliminary report. In Bateman JE, and Welsh RP (eds): Surgery of the Shoulder. Philadelphia: BC Decker, 1984, pp 111–116.

392. Norris TR, Bigliani LU, and Harris E: Complications following the modified Bristow repair for shoulder instability. American Shoulder and Elbow Surgeons 3rd Open Meeting, San Francisco, 1987.

393. Norwood LA: Posterior shoulder approach. Clin Orthop (201):167–72, 1985.

394. Norwood LA: Treatment of acute shoulder dislocations. Ala Med 54(6):30–36, 1984.

395. O'Conner SJ: Posterior dislocation of the shoulder. Arch Surg 72:479–491, 1956.

396. O'Conner SJ, and Jacknow AS: Posterior dislocation of the shoulder. J Bone Joint Surg 37A:1122, 1955.

397. O'Driscoll SW, and Evans DC: The DuToit staple capsulorrhaphy for recurrent anterior dislocation of the shoulder: twenty years of experience in six Toronto hospitals. American Shoulder and Elbow Surgeons 4th Open Meeting, Atlanta, 1988.

398. Older MWJ: Arthroscopy of the shoulder joint. J Bone Joint Surg 58B:253, 1976.

399. Olsson O: Degenerative changes of the shoulder joint and their connection with shoulder pain. Acta Chir Scand [Suppl] 181:1–130, 1953.

400. Onabowale BO, and Jaja MOA: Unreduced bilateral synchronous shoulder dislocations. Niger Med J 9:267–271, 1979.

401. Oppenheim WL, Dawson EG, Quinlan C, and Graham SA: The cephaloscapular projection. A special diagnostic aid. Clin Orthop (195):191–193, 1985.

402. Osmond-Clarke H: Habitual dislocation of the shoulder. The Putti-Platt operation. J Bone Joint Surg 30B:19–25, 1948.

403. Oudard P: La luxation recidivante de l'épaule (variété antero-interne) procede operatoire. J Chir 23:13, 1924.

404. Ovesen J, and Nielsen S: Experimental distal subluxation in the glenohumeral joint. Arch Orthop Trauma Surg 104(2):82–84, 1985.

405. Ovesen J, and Nielsen S: Stability of the shoulder joint: cadaver study of stabilizing structures. Acta Orthop Scand 56:149–151, 1985.

406. Ovesen J, and Nielsen S: Anterior and posterior shoulder instability. A cadaver study. Acta Orthop Scand 57(4):324–327, 1986.

407. Ovesen J, and Nielson S: Posterior instability of the shoulder. A cadaver study. Acta Orthop Scand 57(5):436–439, 1986.

408. Ovesen J, and Söjbjerg JO: Lesions in different types of anterior glenohumeral joint dislocation. An experimental study. Arch Orthop Trauma Surg 105(4):216–218, 1986.

409. Ovesen J, and Söjbjerg JO: Posterior shoulder dislocation. Muscle and capsular lesions in cadaver experiments. Acta Orthop Scand *57*(6):535–536, 1986.

410. Ovesen J, and Söjbjerg JO: Transposition of coracoacromial ligament to humerus in treatment of vertical shoulder joint instability: clinical applicability of experimental technique. Arch Orthop Trauma Surg *106*:323–326, 1987.

411. Ozaki J: Pathogenesis of the loose shoulder. Rinsho Shinkei-gabu *16*:1161, 1981.

412. Paavolainen P, Bjorkenheim JM, Ahovuo J, and Slatis P: Recurrent anterior dislocation of the shoulder. Results of Eden-Hybinette and Putti-Platt operations. Acta Orthop Scand *55*(5):556–560, 1984.

413. Pagden D, Halaburt AS, Wiroszo R, and Karyn A: Posterior dislocation of the shoulder complicating regional anesthesia. Anesth Analg *65*(10):1063–1065, 1986.

414. Palmer I, and Widen A: The bone block method for recurrent dislocation of the shoulder joint. J Bone Joint Surg *30B*:53, 1948.

415. Pappas AM, Goss TP, and Kleinman PK: Symptomatic shoulder instability due to lesions of the glenoid labrum. Am J Sports Med *11*:279–288, 1983.

416. Parisien JS: Shoulder arthroscopy technique and indications. Bull Hosp Joint Dis *43*:56–69, 1983.

417. Parisien VM: Shoulder dislocation: an easier method of reduction. J Maine Med Assoc *70*:102, 1979.

418. Parrish GA, and Skiendzielewski JJ: Bilateral posterior fracture-dislocations of the shoulder after convulsive status epilepticus. Ann Emerg Med *14*(3):264–266, 1985.

419. Parsons SW, and Rowley DI: Brachial plexus lesions in dislocations and fracture dislocation of the shoulder. J R Coll Surg Edinb *31*(2):85–87, 1986.

420. Pascoet G, Jung F, Foucher G, and Kehr P: Treatment of recurrent dislocation of the shoulder by preglenoid artificial ridge using the Latarjet-Vittori technique. J Med Strasbourg *6*:501–504, 1975.

421. Pasila M, Jaroma H, Kiviluoto O, et al: Early complications of primary shoulder dislocations. Acta Orthop Scand *49*:260–263, 1978.

422. Pasila M, Kiviluoto O, Jaroma H, and Sundholm A: Recovery from primary shoulder dislocation and its complications. Acta Orthop Scand *51*:257–262, 1980.

423. Patel MR, Pardee ML, and Singerman RC: Intrathoracic dislocation of the head of the humerus. J Bone Joint Surg *45A*:1712–1714, 1963.

424. Paton DF: Posterior dislocation of the shoulder; a diagnostic pitfall for physicians. Practitioner *223*:111–112, 1979.

425. Pavlov H, Warren RF, Weiss CB Jr, and Dines DM: The roentgenographic evaluation of anterior shoulder instability. Clin Orthop (194):153–158, 1985.

426. Payne RE: Involuntary anterior recurrent subluxation of the shoulder. Clin Orthop *126*:311, 1977.

427. Peiro A, Ferrandis R, and Correa F: Bilateral erect dislocation of the shoulders. Injury *6*:294, 1975.

428. Percy LR: Recurrent posterior dislocation of the shoulder. J Bone Joint Surg *42B*:863, 1960.

429. Perniceni B, and Augereau A: Treatment of old unreduced anterior dislocations of the shoulder by open reduction and reinforced rib graft: discussion of three cases. Ann Chir *36*:235–239, 1983.

430. Perthes G: Uber Operationen bei Habitueller Schulterluxation. Deutsch Ztschr Chir *85*:199–227, 1906.

431. Pettersson G: Rupture of the tendon aponeurosis of the shoulder joint in anterior inferior dislocation. Acta Chir Scand (Suppl.)*77*:1–187, 1942.

432. Pilz W: Zur Rontgenuntersschung der Habituellen Schulterverrenkung. Arch Klin Chir *135*:1–22, 1925.

433. Pinzur MS, and Hookins GE: Biceps tenodesis for painful inferior subluxation of the shoulder in adult acquired hemiplegia. Clin Orthop *May* (206):100–103, 1986.

434. Poppen NK, and Walker PS: Normal and abnormal motion of the shoulder. J Bone Joint Surg *58A*:195, 1976.

435. Poppen NK, and Walker PS: Forces at the glenohumeral joint in abduction. Clin Orthop *135*:165–170, 1978.

436. Post M: The Shoulder. Surgical and Non-surgical Management. Philadelphia; Lea & Febiger, 1978.

437. Pritchett JW, and Clark JM: Prosthetic replacement for chronic unreduced dislocations of the shoulder. Clin Orthop (216):89–93, 1987.

438. Protzman RR: Anterior instability of the shoulder. J Bone Joint Surg *62A*:909–918, 1980.

439. Quigley TB, and Freedman PA: Recurrent dislocation of the shoulder. Am J Surg *128*:595–599, 1974.

440. Rafii M, Firooznia H, Bonamo JJ, et al: CT arthrography of capsular structures of the shoulder. AJR *146*(2):361–367, 1986.

441. Rafii M, Firooznia H, Bonamo JJ, et al: Athlete shoulder injuries: CT arthrographic findings. Radiology *162*(2):559–564, 1987.

442. Randelli M, and Gambrioli PL: Glenohumeral osteometry by computed tomography in normal and unstable shoulders. Clin Orthop *208*:151, 1986.

443. Randelli M, and Gambrioli PL: Recurrent instability of the glenohumeral joint. Ital J Orthop Traumatol *11*(1):107–117, 1985.

444. Randelli M, Ocella F, and Gambrioli PL: Clinical experience with double contrast medium computerized tomography (arthro-CT) in instability of the shoulder. Ital J Orthop Traumatol *12*(2):151–158, 1986.

445. Rao JP, Francis AM, Hurley J, and Daczkewycz R: Treatment of recurrent anterior dislocation of the shoulder by duToit staple capsulorrhaphy. Results of long-term follow-up study. Clin Orthop *204*:169, 1986.

446. Reeves B: Acute anterior dislocation of the shoulder. Ann R Coll Surg Engl *43*:255, 1969.

447. Reeves B: Arthrography in acute dislocation of the shoulder. J Bone Joint Surg *48B*:182, 1968.

448. Reeves B: Experiments on the tensile strength of the anterior capsular structures of the shoulder region. J Bone Joint Surg *50B*:858, 1968.

449. Renstrom P: Swedish research in sports traumatology. Clin Orthop (191):144–158, 1984.

450. Respet PB: A practical technique for reducing shoulder dislocations. J Musculoskeletal Med *6*:29–35, 1988.

451. Richards RR, Waddell JP, and Hudson MB: Shoulder arthrodesis for the treatment of brachial plexus palsy: a review of twenty-two patients. American Shoulder and Elbow Surgeons 3rd Open Meeting, San Francisco, 1987.

452. Rob CG, and Standeven A: Closed traumatic lesions of the axillary and brachial arteries. Lancet *1*:597–599, 1956.

453. Robertson R, and Stack WJ: Diagnosis and treatment of recurrent dislocation of the shoulder. J Bone Joint Surg *29*:797–800, 1947.

454. Roca LA, and Ramos-Vertiz JR: Luxacion erecta de hombro. Rev San Mil Arg *61*:135, 1962.

455. Rockwood CA: Part 2: Dislocations about the shoulder. *In* Rockwood CA, and Green DP (eds): Fractures, 2nd ed, vol. 1. Philadelphia: JB Lippincott, 1984.

456. Rockwood CA Jr: Subluxation of the shoulder—the classification, diagnosis and treatment. Orthop Trans *4*:306, 1979.

457. Rockwood CA Jr, Burkhead WZ Jr, and Brna J: Subluxation for the glenohumeral joint; response to rehabilitative exercise in traumatic vs. atraumatic instability. American Shoulder and Elbow Surgeons 2nd Open Meeting, New Orleans, 1986.

458. Rokous JR, Feagin JA, and Abbott HG: Modified axillary roentgenogram. A useful adjunct in the diagnosis of recurrent instability of the shoulder. Clin Orthop *82*:84–86, 1972.

459. Romanes GJ: Upper and lower limbs. *In* Cunningham's Manual of Practical Anatomy, 13th ed. London: Oxford University Press, 1966, pp 75–76.

460. Roston JB, and Haines RW: Cracking in the metacarpophalangeal joint. J Anat *81*:165–173, 1947.

461. Rowe CR: Prognosis in dislocations of the shoulder. J Bone Joint Surg *38A*:957–977, 1956.

462. Rowe CR: Instabilities of the glenohumeral joint. Bull Hosp Joint Dis *39*:180–186, 1978.

463. Rowe CR: Acute and recurrent anterior dislocations of the shoulder. Orthop Clin North Am *11*:253–269, 1980.

464. Rowe CR: Failed surgery for recurrent dislocations of the shoulder. Instr Course Lect 34:264–267, 1985.

465. Rowe CR, Patel D, and Southmayd WW: The Bankart procedure—a study of late results (proceedings). J Bone Joint Surg 59B:122, 1977.

466. Rowe CR, Patel D, and Southmayd WW: The Bankart procedure—a long-term end-result study. J Bone Joint Surg 60A:1–16, 1978.

467. Rowe CR, Pierce DS, and Clark JG: Voluntary dislocation of the shoulder. A preliminary report on a clinical, electromyographic, and psychiatric study of 26 patients. J Bone Joint Surg 55A:445–460, 1973.

468. Rowe CR, and Sakellarides HT: Factors related to recurrences of anterior dislocations of the shoulder. Clin Orthop 20:40, 1961.

469. Rowe CR, and Yee LBK: A posterior approach to the shoulder joint. J Bone Joint Surg 26A:580, 1944.

470. Rowe CR, and Zarins B: Recurrent transient subluxation of the shoulder. J Bone Joint Surg 63A:863–872, 1981.

471. Rowe CR, and Zarins B: Chronic unreduced dislocations of the shoulder. J Bone Joint Surg 64A:494–505, 1982.

472. Rowe CR, Zarins B, and Ciullo JV: Recurrent anterior dislocation of the shoulder after surgical repair. Apparent causes of failure and treatment. J Bone Joint Surg 66A:159, 1984.

473. Rozing PM, De Bakker HM, and Obermann WR: Radiographic views in recurrent anterior shoulder dislocation. Comparison of six methods for identification of typical lesions. Acta Orthop Scand 57(4):328–330, 1986.

474. Rubenstein J: The bent screw: a sign of postoperative recurrent dislocation. J Can Assoc Radiol 38(1):20–22, 1987.

475. Rubin SA, Gray RL, and Green WR: Scapular Y—a diagnostic aid in shoulder trauma. Radiology 110:725–726, 1974.

476. Rupp F: Ueber ein Vereinfachtes Operationverfahren bei Habitueller Schulterluxatuion. Deutsch Z Chir 198:70–75, 1926.

477. Russell JA, Holmes EM III, Keller DJ, et al: Reduction of acute anterior shoulder dislocations using the Milch technique: a study of ski injuries. J Trauma 21(9):802–804, 1981.

478. Saha AK: Mechanism of shoulder movements and a plea for the recognition of "zero position" of glenohumeral joint. Indian J Surg 12:153–165, 1950.

479. Saha AK: Theory of Shoulder Mechanism. Springfield, IL: Charles C Thomas, 1961.

480. Saha AK: Anterior recurrent dislocation of the shoulder: treatment by latissimus dorsi transfer with follow-up in 22 cases. J Int Coll Surg 39:361–373, 1963.

481. Saha AK: Anterior recurrent dislocation of the shoulder. Acta Orthop Scand 39:479–493, 1967.

482. Saha AK: Surgery of the paralysed and flail shoulder. Acta Orthop Scand (Suppl) 97:5–90, 1967.

483. Saha AK: Dynamic stability of the glenohumeral joint. Acta Orthop Scand 42:491–505, 1971.

484. Saha AK: Mechanics of elevation of glenohumeral joint: its application in rehabilitation of flail shoulder in upper brachial plexus injuries and poliomyelitis and in replacement of the upper humerus by prosthesis. Acta Orthop Scand 44:668, 1973.

485. Saha AK, Bhadra N, and Dutta SK: Latissimus dorsi transfer for recurrent dislocation of the shoulder. Acta Orthop Scand 57(6):539–541, 1986.

486. Saha AK, Das NN, and Chakravarty BF: Treatment of recurrent dislocation of shoulder: past, present, and future: studies on electromyographic changes of muscles acting on the shoulder joint complex. Calcutta Med J 53:409–413, 1956.

487. Samilson RL, and Prieto V: Dislocation arthropathy of the shoulder. J Bone Joint Surg 65A:456–460, 1983.

488. Sarma A, Savanchak H, Levinson ED, and Sigman R: Thrombosis of the axillary artery and brachial plexus injury secondary to shoulder dislocation. Conn Med 45:513–514, 1981.

489. Saxena K, and Stavas J: Inferior glenohumeral dislocation. Ann Emerg Med 12(11):718–720, 1983.

490. Schlemm F: Ueber die Verstarkungsbander am Schultergelenk. Arch Anat Physiol Wissenschaft Med 22:45, 1853.

491. Schroder HA, and Fristed PB: Recurrent dislocation of the shoulder. The Alvik modification of the Eden-Hybinette operation. Acta Orthop Scand 56:396, 1985.

492. Schüller M: Berlin Klin Wochenschr 33:760, 1896.

493. Schulz TJ, Jacobs B, and Patterson RL: Unrecognized dislocations of the shoulder. J Trauma 9:1009–1023, 1969.

494. Schwartz RR, O'Brien SJ, Warren RF, and Torzilli PA: Capsular restraints to anterior-posterior motion in the shoulder. American Shoulder and Elbow Surgeons 4th Open Meeting, Atlanta, 1988.

495. Scott DJ Jr: Treatment of recurrent posterior dislocations of the shoulder by glenoplasty. J Bone Joint Surg 49A:471, 1967.

496. Scougall S: Posterior dislocation of the shoulder. J Bone Joint Surg 39B:726–732, 1957.

497. Segal D, Yablon IG, Lynch JJ, and Jones RP: Acute bilateral anterior dislocation of the shoulders. Clin Orthop 140:21–22, 1979.

498. Seltzer SE, and Weissman BN: CT findings in normal and dislocating shoulders. J Can Assoc Radiol 36(1):41–46, 1985.

499. Sergio G: Recurrent anterior dislocation of the shoulder joint. A modification of Bankart's capsuloplexy. Notes on the surgical technique. Ital J Orthop Traumatol 9:469, 1983.

500. Sever JW: Obstetrical paralysis. Surg Gynecol Obstet 44:547–549, 1927.

501. Sever JW: Fracture of the head of the humerus: treatment and results. N Engl J Med 216:1100–1107, 1937.

502. Shively J, Johnson J: Results of modified Bristow procedure. Clin Orthop 187:150, 1984.

503. Shuman WP, Kilcoyne RF, Matsen FA, et al: Double-contrast computed tomography of the glenoid labrum. AJR 141:581–584, 1983.

503a. Sidles JA, Harryman DT, Simkin PA, et al: Passive and active stabilization of the glenohumeral joint. J Bone Joint Surg (submitted for publication, 1989).

504. Simkin PA: Structure and function of joints. In Schumacher HR(ed): Primer on the Rheumatic Diseases, 9th ed. Atlanta: Arthritis Foundation, 1988, Chap. 11.

505. Simonet WT, and Cofield RH: Prognosis in anterior shoulder dislocation. Paper presented to American Orthopaedic Society for Sports Medicine, Homestead, VA, March 1983.

506. Simonet WT, and Cofield RH: Prognosis in anterior shoulder dislocation. Am J Sports Med 12:19–24, 1984.

507. Singson RD, and Bigliani L: CT arthrographic patterns in recurrent glenohumeral instability. AJR 149(4):749–753, 1987.

508. Singson RD, Feldman F, Bigliani LU, and Rosseberg Z: Recurrent shoulder dislocation after surgical repair: double-contrast CT arthography (work in progress). Radiology 164(2):425–428, 1987.

509. Sisk TD: Campbell's Operative Orthopaedics, 6th ed. St. Louis: CV Mosby, 1980, pp 662–670.

510. Sisk TD, and Boyd HB: Management of recurrent anterior dislocation of the shoulder. DuToit-type or staple capsulorrhaphy. Clin Orthop 103:150, 1974.

511. Speed K: Fractures and Dislocation, 4th ed. Philadelphia: Lea and Febiger, 1942.

512. Staffel F: Verh Dtsch Ges Chir, 24(2):651–656, 1895.

513. Stein E: Case report 374: posttraumatic pseudoaneurysm of axillary artery. Skeletal Radiol. 15(5):391–393, 1986.

514. Steenburg RW, and Ravitch MM: Cervicothoracic approach for subclavian vessel injury from compound fracture of the clavicle: considerations of subclavian axillary exposures. Ann Surg 157:839–846, 1963.

515. Stener B: Dislocation of the shoulder complicated by complete rupture of the axillary artery. J Bone Joint Surg 39B:714–717, 1957.

516. Stevens JH: Brachial plexus paralysis. In Codman, EA: The Shoulder. New York: G. Miller, 1934.

517. Stimson LA: Fractures and Dislocations, 3rd ed. Philadelphia: Lea Brothers, 1900.

518. Stimson LA: A Practical Treatise on Fractures and Dislocations, 7th ed. Philadelphia: Lea and Febiger, 1912.

519. Stromovist B, Wingstrand H, and Egund N: Recurrent shoulder dislocation and screw failure after the Bristow-Latarjet procedure. A case report. Arch Orthop Trauma Surg 106(4):260–262, 1987.

520. Stromsoe K, Senn E, Simmen B, and Matter P: Rezidivhaufigkeit nach Erstmaliger Traumatischer Schulter-luxation. Helv Chir Acta 47:85–88, 1980.

521. Stufflesser H, and Dexel M: The treatment of recurrent dislo-

cation of the shoulder by rotation osteotomy with internal fixation. Ital J Orthop Traumatol 39(2):191, 1977.

522. Sweeney JH, Mead NC, and Dawson WJ: Fourteen years' experience with the modified Bristow procedure. Paper presented to Annual Meeting of American Academy of Orthopaedic Surgeons, San Francisco, CA, March 1–6, 1975.

523. Symeonides PP: The significance of the subscapularis muscle in the pathogenesis of recurrent anterior dislocation of the shoulder. J Bone Joint Surg 54B:476–483, 1972.

524. Tagliabue D, and Esposito A: L'intervento di Latarjet nella lussazione recidivante di spalla-dello sportivo. Ital J Orthop Traumatol 2:91–100, 1980.

525. Taketomi Y: Observations on subluxation of the shoulder joint in hemiplegia. Phys Ther 55:39–40, 1975.

526. Thomas MA: Posterior subacromial dislocation of the head of the humerus. AJR 37:767–773, 1937.

526a. Thomas SC, and Matsen FA III: An approach to the repair of avulsion of the glenohumeral ligaments in the management of traumatic anterior glenohumeral instability. J Bone Joint Surg 71A(4):506–513, 1989.

527. Thomas TT: Habitual or recurrent anterior dislocation of the shoulder. Am J Med Sci 137:229–246, 1909.

528. Thomas TT: Habitual or recurrent dislocation of the shoulder: forty-four shoulder operations in 42 patients. Surg Gynecol Obstet 32:291–299, 1921.

529. Thompson FR, and Winant WM: Unusual fracture-subluxations of the shoulder joint. J Bone Joint Surg (Am) 32:575–582, 1950.

530. Thompson FR, and Winant WM: Comminuted fractures of the humeral head with subluxation. Clin Orthop 20:94–96, 1961.

531. Tibone JE, Prietto C, Jobe FW, et al: Staple capsulorrhaphy for recurrent posterior shoulder dislocation. Am J Sports Med 9:135–139, 1981.

532. Tietjen R: Occult glenohumeral interposition of a torn rotator cuff. J Bone Joint Surg 64A:458–459, 1982.

533. Tijmes J, Loyd HM, and Tullos HS: Arthrography in acute shoulder dislocations. South Med J 72:564–567, 1979.

534. Tobis JS: Posthemiplegia shoulder pain. NY State J Med 57:1377–1380, 1957.

535. Torg JS, Balduini FC, Bonci C, et al: A modified Bristow-Helfet-May procedure for recurrent dislocations and subluxation of the shoulder: report of 212 cases. J Bone Joint Surg 69(6):904–913, 1987.

536. Townley CO: The capsular mechanism in recurrent dislocation of the shoulder. J Bone Joint Surg 32A:370–380, 1950.

537. Trillat A: Traitement de la luxation recidivante de l'épaule: considerations, techniques. Lyon Chir 49:986, 1954.

538. Trillat A, and Leclerc-Chalvet F: Luxation Recidivante de L'Épaule. Paris: Masson, 1973.

539. Trimmings NP: Haemarthrosis aspiration in treatment of anterior dislocation of the shoulder. J R Soc Med 78(12):1023–1027, 1985.

540. Tullos HS, Bennett JB, and Braly WG: Acute shoulder dislocations: factors influencing diagnosis and treatment. Instr Course Lect 33:364–385, 1984.

541. Turkel SJ, Panio MW, Marshall JL, and Girgis FG: Stabilizing mechanisms preventing anterior dislocation of the glenohumeral joint. J Bone Joint Surg 63A(8):1208–1217, 1981.

542. Tuszynski W: Anterior dislocation of the shoulder complicated by temporary brachial paresis. Chir Narzadow Ruchu Orthop Pol 46:129–131, 1981.

543. Unsworth A, Dowson D, and Wright V: "Cracking joints": a bioengineering study of cavitation in the metacarpophalangeal joint. Ann Rheum Dis 30:348, 1971.

544. Uhthoff HK, and Piscopo M: Anterior capsular redundancy of the shoulder: congenital or traumatic? An embryological study. J Bone Joint Surg 67(3):363–366, 1985.

545. Valls J: Acrylic prosthesis in a case with fracture of the head of the humerus. Bal Soc Orthop Trauma 17:61, 1952.

546. Van der Spek K: Rupture of the axillary artery as a complication of dislocation of the shoulder. Arch Chir Neerl 16:113–118, 1964.

547. Vander Ghirst M, and Houssa R: Acrylic prosthesis in fractures of the head of the humerus. Acta Chir Belg 50:31, 1951.

548. Vastamaki M, and Solonen KA: Posterior dislocation and fracture-dislocation of the shoulder. Acta Orthop Scand 51:479–484, 1980.

549. Vegter J, and Marti RK: Treatment of posterior dislocation of the shoulder by osteotomy of the neck of the scapula. J Bone Joint Surg 63:288, 1981.

550. Verrina F: Para-articular ossification following simple dislocation of the shoulder. Minerva Orthop 210:480–486, 1975.

551. Vezina JA, and Beauregard CG: An update of the technique of double-contrast arthrotomography of the shoulder. J Can Assoc Radiol 36(3):176–182, 1985.

552. Vichard P, and Arnould D: Les luxations-fractures posterieures de l'épaule. Rev Chir Orthop 67:71–77, 1981.

553. Waldron VD: Dislocated shoulder reduction—a simple method that is done without assistants. Orthop Rev 11:105–106, 1982.

554. Warren RF: Instability of shoulder in throwing sports. Instr Course Lect 34:337–348, 1985.

555. Warren RF, Kornblatt IB, and Marchand R: Static factors affecting posterior shoulder instability. Orthop Trans 8:1–89, 1984.

556. Watson-Jones R: Dislocation of the shoulder joint. Proc R Soc Med 29:1060–1062, 1936.

557. Watson-Jones R: Recurrent dislocation of the shoulder. J Bone Joint Surg 30B:6–8, 1948.

558. Watson-Jones R: Fractures and Joint Injuries, 4th ed. Baltimore: Williams & Wilkins, 1957.

559. Weber BG: Operative treatment for recurrent dislocation of the shoulder. Injury 1:107–109, 1969.

560. Weber BG, Simpson LA, and Hardegger F: Rotational humeral osteotomy for recurrent anterior dislocation of the shoulder associated with a large Hill-Sachs lesion. J Bone Joint Surg 66A:1443, 1984.

561. Weitbrecht J: Syndesmology; or, a Description of the Ligaments of the Human Body (trans E. B. Kaplan). Philadelphia: WB Saunders, 1969.

562. Wenner SM: Anterior dislocation of the shoulder in patients over 50 years of age. Orthopaedics 8(9):1155–1157, 1985.

563. West EF: Intrathoracic dislocation of the humerus. J Bone Joint Surg 31B:61–62, 1949.

564. White ADN: Dislocated shoulder—a simple method of reduction. Med J Aust 2:726–727, 1976.

565. Wickstrom J: Birth injuries of the brachial plexus: treatment of defects in the shoulder. Clin Orthop 23:187–196, 1962.

566. Wiley AM, and Austwick DH: Shoulder Surgery Through the Arthroscope. Toronto: Department of Surgery, University of Toronto and Toronto Wester Hospital, 1982.

567. Wiley AM, and Older MWJ: Shoulder arthroscopy. J Sports Med 8:31–38, 1980.

568. Wilson JC, and McKeever FM: Traumatic posterior (retro-glenoid) dislocation of the humerus. J Bone Joint Surg 31A:160–172, 1949.

569. Wong-Pack WK, Bobechko PE, and Becker EJ: Fractured coracoid with anterior shoulder dislocation. J Can Assoc Radiol 31:278–279, 1980.

570. Yadav SS: Bilateral simultaneous fracture-dislocation of the shoulder due to muscular violence. J Postgrad Med 23:137–139, 1977.

571. Yoneda B, Welsh RP, and MacIntosh DL: Conservative treatment of shoulder dislocation in young males (proceedings). J Bone Joint Surg 64B:254–255, 1982.

572. Zachary RB: Transplantation of teres major and latissimus dorsi for loss of external rotation at the shoulder. Lancet 2:757–761, 1947.

573. Zarins B, and Rowe CR: Current concepts in the diagnosis and treatment of shoulder instability in athletes. Med Sci Sports Exerc 16(15):444–448, 1984.

574. Zimmerman LM, and Veith I: Great Ideas in the History of Surgery: Clavicle, Shoulder, Shoulder Amputations. Baltimore: Williams & Wilkins, 1961.

575. Zizzi F, Frizziero L, Facchini A, and Zini GL: Artroscopia della spalla: indicazioni e limiti. Reumatismo 33:429–432, 1981.

576. Zuckerman JD, and Matsen FA: Complications about the glenohumeral joint related to the use of screws and staples. J Bone Joint Surg 66A:175, 1984.

Index

Note: Page numbers in *italics* refer to illustrations; page numbers followed by a t refer to tables.

A

Abbott-Saunders procedure, in biceps tendon dislocation, 824
Abduction, after humeral resection, 906
  biceps tendon motion in, 805, 807–808
  fatigue development in, 1096–1097, *1097–1098*
  in brachial plexus injury of newborn, 1039, *1040*, 1041
  in frozen shoulder, 841–842, 842t
  in swimming strokes, 988–989
  ligament position in, 20, *20*
  maximum torque in, 242, 242t, *243*
  measurement of, 164, *172*
  muscles of, testing of, 164, *165*
  supraspinatus tendon hypovascularity in, 648
Abduction transfer procedure, in brachial plexus injury of newborn, 1050–1051
Accessory spinal nerve. See *Spinal accessory nerve.*
Acromial artery, anatomy of, 42, *79*, 80
Acromioclavicular capsule, anatomy of, 211, *211*
Acromioclavicular joint, abnormality of, in impingement syndrome, 627t
  anatomy of, 42–43, *43*, 210–211, *210–211*, *478*, 1010, *1010*
    surgical, 413–420, *414–420*
  anesthetic injection into, diagnostic, 174
  arthritis of. See under *Arthritis.*
  arthrodesis of, 414–415
  arthroscopy of, 262
  articular surface of, 210, *210*, 413
  biomechanics of, 210–212, *210–212*
  blood supply of, 42
  constraints on, 211–212, *212*
  cyst of, 468
  debridement of, 452, *453*
  degenerative arthritis of, acromioplasty failure in, 636
  discs of, 42, 414
  dislocation of, 419, *419*. See also subhead: *injury of, types III to*
    VI.
    historical aspects of, 413
    in sports, 987
    mechanism of, *418–419*, 419–420, *421*
    subacromial, 434
    subcoracoid, 434, *434*
  disorders of, versus frozen shoulder, 852
  embryology of, 10, *11*
  forces on, direct, 420–421, *421*
    indirect, 422, *422*
  impingement of, on rotator cuff. See *Impingement syndrome.*
  inclination of, 413, *414*
  injury of, chronic, treatment of, 446–447, *448*, 460–463, *460–*
    462

Acromioclavicular joint *(Continued)*
  classification of, 422–425, *423*
  complications of, after nonoperative treatment, 465–466
    after operation, 464–465, *467*
    in acute injury, 463–466, *465*
  coracoid fracture with, treatment of, 444, *444–445*
  direct force in, 420, *421*
  historical aspects of, 413
  in sports, 986–987
  incidence of, 425
  indirect force in, 422, *422*
  injuries associated with, 463–464
  mechanism of, 420–422, *421–422*
  prognosis of, 463
  Rockwood classification of, 1020, *1021*
  symptoms of, 425–426, *425–427*
  treatment of, 434–447
    approaches to, 435, 437
    biomechanics of, 442–443
    Bosworth screw in, 440–443, *441*, 454, *454*
    chronic, 446–447, *448*, 460–463, *460–462*
    complications of, *450*, 464–467, *467*
    coracoclavicular ligament repairs in, 438t, 440–443, *441–442*
    Dacron graft in, 441–442, *442*
    distal clavicle excision in, 438t, 443, *443*, 446, 457, 460
    dynamic muscle transfer in, 438t, 443–444, 446–447, *448*
    extra-articular fixation in, 440–443, *441–442*, 457
    historical review of, 436–437
    intra-articular repairs in, 438t, 439–440, *439–440*, 442–443,
      457
    ligament reconstruction in, 447
    nonoperative, 435–438, *435*, *437*, 437t, 445, 447–449, *450–*
      451
    operative. See specific technique.
    postoperative care in, 440, 455, *456–457*
    screw fixation in, 440–443, *441*, 452, *453–457*, 454–455
    skillful neglect in, 437–438
    sling in, 435, *435*, 437–438, *437*, 437t, 447–449, *450–451*
    type I, 435, 447–448
    type II, 435–436, *435*, 448–449, *449*
    type III, 436–445, 437t–438t, *437–445*, 449–455, *450–455*
    type IV, 445, *446*, 455, *455*, 457
    type V, 445, *446*, 455, 457, *458*
    type VI, 445–446, *447*, 455, 457, *459*
    wire loops in, 441–442, *441*
    with coracoid process fracture, 444, *444–445*
  type I, 422–424, *423*
    symptoms of, 425
    treatment of, 435, 447–448
    x-ray evaluation of, 431
  type II, 422–424, *423*

i

Acromioclavicular joint (Continued)
 prognosis of, 463
 symptoms of, 425
 treatment of, 435–436, 435, 448–449, 449
 x-ray evaluation of, 431–432, 431
 type III, 422–424, 423
  joint motion in, 415, 416
  prognosis of, 463
  symptoms of, 425–426, 425
  treatment of, 449–455, 450–455
  x-ray evaluation of, 431–433, 432–433
 type IV, 422, 423, 424
  prognosis of, 463
  symptoms of, 426, 426
  treatment of, 445, 446, 455, 455, 457
  x-ray evaluation of, 433, 433
 type V, 422, 424–425, 423
  prognosis of, 463
  symptoms of, 426, 426–427
  treatment of, 445, 446, 455, 457, 458
  x-ray evaluation of, 433–434, 434
 type VI, 422–425, 423
  prognosis of, 463
  symptoms of, 426
  treatment of, 445–446, 447, 455, 457, 459
  x-ray evaluation of, 434, 434
 innervation of, 42
 instability of, management of, 213, 214
 ligaments of, 42–43, 43, 211, 211. See also Acromioclavicular
   ligament(s); Coracoclavicular ligament.
 loose body in, 429
 motion of, 211–212, 212–213, 414–415, 416–418
 osteoarthritis of, 1095
 osteophytes of, rotator cuff tears in, 651
 palpation of, 157
 pseudodislocation of, 375, 375
 separation of, 386
  misdiagnosis of, 378
  with clavicular fracture, 381, 381
 shape of, 413, 414
 size of, 413
 sprain of, 420–421. See also subhead: injury of, type I; type II.
  mechanism of, 420–421
 x-ray evaluation of, 426–434
  anteroposterior views in, 427, 428–429
  exposure for, 427, 428
  in type I injury, 431
  in type II injury, 431–432, 431
  in type III injury, 431–433, 432–433
  in type IV injury, 433, 433
  in type V injury, 433–434, 434
  in type VI injury, 434, 434
  lateral views in, 427, 429
  problems with, 426–427, 428
  stress type, 427, 429, 430, 431
Acromioclavicular ligament(s), anatomy of, 211, 211, 414, 415, 796
 as constraint, 211–212, 212
 disruption of. See also Acromioclavicular joint, injury of, types II
   to VI.
 in panclavicular dislocation, 375
 function of, 420
 ossification of, 464
 reconstruction of, 439–440, 447
Acromion, abnormality of, in brachial plexus injury of newborn,
   1041
 in impingement syndrome, 627t
 anatomy of, 44–45, 45, 279–280, 280, 336
  comparative, 3, 4
  impingement syndrome and, 625–626, 626
 bipartite (os acromiale), 111–113, 112–113, 340, 342, 342–343
 double, 111, 111
 fracture of, 354–356, 355–357, 361
  in children, 1028
 hooked, 625–626, 626

Acromion (Continued)
 impingement of, on rotator cuff. See Impingement syndrome.
 morphology of, 45, 45
 ossification of, 11, 112, 112, 342, 343
 palpation of, 157
 shape variation in, 625–626, 626
 spurs of, 625
  x-ray evaluation of, 196, 197
 unfused, 45, 45–46
Acromionectomy, in biceps tendon lesions, 828, 828
 radical, in impingement syndrome, 635, 635
Acromioplasty, arthroscopic, in impingement syndrome, 263–264,
   269, 269
  in rotator cuff tear, 270
  postoperative regimen in, 270
  results of, 270
 in biceps tendon lesions, 828–829, 828–829
 in calcifying tendinitis, 786
 in impingement syndrome, 634–636, 965
  arthroscopic, 263–264, 269, 269, 634–635
  failure of, 635–636, 642
  findings in, 634
  indications for, 634
  purpose of, 634
  results of, 634–636
  scarring in, 636
  technique for, 639, 639–642
 in rotator cuff tears, 663
Acrylic shoulder prosthesis, 679, 680
Acupuncture, historical aspects of, 34
Adams view, in x-ray evaluation, 187
Addicts, drug, septic arthritis in, 929, 933–934
Adduction, biceps tendon motion in, 807
 maximum torque in, 242, 242t, 243
Adenocarcinoma, metastatic, incidence of, 892
Adhesion/cohesion mechanism, in glenohumeral joint stability,
   536–537
Adhesive capsulitis, arthrography in, 818, 819
 arthroscopy in, 264, 851
 biceps tendon lesions with, 821
 definition of, 840
 frozen shoulder and, 837, 842–843, 843t
 in humeral fracture, 328
 versus biceps tendon lesions, 822–823
Adipose tissue, anatomy of, 59, 84–88, 87–88
Adson's maneuver, 173, 173
 in thoracic outlet syndrome, 769–770
Aerobic exercise, in impingement syndrome, 638
Age, calcifying tendinitis and, 776, 778–779
 frozen shoulder and, 844
 glenohumeral dislocation and, 568
 impairment evaluation and, 1105
 rotator cuff tears and, 650–654
 tumor distribution and, 892, 894
 versus joint stability, 227–228, 228
Alexander view, in x-ray evaluation, 193, 194, 427, 429
Alkaline phosphatase levels, in tumor diagnosis, 898
Allograft, after limb sparing surgery, 909, 910–911
Alveolar tissue, loose, anatomy of, 85–86, 86–87
AMBRI syndrome, in glenohumeral instability, 151–152, 541, 576,
   576t
 treatment of, 605–608, 606–608
Amelia, adaptation to, 952
American Academy of Orthopaedic Surgeons guidelines, for im-
   pairment evaluation, 1104
 for joint motion measurement, 160, 160t
American Medical Association, impairment evaluation guidelines
   of, 1104
American Society of Shoulder and Elbow Surgeons, humeral frac-
   ture treatment evaluation system of, 284
Aminoglycosides, in bone/joint infections, 934–935, 934t
Ampicillin, in bone/joint infections, 934t, 1081
Amputation, 940–960
 bilateral, adaptation to, 952

Amputation *(Continued)*
    prosthetic management in, *954–955*, 956
  claviculectomy in, 941, 951–952, *952*
  disarticulation, 940, 943, *943–944*, 945
  distal extremity preservation in, 940
  forequarter, 940, 945–949
    anterior approach, 945, *946*, 947
    closed (scapulothoracic dissociation), 361–362, *362*
    posterior approach, 947, *948*, 949
  in arterial injury, 81–82
  in Ewing's sarcoma, 913
  in tumor, 905
  incidence of, 940
  indications for, 941
  interscapulothoracic resection in, 949, *950*
  pain after, 959–960
  postural abnormalities after, 956, 959
  prosthesis for, 952–956
    body-powered, 953–954, *953–956*
    cosmetic, 953, *953*
    externally powered, 954, 956, *957–959*
  scapulectomy in, 941, 949, *951*, 952
  scoliosis after, 956
  through humerus, 940
    at surgical neck, 941, *942*, 943
  Tikhor-Linberg, 907, *908*, 940–941
  types of, 940–941, 949, *950*
  versus limb sparing surgery, 915
Amspacher procedure, in acromioclavicular joint repair, 451–455, *453–457*
Amstutz technique, in prosthetic arthroplasty, 722
Analgesia, in frozen shoulder, 853–854, 858
  patient-controlled, 256
  postoperative, 256
Anatomy. See also specific structure.
  arthroscopic, 259–262, *259–261*, 266–267, *266*, 270–272, *271–272*
  bony, 12–15, *13–14*
  comparative, 1–5, *1–5*
    of biceps tendon, 797, *798*
    of intertubercular groove, 797, *798*
    of scapula, 797, *798*
  developmental, in embryonic period, 6–9, *6–10*
    in fetal period, 9–10, *11*
    of biceps tendon, 799, *799*
    of glenohumeral joint, 799, *799*
    phylogenetic, 1–5, *1–5*
  historical aspects of, 34–38, *36–39*
  of acromioclavicular joint, 42–43, *43*, 210–211, *210–211*, 413–420, *414–420*, 478, 1010, *1010*
  of adipose tissue, *59*, 84–88, *87–88*
  of arteries, 78–82, *79*, *81–82*
  of biceps tendon. See under *Biceps tendon.*
  of blood vessels, 76–83, *77–79*, *81–83*
  of brachial plexus. See under *Brachial plexus.*
  of bursae, 27, *27*, *59*, 88–89, *89*
  of capsule, 15–17, *15–16*, 227–228, *229*
  of clavicle, 41–42, *41–42*, 368–370, *368–369*
    comparative, 2, *2*, 4
    developmental, 10–11, *11*, 1007, 1009
  of compartments, 83–85, *84–85*, 875, *876*, 877
  of fascial spaces, 85–87, *86–87*
  of humerus, 46–49, *47–48*, 262, 279–281, *279–280*, 991–992
    comparative, *3–4*, 4
    developmental, 12, *12*, 991
  of landmark muscles, 65–66, *65*
  of ligaments, 17–27, *17–26*, 209, *209*, 211, *211*, 227–231, *228–232*
    arthroscopic, 260–262, *260–261*
    scapulohumeral, 533–534, *533–534*
  of lymphatic drainage, 82–83, *83*
  of microvasculature, 28–30, *28–30*
  of muscles, 49–66
    axiohumeral, 5
    axioscapular, 5

Anatomy *(Continued)*
    glenohumeral, 57–63, *58–62*
    landmark, 65–66, *65*
    multiple joint, 62–63, *63–65*
    scapulohumeral, comparative, 5, *5*
    scapulothoracic, 54–57, *54–58*
  of nerves, 30–31, *30–31*, 66–76
    brachial plexus, 67–74, *68–75*
    cranial XI, 74–76, *76*
    function and, 66–67, *67*
    intercostal brachial, 76
    supraclavicular, 76, *76*
  of rotator cuff, 262, 279–280, *279*
  of scapula, 43–46, *44–46*, 279–280, *280*, 336–336, *335*, *338*
    comparative, 2, *3–4*, 4, 797, *798*
    developmental, 11–12, *11*, 1025, *1025*
  of skin, 89–92, *90–92*
  of sternoclavicular joint, 39–41, *40–41*
  of subacromial space, 262
  of surgical planes, 85–87, *86–87*
  of veins, 82
Anesthesia, 246–257
  anesthesiologist visit before, 246–247
  cardiovascular monitoring in, 248
  choice of, 249
  diagnostic tests before, 247
  general, in arthroscopy, 265
    indications for, 249
  historical aspects of, 246
  in frozen shoulder manipulation, 856–857
  in glenohumeral dislocation reduction, 570
  local, in injection tests, *172*, 174, 821–823
  medical conditions affecting, 247
  monitoring in, 248
  muscle relaxants with, 248
  oxygen administration with, 248
  pain management after, 256
  positioning for, 248
  postoperative management of, 255
  premedication and, 247–248
  preoperative considerations in, 246–248
  regional, acrylic bone cement problems in, 255
    advantages of, 249
    block onset in, 250, 252
    blood loss reduction with, 249
    brachial plexus block in, 250–255, 250t, *251–254*, 252t
    cervicothoracic epidural block in, 255
    compartment anatomy and, 84–85, *85*
    complications of, 252–253, *254*
    cutaneous paresthesia in, 252, *253*
    drugs for, 250, 252t
    for bone graft donor site, 255
    in arthroscopy, 265
    in calcifying tendinitis analgesia, 786
    induction of, time for, 249
    interscalene brachial plexus block in, 250–255, 250t, *251–254*, 252t
    needle placement in, 250, 252, *252*
    nerve stimulator in, 250, 250t, *251*, 252
    postoperative analgesia from, 249
    sedation with, 249
    subclavian perivascular block in, 250
    supraclavicular block in, 249–250
  respiratory monitoring in, 248
  sedation with, 248
  venous access in, 248
Aneurysmal bone cyst, 885, *895*
Angiosome, 53–54, *53*
  cutaneous representation of, 77
Ankylosing spondylitis, versus frozen shoulder, 852
Antebrachial cutaneous nerve, medial, anatomy of, *68*, 72, 92
Anteroposterior views, in x-ray evaluation, of acromioclavicular joint, 190, *193*, 427, *428–429*
  of glenohumeral joint, 179, *179–180*, 552–554, *552–554*

Anteroposterior views (*Continued*)
  of humeral fracture, 287–288, *287*
  of impingement syndrome, 196
    stress type, 190, *193*
Antibiotics, in bone/joint infections, 933–936, 934t, 1076, 1081–
    1082
  in beads, 935
  prophylactic, 936
Antisepsis, historical review of, 920–921
AO buttress plate and screw, in proximal humeral fracture, 297,
    298
AO classification, of humeral fractures, 283–284
Aorta, pin migration into, 519
Apical lymph nodes, anatomy of, 83, *83*
Apical oblique view, in x-ray evaluation, 185, *186*, 560
Apophysitis, of coracoid process. See *Impingement syndrome.*
Apprehension, definition of, 541
  in dislocation, 152
Apprehension test, in glenohumeral joint assessment, 169–170,
    170–171, 550, *550*, 964–965, *964–965*
Arcuate artery, anatomy of, 280, *280*
Arm, motion of. See *Abduction*; *Adduction*; *Elevation*; *Extension*;
    Flexion; *Rotation.*
Arteriography, in tumor assessment, 898
Artery(ies). See also specific artery.
  anatomy of, 78–82, *79*, *81–82*
  anomalies of, 80–81
  collateral circulation of, 81–82, *81–82*
  obstruction of, torticollis and, 1060
Arthritis, after acromioclavicular joint repair, 442
  after clavicular fracture, 391–392
  degenerative. See also *Osteoarthritis.*
    occupational, 1095
    of acromioclavicular joint, 467
    versus impingement syndrome, 632, *633*
  neuropathic, of glenohumeral joint, versus degenerative arthritis,
    700–701, *700*
  versus frozen shoulder, 852
  of acromioclavicular joint, 467–468, 1083
    degenerative, 467, 636
    glenohumeral arthritis with, 702
    impingement syndrome and, *631*
    in sports, 986
    occupational, 1095
    post-traumatic, 391–392
    rheumatoid, 467–468
    septic, 468, 925, 1083
    versus impingement syndrome, 632
    versus rotator cuff tears, 661–662
  of glenohumeral joint, acromioclavicular arthritis with, 702
    arthrography of, 702
    clinical evaluation of, 701–703
    differential diagnosis of, 700–701, *700*
    laboratory studies in, 702
    pathoanatomy of, in osteoarthritis, 687–688, *687–688*, 689t
      in rheumatoid arthritis, 688–691, *689–694*, 690t
    systemic disease and, 699, *700*
    treatment of, arthrodesis as, 705–707, 705t, *706–713*, 707t,
        711, 711t
      conservative, 703
      methods for, 703, 703t
      osteotomy as, 711–712
      prosthetic arthroplasty as. See *Prosthetic arthroplasty.*
      resection arthroplasty as, 704–705, *705*
      surgical indications in, 686–687, 686t–687t
      synovectomy as, 703–704, *704*
    versus biceps tendon lesions, 823
    versus rotator cuff tears, 661–662
    x-ray evaluation of, 702
  of sternoclavicular joint, 487–489, *487–488*, 1083
    treatment of, 504, *506–507*, 516, 517
  postmenopausal, of sternoclavicular joint, 488–489, *489*, 504, *507*
  psoriatic, versus frozen shoulder, 852
  septic. See *Septic arthritis.*
  rheumatoid. See *Rheumatoid arthritis.*

Arthritis (*Continued*)
  "the syndrome" in, 691, *694*
  traumatic, after clavicular fracture, 391–392
    of glenohumeral joint, 694, *694–696*, 694t
      prosthetic arthroplasty in, 736–738, 737t–738t
    versus frozen shoulder, 852
  versus frozen shoulder, 852
  versus tumor, 900, 900t
Arthrocentesis, in septic arthritis, 933
Arthrodesis, after glenohumeral resection, 906
  after humeral resection, 906
  after limb sparing surgery, 908, *909*, 911
  after rotator cuff tear repair, 672
  of acromioclavicular joint, 414–415
  of glenohumeral joint, arm position for, 706, *706*
    biomechanics of, 224, *224–225*
    casting in, 711, *713*
    complications of, 707, 711, 711t
    extra-articular, 706–707, 707t, *708*, *710*
    in brachial plexus injury, 763–764, 1052
    in prosthesis failure, 742–743
    indications for, 705–706, 705t
    intra-articular, 706–707, *707–708*, 707t, *710*
    techniques for, 706–707, *707–712*, 707t
  of sternoclavicular joint, 502, *503*
Arthrography, distention, 856
  in biceps tendon lesions, 818, *818–819*
  in frozen shoulder, 850–851, *850*, 856
  in glenohumeral arthritis, 702
  in glenohumeral instability, 561
  in humeral head compression fracture, 188, *189*
  in impingement syndrome, 629, *630–631*
  in infections, 931
  in neurological disorders, 753
  in rotator cuff evaluation, 199, *199*
  in rotator cuff tears, 658–659, *658–659*, 666
Arthrogryposis, 1072–1074, *1072–1073*
Arthropathy, crystal, 696–697
  cuff-tear, 654, 660, *660*, 672–673, 696–697, *697*
  of sternoclavicular joint, 488, *488*
Arthroplasty, after limb sparing surgery, 908, *909–910*, 910–911
  cup, 713–714, *714*, 737, 737t
    complications of, 741t
  four-in-one, 827
  of humeral head (hemiarthroplasty), 712–714, *713–714*
    after limb sparing surgery, *909–910*, 910
    complications of, 740, 740t
    results of, 736–738, 737t
  prosthetic. See *Prosthetic arthroplasty.*
  resection, in glenohumeral arthritis, 704–705, *705*
Arthropneumotomography, in rotator cuff tears, 659
Arthroscopy, 258–277
  acromioplasty in, 269–270, *269*
  anatomic considerations in, 258–262
    biceps tendon, 259, *259*
    capsular ligaments, 260–262, *260–261*
    glenohumeral ligaments, 271
    glenoid labrum, 259–260, *259–260*, 270–271, *271*
    humeral head, 262, 271–272, *272*
    rotator cuff, 262
    subacromial space, 262
    subscapularis tendon, 261, *261*
  anesthesia for, 265
  brachial plexus injury in, 756
  debridement in, 263–264, *271*, *272*–273
  diagnostic, 266–268, *266–267*
  equipment for, 264–265
  historical aspects of, 258
  in adhesive capsulitis, 264
  in biceps tendon lesions, 820, 827–828
  in degenerative disease, 264
  in frozen shoulder, 851, 858
  in glenohumeral instability, 562, 584, *585*

Arthroscopy *(Continued)*
  in impingement syndrome, 263–264, *263*, 268–269, *269*, 634–635
  in inflammatory disease, 264
  in instability, 262–263, 270–273, *271–273*
  in rheumatoid arthritis, 704, *704*
  in rotator cuff lesion, 269–270
  in sepsis, 264
  in sports medicine, 976
  indications for, 262–264, *263*
  irrigation equipment for, 264–265
  loose bodies in, 272
  operating room set-up for, 264–265
  patient positioning for, 265–266, *265–266*
  portals for, anterosuperior, *267*, 268
    lateral (subacromial), *266*, 268
    placement of, 266–267, *266–267*
    posterior, *266*, 268
    superior, *266*, 268
  primary joint examination in, 267–268
  stabilization procedures in, 273–276
    biodegradable tack in, 276
    fixation devices for, 273–274, *273*
    postoperative regimen in, 276
    suture technique in, 274–276, *274–275*
  traction in, 265
Arthrotomography, in humeral head compression fracture, 188
  in rotator cuff evaluation, 199, 659
Arthrotomy, in glenohumeral joint drainage, 1082, *1083*
  in septic arthritis, 933
Aspiration, in osteomyelitis, 1076
  in septic arthritis, 933
Athletic activity. See *Sports medicine; Throwing.*
Atlantoaxial subluxation, versus torticollis, 1062–1063
Attrition tendinitis, 810, *810*, 830
Auricular nerves, anatomy of, 76
Autoimmune disorders, brachial plexus neuropathy as, 772
  frozen shoulder as, 849
Autonomic nerves, in brachial plexus, 72–73
  of blood vessels, 77
Avascular necrosis, of humeral head, 290, *291*, 323, *324*
  AO classification and, 283–284
  versus frozen shoulder, 852
Axillary artery, aberrant brachial plexus relationships with, 132, *133*
  anatomy of, *61*, 79–80, *79*
    in coracobrachialis, 63
    in glenohumeral dislocation, 564–565, *565*
    mobility adaptations, 77
  anomalies of, 81
  collateral circulation of, 81, *81–82*
  injury of, 82
    in clavicular fracture, 383
    in glenohumeral dislocation, 564–566
    in humeral fracture, 285, 290
    in reduction procedure, 565–566
    in screw fixation, 586
    mechanism of, 565
    prognosis of, 566
    symptoms of, 566
    treatment of, 566
  occlusion of, in sports, 987–988
Axillary lateral view, in x-ray evaluation, 179, 181, *181*, 190
  of acromioclavicular joint, 427, *429*
Axillary lymph nodes, anatomy of, 83, *83*
  dissection of, 82
Axillary nerve, anatomy of, 30–31, *30–31*, *61*, *68*, 70–71, *280*, 281, 336, *337*, 532–533, *532*, 566, 765–766
  in deltoid innervation, 58–59
  in teres minor innervation, 61
  injury of, 766–767, *766–767*
    diagnosis of, 567
    exploration of, 766–767
    in glenohumeral dislocation, 566–568
    in glenohumeral stabilization procedures, 586

Axillary nerve *(Continued)*
    in humeral fracture, 281, 285, 290–291
    in humeral resection, 906
    in quadrilateral space, 987
    in surgery, 756, 766, *767*
    in tumor resection, 877
    incidence of, 567
    mechanism of, 566–567, *567*
    prognosis for, 567, 766
    treatment of, 567
  protection of, in surgery, *594*, 596
Axillary pouch, arthroscopic portal for, 266, 268
  of inferior glenohumeral ligament, 18, *19*, *21–25*, 24, 260–262, *261*
Axillary sheath, anatomy of, 84–85, *84–85*
Axillary space, anatomy of, 84–88, *87*
Axillary vein, anatomy of, 82
  injury of, in glenohumeral dislocation, 564, 566
  thrombosis of, 988
Axillary vessels, clavicular protection of, 372
Axillary views, in x-ray evaluation, modified, 183–184, *184*
  of glenohumeral instability, 555–556, *556–559*
  of humeral fracture, 287–288, *287*
  of impingement syndrome, 629
Axillopectoral muscle, 124–125, *125*
Axiohumeral muscles. See also specific muscle.
  comparative anatomy of, 5
Axioscapular muscles. See also specific muscle.
  comparative anatomy of, 5
Axonotmesis, 566, 756

B

Bacteremia, in septic arthritis, 489, *490*, 923
Bacteria, activity of, 920
    in osteomyelitis, *935*
    intra-articular, 925–928, *927*
    surface adhesion/colonization, 924–928, *927–928*
  antibiotic susceptibility of, 934, 934t, 936
  culture of, in synovial fluid, 930–931, 931t
  drug addict–related, 929
  prevalence of, 928–929
Ball-in-socket shoulder prosthesis. See under *Prosthetic arthroplasty.*
Bankart lesion, 529, 1002, *1003*, 576. See also *TUBS syndrome.*
  arthroscopic repair of, 584, *585*
Bankart procedure, in glenohumeral instability, 577, 579, 588–592, *588–591*
  complications of, 585
  recurrent, 530
Baseball, throwing in. See *Throwing.*
Basiacromion, anatomy of, 45, *45*, *112*, *343*
Basilia, in fish fin, 1–2, *2*
Bell, nerve of. See *Thoracic nerve, long.*
Benign tumors. See under *Tumor(s).*
Biceps instability test, 813–814, *814*
Biceps muscle. See also *Biceps tendon.*
  anatomy of, 64, 793–794, *793–795*
    comparative, 5
  blood supply of, 64
  force generation by, 235t
  function of, 64
  innervation of, 64
  insertion of, *45*, 46, 64, 793, *793–794*
  origin of, 64, 793, *793*
  palpation of, 157, 159, *159*
  rupture of, 869–871, *870*
  scapular attachment of, *45*, 46, 335, *335–336*
  testing of, 166t
  transfer of, in acromioclavicular joint injury, 443–444, 446
Biceps reflex, testing of, 167
Biceps tendinitis, anatomical considerations in, 47–48, *48*

Biceps tendinitis (Continued)
  arthrography in, 818
  attrition, 810, 810, 830
  calcifying tendinitis with, 785
  clinical presentation of, 812–815, 812–814
  complications of, 820–821
  differential diagnosis of, 821–824
  historical review of, 792–793
  impingement, 808–809, 809, 827–829, 828–829
  in swimmers, 988
  incidence of, 810–811
  intertubercular groove condition in, 799, 801, 803
  occupational, 1094–1095
  pathoanatomy of, 799, 801, 802–805
  pathology of, 799, 800, 808
  physical examination in, 812–815, 812–814
  primary, 808, 827
  secondary, 808
  treatment of, conservative, 824
    corticosteroids in, 830
    in attrition type, 830
    in impingement type, 827–829, 828–829
    in primary type, 827
    keyhole tenodesis in, 826, 826
    operative, 827
  versus glenohumeral instability, 822
  versus impingement syndrome, 632, 821–822
  x-ray evaluation of, 200, 202, 816–817, 816–817
Biceps tendon, anatomy of, 48, 64, 259, 259, 533, 792, 793–794,
      793–798, 796–797
    comparative, 797, 798
    developmental, 799, 799
    functional, 805, 806–807, 807
    impingement syndrome and, 625
    pathological, 799, 800–801
  arthroscopy of, 259, 259
  attrition of, 810, 810, 830
  blood supply of, 794
  dislocation of, 791
    arthrography in, 818, 818
    complications of, 820–821
    etiology of, 811, 811
    historical review of, 791
    incidence of, 811
    mechanism of, 794
    pathoanatomy of, 799, 800
    treatment of, 824–827, 825–826, 829, 830
  electromyography of, 807–808
  evaluation of, 171
  extra-articular portion of, 793–794
  function of, 805, 806–807, 807–808
  hypovascular zone of, 811, 811
  instability of, clinical presentation of, 812–815, 812–815
    physical examination in, 812–815, 812–815
    treatment of, 826, 826, 829–830, 829
  intra-articular portion of, 793–794, 794
  lesions of. See also specific lesion, e.g., Biceps tendinitis.
    arthrography of, 818, 818–819
    arthroscopy of, 820, 827
    classification of, 808–810, 809–810
    clinical presentation of, 812–815, 812–815
    concomitant injuries, 816
    diagnosis of, 821
    differential diagnosis of, 821–824
    historical review of, 791–793, 792–793
    magnetic resonance imaging of, 820
    physical examination in, 821
    prevention of, 811–812
    treatment of, coracoid process tenodesis in, 825, 825
      groove tenodesis in, 825, 825
      Hitchcock procedure in, 825, 825
      keyhole tenodesis in, 826, 826
      keystone tenodesis in, 825–826
      Lippmann procedure in, 824, 824

Biceps tendon (Continued)
      operative, 824–827, 824–826, 830–832, 831
        postoperative care in, 824–827, 824–826, 832
    ultrasonography of, 818, 820
    x-ray evaluation of, 816–817, 816–817
  misunderstandings about, 791
  motion of, 805, 806–807, 807
  osseous structures near, 796–797, 797–798
  rotator cuff function and, 648, 649, 650
  rotator cuff tear effects on, 654, 655
  rupture of, clinical presentation of, 815, 815
    complications of, 820–821
    concomitant injuries and, 816
    etiology of, 811
    in rotator cuff tear, 654
    incidence of, 811
    intertubercular groove condition in, 799, 801, 803
    nontreatment of, 821
    pathoanatomy of, 799, 801, 802–805
    treatment of, 824, 826, 826, 830–832, 831
  soft-tissue restraint on, 794, 795–796, 796
  subluxation of, 809, 810
    differential diagnosis of, 821–824
    incidence of, 810–811
    versus glenohumeral subluxation, 822
  supraglenoid tubercle insertion of, 15
  synovial sheath of, 796
  tendinitis of. See Biceps tendinitis.
  tenosynovitis of, 799, 800–801, 810–811
    treatment of, 825, 825
  tensile strength of, 794
  transfer of, in glenohumeral instability, 584
Bicipital artery, anatomy of, 64
Bicipital groove. See Intertubercular groove.
Bicipital groove view, in x-ray evaluation, 816–817, 817
Bickel shoulder prosthesis, 680, 681
Billington yoke, in clavicular fracture, 394
Biodegradable tack, in arthroscopic stabilization, 276
Biologic graft, in rotator cuff tears, 663
Biomechanics, 208–245. See also Motion of joint.
  articular surfaces and, 218–220, 219–221
  center of rotation, 215–216, 216, 222, 223
    clinical relevance of, 222, 223–225, 224
  constraints and, 226–234
    articular, 219, 226–227, 226–227
    barrier effect in, 232
    capsular, 227–228, 227–229
    clinical relevance of, 232, 234, 234–235
    coracohumeral ligament, 227, 228
    dynamic, 226t, 230, 231–232, 233
    glenohumeral ligaments, 228–231, 229–232
    ligamentous, 227–231, 227–232
    static, 219, 226–232, 226–232, 226t
    sternoclavicular joint ligaments, 208–210, 209
    types of, 226, 226t
  Dempster concept of stability in, 229, 230
  external rotation of humerus, 220, 221–222, 222
  glenohumeral forces in, 239–240, 239–241
  glenohumeral index in, 226
  in resting posture, 218
  in workplace, 1093, 1096–1098, 1096–1099, 1098t
  joint pressure determination in, 241, 242
  joint reaction force in, 240, 241, 242
  maximum torque in, 242–243, 242t, 243
  muscle forces in, 234–235, 235t, 236–239, 238–239
    clinical relevance of, 225, 230, 238, 243
  occupational, 1093, 1096–1098, 1096–1099, 1098t
  of acromioclavicular joint, 210–212, 210–212
  of arm elevation, 219–220, 220–221
  of clavicle, 212, 213
  of glenohumeral joint, 213–218, 214–217
  of glenoid articular surface, 218–219, 219
  of humeral articular surface, 218, 219
  of occupational cervicobrachial disorder, 1093

Biomechanics *(Continued)*
  of scapula, 218, *218*
  of scapulothoracic joint, 213–216, *214–216*
  of sternoclavicular joint, 208–210, *209*
    clinical relevance of, 212–213, *214*
  of swimming, 988–989
  of throwing, 961–963, *962*
  radiography and, 222, *223*
  rigid body spring concept in, 242
  screw displacement axis in, 216–218, *217*, 222, *223*
  terminology of, 208, 208t
Biopsy, 901–903, 913–914
  complications of, 901
  contamination of, 902
  incisional (open), 901–903, *902*
  marginal (excisional), 902
  needle (closed), 901–903
  of humerus, 901–902, *902*
  of lymph nodes, spinal accessory nerve injury in, 759, *761*
Bipartate acromion, 111–113, *112–113*, 340, 342, *342–343*
Bipolar shoulder prosthesis, 737, 737t, 739t, 741t
  for hemiarthroplasty, 713, *714*
Birth injury, clavicular fracture. See *Clavicular fracture, at birth.*
  humeral fracture, 992
  of brachial plexus. See *Brachial plexus injury of newborn.*
  shoulder dislocation, 123–124, *124*
Birth palsy. See *Brachial plexus injury of newborn.*
Blastema, 6, 8
Blastomyces, in bone/joint infection, 929
Bleb theory, in scapular failure of descent, 106–107
Blood dyscrasia, versus tumor, 900t, 901
Blood pressure monitoring, during anesthesia, 248
Blood supply. See specific structure.
Blood vessels. See also specific vessel.
  anatomy of, 76–83, *77–79*, *81–82*
    adaptations of, for high mobility region, 77, *77–78*
    arteries, 78–82, *79*, *81–82*
    in collateral circulation, 81–82, *81–82*
    in cutaneous circulation, 89, *90*, 91
    in lymphatic circulation, 82–83
    veins, 82
  autonomic control of, 77
  evaluation of, 173, *173*
  injury of, in humeral fracture, 290
  of muscle, classification of, 53, *53*
  of skin, 89, *90*, 91
  pin migration into, 519, 521
Blount procedure, in brachial plexus injury of newborn, 1051, *1051*
Bohler brace, in clavicular fracture, *392*
Bone, anatomy of. See specific bone.
  bacterial colonization on, 924–925
  blood supply of, infection and, 921, *922*
  calcifying tendinitis penetration into, 785
  dysplasia of, versus tumor, 900–901, 900t
  fibrous dysplasia of, 885, *886*
  infection of. See *Osteomyelitis.*
  microstructure of, 923
  rheumatoid arthritis effects on, 690, *691–691*, 690t
  tendon insertion in, direct/indirect, 51, *52*
  tumors of, 879–880, *881*, 884–885, *884*, *886–887*
    historical review of, 874–875
Bone block. See *Bone graft.*
Bone cement, application of, in prosthetic arthroplasty, 718, *720*, 721
  complications with, 255
Bone cyst, aneurysmal, 885, 895
  simple (unicameral), 884–885, *884*, *895*, 992
Bone graft, donor site anesthesia for, 255
  in clavicular nonunion, 396–397, *397*, 402–404, 406, *406–407*
  in glenohumeral instability, 580, 598–599
  in glenohumeral joint arthrodesis, 707, *711*
  in prosthetic arthroplasty, 718, *720–721*, 721
  in reconstruction after limb sparing surgery, *909*, 910–911
  in scapulothoracic fusion, 761

Bone ingrowth system, in prosthetic arthroplasty, 718, *719*
Bone scan, in frozen shoulder, 849–850
  in osteomyelitis, 1075
  in sternoclavicular joint disorders, 196
  in tumor follow-up, 895
Bosworth screw, in acromioclavicular joint repair, 440–443, *441*, 454, *454*
Boyd-Sisk procedure, in glenohumeral instability, 598
Boytchev procedure, in glenohumeral instability, 584
Brachial artery, anatomy of, *79*
  collateral circulation of, *81–82*
Brachial birth palsy. See *Brachial plexus injury of newborn.*
Brachial cutaneous nerve, anterior, anatomy of, 70–71
  lateral, anatomy of, 70
  medial, anatomy of, *68*, 72, *90*, 91–92
    anomalous, 74
  upper lateral, anatomy of, 91
Brachial neuritis. See under *Brachial plexus.*
Brachial plexus, aberrant arterial relationships in, 132–133, *133*
  anatomy of, 67–74, *68–75*, 751, *752*
    at clavicle level, 369, *369*
    stretching injury and, 67, *1036*
  autonomic fibers in, 72–73
  avulsion of, during birth, 1034–1035, *1035*, 1037, *1037*, 1037t
  blood supply of, 72, *72*
  clavicular protection of, 372
  collaterals in, 74, *75*
  common origin in, 74, *75*
  cords of, 68–72, *68–69*
    lateral, *68*, 69–70
    medial, *68*, 71–72
    posterior, *68*, 70–71
  distal take off in, 74, *75*
  duplication of nerve in, 74, *75*
  embryology of, 73
  glenohumeral joint innervation by, 30–31
  gross anatomy of, 67–68
  idiopathic neuropathy of, 771–772
  imaging of, 73, *73*
  injury of, 761–765
    at birth. See *Brachial plexus injury of newborn.*
    causes of, 761–762
    closed, 761–762
    compression, 390–391, *391*, 764
    evaluation of, 762
    exercise in, 762
    flail arm in, 762
    glenohumeral joint arthrodesis in, 763–764
    in clavicular fracture, 378, 382, 390–391, *391*, 764–765
    in glenohumeral dislocation, 567
    in glenohumeral stabilization procedures, 586
    in humeral fracture, 285, 290–291
    in surgery, 756
    infraclavicular, 764
    muscle transfer in, 763
    nerve graft in, 762–763, *763*
    prognosis of, 762
    root avulsion in, 762
    subclavicular, 764–765
    traction, 762
    treatment of, 751, 762–764, *763*
    versus musculocutaneous nerve injury, 767–768
  loops in, 74, *75*
  median nerve entrapment in, in Parsonage-Turner syndrome, 132–133, *133*
  multiple nerve origin in, 74, *75*
  muscular bands near, in thoracic outlet syndrome, 136–137
  neuritis of, versus biceps tendon lesions, 823
    versus impingement syndrome, 632
    versus rotator cuff tears, 661
  neurosarcoma of, 875
  postanesthetic palsy of, 253, 255
  prefixed, 73–74, *75*

Brachial plexus *(Continued)*
  proximal take off in, 73–74
  regional anesthesia of, 250, 250t, *251–254*, 252–253, 252t, 255
    anatomical considerations in, 84–85, *84–85*
    in arthroscopy, 265
  repair of, in birth injury, 1052–1053, *1053*
  roots of, 68, *68*
  scalene triangle structures and, *65*
  stretching of, during birth, 1034–1035, *1035*, 1037, *1037*, 1037t
  subscapularis-teres-latissimus muscle penetration of, *126*, 126
  substitutions in, 74, *75*
  trunks of, 68, *68*
  tumor of, imaging of, 898
  variants of, 73–74, *73*, *75*
Brachial plexus injury of newborn, 1033–1055
  arthrodesis in, 1052
  bilateral, 1043, 1043t
  breech delivery and, 1043, 1043t
  classification of, 1037, 1037t
  clavicular fracture in, 1044
  clinical presentation in, 1044
  contractures in, 1039, *1040–1041*, 1041
  diagnosis of, 1044–1045, *1045*
  differential diagnosis of, 1044
  elbow deformity in, 1041–1042, *1041–1043*, 1052
  electrical stimulation in, 1046
  electromyography in, 1044
  etiology of, 1034–1035, *1035*
  exercise in, 1046, 1053–1054, *1054*
  facial nerve injury in, 1037
  forearm deformity in, treatment of, 1052
  fracture with, 1038
  gender distribution in, 1043, 1043t
  histamine response in, 1045, *1045*
  historical review of, 1033–1034, *1034*
  humeral fracture in, 1044
  incidence of, 1033, 1033t, 1043–1044, 1043t, *1044*
  internal rotation procedures in, 1052, *1052*
  manipulation in, 1046
  muscle weakness/paralysis in, *1036*, 1038–1039, *1038–1039*
  myelography in, 1044–1045
  nerve injury in, 1038, 1052–1053, *1053*
  pathogenesis of, 1034–1035, *1035*
  pathology of, 1035–1042
    anatomical location and, 1035, *1036*
    conditions associated with, 1037–1038
    microscopic, 1035, 1037, *1037*, 1037t
    secondary effects of, 1038–1043, *1036*, *1038–1043*
  prognosis for, 1045–1046, 1045t
  radiographic changes in, 1042
  recovery from, 1045–1046, 1045t
  risk factors for, 1043–1044, *1044*
  side affected in, 1043, 1043t
  soft tissue release in, 1047–1048
  spasticity in, 1038
  splinting in, 1046–1047, *1047–1048*
  tendon transfer in, 1048, *1049–1052*, 1051–1052
  torticollis and, 1037–1038, 1059
  treatment of, early, 1053–1054, *1054*
    late, 1054–1055, *1054–1055*
    nonoperative, 1046–1047, *1047–1048*
    operative, 1047–1048, *1049–1055*, 1050–1055
Brachioradialis muscle, motion of, in musculocutaneous nerve injury, 767–768, *767*
  testing of, 167
Brachioradialis reflex, testing of, 167
Brain disorders, frozen shoulder and, 751, 845
  torticollis in, 1064, *1064*
Brisement, in frozen shoulder, 856
Bristow-Helfet procedure, in glenohumeral instability, 580–581, *582–583*
Bristow procedure, 972, *973–976*, 976
  complications of, 585–586, 972
  musculocutaneous nerve injury in, 756

Bupivacaine, in postoperative analgesia, 597
  in regional anesthesia, 250, 252t
  in snapping scapula, 363
Burrows procedure, in sternoclavicular joint repair, 502, *502*
Bursa(e). See also specific bursa, e.g., *Subacromial-subdeltoid bursa.*
  anatomy of, 27, *27*, 88–89, *89*
    infection spread and, 921–922, *922*
  subscapular, 363
Bursectomy, arthroscopic, 269
Bursitis, of rotator cuff, versus rotator cuff tears, 661
  versus frozen shoulder, 852
  versus impingement syndrome, 632
Bursitis calcarea subacromialis. See *Impingement syndrome.*
Bursography, in calcifying tendinitis, 783
  in rotator cuff tears, 659
  subacromial, 199
Buttress plate and screw, in proximal humeral fracture, 297, *298*

C

Caffey's disease, versus osteomyelitis, 1080
Caird, F. M., on glenohumeral instability, 527
Calcification, dystrophic, in arthropathy, 784
  in chondroblastoma, 882
  in Milwaukee shoulder, 776
  of acromioclavicular ligament, 464
  of coracoclavicular ligament, 114, 464
  of rotator cuff tendons, asymptomatic, 775
  versus calcifying tendinitis, 776, 785
Calcifying tendinitis, 774–790
  acute, symptoms of, 782
    x-ray appearance of, 784
  age distribution of, 776, 778–779
  anatomic considerations in, 774–775, *775*
  animal models for, 788
  bilateral, 776
  bursography in, 783
  calcific stage of, 780–781, *780–781*
  calcium granuloma in, 777, *777*
  chondrocytes in, 776–777, *776–777*
  chronic, symptoms of, 782
    x-ray appearance of, 784, *784*
  classification of, 776
  clinical presentation of, 781–783, *781–782*
  complications of, 785
  corticosteroids in, 786–787
  cyclic nature of, 780–782, *780–781*
  differential diagnosis of, 785
  disruption phase of, 781
  formative phase of, 780, *780–781*
  frozen shoulder and, 783, 837
  healing stage of, 777–778, *777–780*
  hip calcification with, 776
  historical review of, 774
  impingement syndrome with, 629, *631*, 782, *782*
  incidence of, 775–776
  increment phase of, 781
  laboratory investigations in, 785
  lavage treatment in, 788
  morphology of, 780, *781*
  occupational role in, 776
  pathogenesis of, 778–781, *780–781*
  pathology of, 776–778, *776–780*
  pathophysiology of, 780, *781*
  phases of, 780–781, *780–781*
  postcalcific stage of, 780, *780–781*
  precalcific stage of, 780, *780–781*
  recurrence of, after surgical treatment, 785
  resorptive phase of, 780–782, *780–782*
    x-ray evaluation in, 783–784, *783–784*

Calcifying tendinitis *(Continued)*
 tissue typing (HLA) in, 785
 treatment of, 786–788
  injection technique, 788
  nonoperative, 785–787, *787*
  operative, 786–788
  radiotherapy, 786
 ultrasonography in, 785
 versus frozen shoulder, 852
 versus impingement syndrome, 632
 "wear and tear" theory of, 778
 x-ray evaluation of, 200, *201*, 783–785, *783*
 xerography in, 783, *783*
Calcium granuloma, in calcifying tendinitis, 777, *777*
Calcium phosphate, in crystal arthropathy, 697
California Division of Industrial Accidents, impairment evaluation
  guidelines of, 1104–1105
Cancer. See *Sarcoma*; *Tumor(s), malignant.*
Candida albicans, in bone/joint infections, 929
 in children, 1081
Capsular ligament(s). See also specific ligament, e.g., *Glenohumeral ligament; Sternoclavicular ligament(s).*
 anatomy of, *478, 479, 480*
 anterior, function of, 209
 as constraint, 210
 function of, 209, *479, 480*, 537–538
 laxity of, in throwing athlete, 966, *966*
 posterior, function of, 209
Capsular shift procedure, in glenohumeral instability, 606–609,
  606–608, 612, *612*
Capsule, anatomy of, 15–17, *15–17*, 227–228, *229*, 840, *840*
 anterior, anatomy of, *539*
  defects of, in glenohumeral instability, 527
 biochemical constitution of, 227
 function of, in stability, 537–538
 osteoarthritic changes in, 689t
 reconstruction of, 577–578, *578*, 592, *593–595*, 596–597, *610–
  611*, 977–978, *977–982*, 981–982. See also *Capsulorrhaphy.*
  anterior, 234, *234*
 release of, in frozen shoulder, 858–859
 rheumatoid arthritis effects on, 690t, 691, *693*
 stretching exercise for, 967, *969*
 tearing of, in manipulation of frozen shoulder, 857
 tensile strength of, versus age, 228, *228*
Capsulite retractile, as synonym for frozen shoulder, 839
Capsulitis, adhesive. See *Adhesive capsulitis.*
 early, 842, 832t
 irritative, 842, 843t
Capsulolabral reconstruction, in glenohumeral instability, 977–978,
  977–982, 981–982
Capsulorrhaphy, in posterior instability, 983–986, *984–986*
 staple, 577–578, *578*, 585–586
Caput obstipum. See *Torticollis.*
Carbon fiber prosthesis, in rotator cuff tears, 663
Carcinoma, versus sarcoma, 877
Cardiac arrest, from bone cement monomer, 255
Cardiovascular disorders, anesthesia and, 247
 frozen shoulder and, 845
Cardiovascular monitoring, during anesthesia, 248
Carotid artery, compression of, in sternoclavicular joint dislocation, 517
 obstruction of, in clavicular fracture, 391
Carpal tunnel syndrome, versus biceps tendon lesions, 823–824
Cartilage, bacterial colonization on, 924–925, *925*
 destruction of, in infection, 925, *925*
  in radiotherapy, *700*
 microanatomy of, 922–923, *924*
 rheumatoid arthritis effects on, 690–691, 690t, *692–694*
 surface characteristics of, 924–925, *925*
 tumors of, benign, 880, 882, *882*
  malignant, 882, *883*, 884
Cartilage rays, in fish fin, 1–2, *2*
Casting. See also specific disorder and procedure.
 in acromioclavicular joint injury, 435

Casting *(Continued)*
 in glenohumeral joint arthrodesis, 711, *713*
 in humeral fracture, 296
Catching, of joint, as chief complaint, 153
Caudal tilt view, in x-ray evaluation, 196, *197–198*
 of biceps tendon lesions, 817, *817*
Cefaclor, in osteomyelitis, 1076
Cefazolin, prophylactic use of, 936
Cefotoxitin, in bone/joint infections, 934t
Ceftraxone, in bone/joint infections, 934t
Cefuroxime, in bone/joint infections, 934t, 1081
Cement, application of, in prosthetic arthroplasty, 718, *720*, 721
 complications with, 255
Center of rotation. See *Instantaneous center of rotation.*
Central lymph nodes, anatomy of, 83, *83*
Cephalexin, in osteomyelitis, 1076
Cephalic tilt view, in x-ray evaluation, 194–195, *195*
 of clavicular fracture, 1017, *1018*
 of sternoclavicular joint, 492–493, *493–494*
Cephalic vein, anatomy of, 82
Cephaloscapular projection, in x-ray evaluation, 560
Cephalosporins, in bone/joint infections, 934t, 1076, 1081
Cerebrovascular accident, frozen shoulder and, 845
 neuromuscular disorders in, 770–771
Cervical artery, transverse, anatomy of, 78, *79*
 in levator scapulae, 56
 in trapezius, 55
Cervical ganglion, anatomy of, 72
Cervical lymph nodes, deep, anatomy of, 83, *83*
Cervical radiculopathy, clinical presentation of, 751
 versus impingement syndrome, 632
Cervical rib resection, in thoracic outlet syndrome, 770
Cervical spine, disc calcification in, versus torticollis, 1062
 disorders of, torticollis in, 1063, *1064*
  versus frozen shoulder, 852
  versus shoulder disorders, 176
  with frozen shoulder, 845
  with glenohumeral arthritis, 702
 examination of, 174–176, *176*, 751
 fracture of, neurological disorders in, 751
 rheumatoid arthritis of, anesthesia and, 247
Cervical spondylosis, versus rotator cuff tears, 661
Cervicothoracic epidural block, 255
Charnley procedure, in glenohumeral joint arthrodesis, 709, *711*
Chemotherapy, in chondrosarcoma, 912
 in Ewing's sarcoma, 913
 in high-grade malignancy, 914–915
 in osteosarcoma, 912–913
 in soft tissue sarcoma, 913, 915
 preoperative, 914–915
Cheroarthropathy, frozen shoulder and, 845
Chest injury, in humeral fracture, 285, 291
Children. See also *Infants.*
 acromial fracture in, 1028
 arthrogryposis in, 1072–1074, *1072–1073*
 clavicular fracture in, 1007–1025
  anatomical considerations in, 1007, 1009–1010, *1009–1010*
  lateral, 1019–1020, *1021–1024*, 1024–1025
  mechanism of injury in, 376
  medial, 1016–1017, *1016–1018*
  middle (shaft), 1010–1016, *1011–1015*
  treatment of, 392, *393*, 398–400, *398–400*
 congenital anomalies in. See *Congenital anomalies.*
 coracoid process fracture in, *1027*, 1028
 glenohumeral instability in, 1002–1007
  anatomical considerations in, 1002–1003, *1003*
  classification of, 1003
  etiology of, 1003
  incidence of, 1003
  mechanism of injury in, 1003–1004, *1004*
  recurrence of, 1005–1006
  symptoms of, 1004–1005, *1005*
  treatment of, 1005–1008, *1008*
  x-ray evaluation of, 1005, *1006–1007*

Children *(Continued)*
  glenoid fracture in, *1027,* 1028
  humeral fracture in, 991–1002
    anatomical considerations in, 991–992
    classification of, 992, *993*
    complications of, 1002, *1002*
    incidence of, 992
    mechanism of injury in, 992
    symptoms of, 993
    treatment of, 993, *994–1001,* 995, 1002
    x-ray evaluation of, 993
  osteomyelitis in, 926, 1074–1080
    diagnosis of, 1075
    incidence of, 1074
    neonatal, 1078, 1080, *1080*
    of clavicle, 1078, *1079*
    of humerus, 1075–1078, *1077–1078*
    of scapula, 1078
    organisms in, 1074, 1076
    pathogenesis of, 1074–1075
    treatment of, 1075–1076, 1078
  scapular fracture in, 1025, *1025–1027,* 1028
  septic arthritis in, 934, 1080–1083, *1083*
  torticollis in. See *Torticollis.*
China, early anatomical studies in, 34
Chlorprocaine, in regional anesthesia, 252t
Choke arterioles, 53
Chondroblastoma, 882, *895*
Chondrocytes, collagen production by, 923
  in calcifying tendinitis, 776–777, *776–777*
Chondroepitrochlear muscle, 126
Chondroma/chondromatosis, periosteal, 882, *895*
  synovial, 884
Chondrosarcoma, 882, *883,* 884, *895*
  age distribution of, *894*
  secondary, 880, 882, *883*
  treatment of, 912, 914
Circulus articuli vasculosus, 921
Circumflex scapular artery, anatomy of, *61, 79,* 80
  collateral circulation of, *81*
Clasp-like cranial margin of scapula, 111, *111*
Clavicle, absence of, 370–371, *371*
  anatomy of, 368–370, *368–369,* 1009
    comparative, 2, *2,* 4, 370
    developmental, 10–11, *11,* 1007, 1009
  arm stability contribution of, 371
  bifid, neurovascular compression and, 390–391, *391*
  biomechanics of, 212, *213*
  brachial plexus proximity to, 369, *369*
  cleidocranial dysostosis and, 99–101, *99–101*
  congenital anomalies of, 99–103, *99–104*
  congenital fossa of, 128, *128*
  cosmetic function of, 372
  cross-sectional view of, *368,* 369
  curvature of, 368–369, *368*
    motion relationships of, 372
  deformity of, in brachial plexus injury of newborn, 1041
  deltoid muscle detachment from. See *Acromioclavicular joint, injury of, types III to VI.*
  distal, excision of, in acromioclavicular joint injury, 443, *443,* 446, 457, 460–462, *460–462*
  duplicated, 103, *103*
  embryology of, 100–103, 368
  epiphysis of, 41
    anatomy of, *481,* 482
    injury of, 509–511, *510–513*
  fascial arrangement about, 370
  floating (panclavicular dislocation), 375, 380
  foramina of, 103, *103–104*
  fracture of. See *Clavicular fracture.*
  frontal view of, 368, *368*
  function of, 370–372, *371,* 1009
  growth of, 10–11, *11*
  interior structure of, 369

Clavicle *(Continued)*
  joints of, 369, *369.* See also *Acromioclavicular joint; Sternoclavicular joint.*
  medial, excision of, in sternoclavicular joint injury, 502
    osteotomy of, in sternoclavicular joint injury, 502
    resection of, 504, *506*
    x-ray evaluation of, 193–196, *194–196*
  motion of, 212, *213,* 371–372, *371*
  muscle attachments of, 372
  muscle transfer to, in acromioclavicular joint injury, 443–444, 446
  name derivation of, 368
  neurovascular protection by, 372
  ossification of, 10–11, *11,* 368, 1007, 1009
  osteitis of, 488
  osteolysis of, 464, *465*
  osteomyelitis of, 924, 926
  osteotomy of, in sternoclavicular dislocation, 502
  palpation of, 157
  periosteal injury of, 424, 510–511, *511–512*
  protective function of, 383
  pseudarthrosis of, 386
    congenital, 101–103, *102*
    versus fracture, 1011, *1012*
  resection of, 940, 949, *950.* See also *Claviculectomy.*
    in neurovascular compression, 397
    in post-traumatic arthritis, 391–392
  respiratory function involvement of, 372
  structures adjoining, 42
  superior view of, 368, *368*
  surgical anatomy of, 370
  transposition of, in phocomelia, 120, *121*
  trapezius muscle detachment from. See *Acromioclavicular joint, injury of, types III to VI.*
  traumatic floating (panclavicular dislocation), 375, 380
  tumors of, 895
  weightlifter's, 374
Clavicular artery, anatomy of, *79,* 80
Clavicular fracture, acromioclavicular joint injury with, 463
  acromioclavicular separation and, 388
  arthritis after, 391–392
  articular surface, 380
  at birth, 1011
    clinical presentation of, 377–378, *378*
    mechanism of, 376
    treatment of, 392, 398
    ultrasonography in, 384
  blood vessel injury in, 383
  bone excision in, 394
  brachial plexus injury with, 378, 764–765
  classification of, 372–375, *373–375*
    in children, 1016–1017, *1016,* 1019–1020, *1021–1023*
    in distal fracture, *1010,* 1019–1020, *1021–1023*
    in medial fracture, 1016–1017, *1016*
  cleidocranial dysostosis and, 387
  clinical presentation of, 377–383
    at birth, 377–378, *378*
    in adults, 379–380, *380*
    in children, 378–379, *378–379*
    injuries associated with, 380–383, *381–382*
  complications of, 1016
    arthritis, 391–392
    malunion, 390
    neurovascular, 390–391, *390,* 397
    nonunion, 387–390, *388–390,* 395–397, *395, 397,* 404, *404–408,* 406, 408
  compound, 379, *380*
  computed tomography in, 1017, *1018*
  congenital pseudarthrosis and, 387
  differential diagnosis of, 386–387
  displacement of, *373*
    versus nonunion, 388
  distal (lateral), 373–375, *374–375*
    classification of, *1010,* 1019–1020, *1021–1023*

Clavicular fracture *(Continued)*
  in children, *1010*, 1019–1020, *1021–1024*, 1024–1025
  incidence of, 1019
  mechanism of, 376, 1019
  nonunion of, 387–388
  symptoms of, 1020
  treatment of, 400, *400*, 402–404, *402–403*, 1020, 1024–1025, *1024*
  x-ray evaluation of, 189–190, *191–194*, 193, 384–385, *385–386*, 1020, *1024*
  figure-of-eight bandage in, 393, *393–394*, 398–401, *401*
  Group I. See subhead: *middle (shaft)*.
  Group II. See subhead: *distal (lateral)*.
  Group III. See subhead: *medial (proximal)*.
  healing of, 1010, *1010*
  historical review of, 367–268
  immobilization of, versus nonunion, 387
  in brachial plexus injury of newborn, 1037, 1044
  in children, distal (lateral), *1010*, 1019–1020, 1024–1025, *1024*
    mechanism of injury in, 376
    medial (proximal), 1016–1017, *1016–1018*, 1019
    middle (shaft), 1010–1016, *1011–1015*
    treatment of, 398–400, *398–400*
  incidence of, 367, 376–377
    distal, 1019
    in children, 1010, 1016, 1019
    medial, 1016, *1016*
    middle (shaft), 1010
  injuries associated with, 380–383, *381–382*
  intramedullary fixation in, 395–397, *395*, 401–403, *403*, 408, *408*
  location of, versus nonunion, 387–388
  malunion in, 390
  mechanism of injury in, 376–377
    distal, 1019
    in children, 1010–1011, 1016, 1019
    medial, 1016
    middle (shaft), 1010–1011
  medial (proximal), 373, 375
    in children, 1016–1017, *1016–1018*, 1019
    mechanism of, 376
    treatment of, 400, 404
    x-ray evaluation of, 385–386
  middle (shaft), 373, *373–374*
    complications of, 1016
    in children, 1010–1016, *1011–1015*
    incidence of, 1010
    mechanism of, 376, 1010–1011
    symptoms of, 1011–1012, *1011–1012*
    treatment of, 401, 1012, *1013–1015*, 1015
    x-ray evaluation of, 189, *190*, 383–384, *383–384*, 1012, *1012*
  neurovascular complications in, 382, *382*, 390–391, *390*, 397
  nonunion in, 387–390, *388–390*, 395, 1016
    treatment of, 395–397, *397*, 404, *404–408*, 406, 408
  open, treatment of, 1016
  open fixation of, 394–396, *395*, *397*, 401–402
    after nonunion, 404, *404–408*, 406, 408
    in distal fracture, 402–404, *402–403*
    nonunion caused by, 388, *388*
  panclavicular dislocation and, 375, 380
  pathologic, 377, *377*
  pneumothorax in, *381*, 382
  postoperative care in, 397
  refracture after, 387
  remodeling in, 1015
  severity of, versus nonunion, 387
  shaft. See subhead: *middle (shaft)*.
  skeletal injuries with, 381–382, *381*
  soft tissue interposition in, 388
  sternoclavicular dislocation and, 387
  symptoms of, distal, 1020
    in children, 1011–1012, *1011–1012*, 1017, *1017*, 1020
    medial, 1017, *1017*
    middle (shaft), 1011–1012, *1011–1012*
  treatment of, 392–397

Clavicular fracture *(Continued)*
  at birth, 392, 398
  closed reduction, 392–394, *392*, *394*, 399, *399*, 401, *401*
    in adults, 393–395, *393–396*
    in children, 392, *393*, 398–400, *398–400*, 1012, *1013–1015*, 1015–1016, 1020, 1024–1025, *1024*
    in distal fracture, 400, *400*, 402–404, *402–403*, 1020, 1024–1025, *1024*
    in medial fracture, 400, 404, 1017–1018, *1018*
    in middle (shaft) fracture, 401, 1012, *1013–1015*, 1015
    in neurovascular complications, 397
    in nonunion, 395–397, *397*
    open, 1016
    open fixation in, 401–402
    recumbency in, 399–400, *399*
  ultrasonography in, 384
  weightlifter's, 374
  x-ray evaluation of, in children, 1012, *1012*, 1017, *1018*, 1020
    in distal fracture, 384–385, *385–386*, 1020, *1024*
    in medial fracture, 385–386, 1017, *1018*
    in middle (shaft) fracture, 383–384, *383–384*, 1012, *1012*
    in nonunion, 388, *388–390*
Clavicular reflex, testing of, 167
Claviculectomy, 941, 951–952, *952*. See also *Clavicle, resection of*.
  in clavicular nonunion, 396
Clavipectoral fascia, anatomy of, 87–88, *88*, 532
Cleidocranial dysostosis, 99–101, *99–101*, 386
  versus clavicular fracture, 1011–1012
Cleitrum, 1
Clindamycin, in bone/joint infections, 934, 1076
Clinical evaluation, 149–177. See also *specific disorder*.
  chief complaints in, catching, 153
    deformity, 153, *153*
    instability, 151–152
    pain, 150–151, *151*
    paresthesia, 153
    stiffness, 152–153
    weakness, 153
  history in, 149–153, *153*
  in acute injury, 153
  interview in, 149–150
  physical examination in. See *Physical examination*.
Coccidioidomycosis, 929, 1076, *1077*
Codman, E. A., on impingement syndrome, 623–624
  on infection, 921
Codman classification, of humeral fractures, 278, 282, *282*
Codman exercise, in humeral fracture, 318, *320*
Codman's paradox, 214, *214–215*
Codman's tumor (chondroblastoma), 882
Cofield shoulder prosthesis, for hemiarthroplasty, 713
  for total arthroplasty, 722, 731, *732*
Cofield technique, in total arthroplasty, 722–735, *723–735*
Cohesion, of glenohumeral joint, 536
Collagen, at tendon insertion, 51, *52*
  in articular cartilage, 923, *924*
  in inferior glenohumeral ligament, 23, *23–26*
  types of, 15, *15*
Collagenase production, by bacteria, 925
Collateral circulation, anatomy of, 81–82, *81–82*
Collum obstipum/distortum. See *Torticollis*.
Comparative anatomy. See under *Anatomy*.
Compartment(s), anatomy of, 875, *876*, 877
  adipose tissue and, *84–88*, 87–88
  compression and, 84, *84*
  infection spread and, 84
  regional anesthesia and, 84–85, *84–85*
  surgical planes and, 85–87, *86–87*
  tumor growth and, 83–84
  tumor containment/escape and, 877–878, *877t–878t*
Compartment syndrome, anatomy of, 84, *84*
  with triceps rupture, 868
Compensation cases. See *Workmen's compensation*.
Compression plate, in clavicular fracture fixation, 396–397, *397*, 404, *404–406*, 406

Compression plate *(Continued)*
  in scapulothoracic fusion, 761
Compression test, in cervical spine examination, 175, *176*
Computed tomography, in acromioclavicular joint disorders, 193
  in anterior instability, 185
  in clavicular fracture, 1017, *1018*
  in glenohumeral instability, 561, *561*
  in glenohumeral joint injury, 184
  in humeral fracture, 188, *189*, 288–289, *288*
  in infections, 931
  in osteomyelitis, 1075
  in rotator cuff evaluation, 199, 659–660
  in sternoclavicular joint disorders, 196, *196*, 495, *496*
  in tumors, 879, 897–898
Congenital anomalies, 98–148
  amputation in, 941
  axillopectoral muscle, 124–125, *125*
  bicipital groove aberrations, 122–123, *123*
  brachial palsy. See *Brachial plexus injury of newborn.*
  chondroepitrochlear muscle, 126, *126*
  clasp-like cranial margin of scapula, 111, *111*
  cleidocranial dysostosis, 99–103, *99–101*
  coracobrachialis muscle, *131*, 132
  coracoclavicular joint/bar, 113–115, *115–116*
  coracoclaviculosternal muscle, 127
  coracocostosternale vestigiale bone, 116
  costocoracoid band, 115–116
  costovertebral bone, 116, *117*
  deltoid muscle, 127–128
  dimple formation, 128, *128*
  dislocation, 123–124, *124*
  dorsal scapular nerve compression, 133–134, *133–134*
  duplicated clavicle, 103, *103*
  embryologic aspects of, 10
  glenohumeral dysplasias, 120–124, *121–124*
  glenohumeral instability, 541
  glenoid dentation, 117–118, *118–119*
  glenoid hypoplasia, 122, *122*
  Holt-Oram syndrome, 109–111
  infrascapular bone, 116–117, *117*
  median nerve compression, 132–133, *133*
  middle suprascapular nerve foramina, 103, *103–104*
  Möbius syndrome, 130
  neurovascular, 132–137, *133–142*, 143
  of acromion, 111–113, *111–113*
  of clavicle, 99–103, *99–104*
  of coracoid process, 111, *111*
  of humerus, 121–122, *121*
  of muscle, 124–132
    abnormal insertion, 131–132, *131*
    absent, 129–131, *129–130*
    extra, 124–127, *125–126*, 128
    fibrous contracture, 127–128, *128*
  Parsonage-Turner syndrome, 132–133, *133*
  pectoralis major muscle, 129–130, *129–130*
  pectoralis minor muscle, 131–132, *1131*
  phocomelia, 118–120, *119–121*
  Poland's syndrome, 129–130, *129–130*
  pseudarthrosis of clavicle, 101–103, *102*, 386
  rhomboid muscles, 130–131
  scapula. See under *Scapula.*
  Sprengel's deformity, 103–109, *104–107*, 105t, *109–110*
  sternalis muscle, 125–126, *125*
  sternoclavicular joint dislocation, 487, 504
  subscapularis-teres-latissimus muscle, 126–127, *126*
  suprascapular nerve compression, 134–136, *135–136*
  thoracic outlet compression syndrome, 136–137, *138–142*, 143
  transverse scapular ligament ossification, 111
  trapezius muscle, 130–131
Conoid ligament, anatomy of, 211, *211*, 415, 418, *418*, 796
  as constraint, 211–212, *212*
  rupture of, in clavicular fracture, 374, *374*
  size of, 419
Conoid tubercle, anatomy of, 41, *42*

Constraints, on shoulder motion. See under *Biomechanics*; specific joint.
Contractures, in brachial plexus injury of newborn, 1039, *1040–1041*, 1041
  treatment of, 1054, *1054–1055*
  of deltoid muscle, 127–128
Conversion reaction, neurological disorders and, 757–758
Convulsion, humeral fracture in, 285
Cooper, Sir Astley, on posterior glenohumeral instability, 530–531
  on sternoclavicular joint injury, 477
Coordination testing, in neurological disorders, 758
Coracoacromial arch, anatomy of, 279–280, *280*, 532, 624, *624–625*
  arthroscopy of, 262
  in impingement syndrome, 624, *624–625*, 626–627, 627t
Coracoacromial ligament, anatomy of, 43, 45, *45*, 796
  impingement of, on rotator cuff. See *Impingement syndrome.*
  transfer of, in acromioclavicular joint injury, 446–447, *448*, 461–463, *462*
Coracobrachialis bursa, anatomy of, 89
Coracobrachialis muscle, anatomy of, 62–63
  blood supply of, 63
  force generation by, 235t
  function of, 62
  humeral insertion of, 48
  innervation of, 62–63
  insertion of, 62
  multiple insertions of, 132
  origin of, 62
  rupture of, 871–872
  scapular attachment of, 335, *335*
  testing of, 166t
  transfer of, in acromioclavicular joint injury, 443–444, 446
Coracoclavicular bar, 42–44, 113–115
  classification of, 114
  clinical findings in, 113–114, *115–116*
  embryology of, 114
  excision of, 114–115
  in acromioclavicular injury, 464
  motion in, 415, *416*
Coracoclavicular joint, 114–115, *115–116*, 420, *420*
Coracoclavicular ligament. See also *Conoid ligament*; *Trapezoid ligament.*
  anatomy of, 211, *211*, 415, 418, *418*, 796
  calcification of, 114
  disruption of. See *Acromioclavicular joint, injury of, types III to VI.*
  function of, 42, 418
  ossification of, 464
  reconstruction of, 439–440, 447
    historical aspects of, 436
    in acromioclavicular joint injury, 452, *453*, 461, *461*
Coracoclavicular screw, in acromioclavicular joint repair, 446, 454, *454–455*
  motion effects of, 414–415, *417*
Coracoclaviculosternal muscle, 127
Coracocostosternale vestigiale bone, 116
Coracoglenoid ligament, anatomy of, 43
Coracohumeral ligament, anatomy of, 15–16, *16*, *19*, 228, 533–534, *533*, 538, 794, 795–796
  function of, 227, 228, 538
  in biceps tendon stabilization, 794, *795–796*
  rupture of, biceps tendon subluxation in, 809, *810*
Coracoid process, anatomy of, 43, 336
    comparative, *3–4*, 4
  anomalies of, 43–44
    in impingement syndrome, 627t
  apophysitis of. See *Impingement syndrome.*
  as landmark, 532
  biceps tendon suture to, 825, *825*
  connection of, to first rib, 115–116
    to sternum, 116
  coracoclavicular bar on. See *Coracoclavicular bar.*
  deformity of, in brachial plexus injury of newborn, 1041

Coracoid process *(Continued)*
double, 111, *111*
embryology of, 114
fracture of, 339, *341*, 357–359, *358–359*, 361, 432–433, *432*
acromioclavicular joint injury with, 444, *444–445*
in children, *1027*, 1028
nonunion of, 464
versus clavicular fracture, 1020, *1023*
impingement of, on rotator cuff. See *Impingement syndrome.*
muscle transfer involving, in glenohumeral instability, 584
ossification of, 11, *11*
transfer of, in glenohumeral instability, 580–581, *582–583*, 584
Coracoiditis. See *Impingement syndrome.*
Corticosteroids, adverse effects of, 633, 697, *698–699*
in biceps tendinitis, 830
in calcifying tendinitis, 786–787
in frozen shoulder, 854–857
in impingement syndrome, 633
in rotator cuff tears, 662
Cosmesis, clavicle role in, 372
in amputation prosthesis, 953, *953*
in sternoclavicular joint injury, 517
Costocervical artery, collateral circulation of, *82*
Costoclavicular ligament, anatomy of, *478*, 479
anterior, anatomy of, 40, *40*, 209, *209*
function of, 209
as constraint, 210
clavicular impression for, 41, *42*
function of, 209, 479
posterior, anatomy of, 40, *40*, 209, *209*
function of, 209
Costoclavicular space, anatomy of, 369
Costoclavicular syndrome, in clavicular fracture, 391
Costocoracoid band, congenital, 115–116
Costovertebral bone, 116, *117*
Cranial nerve XI. See *Spinal accessory nerve.*
Crank test, in glenohumeral joint assessment, 169–170, *170*, 550, *550*
Craquemont (scapular sound), 362
Creatine kinase levels, in occupational cervicobrachial disorder, 1092
Crepitus, scapulothoracic. See *Snapping scapula.*
"Critical zone," of rotator cuff, 28, *29*
Cryosurgery, in tumor treatment, 912, 914
Cryptococcosis, of acromioclavicular joint, 468
Crystal arthropathy, 696–697
Cuff tear arthropathy, 654, 660, *660*, 672–673, 696–697, *697*
"Cuff tendinitis," 653
Cumulative trauma disorder. See *Occupational cervicobrachial disorder.*
Cup arthroplasty, 713–714, *714*, 737, 737t
complications of, 741t
Cyst, bone, aneurysmal, 885, *895*
simple (unicameral), 884–885, *884*, *895*
humeral fracture in, 992
in rotator cuff tears, 656, *656*
of acromioclavicular joint, 468

D

Dacron graft, in acromioclavicular joint repair, 441–442, *442*
in scapular stabilization, 761
DANA shoulder prosthesis, for hemiarthroplasty, 713
for total arthroplasty, 717–718, *717*
results of, 737–738, 737t, 739t
De Fabrica Corporis Humani (Vesalius), 36, *37*
"Dead arm syndrome," 759
Dead meridian plane, 218
deAnquin test, in biceps lesions, 814, *814*
Debridement, arthroscopic, in instability, 272–273
in rotator cuff tear, 263–264
in bone/joint infections, 935

Debridement *(Continued)*
in impingement syndrome, 965
in rotator cuff tears, 665
of acromioclavicular joint, 452, *453*
Deformity, as chief complaint, 153, *153*
evaluation of, 156, *156*
Degenerative disease, occupational, 1095
of acromioclavicular joint, 467
versus impingement syndrome, 632, *633*
versus tumor, 900, 900t
Deltoid artery, anatomy of, 79–80, *79*
collateral circulation of, *81–82*
Deltoid compartment, anatomy of, 875, 877
Deltoid muscle, anatomy of, 57–59, *58–59*, 866–867
comparative, 5, *5*
in glenohumeral joint surgery, 532
atrophy of, in brachial plexus injury of newborn, 1039, *1040*
blood supply of, 59
compartment syndrome of, 84, *84*
contracture in, fibrous, 127–128
from drug injection, 127–128
deficiency of, elevation and, 243
denervation of, in rotator cuff tear repair, 672
detachment of, from clavicle. See *Acromioclavicular joint, injury of, types III to VI.*
electrical stimulation of, snapping scapula in, *750*
fibrous contracture of, 127–128
force generation by, 235t
function of, 50, 58, 59
hand position/load and, 1094
in elevation, 235, 237–239, *237–239*, 241, 242
with supraspinatus muscle, 235, *237–239*, 238–240, *241*, 242
humeral attachment of, 48, 280
incision in, for humeral fracture treatment, 305, *307*
injury of, axillary nerve injury in, 766
innervation of, 59
insertion of, 51, *52*, 57
internal structure of, 58, *58*
origin of, 41, *41*, 57
paralysis of, 59, 767
release of, in contracture, 128
repair of, in acromioclavicular joint injury, 452, *453*
resection of, in bone tumor, 906, *907*
rupture of, 866–867
scapular attachment of, 45, 46, 335, *336–337*
splitting of, 532
strain of, 866–867
testing of, 164, 166t
Deltoid splitting incision, anatomy of, 86
Deltoid tendon failure, in rotator cuff tear repair, 672
Deltoidalgia. See *Impingement syndrome.*
Deltopectoral approach, for humeral fracture treatment, 305, *308*
Deltopectoral groove, anatomy of, 58
Deltotrapezius muscle fascia, repair of, in acromioclavicular joint repair, *453*, 455
Dempster concept of stability, 229, *230*
Dentition, abnormal, in cleidocranial dysostosis, 99
Depression, at sternoclavicular joint, 210
Dermatomes, mapping of, *752*
Diabetes mellitus, anesthesia and, 247
frozen shoulder and, 844–845
Diaphysis, embryology of, 10
Diastematomyelia, in Sprengel's deformity, 105–106, 105t
Diathermy, in frozen shoulder, 854
Dicloxacillin, in osteomyelitis, 1076
Didiee view, in x-ray evaluation, 187, 560
Dimple formation, 128, *128*
Disability, evaluation of, in occupational disorders, 1103–1105
Disability Evaluation Under Social Security, 1104
Disarticulation, of shoulder, 940, 943, *943–944*, 945
Dislocation. See also under specific joint e.g., *Acromioclavicular joint; Sternoclavicular joint.*
arthritis after, 694, *694–695*, 694t
congenital, 123–124, *124*

Dislocation *(Continued)*
  diagnosis of, 151–152
  of scapula, 361
  panclavicular, 375, 380
  terminology of, 424
  with fracture. See *Humerus, fracture dislocation of.*
Distention arthrography, in frozen shoulder, 856
Distraction test, in cervical spine examination, 175, *176*
Drawer test, in glenohumeral instability, 547–548, *548*, 1005, *1005*
Drug(s), injection of, deltoid muscle contracture in, 127–128
Drug addicts, septic arthritis in, 929, 933–934
Duchenne, G. B., anatomical studies of, 37–38, *37*
  neuromuscular studies of, 750, *750*
Duplay, on impingement syndrome, 623
Dupuytren, clavicular fracture treatment of, 367–368
DuToit staple capsulorrhaphy, in glenohumeral instability, 577–578, *578*, 585–586
Dynamic muscle transfer, in acromioclavicular joint injury, 443–444, 446, 457

E

Ectoderm, structures arising from, 6, *7*, 8
Edema, in compartment syndrome, 84
Eden-Hybbinette procedure, in glenohumeral instability, 580
Eden-Lange procedure, in spinal accessory nerve palsy, 760
Effort thrombosis, 988
  in thoracic outlet syndrome, 137, *141*
Eikenella corrodens, antibiotic susceptibility of, 934t
Elbow, deformity of, in brachial plexus injury of newborn, 1041–1042, *1041–1042*, 1052
  injury of, triceps muscle rupture in, 868
Electrical shock, glenohumeral instability in, 544, *545*
  humeral fracture in, 285
Electrical stimulation, in brachial plexus injury of newborn, 1046
Electrogoniometer, in motion measurement, 215
Electromyography, historical aspects of, 37–38, *37*
  in biceps tendon motion, 807–808
  in brachial plexus injury of newborn, 1044
  in muscle fatigue measurement, 1102
  in neurological disorders, 754, *754*
Elevation, acromioclavicular joint motion in, 414–415
  biceps tendon motion in, 805, *806*
  clavicular motion in, 371–372, *371*
  glenohumeral joint action in, 219–220, *220–221*
  glenohumeral joint forces in, 239–240, *239–241*
  in frozen shoulder, 841–842, 842t
  measurement of, in range of motion assessment, 160, *162*
  muscle function in, 235, *237–238*, 238–239
  of clavicle, 212, *213*
  provocative testing of, 173
  rotator cuff blood flow in, 625
  sternoclavicular joint motion in, 210
  weakness in, in rotator cuff tear repair, 672
Embryology, 6–10. See also specific structure.
  congenital malformations and, 10
  embryonic period in, 6–9, *6–10*
  fetal period in, 6, 9–10, *11*
  germ layers in, 6
Emphysema, pulmonary, frozen shoulder and, 845
  subcutaneous, in sternoclavicular joint dislocation, *518*, 519
Employment-related disorders. See *Occupational disorders.*
Enchondroma, 882, *883*, 895
Enders nail, in humeral fracture fixation, 297, *300*
Endoderm, structures arising from, 6, *8*
Endoneurium, structure of, 66
Endotracheal tube, in general anesthesia, 249
English-Macnab shoulder prosthesis, 715, *716*
  complications of, 742
  results of, 739t, 740
Enneking classification, of tumors, 877–879, 877t–878t
Enterococcus, antibiotic susceptibility of, 934t

Eosinophilic granuloma, versus tumor, 900t, 901
Epidural block, cervicothoracic, 255
Epineurium, structure of, 66, *67*
Epiphyseal fracture. See *Children, humeral fracture in.*
Epiphysis, embryology of, 10–11, *11*
  of clavicle, anatomy of, *481*, 482
    injury of, 502, *503*, 504, 509–511, *510–513*
  of scapula, 340, *341–342*
Epithelioid sarcoma, 892
Erb-Duchenne paralysis, 1033–1034. See also *Brachial plexus injury of newborn.*
Ergonomics. See *Occupational disorders.*
Escherichia coli, in bone/joint infection, 929
Esophagus, injury of, in sternoclavicular joint injury, 517
Eulenburg's deformity. See *Sprengel's deformity.*
Eulerian angle system, 216, *217*
Ewing's sarcoma, 887, *889*
  age distribution of, *894*
  chemotherapy in, 914–915
  location of, 875
  pathological fractures in, 898–899
  treatment of, 913–915
Exercise, aerobic, in impingement syndrome, 638
  in biceps tendon protection, 811–812
  in brachial plexus injury, 762
  in brachial plexus injury of newborn, 1046, 1053–1054, *1054*
  in calcifying tendinitis, 785, 787
  in capsulolabral reconstruction, 981–982, *982*
  in clavicular fracture, 397
  in frozen shoulder, 854, 858–859
  in glenohumeral instability, 573, 574t, 576–577, 609, *610–611*, 971, 1007, *1008*
    recurrent, 587–588, *587*, 588t
  in humeral fracture, 292, 318, *320–322*, 323
  in impingement syndrome, 636–638, *637–638*
  in posterior capsulorrhaphy, 984–986
  in prosthetic arthroplasty, 736
  in rotator cuff rehabilitation, 967, *967–970*, 969
  in rotator cuff tears, 664
  in stroke shoulder, 771
  in thoracic outlet syndrome, 770
  strengthening, for frozen shoulder, 854, 859
    for rotator cuff, 967, *970*, 1007, *1008*
  stretching, in frozen shoulder, 854, 859
    in rotator cuff rehabilitation, 967, *967–969*
    in torticollis, 1065, 1071
  throwing activities in, 982, *982*
Exostosis, in osteochondroma, 880, 882, *882*
  of humerus, *895*
Extension, in swimming strokes, 988–989
  maximum torque in, 242, *243*
"Eyebrow" sign, in impingement syndrome, 629, *629*

F

Facial nerve injury, in brachial plexus injury of newborn, 1037
Facioscapulohumeral dystrophy, 761
  diagnosis of, 754–755, *754*
Fairbank splint, elbow deformity from, 1041–1042, *1042–1043*
  in brachial plexus injury of newborn, 1046–1047, *1047–1048*
Falciform ligament, in biceps tendon stabilization, 794, *795*
Falls, acromioclavicular joint injury in, 422, *422*
  clavicular fracture in, 376–377
  humeral fracture in, 284, 992
  pectoralis major muscle rupture in, 864
  triceps muscle rupture in, 868
Fascial graft, in deltoid muscle repair, 867
  in glenohumeral stabilization, 584
  in spinal accessory nerve palsy, 760–761
  in sternoclavicular joint repair, 502
Fascial spaces, anatomy of, 85–86, *86–87*

Fatigue, biomechanics of, 1093, 1096–1098, *1096–1099*, 1098t
   in occupational disorders, 1091–1092, 1094
   in throwing, 963
Fenlin shoulder prosthesis, 680, *682*
Fentanyl, in regional anesthesia, 250
Ferkel procedure, in torticollis, 1068, *1069*
Fetal development theory, in torticollis, 1059
Fibrodysplasia ossificans progressiva, versus torticollis, 1064
Fibroma, nonossifying, of bone, 885, *887*
Fibromatosis, 891–892
Fibromatosis colli. See *Torticollis.*
Fibrosis, of deltoid muscle, 127–128
   of sternocleidomastoid muscle, 1061–1062, *1061*
Fibrositis, in occupational cervicobrachial disorder, 1092
   snapping scapula in, 362
   treatment of, 1102
   versus frozen shoulder, 853
Fibrous dysplasia, 885, *886, 895*
   pathological fractures in, 899
   versus tumor, 900–901, 900t
Fibula, transplantation of, in phocomelia, 119, *120*
Figure-of-eight bandage/sling, in clavicular fracture, 393, *393–394,*
   398–401, *401*, 1012, 1015, *1015*
   in sternoclavicular joint injury, 507
Figure-of-eight tension band fixation, in humeral fracture, 297,
   299
Figure-of-eight wiring, in humeral fracture, 310–311
Fish, fin structure of, 1–2, *1–2*
Fisk view, in x-ray evaluation, 200, *202*, 816, *816*
Flail shoulder, after limb sparing surgery, 908
Flexion, biceps tendon motion in, 807–808
   fatigue development in, 1096, *1096*
   in swimming strokes, 988–989
   maximum torque in, 242, *243*
Flexor muscles, testing of, 164
Floating clavicle (panclavicular dislocation), 375, 380
Floating socket shoulder prosthesis, 680, *684*
Flower, W. H., on glenohumeral instability, 526–527
Fluoroscopy, in glenohumeral instability, 561–562
Foot deformity, in cleidocranial dysostosis, 100
Forces, in acromioclavicular joint, direct, 420–421, *421*
    indirect, 422, *422*
   in throwing, 962–963
   joint reaction, 240, *241*, 242
   muscular, 49–50, *49–50*, 234–235, 235t, *236–239*, 238–239
    versus muscle orientation, 235, *236–237*
    versus muscle size, 235, 235t
    versus muscular activity, 235, *237–239*, 238–239
   on glenohumeral joint, 234–235, 235t, *236–239*, 239–240, *239–241*
Forearm deformity, in brachial plexus injury of newborn, 1052
Foreign body, bacterial colonization on, 925, 927
Forequarter amputation. See under *Amputation.*
Fossa, congenital, 128, *128*
Fossa axillaris, 6
Four-in-one arthroplasty, 827
Fracture, after arthrodesis, 707
   at birth. See *Clavicular fracture, at birth.*
   epiphyseal. See *Children, humeral fracture in; Epiphysis.*
   glenohumeral arthritis after, 694, 694t, 696, *696*
   impression. See under *Humeral fracture.*
   in glenohumeral dislocation, 562, *562–564,* 568–569, *569*, 572
   in prosthetic arthroplasty, 741–742, 741t
    revision in, 743–744, 743t
   malunion of. See *Malunion.*
   nerve injury in, 756
   nonunion of. See *Nonunion.*
   of acromion, 354–356, *355–357,* 361
    in children, 1028
   of clavicle. See *Clavicular fracture.*
   of glenohumeral joint, x-ray evaluation of, 178–184, *179–184*
   of humerus. See *Humeral fracture.*
   of rib, versus frozen shoulder, 852
   with clavicular fracture, 381–382, *381*

Fracture *(Continued)*
   of scapula. See *Scapular fracture.*
   pathological, in metastatic disease, 898–899, *899*
    of clavicle, 377, *377*
    of humerus, 284, 286
   refracture after, in clavicle, 387
   stress, in throwing, 992, *993*
Froimson procedure (keyhole tenodesis), in biceps tendon lesions,
   826, *826*
Froissemant (scapular sound), 362
Froittemant (scapular sound), 362
Frozen shoulder, 837–862
   adhesive capsulitis form of, 842–843, 843t
   age distribution of, 844
   anatomy of, 839–840, *841*
   arthrography in, 850–851, *850*
   arthroscopic surgery in, 858
   autoimmune hypothesis in, 849
   biomechanics of, 222, 224, *225*
   brain tumor as cause of, 751
   calcifying tendinitis and, 783, 785
   cervical disc disease with, 845
   classification of, 842–843, 843t
   clinical examination in, 845–846
   clinical presentation in, 846–849, *847–848*
   coexistent disorders with, 837
   complications of, 851
   definition of, 837
   diabetes mellitus and, 844–845
   diagnostic criteria for, 841–842, 842t
   differential diagnosis of, 851–853, 851t
   distention arthrography in, 856
   early capsulitis form of, 842, 843t
   exclusion criteria for, 837
   exercise in, 854, 858–859
   hematologic tests in, 849
   historical review of, 837–839
   in immobilization, 844
   in stroke, 771
   incidence of, 843–844
   injection protocols for, 854–856, 858
   intracranial pathology and, 845
   intrathoracic disorders and, 845
   irritative capsulitis form of, 842, 843t
   laboratory tests in, 849
   manipulation in, 856–857, 859–860
   mechanism of injury in, 844
   myofascial pain syndrome and, 844
   myofascial trigger point injection in, 856
   painful phase of, 846
   painful stiff shoulder form of, 843, 843t
   pathology of, 840–841, *841*
   personality disorders and, 845
   physiotherapy in, 854, 859
   post-traumatic stiff shoulder form of, 842, 843t
   predisposing factors in, 844–845
   prevention of, 853
   primary, 842, 843t, 846–848, *847*
   radionuclide scan in, 849–850
   radiotherapy in, 858
   range of motion in, 845–846
   secondary, 842, 843t, 848
   stellate ganglion block in, 858
   stiffening phase of, 846–847, *847*
   symptom duration in, 848–849, *848*
   systemic steroid therapy in, 857
   terminology of, 837
   thawing phase of, 847–848
   thyroid disorders and, 845
   traction in, 858
   trauma and, 845
   treatment of, 853–860
    alternatives for, 853, 853t
    distention arthrography in, 856

Frozen shoulder *(Continued)*
    exercise in, 854, 858–859
    injection protocols for, 854–856, 858
    manipulation in, 856–857, 859–860
    Murnaghan protocol for, 858–860
    myofascial approach to, 856
    objectives of, 853
    physiotherapy in, 854, 859
    radiotherapy in, 858
    stellate ganglion block in, 858
    surgical, 858, 860
    systemic steroids in, 857
    traction in, 858
  versus impingement syndrome, 627, 632
  versus rotator cuff tears, 661
  x-ray evaluation of, 849
Fulcrum test, in glenohumeral joint assessment, 170, *170*, 550, *550*
Fungal infections, 928–929, 1076, *1077*
Fusion. See *Arthrodesis*.

G

Gait, observation of, 154
Galen, anatomical studies of, 35–37
  as sports physician, 961
Gallie procedure, in glenohumeral instability, 584
Gallium–67 scan, in osteomyelitis, 1075
Gangrene, in arterial injury, 82
Garth view, in x-ray evaluation, 187
Gaucher's disease, 888
Gentamicin, in bone/joint infections, 934t, 935
Gern procedure, in acromioclavicular joint injury, 443, *443*
"Geyser sign," in impingement syndrome, *631*
  in rotator cuff tear, 659, *659*
Giant cell tumor, 885, *895*, 912, 914
Giant osteoid osteoma (osteoblastoma), 879
Glenohumeral dislocation, acute, treatment of, anterior, 569–573,
        572–573, 574t, *576*
      posterior, 573–575
  anterior, capsular changes in, 562
    clinical presentation of, 544
    fractures in, 562, *562–564*, 564
    incidence of, 1003
    ligament changes in, 562
    mechanism of injury in, 1003–1004
    neural injuries in, 566–568, *567*
    postreduction management of, 571
    recurrence, 568–569
    rotator cuff tears in, 564
    subscapularis muscle rupture in, 872
    surgery in, 571–572
    treatment of, acute traumatic, 569–570
      chronic traumatic, 570–571
      management after, 571
      Matsen method of, 572–573, *572*
      Rockwood method of, 573, *573*
      surgical, 571–572
    vascular injuries in, 564–566, *565*
  arthritis after, 694, 694t, *694–695*
  atraumatic, 1004
    treatment of, 1006–1007, *1008*
  bilateral, clinical presentation of, 546–547
  chronic, treatment of, 570–571, 575
  classification of, in children, 1003
  clinical presentation of, 544, 546–547, *546*
  etiology of, in children, 1003
  fracture in, 572
  in prosthetic arthroplasty, 741–742, 741t
  incidence of, 543
  inferior (luxio erecta), clinical presentation of, *543*, 546
    definition of, 543, *543*
    incidence of, 1003

Glenohumeral dislocation *(Continued)*
    mechanisms of, 544
  intrathoracic, definition of, 542
  Matsen anterior reduction method in, 572–573, *572*
  mechanisms of, 544, *545*
    in children, 1003–1004, *1004*
  posterior, clinical presentation of, 544, 546–547, *546*
    complications of, 569, *569*
    definition of, 542–543, *542*
    fractures in, 569, *569*
    incidence of, 543, 1003
    mechanism of injury in, 1004
    postreduction management in, 574–575
    surgery in, 575
    symptoms of, 1004
    treatment of, 573–575, *576*
  recurrent, 1005–1006
    after acute trauma, 568–569
    clinical presentation of, 547–551, *548–551*
    historical review of, 529, *529*
    immobilization and, 568
  Rockwood anterior reduction method in, 573, *573*, 574t
  soft tissue interposition in, 572
  subclavicular, definition of, 542
  subcoracoid, definition of, 541, *542*
  subglenoid, definition of, 541
  superior, definition of, 543
  symptoms of, in children, 1004, *1005*
  treatment of, anesthesia for, 570
    closed reduction, 1005–1007, *1008*
    exercise in, 573, 574t
    Hippocratic technique in, 570
    in children, 1005–1007, *1008*
    Kocher technique in, 526, *527*, 529–530, 570
    leverage methods in, 570
    Milch technique in, 570
    Steinmann pins in, 574–575
    Stimson technique in, 570
    traction methods in, 570, 572–573, *572*, 574t
  versus frozen shoulder, 852
  voluntary, 1004, *1004*
    atraumatic causes of, 547, *548*
  x-ray evaluation of, 178–184, *179–184*
    in children, 1005, *1006–1007*
Glenohumeral index, 226
Glenohumeral instability, 526–622. See also *Glenohumeral dislocation*; *Glenohumeral joint, subluxation of*.
  acute, definition of, 541
    historical review of, 529–530
  AMBRI syndrome in, 541, 576, 576t
    treatment of, 605–608, *606–608*
  anatomical considerations in, 1002–1003, *1003*
  anterior, definition of, 541–542, *542*
    exercise in, 971
    historical review of, 530
    rehabilitation in, 971
  anterior capsule defects in, historical review of, 527
  apprehension in, 541
  apprehension test in, 169–170, *170–171*, 550, *550*
  arthrography in, 561
  arthroscopy in, 262–263, 270–273, 562, 976
    anatomic considerations in, 270–272, *272*
    diagnostic, 270
    labral debridement in, 272–273
    treatment techniques for, 272–273
  atraumatic. See also subhead: *AMBRI syndrome in*.
    definition of, 541
    mechanisms of, 543
    treatment of, 608–609, *610–612*, 612
  bilateral, 540, *540*. See also subhead: *AMBRI syndrome in*.
  Bristow operation in, 972, *973–976*, 976
  capsulolabral reconstruction in, 977–978, *977–982*, 981–982
  causes of, 541, 547
  chronic, definition of, 541

Glenohumeral instability (Continued)
  chronology of, 541
  classification of, 541–543, 542–543
  clinical presentation of, in dislocation, 544, 546–547, 546
    in recurrence, 547–551, 548–551
  computed tomography in, 561, 561
  congenital, definition of, 541
  crank test in, 169–170, 170, 550, 550
  degree of, 541
  differential diagnosis of, 569
  directions of, 541–543, 542–543
  dislocation. See Glenohumeral dislocation.
  drawer test in, 547–548, 548, 1005, 1005
  essential lesion in, historical review of, 529, 529
  exercise in, 971, 1007, 1008
  fixed abnormalities in, x-ray evaluation of, 557, 559
  fluoroscopy in, 561–562
  fulcrum test in, 550, 550
  genetic predisposition to, 540, 540
  historical review of, acute traumatic dislocation and, 529–530
    anterior capsule defects and, 527
    anterior instability and, 530
    early descriptions of, 526, 527–528
    essential lesion in, 529, 529
    humeral head defect in, 526–527
    posterior instability and, 530–531
    rotator cuff injuries in, 527
  humeral head defect in, 526–527, 559–561, 560
  in children. See under Children.
  in prosthetic arthroplasty, 741–742, 741t, 744
  in rheumatoid arthritis, 691, 693
  in sports. See under Sports medicine.
  in swimming, 989
  incidence of, 543
    in children, 1003
  inferior, treatment of, 605–608, 606–608
  involuntary, 609
    definition of, 541
    treatment of, 609
  jerk test in, 550, 550–551
  ligamentous laxity in, 547
  locked, definition of, 541
  mechanisms of, 543–544
  multidirectional. See also subhead: AMBRI syndrome in.
    treatment of, 605–609, 606–608, 610–612, 612
  neuromuscular causes of, 541
  physical examination in, 543, 544–551, 546, 548–551
  posterior, capsulorrhaphy in, 983–986, 984–986
    historical review of, 530–531
    in athlete, 983–986, 984–986
    treatment of, 530–531, 983–986, 984–986
  push-pull test in, 551, 551
  recurrent, after surgical repair, 585–586
    atraumatic causes of, 547
    definition of, 541
    diagnostic failures in, 586
    essential lesion in, 529
    traumatic causes of, 547
    treatment of, 575–612
      anterior, 575–598, 576t, 578–595, 588t, 610–611
      arthroscopy in, 584, 585
      Bankart procedure in, 530, 577
      bone block in, 580, 598–599, 599
      Boyd-Sisk procedure in, 598
      Boytchev procedure in, 584
      Bristow-Helfet procedure in, 580–581
      capsular repairs in, 577–578, 578
      complications of, 585–587, 605
      coracoid transfer in, 580–581, 582–583, 584
      diagnostic failures and, 586
      DuToit capsulorrhaphy in, 577–578, 578
      Eden-Hybbinette procedure in, 580
      exercise in, 587–588, 587, 588t
      Gallie procedure in, 584

Glenohumeral instability (Continued)
      glenoid osteotomy in, 584, 598–599, 599
      hardware complications in, 586
      Henderson procedure in, 530
      historical review of, 530
      humeral osteotomy in, 584
      in misdiagnosis, 586
      infection after, 585
      inferior, 588t, 605–612, 606–608, 610–612
      Latarjet procedure in, 581, 582–583
      limited motion after, 586–587
      Magnuson-Stack procedure in, 579–580, 580
      Matsen method in inferior instability, 588t, 605–608, 606–608
      Matsen method in posterior instability, 599, 600, 601
      Matsen method in traumatic anterior instability, 587–592, 587–591, 588t
      multidirectional, 588t, 605–612, 606–608, 610–612
      muscle-sling myoplasty in, 530
      neurovascular injury in, 586
      Nicola procedure in, 530, 584
      nonoperative, 576–577, 598, 610–611
      operative, procedures for, 577. See also specific procedure.
      Oudard procedure in, 580
      posterior, 598–605, 599–604
      postoperative management in, 584–585
      Putti-Platt procedure in, 578–579
      recurrent instability after, 585–586
      reverse Putti-Platt procedure in, 598
      Rockwood method in multidirectional instability, 606, 608–610, 610–612, 612
      Rockwood method in traumatic instability, 592, 593–595, 596–598, 610–611
      Rockwood method of posterior reconstruction, 601, 602–604, 605
      Saha procedure in, 584
      staple capsulorrhaphy in, 577–578, 578
      subscapularis muscle procedures in, 578–580, 580
      Trillat procedure in, 580
      x-ray evaluation of, 556–561, 559–561, 559–560
  relocation test in, 964–965, 964–965
  rotator cuff injuries in, historical review of, 527
  secondary to impingement, 965, 966
  stabilization procedures for, arthroscopic, 273–276, 273–275
  subluxation of. See Glenohumeral joint, subluxation of.
  sulcus sign/test in, 548, 549, 550, 1005
  traumatic. See also subhead: TUBS syndrome in.
    definition of, 541
    mechanisms of, 543–544, 545
  treatment of, Bristow operation in, 972, 973–976, 976
    capsulolabral reconstruction, 977–978, 977–982, 981–982
    exercise in, 576–577, 609, 610–611
    "handshake" cast in, 575
    historical review of. See subhead: historical review of.
    in recurrent instability. See under subhead recurrent.
    incision for, 531–532, 531–532
    operative, 571–572, 574–575
  TUBS syndrome in, 541, 576, 576t
    operative treatment of, 588–592, 588–591
  versus biceps tendinitis, 822
  versus impingement syndrome, 632
  versus rotator cuff tears, 662
  voluntary, 606, 608–609
    definition of, 541
    treatment of, 609
  with secondary impingement, 966, 966
  without secondary impingement, 966–967, 966
  x-ray evaluation of, 551–561
    anteroposterior view in, 552–554, 552–554
    axillary view in, 555–556, 556–559
    goals of, 551–552
    in children, 1005
    in scapular plane, 553–556, 553–559
    lateral view in, 554–555, 555–556

Glenohumeral instability *(Continued)*
  transthoracic view in, 553
Glenohumeral joint. See also *Glenoid*; *Humeral head*.
  anatomy of, 531–534, *539*
    arthroscopic, 258–262, *259–261*
    bony, 12–15, *13–14*
    bursae of, 27, *27*
    capsule, 15–17, *15–17*
    clavipectoral fascia, 532
    coracoacromial arch, 532
    developmental, 799, *799*
    in frozen shoulder, 839–840, *840*
    instability and, 1002–1003, *1003*
    ligaments, 17–27, *17–26*, 533–534, *533–534*. See also specific
      ligament.
    muscles, 532
    nerve zone, 532–533, *533*
    rotator cuff. See *Rotator cuff*.
    skin, 531–532, *531–532*
  anesthetic injection into, diagnostic, 174
  arthritis of. See under *Arthritis*.
  arthrodesis of. See under *Arthrodesis*.
  arthroscopy of. See *Arthroscopy*.
  biomechanics of, 213–218, *214–217*
  clinical evaluation of, in arthritis, 701–703
  computed tomography of, 184
  dislocation of. See *Glenohumeral dislocation*.
  drainage of, 1082, *1083*
  dysplasia of, 120–124, *121–123*
  forces at, 239–240, *239–241*
  fracture near, arthritis after, 694, 694t, 696, *696*
  fracture of, x-ray evaluation of, 178–184, *179–184*
  function of, 534
  hemiarthroplasty of, 712–714, *713–714*
    after limb sparing surgery, *909–910*, 910
    complications of, 740, 740t
    results of, 736–738, 737t
  implants for. See *Prosthetic arthroplasty*.
  injection therapy of, 854–856
  innervation of, 30–31, *30–31*
  instability of. See *Glenohumeral instability*.
  intra-articular compartment of, anatomy of, 875
    pressure in, 535–536
  joint reaction force in, *241*, 242
  manipulation of, in frozen shoulder, 856–857
  motion of, 213–218, *214–217*, 805, *806–807*, 807
    Codman's paradox and, 214, *214–215*
    in arthritis, 701–702
    in frozen shoulder, 841–842, 841t
    measurement of, 214–215
    terminology of, 215–216, *216*
    three-dimensional, 216–218, *217*
  muscle forces on, 234–235, 235t, *236–239*
  neoplasia of, 701, *701*
  neuropathic arthritis of, 700–701, *700*
  osteoarthritis of, clinical manifestations of, 701
    occupational, 1095
    pathoanatomy of, 687–688, *687–688*, 689t
    prosthetic arthroplasty in, 736–749, 737t–738t
  osteotomy near. See under *Osteotomy*.
  physical examination of, in arthritis, 701–702
  prosthetic arthroplasty of. See *Prosthetic arthroplasty*.
  pseudodislocation of, 1004
  radiography of, 222, *223*
  radiotherapy near, effects of, 699, *700*
  recesses of, 840, *840*
  replacement of. See *Prosthetic arthroplasty*.
  resection arthroplasty of, 704–705, *704*, 906, *907*, 908
  resting posture of, 218
  rheumatoid arthritis of, clinical evaluation in, 702–703
    pathoanatomy of, 688–691, *689–694*, 690t
    prosthetic arthroplasty in, 736–738, 737t–738t
  screw displacement axis of, 222, *223*
  septic arthritis of, 700, 925

Glenohumeral joint *(Continued)*
  in children, 934, 1080–1082, *1083*
    symptoms of, 929
  stability of, active mechanisms in, 538–539
    adhesion/cohesion mechanism in, 536–537
    articular contribution to, *219*, 226–237, *226*
    assessment of, 167–170, *168–171*
    bony restraints in, 538
    capsular restraints in, 537–538
    finite joint volume in, 535–536
    glenoid labrum detachment in, 538, *539*
    joint conformity and, 534–535, *535*
    ligament contribution to, 227–231, *227–229*, 533, 537–538
    passive mechanisms in, *533–535*, 534–538
    versus age, *227–228*, 228
  subluxation of, in stroke, 771
    mechanism of injury in, in children, 1004, *1004*
    symptoms of, 1005, *1005*
    versus biceps tendon lesions, 822
    x-ray evaluation of, 178–184, *179–184*
  surfaces of, classification of, 12, 14
  synovectomy of, 703–704, *704*
  synovial membrane of, 840
  systemic disease effects on, 699, *700*
  translation testing of, 167–169, *168–169*
  traumatic arthritis of, prosthetic arthroplasty in, 736–738, 737t–738t
  volume of, 535–536
  x-ray evaluation of, in arthritis, 702
Glenohumeral ligament, anatomy of, 228–229, *229*
  variations in, 537
  anterior, anatomy of, 537
  anteroinferior, anatomy of, 533, *534*
  anteromedial, anatomy of, 533, *534*
  inferior, anatomy of, 18–27, *19–27*, 229, 230, 260–261, *261*, 271,
    537
    anterior band of, 20–21, *20–21*, 23, *23*, *26*
    anterior capsule of, 23, *23*
    arthroscopy of, 260–261, *261*
    axillary pouch of, 18, *19*, 21–25, *24*
    deficiency of, 271
    function of, 230, *230*, 537–538
    histology of, 21, 23, *23–26*
    posterior band of, 20–21, *20–26*, 23
    posterior capsule of, 23, *23–25*
    superior band of, 18, *19*
    thickness of, 21, *21*, 23, *23–24*
  middle, anatomy of, 18, *18–19*, 229, *229*, 260, 533, *533*, 537
    arthroscopy of, 260
    function of, 229, *230*, 262, 537–538
    normal variations in, 260
  posteroinferior, anatomy of, 533
  superior, anatomy of, 17–18, *18–19*, 229, 260, *260*, 533, *533*, 537
    arthroscopy of, 260, *260*
    function of, 229, *230*, 261–262
Glenohumeral muscles. See also specific muscle.
  anatomy of, 57–63, *58–62*
Glenohumeral ratio, 219
Glenoid. See also *Glenohumeral joint; Glenoid fossa; Glenoid labrum*.
  anatomy of, 279
    arthroscopic, 270–271, *271*
  articular surface of, 218–219, *219*
  bone graft in, for prosthetic arthroplasty, 718, *720*
  dentated, 117–118, *118*
  dislocation at, in prosthetic arthroplasty, 744
  dysplasia of, versus scapular fracture, 342–343, *344*
  excision of, in glenohumeral arthritis, 704–705, *705*
  fracture of, in children, *1027*, 1028
    in glenohumeral dislocation, 562, *562*
    intra-articular, 345–353, *347–353*
    neck, 343–345, *344–346*
  hypoplasia of, 122, *122*
    stability and, 226, *226*

Glenoid *(Continued)*
  indented, 117–118, *119*
  loosening of, in prosthetic arthroplasty, 715, *716*, 741–744, 741t, 743t
    in rotator cuff deficiency, 243, *243*
  neck of, fracture of, 343–345, *344–346*
    osteotomy of, 584
  osteoarthritic changes in, 688, *688*, 689t
  osteotomy of, biomechanics of, 234, *234*
    in arthritis, 711–712
    in glenohumeral instability, 598–599, *599*, 601, *603*, 605
  prosthesis for, placement of, 729, *729–735*, 731–734
  retroversion of, versus stability, 534, *535*
  rim of, fracture of, in glenohumeral dislocation, 569, *569*, 572
  shape of, versus stability, 534–535, *535*
  spurs on, in throwing athlete, 986
  x-ray evaluation of, 184–185, *185–186*
Glenoid fossa, anatomy of, 12, *13–14*, 14
    comparative, 2, *3*
  angle of, with scapula, 12, *14*
  ossification of, 11–12, 340
  void in, in instability, 553
Glenoid labrum, anatomy of, 14, *14*, 259–260, *259–260*, 538, *539*
    arthroscopic, 270–271, *271*
  arthroscopic debridement of, 272–273
  arthroscopy of, 259–260, *259–260*
  blood supply of, 28, 30, *30*
  disruption of, 259–260, 272–273
  embryology of, 8, *9*, 10
  function of, 259–260, *260*
    in stability, 226, 538
  injury of, in swimming, 989
    in throwing, 965, *966*
    versus biceps tendon subluxation, 822
  reconstruction of, in glenohumeral instability, 977–978, *977–982*, 981–982
  tensile strength of, versus age, 228, *228*
Glenoid sign, vacant, 552
Glycosaminoglycans, in articular cartilage, 923
Goniometer, in motion measurement, 215
Gram-negative bacilli, in joint/bone infections, 929, 934t
Granuloma, eosinophilic, versus tumor, 900t, 901
  in calcifying tendinitis, 777, *777*
Granulomatous infection, of bone, 1076
Gray rami communicans, anatomy of, 72
Greater scapular notch (spinoglenoid notch), anatomy of, 43
Green procedure, in Sprengel's deformity, 108
Gross, S. W., on sarcoma, 874
Ground substance, in articular cartilage, 923
Guides to the Evaluation of Permanent Impairment, 1104

H

Haemophilus influenzae, antibiotic susceptibility of, 934t
  in bone/joint infections, 928–929, 1074, 1076
  in children, 1081
Halstead's test, 173
Hand deformity, in cleidocranial dysostosis, 100
  in Poland's syndrome, 129–130, *129*
Hanging cast, in humeral fracture, 296
Hand-Schüller-Christian disease, versus tumor, 900t, 901
Healing, of clavicular fracture, 1010, *1010*
Heart. See also *Cardiovascular disorders.*
  pin migration into, 519
Helbig classification, of frozen shoulder, 842–843, 843t
Hemangioma, 891
Hematologic disorders, versus tumor, 900t, 901
Hematoma, in biceps muscle rupture, 868–869
  in pectoralis major muscle rupture, 866
  torticollis and, 1060
Hemiarthroplasty, of glenohumeral joint, 712–714, *713–714*
  after limb sparing surgery, *909–910*, 910

Hemiarthroplasty *(Continued)*
  complications of, 740, 740t
    in rotator cuff arthropathy, 660–661, *661*
  results of, 736–738, 737t
Hemiplegia, frozen shoulder and, 845
Hemophilia, versus tumor, 900t, 901
Hemorrhage, into joint, infection and, 923
Hemothorax, in clavicular fracture, 382
Henderson procedure, in recurrent glenohumeral instability, 530
Heredity, torticollis and, 1059–1060
Hermodsson, I., on glenohumeral instability, 527
Hermodsson view, in x-ray evaluation, 187, 559
Herophilus, anatomical studies of, 35
Heuter sign, in biceps lesions, 814
"High shoulder," after amputation, 956, 959
Hill-Sachs lesion, 271–272, *272*, 562, 1005, *1006–1007*
  reverse, 189, *189*, 531, 569, *569*
  x-ray evaluation of, 185, 187, *187*
Hill-Sachs view, in x-ray evaluation, 559
Hilton's law, 30
Hip deformity, in cleidocranial dysostosis, 100
  torticollis and, 1059
Hippocrates, anatomical studies of, 34–35
  on acromioclavicular joint injury, 413
  on clavicular fracture, 367
  on dislocation treatment, 526, *528*
  on glenohumeral dislocation reduction, 570
  on proximal humerus fixation, 278
Histamine response, in brachial plexus injury of newborn, 1045, *1045*
Histiocytoma, malignant fibrous, 892
  age distribution of, *894*
Histiocytosis, versus tumor, 900t, 901
History, and physical examination, 149–153, *151, 153*
Hitchcock procedure, in biceps tendon lesions, 824–825, *825*, 827
Hobbs view, in x-ray evaluation, 492, *492*
Holt-Oram syndrome, 109–111
Hooded component system. See under *Prosthetic arthroplasty.*
Horner's syndrome, diagnosis of, 167
  in brachial plexus injury of newborn, 1037
  in regional anesthesia, 252
Huang-Ti Nei Ching Su Wen, anatomical studies of, 34
Hughes-Neer rehabilitation program, after prosthetic arthroplasty, 735–736
Humeral circumflex artery(ies), aberrant brachial plexus relationships with, 132–133, *133*
  anterior, anatomy of, 28, *28*, 61, *79*, 80, 280, *280*
    collateral circulation of, *81–82*
  posterior, anatomy of, 28, *28*, 30, 61, *79*, 80, 91
    anomalies of, 81
    collateral circulation of, *81–82*
    in deltoid, 58–59
Humeral compartments, anatomy of, 875
Humeral fracture, 278–334
  adhesive capsulitis in, 328
  anatomic neck, 283, *283*
    closed reduction of, 292
    open reduction of, 297, 309
  anatomical considerations in, 991–992
  angular displacement in, 288
  AO buttress plate and screw in, 297, *298*
  AO classification of, 283–284
  arthritis after, 696, *696*
  avascular necrosis in, 290, *291*, 323, *324*
    AO classification and, 283–284
  brachial plexus injury in, 290–291
  casting of, 296
  chest injury in, 291
  classification of, 278, 281–284, *282–283*, 992, *993*
  clinical presentation of, 285, *286*
  closed reduction of, 997–998, *998*
    complications of, 292
    guidelines for, 292
    in four-part fractures, 295

Humeral fracture *(Continued)*
    in impression fractures, 295–296
    in minimal displacement, 309
    in three-part fractures, 294–295
    in two-part fractures, 292, *293–295*, 294, 309–310
    percutaneous pinning after, 296
  comminuted, treatment of, 296, 311, *311*
  complications of, 289–291, *289–291*, 323, *324–328*, 327–328, 1002, *1002*
  computed tomography of, 288–289, *288*
  differential diagnosis of, 286
  early motion after, 292
  Enders nail fixation in, 297, *300*
  etiology of, 284–285
  figure-eight tension band fixation of, 297, *299*
  figure-eight wiring in, 310–311
  four-part, 283, *283*
    avascular necrosis in, *291*
    closed reduction of, 295
    open reduction of, 303, *304*
    treatment of, 312–313, *315–317*
  greater tuberosity, 283, *283*
    closed reduction of, 294, *294–295*
    in glenohumeral dislocation, 572
    open reduction of, 297, *301–302*
    treatment of, 311–312, *311–312*
  head-splitting, 283, *283*, 318, *319*
  historical aspects of, 278–279
  immobilization in, 292
  impression, 283, *283*
    closed reduction of, 295–296
    treatment of, 318, *319*
  in brachial plexus injury of newborn, 1037, 1044
  in children. See under *Children.*
  in infants, 995, *995*
  incidence of, 284
    in children, 992
  internal fixation of, 296–297, *298–302*, 303, *304–306*, 305
  lesser tuberosity, 283, *283*
    closed reduction of, 294, *295*
    open reduction of, 297
    treatment of, 312
  malunion of, 289, *290*, 323, *326*, 327–328
    impingement syndrome in, *630*
  mechanism of injury in, 284–285
    in children, 992
  minimal displacement of, 282–283, 309
  myositis ossificans in, 291
  neck shaft angle in, 288
  Neer classification of, 282–283, *283*
  nerve injury in, *280*, 281
  nonunion of, 288–289, *288–289*, 323, *325*
  open, treatment of, 998
  open reduction of, 296–309
    approaches for, 305, *307–308*, 309
    historical aspects of, 278, 296–297, *298–302*
    in four-part fractures, 303, *304*
    in three-part fractures, 297, *302*, 303, 312, *313–314*
    in two-part fractures, 297, *298–302*, 309–312, *311–312*
    replacement prosthesis in, 303, 305, *305*
  osteoporosis and, 284
  pathological, 284, 286, 898, *899*
  percutaneous pinning in, 296, 310, *310*, 997, *999*
  plaster splint/cast in, 296
  prosthesis failure in, *327–328*, 328
  radiographic evaluation of, 286–289, *287–289*
  rehabilitation in, 318, *320–322*, 323
  replacement prosthesis in, 303, 305, *305*
  Rush rod technique in, 297, *302*
  skeletal traction in, 296
  soft tissue interposition in, 998, *1001*
  splinting of, 296
  surgical approaches to, 305, *307–308*, 309
  surgical neck, 283, *283*

Humeral fracture *(Continued)*
    closed reduction of, 292, *293*, 294
    open reduction of, 297, *298–299*, 309–310
  symptoms of, in children, 993
  three-part, 283, *283*
    closed reduction of, 294–295
    open reduction of, 297, *302*, 303
    treatment of, 312, *313–314*
  treatment of, 993, *994–1001*, 995, 1002. See also under specific
    type of fracture, e.g., *two-part anatomical neck.*
    closed reduction. See subhead: *closed reduction of.*
    in children, 993, *994–1001*, 995, 1002
    in infants, 995, *995*
    operative. See subhead: *open reduction of.*
    percutaneous pinning, 997, *999*
    results rating system for, 284
  two-part anatomical neck, closed reduction of, 292
    open reduction of, 297
    treatment of, 309
  two-part greater tuberosity, 283, *283*
    closed reduction of, 294, *294–295*
    open reduction of, 297, *301–302*
    treatment of, 311–312, *311–312*
  two-part lesser tuberosity, 283, *283*
    closed reduction of, 294, *295*
    open reduction of, 297
    treatment of, 312
  two-part surgical neck, closed reduction of, 292, *293*, 294
    open reduction of, 297, *298–299*
    percutaneous pinning of, 296
    treatment of, 309–311, *309–311*
  x-ray evaluation of, in children, 993
Humeral head, absence of, 121–122
  anatomy of, 12, *13*, 279, *279*
    arthroscopic, 271–272, *272*
  angle of inclination of, 12, *13*
  arthroscopy of, 262, 271–272, *272*
  articular surface of, compression of, 231–232
  avascular necrosis of, versus frozen shoulder, 852
  center of rotation of, 222, *223*
  defects of, in instability, 526–527
  displacement of, rotator cuff tears in, 656, *657*
  fracture of, compression, with anterior dislocation, 185, 187, *187*
    in glenohumeral dislocation, 562, *563–565*, 564, 568–569
  Gaucher's disease of, 888
  Hill-Sachs lesion of. See *Hill-Sachs lesion.*
  hypovascular zone of, 921
  loosening of, in prosthetic arthroplasty, 741–742, 741t
  migration of, in rotator cuff deficiency, 224, *225*
  osteoarthritic changes in, 687, 688, 689t
  osteonecrosis of, pathoanatomy of, 697, *698–699*, 699
    prosthetic arthroplasty of, 736–737, 737t
    versus frozen shoulder, 852
  palpation of, 157, *158*
  pectoralis minor muscle insertion into, 131–132, *131*
  prosthesis for, in fracture, 303, 305, *305*, 312, *315–317*, 316
    failure of, *327–328*, 328
  retroversion angle of, 793, *793*
  retroversion of, 121
  x-ray evaluation of, 559–561, *560*
Humeral ligament, transverse, anatomy of, 16, *16*, 794, *796*
  transverse (intertubercular ligament), 47
Humeral scapular circumflex artery, posterior, in teres minor, 61
Humeroscapular periarthritis. See *Impingement syndrome.*
Humerus, abnormality of, in impingement syndrome, 627t
  anatomic neck of, anatomy of, 47, *47*, 279, *279*
    fracture of. See *Humeral fracture.*
  anatomy of, 46–49, *47–48*, 279–281, *279–280*
    comparative, *3–4*, 4
    developmental, 12, *12*, 991
    surgical, 991–992
  arterial ring around, 921
  articular surface of, 218, *219*
  bicipital groove of. See *Intertubercular groove.*

Humerus *(Continued)*
  biopsy of, 901–902, *902*
  blood supply of, 280–281, *280*
    infection and, 921
  bone cyst of, aneurysmal, 885
    simple (unicameral), 884–885, *884*
  bone graft of, in prosthetic arthroplasty, 721, *721*
  chondroblastoma of, 882
  chondrosarcoma of, *883*
  Codman's paradox and, 214, *214–215*
  dysplasia of, 120–122, *121*
  embryology of, 6, *8*
  enchondroma of, 882, *883*
  Ewing's sarcoma of, 887, *889*
  fibrous dysplasia of, 885, *886*
  fracture dislocation of, 283, *283*, 305, *306*, 313, 316, *317*
    clinical presentation of, 285, *286*
    delayed diagnosis of, *288*
    four-part, 316, *317*
    myositis ossificans in, 291
    three-part, 316
    treatment of, 305, *306*, 313, 316, *317*
    two-part, 313, 316
  fracture of. See *Humeral fracture.*
  giant cell tumor of, 885
  greater tuberosity of, anatomy of, 279, *279*
    fracture of. See under *Humeral fracture.*
  head of. See *Humeral head.*
  hemiarthroplasty of. See *Hemiarthroplasty.*
  innervation of, *280*, 281
  intertubercular groove of. See *Intertubercular groove.*
  lengthening procedure for, in phocomelia, 119–120, *120–121*
  lesser tuberosity of, anatomy of, 279, *279*
    fracture of, 283, *283*, 294, *295*, 297, 312
  limb salvage surgery of. See *Limb spining surgery.*
  medullary canal preparation of, in prosthetic arthroplasty, 727, *728*
  muscle attachments of, 279–280, *279*. See also *Rotator cuff.*
  ossification of, 12, *12*, 991
  osteochondroma of, 880, *882*
  osteoid osteoma of, 879
  osteomyelitis of, 926
    diagnosis of, 1075
    in children, 1075–1076
    spread of, 924
    treatment of, 1075–1076
  osteosarcoma of, 880, *881*
  osteotomy of, in arthrogryposis, 1073–1074, *1073*
    in brachial plexus injury of newborn, 1051–1052, *1051*, 1054–1055, *1055*
    in glenohumeral instability, 584
  Paget's disease of, 888, *890*, 891
  periosteal chondroma of, 882
  physis of, anatomy of, 991
    closure of, 991
    development of, 991
  prosthesis for. See *Prosthetic arthroplasty.*
  pseudodislocation of, 995, *995*
  replacement of (hemiarthroplasty), 712–714, *713–714*
    after limb sparing surgery, *909–910*, 910
    complications of, 740, 740t
    in rotator cuff arthropathy, 660
    results of, 736–738, 737t
  resection of, 906, *907*, 940, 949, *950*
    with scapula, *907*, 908
  rotation of, 220, *221–222*, 222
    in brachial plexus injury of newborn, 1039, 1041, *1041*
  rotator cuff tear effects on, 654, *655*
  shaft of, anatomy of, 279, *280*
  shortening of, in fracture, 1002
  surgical neck of, amputation through, 941, *942*, 943
    anatomy of, 47, 279, *279*
    fracture of. See under *Humeral fracture.*
  tubercles of, anatomy of, 46–47, *47*, 279, *279*

Humerus *(Continued)*
  tumors of, location of, 895, *895*
  varus deformity of, 49, 121, *121*
Humphry, G. M., on joint adhesion/cohesion, 536
Hydrocortisone, in frozen shoulder, 855
Hydrostatic pressure, negative, stabilizing effect of, 234, *235*
Hyperabduction syndrome test, 173
Hyperesthesia, in neurological disorders, 757
Hypertension, anesthesia and, 247
Hyperthyroidism, frozen shoulder and, 845
Hypotension, from bone cement monomer, 255
  in sternoclavicular joint dislocation, *518*, 519
Hypovascular "critical zone," of rotator cuff, 28, *29*
Hysteria, neurological disorders in, 757–758
  versus frozen shoulder, 853

I

Ideberg classification, of scapular fractures, 345, *348–353*, 349–350
Iliac crest, bone graft harvesting from, anesthesia for, 255
Immobilization, frozen shoulder and, 844
  in clavicular fracture, 387
  in humeral fracture, 292
  in septic arthritis, 934
Immunization, brachial plexus neuropathy in, 772
Immunodeficiency, infection susceptibility in, 920
Impairment, evaluation of, in occupational disorders, 1103–1105
Impingement sign, in pain diagnosis, 170–171, *172*
Impingement syndrome, 623–646
  acromioplasty in, 634–636, *635*, 639, *639–642*
    failure of, 642
  activity modification in, 637–638
  acute, treatment of, 633
  aerobic exercise in, 638
  anatomy of, 624–626, *624–626*
  arthrography in, 629, *630–631*
  arthroscopy in, 263–264, *263*, 268–269, *269*
  causes of, 626–627, 627t
  classification of, 626, 627t
  clinical presentation of, 629
  complications of, 632
  conditions associated with, 629, *630–631*
  coracoid, versus biceps tendon lesions, 823
  corticosteroids in, 633
  definition of, 623
  diagnosis of, 965–967
  differential diagnosis of, 632–633, *633*
  flexibility restoration in, 637, *637*
  functional, 627t
  historical review of, 623–624
  imaging techniques in, 629, *629–631*, 632
  in prosthetic arthroplasty, 741, 741t
  in rheumatoid arthritis, 703
  in swimming, 989
  in throwing athletes, 965–967, *966*
  incidence of, 626–627
  mechanisms of injury in, 626–629, 627t, *628*
  occupational causes of, 626–627
  pathology of, 623–624
  prevention of, 627, 629
  range of motion in, 629
  rotator cuff tears in, 632, 651. See also *Rotator cuff.*
  self-perpetuating nature of, 627
  stages of, 624
  strength restoration in, 637–638, *638*
  structural, 627t
  treatment of, 965–967, *966*
    in failed acromioplasty, 653
    Jackins Program in, 636–638, *637–638*
    nonoperative, 633–634, 636–638, *637–638*
    operative, 634–636, *635*, 638–639, *639–642*, 642
  versus biceps tendinitis, 821–822

Impingement syndrome *(Continued)*
    workmen's compensation cases of, 636
    x-ray evaluation of, 196, *197–199,* 199–200
Impingement tendinitis, 808–809, *809,* 827–829, *828–829*
Impingement test, in pain diagnosis, 170–171, *172,* 174
Implants, for arthroplasty. See *Prosthetic arthroplasty.*
Impression fracture, of proximal humerus. See under *Humeral*
       fracture.
Incision. See also specific procedure.
    for glenohumeral surgery, 531–532, *531–532*
    skin tension lines and, *91–92,* 92
India, early anatomical studies in, 34
Indium scan, in infection, 931, 1075
Industry, disorders associated with. See *Occupational disorders.*
Infants, birth injuries of. See also *Brachial plexus injury of new-*
       born; Clavicular fracture, at birth.
    shoulder dislocation, 123–124, *124*
    bone scan in, 1075
    clavicular fractures in, 1011–1012
    humeral fractures in, incidence of, 992
       mechanism of injury in, 992
       treatment of, 995, *995,* 998
       x-ray evaluation of, 993
    Moro reflex testing in, 167
    osteomyelitis in, 1078, 1080, *1080*
Infection, bacterial colonization in, 926–928, *927–928*
    compartment anatomy and, 84
    fungal, 928–929, 1076, *1077*
    granulomatous, of bone, 1076
    in glenohumeral stability surgery, 585
    in joint replacement. See under *Prosthetic arthroplasty.*
    in pectoralis major muscle rupture, 866
    in rotator cuff tear repair, 672
    of bone. See *Osteomyelitis.*
    of joint. See *Septic arthritis.*
    polymicrobial (mixed), 929
    prosthesis revision in, 743, 743t
    torticollis and, 1059
    versus tumor, 900, 900t
    viral, brachial neuritis in, 823
       in septic arthritis, 930
       long thoracic nerve palsy in, 768
Inferior glenohumeral ligament complex, anatomy of, 20–21, *20–21*
Inflammation, versus tumor, 900, 900t
    x-ray evaluation of, 202
Infrascapular bone, 116–117, *117*
Infraspinatus muscle, anatomy of, 60, *60,* 647
    comparative, 5, *5*
    atrophy of, in suprascapular nerve compression, 987
    denervation of, in rotator cuff tear repair, 672
    force generation by, 235t
    function of, 60
       hand position/load and, 1094–1095
    humeral attachment of, 47, *279,* 280, 625
    insertion of, 60, *60*
    origin of, 60, *60*
    scapular attachment of, *45, 46,* 335, *336–337*
    strengthening exercise for, 969, *970*
    testing of, 166t
    weakness of, in brachial plexus injury of newborn, 1039, *1040*
       in suprascapular nerve injury, 765, *765*
Infraspinatus tendon, anatomy of, 774
    blood supply of, 774–775
    calcifying tendinitis of, 784, *784*
    hypovascular zone of, 775
    tendinitis of, occupational, 1094–1095
    transfer of, in rotator cuff tears, 663
Infraspinous fossa, comparative anatomy of, *3,* 4
Infraspinous index, 2, *3*
Injection, of drugs, deltoid muscle contracture in, 127–128
Injection tests, *172,* 174
    of biceps tendon lesions, 821–823
Injection therapy, in frozen shoulder, 854–856, 858
Injury. See also specific structure.

Injury *(Continued)*
    acute, evaluation of, 153
Inspection, in physical examination, 155–157, *156–157,* 175
Instability. See also specific joint; *Dislocation.*
    anterior, 152
       x-ray evaluation of, 184–185, *185–186*
    as chief complaint, diagnosis in, 151–152
    degree of, 152
    direction of, 152
    disability related to, 152
    involuntary, 152
    posterior, 152
       x-ray evaluation of, 189, *189*
    voluntary, 152
Instantaneous center of rotation, 215–216, *216*
    of humeral head, 222
    of scapula, 222, *223*
Interclavicular ligament, anatomy of, 40, *40,* 209, *209,* 478, 479
    function of, 209, *209*
    posterior, as constraint, 210
Intercostal arteries, collateral circulation of, *82*
Intercostal brachial nerve, anatomy of, 76
    anomalous, 74
Intercostal nerves, anterior, anatomy of, 91
    lateral cutaneous branches of, anatomy of, 91
Internal fixation, in arthrodesis, 911
    in glenohumeral joint arthrodesis, 707, *708, 710*
    of metastatic bone lesions, 898–899, *899*
    of proximal humerus fracture. See *Humeral fracture, open reduc-*
      tion of.
Internal rotation procedures, in brachial plexus injury of newborn,
      1052, *1052*
Interosseus nerve, posterior, entrapment of, versus biceps tendon
      lesions, 823–824
Interscalene block, 250–255, 250t, *251–254,* 252t
    in arthroscopy, 265
Interscapulothoracic resection (Tikhor-Linberg procedure), 940–
      941, 949, *950*
Intertubercular (bicipital) groove, anatomy of, 46–48, *47–48,* 279,
      279, 793, *793,* 796–798, *797–798, 907,* 908, *279, 279*
    comparative, 797, *798*
    anesthetic injection into, diagnostic, 174
    angulation of, 123, *123*
    biceps tenodesis in (Hitchcock procedure), 824–825, *825*
    congenital aberration of, 122–123, *123*
    in biceps tendon lesions, 799, 801, *802–803*
    measurements of, 796–797, *798*
    spurs on, 122–123, *123*
       in biceps tendinitis, 801, *803–805*
    stenosis, biceps tendon attrition in, 810, *810*
    ultrasonography of, 818, *820*
Intertubercular (transverse humeral) ligament, anatomy of, 16, *16,*
      47, 794, *796*
Intra-articular disc ligament, anatomy of, 478–479, *478*
    function of, 478–479
Intrafragmentary screw fixation, in clavicular fracture, 396
Intramedullary fixation, of clavicular fracture, 395–397, *395,* 401–
      403, *403,* 408, *408*
    of humeral fracture, 297
Intrathoracic dislocation, of glenohumeral joint, 541
Intrathoracic disorders, frozen shoulder and, 845
Intrauterine factors, in torticollis, 1060–1061
"Iron cross" maneuver, muscular action in, 51
Irritative capsulitis, 832t, 842
Ischemic heart disease, frozen shoulder and, 845
Isoelastic shoulder prosthesis, 714, 737, 737t, 741t

J

Jackins Program, in impingement syndrome treatment, 636–638,
    637–638

Japanese Association of Industrial Health, occupational cervicobrachial disorder classification of, 1101, 1101t
Jerk test, in glenohumeral instability, 550, *550–551*
Joessel, D., on glenohumeral instability, 527
Joint. See also specific joint.
    anatomy of. See specific joint.
    constraints of. See *Biomechanics, constraints and.*
    functions of, 39
    hemorrhage into, infection and, 923
    infection of. See *Septic arthritis.*
    motion of. See *Motion of joint.*
    pressure determination in, *241,* 242
    quality of movement of, assessment of, 159, *160*
    range of motion of. See *Range of motion.*
    transitional zone of, 921
Joint reaction force, 240, *241,* 242
Jugular vein, anterior, anatomy of, 483, *483*
    internal, injury of, in clavicular fracture, 369, *369,* 383

K

Kay classification, of frozen shoulder, 842, 843t
Kenny Howard sling, in acromioclavicular joint injury, 435, *435*
Kessel shoulder prosthesis, 680, *683*
    complications of, 742
    results of, 739t, 740
Keyhole tenodesis, in biceps tendon lesions, 826, *826*
Keystone tenodesis, in biceps tendon lesions, 825–826
Kidney abnormality, in Sprengel's deformity, 105–106, 105t
Kirschner modification, of Neer prosthesis, 722
Kirschner wires, in clavicular fracture fixation, *395,* 396, *402*
    migration of, 464–465
Klippel-Feil syndrome, in Sprengel's deformity, 105–106, 105t, *106*
Klumpke paralysis, 1034. See also *Brachial plexus injury of newborn.*
Knowles pins, in clavicular fracture fixation, 396, 402–403, *403,* 408, *408*
Kocher classification, of humeral fractures, 278, 281, *282, 278*
Kocher technique, in glenohumeral instability, 526, *527,* 529–530, *570*
Kölbel shoulder prosthesis, 680, *683*
König procedure, in Sprengel's deformity, 108

L

Laceration brachial birth palsy. See *Brachial plexus injury of newborn.*
Lamina obscurans/splendins, in articular cartilage, 923, *924*
Landmark muscles. See also specific muscle: *Omohyoid; Scalenus; Sternocleidomastoid.*
    anatomy of, 65–66, *65*
Langer's arm arch (axillopectoral muscle), 124–125, *125*
Langer's lines, *91–92,* 92
Larrey procedure, in shoulder disartication, 943, *943–944,* 945
Laryngeal nerve block, in regional anesthesia, 252
Latarjet procedure, in glenohumeral instability, 581
Lateral lymph nodes, anatomy of, 83, *83*
Lateral view, in x-ray evaluation, 287–288, *287*
Latissimus dorsi muscle, anatomy of, *62,* 63–64
    comparative, 5
    blood supply of, 64
    force generation by, 235t
    function of, 64
    humeral insertion of, 48
    innervation of, 64
    insertion of, *62,* 64
    origin of, *62,* 63–64
    scapular attachment of, *45,* 335, *336–337*
    testing of, 166t

Latissimus dorsi muscle *(Continued)*
    transfer of, in glenohumeral instability, 584
Leonardo da Vinci, anatomical studies during, 35–36, *36*
L'Episcopo procedure, in brachial plexus injury of newborn, 1048–1050, *1049–1050*
Letterer-Siwe disease, versus tumor, 900t, 901
Levator scapulae muscle, anatomy of, 55–56, *55–56*
    comparative, 5
    function of, 56, *56*
    scapular attachment of, *45,* 46, 335, *336–337*
    testing of, 166t
Levator scapulae tendon transfer, in spinal accessory nerve palsy, 760
Lidocaine, in biceps tendon lesion diagnosis, 821–823
    in regional anesthesia, 250, 252t
    at bone graft donor site, 255
Ligaments. See also specific ligament and joint.
    anatomy of, 15–27, *15–27,* 209, *209,* 211, *211,* 227–231, *228–232, 796*
    arthroscopic, 260–262, *260–261*
    laxity of, in throwing athlete, 966, *966*
Limb bud, 6, *7–8,* 8
Limb sparing surgery, historical review of, 874–875
    in sarcoma, 905–906, *907,* 908
    in tumor treatment, 915
    reconstruction after, 908–911, *909–910*
Lipoma, 891, 895
Liposarcoma, 892, *894,* 895
Lippmann procedure, in biceps tendon lesions, 824, *824*
Lippmann test, in biceps lesions, *812,* 814
Littlewood procedure, in forequarter amputation, 947, *948,* 949
Liverpool shoulder prosthesis, 680, *682*
    complications of, 742
    results of, 739t, 740
Load and shift test, of glenohumeral joint stability, 167–169, *168–169*
Long deltopectoral approach, for humeral fracture treatment, 305, *308*
Loose bodies, arthroscopy of, 272, *272*
Ludington test, 171, 814, *814*
Lundberg classification, of frozen shoulder, 842–843, 843t
Lung, clavicular protection of, 372
Luschka's tubercle, in snapping scapula, 363
Luxio erecta injury, 543, *543,* 546, 1003
Lymph nodes, anatomy of, 82–83, *83*
    biopsy of, spinal accessory nerve injury in, 759, *761*
    dissection of, 82

M

McLaughlin procedure, in glenohumeral dislocation, 574–575
Magnetic method, in motion measurement, 215
Magnetic resonance imaging, in biceps tendon lesions, 820
    in neurological disorders, 754
    in osteomyelitis, 932
    in rotator cuff lesions, 200, 659–660
    in tumors, 879, 897–898
Magnuson-Stack procedure, in glenohumeral instability, 579–580, *580,* 585–586
Malgaigne, clavicular fracture treatment of, 368
Malignancy. See also under *Tumor(s).*
    versus frozen shoulder, 852
Malignant fibrous histiocytoma, 892, *894*
Malingering, neurological disorders and, 757–758
    versus frozen shoulder, 853
Malunion, of clavicular fracture, 390
    of humeral fracture, 289, *290,* 323, *326,* 327–328, 1002, *1002*
Mammary artery, internal, collateral circulation of, *82*
Manipulation, in brachial plexus injury of newborn, 1046
    in frozen shoulder, 856–857, 859–860
Mankoff's sign, in pain evaluation, 757

Manual for Orthopaedic Surgeons in Evaluating Permanent Physical Impairment, 1104

Margin, of tumors. See under *Tumor(s)*.

Massage, in brachial plexus injury of newborn, 1046

Matsen Four Star exercise program, in recurrent glenohumeral instability, 587–588, *587*, 588t

Matsen method, in glenohumeral instability, closed reduction, 572–573, *572*
  inferior, 605–608, *606–608*
  multidirectional, 605–608, *606–608*
  operative, 588–592, *588–591*, 599, *600*, 601
  recurrent posterior, 599, *600*, 601
  recurrent traumatic, 588–592, *588–591*

Mayer procedure, in brachial plexus injury of newborn, 1050

Mazas shoulder prosthesis, 680, *685*, 715

Median nerve, anatomy of, 68, 69–72
  compression of, in Parsonage-Turner syndrome, 132–133, *133*

Mepivacaine, in regional anesthesia, 250, 252t
  at bone graft donor site, 255

Mesoacromion, anatomy of, 45, *45–46*, 112, *343*
  impingement syndrome and, 625

Mesoderm, structures arising from, 6, *7–8*, 8

Meta-acromion, anatomy of, 45, *45*, 112, *343*
  impingement syndrome and, 625

Metabolic disorders, versus tumor, 900t, 901

Metastasis, 878
  chemotherapy in, 915
  from adenocarcinoma, incidence of, 892
  pathological fracture in, 898–899, *899*

Methohexital, in regional anesthesia, 250

Methyl prednisolone, in frozen shoulder, 855

Methylmethacrylate cement, application of, in prosthetic arthroplasty, 718, *720*, 721
  complications with, 255

Metson test, in biceps lesions, 812, *812*

Meyer, supratubercular bony ridge of, 122–123, *123*

Michael Reese shoulder prosthesis, 715, *715*
  complications of, 742
  placement of, 722, *723*
  results of, 739t, 740

Midazolam, in regional anesthesia, 250

Milch technique, in glenohumeral dislocation reduction, 570

Milwaukee shoulder, 696–697, *697*
  calcification in, 776

Minnesota Medical Association, impairment evaluation guidelines of, 1104

Mobilization techniques, in frozen shoulder, 854

Möbius syndrome, 130

Moloney's line, in x-ray evaluation, 553

Monitoring, during anesthesia, 248

Monospherical shoulder prosthesis, 739t
  complications of, 741
  for hemiarthroplasty, 713
  for total arthroplasty, 717–718, *717*

Moro reflex, testing of, 167

Motion of joint. See also specific joint and type of motion, e.g., *Elevation*; *Rotation*.
  description of, 215–216, *216*
  measurement of, 214–218, *217*
  planar, 215–216, *216*
  rolling, 216, *216*
  sliding, 215, *216*
  spinning, 216, *216*
  terminology of, 215–216, *216*

Motor system, evaluation of, 758

Multipennate muscle, 49

Multiple joint muscles. See also specific muscle: *Biceps*; *Latissimus dorsi*; *Pectoralis major*; *Triceps*.
  anatomy of, 62–63, *63–65*

Multiple myeloma, 885, 887, *888*
  age distribution of, *894*
  incidence of, 892
  laboratory tests in, 898

Mumford procedure, in acromioclavicular joint injury, 443, *443*, 987

Muscle(s). See also specific muscle.
  activity of, versus force generation, 235, *237–239*, 238–239
  anatomy of, 49–66
    comparative, 5, *5*
    glenohumeral, 57–63, *58–62*
    landmark, 65–66, *65*
    multiple joint, 62–63, *63–65*
    scapulothoracic, 54–57, *54–58*
  angiosome concept and, 53–54, *53*
  attachment of, to bone, 51, *52*
  blood vessels of, 53–54, *53*
  centroid determination in, versus force generation, 235, *237–239*, 238–239
  clavicular attachments of, 372
  congenital anomalies of. See under *Congenital anomalies*.
  disorders of, torticollis and, 1060
  excursion of, 49–50, *49*
  fatigability of, in occupational disorders, 1091–1092
  forces generated by, 49–50, *49–50*
    on glenohumeral joint, 234–235, 235t, *236–239*
  function of, 50–51, *50–51*
  imbalance of, after amputation, 956
  innervation of, 53–54, *53*, *753*
  multipennate, 49
  orientation of, versus force generation, 235, *236–237*
  palpation of, 159
  parallel fiber arrangement in, 49, *49*
  pennate, 49, *49*
  release of, in stroke shoulder, 771
  rupture of, 863–873
    biceps, 869–871, *870*
    causes of, 863
    coracobrachialis, 871–872
    deltoid, 866–867
    pectoralis major, 864–866, *865*
    principles of, 863–864
    serratus anterior, 871
    site of, 863–864
    subscapularis, 872
    triceps, 867–869
  scapular attachments of, 335–336, *335–337*
  size of, versus force generation, 235, 235t
  splitting of, 51, 53, *53*
  stabilizing action of, 50–51, *50*, 231, *233*
  static load measurements of, in occupational disorders, 1090, *1091*
  strain of. See specific muscle.
  testing of, 164–166, 164t–165t
    in arthritis, 702
    in neurological disorders, 758
  tightening of, in stabilization, 234, *234*
  transfer of, in acromioclavicular joint injury, 443–444, 446, 457
    in brachial plexus injury, 763
  trigger points in, frozen shoulder and, 844, 856
  wasting of, evaluation of, 155–156, *156*
  weakness of, in brachial plexus injury of newborn, *1036*, 1037–1038, *1038–1039*

Muscle buds, in fish fin, 1

Muscle fibers, anatomy of, 49, *49*
  internal arrangement of, 49, *49*
  rupture of, in occupational cervicobrachial disorder, 1092

Muscle relaxants, in glenohumeral dislocation reduction, 570
  with anesthesia, 248

Muscle-sling myoplasty, in recurrent glenohumeral instability, 530

Muscular dystrophy, 761
  arthrogryposis as, 1072–1074, *1072–1073*
  electromyography in, 754

Musculocutaneous nerve, anatomy of, 30–31, *30*, 68, 70, *70*, 280, 281, 533
  in biceps innervation, 64
  injury of, 767–768, *767*

Musculocutaneous nerve *(Continued)*
   in biceps muscle rupture, 870
   in Bristow procedure, 756
   in glenohumeral stabilization procedures, 586
   in humeral fracture, 281, 291
Musculotendinous cuff. See *Rotator cuff.*
Muybridge, Eadweard, photographic studies of, 38, *38*
Myalgia, in occupational disorders. See *Occupational cervicobrachial disorder.*
Mycobacterium kansasii, in septic arthritis, 930
Mycobacterium tuberculosis, in bone/joint infection, 929
Myelography, in brachial plexus injury of newborn, 1044–1045
Myeloma, multiple. See *Multiple myeloma.*
Myoelectric prosthesis, 956, *958*
Myofascial pain syndrome, frozen shoulder and, 844, 856
Myofibrositis, in occupational cervicobrachial disorder, 1092
   treatment of, 1102
Myopathy, in torticollis, 1060
Myositis ossificans, 879–880
   in humeral fracture, 291
Myotomy, in torticollis, 1067–1068, *1068,* 1071

N

Nafcillin, in bone/joint infections, 934t, 935, 1076, 1081
Neck. See also *Cervical spine.*
   deformity of. See *Torticollis.*
   pain in. See *Occupational cervicobrachial disorder.*
Necrosis, avascular. See *Avascular necrosis.*
Needle aspiration, in osteomyelitis, 1076
   in septic arthritis, 933, 1082
Neer, Charles, on impingement syndrome, 624
   "the syndrome" described by, in arthritis, 691, *694*
Neer classification, of humeral fractures, 278, 281–283, *283*
Neer criteria, for humeral fracture treatment evaluation, 284
Neer procedure, in prosthetic arthroplasty, 718, *720–721,* 721
Neer prosthesis, for humeral head, 303, 305, *305,* 312, *315–317,*
      316, 678–679, *679,* 712–713, *713,* 736, 737t
   failure of, *327–328,* 328
   for total replacement, 680, *685,* 716–718, 718t
      complications of, 741, 741t
         Kirschner modification of, 722
      results of, 738–739, 738t–739t
      revision of, 742–743, 743t
Neer-Horowitz classification, of humeral fractures, 992
Negative pressure, in joint, stabilizing effect of, 234, *235*
Neisseria gonorrhoeae, antibiotic susceptibility of, 934t
   in intra-articular infection, 925–926, 929, 934
      in children, 1081
Neoplasia. See also *Tumor(s);* specific disorder.
   amputation in, 941, 945
   interscapulothoracic resection in, 940, 949, *950*
   of glenohumeral joint, versus degenerative arthritis, 701, *700*
   scapulectomy in, 949, 951, *951*
Nerve(s). See also specific nerve.
   blood supply of, 66–67, *67*
   fascicular structure of, 66
   function of, 66
   injury of, classification of, 755–757
      crush (axonotmesis), 566, 756
      in humeral fracture, *280,* 281
      in regional anesthesia, 253
      in surgery, 756
      in traumatic limb loss, 959
      mild (neurapraxia), 265, 566, 755–756
      mode of, 756
      prosthesis revision in, 743
      severe (neurotmesis), 567
      traction (axonotmesis), 566, 756
   microanatomy of, 66–67, *67*
   of glenohumeral joint, 30–31, *30–31*
   of skin, *90,* 91–92

Nerve(s) *(Continued)*
   peripheral, entrapment of, versus biceps tendon lesions, 823–824
Nerve block. See *Anesthesia, regional.*
Nerve conduction velocity, in neurological disorders, 754
   in thoracic outlet syndrome, 770
Nerve roots, dermatomes of, 751, *752*
   injury of, avulsion, 762
      in clavicular fracture, 382
      in regional anesthesia, 253
      myelography in, 1044–1045
   muscles supplied by, 751, *753*
   stretching of, in birth injury, 1035, *1035–1036*
Nerve stimulator, in regional anesthesia induction, 250, 250t, *251,*
     252
Neurapraxia, 566, 755–756
   after arthroscopy, 265
Neuritis, brachial, versus biceps tendon lesions, 823
      versus impingement syndrome, 632
Neurological examination, 165–167, 166t, 175, 751, 757–758
Neurological problems, 750–773. See also specific disorder and
     nerve.
   anatomical considerations in, 751, *752–753*
   arthrography in, 752
   brachial plexus injury. See *Brachial plexus, injury of.*
   classification of, 755–757
   clinical presentation of, 751, *752–753*
   differential diagnosis of, 757–758
   electromyography in, 754
   functional versus organic, 757–758
   glenohumeral instability in, 541
   historical aspects of, 750–751, *750*
   laboratory evaluation in, 754–755, *754*
   magnetic resonance imaging in, 754
   muscular dystrophy, 761
   nerve conduction velocity in, 754
   organic versus functional, 757–758
   physical examination in, 751, 757–758
   poliomyelitis, 750–751
   referred pain and, 751
   spinal accessory nerve palsy, 759–761, *760–761*
   stroke shoulder, 770–771
   thoracic outlet syndrome. See *Thoracic outlet syndrome.*
   torticollis and, 1060
   treatment of, 758–759
   ultrasonography in, 753–754
   x-ray evaluation of, 751, 753–754, *753–754*
Neuropathic arthritis, of glenohumeral joint, 700–701, *700*
   versus frozen shoulder, 852
Neurosarcoma, 875
Neurotmesis, 567, 756
Neviaser classification, of frozen shoulder, 843, 843t
Nicola procedure, in glenohumeral instability, 584
   recurrent, 530
Night pain, in bony tumors, 895
Nonossifying fibroma, of bone, 885, *887*
Nonretentive shoulder prosthesis, 680, *685,* 715, 739t
Nonsteroidal anti-inflammatory drugs, in frozen shoulder, 854
Nonunion, in osteomyelitis, 1076–1077, *1078*
   of clavicular fracture, 387–390, 1016
      incidence of, 387
      physical examination in, 390
      predisposing factors in, 387–388, *388*
      symptoms of, 389–390
      treatment of, 395–397, *397,* 404–408, *404–408*
      x-ray evaluation of, 388–389, *388–389*
   of coracoid process fracture, 464
   of humeral fracture, 288–289, *288–289,* 323, *325,* 1002
Nullmeridianebene, 218

O

Ober procedure, in Sprengel's deformity, 108
Obesity, anesthesia and, 247

Obstetric paralysis. See *Brachial plexus injury of newborn.*
Occipital artery, in sternocleidomastoid, 65
Occupational cervicobrachial disorder, 1088–1093
    Australian epidemic of, 1090
    classification of, 1101–1102, *1101*, 1101t–1102t
    constitutional symptoms in, 1089
    creatine kinase levels in, 1092
    definition of, 1088
    differential diagnosis of, 1100
    epidemiology of, 1088–1090
    etiology of, 1090–1093, *1091*, *1093*
    fatigue measurement in, 1102
    Grades I to III, *1101*, 1102, 1102t
    in assembly-line workers, 1091–1092, *1093*
    in cash register operators, 1089
    in keyboard operators, 1089–1090, *1091*, 1092
    in musicians, 1089
    interstitial myofibrositis in, 1092
    muscle fiber rupture in, 1092
    myalgia in, 1090
    organic theory of, 1090, *1091*
    pre-employment screening for, 1100
    psychologic factors in, 1090
    static muscle load measurements in, 1090, *1091*, 1092
    stress sources in, 1103
    thoracic outlet syndrome and, 1089–1090
    treatment of, 1100–1103, *1101*, 1101t–1102t
    video analysis of, 1093
    weightlifting and, 1089
Occupational disorders, 1088–1108. See also *Sports medicine; Throwing.*
    biceps lesions, 811
    biomechanics of, 1093, 1096–1098, *1096–1099*, 1098t
    calcifying tendinitis, 776
    classification of, 1088
    degenerative arthritis, 1095
    evaluation of impairment in, 1103–1105
    in video display terminal work, 1098
    incidence of, 1088
    job rotation and, 1098–1099
    occupational cervicobrachial disorder. See *Occupational cervicobrachial disorder.*
    pre-employment screening for, 1099–1100
    prevention of, 1095–1100
        efficacy of, 1100
        exercise in, 811–812
        training in, 1100
        work method design in, 1098–1099
        worker selection in, 1099–1100
        workplace design in, 1096–1098, *1096–1099*, 1098t
    rest breaks and, 1098–1099
    shoulder load in, 1093, 1096–1098, *1096–1097*, 1098t
    tendinitis, 1093–1095, *1094*
    treatment of, 1100–1103, *1101*, 1101t–1102t
Occupational Repetition Strain Advisory Committee, occupational cervicobrachial disorder classification of, 1101, 1102t
Ocular torticollis, 1063, *1063–1064*
Oligohydramnios, torticollis and, 1059
Omohyoid muscle, anatomy of, 65–66
    scapular attachment of, *45*, 46, *335–336*
Omovertebral bone, in Sprengel's deformity, 106, *107*
    removal of, 109
Operating room, arrangement of, *254*
Os acromiale (bipartite acromion), 111–113, *112–113*, 340, 342, *342–343*, 1025, *1025*
Os subclaviculare (duplicated clavicle), 103, *103*
Oscillating veins, 54
Osseous tumors. See under *Tumor(s).*
Ossification, 10–12, *11–12*
    of acromion, 112, *112*, 342, *343*, 625–626
    of clavicle, 368
    of humerus, 991

Ossification *(Continued)*
    of scapula, 340, *341–342*
Osteitis, of sternoclavicular joint, 488, 504
Osteitis deformans (Paget's disease), 888, *890*, 891
Osteoarthritis, of acromioclavicular joint, occupational, 1095
    of glenohumeral joint, after Putti-Platt procedure, 579
        clinical manifestations of, 701
        occupational, 1095
        pathoanatomy of, 687–688, *687–688*, 689t
        prosthetic arthroplasty in, 736–738, 737t–738t
    of sternoclavicular joint, 487–488, *487*, 504, *506*
    versus frozen shoulder, 852
Osteoblastoma, 879
Osteochondroma/osteochondromatosis, 880, 882, *882*, 884
    of scapula, crepitus in, 362, *363–364*
        neurological disorders in, *753*
    versus frozen shoulder, 852
Osteoid osteoma, 879, *895*
Osteolysis, of clavicle, 464, *465*
Osteoma, osteoid, 879, *895*
Osteomalacia, versus tumor, 900t, 901
Osteomyelitis, anatomical considerations in, 921, 923
    antibiotics in, 934, 934t, 936, 1076
    bone scan in, 1075
    classification of, 923–924, 923t
    clinical presentation of, 928, *929*
    complications of, 932
    computed tomography in, 931, 1075
    contiguous, 926
    debridement in, 936
    hematogenous, 924, 926, 1074–1080, *1077–1080*
    historical review of, 920–921
    in children. See under *Children.*
    in metaphyseal zone, 921, *922*
    incidence of, in children, 1074
    intramedullary pressure in, 1074–1075
    magnetic resonance imaging of, 932
    neonatal, 1078, 1080, *1080*
    nonunion in, 1076–1077, *1078*
    of clavicle, 924, 926
    of glenoid, resection arthroplasty in, 704–705
    of humerus, 926
        diagnosis of, 1075
        in children, 1075–1076
        spread of, 924
        treatment of, 1075–1076
    of scapula, 924, 926, *929*
    pathogenesis of, 920, 924–926, 926t, *935*
        in children, 1074–1075
        in neonatal type, 1078, 1080, *1080*
    pathogens in, 928–929
        in children, 1074
        in neonatal type, 1080, *1080*
    physeal arrest in, 1076, *1077*
    recurrence of, 1076
    spread of, 924
    susceptibility to, 920
    treatment of, 934, 934t, *935*, 936
    ultrasonography of, 931
    vascular injury in, 1077–1078
    versus tumor, 900, 900t
    x-ray evaluation of, 931, 1075
Osteonecrosis, of humeral head, pathoanatomy of, 697, *698–699*, 699
    prosthetic arthroplasty of, 736, 737t
    versus frozen shoulder, 852
Osteoporosis, in humeral fractures, 284
    versus tumor, 900t, 901
Osteoporosis circumscripta (Paget's disease), 888, *890*, 891
Osteosarcoma, 880, *881*
    age distribution of, *894*
    biopsy in, 913
    chemotherapy in, 914–915
    incidence of, 892

Osteosarcoma *(Continued)*
  location of, 875
  of humerus, *895*
  Pagetoid, *890*, 891
  secondary, 880
  treatment of, 912–915
Osteotomy, near glenohumeral joint, in arthritis, 711–712
  of glenoid, biomechanics of, 234, *234*
    in glenohumeral instability, 584, 588–589, *599*, 601, *603*, 605
  of humerus, in arthrogryposis, 1073–1074, *1073*
    in brachial plexus injury of newborn, 1051–1052, *1051*, 1054–1055, *1055*
    in glenohumeral instability, 584
Oudard procedure, in glenohumeral instability, 580
Outlet view, in x-ray evaluation, 817, *817*
Overhead exercise test, in thoracic outlet syndrome, 769
Oxacillin, in bone/joint infections, 935
Oxygen therapy, during anesthesia, 248

P

Paget's disease, 888, *890*, 891
Paget-Schroetter syndrome, in thoracic outlet syndrome, 137, *141*
  versus tumor, 900–901, 900t
Pain, after amputation, 959–960
  as chief complaint, 150–151, *151*
  causes of, 150
  diagnosis of, impingement test in, 170–171, *172*
  in acromioclavicular joint injury, 425–426
  in bony tumors, 895
  in brachial plexus neuropathy, 771–772
  in calcifying tendinitis, *780–781*, 781–782
  in clavicular fracture nonunion, 389–390
  in frozen shoulder, 841–842, 842t, 846
  in glenohumeral arthritis, 701
  intensity of, 151
  localization of, 150, *151*
  night, 150
    in bony tumors, 895
  postoperative, management of, 256
  referred, 751
    diagnostic problems in, 751
    versus frozen shoulder, 852
  types of, 150
Painful arc, in calcifying tendinitis, 782
  in impingement test, 170–171, *172*
Palpation, in physical examination, 157, *158*, 159, 175
Panclavicular dislocation, 375, 380
Parachuting, biceps muscle rupture in, 869
Parallel fiber arrangement, in muscle, 49, *49*
Paralysis, in Parsonage-Turner syndrome, 132–133
  obstetric. See *Brachial plexus injury of newborn.*
  of deltoid muscle, 59
  of trapezius muscle, 54–55
Paresthesia, as chief complaint, 153
Parham support, in clavicular fracture, *392*
Parosteal osteosarcoma, 880
Paroxysmal torticollis of infancy, 1064
Parsonage-Turner syndrome, 132–133, *133*, 823
Pathological fracture. See under *Fracture.*
Patient-controlled analgesia, postoperative, 256
Péan prosthetic shoulder, 678, *678*
Pectoral artery, anatomy of, 79, *79*
  in pectoralis major, 63
Pectoral compartment, anterior, anatomy of, 875
Pectoral nerve, lateral, anatomy of, *68*, 69–70
  in pectoralis major innervation, 63
  medial, anatomy of, *68*, 71–72
    anomalous, 74
    in pectoralis major innervation, 63
    in pectoralis minor innervation, 57
Pectoral nodes, anatomy of, 83, *83*

Pectoralis major muscle, absence of, 63, 129–130, *129–130*
  anatomy of, 63, *63*, 794, *795*, 864
    comparative, 5
  blood supply of, 63
  chondroepitrochlear muscle origin in, 126
  clavicular attachment of, 372
  contracture of, in brachial plexus injury of newborn, 1039, *1040*
  deficiency of, 129–130, *129–130*
  embryology of, 130
  force generation by, 235t
  function of, 63
  humeral attachment of, 48, *279*, 280
  in biceps tendon stabilization, 794, *795*
  innervation of, 63
  insertion of, 63, *63*
  origin of, 41, *41*, 63, *63*
  rupture of, 864–866, *865*
  strain of, 864–866
  testing of, 166t
Pectoralis major tendon transfer, in long thoracic nerve palsy, 768, *769*
Pectoralis minor muscle, absence of, 57
  anatomy of, 57, *57*
    comparative, 5
  blood supply of, 57
  embryology of, 130
  function of, 57
  innervation of, 57
  insertion of, 57, *57*, 131–132, *131*
  origin of, 57, *57*
  scapular attachment of, *45*, 46, 335, *335*
  testing of, 166t
Pectoralis minor tendon transfer, in long thoracic nerve palsy, 768
Pectoralis reflex, testing of, 167
Pediatric patients. See *Children*; *Congenital anomalies*; *Infants.*
Pelvic reconstruction plate, in glenohumeral joint arthrodesis, 707, *710*
Pelvis, abnormal, in cleidocranial dysostosis, 100
Penicillins, in bone/joint infections, 934t, 1081
Pennate muscle, 49, *49*
Pepsinum purissimum, in torticollis, 1065
Percutaneous pins, in humeral fracture, 296, 310, *310*, 997, *999*
Periarthritis humeroscapularis. See *Impingement syndrome.*
Periarthritis scapulo humerale. See *Frozen shoulder.*
Perineurium, structure of, 66, *67*
Periosteal chondroma, 882, *895*
Periosteal osteosarcoma, 880
Periosteum, tendon insertion in, 51, *52*
Peritendinitis calcarea. See *Calcifying tendinitis.*
Personality, periarthritis, in frozen shoulder, 845
Perthes, G., on glenohumeral instability, 529–530, *529*, 577
Perthes lesion, 1002, *1003*
Petrie procedure, in Sprengel's deformity, 108
Pettersson, G., on impingement syndrome, 623–624
Phantom pain, after amputation, 959–960
Phemister, D. B., limb salvage surgery of, 874–875
Phocomelia, 118–120, *119–121*
  amputation in, 941
Phrenic nerve block, in regional anesthesia, 252, *254*
Phrenic nerve paralysis, in brachial plexus injury of newborn, 1037
Physeal region. See *Epiphysis.*
Physical examination, 153–174
  Adson's maneuver in, 173, *173*
  anesthetic injection techniques in, *172*, 174
  apprehension tests in, 169–170, *170–171*
  attitude of shoulder in, 155
  benefits of, 154
  biceps evaluation in, 171, *173*
  cervical spine evaluation in, 174–176, *176*
  compression test in, 175, *176*
  deformity in, *153*, 156, *156*
  dynamic factors in, 154–155
  format for, 154, 154t

Physical examination *(Continued)*
  general condition assessment in, 173–174
  glenohumeral translation test in, 167–169, *168–169*
  gown for, 155, *155*
  Halstead's test in, 173
  history and, 149–153, *151, 153*
  hyperabduction syndrome test in, 173
  impingement tests in, 170–172, *172*
  in arthritis, 701–702
  in biceps lesions, 812–815, *812–815*, 821
  in frozen shoulder, 845–846
  in glenohumeral instability, 544–551, *546, 548–551*
  in neurological disorders, 751, 757–758
  initial impression in, 154–155, *155*
  inspection in, 155–157, *156–157*, 175
  joint motion assessment in, 159–164
    abduction in, 164, *172*
    external rotation in, 162, *163*
    internal rotation in, 162, 164, *164*
    measurement of, 160, 160t–161t
    movement quality in, 159, *160*
    position for, 159–160
    recording of, 160, 160t–161t
    total elevation in, 160, *162*
  muscle features in, 155–156, *156*
  muscle testing in, 164–166, 164t–166t, *165*
  neurological, 165–167, 166t, 175
  palpation in, 157–159, *158–159*, 175
  provocative elevation testing in, 173
  range of motion assessment in, 159–164, 160t–161t, *162–164, 172*
  reflex testing in, 166–167
  sensory testing in, 166
  skin inspection in, 157
  Spurling's test in, 175, *176*
  stability assessment in, 167–170, *168–173*
  static factors in, 154
  strength testing in, 164–165, 164t–165t, *165*
  swelling in, 156, *157*
  symptomatic translation in, 169–170
  vascular examination in, 173, *173*
Physiotherapy. See also *Exercise.*
  in frozen shoulder, 854, 859
Pigmented villonodular synovitis, 884
Pins, in acromioclavicular joint repairs, 439, *439–440*, 457
  in clavicular fracture fixation, 396, 402–403, *403*, 408, *408*
  migration of, 464–465, *467*, 519, 521
  percutaneous, in humeral fracture, 296, 310, *310*, 997, *999*
Pitching. See *Throwing.*
Plagiocephaly, in torticollis, 1062, 1065, *1066*
"Plane type" of joint, acromioclavicular joint as, 210, *210*
Plasmacytoma, 887, 898
Plate fixation. See also *Compression plate.*
  in glenohumeral joint arthrodesis, 707, *710–711*
Pleural lesions, versus neurological disorders, 753, *754*
Pneumococcus, in bone/joint infections, 1076
Pneumothorax, in clavicular fracture, *381*, 382
  in humeral fracture, 285
  in regional anesthesia, 252, *254*
"Poise of the shoulder," ligament function in, 479, *480*
Poland's syndrome, 129–130, *129–130*
Poliomyelitis, muscle studies in, 750
Portals, for arthroscopy. See under *Arthroscopy.*
Position, for arthroscopy, 265–266, *265–266*
  for surgery, 248
Post technique, in prosthetic arthroplasty, 722, *723*
Postganglionic fibers, in brachial plexus, 72
Postmenopausal arthritis, of sternoclavicular joint, 488–489, *489*, 504, *507*
Postoperative care, anesthetic complications and, 255
Post-traumatic arthritis. See *Traumatic arthritis.*
Posture, after amputation, 956, 959
Preacromion, anatomy of, 45, *45, 112, 343*
  impingement syndrome and, 625
Prednisolone, in frozen shoulder, 854

Preganglionic fibers, in brachial plexus, 72
Premedication, with anesthesia, 247–248
Procaine, in frozen shoulder, 856
Profunda artery, anatomy of, *79*
  collateral circulation of, *81–82*
  in triceps, 65
Prosthesis, in amputation. See under *Amputation.*
Prosthetic arthroplasty, acrylic prosthesis in, 679, *680*
  after limb sparing surgery, 908, *909–910*, 910–911
  anatomical (unconstrained) systems in, 680, *686*, 686t, *716*, 717–718, 718t
    failure of, 742–744, 743t
  ball-in-socket (constrained) system in, 680, *682–683*, 686, 686t
    complications of, 742
    failure of, 744
  Bickel prosthesis in, 680, *681*
  biomechanics of, 224
  bipolar prosthesis in, 713, *714*, 737, 737t, 739t, 741t
  bone cement problems in, 255
  bone graft in, glenoid, 718, *720*
    humeral, 721, *721*
  bone ingrowth system in, 718, *719*
  Cofield prosthesis in, 713, 722, 731, *732*
  complications of, 740–742, 740t–741t
  component loosening in, 743–744, 743t
  composite reconstruction in, *909–910*, 910
  constrained (ball-in-socket) system in, 680, *682–683*, 686, 686t
    complications of, 742
    failure of, 744
  cup, 713–714, *714*, 737, 737t
    complications of, 741t
  DANA prosthesis in. See *DANA shoulder prosthesis.*
  draping method for, 723, *723*
  English-Macnab prosthesis in, 715, *716*, 739t, 740, 742
  exercise after, 736
  failure of, 742–745, 743t
  Fenlin prosthesis in, 680, *682*
  floating socket prosthesis in, 680, *684*
  fracture in, 743–744, 743t
  glenohumeral instability in, 744
  glenoid component placement in, 729, *729–735*, 731–734
  glenoid condition in, 727, 729, *729*
  glenoid loosening in, 715, *716*
  hemiarthroplasty, 712–714, *713–714*, 736–738, 737t
    after limb sparing surgery, *909–910*, 910
    complications of, 740, 740t
  historical review of, 678–680, *678–686*, 679, 686t
  hooded component (semiconstrained) systems in, 680, *686*, 686t, 715–717, *716–717*, 742
  humeral canal preparation in, 727, *728*
  humeral component placement in, 735
  humeral head prosthesis in, 303, 305, *305*, 312, *315–317*, 316
    failure of, *327–328*, 328
  humeral osteotomy in, 726, *727*
  in osteoarthritis, 736–737, 737t
  in osteonecrosis, 736–737, 737t
  in rheumatoid arthritis, 736–737, 737t
  in rotator cuff arthropathy, 660
  in rotator cuff repair failure, 673
  in scapulectomy, 911
  in traumatic arthritis, 736, 737t
  indications for, 686–687, 686t–687t
  infection in, 743, 743t, 925
    bacterial adhesion in, 927–928, *927–928*
    resection arthroplasty and, 704, *705*
    symptoms of, 929–930
    treatment of, 936–937
  isoelastic prosthesis in, 714, 737, 737t, 741t
  Kessel prosthesis in, 680, *683*, 739t, 740, 742
  Kölbel prosthesis in, 680, *683*
  Liverpool prosthesis in, 680, *682*, 739t, 740, 742
  Mazas prosthesis in, 680, *685*, 715
  mechanical failure in, 744

Prosthetic arthroplasty (Continued)
  Michael Reese prosthesis in, 715, 715, 722, 723, 739t, 740, 742
  modular system in, 714
  monospherical prosthesis in, 713, 717–718, 717, 739t, 741
  Neer prosthesis in. See Neer prosthesis.
  nerve injury in, 743
  nonretentive prosthesis in, 680, 685, 715, 739t
  operative approaches in, Amstutz technique, 722
    Cofield technique, 722–735, 723–735
    Neer technique, 718, 720–721, 721
    Post technique, 722, 723
  prosthetic design criteria in, 679, 680
  rehabilitation after, 735–736
  revision of, 742–745, 743t
  rotator cuff tears in, 743–744, 743t
  St. Georg prosthesis in, 680, 680, 715, 716, 739t, 741–742
  semiconstrained (hooded component) systems in, 680, 686, 686t,
    715–717, 716–717, 742
  soft-tissue repair in, 721
  Stanmore prosthesis (metal-on-metal) in, 714–715, 715, 739t,
    740, 742
  Swanson prosthesis in, 713, 714, 737, 737t
  total, complications of, 741–742, 741t
    infection in, 929–930
    operative approaches for, 718, 720–721, 721–735, 723–735
    radiography of, 738–739, 739t
    results of, 738–740, 738t–739t
    systems for, 678–680, 678–686, 679t, 686t, 714–718, 715–717,
      718t, 719
  trispherical prosthesis in, 680, 684, 715, 739t, 740
  unconstrained (anatomical) systems in, 680, 686, 686t, 716, 717–
    718, 718t
    failure of, 742–744, 743t
  Zippel prosthesis in, 680, 681
Prosthetic graft, in rotator cuff tears, 663–664
Proteoglycan, in articular cartilage, 923
Protrusion, at sternoclavicular joint, 210
Provocative elevation testing, 173
Pseudarthrosis, after glenohumeral arthrodesis, 711t
  of clavicle, 386
    congenital, 101–103, 102
    versus fracture, 1011, 1012
Pseudocyst formation, in pectoralis major muscle rupture, 866
Pseudomalignant myositis ossificans, 880
Pseudomonas aeruginosa, antibiotic susceptibility of, 934t
  in bone/joint infection, 920, 929
Psoriatic arthritis, versus frozen shoulder, 852
Psychogalvanic response, in neurological testing, 758
Psychologic factors, in frozen shoulder, 845
  in occupational cervicobrachial disorder, 1090
Pulmonary artery, pin migration into, 519
Pulmonary function, anesthesia and, 247
  clavicular role in, 372
  frozen shoulder and, 845
  monitoring of, during anesthesia, 248
Pulses, evaluation of, 173, 173
Push-pull test, in glenohumeral instability, 551, 551
Putti procedure, in Sprengel's deformity, 108
Putti-Platt procedure, 578–579
  complications of, 585–587
  reverse, 598

Q

Quadrangular/quadrilateral space, anatomy of, 70–71, 71, 533
Quadrilateral space syndrome, 987

R

Radial, in fish fin, 1–2, 2
Radial head fracture, with triceps rupture, 868

Radial nerve, anatomy of, 68, 71
  anomalous, 74
  in triceps innervation, 65
Radiculopathy, cervical, clinical presentation of, 751
    versus impingement syndrome, 632
Radiography. See also X-ray evaluation.
  biomechanics and, 222, 223
Radionuclide scan. See also Bone scan.
  in frozen shoulder, 849–850
Radiotherapy, bone graft effects of, 911
  complications of, 699, 700
  in calcifying tendinitis, 786
  in Ewing's sarcoma, 913, 915
  in frozen shoulder, 858
  in soft tissue sarcoma, 913
Range of motion, assessment of, 159–164, 160t–161t, 162–164,
    172, 175
  in frozen shoulder, 846
  joint function in, 39
Recumbency, long thoracic nerve palsy in, 768
Reduction, of fractures. See specific bone.
Reeves classification, of frozen shoulder, 842, 843t
Reflex sympathetic dystrophy, 771
  versus frozen shoulder, 853
Reflexes, testing of, 166–167
Refracture, of clavicle, 387
Regional anesthesia. See under Anesthesia.
Rehabilitation. See specific disorder; Exercise.
Relaxed skin tension lines, 91–92, 92
Relocation test, in instability, 964–965, 964–965
Renaissance, anatomical studies during, 35–36, 36–37
Renal osteodystrophy, 900t, 901
Repetitive stress injury. See Occupational cervicobrachial disorder.
Replacement arthroplasty. See Prosthetic arthroplasty.
Resection arthroplasty, in glenohumeral arthritis, 704–705, 705
Reticuloendothelial tumors, 885, 887
Retraction, at sternoclavicular joint, 210
Revision, of prosthetic arthroplasty, 742–745, 743t
Rhabdomyosarcoma, 892
Rheumatoid arthritis, anesthesia and, 247
  arthroscopy in, 264
  complications of, 691
  dry form of, 689, 689
  multiple joint involvement in, 702–703
  of acromioclavicular joint, 467–468
  of glenohumeral joint, pathoanatomy of, 688–689, 689–694,
    690t
    prosthetic arthroplasty in, 736–738, 737t–738t
  of sternoclavicular joint, 488, 488, 504
  resorptive form of, 690, 690
  septic arthritis in, 930
  serratus anterior muscle rupture in, 871
  synovectomy in, 703–704, 704
  versus frozen shoulder, 852
  wet form of, 689–690, 690
Rhomboid ligament. See Costoclavicular ligament.
Rhomboid major/minor muscles, absence of, 130–131
  anatomy of, 55, 55
    comparative, 5
  scapular attachment of, 45, 46, 335, 336–337
  testing of, 166t
Rhomboid tendon transfer, in spinal accessory nerve palsy, 760
Rib(s), abnormalities of, in Sprengel's deformity, 105–106, 105t
  cervical, resection of, in thoracic outlet syndrome, 137
  connection of, to coracoid process, 115–116
    to vertebra, 116, 117
  exostosis of, in snapping scapula, 362
  fracture of, versus frozen shoulder, 852
    with clavicular fracture, 381–382, 381
  resection of, in thoracic outlet syndrome, 143, 770
Rigid body spring concept, in biomechanics, 242
"Rim rent," in rotator cuff, 651–652, 651–652
Robinson procedure, in Sprengel's deformity, 108

Rockwood classification, of clavicular/acromioclavicular region, 1020, *1021–1023*
Rockwood method, in acromioclavicular joint repair, 451–455, *453–457*
  in glenohumeral instability, anterior, 573, *573*
    atraumatic, 608–609, *610–612*, 612
    closed reduction, 573, *573*
    multidirectional, 608–609, *610–612*, 612
    posterior reconstruction, 601, *602–604*, 605
    traumatic, 592, *593–595*, 596–597, *610–611*
  in glenohumeral joint drainage, 1082, *1083*
Rodrigues, on sternoclavicular joint injury, 477
Rolling motion of joint, 216, *216*
Roos procedure, in thoracic outlet syndrome treatment, 137, 143
Roos test, in thoracic outlet syndrome, 137
Rotation, assessment of, 162, *163–164*, 164
  biceps tendon motion in, 805, 807
  in arthrogryposis, 1072–1074, *1072–1073*
  in frozen shoulder, 841–842, 842t
  in swimming strokes, 988
  instantaneous center of, 215–216, *216*
    of humeral head, 222
    of scapula, 222, *223*
  maximum torque in, 242, *243*
  muscles of, testing of, 164
  of acromioclavicular joint, 211–212
  of clavicle, 212, *213*, 371–372
  of glenohumeral joint, 216–218, *217*
  of humerus, external, 220, *221–222*, 222
  of scapula, clavicular role in, 372
    in arm elevation, 220, *221*
  of sternoclavicular joint, 210
  synchronous scapuloclavicular, 415, *456*
  terminology of, 214
Rotator cuff. See also specific muscles: *Infraspinatus*; *Subscapularis*; *Supraspinatus*; *Teres minor.*
  acromion shape and, 45, *45*
  anatomy of, 17, *17*, 279, 280, 533, 647–648, *649*, 650
    impingement syndrome and, 624–625, *625*
  arthroscopy of, 262
  blood supply of, 28, *28–29*, 281, 625, 647–648
  bursitis of, versus rotator cuff tears, 661
  calcifying tendinitis of. See *Calcifying tendinitis.*
  "critical zone" of, 625, 648, 774–775, *775*
  freeze-dried, in tear repair, 663
  function of, 625, 648, *649*, 650
    in humeral head depression, *649*, 654
    stabilizing, 231
  hypovascular zone of, 28, *29*, 625, 648, 774–775, *775*
  impingement on. See *Impingement syndrome.*
  lesions of, acromioclavicular joint cyst with, 468
    exercise in, 967, *967–970*, 969
    glenoid loosening in, 243, *243*
    humeral head translation in, 224, *225*
    in aging, 776, 778–779
    in athlete, 967, *967–970*, 969
    in rheumatoid arthritis, 690–691, *692–693*, 690t
    rehabilitation program for, 967, *967–970*, 969
  resection of, in bone tumor, 906
  strengthening exercise for, 967, *970*, 1007, *1008*
  stretching exercise for, 967, *967–969*
  supraspinatus insertion in, histology of, 648
  tears of. See *Rotator cuff tears.*
  tendinitis of. See also *Calcifying tendinitis.*
    occupational, 1093–1095
    versus rotator cuff tears, 661
  tendons of, anatomy of, 647–648, 774–775, *775*
    blood supply of, 774–775, *775*
    fiber interdigitation in, 648
    strain of, versus impingement syndrome, 632
    strength of, 651
  tensile strength of, versus age, 228, *228*
  ultrasonography of, 629

Rotator cuff *(Continued)*
  weakness of, impingement syndrome and, 627, *628*
  x-ray evaluation of, 196, *197–199*, 199–200
Rotator cuff tears, acromial abnormalities in, 651
  acromioclavicular joint osteophytes in, 651
  acute, definition of, 650
    treatment of, 657, 665
  acute extension of, definition of, 650
  age and, 650–654
  anatomical considerations in, 647–648, *649*, 650
  arthrography in, 658–659, *658–659*, 666
  arthropathy in, 654, *655*, 660, *660*, 672–673
  arthropneumotomography in, 659
  arthroscopy in, 269, *269*
  arthrotomography in, 659
  biceps tendon changes in, 654, *655*
  biceps tendon lesions with, 820–821
  biceps tendon motion in, 807–808
  bipartate acromion with, 112–113, *112–113*
  bursography of, 659
  chronic, definition of, 650
  classification of, 650
  clinical presentation of, 654–656
  complications of, 660–661, *660–661*
  computed tomography of, 659–660
  "creeping tendon ruptures" in, 653
  "cuff tendinitis" and, 653
  cyst formation in, 656, *656*
  degenerative change and, 652–653
  differential diagnosis of, 661–662
  electromyography in, 807–808
  end stage of, 654
  full-thickness, clinical manifestations of, 655
    definition of, 650
    incidence of, 650
    mechanism of, 652
    treatment of, 663
  "geyser sign" in, 659, *659*
  glenohumeral instability in, 527
  healing impairment in, 654
  historical review of, 647
  history in, 654–656
  humeral head displacement in, 656, *657*
  imaging evaluation in, 629, *630–631*, 656–660, *656–659*, 666
  in acromial fracture, 354, *360*
  in glenohumeral dislocation, 564
  in impingement syndrome, 263–264, *263*, 828–829, *829*
  in osteoarthritis, 688, 689t
  in prosthetic arthroplasty, 741, 741t
    revision in, 743–744, 743t
  in rheumatoid arthritis, 691, *692–693*, 702
  in throwing, 651–652, *651–652*
  incidence of, 650–651
  injuries associated with, 654, *655*
  irreparable, 660–661, *661*
  magnetic resonance imaging in, 200, 659–660
  massive, 656, *657*, 660–661, *661*
    treatment of, 663–664, 671
  mechanism of, 651–654, *651–652*
  Milwaukee shoulder and, 696–697
  occupational, 1093–1095
  partial-thickness, arthrography of, 659, *659*
    clinical manifestations of, 655
    definition of, 650
    incidence of, 650
    mechanism of, 652
    treatment of, 663
  patient evaluation in, 665–666
  physical findings in, 656
  position of, 650
  progression/propagation of, 653, 660, *660*
  "rim rent" in, 651–652, *651–652*
  size of, versus treatment results, 664
  small, imaging of, 656, *656*

Rotator cuff tears *(Continued)*
  treatment of, 662–672
    anterior acromioplasty approach in, 663
    biologic grafts in, 663
    decompression and debridement in, 665
    exercise in, 664, 666
    goals of, 662
    nonoperative, 662, 666
    nonsteroidal anti-inflammatory drugs in, 666
    operative, 662–664
      approaches for, 663–664
      failure of, 665, 672–673
      indications for, 662–663, 667
      management after, 671–672
      results of, 664–665, 672
      technique for, 667, *668–670*, 671
    patient evaluation in, 665–666
    prosthetic materials in, 663–664
    rest in, 666
    return to activity after, 666–667
    subscapularis transfer in, 663, 671
    tendon advancement in, 663
    tendon-to-tendon repair in, 663
    theoretical aspects of, 665
  ultrasonography of, 199–200, 656–658, *657–658*, 666
  versus impingement syndrome, 632
Rotator interval, anatomy of, 533
  definition of, 27
Rouleaux's method, in joint motion description, 215, *216*
Round cell lesions, of humerus, *895*
Rupture, of musculotendinous unit. See under *Muscle(s)*, and specific structure, e.g., *Biceps tendon.*
Rush rod technique, in proximal humeral fracture, 297, *302*

S

Saha procedure, in glenohumeral instability, 584
St. Georg shoulder prosthesis, 680, *680*, 715, *716*
  complications of, 741–742
  results of, 739t
Salmonella, antibiotic susceptibility of, 934t
Salter-Harris fracture classification, clavicular, 1016–1017, *1016*
  humeral, 992
Sandifer's syndrome, versus infantile torticollis, 1063–1064
Sarcoma, age distribution of, 892, *894*
  anatomical considerations in, 875, *876*, 877
  biopsy of, 892, 901–903, *902*, 913–914
  chondrosarcoma, 882, *883*, 884, 912
  clinical presentation of, 895–896
  epithelioid, 892
  Ewing's. See *Ewing's sarcoma.*
  historical review of, 874–875
  limb salvage surgery in, 905–906, *907*, 908
  liposarcoma, 892, *894*, 895
  neurosarcoma, 875
  osteosarcoma, 880, *881*, 912–913
    location of, 875
  Pagetoid, *890*, 891
  soft tissue, 892, 892t, *893*, 913, 915
    clinical presentation of, 892t, 895
    incidence of, 892
    treatment of, 915
  staging of, 877–879, 877t–878t
  surgical margins of, 903, *904*, 905, 905t
  symptoms of, 892t
  synovial, 892
    age distribution of, *894*
  treatment of, 912–915
  versus carcinoma, 877
Sayre bandage, in clavicular fracture, 393, *393*
Scalene block, 250–255, 250t, *251–254*, 252t
  in arthroscopy, 265

Scalene triangle, anatomy of, 65, *65*
Scalenectomy, anterior, in dorsal scapular nerve compression, 134
Scaleneotomy, anterior, in thoracic outlet syndrome, 137
Scalenus anterior muscle, anatomy of, 65, *65*
Scalenus medius muscle, anatomy of, 65, *65*
  dorsal scapular nerve compression by, 134
Scalenus minimus muscle, dorsal scapular nerve compression by, 134
Scapula, abnormality of, in cleidocranial dysostosis, 100
  in impingement syndrome, 627t
  absence of, 118–120
  acromial process of. See *Acromion.*
  anatomy of, 43–46, *44–46*, 335–336, *335–338*
    comparative, 2, *3–4*, 4, 797, *798*
    cross-sectional, *44*
    developmental, 11–12, *11*, 1025, *1025*
  center of rotation of, 222, *223*
  clasp-like margin of, 111, *111*
  congenital fossa of, 128, *128*
  coracoclavicular bar on. See *Coracoclavicular bar.*
  coracocostosternale vestibiale bone of, 116
  coracoid process of. See *Coracoid process.*
  costocoracoid band on, 115–116
  dislocation of, 361
    anterior, 424. See also *Acromioclavicular joint, injury of, type IV.*
    in children, 1028
  dissection of, 364
  dysplasia of, versus scapular fracture, 342–343, *344*
  elevation of, in Sprengel's deformity, 103–109, *104–107*, 105t, *109–110*
    muscular action in, 50–51, *51*
  embryology of, 8,, 106–107, *107*, 114
  epiphyseal lines of, 340, *341–342*
  foramina of, versus scapular fracture, 343
  forward fixation of (costocoracoid band), 115–116
  fracture of. See *Scapular fracture.*
  function of, 335–336
  glenoid region of. See *Glenoid.*
  injury of, etiology of, 335
  ligaments of, anatomy of, 43, 45, *45*
  motion of, 218, *218*, 839
    versus frozen shoulder, 852
  multiple myeloma in, 887, *888*
  muscle attachments of, 335–336, *335–337*
  notched edge of, 43, 117, *118*, 336
  ossification of, 11–12, *11*, 340, *341–342*, 1025, *1025*
    accessory center in, 116–117
  osteochondroma of, crepitus in, 362, *363–364*
    neurological disorders in, *753*
  osteoid osteoma of, 879
  osteomyelitis of, 924, 926, *929*
  palpation of, 159
  prosthetic replacement of, 911
  pseudowinging of, in snapping scapula, 362–363
  ptosis of, in thoracic outlet syndrome, 769–770, *769*
  regional anesthesia for, 249
  resection of, *907*, 908, 940, 949, *950*. See also *Scapulectomy.*
    reconstruction after, 911
  resting posture of, 218, *218*
  rotation of, clavicular role in, 372
    in Holt-Oram syndrome, 109–111
  snapping, 362–364, *363–364*
    in deltoid electrical stimulation, *750*
    in serratus anterior paralysis, *750*
    versus impingement syndrome, 632–633
    versus rotator cuff tears, 661
  sounds of, 362
  spine of, anatomy of, 44
  suspension of, in spinal accessory nerve palsy, 760–761, *761*
  swallow tail malformation of, 117, *118*
  tumors of, 895
  violent displacement of, 361–362, *362*

Scapula *(Continued)*
  winging of, contractural (Putti sign), 1039, 1041, *1041*
    evaluation of, 156, *156*
    in deltoid muscle contracture, 127–128
    in serratus anterior muscle rupture, 871
    in snapping scapula, 362
Scapular artery, circumflex, anatomy of, 30
  dorsal, anatomy of, 78–79
    collateral circulation of, *81*
    in levator scapulae, 56
    in trapezius, 55
Scapular compartment, posterior, anatomy of, 875
Scapular fracture, acromial, 354–356, *355–357*, 361
  acromioclavicular separation in, 358–359, *358*
  anatomical considerations in, 1025, *1025–1026*
  avulsion, 359
  body, 353–354, *354–355*, 360
  causes of, 353
  classification of, 336, 338, *348*, 1025
  clinical presentation of, 338
  comminuted, *347*, 353, *354*
  complications of, 338–339
  coracoid, 339, *341*, 357–359, *358–359*, 361
  differential diagnosis of, 339–343, *339–344*
  etiology of, 335
  extra-articular (glenoid neck), 343–345, *344–346*, 360
  fatigue, 357–358, *359*
  glenoid (intra-articular), 345–353, *347–353*, 360–361
  glenoid neck (extra-articular), 343–345, *344–346*, 360
  in children, 1025, *1025–1027*, 1028
  incidence of, 335
  injuries associated with, 335, 338–339
  mechanism of, *1026*, 1028
  nonunion of, 356, *356–357*
  snapping scapula in, 363
  stable, 345, *346*
  treatment of, 1028
    acromial, 354–356, *355–357*, 361
    body, 360
    coracoid, 361
    glenoid (intra-articular), 345–353, *347–353*, 360–361
    glenoid neck (extra-articular), 343–345, *344–346*, 360
    in body fracture, 354
    results of, 359–360
  type I (anterior avulsion), 345, 349–350, *349*
  type II (transverse/oblique), 350, *350–351*
  type III (oblique through glenoid), 350, *351–352*
  type IV (horizontal glenoid), 350
  type V (combination), 350, *352–353*, 353
  unstable, 345, *346*
  x-ray evaluation of, 200, *200*, 339–340, *339–341*
Scapular ligament, transverse, anatomy of, 43
  congenital ossification of, 111
Scapular nerve, dorsal, anatomy of, *68–69*, 69
  compression of, congenital, 133–134, *133–134*
  in levator scapulae innervation, 56
  in rhomboids, 55
Scapular outlet view, in x-ray evaluation, 196, *198*, 199
Scapular plane views, in x-ray evaluation, 552–556, *552–559*
Scapular reflex, testing of, 167
Scapular sign of Putti, 1039, 1041, *1041*
Scapulectomy, 941, 949, 951, *951*. See also *Scapula, resection of.*
  reconstruction after, 911
Scapuloclavicular injury. See *Acromioclavicular joint, injury of.*
Scapuloclavicular rotation, synchronous, 415, *456*
Scapulohumeral ligaments, anatomy of, 533–534, *533–534*
Scapulohumeral muscles. See also specific muscle.
  anatomy of, 54–57, *54–58*
    comparative, 5, *5*
Scapulohumeral resection, *907*, 908
Scapulolateral view, in x-ray evaluation, 181–183, *181–183*
    Alexander modification of, 193, *194*
    of acromioclavicular joint, 427, *429*
    of glenohumeral instability, 554–555, *555–556*

Scapulolateral view *(Continued)*
    of humeral fracture, 287–288, *287*
Scapulopexy, in spinal accessory nerve palsy, 760–761, *761*
Scapulothoracic crepitus. See *Snapping scapula.*
Scapulothoracic dissociation, 361–362, *362*
Scapulothoracic fusion, in spinal accessory nerve palsy, 761
Scapulothoracic joint, biomechanics of, 213–216, *214–216*
  motion of, 219–220, *220–221*
Scapulothoracic rhythm, 219–220, *220–221*
Scarring, in rotator cuff tear repair, 672
Schwann cells, 66
Sclerosis, subacromial, 629, *629*
Scoliosis, after amputation, 956
  in Sprengel's deformity, 105–106, 105t
Screw displacement axis, 216–218, *217*, 222, *223*
Screw fixation, in acromioclavicular joint repair, 440–443, *441*, 452, *453–457*, 454
    removal of, 455, *457*
  in clavicular fracture, 396
  in glenohumeral joint arthrodesis, 707, *707–708*
  in glenohumeral stabilization, 570–581, *582–583*, 586
Sedation, in regional anesthesia, 249–250
Seddon classification, of nerve injury, 755–757
Seizure, glenohumeral instability in, 544, *545*
  humeral fracture in, 285
Sensory testing, 166, 757–758
Sepsis. See *Infection; Osteomyelitis; Septic arthritis.*
Septic arthritis, after total joint replacement, 929–930, 936–937
  anaerobic, 931
  anatomical considerations in, 921–923, *922*, *924*
  antibiotics in, 933–934, 934t, 936, 1081–1082
  arthrography in, 931
  arthroscopic debridement in, 264
  arthrotomy in, 933
  cell biology of, 922–923, *924*
  classification of, 923–924, 923t
  clinical presentation of, 929–930
  complications of, 932, *933*, 1082
  computed tomography in, 931
  debridement in, 936
  diagnosis of, in children, 1081
  differential diagnosis of, 930
  gonococcal, 934
    in children, 1081
  historical review of, 920–921
  immobilization in, 934
  in children, 934, 1080–1083, *1083*
  in drug addicts, 929, 933–934
  in rheumatoid arthritis, 930
  incidence of, 926, 926t
    in children, 1080–1081
  laboratory evaluation of, 930–931, 931t
  microanatomy of, 922–923, *924*
  microbial adhesion in, 926–928, *927–928*
  monoarticular, 930
  needle aspiration in, 933, 1082
  of acromioclavicular joint, 468, 925, 1083
  of glenohumeral joint, 925
    in children, 1080–1082, *1083*
    symptoms of, 929
    versus degenerative arthritis, 700
  of sternoclavicular joint, 489, *490*, 925–926, 1083
    symptoms of, 929
    treatment of, 504, 507, 517
  organisms causing, in children, 1081
  passive range of motion in, 934
  pathogenesis of, 920, 923–926, *925*
  pathogens in, 928–929
  polymicrobial (mixed), 929
  predisposing factors in, 933
  prophylaxis of, 936
  resection arthroplasty in, 704–705, *705*
  routes of infection in, 920–921, *922*
  susceptibility to, 920

Septic arthritis *(Continued)*
  synovial fluid analysis in, 930–931, 931t
  treatment of, 932–934, 934t, 936–937
    in children, 1081–1082, *1083*
  ultrasonography in, 931
  versus frozen shoulder, 852
  x-ray evaluation in, 931, *931–932*
Serendipity view, in x-ray evaluation, 194–195, *195*
  of clavicular fracture, 1017, *1018*
  of sternoclavicular joint disorders, 492–493, *493–494*
Serratus anterior muscle, anatomy of, 56–57, *56*
  comparative, 5
  blood supply of, 57
  function of, 56–57
    in elevation, 239
  innervation of, 57
  insertion of, 56, *56*
  origin of, 56
  paralysis of, in long thoracic nerve palsy, 768
    snapping scapula in, *750*
  rupture of, 871
  scapular attachment of, *45*, 46, 335, *335–336*
  testing of, 166t
Sever brace, in brachial plexus injury of newborn, 1046–1047, *1047*
Sever procedure, in brachial plexus injury of newborn, 1048
Shoulder forward view (Alexander view), in x-ray evaluation, 193, *194*, 427, *429*
Shoulder girdle. See *Muscle(s)*.
Shoulder spica cast, in humeral fracture, 296
Shoulder-hand syndrome, 838
  versus frozen shoulder, 853
Shrock procedure, in Sprengel's deformity, 108
Simple bone cyst, 884–885, *884*, *895*, 992
Sitting position, for surgery, 248
Skeletal traction, in humeral fracture, 296
Skin, anatomy of, 89–92, *90–92*
  circulation of, 89, *90*, 91
  innervation of, 91–92
  inspection of, 157
  relaxed tension lines in, *91–92*, 92
  sensation in, 91–92, 166
Skull, deformities of, in cleidocranial dysostosis, 99, *99*
Sliding motion of joint, 215, *216*
Sling, in acromioclavicular joint injury, 435, *435*, 437–438, *437*, 437t, 447–449, *450–451*
  in clavicular fracture, 392–393, *393*
Snapping scapula, 362–364, *363–364*
  in deltoid electrical stimulation, *750*
  in serratus anterior paralysis, *750*
  versus impingement syndrome, 632–633
  versus rotator cuff tears, 661
Social Security Administration, impairment evaluation guidelines of, 1104
Society of American Shoulder and Elbow Surgeons, joint motion measurement guidelines of, 160, 161t
Soft tissue release, in brachial plexus injury of newborn, 1047–1048
"Sourcil" sign, in impingement syndrome, 629, *629*
Spasticity, in brachial plexus injury of newborn, 1038
Speed test, 171, 813, *813*
Spinal accessory nerve, anatomy of, 74–76, *76*, 759
    in sternocleidomastoid muscle, *1057*, 1058
  in levator scapulae innervation, 56
  in sternocleidomastoid innervation, 65
  in trapezius innervation, 55
  palsy of, 759–761, *760–761*
Spinal block, in regional anesthesia, 253
Spinal nerves, dorsal rami of, anatomy of, *90*, 91
Spine, abnormal, in cleidocranial dysostosis, 100
  cervical. See *Cervical spine*.
  dysraphism of, in Sprengel's deformity, 105–106, 105t
Spinning motion of joint, 216, *216*
Spinoglenoid notch, of scapula, anatomy of, 43
Splinting, elbow deformity from, 1041–1042, *1042–1043*
  in brachial plexus injury of newborn, 1046–1047, *1047–1048*

Splinting *(Continued)*
  in humeral fracture, 296
Spondylosis, cervical, versus rotator cuff tears, 661
Sports medicine. See also *Throwing*.
  acromioclavicular joint problems in, 986–987
  activity modification in, in impingement syndrome, 638
  glenohumeral instability in, 963–983
    arthroscopy in, 976
    Bristow operation in, 972, *973–976*, 976
    capsulolabral reconstruction in, 977–978, *977–982*, 981–982
    classification of, 965–967, *966*
    posterior, 983–986, *984–986*
    rehabilitation program for, 971
    relocation test in, 964–965, *964–965*
  glenoid spurs in, 986
  historical review of, 961
  impingement syndrome in, 627, 638, 963–967, *966*
  in swimming, 988–989
  neurologic problems in, 987
  rotator cuff problems in, rehabilitation program for, 967, *967–970*, 969
  stress fracture in, 992, *993*
  treatment goals in, 961
  vascular problems in, 987–988
Sprain, of acromioclavicular joint, 420–421
  of sternoclavicular joint, 486, 491, 495, 507
Spray and stretch program, in frozen shoulder, 856
Sprengel's deformity, 103–109
  anomalies associated with, 105–106, 105t, *106*
  clinical findings in, 104, *104–105*
  conservative treatment of, 107
  grading system for, 107
  inheritance of, 104–105
  pathology of, 106–107, *107*
  snapping scapula in, 363
  surgery for, indications for, 107–108
    procedures for, 108–109, *110*
  Woodward procedure in, 108–109, *110*
Spurling's test, in cervical spine examination, 175, *176*
  in thoracic outlet syndrome, 137
Stability. See also *Biomechanics, constraints and*; *Instability*; specific joint.
  central concept of, 232
  clinical relevance of, 232, 234
  testing for. See under *Glenohumeral joint*.
Staging, of tumors, 877–879, 877t–878t
Stanmore shoulder prosthesis, 714–715, *715*
  complications of, 742
  results of, 739t, 740
Staphylococcus, in bone/joint infections, in children, 1081
  in neonates, 1080, *1080*
Staphylococcus aureus, 920
  antibiotic susceptibility of, 934t
  collagenase production by, 925
  in bone/joint infections, 929
  surface adhesion of, 924–925
Staphylococcus epidermidis, in bone/joint infections, 929, 1074
  pathogenic transformation of, 920
  surface adhesion of, 924–925
Staple capsulorrhaphy, in glenohumeral instability, 577–578, *578*, 585–586
Staples, migration of, 586
Statue of Liberty (Fairbank) splint, elbow deformity from, 1041–1042, *1042–1043*
  in brachial plexus injury of newborn, 1046–1047, *1047–1048*
Steel maneuver, in closed reduction, 1005
Steindler, Arthur, kinesiology studies of, 750
Steinmann pins, in acromioclavicular joint repairs, 439, *439–440*
  in clavicular fracture fixation, 396, 402
  in glenohumeral dislocation, 574–575
  in glenohumeral joint arthrodesis, 707, *708*, *710*, 711
  migration of, 464–465, *467*, 519, 521
Stellate ganglion block, in frozen shoulder, 858
Stereometric method, in motion measurement, 215

Sternalis muscle, 125–126, *125*
Sternoclavicular dislocation, 386
  acute, 486
  anterior, *484*, 486, *493*
    incidence of, 490–491
    mechanism of, 484, *485*
    symptoms of, 491, *493*
    treatment of, 496–497, 507–508, 514, *514*
    unreduced, 514, *514–515*
  bilateral, 491, 519, *519–520*
  misdiagnosis of, 379
  posterior, *484*, 486, *494*, *499*
    complications of, 517, *517–519*
    death from, 510
    incidence of, 490–491
    mechanism of, 484, *485*
    symptoms of, 491
    treatment of, 497, *498–501*, 500–501, 508–509, *509*, 514
    unreduced, 514
  recurrent, 486, 501–502, *502*, 511
  spontaneous, 486–487, 504, *505*, 514, 517
  symptoms of, 491, *493*
  treatment of, abduction traction technique, 497, *498–499*
    adduction traction technique, 497
    arthrodesis, 502, *503*
    clavicular osteotomy/resection, 502
    closed reduction, 496–497, *498–501*, 500
    coracoclavicular ligament reconstruction, 502, *502*
    fascial loop, 502
    in anterior dislocation, 496–497, 507–508, 514, *514*
    in posterior dislocation, 497, *498–501*, 500–501, 508–509, *509*, 514
    in recurrence, 501–502, *502*, 511
    in spontaneous dislocation, 504, *505*, 514, 517
    operative, 500–502, *500–503*
    postreduction care in, 497, 500
    subclavius tendon in, 502, *502*
    unreduced, 501–502, *502*, 514, *514*
  unreduced, 486, 501–502, *502*, 514, *514*
Sternoclavicular joint, anatomy of, 39–41, *40–41*, 208–209, *209*, 477–479, *478*, *480*, 1009, *1009*
    surgical, 477–483, *478*, *480–483*
  arthritis of, 487–489, *487–489*
    treatment of, 504, *506–507*, *516*, 517
  arthrodesis of, 502, *503*
  arthropathy of, 488, *488*
  articular surface of, 208, *209*, 477–478
  atraumatic problems of, 486–489, *487–490*
    treatment of, 504, *505–507*, 507, 514, *516*, 517
  biomechanics of, 208–210, *209*
    clinical relevance of, 212–213, *214*
  blood supply of, 40–41
  clavicular displacement in, 504
  clavicular epiphysis and, anatomy of, *481*, 482
    injury of, 502, *503*, 504, 509–511, *510–513*
  congenital problems of, treatment of, 504
  constraints on, *209*, 210
  disc of, 40, *40*
  dislocation of. See *Sternoclavicular dislocation.*
  hyperostosis of, 488, 504
  infection of, 489, *490*, 504, 507, 517, 925–296, 929, 1083
  injury of. See also subheads: *sprain of*; *subluxation of*; *Sternoclavicular dislocation.*
    causes of, 484, 486, 486–489, *487–490*
    classification of, anatomy-based, 486, *493–494*, *499*
      etiology-based, 486–489, *487–490*
    complications of, 517, *517–519*, 519
    computed tomography in, 495, *496*
    direct force in, 484, *484*
    historical review of, 477
    incidence of, 489–491
    indirect force in, 484, *485*
    mechanism of, 483–485, *484–486*

Sternoclavicular joint *(Continued)*
    symptoms of, 491, *493*
    tomography in, 493, 495, *495*
    treatment of, atraumatic, 504, *505–507*, 507
      closed reduction, 507–508, *509*
      complications of, 519, 521
      in dislocation, 496–497, *498–503*, 500–502, 507–509, *509*
      in sprain, 495, 507
      in subluxation, 495–496, 507
      operative, 508–509, 514, 517, 519, 521
      physeal, 502, *503*, 504
      postreduction care in, 508
    x-ray evaluation of, 491–495, *492–496*
  innervation of, 41
  instability of, inherent, 478
    management of, 212–213
  ligaments of, 208–209, *209*. See also specific ligament, e.g., *Costoclavicular ligament.*
    anatomy of, 40, *40*, 478–479, *478*, *480*
  meniscus of, 209, *209*
  motion of, 40, *209*, 210, 212, *213*, 1009
  osteitis of, 488, 504
  osteoarthritis of, 487–488, *487*
  palpation of, 157, *158*, 157, *158*
  post-traumatic arthritis of, 391–392
  postmenopausal arthritis of, 488–489, *489*
  range of motion of, 479, *481*, 482
  rheumatoid arthritis of, 488, *488*
  separation of, with clavicular fracture, 381
  septic arthritis of, 489, *490*, 504, 507, 517, 925–926, 929, 1083
  sprain of, 486
    symptoms of, 491
    treatment of, 495, 507
  structures near, 41, *41*, 482–483, *483*
  subluxation of, 486
    spontaneous, 486–487, *487*, 504, *505*, 514, 517
    symptoms of, 491
    treatment of, 495–496, 504, *505*, 507, 514, 517
  syphilis effects on, 489
  x-ray evaluation of, 193–196, *194–196*
Sternoclavicular ligament(s), anterior, anatomy of, 40, *40*
    as constraint, 210
  disruption of, in panclavicular dislocation, 375
  function of, 209, *209*
    in clavicular stability, 421
  posterior, anatomy of, 40, *40*
    as constraint, 210
Sternocleidomastoid muscle, absence of, versus torticollis, 1064
  anatomy of, 65, 1056, *1057–1058*, 1058
  blood supply of, 65, 1058, *1058*
  clavicular attachment of, 372, 1056, *1057*, 1058
  deformity of, after torticollis correction, 1068–1069, *1069–1070*, 1071
  function of, 1058
  hematoma of, torticollis and, 1060
  innervation of, 65, 1058, *1058*
  insertion of, 65
  myotomy of, in torticollis, 1067–1068, *1068*
  origin of, *41*, 42, 65
  resection of, in torticollis, 1066–1067, *1066–1067*
  sternal head of, 1056, *1057*
Sternohyoid muscle, origin of, 42, *42*
Sternomastoid muscle, anatomy of, 1056, *1057*
  embryology of, 131
  testing of, 166t
Sternomastoid tumor, in torticollis. See *Torticollis (infantile).*
Sternum, connection of, to coracoid process, 116
Stiffness, as chief complaint, 152–153
  in stroke shoulder, 771
  of posterior capsule, impingement syndrome and, 627, *628*
  versus impingement syndrome, 632
Stimson maneuver, in closed reduction, 570, 1005
Strain, muscular. See specific muscle.
Strength, testing of, 164–165, 165t

Strengthening exercise, for frozen shoulder, 854, 859
  for rotator cuff, 967, 970, 1007, *1008*
Streptococcus, antibiotic susceptibility of, 934t
  in bone/joint infections, 929, 1076, 1074
    neonatal, 1080, *1080*
Stress, in occupational cervicobrachial disorder, 1103
Stress fracture, of humerus, 992, *993*
Stress view, in x-ray evaluation, 190, *193, 557–558*
Stretching exercise. See under *Exercise.*
Stripp axillary lateral view, in x-ray evaluation, 183
Stroke, frozen shoulder and, 845
  neuromuscular disorders in, 770–771
Stryker notch view, in x-ray evaluation, 187, *188*
  of acromioclavicular joint, 433, *433*
  of clavicular fracture, 1020, *1024*
  of glenohumeral instability, 559–560, *560*
Study Group for the Problem of Osteosynthesis (AO) classification, of humeral fractures, 283–284
Subacromial bursography, 199
Subacromial crowding, in impingement syndrome, 627, *628*
Subacromial decompression, in impingement syndrome, 639, *639–642*
  in rotator cuff tear, 264
Subacromial impingement. See *Impingement syndrome.*
Subacromial sclerosis, 629, *629*
Subacromial space, anesthetic injection into, diagnostic, *172, 174*
  arthroscopy of, 262, *266, 268–269*
Subacromial-subdeltoid bursa, anatomy of, 27, 88, *89,* 280
  impingement syndrome and, 624
  injection therapy of, 855
  rheumatoid arthritis of, 690, *690,* 690t, 702
Subclavian artery, anatomy of, 78, *79*
  collateral circulation of, 81, *81–82*
  in brachial plexus supply, 72, *72*
  injury of, 81–82
    in clavicular fracture, 382–383, *382*
    in sternoclavicular joint dislocation, 517
  obstruction of, in clavicular fracture, 391
  pin migration into, 519
Subclavian nerve, anatomy of, 69
  in subclavius muscle, 57
Subclavian perivascular block, 250
Subclavian vein, anatomy of, 82
  injury of, in clavicular fracture, 382–383, *382*
  obstruction of, in clavicular fracture, 391
  thrombosis of, 988
Subclavian vessels, clavicular protection of, 372
Subclavicular dislocation, of glenohumeral joint, 541
Subclavius muscle, anatomy of, 57, *58*
  blood supply of, 57
  clavicular attachment of, 41, *41,* 372
  function of, 57
  innervation of, 57
  insertion of, 57, *58*
  origin of, 57, *58*
  testing of, 166t
Subclavius tendon, in sternoclavicular joint repair, 502, *502*
Subcoracoid dislocation, of glenohumeral joint, 541, *542*
Subdeltoid bursa. See *Subacromial-subdeltoid bursa.*
Subglenoid dislocation, of glenohumeral joint, 541
Subluxation. See also specific joint.
  diagnosis of, 151–152
Subscapular artery, aberrant brachial plexus relationships with, 132–133, *133*
  anatomy of, 28, 30, *61, 79, 80*
  anomalies of, 81
  collateral circulation of, *81–82*
  in subscapularis, 61–62
  in teres major innervation, 62
Subscapular bursitis, 363
Subscapular compartment, anatomy of, 875
Subscapular nerve, anatomy of, 30–31
  anomalous, 74

Subscapular nerve *(Continued)*
  lower, anatomy of, *68,* 70
    in subscapularis innervation, 61
    in teres major innervation, 62
  upper, anatomy of, *61, 68,* 70
    in subscapularis innervation, 61
Subscapular nodes, anatomy of, 83, *83*
Subscapular vein, anatomy of, 82
Subscapularis bursa, anatomy of, 27, *27,* 88
  variations in, 27, *27*
Subscapularis muscle, anatomy of, 61–62, *61,* 647, *795*
  comparative, 5
  blood supply of, 61–62
  contracture of, in brachial plexus injury of newborn, 1039, *1040*
  denervation of, in rotator cuff tear repair, 672
  force generation by, 235t
  function of, 61
  humeral attachment of, 47, *279,* 280, *625*
  innervation of, 61
  insertion of, 61
  origin of, 61
  procedures involving, in glenohumeral instability, 578–580, *580*
  rupture of, 872
  scapular attachment of, *45,* 46, 335, *335*
  strengthening exercise for, 969, *970*
  testing of, 166t
  trigger points in, frozen shoulder and, 844, 856
Subscapularis recess, anatomy of, *61*
Subscapularis tendon, anatomy of, 261, *261*
  arthroscopy of, 261, *261*
  degeneration of, in biceps dislocation, 799, *800*
  function of, 261
  hypovascular zone of, 775
  transfer of, in glenohumeral instability, 579–580, *580*
  in rotator cuff tears, 663, 671
Subscapularis-teres-latissimus muscle, 126–127, *126*
Sulcus sign/test, 168, *169,* 548, *549,* 550, 1005
Sunderland classification, of nerve injury, 756
Superior deltoid approach, for humeral fracture treatment, 305, *307*
Supraclavicular block, 249–250
Supraclavicular nerve, anatomy of, 76, *76, 90,* 91
Suprahumeral artery, anatomy of, 28
Suprascapular artery, anatomy of, 28, *28,* 78, *79*
  collateral circulation of, *81*
  in infraspinatus muscle, 60
  in subclavius muscle, 57
  in supraspinatus muscle, 60
  injury of, in clavicular fracture, 383
Suprascapular nerve, anatomy of, 30–31, *30–31, 68–69,* 69, 135, *135,* 280, 281, 336, *337*
  anesthetic injection into, diagnostic, 174
  clavicular foramina for, 103, *103–104*
  compression of, congenital, 134–136, *135*
    in sports, 987
    versus rotator cuff tears, 661
  in infraspinatus innervation, 60
  in supraspinatus innervation, 60
  injury of, compression, 765, *765*
    in clavicular fracture, 764
    in humeral fracture, 291
  repair of, 762
  versus impingement syndrome, 632
  versus rotator cuff tears, 661
Suprascapular notch, anatomy of, 43, 135–136, *135–136*
  anomalies of, 135–136, *136*
Suprascapular tendon, blood supply of, 774–775
Supraspinatus fossa, congenital, 128, *128*
Supraspinatus muscle, anatomy of, 58–59, *59,* 647, *795*
  comparative, 5, *5*
  blood flow to, compromise of, 625
  blood supply of, 60
  deficiency of, elevation and, 238, 243
  denervation of, in rotator cuff tear repair, 672

Supraspinatus muscle (Continued)
  force generation by, 235t
  function of, 59–60
    in elevation, 235, 237–238, 238–240, 241, 242
    with deltoid muscle, 235, 237–238, 238–240, 241, 242
  humeral attachment of, 47, 279, 280, 625
  innervation of, 60
  insertion of, 51, 52, 59, 60
  origin of, 59, 60
  scapular attachment of, 45, 46, 335, 336
  strengthening exercise for, 969, 970
  testing of, 164, 165, 166t
  weakness of, in suprascapular nerve injury, 765, 765
Supraspinatus outlet, 60
Supraspinatus tendon, anatomy of, 774–775, 775
  blood supply of, 774–775, 775
  calcification in, 775. See also Calcifying tendinitis.
  embryology of, 775, 775
  fibrocartilage pad of, 648
  hypovascular zone of, 647–648, 774–775, 775
  insertion of, histology of, 648
  tendinitis of, occupational, 1093–1095
  transfer of, in rotator cuff tears, 663
Supratubercular ridge, 122–123, 123
  in biceps tendon lesions, 801, 804
Surgical planes, anatomy of, 85–86, 86–87
Sustruta, anatomical studies of, 34
Sutures, in arthroscopic stabilization, 274–276, 274–275
  in clavicular fracture fixation, 396
  in collagen-rich structures, 51, 52
"Swallow tail" malformation, of scapula, 117, 118
Swanson shoulder prosthesis, 737, 737t
  for hemiarthroplasty, 713, 714
Swelling, evaluation of, 156
Swimming, overuse syndrome in, 988–989
Sympathetic nervous system, in brachial plexus, 72–73
Syndactyly, in Poland's syndrome, 129–130
Synovectomy, arthroscopic, in rheumatoid arthritis, 264
  in glenohumeral arthritis, 703–704, 704
Synovial fluid analysis, in septic arthritis, 930–931, 931t, 1081
Synovitis, in rheumatoid arthritis, 690t, 691, 691, 693–694
  pigmented villonodular, 884
Synovium, dysplasia of, 884
  microanatomy of, 922–923, 924
  sarcoma of, 892, 894
Syphilis, sternoclavicular joint manifestations of, 489

T

Tack, biodegradable, in arthroscopic stabilization, 276
Tangential lateral view, in x-ray evaluation. See Scapulolateral view.
Taylor clavicle support, 392
Technetium–99m scan, in frozen shoulder, 849–850
  in infection, 931
  in osteomyelitis, 1075
Teeth, abnormal, in cleidocranial dysostosis, 99
Teflon prosthesis, in rotator cuff tears, 663–664
Telangiectatic osteosarcoma, 880
Temporomandibular joint, rheumatoid arthritis of, anesthesia and, 247
Tendinite calcifante. See Calcifying tendinitis.
Tendinitis, biceps. See Biceps tendinitis.
  calcific. See Calcifying tendinitis.
  impingement test in, 170–171, 172
  in welders, 1093–1094, 1094
  infraspinatus, 1094–1095
  occupational, 1093–1095
  of rotator cuff, 1093–1095
    versus rotator cuff tears, 661
  supraspinatus, 1093–1095
  uncalcified. See Frozen shoulder.

Tendinitis (Continued)
  versus frozen shoulder, 852
Tendon(s). See also specific tendon.
  calcification of. See Calcifying tendinitis.
  insertion of, direct/indirect, 51, 52
  lesions of, versus impingement syndrome, 629
  rupture of. See Muscle(s), rupture of.
  splitting of, 51, 53
  transfer of, in brachial plexus injury of newborn, 1048–1052, 1049–1051
Tenosynovitis, of biceps tendon, 799, 800–801, 810–811
Tension band wiring, glenohumeral joint arthrodesis, 707, 708
Teres major muscle, anatomy of, 62, 62
  comparative, 5
  blood supply of, 62
  force generation by, 235t
  function of, 51, 51, 62
  humeral insertion of, 48
  innervation of, 62
  insertion of, 62, 62
  origin of, 62, 62
  scapular attachment of, 45, 46, 335, 336
  testing of, 166t
Teres minor muscle, anatomy of, 60–61, 60, 647
  comparative, 5
  force generation by, 235t
  function of, 61
  humeral attachment of, 47, 280, 625
  insertion of, 60, 60
  origin of, 60, 60
  scapular attachment of, 45, 46, 335, 336
  strengthening exercise for, 969, 970
  testing of, 166t
Teres minor tendon, anatomy of, 774
  blood supply of, 774
  transfer of, in rotator cuff tears, 663
Thalamic pain syndrome, 771
"The syndrome," in arthritis, 691, 694
Theraband, glenohumeral instability exercises and, 609, 610
Thoracic artery(ies), lateral, aberrant brachial plexus relationships with, 132, 133
  absence of, 81
  anatomy of, 79, 80
  anomalies of, 80
  collateral circulation of, 82
  in serratus anterior, 57
  posterior, in pectoralis minor, 57
  superior, anatomy of, 79
    collateral circulation of, 82
Thoracic nerve, lateral anterior, anatomy of, 69
  long, anatomy of, 68–69, 69–70
    in serratus anterior innervation, 57
    palsy of, 768
Thoracic outlet syndrome, 768–770
  anatomical considerations in, 136–137, 138–142, 768–769
  classification of, 137, 138–142
  clinical manifestations of, 137, 769–770, 769–770
  congenital, 136–137, 138–142, 143
  diagnosis of, 137, 769–770, 769–770
  in sternoclavicular joint dislocation, 517
  occupational cervicobrachial disorder and, 1089–1090
  treatment of, 137, 143, 770
  versus biceps tendon lesions, 823
  x-ray evaluation of, 751
Thoracoacromial artery, anatomy of, 28, 29, 79, 79
  clavicular branch, 57
  deltoid branch, 58–59, 63
  pectoral branch, 57
Thoracoacromial axis/trunk, anatomy of, 79, 80
  collateral circulation of, 81–82
Thoracodorsal artery, anatomy of, 79, 80
  collateral circulation of, 81
  in latissimus dorsi innervation, 64
  in serratus anterior, 57

Thoracodorsal nerve, anatomy of, *68*, 70
  in latissimus dorsi innervation, 64
Thrombosis, effort, in thoracic outlet syndrome, 137, *141*
  in clavicular fracture, 383
  of axillary vein, 988
Throwing, acceleration phase of, *962*, 963
  anticocking phase of, 963
  biceps tendon lesions in, 810–811
  biceps tendon motion in, 808
  biomechanics of, 961–963, *962*
  deltoid muscle rupture in, 867
  early cocking phase of, 962–963, *962*
  fatigue in, 963
  faulty technique in, biomechanical effects of, 963
  follow-through phase of, *962*, 963
  glenohumeral instability in, 963–983
    arthroscopy in, 976
    Bristow operation in, 972, *973–976*, 976
    capsulolabral reconstruction in, 977–978, *977–982*, 981–982
    classification of, 965–967, *966*
    posterior, 983–986, *984–986*
    rehabilitation program for, 971
    relocation test in, 964–965, *964–965*
  glenoid labrum tears in, 822
  glenoid spurs and, 986
  impingement syndrome in, rehabilitation of, 633–634
  in exercise program, 982, *982*
  late cocking phase of, *962*, 963
  neurological problems in, 987
  overuse syndrome in, 964
  pathologic mechanisms in, 962–963
  phases of, 962–963, *962*
  quadrilateral space syndrome in, 987
  rotator cuff tears in, 651–652, *651–652*
  scapular elevation motion in, 50–51, *51*
  stabilizing mechanisms in, 964
  stress fracture in, 992, *993*
  subscapularis muscle action in, 61
  suprascapular nerve compression in, 987
  triceps action in, 65
  vascular problems in, 987–988
  versus activities of daily living, 961
  whole body use in, 962–963, *962*
  wind-up phase of, 962, *962*
Thyrocervical trunk, anatomy of, 78, *79*
  collateral circulation of, *81–82*
Thyroid artery, superior, in sternocleidomastoid, 65
Thyroid disorders, frozen shoulder and, 845
Tightness, versus impingement syndrome, 629
Tikhor-Linberg procedure, *907*, 908, 940–941, 949, *950*
Tobramycin, in bone/joint infections, 934t, 935
Tomography, in sternoclavicular joint disorders, 196, 493, 495, *495*
Torque, maximum, of shoulder, 242–243, 242t, *243*
Torticollis (infantile), 1055–1071
  anatomical considerations in, 1056, *1057–1058*, 1058
  arterial obstruction in, 1060
  bilateral, 1055, 1059
  brachial plexus injury and, 1037–1038, 1059
  breech presentation and, 1059–1060
  classification of, 1055–1056, 1056t
  clinical appearance of, 1062–1064, *1062–1064*
  clinical course of, 1064–1065, *1065*
  conditions associated with, 1059
  definition of, 1055
  diagnosis of, 1062, *1062*
  differential diagnosis of, 1062–1064, *1062–1064*
  etiology of, 1059–1061
  exostosis development in, 1061, *1062*
  facial asymmetry in, 1062, 1065, *1065*, 1071
  fetal development defects in, 1059
  hematoma in, 1060
  hereditary factors in, 1059–1060
  hip dislocation with, 1059

Torticollis (infantile) *(Continued)*
  historical review of, 1055
  in twins, 1060
  incidence of, 1058–1059
  infection in, 1059
  intrauterine factors in, 1060–1061
  lateral band persistence in, 1068–1069, *1069–1070*, 1071
  myogenic lesions and, 1064
  myopathy in, 1060
  myotomy in, 1071
  neurogenic theory of, 1060
  oligohydramnios and, 1059
  osseous lesions in, 1063, *1064*
  paroxysmal, 1064
  pathology of, 1061, *1061*
  plagiocephaly in, 1062, 1065, *1066*
  posterior fossa tumors in, 1064, *1064*
  prenatal, 1060–1061
  Sandifer's syndrome and, 1063–1064
  stretching exercise in, 1065, 1071
  tractor cap in, 1067–1068, *1068*
  treatment of, complications of, 1068–1069, *1069–1070*, 1071
    in infant, 1071
    in older child, 1071
    myotomy, 1067–1068, *1068*
    nonoperative, 1065, *1066*
    recurrence after, 1071
    resection of tumor in, 1066–1067, *1066–1067*
    results of, 1071
  tumor form of, 1061–1062, 1064–1065, *1065*
  venous occlusion in, 1060
  versus ocular form, 1063, *1063*
  wryneck form of, 1061–1062, 1065
Torticollis (late onset–acquired), 1055, 1056t
Total elevation measurement, in range of motion assessment, 160, *162*
Total joint replacement. See under *Prosthetic arthroplasty.*
Trachea, injury of, in sternoclavicular joint injury, 517, *518*, 519
Traction, in arthroscopy, 265
  in frozen shoulder, 858
  in humeral fracture, 296
Transcutaneous electrical stimulation, after amputation, 959–960
Transscapular view, in x-ray evaluation. See *Scapulolateral view.*
Transthoracic view, in x-ray evaluation, 553
Trapezius muscle, absence of, 130–131
  anatomy of, 54–55, *54*
    comparative, 5
  blood supply of, 55
  clavicular attachment of, 41, *41*, 372, 374, *374*
  clavicular penetration of, 445, *446*
  detachment of, from clavicle. See also *Acromioclavicular joint, injury of, types III to VI.*
  embryology of, 131
  fatigue of, in occupational disorders, 1091–1092
  function of, 54
    in clavicular stability, 421
    in elevation, 238–239
  innervation of, 55
  insertion of, 54, *54*
  origin of, 54, *54*
  paralysis of, 54–55
    in spinal accessory nerve injury, 759–761, *760–761*
  repair of, in acromioclavicular joint injury, 452, *453*
  scapular attachment of, *45*, 46, 335, *336–337*
  testing of, 166t
Trapezoid ligament, anatomy of, 211, *211*, 415, 418, *418*, 796
  as constraint, 211–212, *212*
  size of, 419
Trapezoid line, anatomy of, 41, *42*
Trauma, amputation in, 941
  frozen shoulder and, 845
  versus tumor, 900, 900t
Trauma axillary lateral view, in x-ray evaluation, 183–184, *184*
Trauma series, of x-rays, 178–184, *179–184*

Trauma series *(Continued)*
　　in humeral fracture, 287–288, *287*
Traumatic arthritis, after clavicular fracture, 391–392
　　of glenohumeral joint, 694, *694–696*, 694t
　　　prosthetic arthroplasty in, 736–738, 737t–738t
　　versus frozen shoulder, 852
Triamcinolone, in frozen shoulder, 858
Triceps muscle, anatomy of, 64–65, *795*, 868
　　comparative, 5
　　blood supply of, 65
　　force generation by, 235t
　　function of, 65
　　innervation of, 65
　　insertion of, 64
　　origin of, 64–65
　　rupture of, 867–869
　　scapular attachment of, *45*, 46, *335–336*, 336
　　testing of, 166t
Triceps reflex, testing of, 167
Triceps tendon, anatomy of, 64
Trigger points, frozen shoulder and, 844, 856
Trillat procedure, in glenohumeral instability, 580
Trimethoprim-sulfamethoxazole, in bone/joint infections, 934t
Trispherical shoulder prosthesis, 680, *684*, 715, 739t, 740
"Trough line," in glenohumeral instability, 553
Tuberculosis, frozen shoulder and, 845
　　of acromioclavicular joint, 468
TUBS syndrome, 151–152, 541, 576, 576t
　　operative stabilization in, 588–592, *588–591*
Tumor(s). See also *Neoplasia.*
　　amputation in. See *Amputation.*
　　anatomical considerations and, 875, *876*, 877
　　aneurysmal bone cyst, 885, *895*
　　benign, aggressive, 911–912
　　　cartilaginous, 880, 882, *882*
　　　osseous, 879–880, 911–912
　　　soft tissue, 891–892
　　　staging of, 877t, 878
　　biopsy of, 901–903, *902*, 913–914
　　brain, torticollis in, 1064, *1064*
　　cartilaginous, benign, 880, 882, *882*
　　　malignant, 882, *883*, 884
　　chest wall involvement of, 898
　　chondroblastoma, 882, *895*, 912, 914
　　chondrosarcoma, 882, *883*, 884
　　　secondary, 880, 882, *883*, *894–895*
　　clinical presentation of, 892t, 895–896
　　compartment anatomy and, 83–84
　　compartmentalization of, 877–878, 877t–878t
　　computed tomography of, 879, 897–898
　　density of, 897–898
　　differential diagnosis of, 899–901, *900*, 900t
　　encapsulated, 877t, 878
　　enchondroma, 882, *883*, 895
　　Ewing's sarcoma. See *Ewing's sarcoma.*
　　fibromatosis, 891–892
　　fibrous dysplasia, of bone, 885, *886*
　　follow-up protocol for, 895
　　Gaucher's disease, 888
　　giant cell, of bone, 92, 885, *895*
　　hemangioma, 891
　　high-grade, 877–878, 877t, 912–913
　　histologic grading of, 878
　　historical review of, 874–875
　　incidence of, 892, *894*, 895
　　intra-articular, 875
　　laboratory evaluation of, 898
　　limb salvage surgery in, 905–908, *907*
　　lipoma, 891, 895
　　liposarcoma, 892, *894*, 895
　　location of, 897
　　low-grade, 877–878, 877t, 912
　　magnetic resonance imaging of, 879, 897–898

Tumor(s) *(Continued)*
　　malignant. See also *Sarcoma.*
　　　cartilaginous, 882, *883*, 884
　　　high-grade, 912–913
　　　low-grade, 912
　　　osseous, 880, *881*, 912–913
　　　soft tissue, 892, 892t, *893*, 913
　　margins of, 878–879, 903–905
　　　definition of, 903
　　　growth rate and, 897
　　　in limb salvage surgery, *904*, 905t
　　　intracapsular (intralesional), 903, *904*, 905, 905t
　　　marginal, 903, *904*, 905t
　　　radical, 903, *904*, 905t
　　　types of, 903–904, *904*, 905t
　　　wide, 903, *904*, 905t
　　metastasis from. See *Metastasis.*
　　multiple myeloma, 885, 887, *888*, 892, *894*, 898
　　myositis ossificans, 291, 879–880
　　nonossifying fibroma of bone, 885, *887*
　　osseous, 884–885, 884, *886–887*
　　　benign, 879–880, 911–912
　　　malignant, 880, *881*, 912–913
　　osteoblastoma, 879
　　osteochondroma. See *Osteochondroma.*
　　osteoid osteoma, 879, *895*
　　osteosarcoma. See *Osteosarcoma.*
　　Paget's disease, 888, *890*, 891, 900–901, 900t
　　pathological fractures and, 898–899, *899*
　　periosteal chondroma, 882
　　recurrence of, 878–879
　　reticuloendothelial, 885, 887, *888–889*
　　simple bone cyst, 884–885, *884*, *895*
　　soft tissue, benign, 891–892
　　　malignant, 892, 892t, *893*, 913
　　staging of, 877–879, 877t–878t
　　sternomastoid, in torticollis. See *Torticollis (infantile).*
　　surgical site classification of, 878, 878t
　　synovial dysplasia, 884
　　treatment of. See also specific disorder.
　　　chemotherapy in, 912–915
　　　glenohumeral resection in, 906, *907*, 908
　　　humeral resection in, 906, *907*
　　　in aggressive benign lesion, 911–912, 914
　　　in high-grade malignancy, 912, 914–915
　　　in low-grade malignancy, 912, 914
　　　limb salvage surgery in, 905–908, *907*
　　　operative, 914
　　　planning in, 879
　　　reconstructive procedures for, 908–911, *909–910*
　　　scapular resection in, *907*, 908
　　　scapulohumeral resection in, *907*, 908
　　x-ray evaluation of, 200, 202, 897–898

U

Ulnar collateral nerve, anatomy of, 71
Ulnar nerve, anatomy of, 68, *72*
　　anomalous, 74
　　injury of, in clavicular fracture, 382
　　neuritis of, versus biceps tendon lesions, 823–824
Ultrasonography, in biceps tendon lesions, 818, *820*
　　in calcifying tendinitis, 785
　　in clavicular fracture, 398
　　in infections, 931
　　in neurological disorders, 753–754
　　in rotator cuff disorders, 199–200, 629, 656–658, *657–658*, 666
Ultrasound treatment, in frozen shoulder, 854
"Uncalcified tendinitis." See *Frozen shoulder.*
Unicameral (simple) bone cyst, 884–885, *884*, *895*, 992
Utah arm, 956, *958*

V

Vacant glenoid sign, 552
Valsalva's maneuver, in cervical spine examination, 175–176
Vancomycin, in bone/joint infections, 934t
Vein(s). See also specific vein, e.g., *Axillary vein.*
    access to, in anesthesia, 248
    anatomy of, 82
    occlusion of, torticollis and, 1060
    of muscles, 53–54
    oscillating, 54
Velpeau axillary lateral view, in x-ray evaluation, 288
Velpeau axillary view, in x-ray evaluation, 183, *184*, 556, *559*
Velpeau bandage, in clavicular fracture, *392*, 393
Velpeau sling, in humeral fracture, 296
Vertebra, connection of, to rib, 116, *117*
Vertebral artery, anatomy of, 78
    collateral circulation of, *82*
    in brachial plexus supply, 72, *72*
    regional anesthetic effects on, 252–253
Vesalius, anatomical studies of, 36, *37*
Vibration sense, evaluation of, 758
Video Registration and Analysis system, in occupational cervico-brachial disorder, 1093
Viral infection, brachial neuritis in, 823
    in septic arthritis, 930
    long thoracic nerve palsy in, 768
Voice changes, in sternoclavicular joint dislocation, 517, *517*

W

Watson-Jones classification, of humeral fractures, 281–282
Weakness, as chief complaint, 153
Weaver-Dunn procedure, in acromioclavicular joint injury, 443
Weightlifter's clavicle, 374
Weightlifting, biceps muscle rupture in, 869, *869*
    occupational cervicobrachial disorder and, 1089
    pectoralis major muscle rupture in, 864
West Point view, in x-ray evaluation, 184–185, *185*, 557, *559*
White rami communicans, anatomy of, 72
Whitman procedure, in spinal accessory nerve palsy, 760
Wilkinson procedure, in Sprengel's deformity, 108
Wires and wiring. See also *Kirschner wires.*
    in acromioclavicular joint repair, 441–442, *441*
    tension band, in glenohumeral joint arthrodesis, 707, *708*
Withers classification, of frozen shoulder, 842, 843t
Woodward procedure, in Sprengel's deformity, 108–109, *110*
Worker's Compensation Permanent Partial Disability Schedule, 1104
Workmen's compensation, disability evaluation for, 1103–1105
    impingement syndrome and, 636
    neurological disorders and, 757
    occupational cervicobrachial disorder and, 1090
Workplace disorders. See *Occupational disorders.*
Wright's maneuver, in thoracic outlet syndrome, 769, *770*
Wryneck. See *Torticollis.*

X

X-ray evaluation, 178–207. See also *Arthrography; Computed to-mography; Ultrasonography;* specific disorder.
    Adams view in, 187
    Alexander view in, 193, 427, *429*
    anteroposterior views in, 190, *193*, 196
        in acromioclavicular joint disorders, 427, *428–429*
        in clavicular disorders, 383–384, *383–384*
        in glenohumeral instability, 552–554, *552–554*
        in humeral fracture, 287–288, *287*

X-ray evaluation *(Continued)*
        stress type, 190, *193*
    apical-oblique view in, 185, *186*, 560
    axillary lateral view in, 179, 181, *181*, 190, 427, *429*
    axillary view in, in glenohumeral instability, 555–556, *556–559*
        in humeral fracture, 287–288, *287*
    bicipital groove view in, *816–817*, 817
    caudal tilt view in, 196, *197–198*, 817, *817*
    cephalic tilt view in, 194–195, *195*
        in clavicular fracture, 1017, *1018*
        in sternoclavicular joint disorders, 492–493, *493–494*
    cephaloscapular view in, 560
    Didiee view in, 560
    Fisk view in, 200, *202*, 816, *816*
    Hermodsson view in, 559
    Hill-Sachs view in, 559
    Hobbs view in, 492, *492*
    in acromioclavicular joint disorders, 189–193, *191–194*
    in biceps tendon lesions, 200, *202*, 816–817, *816–817*
    in brachial plexus injury of newborn, 1042
    in calcifying tendinitis, 200, *201*, 783–785, *782–784*
    in clavicular disorders, 1020, *1024*
        distal, 189–193, *191–194*, 384–385, *385–386*
        in children, 1012, *1012*, 1017, *1018*
        medial, 193–196, *194–196*, 385–386
        nonunion, 388–389, *388–389*
        shaft, 189, *190*, 383–384, *383–384*
    in frozen shoulder, 849
    in glenohumeral arthritis, 702
    in glenohumeral instability, 178–189, 551–561, *556–559*, 1005
        anterior, 184–188, *185–189*
        dislocation, 178–184, *179–184*
        fractures, 178–184, *179–184*
        goals of, 551–552
        posterior, 189, *189*
        recurrent, 556–557, 559–561, *559–560*
        subluxation, 178–184, *179–184*
    in humeral fracture, 286–289, *286–289*
        in children, 993
    in humeral head disorders, 185, 187, *187*, 559–561, *559–560*
    in impingement syndrome, 196, *197–199*, 199–200, 629, *629–631*, 632
    in inflammatory disorders, 202
    in muscle rupture. See specific muscle.
    in neurological disorders, 751, *753–754*, 754
    in osteomyelitis, 1075
    in prosthetic arthroplasty, 738–739, 739t
    in rotator cuff disorders, 196, *197–199*, 199–200, 656, *656–657*
    in scapular injury, 200, *200*, 339–340, *339–341*
    in septic arthritis, 930–931, *931–932*
    in sternoclavicular joint disorders, 193–196, *194–196*, 491–495, *492–496*
    in tumors, 200, 202, 897–898
    lateral view in, 287–288, *287*
    modified axillary views in, 183–184, *184*
    number of views for, 178, *179*
    reduced voltage technique in, 190, *191*
    rolled cassette for, 181, *181*
    scapular outlet view in, 196, *198*, 199
    scapulolateral view in, 181–183, *181–183*
        in glenohumeral instability, 554–555, *555–556*
        in humeral fracture, 287–288, *287*
        of acromioclavicular joint, 427, *429*
    serendipity view in, 194–195, *195*
        in clavicular fracture, 1017, *1018*
        in sternoclavicular joint disorders, 492–493, *493–494*
    stress views in, 190, *193*
        in glenohumeral instability, 557–558
        of acromioclavicular joint, 427, 429, *430*, 431
    Stripp axillary lateral view in, 183
    Stryker notch view in, 187, *188*
        in clavicular fracture, 1020, *1024*
        in glenohumeral instability, 559–560, *560*
        of acromioclavicular joint, 433, *433*

Stryker notch view in *(Continued)*
    subacromial bursography in, 199
    supraspinatus outlet view in, 629, *630*
    transthoracic view in, in glenohumeral instability, 553
    trauma axillary lateral view in, 183–184, *184*
    trauma series in, 178–184, *179–184*, 287–288, *287*
    true anteroposterior view in, 179, *179–180*
    Velpeau axillary view in, 183, *184*, 288, 556, *559*
    West Point view in, 184–185, *185*, 557, *559*
    Zanca view in, 190, *191–192*, 427, *428–429*
Xerography, in calcifying tendinitis, 783, *783*
Xylocaine. See *Lidocaine.*

Y

Y lateral view, in x-ray evaluation. See *Scapulolateral view.*
Yergason sign/test, 171, *173*, 813, *813*

Z

Zachary procedure, in brachial plexus injury of newborn, 1050
Zanca view, in x-ray evaluation, 190, *191–192*, 427, *428–429*
Zancolli classification, of contractures, in brachial plexus injury of
    newborn, 1039, 1041
Zancolli procedure, in brachial plexus injury of newborn, 1050,
    1050, 1052, *1052*
Zippel shoulder prosthesis, 680, *681*